Liver, Gall Bladder, and Bile Ducts

GASTROINTESTINAL SURGERY LIBRARY

Abdominal Trauma, Peritoneum, and Retroperitoneum
Aditya Nanavati and Sanjay Nagral

Appendix, Colon, and Rectum
Parul J. Shukla, Jeffrey Milsom, and Kota Momose

Duodenum and Small Bowel
John A. Windsor, Sanjay Pandanaboyana, and Anil K. Agarwal

Liver, Gall Bladder, and Bile Ducts
Mohamed Rela and Pierre-Alain Clavien

Oesophagus and Stomach
Matthias Reeh and Jakob R. Izbicki

Pancreas
Shailesh V. Shrikhande and Markus W. Büchler

Liver, Gall Bladder, and Bile Ducts

EDITED BY

Mohamed Rela
Chancellor, Bharath Institute of Higher Education and Research (BIHER), and Chairman, Dr. Rela Institute and Medical Centre, Chennai, India

Pierre-Alain Clavien
Professor and Chairman, Department of Surgery and Transplantation, University Hospital, Zürich, Switzerland

SERIES EDITORS

Samiran Nundy
Emeritus Consultant, Sir Ganga Ram Hospital, New Delhi, India

Dirk J. Gouma
Emeritus Professor of Surgery, Amsterdam University Medical Centre, Amsterdam, The Netherlands

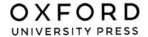

OXFORD
UNIVERSITY PRESS

Great Clarendon Street, Oxford, OX2 6DP,
United Kingdom

Oxford University Press is a department of the University of Oxford.
It furthers the University's objective of excellence in research, scholarship,
and education by publishing worldwide. Oxford is a registered trade mark of
Oxford University Press in the UK and in certain other countries

© Oxford University Press 2023

The moral rights of the authors have been asserted

First edition published in 2023

All rights reserved. No part of this publication may be reproduced, stored in
a retrieval system, or transmitted, in any form or by any means, without the
prior permission in writing of Oxford University Press, or as expressly permitted
by law, by licence or under terms agreed with the appropriate reprographics
rights organization. Enquiries concerning reproduction outside the scope of the
above should be sent to the Rights Department, Oxford University Press, at the
address above

You must not circulate this work in any other form
and you must impose this same condition on any acquirer

Published in the United States of America by Oxford University Press
198 Madison Avenue, New York, NY 10016, United States of America

British Library Cataloguing in Publication Data
Data available

Library of Congress Control Number: 2023935533

ISBN 978–0–19–286245–7

DOI: 10.1093/med/9780192862457.001.0001

Printed and bound by
CPI Group (UK) Ltd, Croydon, CR0 4YY

Oxford University Press makes no representation, express or implied, that the
drug dosages in this book are correct. Readers must therefore always check
the product information and clinical procedures with the most up-to-date
published product information and data sheets provided by the manufacturers
and the most recent codes of conduct and safety regulations. The authors and
the publishers do not accept responsibility or legal liability for any errors in the
text or for the misuse or misapplication of material in this work. Except where
otherwise stated, drug dosages and recommendations are for the non-pregnant
adult who is not breast-feeding

Links to third party websites are provided by Oxford in good faith and
for information only. Oxford disclaims any responsibility for the materials
contained in any third party website referenced in this work.

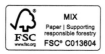

Foreword to the Gastrointestinal Surgery Library

We are currently led to believe that textbooks are déclassé. Information is no longer gathered other than online through PubMed or Google and their equivalents. This is not so. First, much of the world, especially in low- and middle-income countries, still derives scholarly information from textbooks; and secondly, we ignore the obvious, where does the online information come from? Certainly, for a narrow, topic-specific search we can immediately reach for PubMed, but where does generic broad disease-based topic information come from? Is it possible to educate our current and future surgeons on Wikipedia alone? Truth is hard to find, truth in surgery even harder. We surgeons, like the rest of the world, find it easy to fall back on the confirmation biases of our already held beliefs. We all still struggle with 'we do this this way, because that is the way we have always done so'. Only in recent decades have surgeons moved from numerator doctors remembering the energizing success and the damaging failure to provide denominators for our actions. How to find the truth or even the facts is a great challenge in our information overloaded society. Clinical trials in the discipline of surgery are hard to do, and even harder where equipoise does not exist. Our best recourse is to begin with those leading their respective fields, often in academic environments where challenge and controversy are healthy endeavours. A culture where the student becomes the conscience of the professor is what academia should be about.

Where can we go to look for the most current validated information? Where can our trainees go beyond their immediate environment? Nowhere is this more important as we become a global surgical society. The low- and middle-income countries look to the high-income countries for leadership and guidance, but is that correct? What we do in tertiary institutions may well not serve our colleagues in resource poor countries. This should be a two-way street; what can we in tertiary centres learn from less privileged but equally demanding societies? We embrace technology for technology's sake, we think little of value but only of perceived benefit. What an opportunity to embrace excellence and define the greater benefit for the greatest number.

The *Gastrointestinal Surgery Library* series has taken on this Herculean task.

The lead editors, Professor Samiran Nundy from New Delhi and Professor Dirk J. Gouma from Amsterdam, have the stature and fortitude to lead this challenge. A mammoth text focused on a global readership in print, eBook, and online editions. To do this they have assembled a cadre of volume editors from six countries. The volume editors have then recruited leaders within the gastrointestinal surgical fraternity from several more countries to address global problems in gastrointestinal surgery, from oesophagus to anus and all tissues and viscera that surround the alimentary tract. Together, they provide a comprehensive umbrella that most will find weatherproof, but not impermeable.

Sir Murray F. Brennan
Memorial Sloan Kettering Cancer Center
New York, USA

Contents

Introduction from the Series Editors ix
Introduction from the Volume Editors xi
About the Series Editors xiii
About the Volume Editors xv
Acknowledgement xvi
Abbreviations xvii
Contributors xxi

SECTION 1 The liver
PART 1 Anatomy and physiology

1. **Surgical anatomy of the liver** 3
   Ashwin Rammohan and Mohamed Rela

2. **Applied physiology of the liver** 12
   Bruno Stieger and Joachim C. Mertens

3. **Liver regeneration** 17
   Bostjan Humar and Rok Humar

4. **Perioperative management and nutrition in patients with liver and biliary tract disease** 30
   Akila Rajakumar, Ilankumaran Kaliamoorthy, and Rathnavel G. Kanagavelu

PART 2 Investigations

5. **Liver function tests and assessment of liver function** 40
   Omar Y. Mousa and Patrick S. Kamath

6. **Imaging: ultrasound, computed tomography, magnetic resonance imaging, nuclear medicine, and angiography** 49
   Guido Costa, Ezio Lanza, Matteo Donadon, and Guido Torzilli

PART 3 Infectious disease of the liver

7. **Bacterial and parasitic infections of the liver** 59
   Chandan Kumar Kedarisetty, Mayank Jain, Thamarai S. Selvan, Varanasi Y. Bhargav, and Jayanthi Venkataraman

8. **Fatty liver in liver surgery** 67
   Nicolas Goldaracena and Lucas McCormack

9. **Cystic lesions of the liver** 73
   David Martin and Emmanuel Melloul

10. **Benign liver tumours** 87
    Sadhana Shankar, Evangelia Florou, and Parthi Srinivasan

11. **Modern management of liver trauma** 114
    Philip C. Müller, Valentin Neuhaus, Thomas Pfammatter, and Henrik Petrowsky

PART 4 Aetiology and management of portal hypertension

12. **Extrahepatic portal venous obstruction, idiopathic non-cirrhotic portal fibrosis, and hepatic venous outflow tract obstruction** 124
    Mohammad Qasim Khan and Patrick S. Kamath

13. **Medical management of portal hypertension and its complications** 137
    Mohammad Qasim Khan and Patrick S. Kamath

14. **Interventional radiological and surgical treatment of portal hypertension** 146
    Mohammad Qasim Khan and Patrick S. Kamath

PART 5 Vascular diseases of liver

15. **Budd–Chiari syndrome, veno-occlusive disease, and secondary vascular diseases of the liver** 152
    Patricia Sánchez-Velázquez and Fernando Burdío

PART 6 Neoplasms of liver

16. **Treatment of hepatocellular carcinoma: a surgical perspective** 162
    Vincenzo Mazzaferro, Michele Droz dit Busset, and Matteo Virdis

Contents

17. **Cholangiocarcinoma** 176
    Mohamed Rela and Mettu Srinivas Reddy

18. **Primary neoplasms of the liver: hepatoblastoma** 187
    Paolo Muiesan,[†] Andrea Schlegel, Chiara Grimaldi, and Kejd Bici

19. **Primary neoplasms of the liver: other neoplasms** 204
    Jan Lerut and Quirino Lai

20. **Secondary neoplasms of the liver** 217
    Pål-Dag Line

PART 7 Liver resection and transplantation

21. **Principles and techniques of liver resection** 223
    Philipp Kron and J. Peter A. Lodge

22. **Liver transplantation: general principles** 232
    Greg J. McKenna

23. **Paediatric liver transplantation** 247
    Mureo Kasahara

24. **Live donor liver transplantation** 259
    Michele Finotti and Giuliano Testa

PART 8 Non-operative management and long-term outcomes

25. **Non-operative management of liver lesions** 273
    T. Deepa Shree and Sandeep Botcha

26. **Long-term outcomes following liver surgery** 286
    Yasuhito Iwao and Nigel D. Heaton

SECTION 2 The gall bladder and bile ducts
PART 9 Diagnostic and therapeutic approaches for the biliary tree and gall bladder

27. **Non-invasive imaging of the biliary tract** 301
    Daniela Husarik and Cäcilia S. Reiner

28. **Endoscopic diagnostic and treatment modalities of the biliary system** 311
    Christoph Gubler and Frans Oliver The

29. **Percutaneous biliary imaging and interventions** 323
    Mathilde Vermersch, Alban Denys, and Naik Vietti Violi

[†] It is with regret that we report the passing of Paolo Muiesan during the writing of this volume.

30. **Laparoscopic liver surgery** 336
    Christian Hobeika, François Cauchy, and Olivier Soubrane

31. **Pathogenesis and natural history of gallstones** 348
    Veena Bheeman, Royce P. Vincent, and Ameet G. Patel

PART 10 Specific conditions of the gall bladder

32. **Acute and chronic cholecystitis** 361
    Claire Goumard and Olivier Scatton

33. **Post-cholecystectomy biliary injury** 366
    Kayvan Mohkam, Jean-Yves Mabrut, Agnès Rode, and Mickaël Lesurtel

34. **Biliary fistula, gallstone ileus, and Mirizzi syndrome** 376
    Martin Palavecino and Juan Pekolj

35. **Benign and malignant lesions of the gall bladder** 391
    Anil K. Agarwal and Raja Kalayarasan

36. **Medical and innovative therapies for biliary malignancies** 415
    Sudha Kodali, Joy V. Nolte Fong, and R. Mark Ghobrial

PART 11 The intrahepatic and extrahepatic bile ducts

37. **Biliary atresia** 423
    Priya Ramachandran

38. **Neonatal cholestasis syndrome** 433
    Priya Ramachandran

39. **Acute cholangitis, recurrent cholangitis, and management of common bile duct calculi** 437
    Haitham Triki and Karim Boudjema

40. **Cystic diseases of the biliary system** 446
    Stefan Heinrich

41. **Primary sclerosing cholangitis** 453
    James Neuberger

42. **Malignant lesions of the extrahepatic biliary system** 458
    Philippe Compagnon, Andrea Peloso, and Christian Toso

Index 477

Introduction from the Series Editors

Gastrointestinal (GI) surgery is performed for a range of benign and malignant diseases, in both the elective and emergency settings. Although there are many textbooks related to GI surgery most of them are addressed to a predominantly Western readership or deal with individual organs or organ systems.

We have strived to create a comprehensive *Gastrointestinal Surgery Library* in which each of these six books deals with a specific organ and is edited by internationally recognized experts from both the developed as well as the developing countries. We thus have 14 editors and 350 contributors from 24 different countries from as far afield as Argentina and New Zealand.

The *Gastrointestinal Surgery Library* will, we hope, serve as reference manuals on this important subject and will cater to a global audience. The inclusion of experts across the world to edit the individual volumes and contribute to the chapters will also result in the description of effective management protocols which are relevant to both economically developed and developing nations.

Samiran Nundy
Dirk J. Gouma

Introduction from the Volume Editors

> To study the phenomena of disease without books is to sail an uncharted sea.
>
> Sir William Osler (1849–1919)

The mastery of hepatobiliary surgery requires one to be an accomplished surgical craftsman with an in-depth knowledge of anatomy and physiology, a capable internist, and a skilled radiologist. With exponential developments in technology and an improved understanding of disease processes, most complex hepatobiliary problems are best managed by securing the opinion of experts from all the interrelated disciplines. While compiling this book, we attempted to parallel that dialogue by collating the expertise and experience of all these disciplines and distilling it down into one volume.

This book aims to cover an area of surgical practice and to be available for consultation, not merely in hospital or medical school libraries, but also and more importantly in the surgeon's own office or study. We aspire to provide a comprehensive coverage of the subject matter, so that the readers can feel confident that in turning to it they will, as a rule, be able to obtain good advice and not too often encounter disconcerting hiatuses. To offer such an assurance, we have carefully selected contributors from around the world. They are experts with decades of wisdom and are recognized masters in their field. Most of them are established educators and have successfully trained generations of young surgeons.

Apart from a thorough analysis of current knowledge, future advances in the field, and a review of relevant literature, this book ensures the presence of high-quality images and illustrations. These images enormously clarify and shorten didactic accounts, breaking the monotony of the text.

We believe that this book provides an updated, new evidence-based look at hepatobiliary surgery. We hope that surgeons of different levels of seniority will benefit from this huge effort combining the work of many experts.

Mohamed Rela
Pierre-Alain Clavien

About the Series Editors

Samiran Nundy was a medical undergraduate in Cambridge and Guy's Hospital London, UK and then trained, first in Medicine at the Hammersmith Hospital, and later in Surgery at Guy's, Addenbrooke's Cambridge, the Hammersmith, and the Massachusetts General Hospital in Boston, USA. He has taught at the universities of Cambridge, London, and Harvard, and returned to the All India Institute of Medical Sciences in 1975 where he eventually became Professor and Head of the Department of Gastrointestinal Surgery. He left AIIMS in 1996 to start the Surgical Gastroenterology and Liver Transplantation Department in the Sir Ganga Ram Hospital, New Delhi, India. His clinical and research interests are in the management of complicated diseases of the liver, bowel, and pancreas, the quality of Indian medical research and publications and health information on the web. He has written or edited 37 books and authored or co-authored 236 research papers. He has been Editor of the *National Medical Journal of India*, *Tropical Gastroenterology*, the *Indian Journal of Medical Ethics*, and the website DrRaxa.com and has served on 24 journal Editorial Boards including the *British Medical Journal*. He is Emeritus Editor of *Current Medicine Research and Practice*, on the Board of Trustees of Sir Ganga Ram Hospital, and President of the All India Institute of Medical Sciences, Rishikesh.

Dirk J. Gouma is Emeritus Professor of Surgery at the Academic Medical Center Amsterdam, the Netherlands. He served as chairman of the department of Surgery and chairman of the division of surgical specialities at the AMC. During his surgical training he worked as fellow at Maastricht University and thereafter as associate professor. He conducted his PhD research program at Maastricht; Hammersmith Hospital London, UK; Massachusetts General Hospital, Boston, USA; and Hermann Hospital, Houston, USA. His clinical and research efforts concentrated on outcome of treatment of hepato-biliary and pancreatic disease as well as evaluation of diagnostic strategies and pathophysiology of obstructive jaundice and biliary drainage. More recently aspects of patient safety programs and quality control such as centralization and development and implementation of checklist are included. He has served as chairman of the scientific committee of the European Surgical Association (ESA), Council member of the United European Gastroenterology (UEG); President of the European-African Hepato-Pancreatico-Biliary Association (E-AHPBA), Secretary general of the IHPBA, and chairman of the European Digestive Surgery (EDS). He was member of the National Health Council, Netherlands; Chairman of the Concilium Chirurgicum (the Dutch advisory board of surgical education training) and member of the Editorial Board of several medical journals. He was supervisor of over 50 PhD fellows and is author/co-author of over 660 publications in peer-reviewed journals (H-index 95) and more than 150 non-peer-reviewed papers and chapters in books.

About the Volume Editors

Professor Mohamed Rela is an acclaimed liver transplant surgeon with over 25 years' experience in the field. He has been a Consultant Surgeon and Professor of Liver Surgery at King's College Hospital, London, UK since 1993 and has been working in India since 2009. He now runs the busiest liver transplantation programme in South India, performing over 250 liver transplants each year. Professor Rela has authored over 500 peer-reviewed publications and a number of book chapters including a chapter in the latest edition of *Gray's Anatomy*. In 2011 he started the annual Master Class in Liver Disease series which is now one of the most popular academic events in South Asia, regularly attended by over 1000 delegates across the world. He is the President-Elect of the International Liver Transplantation Society (ILTS).

Professor Pierre-Alain Clavien is a world-renowned surgeon and researcher. Since 2001 he has led the Department of Surgery at the University Hospital Zürich, Switzerland, and leads the liver research group of the Wyss Institute. He was the first surgeon to receive the most prestigious Swiss scientific prize, Otto Naegeli, for his work on liver transplantation. He developed a classification of complications that holds his name, which is used worldwide as the standard reporting for postoperative morbidity. He has organized several international consensus conferences using an independent jury on liver surgery and innovation including one on how to select a chair of medicine ('International Conference on Selection of Academic Medical Chairs') which has had a worldwide impact on academic medicine. Finally, he was a major player in the Oxford Balliol consortium, which defined the IDEAL framework assessing surgical innovations. In 2020 he was elected as an active member of the National Academy of Medicine of the United States of America.

Acknowledgement

We are grateful to Shri Parmanand Tiwari, Executive, Sir Ganga Ram Hospital, for his help in getting this book together.

Abbreviations

AASLD	American Association for the Study of Liver Diseases
AC	acute cholecystitis
AE	alveolar echinococcosis
AFP	alpha-fetoprotein
AGS	Alagille syndrome
AI	artificial intelligence
AIH	autoimmune hepatitis
AJCC	American Joint Committee on Cancer
ALA	amoebic liver abscess
ALF	acute liver failure
ALP	alkaline phosphatase
ALPPS	associating liver partition and portal vein ligation for staged hepatectomy
ALT	alanine aminotransferase
APC	antigen-presenting cell
APRI	aspartate aminotransferase-to-platelet index
ASA	American Society of Anesthesiologists
ASA-PS	American Society of Anesthesiologists—Physical Status
AST	aspartate aminotransferase
ATP	adenosine triphosphate
BA	biliary atresia *or* bile acid
BASM	biliary atresia–splenic malformation
BCA	biliary cystadenoma
BCAC	biliary cystadenocarcinoma
BCLC	Barcelona Clinic Liver Cancer
BCLS	breast cancer liver secondaries
BD	bile duct
BDI	bile duct injury
BERS	biliary embryonal rhabdomyosarcoma
BFSG	biliary fistulae secondary to gallstones
BRIC	benign recurrent intrahepatic cholestasis
BRTO	balloon-occluded retrograde transvenous obliteration
B-TACE	balloon-occluded transarterial chemoembolization
CA19-9	carbohydrate antigen 19-9
CC/CCA	cholangiocarcinoma
CCK	cholecystokinin
CCM	congenital choledochal malformation
CEA	carcinoembryonic antigen
CECT	contrast-enhanced computed tomography
CHIC	Children's Hepatic tumours International Collaboration
CHIC-HS	Children's Hepatic Tumor International Collaboration–Hepatoblastoma Stratification
CI	confidence interval
CNI	calcineurin inhibitor
COG	Children's Oncology Group
CRCL	colorectal liver secondaries
CRLM	colorectal liver metastasis
CRT	chemoradiotherapy
CT	computed tomography
C-TACE	conventional transarterial chemoembolization
CTP	Child–Turcotte–Pugh
CVS	critical view of safety
dCC/dCCA	distal cholangiocarcinoma
DCS	damage control surgery
DDLT	deceased donor liver transplantation
DEB-TACE	drug-eluting bead transarterial chemoembolization
DFS	disease-free survival
DGE	delayed gastric emptying
DH	diaphragmatic hernias
DOAC	direct-acting oral anticoagulant
DPM	ductal plate malformation
DSRS	distal splenorenal shunt
EASL	European Association for the Study of the Liver
EBD	external biliary drain/drainage
EBV	Epstein–Barr virus
EC	echinococcal cyst
eCCA	extrahepatic cholangiocarcinoma
ECM	extracellular matrix
EFS	event-free survival
EGFR	epidermal growth factor receptor
EHE	epithelioid haemangioendothelioma
EHPVO	extrahepatic portal venous obstruction
EHS	embryonal hepatic sarcoma
ELISA	enzyme-linked immunosorbent assay
ELITA	European Liver and Intestine Transplant Association
ELTR	European Liver Transplant Registry
EN	enteral nutrition
ENBD	endoscopic nasobiliary drainage
ERCP	endoscopic retrograde cholangiopancreatography
EUS-BD	endoscopic ultrasound-guided biliary drainage
FAST	Focused Assessment with Sonography for Trauma
FDG	fluorodeoxyglucose
FHVP	free hepatic venous pressure
FISH	fluorescence in situ hybridization
FLR	future liver remnant
FNA	fine-needle aspiration
FNH	focal nodular hyperplasia

Abbreviations

GB	gall bladder	KPE	Kasai portoenterostomy
GBC	gall bladder cancer/carcinoma	Lap-C	laparoscopic cholecystectomy
Gd-BOPTA	gadobenate dimeglumine	LDLT	living donor liver transplantation
Gd-EOB-DTPA	gadolinium ethoxybenzyl diethylenetriamine pentaacetic acid	LHA	left hepatic artery
		LHD	left hepatic duct
GGT	gamma-glutamyl transpeptidase	LHV	left hepatic vein
GIST	gastrointestinal stromal tumour	LLR	laparoscopic liver resection
GPOH	German Society of Pediatric Oncology and Hematology	LLS	left lateral segment
		LMS	leiomyosarcoma
HAIC	hepatic arterial infusion therapy	LMWH	low-molecular-weight heparin
HAML	hepatic angiomyolipoma	LN	lymph node
HAT	hepatic artery thrombosis	LR	liver regeneration *or* liver resection
HB	hepatoblastoma	LSEC	liver sinusoidal endothelial cell
HBV	hepatitis B virus	LT	liver transplantation
HCA	hepatocellular adenoma	LTWR	length-to-width ratio
HCC	hepatocellular carcinoma	MCN	mucinous cystic neoplasm
HCN-NOS	hepatocellular neoplasm not otherwise classified	MELD	Model for End-Stage Liver Disease
		MELD-Na	Model for End-Stage Liver Disease with sodium
HCV	hepatitis C virus		
HEHE	hepatic epithelioid haemangioendothelioma	MHV	middle hepatic vein
HGF	hepatocyte growth factor	MILS	minimally invasive liver surgery
HIFU	high-intensity focused ultrasound	MIS	minimally invasive surgery
HIHE	hepatic infantile haemangioendothelioma	MODY	maturity-onset diabetes of the young
HMB-45	human melanoma black-45	MR	magnetic resonance
HPB	hepatopancreatobiliary	MRCP	magnetic resonance cholangiopancreatography
HPC	haemangiopericytoma	MRI	magnetic resonance imaging
HPD	hepatopancreatoduodenectomy	MS	Mirizzi syndrome
HR	hazard ratio	MSKCC	Memorial Sloan Kettering Cancer Center
HSC	hepatic stellate cell	mTOR	mammalian target of rapamycin
HSCT	haematopoietic stem cell transplantation	MWA	microwave ablation
HSVN	hepatic small vessel neoplasm	NADH	reduced nicotinamide adenine dinucleotide
HVPG	hepatic venous pressure gradient	NAFLD	non-alcoholic fatty liver disease
HX	hepatectomy	NASH	non-alcoholic steatohepatitis
IBD	inflammatory bowel disease	NBBB	non-selective beta-blocker
ICC	intrahepatic cholangiocellular carcinoma	NCCN	National Comprehensive Cancer Network
iCCA	intrahepatic cholangiocarcinoma	NCS	neonatal cholestasis syndrome
ICOS	inducible T-cell co-stimulator	NET	neuroendocrine tumour
ICU	intensive care unit	NETLS	neuroendocrine tumour with liver secondaries
IDH	isocitrate dehydrogenase	NICE	National Institute for Health and Care Excellence
IEBD	internal–external biliary drain		
IGBC	incidental gall bladder cancer	NK	natural killer
IH	immunohistochemical	NOM	non-operative management
I-HCA	inflammatory hepatocellular adenoma	NRH	nodular regenerative hyperplasia
IHCC	intrahepatic cholangiocarcinoma	NSAID	non-steroidal anti-inflammatory drug
IMCU	intermediate care unit	OCP	oral contraceptive pill
INCPH	idiopathic non-cirrhotic portal hypertension	OS	overall survival
INR	international normalized ratio	PAIR	puncture, aspiration, injection, and re-aspiration
IOC	intraoperative cholangiography		
IOUS	intraoperative ultrasound	PBC	primary biliary cholangitis
IPL	inflammatory pseudotumour of the liver	PBD	preoperative biliary drainage
IPMN-B	intraductal papillary mucinous neoplasm of the bile ducts	pCCA	perihilar cholangiocarcinoma
		PCLD	polycystic liver disease
IPNB	intraductal papillary neoplasm of the bile duct	PCR	polymerase chain reaction
		PEI	percutaneous ethanol injection
IRHV	inferior right hepatic veins	PEP	post-ERCP pancreatitis
IVC	inferior vena cava	PET	positron emission tomography
JPLT	Japanese Study Group for Pediatric Liver Tumors	PFIC	progressive familial intrahepatic cholestasis
KC	Kupffer cell	PHCC	perihilar cholangiocarcinoma

PHITT	Pediatric Hepatic International Tumor Trial	SFSS	small-for-size syndrome
PHLF	post-hepatectomy liver failure	SIOPEL	International Childhood Liver Tumor Study Group
PLTCC	Pediatric Liver Tumor Consensus Classification	SLT	split liver transplantation
PMN	polymorphonuclear neutrophil	SMA	superior mesenteric artery
PN	parenteral nutrition	SMV	superior mesenteric vein
PNF	primary non-function	SNL	survival with native liver
POBD	preoperative biliary drainage	SOS	sinusoidal obstruction syndrome
POSTEXT	POST-Treatment EXTent of the disease	SPECT	single-photon emission computed tomography
PRETEXT	PRE-Treatment EXTent of the tumour	SRTR	Scientific Registry of Transplant Recipients
PS	patient survival	TACE	transarterial chemoembolization
PSC	primary sclerosing cholangitis	TAE	transarterial embolization
PTBD	percutaneous transhepatic biliary drainage	TARE	transarterial radioembolization
PTC	percutaneous transhepatic cholangiography	TB	tuberculosis
PTCD	percutaneous transhepatic cholangiography and drainage	TCR	T-cell receptor
		TGF	transforming growth factor
PTLD	post-transplant lymphoproliferative disorder	TIPS	transjugular intrahepatic portosystemic shunt
PVA	polyvinyl alcohol	TKI	tyrosine kinase inhibitor
PVE	portal vein embolization	TLR	Toll-like receptor
PVT	portal vein thrombosis	TNM	tumour, node, and metastasis
RCT	randomized controlled trial	Treg	T-regulatory
RF	radiofrequency	TSH	two-stage hepatectomy
RFA	radiofrequency ablation	UC	ulcerative colitis
RHA	right hepatic artery	UDCA	ursodeoxycholic acid
RHV	right hepatic vein	UELS	undifferentiated embryonal liver sarcoma
RL	right lobe	UICC	Union for International Cancer Control
SAAG	serum–ascites albumin gradient	ULN	upper limit of normal
SaHCC	sarcomatous hepatocellular carcinoma	UNOS	United Network for Organ Sharing
SAP	serum alkaline phosphatase	USG	ultrasonography
SBP	spontaneous bacterial peritonitis	VEGF	vascular endothelial growth factor
SBRT	stereotactic body radiation therapy	VKA	vitamin K antagonist
SCU	small cell undifferentiated	VOD	veno-occlusive disease
SEER	Surveillance, Epidemiology, and End Results	WDF	well-differentiated fetal
SEMS	self-expandable metal stent	WHVP	wedged hepatic venous pressure

Contributors

Anil K. Agarwal Department of GI Surgery, GB Pant Institute of Medical Education and Research, and MAM College, Delhi University, New Delhi, India

Varanasi Y. Bhargav Department of Hepatology, Sri Ramachandra Institute of Higher Education and Research, Chennai, India

Veena Bheeman Gastroenterology Service, King's College Hospital NHS Foundation Trust, London, UK

Kejd Bici Department of Pediatric Surgery, Meyer Children's Hospital, Florence, Italy

Sandeep Botcha Dr. Rela Institute and Medical Centre, Chennai, India

Karim Boudjema Department of Hepatobiliary and Digestive Surgery, Rennes University Hospital, Rennes, France

Fernando Burdío Department of General and Digestive Surgery, University Hospital of Mar, Barcelona, Spain

François Cauchy Department of HPB Surgery and Liver Transplantation, Beaujon Hospital, Assistance Publique, Hôpitaux de Paris, France; Université de Paris, France

Pierre-Alain Clavien Department of Surgery and Transplantation, University Hospital, Zürich, Switzerland

Philippe Compagnon Division of Transplantation, Department of Surgery, Geneva University Hospitals, Geneva, Switzerland

Guido Costa Department of Hepatobiliary and General Surgery, Humanitas Clinical and Research Center—IRCCS, Rozzano, Milan, Italy; Department of Biomedical Sciences, Humanitas University, Pieve Emanuele, Milan, Italy

Alban Denys Department of Radiology, Lausanne University Hospital, Lausanne, Switzerland

Matteo Donadon Department of Hepatobiliary and General Surgery, Humanitas Clinical and Research Center – IRCCS, Rozzano, Milan, Italy; Department of Biomedical Sciences, Humanitas University, Pieve Emanuele, Milan, Italy

Michele Droz dit Busset HPB Surgery, Hepatology and Liver Transplantation, Istituto Nazionale Tumori, Fondazione IRCCS, Milan, Italy

Michele Finotti Simmons Transplant Institute, Baylor University Medical Center, Dallas, Texas, USA

Evangelia Florou Institute of Liver Studies, King's College Hospital, London, UK

Frans Oliver The Department of Gastroenterology and Hepatology, University Hospital Zürich, Zürich, Switzerland

R. Mark Ghobrial J.C. Walter Jr. Transplant Center, Sherrie and Alan Conover Center for Liver Disease and Transplantation, Weill Cornell Medical College, and Houston Methodist Research Institute, Houston, Texas, USA

Nicolas Goldaracena Abdominal Organ Transplant and Hepatobiliary Surgery, Division of Transplant Surgery, Department of Surgery, University of Virginia Health System, Charlottesville, Virginia, USA

Claire Goumard Department of Hepatobiliary Surgery and Liver Transplantation, Sorbonne Université, Hôpital Pitié-Salpêtrière, Assistance Publique-Hopitaux de Paris, France

Chiara Grimaldi Department of Pediatric Surgery, Meyer Children's Hospital, Florence, Italy

Christoph Gubler Department of Gastroenterology and Hepatology, University Hospital Zürich, Zürich, Switzerland

Nigel D. Heaton Institute of Liver Studies, King's College Hospital NHS Foundation Trust, London, UK

Stefan Heinrich Department of General, Visceral, and Transplantation Surgery, University Hospital of Mainz, Mainz, Germany

Christian Hobeika Department of HPB Surgery and Liver Transplantation, Beaujon Hospital, Assistance Publique, Hôpitaux de Paris, France; Université de Paris, France

Bostjan Humar Swiss Hepato-Pancreato-Biliary Laboratory, Department of Surgery, University Hospital Zürich, Zürich, Switzerland

Rok Humar Research Unit, Department of Internal Medicine, University Hospital Zürich, Zürich, Switzerland

Daniela Husarik Radiology Department, Cantonal Hospital St. Gallen, St. Gallen, Switzerland

Yasuhito Iwao Institute of Liver Studies, King's College Hospital NHS Foundation Trust, London, UK

Mayank Jain Department of Gastroenterology, Arihant Hospital and Research Centre, Indore, India

Raja Kalayarasan Department of GI Surgery, GB Pant Institute of Medical Education and Research, and MAM College, Delhi University, New Delhi, India

Ilankumaran Kaliamoorthy Department of Liver Intensive Care and Anaesthesia, Dr. Rela Institute and Medical Centre, Bharath Institute of Higher Education and Research, Chennai, India

Patrick S. Kamath Division of Gastroenterology and Hepatology, Mayo Clinic Rochester, Minnesota, USA

Rathnavel G. Kanagavelu Department of Liver Intensive Care and Anaesthesia, Dr. Rela Institute and Medical Centre, Bharath Institute of Higher Education and Research, Chennai, India

Mureo Kasahara Organ Transplantation Center, National Center for Child Health and Development, Tokyo, Japan

Chandan Kumar Kedarisetty Department of Hepatology, Sri Ramachandra Institute of Higher Education and Research, Chennai, India

Mohammad Qasim Khan Division of Gastroenterology and Hepatology, Mayo Clinic, Rochester, Minnesota, USA

Sudha Kodali J.C. Walter Jr. Transplant Center, Sherrie and Alan Conover Center for Liver Disease and Transplantation, Weill Cornell Medical College, and Houston Methodist Research Institute, Houston, Texas, USA

Philipp Kron HPB and Transplant Unit, St James's University Hospital, Leeds, UK

Quirino Lai Institute for Experimental and Clinical Research (IREC), Université Catholique de Louvain—UCL, Brussels, Belgium; Hepatobiliary and Organ Transplantation Unit, Sapienza University of Rome, Umberto I Polyclinic of Rome, Rome, Italy

Ezio Lanza Department of Interventional Radiology, Humanitas Clinical and Research Center—IRCCS, Rozzano, Milan, Italy

Jan Lerut Institute for Experimental and Clinical Research (IREC), Université Catholique de Louvain—UCL, Brussels, Belgium

Contributors

Mickaël Lesurtel Department of Digestive Surgery and Liver Transplantation, Croix Rousse University Hospital, Hospices Civils de Lyon, University of Lyon, Lyon, France

Pål-Dag Line Department of Transplantation Medicine, Oslo University Hospital and Institute for Clinical Medicine, University of Oslo, Oslo, Norway

J. Peter A. Lodge HPB and Transplant Unit, St James's University Hospital, Leeds, UK

Jean-Yves Mabrut Department of Digestive Surgery and Liver Transplantation, Croix Rousse University Hospital, Hospices Civils de Lyon, University of Lyon, Lyon, France

David Martin Department of Visceral Surgery, University Hospital CHUV, University of Lausanne, Lausanne, Switzerland

Vincenzo Mazzaferro Department of Oncology and Hemato-Oncology, University of Milan, Milan, Italy; HPB Surgery, Hepatology and Liver Transplantation, Istituto Nazionale Tumori, Fondazione IRCCS, Milan, Italy

Lucas McCormack Liver Surgery and Abdominal Transplantation Unit, Hospital Alema of Buenos Aires, Buenos Aires, Argentina

Greg J. McKenna Texas A&M School of Medicine, Dallas, Texas, USA

Emmanuel Melloul Department of Visceral Surgery, University Hospital CHUV, University of Lausanne, Lausanne, Switzerland

Joachim C. Mertens Department of Gastroenterology and Hepatology, University Hospital Zürich, Zürich, Switzerland

Kayvan Mohkam Department of Digestive Surgery and Liver Transplantation, Croix Rousse University Hospital, Hospices Civils de Lyon, University of Lyon, Lyon, France

Omar Y. Mousa Division of Gastroenterology and Hepatology, Mayo Clinic Rochester, Minnesota, USA; Division of Gastroenterology, Mayo Clinic Health System, Mankato, Minnesota, USA

Paolo Muiesan[†] Liver and Hepato-Pancreato-Biliary (HPB) Unit, Queen Elizabeth and Birmingham Children's Hospitals, Birmingham, UK

Philip C. Müller Swiss HPB and Transplantation Center, Department of Surgery and Transplantation, University Hospital Zürich, Zürich, Switzerland

James Neuberger Liver Unit, Queen Elizabeth Hospital, Birmingham, UK

Valentin Neuhaus Department of Traumatology, University Hospital Zürich, Zürich, Switzerland

Joy V. Nolte Fong Houston Methodist Research Institute, Houston, Texas, USA

Martin Palavecino Hepato-Pancreato-Biliary Surgery Section, and General Surgery Service, Hospital Italiano de Buenos Aires, Argentina

Ameet G. Patel Hepatobiliary and Pancreatic (HPB) Service, King's College Hospital NHS Foundation Trust, London, UK

Juan Pekolj Hepato-Pancreato-Biliary Surgery Section, General Surgery Service, and Liver Transplantation Unit, Hospital Italiano de Buenos Aires, Buenos Aires, Argentina

Andrea Peloso Division of Abdominal Surgery, Department of Surgery, Geneva University Hospitals, Geneva, Switzerland

Henrik Petrowsky Swiss HPB and Transplantation Center, Department of Surgery and Transplantation, University Hospital Zürich, Zürich, Switzerland

Thomas Pfammatter Department of Interventional Radiology, University Hospital Zürich, Zürich, Switzerland

Akila Rajakumar Department of Liver Intensive Care and Anaesthesia, Dr. Rela Institute and Medical Centre, Bharath Institute of Higher Education and Research, Chennai, India

Priya Ramachandran Kanchi Kamakoti Childs Trust Hospital, and Dr. Rela Institute and Medical Centre, Chennai, India

Ashwin Rammohan Institute of Liver Disease and Transplantation, Dr. Rela Institute and Medical Centre, Chennai, India

Mettu Srinivas Reddy Institute of Liver Disease and Transplantation, Gleneagles Global Hospital and Health City, Cheran Nagar, Chennai, India

Cäcilia S. Reiner Institute of Diagnostic and Interventional Radiology, University Hospital Zürich, Zürich, Switzerland

Mohamed Rela Bharath Institute of Higher Education and Research (BIHER), and Dr. Rela Institute and Medical Centre, Chennai, India

Agnès Rode Department of Radiology, Croix Rousse University Hospital, Hospices Civils de Lyon, University of Lyon, Lyon, France

Patricia Sánchez-Velázquez Department of General and Digestive Surgery, University Hospital of Mar, and Institut Hospital del Mar d'Investigacions Mèdiques (IMIM), Pompeu Fabra University, Barcelona, Spain

Olivier Scatton Department of Hepatobiliary Surgery and Liver Transplantation, Sorbonne Université, Hôpital Pitié-Salpêtrière, Assistance Publique-Hopitaux de Paris, France

Andrea Schlegel Liver and Hepato-Pancreato-Biliary (HPB) Unit, Queen Elizabeth and Birmingham Children's Hospitals, Birmingham, UK

Thamarai S. Selvan Department of Hepatology, Sri Ramachandra Institute of Higher Education and Research, Chennai, India

Sadhana Shankar Institute of Liver Studies, King's College Hospital, London, UK

T. Deepa Shree Department of Interventional Radiology, Dr. Rela Institute and Medical Centre, Chennai, India

Olivier Soubrane Department of Surgery, Institut Mutualiste Montsouris, Paris, France

Parthi Srinivasan Institute of Liver Studies, King's College Hospital, London, UK

Bruno Stieger Department of Clinical Pharmacology and Toxicology, University Hospital Zürich, Zürich, Switzerland

Giuliano Testa Simmons Transplant Institute, Baylor University Medical Center, Dallas, Texas, USA

Guido Torzilli Department of Hepatobiliary and General Surgery, Humanitas Clinical and Research Center—IRCCS, Rozzano, Milan, Italy; Department of Biomedical Sciences, Humanitas University, Pieve Emanuele, Milan, Italy

Christian Toso Division of Abdominal Surgery, Department of Surgery, Geneva University Hospitals, Geneva, Switzerland

Haitham Triki Department of Hepatobiliary and Digestive Surgery, Rennes University Hospital, Rennes, France

Jayanthi Venkataraman Department of Hepatology, Sri Ramachandra Institute of Higher Education and Research, Chennai, India

Mathilde Vermersch Department of Radiology, Lausanne University Hospital, Lausanne, Switzerland; Department of Radiology, Valenciennes Hospital, Valenciennes, France; Department of Radiology and Digestive Imaging, Lille University Hospital, Lille, France

Royce P. Vincent Faculty of Life Sciences and Medicine, King's College London, London, UK; Department of Clinical Biochemistry, King's College Hospital NHS Foundation Trust, London, UK

Naik Vietti Violi Department of Radiology, Lausanne University Hospital, Lausanne, Switzerland

Matteo Virdis HPB Surgery, Hepatology and Liver Transplantation, Istituto Nazionale Tumori, Fondazione IRCCS, Milan, Italy

---

[†] It is with regret that we report the passing of Paolo Muiesan during the writing of this volume.

SECTION 1
The liver

Anatomy and physiology

1. Surgical anatomy of the liver 3
   Ashwin Rammohan and Mohamed Rela

2. Applied physiology of the liver 12
   Bruno Stieger and Joachim C. Mertens

3. Liver regeneration 17
   Bostjan Humar and Rok Humar

4. Perioperative management and nutrition in patients with liver and biliary tract disease 30
   Akila Rajakumar, Ilankumaran Kaliamoorthy, and Rathanvel G. Kanagavelu

Investigations

5. Liver function tests and assessment of liver function 40
   Omar Y. Mousa and Patrick S. Kamath

6. Imaging: ultrasound, computed tomography, magnetic resonance imaging, nuclear medicine, and angiography 49
   Guido Costa, Ezio Lanza, Matteo Donadon, and Guido Torzilli

Infectious disease of the liver

7. Bacterial and parasitic infections of the liver 59
   Chandan Kumar Kedarisetty, Mayank Jain, Thamarai S. Selvan, Varanasi Y. Bhargav, and Jayanthi Venkataraman

8. Fatty liver in liver surgery 67
   Nicolas Goldaracena and Lucas McCormack

9. Cystic lesions of the liver 73
   David Martin and Emmanuel Melloul

10. Benign liver tumours 87
    Sadhana Shankar, Evangelina Florou, and Parthi Srinivasan

11. Modern management of liver trauma 114
    Philip C. Müller, Valentin Neuhaus, Thomas Pfammatter, and Henrik Petrowsky

Aetiology and management of portal hypertension

12. Extrahepatic portal venous obstruction, idiopathic non-cirrhotic portal fibrosis, and hepatic venous outflow tract obstruction 124
    Mohammad Qasim Khan and Patrick S. Kamath

13. Medical management of portal hypertension and its complications 137
    Mohammad Qasim Khan and Patrick S. Kamath

14. Interventional radiological and surgical treatment of portal hypertension 146
    Mohammad Qasim Khan and Patrick S. Kamath

Vascular diseases of liver

15. Budd–Chiari syndrome, veno-occlusive disease, and secondary vascular diseases of the liver 152
    Patricia Sánchez-Velázquez and Fernando Burdío

Neoplasms of liver

16. Treatment of hepatocellular carcinoma: a surgical perspective 162
    Vincenzo Mazzaferro, Michele Droz dit Busset, and Matteo Virdis

17. Cholangiocarcinoma 176
    Mohamed Rela and Mettu Srinivas Reddy

18. Primary neoplasms of the liver: hepatoblastoma 187
    Paolo Muiesan,† Andrea Schlegel, Chiara Grimaldi, and Kejd Bici

19. Primary neoplasms of the liver: other neoplasms 204
    Jan Lerut and Quirino Lai

20. Secondary neoplasms of the liver 217
    Pål-Dag Line

Liver resection and transplantation

21. Principles and techniques of liver resection 223
    Philipp Kron and J. Peter A. Lodge

22. Liver transplantation: general principles 232
    Greg J. McKenna

23. Paediatric liver transplantation 247
    Mureo Kasahara

24. Live donor liver transplantation 259
    Michele Finotti and Giuliano Testa

Non-operative management and long-term outcomes

25. Non-operative management of liver lesions 273
    T. Deepa Shree and Sandeep Botcha

26. Long-term outcomes following liver surgery 286
    Yasuhito Iwao and Nigel D. Heaton

1

Surgical anatomy of the liver

Ashwin Rammohan and Mohamed Rela

Introduction

A comprehensive understanding of liver anatomy and its application is a sine qua non for safe liver surgery. Most immediate postoperative biliary and vascular complications can be attributed to technical problems, many of which may be due to a failure of recognition of anomalous anatomy. Relevance of this understanding is apparent in various liver surgeries, which most often are a balance between oncological clearance and preservation of an adequate functional hepatic reserve. A thorough knowledge of liver anatomy is also of paramount importance in liver transplantation (LT), especially in split liver transplantation (SLT), paediatric LT, and living donor liver transplantation (LDLT), where the minimization of complications is intimately associated with anatomical and technical competence.

The anatomy of the liver can be described at three different levels of complexity according to the use that the description serves.[1,2] The first, conventional, level corresponds to the standard extrahepatic anatomy and the traditional eight-segment schema of Couinaud. This serves as a common language between clinicians from different specialties to describe the location of focal hepatic lesions. The second, surgical, level to be applied to anatomical liver resections and transplantations, takes into account the detailed branching of the major vascular pedicles and biliary radicles. The third, histological, level of complexity refers to the microscopic anatomy and bridges the anatomical and physiological perceptions of the liver.

This chapter will present a brief overview of the first and second levels of liver anatomy with a view to providing a comprehensive understanding of its surgical application.

History of hepatic segmentation

Rex (1888), Cantlie (1898), and Serege (1901) classified the liver into left and right sides. Rex, in 1888, advocated the concept of the 'hemiliver' based on the anatomy of the portal venous system and found that the boundary between the right and left hemilivers was located along the line connecting the gall bladder bed and the inferior vena cava (IVC) and that the middle hepatic vein (MHV) indicated the position of this interlobar plane.[3–5] Cantlie independently proposed the same anatomical characteristics and predicted clinical applications of these segments for bleeding control during hepatectomy or portal vein ligation. Therefore, the interlobar line between either side of the hemiliver has eponymously been called the 'Rex–Cantlie line'. The intersegmental borders were further classified by Hjortsjö (1948), Healey (1953), and Couinaud (1954).[3,4,6,7] Healey and Schroy established the current basic concept of gross liver segmentation, which consisted of the left lateral, medial, right anterior, and right posterior areas, each of which was further divided into two parts. Their findings were used by Couinaud in 1954 to further the concept of liver segmentation into eight parts.[7]

Liver segmentation

The terminology of the anatomical divisions is based completely on the internal anatomy and the true definition of segmental anatomy is dictated by the vascular pedicle supplying each part of the liver (Figure 1.1). Thus, the terms 'liver' or 'hemiliver' refer to the first-order division, and the terms 'sector' and 'segment' refer to second- and third-order divisions, respectively. The term 'portal scissura' refers to a plane which divides the liver into its sectors. Interestingly, as discussed below, while each of the portal scissurae has a hepatic vein within it, they may or may not have a portal vein coursing in them.

The three main hepatic veins within the scissurae divide the liver into four sectors, each of which receives a portal pedicle. The main portal scissura contains the MHV and progresses from the middle of the gall bladder bed anteriorly to the left of the IVC posteriorly. The right and left parts of the liver, demarcated by the main portal scissure, are independent in terms of portal vascularization and biliary drainage. These right and left parts of the livers are themselves divided into two by the remaining portal scissurae. These four subdivisions are second order and hence are referred to as sectors. The right portal scissura separates the right liver into two sectors—anteromedial (anterior) and posterolateral (posterior)—with the right hepatic vein (RHV) running along it. The left portal scissura divides the left liver into two sectors, but the left portal scissura does not coincide with the umbilical fissure. Since it does not contain the left hepatic vein (LHV), the umbilical fissure is not a portal scissura; instead it contains a portal pedicle. The left portal scissura is located posterior to the ligamentum teres and within the left liver, along the course of the LHV. Although the description by Couinaud

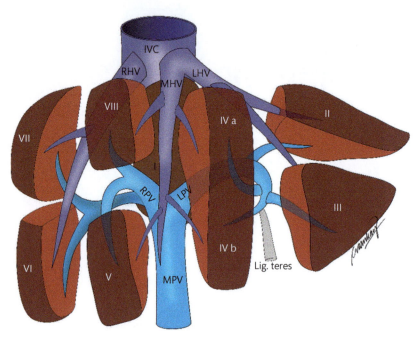

Figure 1.1 Segmentation of the liver. I–VIII, liver segments; IVC, inferior vena cava; LHV, left hepatic vein; Lig. teres, ligamentum teres; LPV, left portal vein; MHV, middle hepatic vein; MPV, main portal vein; RHV, right hepatic vein; RPV, right portal vein.

is widely used, an alternative terminology to ensure uniformity of usage was suggested by a committee of the International Hepato-Pancreatico-Biliary Association in 2000.[8] The main difference is that in the alternative terminology, Couinaud's sectors are referred to as sections. Also, the left medial section is composed of one segment (i.e. segment IV). While the above anatomical descriptions serve as a guide for surgery, it is vital to recognize that there exist an infinite number of anatomical variations in vascular branching patterns as well as segmental size and location that will not always follow textbook definitions.

Hepatic veins

The venous drainage of the liver comprises three main hepatic veins that drain into the suprahepatic part of the IVC, and a multitude of accessory hepatic veins that drain directly into the retrohepatic IVC (Figures 1.1 and 1.2). The RHV, the longest vein in the liver, is single in about 94% of cases and runs in the plane between the anterior and posterior sectors of the right lobe (RL).[9–11] The main trunk is formed by the convergence of an anterior trunk situated in the right portal fissure (draining mainly segments VI and parts of segment V), and a posterior trunk that chiefly drains segment VII and parts of segment VIII. The MHV courses along the Rex–Cantlie line in the principal portal fissure and forms a common trunk with the LHV in about 85% of cases. It drains the central sectors (segments IV, V, and VIII) of the liver, receiving constant tributaries from segment IV on the left, and from segments V and VIII on the right.[5,9–11] It is often the main vein draining the right anterior sector. The LHV arises from the confluence of a transverse vein draining segment II and a sagittal vein draining segment III. It occasionally receives a contribution from segment IV. The main trunk, in the majority of cases, forms a common channel with the MHV and opens into the suprahepatic IVC. Occasionally, it runs as an independent vein of the left lateral segment (LLS), draining separately from the MHV.[5,10,12] Short accessory (inferior) right hepatic veins (IRHVs), not to be mistaken for the caudate lobe veins, drain the dorsal sector of the liver (mainly segments VI and VII) and empty directly into the retrohepatic IVC on its right.

Variations and anomalies

The size of the main RHV determines the number and calibre of accessory hepatic veins. If the RHV is large, it drains most of the right posterior sector resulting in small or absent IRHVs. If the RHV is medium sized, one or more IRHVs, 0.5 ± 1 cm in diameter, drain the posteroinferior segment (segment VI) of the RL directly into the IVC.[2,4,5,10,11] In just under a quarter of livers, however, the RHV is small and short and drains only segment VII, while one or more large IRHVs, up to 1.8 cm in diameter, drain the bulk of the posteroinferior area of the RL (Figure 1.3). In such circumstances the right anterior sector can drain solely into the MHV. The MHV is formed by the union of the segment V and segment IVb veins and drains segments V, VIII, and IV. It receives a variable number of tributaries from each of these segments. Usually, there are up to four major veins (≥0.5 cm in diameter) which drain into the MHV from segments V and VIII. The volume of segment IV draining into the MHV depends on the presence and calibre of the fissural vein. Present in over 60% of people, the fissural or umbilical vein drains variably into the LHV, at the LHV–MHV confluence as a trifurcation or rarely into the cranial part of the MHV. In less than 10% of people the segment III vein crosses the rex recess to join the MHV instead of uniting with the segment II vein.[5,9,12,13]

Implications

A thorough preoperative knowledge of the variations and course of these veins is crucial for safe liver surgery. Formal major anatomical resections of the liver follow the planes in which the RHV and MHV lie. Respecting these planes allows for a relatively bloodless

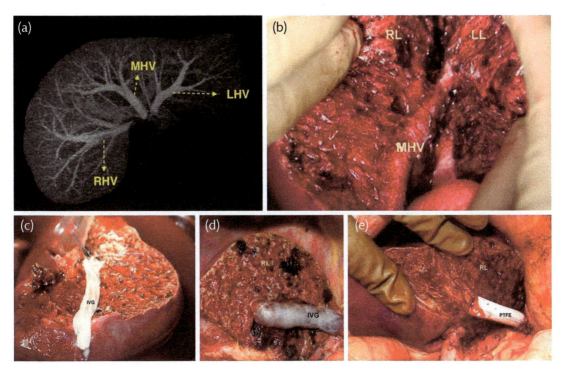

Figure 1.2 Hepatic venous anatomy. (a) Computed tomography scan showing the anatomical configuration of the three main hepatic veins. (b) Intraoperative image during the live donor operation following liver parenchymal transection along the plane of the middle hepatic vein (MHV). (c) Bench reconstruction of venous outflow of the anterior sector (segments V, VIII) in a right lobe graft, using a cadaveric iliac vein graft (IVG). (d) Liver graft post implantation, showing a well-drained anterior sector via the IVG. (e) Synthetic grafts like polytetrafluoroethylene (PTFE) may also be used as conduits to reconstruct the anterior sector venous drainage. LHV, left hepatic vein; LL, left lobe; RHV, right hepatic vein; RL, right lobe.

and complication-free surgery. The commonest form of SLT involves division of the liver into a LLS based on the LHV, and an extended RL based on the MHV and RHV. The line of splitting passes through the watershed zone, and tributaries of the LHV and MHV draining this zone are invariably encountered. These can be ligated without compromising the outflow of the LLS or segment IV. Care is, however, required when dealing with a segment III vein draining into the MHV. This may also be encountered in LLS donations in LDLT. After parenchymal division, the graft's two outflow orifices may be unified via a venoplasty using a vein patch.[5,12] Sometimes, it

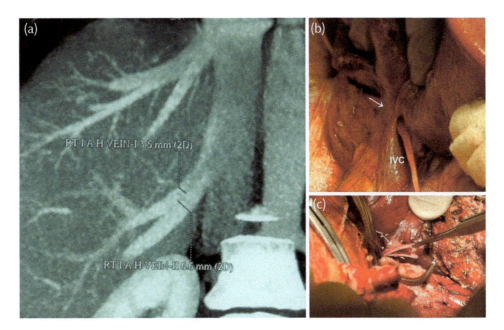

Figure 1.3 Anatomy and surgical implications of the presence of inferior right hepatic veins (IRHVs). (a) Computed tomography scan showing the presence of inferior accessory hepatic (IAH) vein. (b) Intraoperative image in a live donor operation showing the IRHV (white arrow) draining into the inferior vena cava (IVC). (c) Anastomosis of the IRHV (white arrow) to the recipient's IVC during implantation of the liver graft.

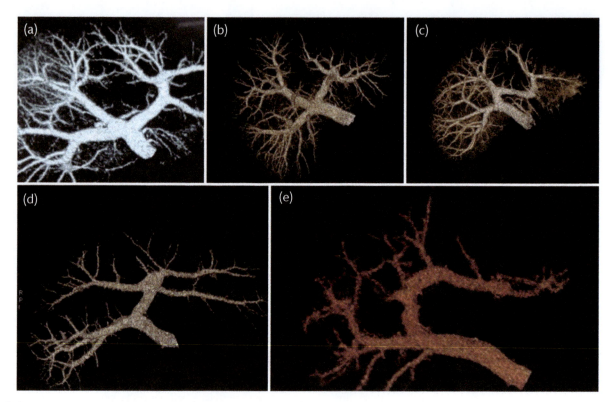

Figure 1.4 Variations in portal venous anatomy (Nakamura classification). (a) Type A anatomy with a short stump of right portal vein. (b) Type B anatomy with trifurcation of the main portal vein. (c, d) Type C and D anatomies with right anterior portal vein arising from the left portal vein. Types B, C, and D will lead to two portal veins in a right lobe liver graft in live donor liver transplantation. These will need to be reconstructed in the recipient. Donor's portal vein stump closures must be done carefully to avoid narrowing the left portal vein. (e) Type E single portal vein supplying the liver. This anatomical variation is an absolute contraindication to liver donation.

may not be possible to reconstruct the outflow into a single opening if the orifices are wide apart, and they will need to be implanted separately onto the recipient's IVC. In very small children, mapping the LHV tributaries aids in anatomically reducing a split LLS graft into a monosegment for LT, thereby overcoming a size discrepancy between donor and recipient.

SLT may also include splitting the whole liver in a manner to provide right and left lobe grafts for two adults. The plane of dissection lies to the right of the MHV to create two grafts of adequate mass for two adult recipients. A not so dissimilar situation is observed in adult LDLTs, where either a right or a left lobe graft is donated by a live related donor. Due to the shared drainage of segments V, VIII, and IV, one of the biggest dilemmas in LDLT is that of the MHV, and the anatomy of the MHV holds the key to RL living donation[14–17] (**Figure 1.2**). While there is centre-to-centre variation in this protocol, traditionally, the MHV was taken with the RL graft. However, with donor safety as paramount, more recently there has been a decisive shift towards retaining the MHV with the donor.[14–18] This leads to venous congestion of segments V and VIII, leading to troublesome bleeding after reperfusion and, more importantly, a compromise of the functional graft liver volume in the recipient. Hence, draining veins of segments V and VIII are reconstructed on the back bench with either prosthetic or cadaveric vein grafts to restore the outflow of the anterior sector (**Figure 1.3**). In some cases, where the left lobe volumes are adequate and the anterior sector veins draining into the MHV cannot be reconstructed, it is not unusual to take most of the MHV with the RL graft.[15,16,19] However, the presence of a fissural vein is necessary for this to be done safely. In RL LDLT grafts, IRHVs, when encountered over 5 mm in size, are implanted separately onto the recipient's IVC[11,20] (**Figure 1.4**).

Finally, congenital absence of the IVC in the recipient, as seen in syndromic biliary atresia, presents unique challenges in paediatric LT. Here, the grafts are either implanted directly onto the cuff of the confluent hepatic veins draining into the right atrium or, in exceptional situations, a new vena cava may be reconstructed using a cadaveric iliac vein.[13]

Portal vein

The main portal vein is created by the confluence of the splenic and superior mesenteric veins behind the neck of the pancreas. It ascends behind the common bile duct and the hepatic artery into the hilum of the liver where it bifurcates into a larger right portal vein and smaller left portal vein. The left branch enters the umbilical fissure and supplies the left liver. The right branch, which has a much shorter extrahepatic course, enters the liver through the hilar plate to divide into the right anterior and the right posterior sectoral branches. The anterior branch curves forward, lies in a vertical plane, and divides into ascending and descending branches for segments V and VIII, respectively. The posterior branch curves posterolaterally, lying in a horizontal plane, and divides similarly for segments VI and VII. The left portal vein is much longer and its course consists of two parts: a transverse part lying at the base of segment IV, and a vertical part that curves anteriorly and to the left as an arch lying in the umbilical fissure where it is joined anteriorly by the round ligament. The anatomy of the left portal venous system is remarkably constant. The segment II vein is usually solitary, whereas segment III can have up to three veins and segment IV a varying number of ascending and descending branches. The caudate lobe is most commonly vascularized by the left branch of the portal vein and only occasionally by the right.

Variations and anomalies

The right portal vein has the most variations (Figure 1.4). A trifurcation of the main portal vein occurs in 10–15% of cases, where the right portal vein immediately divides into two sectoral branches.[21–23] Occasionally, one of the sectoral veins, usually the one supplying the right anterior segments V and VIII, arises from the left portal vein a short distance into its course (type C). A third variation is the caudal shift of the right posterior segments resulting in the right posterior portal vein arising directly from the main portal vein, before its bifurcation.[4,5] In all these circumstances the transverse portion of the left portal vein is usually shorter than normal. Finally, the left portal vein may rarely be absent. In such cases the main portal trunk is undivided as it enters the liver, gives off its right segmental branches and then turns left, to supply branches to the left lobe segments.

Implications

The identification and early ligation of the portal vein in the hilum during liver resectional surgery, especially those for vascular or oncological purposes, helps define the plane of transection and allows for a more bloodless and oncologically precise operation. In subsegmental resections, the portal pedicles are identified ultrasonically or during parenchymal transection and ligated intrahepatically.

Splitting a liver in SLT into an LLS and an extended RL interrupts the portal inflow to segment IV with resultant ischaemia. Whether or not that segment needs to be discarded after a standard split remains a matter of debate.[24–26] In LDLT, for type B or C anatomy, the RL graft invariably has two portal vein stumps. These need to be reconstructed on the bench, using either the recipient's portal vein retrieved from the explanted liver or with a cadaveric vein patch. It is imperative to accurately assess and ensure the lumen and direction of either of the orifices is not compromised during the back-table reconstruction. A particular anomaly which remains an absolute contraindication for SLT and LDLT is the undivided single portal supply to the whole liver (type E)[4,22] (Figure 1.4). On rare occasions, the shortness of the transverse portion of the left portal vein, especially in cases of a trifurcation, may pose difficulties in implantation of the LLS graft. Ligating and dividing a few caudate branches helps overcome this hurdle. The recipient portal vein may be atretic in children with biliary atresia and an interposition or jump graft from the superior mesenteric vein may be necessary to revascularize the graft.[13]

Hepatic artery

The common hepatic artery arises from the coeliac axis and becomes the proper hepatic artery after giving off the gastroduodenal and right gastric arteries. It then branches into the right hepatic artery (RHA) and the left hepatic artery (LHA). The left branch extends towards the base of the umbilical fissure and gives off branches to the caudate lobe and segments II–IV. Often the LHA branches into lateral and medial branches extrahepatically that feed segments II/III and IV, respectively. The segment IV branch can also arise from the RHA and has embryologically been referred to as the middle hepatic artery. The RHA usually passes posterior to the common hepatic duct, although it may pass anteriorly in about 10–20% of cases.[3,5,23] The RHA typically divides into an anterior and posterior branch, which can often be dissected in an extrahepatic location.

Variations and anomalies

The 'standard' anatomy is present in 55–60% of the population. The arterial variations are myriad and so are their classifications. The most commonly used ones are those described by Hiatt et al.[27] and Michels[28] (Figure 1.5). The variations of the hepatic artery can be divided into those of origin, course, and number.

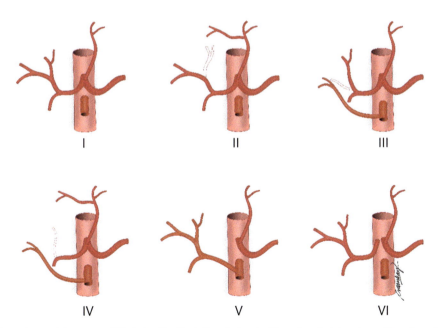

Figure 1.5 Variations in hepatic arterial anatomy (Hiatt classification). Type I: standard hepatic arterial anatomy. Type II: replaced or accessory left hepatic artery (LHA). Type III: replaced or accessory right hepatic artery (RHA). Type IV: replaced or accessory LHA and RHA. Type V: common hepatic artery from superior mesenteric artery. Type VI: common hepatic artery from aorta.

The commonest variation is an aberrant (accessory or replaced) LHA arising from the left gastric artery; this occurs in approximately 25% of cases.[5,23,27] When present this aberrant LHA may provide the whole inflow (replaced) to the LLS in nearly half of the cases. An aberrant (accessory or replaced) RHA from the superior mesenteric artery (SMA) is present in about 17% of cases, and in 12% provides the entire supply of the RL.[5,23,27] The hepatic arterial trunk arises in about 2.5% of people wholly from the SMA and, more rarely, from the left gastric artery or the aorta. When present, the aberrant LHA courses in the hepatogastric ligament to enter the liver anterior to the Arantius ligament. The aberrant RHA from the SMA follows a more posterior course, and lies posterior to the portal vein before coursing anterolaterally to enter the liver.

Implications

Arterial anomalies should readily be recognized during deceased donor multiorgan retrievals. These aberrant arteries, unless precluded due to calibre, will need to be reconstructed. Back-table reconstruction of the aberrant arteries is relatively routine, although it may increase the likelihood of complications. The aberrant RHA is typically anastomosed onto the stump of the gastroduodenal artery, thereby allowing for a single anastomosis in the recipient.

Hepatic arterial reconstructions are much more difficult during LDLT or SLT, as opposed to whole organ transplantation, because the graft arteries are smaller and shorter and, at times, multiple arteries need to be taken with the graft. Double arteries are more commonly seen in left lobe grafts when the segment IV artery arises from the RHA. Two arteries in the RL grafts may occur when there is an accessory RHA from the SMA, or when the anterior and posterior divisions of the RHA occur extrahepatically and these vessels course on either side of the donor's bile duct (Figure 1.6). The second artery may need to be reconstructed in the absence of a pulsatile backflow on division of the smaller of the two arteries, indicating a lack of intraparenchymal arterial overlap. Reconstruction, when indicated, is usually performed on the back-table using the hepatic arterial bifurcation from the recipient's explanted liver—this allows for a single arterial anastomosis in the recipient.

The presence near the hilum of a vascular plexus supplying the extrahepatic and intrahepatic biliary radicals always needs to be kept in mind with a view to minimizing hilar dissection, thereby reducing the incidence of a postoperative ischaemic biliary stricture.

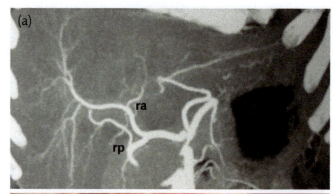
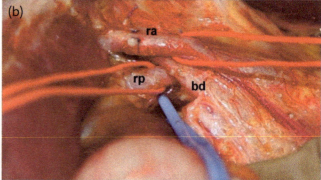
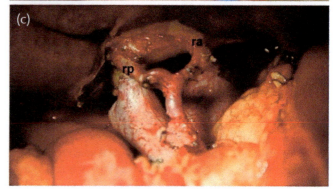

Figure 1.6 Variation in the right hepatic artery which may complicate both donor and recipient operation in a live donor liver transplantation. (a) Computed tomography scan showing extrahepatic bifurcation of right hepatic artery into its right anterior (ra) and posterior (rp) divisions. (b) Intraoperative view showing the ra and rp branches of the right hepatic artery coursing above and below the common bile duct (bd), respectively. This variation leads to two arteries in a right lobe graft. (c) Both arteries (ra and rp) reconstructed in the recipient.

Bile ducts

Biliary drainage follows a remarkably similar anatomical pathway to that of the portal inflow. The right anterior and right posterior sectoral branches combine to form the right hepatic duct, which has a short extrahepatic course before joining the left hepatic duct (LHD) at the biliary confluence to form the common hepatic duct. The LHD courses along the posterior aspect of segment IV.

The arterial supply to the supraduodenal bile duct is predominantly axial (98% related to vessels at its upper and lower ends). On average, eight small vessels, 0.3 mm in diameter, supply the supraduodenal bile duct. The most consistent and functionally important of these vessels are the 3 and 9 o'clock arteries that run along the lateral borders of the common bile duct. Approximately 60% of the vessels that supply the supraduodenal duct run upwards from the gastroduodenal arcade below, while 38% run down, mainly from the RHA. The remaining 2% is a non-axial supply arising from the common hepatic artery.[5,29,30] The arterial inflow to this vascular plexus arises mostly from the retroduodenal artery below and the RHA above. A vascular plexus composed of branches arising directly from the right and left hepatic arteries, surrounds the hilar and intrahepatic bile ducts. This plexus is in direct continuity with that which surrounds the common hepatic and common bile duct. The plexus surrounding the intrahepatic bile ducts is closely associated with the arterial supply of the caudate lobe.[5,29,30]

Variations and anomalies

So many variations of the biliary tree exist that the 'normal' anatomy is present in only about 50% of people. Commonly followed classifications of these variations include those described by Couinaud et al., Huang et al., and Ohkubo et al.[4–6,10,31] (Figure 1.7).

Smadja and Blumgart have classified these variations into six main types.[31,32] In type A (57%) the anatomy is standard. In type B (12%) there is a trifurcation of the common bile duct into the right anterior, right posterior, and left hepatic ducts, with an absence of a demonstrable length of the right hepatic duct. In type C (20%) there is an aberrant drainage of the right segmental ducts into the common hepatic duct. In type D (6%) there is an aberrant drainage of the right segmental ducts into the LHD. The right posterior duct (21%) is more commonly aberrant than the right anterior duct in both types C and D. In type E (3%) there is absence of hepatic duct confluence, there being convergence of two or more ducts from either lobe to form the common hepatic duct. Finally, in type F (2%) there is an absence of the right hepatic duct with ectopic drainage of the right posterior duct into the cystic duct.

Implications

The presence of the standard anatomy in only 50% of individuals is in part one of the reasons for biliary complications following laparoscopic cholecystectomy (covered elsewhere in this book). A thorough preoperative knowledge of the biliary anatomy is imperative before embarking on managing any of these complications. Alterations in the surgical plan for cholangiocarcinoma may be needed based on the variations in biliary anatomy (e.g. type D biliary anatomy) (covered elsewhere in this book).

The incidence of biliary complications is greater after SLT and LDLT than after whole liver transplantation.[33,34] In SLT, the common hepatic duct is invariably allocated to the RL of a split as the only source of its blood supply is from above, from the right hepatic arterial plexus. With RL living donation, pre-donation imaging helps define the anatomy allowing for an accurate and safe division of the RHD. Many centres routinely use intraoperative cholangiograms to further elucidate the anatomy before duct division.[35] It is vital to ensure that the continuity of the donor's biliary system is secured. Particular care must be taken while transecting the caudate lobe as failure to identify transected ducts here may lead to troublesome bile leaks and collections adjacent to the biliary anastomosis resulting in inflammatory strictures. The 'complete hilar encircling' technique ensures that donor bile ducts are isolated along with an intact hilar plate, and are transected in the same plane as the adjacent plate, thereby ensuring the presence of healthy, vascularized tissue around the bile ducts.[35,36] The ducts are transected flush with the liver parenchyma to further

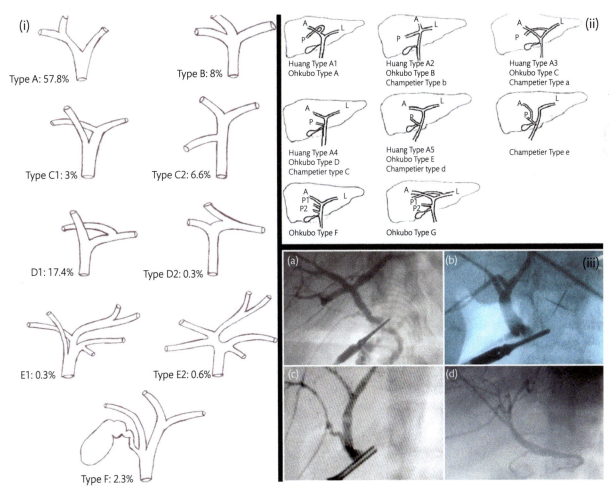

Figure 1.7 Classifications of biliary anatomy. (i) Couinaud classification. (ii) Other classifications. (iii) Intraoperative cholangiogram showing variations in the bile duct anatomy which may make the bile duct reconstruction in liver transplantation more complex. (iii) (a) Standard anatomy, however there is a short stump of the right hepatic duct that may lead to two ducts in the graft. (b, c) Huang A3 and A5 variations which will lead to two bile ducts in the liver graft. (d) Complex biliary anatomy, leading to three or more ducts in a right lobe graft.

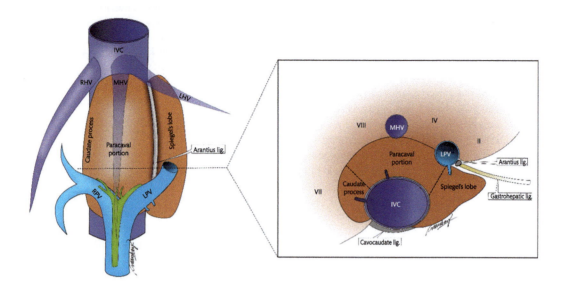

Figure 1.8 Coronal (left) and axial (right) views defining the parts and boundaries of the caudate lobe. II, IV, VII, VIII, segments of the liver; IVC, inferior vena cava; LHV, left hepatic vein; lig, ligament; LPV, left portal vein; MHV, middle hepatic vein; RHV, right hepatic vein; RPV, right portal vein.

reduce the chance of ischaemia. Type B and C anatomical variations lead to two or more ducts in the RL graft. When the ducts are not separated and have an intact hilar plate around them, a single anastomosis may be performed to include the hilar plate in the anastomosis. However, when the duct orifices are far apart, two or more anastomoses onto the recipient duct or a Roux loop may be required.

Anatomy of the caudate lobe

The caudate lobe of the liver wraps around most of the retrohepatic IVC. The posterior and left boundaries of the caudate lobe are well defined. However, the right as well as the roof or anterior boundary of the caudate lies intrahepatically and is more diffuse. The hepatic hilum forms the inferior aspect of the anterior boundary. Superiorly, the anterior boundary of the caudate is formed from left to right by the Arantius ligament, the downstream terminal portions of the three main hepatic veins, and its intervening hepatic parenchyma (segments IV and VIII).

The caudate lobe of the liver is anatomically divided into three parts: Spiegel's lobe (Couinaud's segment I), the paracaval portion (Couinaud's segment IX), and the caudate process (Figure 1.8).[10,37-39] However, for the purpose of surgical anatomy the caudate lobe can be considered as consisting of two parts, Spiegel's lobe on the left and the paracaval portion on the right, which includes the caudate process. The two parts are anatomically separated by a deep notch in about 50% of individuals. The vascular inflow to the caudate lobe is predominately from the left portal pedicle. The caudate lobe and process also receive separate branches from the right and left hepatic arteries in what has been described as an 'arcade' or 'tree' pattern. The venous drainage is predominantly on the left by a single vein in 50% of people and by two or three veins in the rest.[10,37-39] In addition, there may be up to 20 small short venules attaching the caudate lobe to the retrohepatic IVC. This uniqueness of the caudate venous outflow remains the cause of caudate hypertrophy commonly observed in patients with cirrhosis and in Budd–Chiari syndrome. In both these conditions the unimpeded direct venous drainage into the IVC allows for a compensatory hypertrophy of the caudate lobe.

There are usually between one and three bile ducts draining each portion with a maximum of five ducts for the whole caudate.[10,37-39] The majority of Spiegel's lobe ducts drain into the LHD; however, a significant number of variations have been described. Spiegel's ducts may drain into the right posterior sectoral duct, and less commonly into the RHD or even into the confluence of the hepatic ducts. The majority of ducts from the paracaval portion drain into the right posterior sectoral duct, although a significant percentage (27%) of these ducts cross to the opposite system, to drain into the LHD. Biliary leaks from divided and unrecognized caudate ducts cause significant complications after SLT.[10,24,37-39] Cut-surface bile leak following these procedures may be due to a leak from left and right hepatic or right posterior sectoral ducts through the divided ducts of the caudate lobe. Knowledge of the biliary anatomy of the caudate lobe, and attention to securing these ducts, is important in reducing biliary complications in SLT and LDLT.

Conclusion

Liver anatomy can be quite variable. A detailed knowledge of the liver's anatomical structure along with an understanding of anatomical variations and their implications is crucial to good outcomes in hepatobiliary surgery. This chapter provides a foundation for appreciating the anatomy of the liver along with its variants and their relevance in liver resectional surgeries and LT.

REFERENCES

1. Majno P, Mentha G, Toso C, Morel P, Peitgen HO, Fasel JHD. Anatomy of the liver: an outline with three levels of complexity—a further step towards tailored territorial liver resections. *J Hepatol.* 2014;**60**:654–662.

2. Chaib E, Ribeiro MAF, Saad WA, Gama-Rodrigues J. The main hepatic anatomic variations for the purpose of split-liver transplantation. *Transplant Proc*. 2005;**37**:1063–1066.
3. Lowe MC, D'Angelica MI. Anatomy of hepatic resectional surgery. *Surg Clin North Am*. 2016;**96**:183–195.
4. Sakamoto Y, Kokudo N, Kawaguchi Y, Akita K. Clinical anatomy of the liver: review of the 19th Meeting of the Japanese Research Society of Clinical Anatomy. *Liver Cancer*. 2017;**6**:146–160.
5. Deshpande RR, Heaton ND, Rela M. Surgical anatomy of segmental liver transplantation. *Br J Surg*. 2002;**89**:1078–1088.
6. Hjortsjö CH. The topography of the intrahepatic duct systems. *Cells Tissues Organs*. 1950;**11**:559–615.
7. Couinaud C. [Anatomic principles of left and right regulated hepatectomy: technics]. *J Chir (Paris)*. 1954;**70**:933–966.
8. Strasberg SM. Nomenclature of hepatic anatomy and resections: a review of the Brisbane 2000 system. *J Hepatobiliary Pancreat Surg*. 2005;**12**:351–355.
9. Nakamura S, Tsuzuki T. Surgical anatomy of the hepatic veins and the inferior vena cava. *Surg Gynecol Obstet*. 1981;**152**:43–50.
10. Skandalakis JE, Skandalakis LJ, Skandalakis PN, Mirilas P. Hepatic surgical anatomy. *Surg Clin North Am*. 2004;**84**:413–435.
11. Nayak SB, Deepthinath R, Kumar N, et al. Evaluation of numerical and positional variations of the hepatic veins: a cadaveric study. *J Cardiovasc Echogr*. 2016;**26**:5–10.
12. Dar FS, Faraj W, Heaton ND, Rela M. Variation in the venous drainage of left lateral segment liver graft requiring reconstruction of segment III vein with donor iliac artery. *Liver Transplant*. 2008;**14**:576–579.
13. Bartlett A, Rela M. Progress in surgical techniques in pediatric liver transplantation. *Pediatr Transplant*. 2010;**14**:33–40.
14. de Villa VH, Chen CL, Chen YS, et al. Right lobe living donor liver transplantation—addressing the middle hepatic vein controversy. *Ann Surg*. 2003;**238**:275–282.
15. Lo CM. The middle hepatic vein controversy: art and science. *Liver Transplant*. 2018;**24**:870–871.
16. Liu CL, Lo CM, Fan ST. What is the best technique for right hemiliver living donor liver transplantation? With or without the middle hepatic vein? Duct-to-duct biliary anastomosis or Roux-en-Y hepaticojejunostomy? *J Hepatol*. 2005;**43**:17–22.
17. Zhang S, Dong Z, Zhang M, Xia Q, Liu D, Zhang JJ. Right lobe living-donor liver transplantation with or without middle hepatic vein: a meta-analysis. *Transplant Proc*. 2011;**43**:3773–3779.
18. Varghese CT, Bharathan VK, Gopalakrishnan U, et al. Randomized trial on extended versus modified right lobe grafts in living donor liver transplantation. *Liver Transplant*. 2018;**24**:888–896.
19. Fan ST, Lo CM, Liu CL, Wang WX, Wong J. Safety and necessity of including the middle hepatic vein in the right lobe graft in adult-to-adult live donor liver transplantation. *Ann Surg*. 2003;**238**:137–148.
20. Sureka B, Sharma N, Khera PS, Garg PK, Yadav T. Hepatic vein variations in 500 patients: surgical and radiological significance. *Br J Radiol*. 2019;**92**:20190487.
21. Carneiro C, Brito J, Bilreiro C, et al. All about portal vein: a pictorial display to anatomy, variants and physiopathology. *Insights Imaging*. 2019;**10**:38.
22. Kishi Y, Sugawara Y, Kaneko J, Matsui Y, Akamatsu N, Makuuchi M. Classification of portal vein anatomy for partial liver transplantation. *Transplant Proc*. 2004;**36**:3075–3076.
23. Varotti G, Gondolesi GE, Goldman J, et al. Anatomic variations in right liver living donors. *J Am Coll Surg*. 2004;**198**:577–582.
24. Rela M, Heaton ND. Split-liver transplantation. *Br J Surg*. 1998;**85**:881–883.
25. Cherukuru R, Reddy MS, Shanmugam NP, et al. Feasibility and safety of split-liver transplantation in a nascent framework of deceased donation. *Liver Transplant*. 2019;**25**:450–458.
26. Hackl C, Schmidt KM, Süsal C, Döhler B, Zidek M, Schlitt HJ. Split liver transplantation: current developments. *World J Gastroenterol*. 2018;**24**:5312–5321.
27. Hiatt JR, Gabbay J, Busuttil RW. Surgical anatomy of the hepatic arteries in 1000 cases. *Ann Surg*. 1994;**220**:50–52.
28. Michels NA. Newer anatomy of the liver and its variant blood supply and collateral circulation. *Am J Surg*. 1966;**112**:337–347.
29. Chen WJ, Ying DJ, Liu ZJ, He ZP. Analysis of the arterial supply of the extrahepatic bile ducts and its clinical significance. *Clin Anat*. 1999;**12**:245–249.
30. Northover JMA, Terblanche J. A new look at the arterial supply of the bile duct in man and its surgical implications. *Br J Surg*. 1979;**66**:379–384.
31. Deka P, Islam M, Jindal D, Kumar N, Arora A, Negi SS. Analysis of biliary anatomy according to different classification systems. *Indian J Gastroenterol*. 2014;**33**:23–30.
32. Chaib E, Kanas AF, Galvão FHF, D'Albuquerque LAC. Bile duct confluence: anatomic variations and its classification. *Surg Radiol Anat*. 2014;**36**:105–109.
33. Zimmerman MA, Baker T, Goodrich NP, et al. Development, management, and resolution of biliary complications after living and deceased donor liver transplantation: a report from the adult-to-adult living donor liver transplantation cohort study consortium. *Liver Transplant*. 2013;**19**:259–267.
34. Rammohan A, Govil S, Vargese J, Kota V, Reddy MS, Rela M. Changing pattern of biliary complications in an evolving liver transplant unit. *Liver Transplant*. 2017;**23**:478–486.
35. Rammohan A, Reddy MS, Narasimhan G, et al. Live liver donors: is right still right? *World J Surg*. 2020;**44**(7):2385–2393.
36. Rammohan A, Govil S, Vargese J, Kota V, Reddy MS, Rela M. Changing pattern of biliary complications in an evolving liver transplant unit. *Liver Transplant*. 2017;**23**:478–486.
37. Filipponi F, Romagnoli P, Mosca F, Couinaud C. The dorsal sector of human liver: embryological, anatomical and clinical relevance. *Hepatogastroenterology*. 2000;**47**:1726–1731.
38. Abdalla EK, Vauthey JN, Couinaud C. The caudate lobe of the liver implications of embryology and anatomy for surgery. *Surg Oncol Clin N Am*. 2002;**11**:835–848.
39. Jassem W, Heaton ND, Rela M. Reducing bile leak following segmental liver transplantation: understanding biliary anatomy of the caudate lobe. *Am J Transplant*. 2008;**8**:271–274.

2

Applied physiology of the liver

Bruno Stieger and Joachim C. Mertens

Introduction

Within the circulatory system, the liver is situated between the gut and the systemic circulation. Consequently, all substances entering the body via the gut must pass through the liver. The liver therefore represents a second boundary against the outside of the body, specifically the lumen of the gut. This position is reflected by the five key physiological functions of the liver: energy homoeostasis of the body, amino acid homoeostasis, bile formation, biotransformation, and synthesis of plasma proteins.

The histoanatomical subunit of the liver is the liver lobule (Figure 2.1), a several millimetres long hexagonal structure delineated by (six) portal triads with a central vein in the middle. The functional unit of the liver is the acinus, a rhomboid that is delineated by two central veins and two portal triads. The acinus (Figure 2.1) is commonly divided into zone 1 (located around the portal triad) and zone 3 around the central vein while zone 2 is an intermediate area between zones 1 and 3. The acinus receives mixed intestinal and arterial blood from the portal triad (~80% venous blood from a small branch of the portal vein and ~20% arterial blood from a small branch of the hepatic artery), which drains through the central vein. As a consequence, a gradient of oxygen partial pressure exists between the portal triad and the central vein. The aforementioned zones of the liver acinus reflect these different levels of oxygenation. In part due to these different oxygen levels and to different nutrient supply, biochemical processes are not evenly distributed throughout the acinus.[1] For example, the urea cycle is ongoing in the periportal area of the acinus while the final scavenging of ammonium ions (NH_4^+) by glutamine synthase is concentrated in a single cell layer around the central vein. Glycogen synthesis starting from lactate is higher in the periportal area, while glucose-dependent glycogen synthesis is higher in the pericentral area. Reactions of biotransformation similarly occur in different zones of the liver acinus. Cytochrome P450s (CYPs), the key enzymes in biotransformation, show varying expression in the different acinar zones. CYP1A2 and CYP2E1, for example, are highly expressed around the pericentral area and practically absent in the periportal area. This is one factor explaining the extensive pericentral damage, for example, after a paracetamol overdose due to the formation of reactive metabolites. Similarly, ischaemic liver injury typically causes necrosis starting in the centrilobular area.[2]

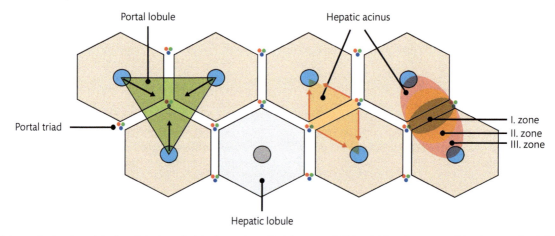

Figure 2.1 Schematic drawing of the liver lobule and of the liver acinus. Red dots: arterial blood; blue dot: venous blood; green dot: bile. Blue arrows depict the general direction of blood flow form the portal triad to the central vein; green arrows depict the general direction of bile flow.

Reproduced from Fontana, Josef, et al. *Functions of Cells and Human Body: Multimedia Textbook.* Liver and Biotransformation of Xenobiotics, under a Creative Commons CC BY-SA 2.0 licence (https://creativecommons.org/licenses/by-sa/2.0/). Available at http://fblt.cz/en/skripta/ix-travici-soustava/5-jatra-a-biotransformace-xenobiotik/

Carbohydrate metabolism

After a meal, serum glucose levels rise in the absorptive phase and, as a consequence, endogenous glucose production is strongly suppressed. This downregulation of endogenous glucose production is mediated by increasing insulin levels. It is important to note that insulin is released from the beta cells of the pancreas directly into the portal circulation. Therefore, the liver is exposed to higher insulin levels than the rest of the organism. At the same time, the liver is the central organ for insulin clearance. To keep the systemic glucose concentration within the physiological range, the liver imports up to one-third of the glucose that arrives in the postprandial portal bloodstream from the gut via glucose transporter 2 (GLUT2) transporters.[3] GLUT2 is an insulin-insensitive, low-affinity, high-capacity glucose transport system, which facilitates movement of glucose across a membrane along its concentration gradient. Hence, GLUT2 can mediate uptake as well as release of glucose from hepatocytes. In the hepatocytes, the enzyme glycogen synthase converts most of the postprandial glucose into glycogen, the storage form of glucose in hepatocytes.[4] During this phase of high glucose blood levels, insulin prevents inactivation of glycogen synthase by phosphorylation and maintains the active, dephosphorylated form. In addition, rising intracellular glucose concentrations drive hepatocellular glucose metabolism towards glycolysis. Glycolysis[5] breaks down glucose into two molecules of pyruvate and each produces two reduced nicotinamide adenine dinucleotide (NADH) and adenosine triphosphate (ATP) molecules. Pyruvate is converted into acetyl coenzyme A and enters the citric acid cycle. The citric acid cycle yields three NAHD, one reduced flavin adenine dinucleotide (FADH$_2$), and one guanosine triphosphate (GTP) (or ATP) molecules.

In the postabsorptive state (i.e. after complete absorption of nutrients in the intestine), the liver supplies the body with energy by releasing glucose back into the circulation. This process is triggered by low serum insulin and high glucagon levels, which activate glucagon-mediated glycogenolysis. In addition, decreasing intracellular glucose levels drive hepatocellular glucose metabolism towards gluconeogenesis. Gluconeogenesis starts from pyruvate and synthesis of glucose occurs essentially by reversal of the enzymatic cascade of glycolysis (the three steps utilize different enzymes) under the consumption of two ATP and NADH molecules. Pyruvate for gluconeogenesis is supplied by lactate or by the glucogenic amino acid alanine. Patients with acute liver failure have a decreased insulin clearance by hepatocytes. This leads to increased systemic insulin levels and to hypoglycaemia. The hypoglycaemia is aggravated by an insulin-mediated downregulation of gluconeogenesis in hepatocytes.[6] Hypoglycaemia due to hepatic failure may require continuous glucose infusion in the acute phase.

While the liver is the primary organ receiving and regulating levels of systemic glucose, it has to be kept in mind that muscles and fat tissue are also involved in maintaining glucose homoeostasis. In fact, muscles can store about four times the amount of glycogen than the liver. Lactate is, among other products, produced by muscles under anaerobic glycolysis, which enters the circulation. The liver metabolizes up to 70% of lactate produced by the body. Lactate, together with glycerol (derived from triglyceride metabolism) and glucogenic amino acids, is used for gluconeogenesis. In critically ill patients, lactate production may increase in the peripheral organs and tissues and at the same time liver perfusion may be reduced to a critical threshold of 25% below normal. As a consequence, lactate clearance by the liver is strongly impaired.

Lipid metabolism

The second major energy source derived from the diet is fat. Fat is digested in the upper small intestine and requires bile as well as pancreatic juice for this process. Bile acids from bile activate pancreatic lipases in the upper small intestine and emulsify dietary fat. The latter allows lipases to access triglycerides and to break them down. The breakdown of triglycerides by lipases results in free fatty acids and 2-monoacylglycerol. Free fatty acids and monoacylglycerols are then taken up into enterocytes. Within enterocytes, monoacylglycerols are remodelled in the endoplasmic reticulum into triglycerides and assembled together with other lipids into chylomicrons. Chylomicrons are composed mainly of triglycerides and are released by enterocytes into the abdominal lymphatic system. This drains via the thoracic duct into the systemic circulation. During the circulation of chylomicrons through the vessels and capillaries, lipoprotein lipase expressed at the surface of the endothelial cells hydrolyses triglycerides and releases fatty acids and glycerol from chylomicrons. Fatty acids are taken up by adipocytes and muscle cells and also by hepatocytes. In hepatocytes, fatty acids are converted into triglycerides and lipid droplets. During triglyceride hydrolysis in the circulation, chylomicrons are converted in chylomicron remnants, which are rich in cholesteryl esters. These remnants are cleared from the circulation by the liver via low-density lipoprotein receptor-related protein l (LPR1).[7] In the periphery, high-density lipoprotein (HDL) is loaded with cholesterol and destined for reverse cholesterol transport to the liver. Other tissues (e.g. steroidogenic tissues) are also supplied with cholesterol by HDL. The liver takes up cholesterol bound to HDL via scavenger receptor SR-BI. In addition to receiving cholesterol from the circulation, the liver synthesizes a considerable amount of cholesterol. Cholesterol, which enters hepatocytes from the circulation, is used for the synthesis of very low-density lipoprotein. This particle is an addition loaded with triglycerides in secreted back into the circulation.[8] Cholesterol produced by biosynthesis in hepatocytes is converted into bile acids and bile salts and secreted into bile. In addition to bile salts, bile contains cholesterol. Export of cholesterol from hepatocytes in the canaliculi requires the concerted action of bile salts and phospholipids in the canaliculus. The regulation of cholesterol homeostasis in hepatocytes is complex: cholesterol biosynthesis is regulated at the transcriptional level by sterol regulatory element binding proteins (SREBPs).[9] SREBPs can also control the extracellular supply of cholesterol by transcriptional regulation of low-density lipoprotein receptor biosynthesis. Biosynthesis of cholesterol is also under positive control by insulin and negative control by glucagon. Any excess of hepatocellular fat is stored in lipid droplets. When the liver is continuously exposed to the fat surplus, the prolonged disposition of lipid droplets will lead to steatosis.[10]

As glucose (sugar) metabolism and lipid metabolism are intimately linked in the liver, any disturbance of this balance can lead to liver disease. This is highlighted in the metabolic syndrome, which is accompanied by non-alcoholic fatty liver disease or non-alcoholic steatohepatitis. In clinics, patients with, for example, intestinal failure or sepsis who require parenteral nutrition are at risk for acute steatosis, cholestasis, or gallbladder sludge (parenteral nutrition-associated liver disease). The composition of the parenteral nutrition and/or excessive total caloric administration is a risk factor for developing this form of liver disease.[11]

Amino acid metabolism

Digestion of proteins in the intestine leads to the absorption of amino acids. Nine of the twenty amino acids used by the body are essential, that is, they cannot be synthesized by humans but have to be provided in the protein part of the diet. As the liver secretes between 10 and 50 g of newly synthesized proteins each day, it needs an adequate supply of amino acids. Amino acids that enter the hepatocytes after a meal cannot be stored. Therefore, they immediately have to be used as building blocks for proteins in biosynthetic processes or are metabolized. The first step of amino acid metabolism typically involves removal of the alpha amino group by aminotransferases and hence leads to generation of NH_4^+. NH_4^+ is detoxified in the liver through the urea cycle.[12] Urea, the end-product of this metabolic amino acid pathway, is then eliminated from the body by the kidneys. Among amino acids, alanine serves a special role. First, this amino acid can be the starting product for gluconeogenesis. Second, in muscles, alanine can be synthesized from glutamate and NH_4^+ and released into the circulation, and as such helps in removing NH_4^+ from amino acid catabolism. Alanine is transported from muscles to the liver, where NH_4^+ is converted into urea. This process is also called the glucose–alanine cycle.

Protein synthesis

Protein synthesis in the liver does not only serve the needs of the organ. The liver synthesizes and secretes a large array of proteins with various functions into the circulation.[13] Albumin and alpha-1-acid glycoprotein (also called orosomucoid) are major plasma constituents and are, together with other proteins, important xenobiotic binding plasma proteins. Further important plasmatic transport proteins mainly provided by the liver are transferrin, ceruloplasmin, transthyretin, vitamin D-binding protein, thyroid-binding globulin or insulin-like growth factor-binding proteins. Fibrinogen and all blood clotting factors except factor VIII are synthesized in the liver. In addition to these, the liver synthesizes and secretes apolipoproteins in the form of lipoprotein particles. Given the large variety and important functions of the secreted proteins, it is not surprising that acute or chronic liver diseases with impaired liver function and protein synthesis swiftly affect the entire organism in a potentially disastrous way. For example, blood clotting factor VII has a half-life of 3–6 hours, illustrating why patients with acute liver failure quickly develop problems with haemostasis.

In chronic severe liver disease, protein synthesis and secretion often become impaired, which can lead to low plasma albumin concentrations. Likewise, the reduced secretion of blood clotting factors leads to altered haemostasis. The international normalized ratio as a surrogate marker of liver protein synthesis is included in common prognostic scores for liver disease (Child–Pugh, Model for End-Stage Liver Disease (MELD)). In some inherited diseases, mutations in genes coding for liver-secreted proteins lead to liver disease. Alpha-1 antitrypsin deficiency is a common inherited disease with a frequency of about 1:3500 live births. Different mutations lead to different clinical phenotypes. The wild-type allele is called *PI*M*, while the two most common mutated alleles are named *PI*S* and *PI*Z*.[14,15] Patients with *PI*MM* alleles typically present with lung disease, while patients with *PI*ZZ* alleles have both liver and lung disease. Mutations of the *PI*Z* type lead to insoluble globular proteins and will over time lead to an accumulation of misfolded proteins in the endoplasmic reticulum of hepatocytes. This results in endoplasmic reticulum stress leading to fibrosis and ultimately to cirrhosis.

Bilirubin metabolism

Once they reach the end of their life span, erythrocytes are broken down by the reticuloendothelial system. Degradation of the haem group releases the metabolic end product bilirubin into the circulation.[16] In addition, other proteins containing a haem group contribute to the serum bilirubin upon their degradation. As bilirubin is practically water insoluble, it is tightly, but reversibly bound to albumin and as such reaches hepatocytes via the blood plasma. Extraction of bilirubin from albumin is poorly understood. Nevertheless, hepatocytes take up bilirubin and conjugate it by the action of UDP-glucuronosyltransferase 1A1 (UGT1A1) with glucuronic acid to form bilirubin mono- and diglucuronide and thereby increase the water solubility of bilirubin. Bilirubin glucuronides are then excreted across the canalicular membrane into bile and are disposed into the intestine. In the intestine, parts of the bilirubin glucuronides are hydrolysed by the gut flora to urobilinogen and bilirubin. These compounds are reabsorbed and bilirubin is again glucuronidated in enterocytes and released into the circulation.

Mutations in the gene coding for UGT1A1 can lead to severe unconjugated hyperbilirubinaemia (Crigler–Najjar disease), which can be fatal. Milder forms such as Gilbert–Meulengracht syndrome can lead to intermittent, benign hyperbilirubinaemia.[17] Some drugs, like atazanavir, can also inhibit UGT1A1, which leads to an unconjugated hyperbilirubinaemia. Mutations in the gene coding for the efflux transporter of bilirubin glucuronides lead to conjugated hyperbilirubinaemia (Dubin–Johnson syndrome). Elevation of serum bilirubin is a symptom of many forms of liver disease and must therefore be considered in the context of additional diagnostic tests to correctly diagnose the underlying condition.

Bile formation

Bile is largely composed of bile salts, lipids, and organic anions. The distribution of organic components in bile is approximately 67% bile salts, 27% phospholipids, 5% cholesterol and protein each, and the remainder bile pigments.[18,19] Bile salts are taurine or glycine conjugates of the primary bile acids cholic acid and chenodeoxycholic acid, which are synthesized in the liver and in humans have a roughly equal molar ratio. In humans, glycine conjugates are the predominant form while taurine conjugates of bile acids are less abundant. Primary bile acids that enter the gut via bile fluid are modified into secondary bile salts by the gut flora.[20] In humans, the predominant secondary bile salt is deoxycholate, which is generated by dehydroxylation of cholate at the 7α position. The synthesis of bile acids is complex and involves (at least) 15 enzymes. After their synthesis, bile acids are conjugated to glycine or taurine and are secreted across the canalicular membrane into primary bile.[21] Generation of bile flow is an osmotically driven process, that is, water follows the secreted bile constituents in a transcellular and paracellular route into the canaliculi. Canalicular bile salt secretion is achieved by the bile salt export pump (BSEP), which generates in an ATP-dependent process a steep bile salt concentration gradient across the canalicular membrane. Other organic anions like bilirubin glucuronides or glutathione and glutathione conjugates are secreted by the multidrug resistance-associated protein 2 (MRP2). These substrates are also osmotically active and hence contribute to the bile flow. Bile salts are responsible for bile salt-dependent bile flow and other organic anions drive bile salt-independent bile flow. In humans, bile salt-dependent bile flow is about four times that of the bile salt-dependent bile flow. Canalicular bile flows into bile ducts, where it is modified by the action of cholangiocytes. Additional secretion by cholangiocytes contributes to the so-called ductular bile flow. Bile reaches the gall bladder via the common bile duct and the cystic duct, where is it concentrated by reabsorption of water. This concentrated bile fluid is then released into the duodenum upon hormonal stimulation particularly following nutrition intake. As mentioned previously, bile is essential for the digestion of fat because amphipathic bile salts emulsify lipids in the gut and facilitate their transport across membranes.

About 95% of the bile salts are reabsorbed in the intestine and transported back to the liver via the portal tract. In the liver, bile salts are largely absorbed into the hepatocytes. Unconjugated bile acids produced in the gut by bacterial deconjugation are taken up into hepatocytes by organic anion transporting polypeptides (OATPs). OATP1B1, OATP1B3, and OATP2B1 proteins are found in human hepatocytes. Their exact transport mechanisms are still not known. Bile acids absorbed into hepatocytes are very efficiently and quickly conjugated again to bile salts. Bile salts from the portal plasma are predominantly absorbed by the sodium taurocholate co-transporting polypeptide (NTCP). This system utilizes both the sodium gradient and the membrane potential of hepatocytes and can therefore take up bile salts against a concentration gradient.

Of note, OATPs are important drug transporters and involved in drug uptake into hepatocytes for metabolism and elimination. Once taken up into hepatocytes, bile salts are secreted again into the canaliculus, where their enterohepatic circulation starts again.

In addition to secretion of organic anions via BESP and MRP2, the canalicular membrane also exports phospholipids and cholesterol into bile. In human bile more than 95% of the phospholipids are phosphatidylcholine or lysophosphatidylcholine, while the remaining phospholipid is almost completely phosphatidylethanolamine. Biliary phospholipid secretion requires the combined action of multidrug resistance protein 3 (MDR3) and canalicular bile salts. MDR3 flips phosphatidylcholine (and probably also the small amount of phosphatidylethanolamine) from the inner to the outer leaflet of the canalicular membrane. The canalicular bile salts release the phospholipids from the outer leaflet of the canalicular membrane into bile due to their detergent properties. MDR3 is an ATP-dependent transporter. In the canaliculus, bile salts and phospholipids form mixed micelles and thereby attenuate the detergent action of bile.

The canalicular secretion of cholesterol is facilitated by the action of the heterodimeric ATP-dependent transporter ABCG5/ABCG8 together with the action of bile salts. Cholesterol is incorporated into mixed micelles in order to keep it in solution in bile. The presence of phospholipids in bile is essential for the prevention of bile duct damage by the toxic detergent action of bile salts.

The appropriate formation of mixed micelles between phospholipids and bile salts is essential for protecting the bile ducts from the toxic action of bile salts.[22] Diseases altering the balance between phospholipid and bile salt concentration in bile cause damage to the bile ducts and may lead to cholangitis with possible destruction of the biliary tree.

The vital function of the canalicular bile salt organic anion and lipid transporters is exemplified by the observation that mutations in the genes coding for these transporters lead to progressive cholestasis with severe liver disease, often already present in childhood. Progressive familial intrahepatic cholestasis (PFIC) type 1, for example, is caused by mutations in the *ATB8B1* gene. ATP8B1 is essential in maintaining the phospholipid equilibrium between the inner and the outer leaflet of the canalicular membrane. PFIC2 is caused by mutations in *ABCB11*, coding for BSEP, and PFIC3 is caused by mutations in *ABCB4*, coding for MDR3. These three rare forms of inherited liver disease often require liver transplantation by a young age.

Conclusion

The liver is not only a second boundary for substances entering the body via the gut but also a central organ controlling energy homoeostasis of the body. This function is complemented by a key role in biotransformation, a process central for the excretion of metabolic end products and of xenobiotics entering the body. As such, the organ is the target of many hormones that balance energy homoeostasis in the body and, in the case of a surplus of energy intake, an important storage organ for excess energy in the form of glycogen or lipid droplets. Bile produced by the liver is essential for the intestinal digestion of fat and therefore is not only a vehicle for the excretion of end products but also for the digestion and absorption of fat, an important energy source.

REFERENCES

1. Ben-Moshe S, Itzkovitz S. Spatial heterogeneity in the mammalian liver. *Nat Rev Gastroenterol Hepatol*. 2019;**16**(7):395–410.
2. Krishna M. Patterns of necrosis in liver disease. *Clin Liver Dis (Hoboken)*. 2017;**10**(2):53–56.
3. Thorens B. GLUT2, glucose sensing and glucose homeostasis. *Diabetologia*. 2015;**58**(2):221–232.
4. Nordlie RC, Foster JD, Lange AJ. Regulation of glucose production by the liver. *Annu Rev Nutr*. 1999;**19**:379–406.
5. Rui L. Energy metabolism in the liver. *Compr Physiol*. 2014;**4**(1):177–197.
6. Sharabi K, Tavares CD, Rines AK, Puigserver P. Molecular pathophysiology of hepatic glucose production. *Mol Aspects Med*. 2015;**46**:21–33.

7. Zanoni P, Velagapudi S, Yalcinkaya M, Rohrer L, von Eckardstein A. Endocytosis of lipoproteins. *Atherosclerosis*. 2018;**275**:273–295.
8. Scheja L, Heeren J. Metabolic interplay between white, beige, brown adipocytes and the liver. *J Hepatol*. 2016;**64**(5):1176–1186.
9. Shimano H, Sato R. SREBP-regulated lipid metabolism: convergent physiology—divergent pathophysiology. *Nat Rev Endocrinol*. 2017;**13**(12):710–730.
10. Seebacher F, Zeigerer A, Kory N, Krahmer N. Hepatic lipid droplet homeostasis and fatty liver disease. *Semin Cell Dev Biol*. 2020;**108**:72–81.
11. Nowak K. Parenteral nutrition-associated liver disease. *Clin Liver Dis (Hoboken)*. 2020;**15**(2):59–62.
12. Morris SM Jr. Regulation of enzymes of the urea cycle and arginine metabolism. *Annu Rev Nutr*. 2002;**22**:87–105.
13. Kuscuoglu D, Janciauskiene S, Hamesch K, Haybaeck J, Trautwein C, Strnad P. Liver—master and servant of serum proteome. *J Hepatol*. 2018;**69**(2):512–524.
14. Stoller JK, Aboussouan LS. Alpha1-antitrypsin deficiency. *Lancet*. 2005;**365**(9478):2225–2236.
15. Stoller JK, Aboussouan LS. A review of alpha1-antitrypsin deficiency. *Am J Respir Crit Care Med*. 2012;**185**(3):246–259.
16. Sullivan JI, Rockey DC. Diagnosis and evaluation of hyperbilirubinemia. *Curr Opin Gastroenterol*. 2017;**33**(3):164–170.
17. Strassburg CP. Hyperbilirubinemia syndromes (Gilbert-Meulengracht, Crigler-Najjar, Dubin-Johnson, and Rotor syndrome). *Best Pract Res Clin Gastroenterol*. 2010;**24**(5):555–571.
18. Esteller A. Physiology of bile secretion. *World J Gastroenterol*. 2008;**14**(37):5641–5649.
19. Boyer JL. Bile formation and secretion. *Compr Physiol*. 2013;**3**(3):1035–1078.
20. Molinero N, Ruiz L, Sanchez B, Margolles A, Delgado S. Intestinal bacteria interplay with bile and cholesterol metabolism: implications on host physiology. *Front Physiol*. 2019;**10**:185.
21. Vaz FM, Ferdinandusse S. Bile acid analysis in human disorders of bile acid biosynthesis. *Mol Aspects Med*. 2017;**56**:10–24.
22. Trauner M, Fickert P, Halilbasic E, Moustafa T. Lessons from the toxic bile concept for the pathogenesis and treatment of cholestatic liver diseases. *Wien Med Wochenschr*. 2008;**158**(19–20):542–548.

3

Liver regeneration

Bostjan Humar and Rok Humar

Introduction

The liver is the largest internal organ and gland of our body. Centrally placed, it receives blood from most of the intestine, the pancreas, and the spleen. The venous blood enters the liver via the portal vein, unites with the blood from the hepatic artery, and flows along the sinusoids to exit the liver via the central vein (Figure 3.1). The vascular system is tightly linked to the functional unit of the liver, the lobule, a hexagonal structure defined by portal triads (portal vein, hepatic artery, and bile duct) at its edges and the central vein in the middle, all permeated through connecting sinusoids (Figure 3.1). The latter are highly differentiated vessels that lack basement membranes but feature fenestrations to optimize exchange between blood and the hepatocytes, the functional epithelial units of the liver. All hepatocytes align along the sinusoids (Figure 3.2), which are formed by liver sinusoidal endothelial cells (LSECs) and provide a habitat to Kupffer cells (KCs, resident macrophages) and hepatic stellate cells (HSCs, pericyte-like cells within the space of Disse).

Both the unique supply of blood and its close contact with hepatocytes are prerequisites for proper liver function. With portal blood as the main inflow, the liver receives all nutrients absorbed by the digestive tract and metabolizes them for their bodily distribution. Thus, the liver secretes various proteins, lipids (as lipoproteins), and glucose released from its glycogen stores into the circulation. Bile acids (BAs) are produced to support the digestive system in the absorption of lipophilic nutrients. Portal blood further imports myriads of xeno- and endobiotics and toxins, many of which are harmful and need neutralization through the liver. Thus, the liver as our 'metabolic headquarters' exerts a vital function, but is continually stressed by toxin exposure—the likely reason why the liver has evolved with a unique regenerative capacity, a prerequisite for prolonged lifespans.

Liver regeneration

The liver can regenerate in response to various injuries including acute tissue loss. Even following removal of 70% of its tissue, the liver rapidly regains its original volume, a process that takes about 2–3 weeks in humans and 1 week in mice. Regrowth following hepatectomy (HX) starts from mature hepatocytes,[1,2] while regeneration after hepatotoxic injury occurs from stem cells[3,4] and will not be discussed here.

The standard model for the study of liver regeneration (LR) is a 70% HX in the mouse,[5] simply performed by ligating off three of the four major liver lobes (i.e. macroscopic liver units). HX induces compensatory overgrowth of the remaining two lobes in the absence of significant injury. Volume is restored within a few days, however slow lobular re-organization is believed to eventually reconstruct the original liver architecture.[6] Immediately following HX, the portal inflow into the remnant roughly triples without changes in the arterial supply. Consequently, portal pressure increases, and the remnant now receives three times more nutrients and other components (such as growth factors) present in the mesenteric blood. Within a few minutes, the urokinase system starts to remodel the extracellular matrix (ECM), a prerequisite for the later repopulation and reorganization of the liver.[7] Bodily glucose provision likewise decreases, causing hypoglycaemia, mobilization of peripheral lipids, and their hepatic accumulation to transient steatosis (Figure 3.3).[8] All these events are associated with the *priming phase* of LR, characterized by marked changes in hepatocellular gene expression. Priming is thought to prepare the remnant for the imminent growth phase, as evinced by an upregulation of cell cycle-related genes but also metabolic/secretory pathways to maintain metabolic function.[9] Notably, similar gene expression alterations also occur following minor resection that induces little replication, illustrating that priming does not commit hepatocytes to enter the cell cycle.[9] Indeed, even laparoscopy without HX can induce some priming.[10] The first growth response to resection, however, is not hyperplasia, but an increase in hepatocyte size.[11,12] Hypertrophy alone is responsible for the regain of volume after minor resection; proliferation will be induced only when tissue loss is major. Hypertrophy therefore is the primal growth mode of LR, while hyperplasia serves to rapidly generate liver mass in more pressing settings.[11]

Following priming, most hepatocytes have entered the cell cycle towards 20 hours post HX and continue with hypertrophic (no S-phase progression) or hyperplastic growth (Figure 3.3). The major parenchymal expansion coincides with the hepatocellular S/M-phase peaking around 32–48 hours after resection.[10,12–15] A second mitotic wave may occur, perhaps in concert with an apoptotic wave to fine tune the number of needed hepatocytes, but overall proliferative activity fades away.[10,16] The proliferation of other liver cells is less

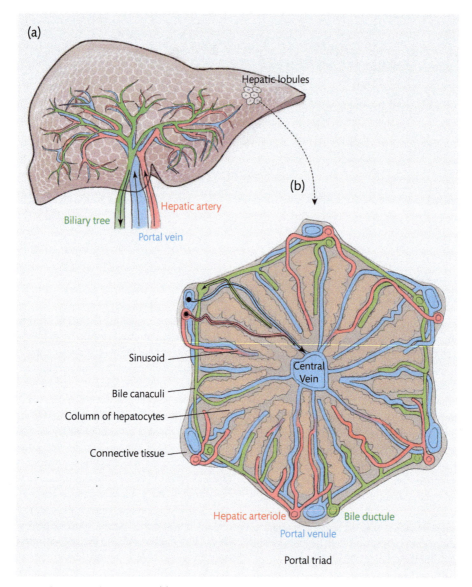

Figure 3.1 Liver architecture and associated vasculature. (a) Schematic drawing of the liver with the biliary, arterial, and portal vein tree. Hepatic lobules are represented through the white hexagon mesh. (b) Schematic drawing of a single hepatic lobule. Solid arrows indicate blood and bile flow directions.

studied; hepatocyte regeneration is thought to trigger overlapping cholangiocyte proliferation[17] and the subsequent angiogenic phase, where LSEC proliferation leads to the reconstitution of the sinusoidal vasculature within 3–4 days.[17–19] KCs and HSCs likely proliferate during the angiogenic phase,[17] given their spatial association with sinusoids. Altogether, the process of LR occurs in an ordered fashion of distinct phases that are, however, interdependent and not strictly separated: priming leads to the proliferative phase that induces the angiogenic phase, which eventually terminates the proliferative phase.

Mechanisms of regeneration

Priming

A profound change following tissue loss is the marked increase in portal blood flowing into the remnant. In response to the pressure increases, sinusoids dilate to enable the surplus blood to pass. Dilatation leads to mechanical stretching of LSECs, which is sensed through endothelial integrin β1 (INGB1) and vascular endothelial growth factor receptor 3 (VEGFR3; marking fenestrated vessels) and elicits the release of hepatocyte growth factor (HGF), a strong hepatocellular mitogen.[20,21] LSECs meanwhile are regarded as an angiocrine niche that provides trophogens to initiate and sustain LR (Figure 3.4): additional HGF is conveyed through the VEGFR2–inhibitor of DNA-binding protein 1 (ID1) signalling axis, which also induces WNT2 production to activate β-catenin in adjacent hepatocytes,[19] an event seen by 5 minutes after HX.[6] Failed VEGFR2–ID1 signalling in LSECs has profound effects, with blunted hepatocyte and LSEC regeneration for at least 28 days.[19] HGF is also released by KCs/HSCs and likewise stimulates β-catenin activity.[22,23] β-catenin not only induces proliferative and metabolic genes but also participates in the activation of the urokinase system (PLAU–PLG–MMP) required for ECM remodelling,[24–26] another early key event.

Mechanisms of regeneration 19

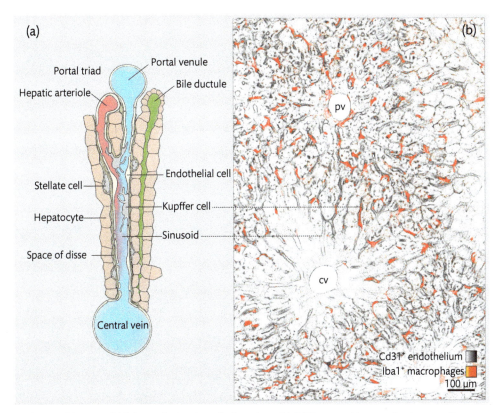

Figure 3.2 Microscopic liver architecture. (a) Schematic drawing of a liver sinusoid. (b) Processed image of an immunofluorescent confocal micrograph of an archived mouse liver section. Kupffer cells and macrophages are stained with an αIba1 antibody (red), while hepatic endothelia (veins and sinusoids) are stained with an αCD31 antibody (grayscale).

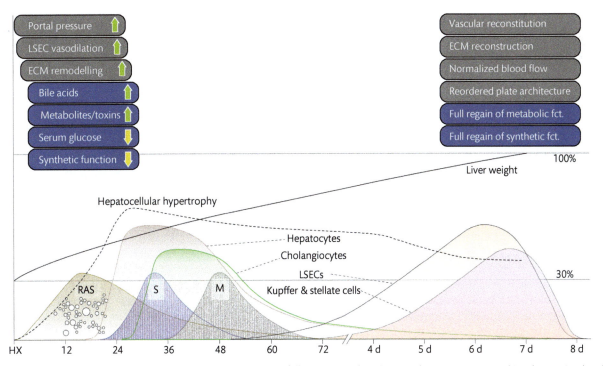

Figure 3.3 Temporal course of key processes during liver regeneration following tissue loss. Boxes indicate processes marking the proximal and distal events during regeneration. Percentages (right y-axis) refer to percentage of liver weight regain after 70% hepatectomy. Time is indicated in hours followed by days and refers to liver regeneration in mice. The dashed line indicates the extent of hepatocellular hypertrophy occurring, while solid lines indicate the main proliferative phases of liver parenchymal and non-parenchymal cells. RAS indicates the peak of regeneration-associated steatosis occurring in hepatocytes after resection. S and M refer to the replication and division peaks of hepatocytes. fct., function.

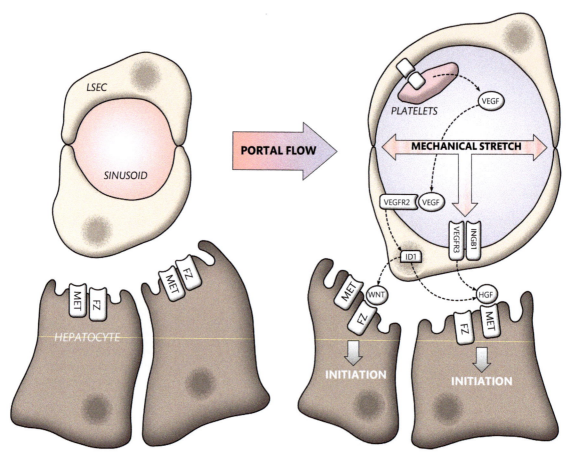

Figure 3.4 The angiocrine niche provides central triggers for the initiation of liver regeneration. Mechanical stretch and the ongoing vasodilation of sinusoids in response to the increased portal inflow induce via INGB1/VEGFR3 the release of the core hepatic trophogen HGF. In parallel, increases in circulating VEGF (through blood import and platelet activation) stimulate the VEGFR2–ID1 axis to provide WNT2 and further HGF. Activation of MET and FZ receptors then initiates the regenerative process in nearby hepatocytes. Note that the signal transmission up- and downstream of INGB1/VEGFR3 is unclarified.

Remodelling frees matrix-bound (inactive) HGF to augment its local availability, but also TGFB1, a strong inhibitor of hepatocyte proliferation, which usually keeps liver at rest by opposing matrix-associated growth factors. Upon its release, TGFB1 is neutralized by serum α2-macroglobulin to unleash the regenerative potential of the liver. Mechanical stress acting on LSECs and KCs/HSCs likely contributes to the activation of the urokinase system and other remodelling proteins.[6] HSCs are particularly important in ECM remodelling, with matrix production as one of their main tasks.[27] The increased blood flow further imports elevated amounts of circulating growth factors per hepatocyte, such as EGF, which originates from duodenal Brunner's glands.[28] Its receptor EGFR is activated around 30 minutes post HX, akin to the HGF receptor MET.[6] Both EGFR and MET are considered key drivers of regeneration; their simultaneous inhibition leads to full abortion of LR, loss in hepatocyte size, and liver decompensation—reflecting the role of EGF and HGF as the core hepatocyte mitogens.[6,21]

An auxiliary, but relevant growth factor is VEGF. Platelets activated by turbulent flow release VEGF (but also HGF/EGF)[29] to elevate initial levels[30–32] in addition to increased VEGF portal inflow.[33] Moreover, platelets release pro-regenerative serotonin,[34] which might enhance local VEGF secretion from LSECs.[35–37] VEGF in turn engages the LSEC VEGFRs to foster their paracrine provision of HGF and WNT2 (Figure 3.4).[19,20,38] VEGF levels steadily rise from 2 hours onwards mostly due to secretion from hepatocytes, fortifying the above pathways but also preparing for the later angiogenic phase.[17,18]

Mutual fortification of regenerative signals seems to be a general principle driving liver regrowth. Norepinephrine, released by adrenal glands and sympathetic nerve endings upon stress, enhances EGFR/MET activities while suppressing those of opposing transforming growth factor (TGF)-B1, with adrenergic receptor inhibition blocking LR.[6,39] Likewise, hepatocyte-derived TGFA promotes EGFR transactivation and later the stimulation of cholangiocytes/non-parenchymal cells.[6] TNFA (secreted by KCs, see below) alone supports the action of mitogens; however, it also stimulates the release of TGFA, with which it acts together to become a mitogenic pair.[6] EGFR activation, in turn, induces early (within 1 hour) NOS3 activity in hepatocytes, which fosters the production of MMP9 and vasodilatory nitric oxide,[40] likely also released by LSECs upon first shear stress after resection.[41,42] Thus, hepatocytes seem to co-operate with LSECs to augment nitric oxide and MMP9 production for proper LSEC vasodilation and ECM remodelling, thereby promoting their own feeding with mitogens.[20]

Overall, the increasing engagement of various growth factor receptors (particularly MET, EGFR, and WNT/FZ) excites downstream

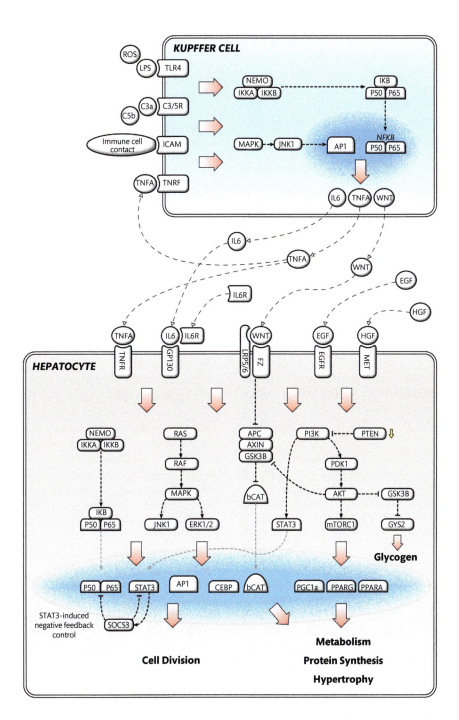

Figure 3.5 Main signalling pathways related to the priming phase and the entry of hepatocytes into the cell cycle. Kupffer cells translate inflammatory signals associated with resection into regenerative stimuli acting on hepatocytes. Liver sinusoidal endothelial cells and other non-parenchymal cells likewise contribute to the priming and progression phases. Due to reasons of graphical clarity, these contributions have not been depicted. With regard to the negative feedback loop between STAT3 and SOCS3, note that SOCS3 inhibitory activities do not act at the transcriptional level but downstream of the incoming receptor signals.

signalling in hepatocytes, with prominent examples being the PI3K–AKT–mTOR, RAS/MAPK–ERK/JNK1, WNT (β-catenin), STAT3, and NFκB pathways (Figure 3.5). Most of these pathways are shared (albeit to varying extents) among the numerous growth receptors, thus individual contributions are hard to deduce. These pathways converge on various transcription factors, of which NFκB, STAT3, AP-1 (FOS/JUN), and CEBPB/A are the classic representatives associated with immediate early gene expression patterns.[7,43] The PI3K–AKT–mTOR pathway, for example, activates STAT3 in one branch, while AKT–mTOR governs protein synthesis and induces metabolic genes via PPARG, PPARA, and PPARGC1A transcriptional regulators.[44] An elegant study demonstrated that STAT3 specifically fosters proliferative programmes, while the AKT–mTOR branch is key to hypertrophic regeneration.[12]

Decisive contributions to priming come from KCs (Figure 3.5).[45] The enhanced portal inflow elevates gut bacterial endotoxins (e.g. LPS) in the remnant, which bind to TLR receptors on KCs.[17,43] Complement components C3a/C5b, likely activated by injury and platelets,[46] also activate KCs through their receptors, and TLRs may additionally be stimulated through hypoxia-derived reactive oxygen species given the tripled inflow of oxygen-poor portal blood. In response, KCs secrete in an NFκB-dependent way IL6 and TNFA, which act on hepatocytes to amplify their STAT, NFκB, and MAPK-JNK1 activities, respectively.[6,17,22,47] KCs likewise contribute to WNT secretion.[23] Adding a layer of complexity, various immune cells contribute to LR either through interaction with KCs or via direct signalling to hepatocytes. Broadly, circulating monocytes, innate lymphoid cells, B cells, T cells, eosinophils, and dendritic cells are thought to promote LR, while the role of natural killer cells appears less straightforward.[23,48–50]

Collectively, the sum of these events prepares the remnant to enter the major growth phase, that is, the wave of parenchymal proliferation peaking 32–48 hours after resection.[10,12–15]

Progression

How priming segues into cell cycle entry and further progression is not understood in detail. The above-described processes lead to the activation of numerous pathways, which synergize to push hepatocytes into G_1. Rather than specific events, the precise orchestration of pathways to an overall activity peak may constitute a plausible trigger point.

Cytokine-induced NFKB/STAT3 and MET/EGFR-induced STAT3 activities, however, are considered central for the initiation of hepatocyte proliferation (Figure 3.5).[7,51] Notably, negative feedback regulation through SOCS3 limits these activities following the onset of proliferation,[51–53] imposing timely order on cell cycle entry. Nonetheless, the precise contributions of pathways to $G_0 \rightarrow G_1$, $G_1 \rightarrow S$ and $G_2 \rightarrow M$ transitions have not been dissected, likely also because of the difficulties in recognizing redundancies and compensatory mechanisms. For example, combined MET/EGFR inhibition blocks all proliferation,[21] akin to the effects of combined MET/WNT blockade.[19] On the other hand, inhibition of only MET, EGFR, or WNT-dependent pathways markedly affects $G_1 \rightarrow S$ and/or G_2/M progression, but has less impact on G_1 entry.[24,54–58] A fair view of LR thus seems that cell cycle entry depends on full cooperation between main mitogenic pathways, whereas sustained activity of a lesser number of pathways is needed for further progression. Of note, many additional pathways are known to participate in LR (e.g. Notch, Hedgehog, FGFs, PDGFs, nuclear receptors, and all the usual pathways regulating cell division and growth).[7,17,23,39,59] Most single pathways act in redundant ways (i.e. their deficiency causes a delay, but not a complete halt) so as to provide LR with the stability required to restore full liver function under suboptimal conditions.

While progression represents the major period of parenchymal expansion,[14] liver weight is already increased 24 hours post HX, thus *before* hepatocytes have entered the cell cycle. This early growth is due to hepatocellular hypertrophy that is cell cycle independent but might relate to increases in metabolic activity (such as increased protein synthesis) required to adapt to the elevated metabolic pressure acting on the small remnant.[11,15,44,60]

Progression–angiogenic period

After the first mitotic peak (48 hours post HX), hepatocellular proliferation starts to decline. This decline overlaps with mounting hyperplasia of non-parenchymal cells, particularly LSECs that start to divide at day 4, reinstalling sinusoidal vasculature within the next 3–4 days.[19] The events associated with LSEC proliferation nicely illustrate the interdependence of cell type-specific regeneration patterns (Figure 3.6).

Early after HX, VEGFR2–ID1 signalling from LSECs provides crucial trophogens (e.g. HGF) for hepatocytes to divide (see 'Priming').[19] In parallel, LSECs downregulate ANGPT2, leading to reduced expression of TGFB1 (the main inhibitor of hepatocyte proliferation) and of VEGFR2 (essential for LSEC proliferation)[61]—conditions that favour hepatocyte over LSEC proliferation.[62] With parenchymal expansion, the increasing rarefaction of vessels causes liver hypoxia, eventually leading to the stabilization of hepatocellular HIF2A. In turn, HIF2A fosters hepatocyte mitosis (via *FOXM1* induction) but also boosts VEGF secretion.[18] Hepatic VEGF levels continue to rise and peak after hepatocyte mitosis,[61] stimulating LSECs to re-elevate ANGPT2. Consequently, TGFB1 and VEGFR2 levels are upregulated to reverse pre-mitotic conditions, now favouring LSEC proliferation.[18,62] With these events, re-vascularization of the regenerating liver is initiated. Therefore, reciprocal control between hepatocytes and LSECs couples the angiogenic phase to successful hepatocyte division, thereby installing spatiotemporal order on the regeneration of the two major liver cell populations. The reconstitution of vasculature likely is a prerequisite for the reconstruction of a normal liver architecture, with each hepatocyte chord realigned between LSECs and cholangiocytes. Overall, LSECs are key to both the initiation and termination of hepatocellular proliferation, highlighting their governing role in LR.[63]

Termination

Termination with recovery of the original liver size is the least understood phase of regeneration. Available data focus on the hepatocellular switch from a proliferative to a resting state.

Hepatocyte identity and function is specified through the differentiation factor HNF4A, which is downregulated early after HX to enable proliferative function. Its re-elevation with the angiogenic phase constitutes an important signal for hepatocytes to stop proliferation and resume hepatic function.[64,65] During the angiogenic phase (see 'Progression—angiogenic period'), LSECs increase the production of TGFB to dampen hepatocellular proliferation. Intriguingly, *TGFB* gene expression from non-parenchymal cells already starts to rise early after HX—possibly a HGF/EGF-induced negative feedback—and peaks with the angiogenic phase.[7,66,67] ECM remodelling keeps most of TGFB in plasma (see 'Priming'), thus away from hepatocytes, which further downregulate TGFBRs to resist its effects.[66] However, the newly produced TGFB promotes angiogenesis and acts on HSCs to stimulate ECM synthesis,[7] central events during late-stage LR. With the repopulation of non-parenchymal cells, the ECM reassumes its original state and binds TGFB back to hepatocytes. TGFB then acts in concert with activin to engage antiproliferative SMAD signalling in hepatocytes,[68] thereby reinstalling tonic inhibition of proliferation as found in resting liver.[66] The ECM also ties down free HGF for its inactivation, and engages integrins and outer membrane proteins such as glypican, which

Mechanisms of regeneration

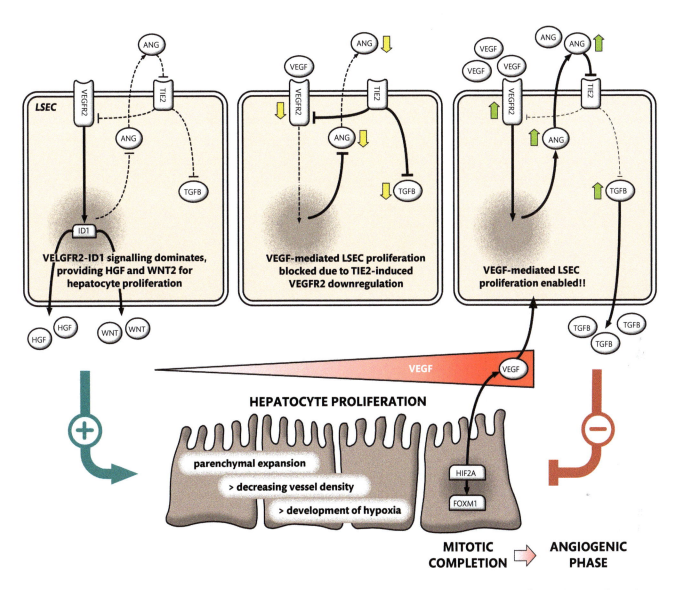

Figure 3.6 Reciprocal control between liver sinusoidal endothelial cells and hepatocytes for an ordered expansion of parenchyma and vasculature. The early dominance of LSEC-derived, hepatocyte-specific regeneration signals leads to parenchymal expansion. The resulting vessel paucity causes liver hypoxia and the activation of HIF2A. On the one hand, HIF2A promotes hepatocellular mitosis to complete parenchymal expansion. On the other hand, HIF2A induces marked VEGF production to initiate the proliferation of LSECs, which in turn change their secretome to terminate parenchymal expansion. ANG and TIE2 stand for angiopoietin 2 and its main receptor, which is inhibited by its ligand.

rely termination signals to hepatocytes.[6,69–71] Both ILK (the kinase transmitting integrin signals) and glypican are connected with the Hippo–Yes-associated protein 1 (YAP1) pathway, the famous organ size restrictor.[70,71] The Hippo pathway is suppressed after HX, losing pro-regenerative YAP1 activity.[72–74] Hippo signalling is reactivated with the restoration of the original liver volume, marking an end-point of liver size recovery.[74]

Thus, the ECM and associated molecules, the Hippo pathway, but also the regain of full metabolic capacity (see 'Metabolic control of LR') are part of a hepatostat that preserves the species-specific ratio of liver-to-body size.[6]

Metabolic control of liver regeneration

Hepatic insufficiency resulting from tissue loss conceivably must be sensed by the body. The loss and recovery of hepatic capacity may therefore generate systemic metabolic responses that aid in the initiation and termination of LR.

After resection, the remaining glycogen stores do not suffice for continuous glucose provision, leading to systemic hypoglycaemia. In response, peripheral fat stores are mobilized, and lipids are transported into the remnant, while hepatocytes undergo partial adipocyte transdifferentiation.[75] The resulting steatosis peaks at 16 hours after HX (i.e. before cell cycle entry) and fades away with successful liver growth.[76–78] Prevention of steatosis (e.g. by suppressing hypoglycaemia) or blocking β-oxidation both inhibit LR, because lipids provide the regenerative fuel.[77,79,80] Therefore, systemic glucose insufficiency generates a regenerative trigger, which adjusts to the energy demands of a growing tissue. As such, the onset of LR may be viewed as a modified fasting response.[81]

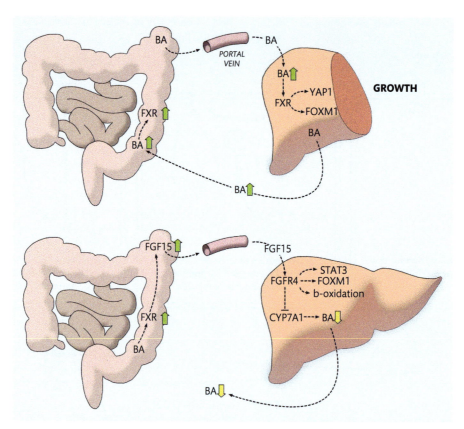

Figure 3.7 The contribution of bile acids (BAs) to the metabolic control of liver regeneration. Circulating from the liver to the gut and back, BAs provide a liver–gut communication axis that aids in the regulation of liver regeneration. Owing to the loss of liver mass after hepatectomy, the circulating pool of BAs increases, activating a range of intestinal and hepatic nuclear receptors. Among these, FXR induces key pathways that balance liver size increases with reduced BA production to eventually return to homeostatic conditions.

A beautiful example of metabolic control is the bodily BA pool that the liver must circulate (Figure 3.7). BAs are reabsorbed by the gut to re-enter the liver via the portal vein. Upon resection, BA influx increases with the portal inflow. To avoid toxic overload, the primary *hepatic* BA sensor FXR is activated and promotes hepatocyte proliferation via YAP1 and FOXM1—adapting liver size to the increased metabolic pressure.[82,83] BAs also stimulate *gut* FXR to induce the secretion of FGF15, which then binds to *hepatic* FGFR4 to support size adaptations (via STAT3/FOXM1 and β-oxidation promotion), but particularly to lower BA production via CYP7A1 downregulation.[82,84–87] In the absence of FGF15, the hepatic BA pool enlarges and so does liver size, leading to hepatomegaly.[82,88] Thus, the restoration of normal BA circulation after resection requires gut–liver communication and is an integral component of the hepatostat.

Indeed, the liver is equipped with a great number of nuclear receptors that each 'sense' a range of specific metabolites and participate—via modulation of gene expression—in the molecular circuits coordinating metabolic with proliferative needs. Their activity regulates BA, lipid, glucose, energy, hormone, and xeno/endobiotic metabolism including detoxification—the key functions of the liver. Deficiencies in, for example, PPARA, PPARG, LXR, PXR, ER, CAR, or RXRA (the heterodimeric partner of many nuclear receptors) all impact LR.[84,89–93] CAR is the classic example of a metabolic sensor; activated by various xeno/endobiotics, bilirubin, or steroid hormones, the transcription factor induces metabolic genes (e.g. for drug/bilirubin clearance), but likewise proliferative genes. In resting liver, strong CAR activation provokes hepatomegaly, illustrating how metabolic strain adapts liver volume to request[94,95]—properties that are likewise essential for the regenerating liver.[13] After tissue loss, the portal inflow imports not only more growth factors, but also more toxins and metabolites. The nuclear receptors react to the metabolic pressure by increasing liver mass along with appropriate enzyme expression, enabling the remnant to cope—a ubiquitous principle behind LR. Vice versa, the body may sense the loss of hepatosynthetic function (e.g. serum albumin) and transmit regenerative signals back to the remnant—however, this area is ill-researched.

Clinical issues related to liver regeneration

Post-hepatectomy liver failure

Radical surgical removal of hepatic tumours rests on the liver's regenerative capacity and still offers the best chance of cure. Up to 75% of liver mass can be removed without major risks for patients. However, liver may not recover if the remnant is too small or of too poor quality, leading to post-hepatectomy liver failure (PHLF), the main cause of death due to liver surgery.[96]

Why small liver remnants fail to recover is unclarified. Excess injury has been proposed, with the massive portal inflow (inversely proportional to remnant volume) damaging the sinusoidal lining and persistently affecting hepatocyte function.[97] Experimental

Clinical issues related to liver regeneration

evidence supports this view, and clinical observations suggest portal pressure can predict PHLF.[97–102] Intriguingly however, extended 86% HX modified to induce little injury *still* provokes typical features of PHLF (metabolic dysfunction, regenerative deficiency, increased mortality), with stalled S/M-phase progression as the underlying cause.[13,14] Therefore, injury is not a prerequisite to PHLF development, but remains an issue in the clinic: unlike the ligation of lobes in mice, tumour resections cut straight through the parenchyma, causing physical injury and bleeding. Bleeding, in turn, inhibits hepatocellular cell cycle activities after HX.[103] Accordingly, perioperative bleeding increases PHLF risks.[104]

Overall, a small remnant faces a conflict between the need for metabolic tasks versus the need to grow, with exaggerated proliferative signals perhaps causing negative feedback inhibition of cell cycle progression.[14,105,106] Likely, the immense metabolic pressure, together with an anaerobic shift due to a blocked arterial buffer response,[96,107] might impair both the metabolic and regenerative capacity already before the onset of proliferation (e.g. via insufficient energy provision).[77]

Background liver disease (i.e. steatosis, fibrosis/cirrhosis, cholestasis, or chemotherapy-related injury) that frequently accompanies common liver malignancies likewise is a risk factor for PHLF, simply because it reduces the metabolic and/or regenerative capacity.[96] Therefore, the *functional* liver volume that remains after resection is key to the regenerative success and defines a physiological limit to LR.

Non-alcoholic fatty liver disease

Typified by the chronic accumulation of lipids within hepatocytes, non-alcoholic fatty liver disease (NAFLD) can progress to steatohepatitis and cirrhosis, representing the commonest cause of chronic liver disease. NAFLD impairs LR and is an increasing burden for liver surgery given its global spread.[108,109] Defective growth factor responses such as EGFR-related signalling have been proposed to slow LR in fatty liver.[109,110] While EGFR promotion indeed can restore normal regenerative capacity,[111,112] EGFR inhibition paradoxically mitigates experimental NAFLD.[113] Therefore, EGFR-related deficiencies in NAFLD patients might be (1) hepatic defence strategies to restrain disease at the expense of regenerative capacity or (2) secondary to a more principal problem. Interestingly, a Western diet rich in omega-6 arachidonic acid favours vasoconstrictive conditions in the liver.[114] The resulting reductions in blood flow might reduce growth factor/metabolite influx post resection, while vessel constriction would counteract the sinusoidal dilation required for LR onset.[20,115] Abnormal energy metabolism might add to impaired LR: in NAFLD, fat is stored rather than burned, and impaired β-oxidation might hinder the provision of regenerative fuel.[77,108] Of note, fructose-induced steatosis (favouring glycolysis)

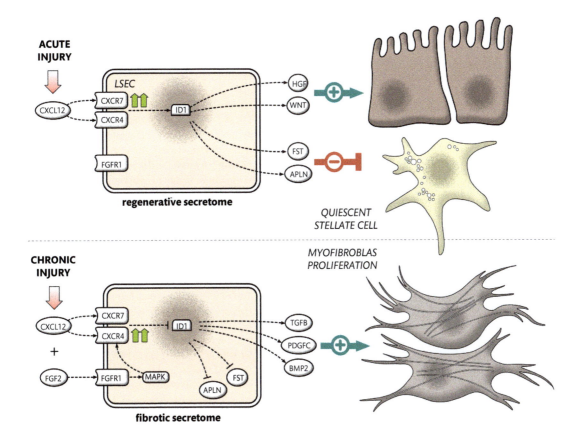

Figure 3.8 The dependency of regenerative versus fibrotic injury responses on intact liver sinusoidal endothelial cells. Upon acute injury, LSECs secrete factors that foster hepatocellular regeneration while keeping stellate cells at quiescence. Chronic injury, by contrast, causes LSEC to de-differentiate, owing either to failed hepatocyte support or to direct impact on LSECs. De-differentiation is accompanied by a switch in the LSEC secretome (regulated through the CXCR4-to-CXCR7 ratio), with upregulation of profibrotic factors at the expense of quiescence promoters. The resulting conditions favour stellate cell activation to proliferative myofibroblasts, while hepatocyte proliferation (i.e. TGFB) is dampened.

seems to markedly impact LR, while high-fat diet-induced steatosis (favouring β-oxidation) does little harm in rats[116]—perhaps mirroring the clinical observation that steatosis, particularly if mild, may not always impair LR.[109]

Fibrosis

Fibrosis, the accumulation of ECM around the sinusoids and portal tracts, is thought to result from chronic injury switching regeneration to scarring, with cirrhosis representing the end stage of fibrotic progression.

In brief, chronic hepatocyte injury impacts neighbouring LSECs (perhaps via reduced VEGF provision), which start to de-differentiate, lose their fenestration, and change their secretome[117-119]: increased secretion of ECM proteins such as fibronectin leads to the formation of a basement membrane and activates HSCs that in turn proliferate, contract to promote LSEC vasoconstriction, and start to deposit ECM, which aggravates LSECs de-differentiation.[120] This self-amplifying cycle is thought to drive fibrotic development. Molecularly, the secretome change is regulated through the CXCR7-to-CXCR4 expression ratio on LSECs (Figure 3.8): *acute* injury induces a high CXCR7-to-CXCR4 ratio, which stimulates pro-regenerative VEGFR2–ID1–HGF/WNT2 signalling via ID1 upregulation. In contrast, *chronic* injury favours a high CXCR4-to-CXCR7 ratio through constitutive FGFR1 engagement, now promoting HSC proliferation via secretion of profibrotic cytokines (TGFB, BMP2, PDGFC).[19,121] Indeed, the pathways (VEGF–NOS3–sGC)[120] required to maintain LSEC fenestration (the key feature of their fully differentiated state) also contribute to the provision of the angiocrine signals (i.e. WNTs) needed for parenchymal regeneration after tissue loss.[19,122] Therefore, early de-differentiation leading to the loss of proper LSEC function is central for the regenerative deficits of fibrotic liver.

Conclusion

The regenerative capacity of the liver is unique among mammalian organs and has attracted tremendous research interest. This chapter cannot do justice to all the relevant studies; however, key findings have been included to illustrate general principles underlying regeneration after tissue loss. Communication with the periphery is essential to sense systemic insufficiencies, providing cues to regrow to the species-specific liver size. Likewise, metabolic overload creates proximal pressure that initiates LR and declines towards the restoration of metabolic capacity. Cooperation among various liver cell types fosters interdependency, where feedback between preceding and succeeding events enables an ordered progression of LR. Here, LSECs have emerged as central players, perhaps reflecting the intimate relationship between blood, hepatocytes, and liver function. Similar principles seem to govern associated molecular circuits, where mutual fortification synergizes to trigger activity peaks that then are dampened by negative feedback. Pathway redundancy underlies LR with stability and the flexibility needed for a successful regrowth also in a changing and adverse environment. The overlay of organ-to-organ, cell-to-cell, and molecule-to-molecule interactions ultimately is required to allow for an efficient and precise recovery of small liver remnants without the loss of vital function—still a miraculous process that will keep challenging future science.

REFERENCES

1. Gu X, Huang D, Ci L, et al. Fate tracing of hepatocytes in mouse liver. *Sci Rep.* 2017;**7**(1):16108.
2. Pu W, Zhang H, Huang X, et al. Mfsd2a+ hepatocytes repopulate the liver during injury and regeneration. *Nat Commun.* 2016;**7**:13369.
3. Itoh T, Miyajima A. Filling a gYap in hepato-biliary tissue integration in liver homeostasis and regeneration. *Cell Stem Cell.* 2019;**25**(1):5–6.
4. Evarts RP, Nagy P, Marsden E, Thorgeirsson SS. A precursor-product relationship exists between oval cells and hepatocytes in rat liver. *Carcinogenesis.* 1987;**8**(11):1737–1740.
5. Higgins RA, Anderson RM. Experimental pathology of the liver. I. Restoration of the liver of the white rat following partial surgical removal. *Arch Pathol.* 1931;**12**:186–202.
6. Michalopoulos GK. Liver regeneration. *J Cell Physiol.* 2007;**213**(2):286–300.
7. Michalopoulos GK. Principles of liver regeneration and growth homeostasis. *Compr Physiol.* 2013;**3**(1):485–513.
8. Rudnick DA, Davidson NO. Functional relationships between lipid metabolism and liver regeneration. *Int J Hepatol.* 2012;**2012**:549241.
9. Riehle KJ, Dan YY, Campbell JS, Fausto N. New concepts in liver regeneration. *J Gastroenterol Hepatol.* 2011;**26**(Suppl 1):203–212.
10. Minocha S, Villeneuve D, Rib L, Moret C, Guex N, Herr W. Segregated hepatocyte proliferation and metabolic states within the regenerating mouse liver. *Hepatol Commun.* 2017;**1**(1):871–885.
11. Miyaoka Y, Miyajima A. To divide or not to divide: revisiting liver regeneration. *Cell Div.* 2013;**8**(1):8.
12. Haga S, Ozaki M, Inoue H, et al. The survival pathways phosphatidylinositol-3 kinase (PI3-K)/phosphoinositide-dependent protein kinase 1 (PDK1)/Akt modulate liver regeneration through hepatocyte size rather than proliferation. *Hepatology.* 2009;**49**(1):204–214.
13. Tschuor C, Kachaylo E, Limani P, et al. Constitutive androstane receptor (Car)-driven regeneration protects liver from failure following tissue loss. *J Hepatol.* 2016;**65**(1):66–74.
14. Lehmann K, Tschuor C, Rickenbacher A, et al. Liver failure after extended hepatectomy in mice is mediated by a p21-dependent barrier to liver regeneration. *Gastroenterology.* 2012;**143**(1):1609–1619.
15. Miyaoka Y, Ebato K, Kato H, Shimizu S, Miyajima A. Hypertrophy and unconventional cell division of hepatocytes underlie liver regeneration. *Curr Biol.* 2012;**22**(13):1166–1175.
16. Sakamoto T, Liu Z, Murase N, et al. Mitosis and apoptosis in the liver of interleukin-6-deficient mice after partial hepatectomy. *Hepatology.* 1999;**29**(2):403–411.
17. Abu Rmilah A, Zhou W, Nelson E, Lin L, Amiot B, Nyberg SL. Understanding the marvels behind liver regeneration. *Wiley Interdiscip Rev Dev Biol.* 2019;**8**(3):e340.
18. Kron P, Linecker M, Limani P, et al. Hypoxia-driven Hif2a coordinates mouse liver regeneration by coupling parenchymal growth to vascular expansion. *Hepatology.* 2016;**64**(6):2198–2209.
19. Ding BS, Nolan DJ, Butler JM, et al. Inductive angiocrine signals from sinusoidal endothelium are required for liver regeneration. *Nature.* 2010;**468**(7321):310–315.
20. Lorenz L, Axnick J, Buschmann T, et al. Mechanosensing by beta1 integrin induces angiocrine signals for liver growth and survival. *Nature.* 2018;**562**(7725):128–132.

21. Paranjpe S, Bowen WC, Mars WM, et al. Combined systemic elimination of MET and epidermal growth factor receptor signaling completely abolishes liver regeneration and leads to liver decompensation. *Hepatology*. 2016;**64**(5):1711–1724.
22. Fazel Modares N, Polz R, Haghighi F, et al. IL-6 trans-signaling controls liver regeneration after partial hepatectomy. *Hepatology*. 2019;(6):2075–2091.
23. Preziosi ME, Monga SP. Update on the mechanisms of liver regeneration. *Semin Liver Dis*. 2017;**37**(2):141–151.
24. Russell JO, Monga SP. Wnt/beta-catenin signaling in liver development, homeostasis, and pathobiology. *Annu Rev Pathol*. 2018;**13**:351–378.
25. Lehwald N, Tao GZ, Jang KY, et al. Beta-catenin regulates hepatic mitochondrial function and energy balance in mice. *Gastroenterology*. 2012;**143**(3):754–764.
26. Sodhi D, Micsenyi A, Bowen WC, Monga DK, Talavera JC, Monga SP. Morpholino oligonucleotide-triggered beta-catenin knockdown compromises normal liver regeneration. *J Hepatol*. 2005;**43**(1):132–141.
27. Yin C, Evason KJ, Asahina K, Stainier DY. Hepatic stellate cells in liver development, regeneration, and cancer. *J Clin Invest*. 2013;**123**(5):1902–1910.
28. Olsen PS, Poulsen SS, Kirkegaard P. Adrenergic effects on secretion of epidermal growth factor from Brunner's glands. *Gut*. 1985;**26**(9):920–927.
29. Murata S, Ohkohchi N, Matsuo R, Ikeda O, Myronovych A, Hoshi R. Platelets promote liver regeneration in early period after hepatectomy in mice. *World J Surg*. 2007;**31**(4):808–816.
30. Kono H, Fujii H, Suzuki-Inoue K, et al. The platelet-activating receptor C-type lectin receptor-2 plays an essential role in liver regeneration after partial hepatectomy in mice. *J Thromb Haemost*. 2017;**15**(5):998–1008.
31. Starlinger P, Haegele S, Offensperger F, et al. The profile of platelet alpha-granule released molecules affects postoperative liver regeneration. *Hepatology*. 2016;**63**(5):1675–1688.
32. Wartiovaara U, Salven P, Mikkola H, et al. Peripheral blood platelets express VEGF-C and VEGF which are released during platelet activation. *Thromb Haemost*. 1998;**80**(1):171–175.
33. Yamamoto C, Yagi S, Hori T, et al. Significance of portal venous VEGF during liver regeneration after hepatectomy. *J Surg Res*. 2010;**159**(2):e37–e43.
34. Lesurtel M, Graf R, Aleil B, et al. Platelet-derived serotonin mediates liver regeneration. *Science*. 2006;**312**(5770):104–107.
35. Kambakamba P, Linecker M, Schneider M, et al. Novel benefits of remote ischemic preconditioning through VEGF-dependent protection from resection-induced liver failure in the mouse. *Ann Surg*. 2018;**268**(5):885–893.
36. Oberkofler CE, Limani P, Jang JH, et al. Systemic protection through remote ischemic preconditioning is spread by platelet-dependent signaling in mice. *Hepatology*. 2014;**60**(4):1409–1417.
37. Furrer K, Rickenbacher A, Tian Y, et al. Serotonin reverts age-related capillarization and failure of regeneration in the liver through a VEGF-dependent pathway. *Proc Natl Acad Sci U S A*. 2011;**108**(7):2945–2950.
38. Shido K, Chavez D, Cao Z, et al. Platelets prime hematopoietic and vascular niche to drive angiocrine-mediated liver regeneration. *Signal Transduct Target Ther*. 2017;**2**:16044.
39. Michalopoulos GK. Liver regeneration after partial hepatectomy: critical analysis of mechanistic dilemmas. *Am J Pathol*. 2010;**176**(1):2–13.
40. Mei Y, Thevananther S. Endothelial nitric oxide synthase is a key mediator of hepatocyte proliferation in response to partial hepatectomy in mice. *Hepatology*. 2011;**54**(5):1777–1789.
41. Asencio JM, Garcia-Sabrido JL, Lopez-Baena JA, et al. Preconditioning by portal vein embolization modulates hepatic hemodynamics and improves liver function in pigs with extended hepatectomy. *Surgery*. 2017;**161**(6):1489–1501.
42. Gracia-Sancho J, Russo L, Garcia-Caldero H, García-Pagán JC, García-Cardeña G, Bosch J. Endothelial expression of transcription factor Kruppel-like factor 2 and its vasoprotective target genes in the normal and cirrhotic rat liver. *Gut*. 2011;**60**(4):517–524.
43. Fausto N. Liver regeneration. *J Hepatol*. 2000;**32**(1):19–31.
44. Laplante M, Sabatini DM. mTOR signaling at a glance. *J Cell Sci*. 2009;**122**(20):3589–3594.
45. Santamaria-Barria JA, Zeng S, Greer JB, et al. Csf1r or Mer inhibition delays liver regeneration via suppression of Kupffer cells. *PLoS One*. 2019;**14**(5):e0216275.
46. Peerschke EI, Yin W, Ghebrehiwet B. Complement activation on platelets: implications for vascular inflammation and thrombosis. *Mol Immunol*. 2010;**47**(13):2170–2175.
47. Iimuro Y, Fujimoto J. TLRs, NF-kappaB, JNK, and liver regeneration. *Gastroenterol Res Pract*. 2010;**2010**:598109.
48. Nachmany I, Bogoch Y, Sivan A, et al. CD11b(+)Ly6G(+) myeloid-derived suppressor cells promote liver regeneration in a murine model of major hepatectomy. *FASEB J*. 2019;**33**(5):5967–5978.
49. Behnke K, Zhuang Y, Xu HC, et al. B cell-mediated maintenance of cluster of differentiation 169-positive cells is critical for liver regeneration. *Hepatology*. 2018;**68**(6):2348–2361.
50. Li N, Hua J. Immune cells in liver regeneration. *Oncotarget*. 2017;**8**(2):3628–3639.
51. Seki E, Kondo Y, Iimuro Y, et al. Demonstration of cooperative contribution of MET- and EGFR-mediated STAT3 phosphorylation to liver regeneration by exogenous suppressor of cytokine signalings. *J Hepatol*. 2008;**48**(2):237–245.
52. Riehle KJ, Campbell JS, McMahan RS, et al. Regulation of liver regeneration and hepatocarcinogenesis by suppressor of cytokine signaling 3. *J Exp Med*. 2008;**205**(1):91–103.
53. Dierssen U, Beraza N, Lutz HH, et al. Molecular dissection of gp130-dependent pathways in hepatocytes during liver regeneration. *J Biol Chem*. 2008;**283**(15):9886–9895.
54. Xu D, Yang F, Yuan JH, et al. Long noncoding RNAs associated with liver regeneration 1 accelerates hepatocyte proliferation during liver regeneration by activating Wnt/beta-catenin signaling. *Hepatology*. 2013;**58**(2):739–751.
55. Factor VM, Seo D, Ishikawa T, et al. Loss of c-Met disrupts gene expression program required for G2/M progression during liver regeneration in mice. *PLoS One*. 2010; (9):5.
56. Natarajan A, Wagner B, Sibilia M. The EGF receptor is required for efficient liver regeneration. *Proc Natl Acad Sci U S A*. 2007;**104**(43):17081–17086.
57. Paranjpe S, Bowen WC, Bell AW, Nejak-Bowen K, Luo JH, Michalopoulos GK. Cell cycle effects resulting from inhibition of hepatocyte growth factor and its receptor c-Met in regenerating rat livers by RNA interference. *Hepatology*. 2007;**45**(6):1471–1477.
58. Tan X, Behari J, Cieply B, Michalopolous GK, Monga SP. Conditional deletion of beta-catenin reveals its role in liver growth and regeneration. *Gastroenterology*. 2006;**131**(5):1561–1572.

59. Caldez MJ, Van Hul N, Koh HWL, et al. Metabolic remodeling during liver regeneration. *Dev Cell.* 2018;**47**(4):425–438.
60. Sinturel F, Gerber A, Mauvoisin D, et al. Diurnal oscillations in liver mass and cell size accompany ribosome assembly cycles. *Cell.* 2017;**169**(4):651–663.
61. Taniguchi E, Sakisaka S, Matsuo K, Tanikawa K, Sata M. Expression and role of vascular endothelial growth factor in liver regeneration after partial hepatectomy in rats. *J Histochem Cytochem.* 2001;**49**(1):121–130.
62. Hu J, Srivastava K, Wieland M, et al. Endothelial cell-derived angiopoietin-2 controls liver regeneration as a spatiotemporal rheostat. *Science.* 2014;**343**(6169):416–419.
63. Poisson J, Lemoinne S, Boulanger C, et al. Liver sinusoidal endothelial cells: physiology and role in liver diseases. *J Hepatol.* 2017;**66**(1):212–227.
64. Huck I, Gunewardena S, Espanol-Suner R, Willenbring H, Apte U. Hepatocyte nuclear factor 4 alpha activation is essential for termination of liver regeneration in mice. *Hepatology.* 2019;**70**(1):666–681.
65. Walesky C, Apte U. Role of hepatocyte nuclear factor 4alpha (HNF4alpha) in cell proliferation and cancer. *Gene Expr.* 2015;**16**(3):101–108.
66. Michalopoulos GK. Hepatostat: liver regeneration and normal liver tissue maintenance. *Hepatology.* 2017;**65**(4):1384–1392.
67. Braun L, Mead JE, Panzica M, Bell GI, Fausto N. Transforming growth factor beta mRNA increases during liver regeneration: a possible paracrine mechanism of growth regulation. *Proc Natl Acad Sci U S A.* 1988;**85**(5):1539–1543.
68. Oe S, Lemmer ER, Conner EA, et al. Intact signaling by transforming growth factor beta is not required for termination of liver regeneration in mice. *Hepatology.* 2004;**40**(5):1098–1105.
69. Greenhalgh SN, Matchett KP, Taylor RS, et al. Loss of integrin alphavbeta8 in murine hepatocytes accelerates liver regeneration. *Am J Pathol.* 2019;**189**(2):258–271.
70. Liu B, Bell AW, Paranjpe S, et al. Suppression of liver regeneration and hepatocyte proliferation in hepatocyte-targeted glypican 3 transgenic mice. *Hepatology.* 2010;**52**(3):1060–1067.
71. Apte U, Gkretsi V, Bowen WC, et al. Enhanced liver regeneration following changes induced by hepatocyte-specific genetic ablation of integrin-linked kinase. *Hepatology.* 2009;**50**(3):844–851.
72. Tschuor C, Kachaylo E, Ungethum U, et al. Yes-associated protein promotes early hepatocyte cell cycle progression in regenerating liver after tissue loss. *FASEB Bioadv.* 2019;**1**(1):51–61.
73. Oh SH, Swiderska-Syn M, Jewell ML, Premont RT, Diehl AM. Liver regeneration requires Yap1-TGFbeta-dependent epithelial-mesenchymal transition in hepatocytes. *J Hepatol.* 2018;**69**(2):359–367.
74. Patel SH, Camargo FD, Yimlamai D. Hippo signaling in the liver regulates organ size, cell fate, and carcinogenesis. *Gastroenterology.* 2017;**152**(3):533–545.
75. Shteyer E, Liao Y, Muglia LJ, Hruz PW, Rudnick DA. Disruption of hepatic adipogenesis is associated with impaired liver regeneration in mice. *Hepatology.* 2004;**40**(6):1322–1332.
76. Abshagen K, Degenhardt B, Liebig M, et al. Liver-specific Repin1 deficiency impairs transient hepatic steatosis in liver regeneration. *Sci Rep.* 2018;**8**(2):16858.
77. Kachaylo E, Tschuor C, Calo N, et al. PTEN down-regulation promotes beta-oxidation to fuel hypertrophic liver growth after hepatectomy in mice. *Hepatology.* 2017;**66**(3):908–921.
78. Huang J, Rudnick DA. Elucidating the metabolic regulation of liver regeneration. *Am J Pathol.* 2014;**184**(2):309–321.
79. Huang J, Schriefer AE, Cliften PF, et al. Postponing the hypoglycemic response to partial hepatectomy delays mouse liver regeneration. *Am J Pathol.* 2016;**186**(3):587–599.
80. Weymann A, Hartman E, Gazit V, et al. p21 is required for dextrose-mediated inhibition of mouse liver regeneration. *Hepatology.* 2009;**50**(1):207–215.
81. Cuenca AG, Cress WD, Good RA, Marikar Y, Engelman RW. Calorie restriction influences cell cycle protein expression and DNA synthesis during liver regeneration. *Exp Biol Med.* 2001;**226**(11):1061–1067.
82. Naugler WE, Tarlow BD, Fedorov LM, et al. Fibroblast growth factor signaling controls liver size in mice with humanized livers. *Gastroenterology.* 2015;**149**(3):728–740.
83. Huang W, Ma K, Zhang J, et al. Nuclear receptor-dependent bile acid signaling is required for normal liver regeneration. *Science.* 2006;**312**(5771):233–236.
84. Shin DJ, Wang L. Bile acid-activated receptors: a review on FXR and other nuclear receptors. *Handb Exp Pharmacol.* 2019;**256**:51–72.
85. Padrissa-Altes S, Bachofner M, Bogorad RL, et al. Control of hepatocyte proliferation and survival by Fgf receptors is essential for liver regeneration in mice. *Gut.* 2015;**64**(9):1444–1453.
86. Cicione C, Degirolamo C, Moschetta A. Emerging role of fibroblast growth factors 15/19 and 21 as metabolic integrators in the liver. *Hepatology.* 2012;**56**(6):2404–2411.
87. Inagaki T, Choi M, Moschetta A, et al. Fibroblast growth factor 15 functions as an enterohepatic signal to regulate bile acid homeostasis. *Cell Metab.* 2005;**2**(4):217–225.
88. Alvarez-Sola G, Uriarte I, Latasa MU, et al. Bile acids, FGF15/19 and liver regeneration: from mechanisms to clinical applications. *Biochim Biophys Acta Mol Basis Dis.* 2018;**1864**(4 Pt B):1326–1334.
89. Xie G, Yin S, Zhang Z, et al. Hepatocyte peroxisome proliferator-activated receptor alpha enhances liver regeneration after partial hepatectomy in mice. *Am J Pathol.* 2019;**189**(2):272–282.
90. Batmunkh B, Choijookhuu N, Srisowanna N, et al. Estrogen accelerates cell proliferation through estrogen receptor alpha during rat liver regeneration after partial hepatectomy. *Acta Histochem Cytochem.* 2017;**50**(1):39–48.
91. Liu HX, Fang Y, Hu Y, Fang J, Wan YJ. PPARbeta regulates liver regeneration by modulating Akt and E2f signaling. *PLoS One.* 2013;**8**(6):e65644.
92. Halilbasic E, Claudel T, Trauner M. Bile acid transporters and regulatory nuclear receptors in the liver and beyond. *J Hepatol.* 2013;**58**(1):155–168.
93. Vacca M, Degirolamo C, Massafra V, et al. Nuclear receptors in regenerating liver and hepatocellular carcinoma. *Mol Cell Endocrinol.* 2013;**368**(1–2):108–119.
94. Blanco-Bose WE, Murphy MJ, Ehninger A, et al. C-Myc and its target FoxM1 are critical downstream effectors of constitutive androstane receptor (CAR) mediated direct liver hyperplasia. *Hepatology.* 2008;**48**(4):1302–1311.
95. Kowalik MA, Saliba C, Pibiri M, et al. Yes-associated protein regulation of adaptive liver enlargement and hepatocellular carcinoma development in mice. *Hepatology.* 2011;**53**(6):2086–2096.
96. van Mierlo KM, Schaap FG, Dejong CH, Olde Damink SW. Liver resection for cancer: new developments in prediction, prevention and management of postresectional liver failure. *J Hepatol.* 2016;**65**(6):1217–1231.
97. Kim DS, Ji WB, Han JH, et al. Effects of splanchnic vasoconstrictors on liver regeneration and survival after 90% rat hepatectomy. *Ann Surg Treat Res.* 2018;**94**(3):118–128.

98. Bogner A, Reissfelder C, Striebel F, et al. Intraoperative increase of portal venous pressure is an immediate predictor of posthepatectomy liver failure after major hepatectomy: a prospective study. *Ann Surg*. 2019;**274**(1):e10–e17.
99. Carrapita JG, Rocha C, Donato H, et al. Portal venous pressure variation during hepatectomy: a prospective study. *Acta Med Port*. 2019;**32**(6):420–426.
100. Marshall KM, He S, Zhong Z, Atkinson C, Tomlinson S. Dissecting the complement pathway in hepatic injury and regeneration with a novel protective strategy. *J Exp Med*. 2014;**211**(9):1793–1805.
101. Ishizaki Y, Kawasaki S, Sugo H, Yoshimoto J, Fujiwara N, Imamura H. Left lobe adult-to-adult living donor liver transplantation: should portal inflow modulation be added? *Liver Transpl*. 2012;**18**(3):305–314.
102. Man K, Fan ST, Lo CM, et al. Graft injury in relation to graft size in right lobe live donor liver transplantation: a study of hepatic sinusoidal injury in correlation with portal hemodynamics and intragraft gene expression. *Ann Surg*. 2003;**237**(2):256–264.
103. Matot I, Nachmansson N, Duev O, et al. Impaired liver regeneration after hepatectomy and bleeding is associated with a shift from hepatocyte proliferation to hypertrophy. *FASEB J*. 2017;**31**(12):5283–5295.
104. Jarnagin WR, Gonen M, Fong Y, et al. Improvement in perioperative outcome after hepatic resection: analysis of 1,803 consecutive cases over the past decade. *Ann Surg*. 2002;**236**(4):397–406.
105. Meier M, Knudsen AR, Andersen KJ, et al. Perturbations of urea cycle enzymes during posthepatectomy rat liver failure. *Am J Physiol Gastrointest Liver Physiol*. 2019;**317**(4):G429–G440.
106. Meier M, Knudsen AR, Andersen KJ, Bjerregaard NC, Jensen UB, Mortensen FV. Gene expression in the liver remnant is significantly affected by the size of partial hepatectomy: an experimental rat study. *Gene Expr*. 2017;**17**(4):289–299.
107. Kohler A, Moller PW, Frey S, et al. Portal hyperperfusion after major liver resection and associated sinusoidal damage is a therapeutic target to protect the remnant liver. *Am J Physiol Gastrointest Liver Physiol*. 2019;**317**(3):G264–G274.
108. Della Fazia MA, Servillo G. Foie gras and liver regeneration: a fat dilemma. *Cell Stress*. 2018;**2**(7):162–175.
109. Allaire M, Gilgenkrantz H. The impact of steatosis on liver regeneration. *Horm Mol Biol Clin Investig*. 2018;**41**:1.
110. Kaltenecker D, Themanns M, Mueller KM, et al. Hepatic growth hormone–JAK2–STAT5 signalling: metabolic function, non-alcoholic fatty liver disease and hepatocellular carcinoma progression. *Cytokine*. 2019;**124**:154569.
111. Zimmers TA, Jin X, Zhang Z, Jiang Y, Koniaris LG. Epidermal growth factor receptor restoration rescues the fatty liver regeneration in mice. *Am J Physiol Endocrinol Metab*. 2017;**313**(4):E440–E449.
112. Collin de l'Hortet A, Zerrad-Saadi A, Prip-Buus C, et al. GH administration rescues fatty liver regeneration impairment by restoring GH/EGFR pathway deficiency. *Endocrinology*. 2014;**155**:2545–2554.
113. Bhushan B, Banerjee S, Paranjpe S, et al. Pharmacologic inhibition of epidermal growth factor receptor suppresses nonalcoholic fatty liver disease in a murine fast-food diet model. *Hepatology*. 2019;**70**(5):1546–1563.
114. El-Badry AM, Jang JH, Elsherbiny A, et al. Chemical composition of hepatic lipids mediates reperfusion injury of the macrosteatotic mouse liver through thromboxane A(2). *J Hepatol*. 2011;**55**(6):1291–1299.
115. Persico M, Masarone M, Damato A, et al. Non alcoholic fatty liver disease and eNOS dysfunction in humans. *BMC Gastroenterol*. 2017;**17**(1):35.
116. Tanoue S, Uto H, Kumamoto R, et al. Liver regeneration after partial hepatectomy in rat is more impaired in a steatotic liver induced by dietary fructose compared to dietary fat. *Biochem Biophys Res Commun*. 2011;**407**(1):163–168.
117. Maretti-Mira AC, Wang X, Wang L, DeLeve LD. Incomplete differentiation of engrafted bone marrow endothelial progenitor cells initiates hepatic fibrosis in the rat. *Hepatology*. 2019;**69**(3):1259–1272.
118. Cordero-Espinoza L, Huch M. The balancing act of the liver: tissue regeneration versus fibrosis. *J Clin Invest*. 2018;**128**(1):85–96.
119. Marrone G, Shah VH, Gracia-Sancho J. Sinusoidal communication in liver fibrosis and regeneration. *J Hepatol*. 2016;**65**(3):608–617.
120. Xie G, Wang X, Wang L, et al. Role of differentiation of liver sinusoidal endothelial cells in progression and regression of hepatic fibrosis in rats. *Gastroenterology*. 2012;**142**(4):918–927.
121. Ding BS, Cao Z, Lis R, et al. Divergent angiocrine signals from vascular niche balance liver regeneration and fibrosis. *Nature*. 2014;**505**(7481):97–102.
122. Duan JL, Ruan B, Yan XC, et al. Endothelial Notch activation reshapes the angiocrine of sinusoidal endothelia to aggravate liver fibrosis and blunt regeneration in mice. *Hepatology*. 2018;**68**(2):677–690.

4

Perioperative management and nutrition in patients with liver and biliary tract disease

Akila Rajakumar, Ilankumaran Kaliamoorthy, and Rathnavel G. Kanagavelu

Introduction

Patients with liver disease and disorders of the biliary system present unique challenges to the perioperative physician. Advances in clinical medicine have improved survival in patients with liver cirrhosis.[1,2] They live longer and develop advanced age-related comorbidities in addition to liver-related risk factors and present to the healthcare team for non-liver surgeries as well as liver resection. Physicians, general surgeons, gastroenterologists, hepatologists, hepatobiliary surgeons and other surgical specialists, anaesthesiologists, and critical care physicians could be presented with the challenges of managing this special group of patients for surgery and postoperative care. A multidisciplinary approach integrating all aspects of perioperative care of these patients is essential to optimize outcomes. A thorough preoperative evaluation, detailed assessment of the need for surgery, and meticulous planning and handling of the intraoperative and postoperative period are required for a smooth recovery phase of these patients. A comprehensive and detailed discussion among the medical professionals and the family is vital and the risks and benefits of surgery should be carefully weighed up before arriving at a consensus decision. Most of the evidence currently available in the literature comes from single-centre experiences of patients without risk-matched controls.

Integrating the knowledge of (1) pathophysiology and altered pharmacokinetics in these patients; (2) perioperative risks, prediction scores, and their optimization whenever possible; and (3) nutritional abnormalities and ways to optimize them for elective surgeries, to available best clinical practice, is essential for successful anaesthetic management of this cohort of patients.

Prediction of perioperative outcomes and planning the timing of surgery

Risk prediction

Prediction of postoperative outcomes is usually made with liver disease severity scores, the Model for End-Stage Liver Disease (MELD) score and Child–Turcotte–Pugh (CTP) scores (more prevalent in the pre-MELD area), age, American Society of Anesthesiologists—Physical Status (ASA-PS) category, invasiveness of surgery, nature of surgery (elective/urgent/emergency), and other associated comorbidities. The scores have been validated in different surgical populations, although with variable levels of evidence.

In general, patients with CTP class A and a few selected cases of class B cirrhosis can undergo non-hepatic surgeries with less risk of hepatic decompensation. CTP class C patients are not considered candidates for elective procedures. In major abdominal surgery, the mortality in CTP class A cirrhosis was reported to be 10%, 30–31% in class B, and 76–82% in class C.[3] Anticipated postoperative complications include liver failure, worsening encephalopathy, bleeding, infection, renal failure, hypoxia, and intractable ascites which can lead to a high risk of mortality.

The MELD score emerged as a better predictor of postoperative outcomes in comparison to the CTP score.[2] In patients with massive ascites, which, by itself, is an independent predictor of poor outcomes, and severe portal hypertension, with well-preserved synthetic function, CTP scores are superior to MELD scores. The risk of mortality increases linearly for MELD scores greater than 8 in patients undergoing abdominal, cardiac, and orthopaedic procedures.[4]

The ASA-PS classification is universally used for risk stratification in surgical populations. The ASA-PS categories have been shown to have a non-linear association with adverse perioperative outcomes.[5] It is a measure of comorbidities and has not been widely proven to be a direct predictor of outcomes in patients with cirrhosis.[6] The Mayo Clinic Postoperative Mortality risk prediction score includes age and ASA category in addition to the MELD score and has been shown to be a better predictor of outcomes in cirrhotic patients in Korea.[7] It has been consistently shown that urgent and emergency operations have more adverse outcomes than elective procedures.[8] Similar trends are also seen in patients with cirrhosis.[9–11] High-risk surgery is defined as intraperitoneal, intrathoracic, or suprainguinal vascular surgery in the general population.[12] In addition to these, hepatobiliary surgery is considered to be a very high-risk procedure in this cohort of patients.

Timing of non-liver surgeries in patients with cirrhosis

The first point to address is to decide whether the patient is a candidate for liver transplantation (LT). If no, then it is important for the entire team and the patient's family to understand that no rescue transplantation can be planned in the event of postoperative deterioration of liver function. If yes, it should be discussed if the procedure can wait until LT. In cases where surgery needs to be performed to maintain the quality of life, it is recommended to complete a pretransplant evaluation and then proceed with surgery. This is more important in patients with a higher risk of perioperative decompensation, MELD score greater than 15, or when the risk stratification models give a predicted postoperative 3-month mortality rate greater than 15%.[13] Avoid or delay until after LT, if possible, all but the most urgent and life-saving procedures in this population.

In cases where living donor LT is feasible, it is advisable to have the donor evaluated and prepared, so that rescue transplantation can be performed in the event of postoperative deterioration of liver function.

Patients for liver resection

The following factors can make liver resection safer in patients with a lower chance of decompensation:

- Absence of significant portal hypertension as evidenced by platelet counts greater than 100,000/μL.[14]
- Absence of venous collaterals on computed tomography imaging and on upper gastrointestinal endoscopy.[15,16]
- Hepatic venous pressure gradient less than 10 mmHg.[17,18]
- Liver stiffness measurement by transient elastography. Studies show varying cut offs from 10 to 22 kPa for the decision on the suitability of liver resection.[19,20]
- Patients with a MELD score less than 7–9 have a good prognosis following liver resection.[21,22]

Of the various strategies available to evaluate preoperative functional liver reserve, the indocyanine green (ICG) clearance test has been extensively studied and ICG retention of greater than 14% at 15 minutes was shown to be associated with a significant increase in post-hepatectomy mortality.[23]

Cholangitis impairs regenerative capacity of the liver post resection and can lead to post-hepatectomy liver failure and other complications.[24–26] Preoperative biliary drainage is often performed in most centres before major hepatectomy to reduce cholestasis, especially in the setting of cholangitis, and it is believed to improve the regenerative capacity of the liver after resection.[27]

Altered pathophysiology in organ systems

Patients with cirrhosis have a hyperdynamic circulation characterized by increased cardiac output, increased heart rate, low systemic vascular resistance, and decreased arterial blood pressure.[28–30] Vascular hyporeactivity is seen amidst the presence of excessive endogenous vasoconstrictors due to diminished baroreceptor reflex sensitivity and therefore the blood pressure remains low.[31–33] Arterial vasodilatation leads to reduced central blood volume thus manifesting as effective hypovolaemia.[34]

Cirrhotic cardiomyopathy is the term applied to the form of cardiac dysfunction in cirrhosis characterized by a blunted contractile response to stress and an altered diastolic relaxation associated with electrophysiological abnormalities, most commonly a prolonged QT interval.[35]

Bilirubin and bile acids are known to cause negative chronotropic effects. It has recently been demonstrated that high concentrations of bile acids are associated with a lower heart rate along with an increased ejection fraction and shortening fraction of the left ventricle.[36] Bile acid overload has a strong association with cirrhotic cardiomyopathy in experimental models. Electrocardiographic and echocardiographic features of cardiomyopathy resolved with reversal of liver injury. The authors refer to this cardiac manifestation as 'cholecardia' to describe the myocardial depressant effects of bile acids.[36]

Respiratory manifestations in patients with liver disease include pleural effusion/hydrothorax, atelectasis due to restrictive effects of pleural effusion and ascites, hepatopulmonary syndrome, and portopulmonary hypertension.[37]

Renal failure is a common complication in cirrhosis. Kidneys are very susceptible to dysfunction even with minor insults in these patients. Hepatorenal syndrome occurs in 20% of patients with ascites.[38] A hyperdynamic circulatory state, the low renal perfusion pressure, and the abnormal neurohumoral regulation—intense activation of the sympathetic nervous system and renin–angiotensin–aldosterone system—contribute to renal dysfunction in these patients.[38–40] After a while, with progressive arterial vasodilatation and a reduction in the systemic vascular resistance, cardiac output reaches a maximal steady state and then starts declining.[41] This has been referred to as the cardiorenal syndrome[6] which results in further decreases in central blood volume and blood pressure and can augment accelerated progression of renal failure.[42,43]

Hyponatraemia is another common problem in these patients. Cirrhotic patients have an impairment in solute free water excretion which can result in hyponatraemia. The main factor responsible is increased production of arginine vasopressin due to the circulatory dysfunction seen in advanced cirrhosis.[44]

Relative adrenal insufficiency has been reported in nearly half of patients with cirrhosis and it seems more prevalent in cirrhotic patients with acute critical illness.[45] Patients with relative adrenal insufficiency have poor survival rates and are at increased risk of developing complications like bleeding and hepatorenal syndrome.[45,46] They have more profound haemodynamic instability and also a poor response to vasopressors.[46] Corticosteroid therapy has been shown to improve survival in critically ill patients with cirrhosis.[45] Relative adrenal insufficiency can be due to the circulating cytokines such as tumour necrosis factor alpha and interleukin-6 which are presumed to impair pituitary responsiveness leading to inadequate cortisol secretion.[47]

The coagulation system in cirrhosis

It has been well recognized that patients with cirrhosis achieve a state of rebalanced coagulation.[48,49] The decreased synthesis of clotting factors is balanced by the decreased synthesis of anticoagulant factors and patients do not bleed as much, as depicted by conventional coagulation test values. In advanced liver disease, they may become thrombophilic due to severe deficiency of protein C.[50]

Platelet counts of 50,000–60,000/μL have been adequate to generate thrombin and therefore this value has been used as the cut off in the general population. But for patients with cirrhosis, against a background of an elevated von Willebrand factor level and activated platelets in circulation,[51,52] this might be a higher target than required.

Perioperative bleeding in these patients can be due to two main factors: (1) portal hypertension related, from collaterals; or (2) mucosal or puncture wound bleeding, due to premature clot dissolution and hyperfibrinolysis—this entity is called accelerated intravascular coagulation and fibrinolysis.[51]

Significant variations in international normalized ratio (INR) values occur in cirrhosis, in different hospitals based on the type of thromboplastin used.[53] Furthermore, the use of fresh frozen plasma to correct a prolonged INR cannot change thrombin production,[54] but it does exacerbate portal hypertension and comes with all associated risk factors. Fibrinogen levels can be more meaningful as a measure of bleeding risk when compared to INR and platelet values.

Altered drug handling in liver disease

Significant changes in drug handling in patients with diseases of the liver and biliary tract include the following:

- There is a larger volume of distribution in patients with ascites, necessitating a higher initial dose for some drugs.
- Lower serum albumin and alpha-1 glycoprotein levels—concern with protein-bound drugs. More unbound drug is available for clinical activity.
- Porto-systemic shunting could increase the oral bioavailability of drugs with intermediate to high hepatic extraction ratios by reducing first-pass metabolism.
- Impaired drug metabolism—phase 1 enzymes are more affected in liver disease than phase 2 enzymes.[55,56] Intra- and extrahepatic cholestasis leads to impaired excretion of drugs and its metabolites, which are eliminated through the biliary system.
- Liver diseases without cirrhosis such as chronic active hepatitis and liver cancer are not generally associated with significant impairment of drug metabolism and elimination.[56]
- Associated renal dysfunction could potentially alter drug pharmacokinetics to a greater extent causing accumulation of metabolites.

There is no single test available to predict hepatic function to assess the elimination capacity of specific drugs.

Anaesthetic drugs in liver disease

Intravenous anaesthetic agents

All intravenous anaesthetic agents should be administered in carefully titrated doses. They can produce precipitous falls in blood pressure because of the circulatory haemodynamics present in patients with cirrhosis. Patients with alcoholic liver disease have increased anaesthetic requirements.

Inhalational anaesthetic agents

Volatile anaesthetic-induced liver injury ranges from an asymptomatic rise in alanine transferase to fulminant hepatic failure. Isoflurane and sevoflurane seem to induce upregulation of haem oxygenase-1[57] and this enzyme catalyses the conversion of haem to biliverdin IX, carbon monoxide, and free iron, which causes a reduction in portal vascular resistance and an increase in hepatic blood flow. Studies have confirmed that isoflurane is a vasodilator and it increases the oxygen supply to the liver.[58] In elective liver resections, a study group observed a beneficial effect of pharmacological preconditioning with sevoflurane.[59] Desflurane is metabolized by cytochrome P450 to only a small degree (<0.02%) and the incidence of reported hepatotoxicity with desflurane is very low compared to other volatile agents.[60,61] Halothane should be avoided as it leads to a significant decrease in hepatic blood flow, oxygen supply, and can cause postoperative liver dysfunction, and immune-mediated halothane hepatitis is a serious concern.

Neuromuscular blocking agents

The higher volume of distribution due to ascites and oedema necessitate higher initial doses of neuromuscular blocking agents. Vecuronium and rocuronium are primarily metabolized by the liver and have a slower onset and longer duration of action.[62-64] Atracurium and cisatracurium are considered to be safer in liver disease as neither of them is metabolized in the liver or the kidney. It is prudent to use neuromuscular monitoring in these patients.

Commonly used analgesics

Paracetamol

Pain management in patients with liver dysfunction is challenging. There is a general tendency to avoid paracetamol in hepatic impairment probably due to the well-known association between paracetamol and liver failure. Paracetamol is mainly metabolized to glucuronide and sulphate and less than 5% is oxidized to a hepatotoxic metabolite, *N*-acetyl-*p*-benzoquinone imine, which is rendered non-toxic by binding with glutathione. Toxicity occurs when glutathione stores are depleted. Studies have shown that short-term therapeutic doses of paracetamol in non-alcoholic liver disease are safer to use.[65-67] However, a review on this subject suggests restricting the dose of paracetamol to 2 g/day in adults owing to changes in pharmacokinetic parameters and to avoid use as much as possible in alcoholic liver disease, where the glutathione level is expected to be low.[68]

Non-steroidal anti-inflammatory drugs (NSAIDs)

Most NSAIDs are eliminated via hepatic metabolism. NSAID usage could lead to multiple complications including renal failure, platelet dysfunction, and bleeding by inhibiting prostaglandins and thromboxane A2 synthesis. NSAIDs could also cause hepatotoxicity by multiple mechanisms, which could be idiosyncratic or dose dependent. Around 10% of all drug-induced liver toxicity is due to NSAIDs.[69] Ibuprofen has the best liver safety profile.

Opioids

The liver is the major site of biotransformation for opioids and patients with liver disease have an increased sensitivity to these drugs.[70] Most of the opioids undergo oxidation except buprenorphine and morphine, which undergo glucuronidation, and remifentanil, which undergoes ester hydrolysis. In cirrhotic patients, oxidation is affected more than glucuronidation and clearance of morphine is decreased and oral bioavailability increased.[70] Lower doses and longer administration intervals should be considered while administering morphine, oxycodone, and hydromorphone to avoid the risk of accumulation. Pethidine, which has toxic metabolites, should be avoided in this population. The analgesic effect of codeine and tramadol will be lower in severe hepatic impairment as these drugs rely on the liver for biotransformation to active metabolites. The kinetics of fentanyl, sufentanil, and remifentanil appear to be unaffected in liver disease and are safer to administer. However, the pharmacokinetic property of continuously infused fentanyl in liver disease is not yet established.

Causes of malnutrition in cirrhosis

The prevalence of poor nutrition in patients with end-stage liver disease and other disorders of the biliary tree is very high and the causes can be grouped into either (a) inadequate supply of nutrients or (b) excessive demand for nutrients. Inadequate supply can be because of (a) decreased synthesis, (b) decreased intake, (c) impaired absorption, and/or (d) excessive losses (Box 4.1).

In patients with chronic liver disease, the dietary intake is often poor due to a variety of causes. Ascites and a raised intra-abdominal pressure, gastroparesis, small intestinal dysmotility, bacterial overgrowth, and chronic inflammation can cause nausea and also early satiety.[71,72] Altered taste and smell perception due to zinc and magnesium deficiency also contributes to poor intake. Madden et al.[73] demonstrated that cirrhotic patients demonstrated higher gustatory thresholds for different tastes. It was also shown that hypomagnesaemia correlates with diminished gustatory acuity. Heiser et al.[74] demonstrated that olfactory function is altered in patients with cirrhosis. A significant correlation was observed between loss of olfactory function and increasing grades of encephalopathy.

Box 4.1 Causes of malnutrition in cirrhosis

- *Decreased synthesis*: transport and carrier protein synthesis affected.
- *Diminished intake*:
  - Early satiety—ascites and raised intra-abdominal pressure.
  - Diminished appetite—impaired olfactory and gustatory function; deficiencies in macronutrients like zinc or magnesium.
  - Encephalopathy—decreased voluntary intake and intermittent periods of nil by mouth status for airway protection in grade 2 or more encephalopathy.
  - Taste considerations—with salt and fluid restriction and specific dietary formulations, some people consider it unpalatable.
  - Inappropriate long-term protein restrictions for fear of encephalopathy.
  - Recurrent hospital outpatient visits—missed meals or starvation for endoscopy.
- *Impaired absorption due to cholestasis, bacterial overgrowth*: disturbance in enterohepatic circulation—altered small bowel mucosa and bacterial overgrowth.
- *Excessive losses*:
  - Recurrent large volume paracentesis.
  - Losses due to overzealous use of diuretics.
  - Lactulose therapy can cause micronutrient losses.
- *Hypermetabolic state*:
  - Hyperdynamic circulation.
  - Increase energy expenditure and demand.
- *Altered metabolism*:
  - Diminished hepatic glycogen stores.
  - Mobilization of glucose from skeletal muscle amino acids.

Most often, due to the restriction of total salt and water intake and the variety of nutritional formulae available in the market, patients perceive food as being unpalatable. Frequent hospital admissions and outpatient visits also cause a disturbance in the regular feeding of these patients. To avoid muscle breakdown, more frequent feeds need to be provided.

In severe cholestasis, intraluminal bile salts are reduced with malabsorption of fat and fat-soluble vitamins. Advanced liver disease associated with cholestasis, bacterial overgrowth, and/or malabsorption causes severe deficiencies of fat-soluble vitamins and other nutrients.[71,72] Alcohol intake with or without liver cirrhosis has been significantly associated with changes in the small bowel mucosa at the cellular level and is associated with changes in enzyme expression at the brush border level which can also contribute to malabsorption.[75]

Resting energy expenditure does not always correlate with predicted energy expenditure in cirrhosis. In one study, 33.8% of patients with cirrhosis were shown to be hypermetabolic and were found to have increased plasma concentrations of catecholamines.[76] Hypermetabolism demonstrated in this group of patients with cirrhosis can contribute to malnutrition if increased demands are not met by adequately increased intake which has been demonstrated in patients with human immunodeficiency virus infection.[77]

In patients with chronic liver disease, hepatic glycogen reserves are reduced. Gluconeogenesis from muscle proteins explains the protein deficiency in these patients. Diminished hepatic glycogen reserves, a lower rate of glucose production in the liver, and a decreased rate of glucose oxidation due to insulin resistance are common in cirrhosis.[78–81] Therefore, these patients do not tolerate prolonged periods of starvation. An overnight fast can simulate conditions similar to prolonged starvation in healthy individuals.[82] Insulin resistance is commonly seen in these patients.[78,79,81] Protein depletion seen in cirrhotic patients is due to the reduced protein synthesis in the muscles coupled with increased protein catabolism accounting for muscle wasting and sarcopenia.[83]

Although malnutrition was thought to be more prevalent in patients with alcoholic liver disease, it was shown that the aetiology of liver disease does not influence the prevalence and severity of malnutrition and protein energy depletion.[84–86] Additional factors such as poor social support and unhealthy living conditions and diet can aggravate the poor nutritional state in patients with alcohol dependence.

With the progression of liver disease, in addition to protein energy depletion causing muscle wasting, there is an increase in total body water and sodium retention. Potassium, magnesium, phosphate, and other intracellular minerals are slowly depleted. Fat-soluble vitamins are found to be profoundly deficient in patients with liver disease and obstructive jaundice is present due to the cholestasis-induced steatorrhoea and malabsorption and bile salt deficiency.[87] Deficiency of water-soluble vitamins is also common in patients with cirrhosis and occurs more frequently in people with alcohol dependence. Derangement of hepatic synthesis of carrier proteins/transport proteins also contributes to the deficiency of vitamins.[88] Zinc and magnesium deficiencies occur due to impaired intake, diuretic losses, and increased losses secondary to malabsorption. They contribute to altered taste perception and magnesium deficiency can cause muscle weakness.[71,88] These nutritional deficiencies and water and sodium retention set in even before other obvious clinical manifestations of liver disease.[86,89] Plasma levels of essential fatty acids and poly unsaturated fatty acids are reduced in cirrhosis and the effects are more pronounced with severe liver disease.[90]

There is a significant proportion of cirrhotic patients who are overweight or obese and they also form a cohort of malnourished patients.[91,92] Weight reduction with monitored dietary intake in terms of reduced carbohydrate and fat intake with preserved protein intake, in addition to graded physical activity, should be recommended.[91]

In patients with acute liver failure with complete or subtotal loss of hepatocellular function, a severe derangement of carbohydrate, protein, and lipid metabolism occurs. Impaired or complete failure of glucose production, impaired lactate clearance, and excessive protein catabolism resulting in hyperaminoacidaemia and hyperammonaemia have been observed.[93]

Optimizing nutritional status

All patients with liver disease presenting for surgery should be thoroughly screened for the presence of malnutrition.[93] Because of the high prevalence of the hypermetabolic state, patients with chronic liver disease and a sedentary lifestyle should receive a total energy supply of 1.3 × resting energy expenditure. As long as cough and swallowing reflexes are intact, patients with mild hepatic encephalopathy should continue to receive oral feeds during any hospital admissions. When the target cannot be achieved by the patient's dietary intake alone, oral nutritional supplements should be considered. Protein restriction should not be performed in hepatic encephalopathy because it can, by itself, increase protein catabolism. Micronutrients should be supplemented in patients based on clinical suspicion or with laboratory-proven deficiency.

The target energy requirement in patients with cirrhosis with malnutrition and muscle depletion should be 30–35 kcal/kg/day and protein 1.2–1.5 g/kg/day. Protein-intolerant patients should receive vegetable proteins or branched chain amino acids at the rate of 0.25 g/kg/day. Strict restrictions on sodium and fluid should be reviewed regularly and attempts made to ensure food is palatable for patients.

Branched chain amino acid-enriched formulas have been shown to be effective in improving body composition in paediatric patients with cholestatic liver disease[94] but a similar effect was not seen in adults when branched chain amino acids were compared with standard nutritional regimens.

Nocturnal feeds improve protein metabolism in cirrhosis.[95] Nutritional therapy should be instituted in patients with non-alcoholic fatty liver disease or steatohepatitis, when oral nutrition is contraindicated, in the event of other concurrent illness with a target energy intake of 25 kcal/kg/day and a target protein of 2–2.5 g/kg/day (ideal body weight to be used instead of actual body weight).

In patients with severe alcoholic steatohepatitis, nutrition therapy is extremely important because of their hypermetabolic state. Enteral or parenteral nutrition (EN or PN) should be initiated promptly with high-density formulae providing 1.5 kcal/mL with vitamins and trace element supplementation. For those patients who cannot be fed for more than 12 hours, intravenous glucose at the rate of 2–3 g/kg/day should be provided.

In patients with acute liver failure, nutritional goals would be to ensure adequate provision of energy by exogenous administration of glucose, lipids, proteins/amino acids, vitamins, and trace elements. In patients with hyperacute disease, it is preferable to defer nutritional protein support for 24–48 hours until hyperammonaemia is controlled. Protein supplementation should be done with monitoring of serum ammonia levels.[93] Otherwise, nutritional therapy principles should be similar to those used for other critically ill patients and PN should be initiated if EN cannot be established within 5–7 days.

In the preoperative period, continue with recommended nutrition goals. It is preferable to implement the enhanced recovery after surgery (ERAS) approach for non-liver as well as liver operations in these patients. It is important to limit periods of unnecessary starvation to avoid gluconeogenesis from protein breakdown. Liver surgeries using ERAS pathways have shown better outcomes in terms of length of hospital stay and other morbidities.[96,97] Carbohydrate-containing clear liquid 2 hours before surgery, and early feeding and early mobilization postoperatively are important components of the ERAS pathway. In patients after LT, feeding should be initiated as early as possible. Feeding initiated in the first 12–24 hours postoperatively has been shown to reduce infection rates.[98]

Negative nitrogen balance persists for a prolonged period after major operations[99,100] and adequate provision of proteins and amino acids is important to ensure nitrogen balance improves. Adequate nutritional support in the postoperative period has achieved beneficial outcomes with improved nitrogen balance and reduced rate of complications in patients undergoing non-transplant surgeries.[101,102] Seven-day nitrogen balance was better with EN than PN regimens.[102] Therefore, it is important to resume energy intake of 30–35 kcal/kg/day and protein 1.2–1.5 g/kg/day once the immediate acute postoperative phase is over. Nasogastric or nasojejunal feeds should be used for early EN with similar indications as in other patients after major surgeries. Specialized nutritional protocols should be available in postoperative units to make optimal use of EN because of the risks associated with PN.

In those patients with hypermetabolism, peak metabolic requirement has been noted on the tenth day post LT.[103] By the end of 12 months post LT, the metabolic state was comparable to other healthy individuals.[99,103] It is important to supply the extra energy requirements in this group of patients. It was seen that patients with hypermetabolism had reduced event-free survival and unfavourable outcomes after LT.[104,105]

Anaesthetic management

It is prudent to integrate knowledge of basic pathophysiology with the planning of perioperative management strategies for patients with liver disease. Because of synthetic dysfunction, these patients have varying degrees of malnutrition which by itself can delay recovery from any surgery in terms of wound healing and mobilization. Coagulopathy and the collaterals from portal hypertension may contribute to major bleeding during or after surgery. Hepatic and the associated renal dysfunction can alter drug disposition and fluid–electrolyte homoeostasis. All these factors can potentially lead to higher morbidity and mortality in these patients. Liver resection is more dangerous because, in addition to these changes, there is further reduction in liver cell mass. Liver decompensation can lead to acute worsening of portal hypertension and thereby cause ascites, hepatic encephalopathy, and bleeding which can lead to the need for prolonged organ support and prolonged intensive care unit stay, increased predisposition to sepsis, and multiorgan failure.

Involvement of a multidisciplinary team from the start and performing surgery in a centre with adequate expertise in handling critically ill patients with cirrhosis are vital requirements. Thorough discussion and informed consent with patient's family is an essential prerequisite.

Detailed analysis of the pathophysiological changes and predicting postoperative problems, understanding altered drug handling, and having a close communication with a multidisciplinary team and family are key to a smooth perioperative course.

Risk minimization and optimization whenever possible

- Control of ascites—diuretics as tolerated. In patients where time is not available for optimization of ascites or in diuretic intolerant patients, preoperative large volume paracentesis, with a pigtail catheter in some cases, should be performed under adequate albumin replacement. For large-volume paracentesis, an albumin infusion of 6–8 g/L of fluid removed appears to improve survival and is recommended.[106]

  This will improve lung function by decreasing the restrictive effect of the distended abdomen and also decrease the chance of aspiration during anaesthesia. In patients undergoing abdominal surgeries, drainage can also help with wound healing by avoiding soakage of incisional sites. Adequate antibiotic prophylaxis for spontaneous bacterial peritonitis as per a local antibiogram needs to be instituted. Pleural drains are placed preoperatively only in patients with significant pleural effusion. Due to lack of evidence, pre-emptive transjugular intrahepatic portosystemic shunt placement cannot be recommended for refractory ascites.
- Control of varices electively to avoid bleeding in the postoperative period whenever needed.
- Management of hepatic encephalopathy—continue prophylactic treatment.
- Continue antiviral medications in patients with chronic viral hepatitis to prevent relapse.
- Continue steroids/supplement with parenteral steroids in autoimmune hepatitis.
- Cardiopulmonary evaluation as in the general surgical population.
- Risk stratification as discussed earlier.

Elective surgeries should be postponed until optimization of the above points has occurred.

Fluid management

It is important to adequately hydrate patients to avoid renal dysfunction in those with obstructive jaundice. In cirrhosis, overzealous fluid administration will only flood the splanchnic system and cause bleeding and other postoperative complications. If required, cardiac output monitoring should be instituted to guide fluid therapy. The response to vasopressors will be poor, especially in patients on beta-blockers for portal hypertension. Kidneys are very susceptible to injury during perioperative stress. Maintenance of adequate perfusion pressure and avoidance of nephrotoxic drugs should be the goals of intraoperative management.

Management of coagulopathy

There are enough data to demonstrate a low risk of bleeding complications for minimally invasive procedures like paracentesis in patients with cirrhosis.[48,107] Despite this, conventional formulas are still being used inappropriately to correct coagulation parameters before any invasive procedure.

Thrombopoietin agonists such as eltrombopag, avatrombopag, and lusutrombopag have been shown to improve platelet counts gradually over a span of 2 weeks at different rates. In a minority of patients, eltrombopag has been shown to be associated with portal vein thrombosis while avatrombopag and lusutrombopag have not shown this effect in the trials performed thus far.[108,109] They are better alternatives to platelet transfusions because the concern of circulatory overload is diminished and they could be used in elective surgeries.

Point-of-care viscoelastic tests such as thromboelastography, rotational thromboelastometry, and Sonoclot have become the standard of care in these patients in order to decide which patients require coagulation correction. They have shown benefit in reducing patients' transfusion needs.[110,111] However, these tests have not been validated for target values in patients with cirrhosis.

Transfusions of blood and blood products carry the risks of exacerbating portal hypertension from volume expansion in patients with cirrhosis in addition to the usual risks of infections due to bacterial and viral contamination, circulatory overload, transfusion-associated lung injury, transfusion reactions, and the risk of developing alloimmunization which can impact the candidacy for LT and receiving further blood transfusions.[112–115]

Fibrinogen levels can be more meaningful, as a measure of bleeding risk, when compared to INR and platelet values.[116] Target values are between 1.0 and 1.5 g/L as seen from other bleeding patients.[117,118] Smaller volumes are sufficient in comparison to fresh frozen plasma and, therefore, might have less impact on portal hypertension.

Prothrombin complex concentrate seems to correct conventional coagulation test values in patients with cirrhosis without any additional adverse events.[119] Prothrombin complex concentrate was more effective than fresh frozen plasma in increasing thrombin generation.[120] In LT, thromboelastometry-guided treatment with fibrinogen concentrate and/or prothrombin complex concentrate did not appear to increase the occurrence of thrombosis and ischaemic events compared to patients who did not receive these concentrates.[121]

The following transfusion thresholds for management of active bleeding or high-risk procedures may optimize clot formation in advanced liver disease: haematocrit greater than or equal to 25%, platelet count greater than 50,000/μL, and fibrinogen greater than 120 mg/dL.[122] The commonly utilized thresholds for INR correction are not supported by evidence.

Regional anaesthesia is a contraindication in the presence of coagulopathy. But in patients with normal coagulation preoperatively, impairment of liver function in the perioperative period can result in coagulopathy which could be a problem with epidural anaesthesia.[123] Delayed removal of the catheter after resolution of coagulopathy is advised in such instances.[124]

It is important to observe these patients in a high dependency unit or intensive care unit for at least 24–48 hours after surgery. Monitoring, pain control, fluid management, feeding, and mobilization should be planned while keeping in mind all the concerns listed.

Conclusion

Patients with diseases of the liver and biliary tract present unique challenges to the perioperative physician. Identifying the challenges and involvement of a multidisciplinary team to decide whether surgery can be offered to the patient are essential. Detailed planning of perioperative strategies and performing these procedures in a centre with expertise in handling critically ill patients with cirrhosis can help achieve better outcomes.

REFERENCES

1. Mokdad AA, Lopez AD, Shahraz S, et al. Liver cirrhosis mortality in 187 countries between 1980 and 2010: a systematic analysis. *BMC Med*. 2014;**12**:145.
2. Befeler AS, Palmer DE, Hoffman M, Longo W, Solomon H, Di Bisceglie AM. The safety of intra-abdominal surgery in patients with cirrhosis: model for end-stage liver disease score is superior to Child-Turcotte-Pugh classification in predicting outcome. *Arch Surg*. 2005;**140**(7):650–654.
3. Friedman LS. Surgery in the patient with liver disease. *Trans Am Clin Climatol Assoc*. 2010;**121**:192–204.
4. Teh SH, Nagorney DM, Stevens SR, et al. Risk factors for mortality after surgery in patients with cirrhosis. *Gastroenterology*. 2007;**132**(4):1261–1269.
5. Dripps RD, Lamont A, Eckenhoff JE. The role of anesthesia in surgical mortality. *JAMA*. 1961;**178**:261–266.
6. Neeff H, Mariaskin D, Spangenberg HC, Hopt UT, Makowiec F. Perioperative mortality after non-hepatic general surgery in patients with liver cirrhosis: an analysis of 138 operations in the 2000s using Child and MELD scores. *J Gastrointest Surg*. 2011;**15**(1):1–11.
7. Kim SY, Yim HJ, Park SM, et al. Validation of a Mayo postoperative mortality risk prediction model in Korean cirrhotic patients. *Liver Int*. 2011;**31**(2):222–228.
8. Mullen MG, Michaels AD, Mehaffey JH, et al. Risk associated with complications and mortality after urgent surgery vs elective and emergency surgery: implications for defining 'quality' and reporting outcomes for urgent surgery. *JAMA Surg*. 2017;**152**(8):768–774.
9. Odom SR, Gupta A, Talmor D, Novack V, Sagy I, Evenson AR. Emergency hernia repair in cirrhotic patients with ascites. *J Trauma Acute Care Surg*. 2013;**75**(3):404–409.
10. Carbonell AM, Wolfe LG, DeMaria EJ. Poor outcomes in cirrhosis-associated hernia repair: a nationwide cohort study of 32,033 patients. *Hernia*. 2005;**9**(4):353–357.
11. Andraus W, Pinheiro RS, Lai Q, et al. Abdominal wall hernia in cirrhotic patients: emergency surgery results in higher morbidity and mortality. *BMC Surg*. 2015;**15**:65.
12. Duceppe E, Parlow J, MacDonald P, et al. Canadian Cardiovascular Society guidelines on perioperative cardiac risk assessment and management for patients who undergo noncardiac surgery. *Can J Cardiol*. 2017;**33**(1):17–32.
13. Northup PG, Friedman LS, Kamath PS. AGA clinical practice update on surgical risk assessment and perioperative management in cirrhosis: expert review. *Clin Gastroenterol Hepatol*. 2019;**17**(4):595–606.
14. Tomimaru Y, Eguchi H, Gotoh K, et al. Platelet count is more useful for predicting posthepatectomy liver failure at surgery for hepatocellular carcinoma than indocyanine green clearance test. *J Surg Oncol*. 2016;**113**(5):565–569.
15. Panicek DM, Giess CS, Schwartz LH. Qualitative assessment of liver for fatty infiltration on contrast-enhanced CT: is muscle a better standard of reference than spleen? *J Comput Assist Tomogr*. 1997;**21**(5):699–705.
16. Shoup M, Gonen M, D'Angelica M, et al. Volumetric analysis predicts hepatic dysfunction in patients undergoing major liver resection. *J Gastrointest Surg*. 2003;**7**(3):325–330.
17. Bruix J, Castells A, Bosch J, et al. Surgical resection of hepatocellular carcinoma in cirrhotic patients: prognostic value of preoperative portal pressure. *Gastroenterology*. 1996;**111**(4):1018–1022.
18. Ripoll C, Groszmann R, Garcia-Tsao G, et al. Hepatic venous pressure gradient predicts clinical decompensation in patients with compensated cirrhosis. *Gastroenterology*. 2007;**133**(2):481–488.
19. Rajakannu M, Coilly A, Adam R, Samuel D, Vibert E. Prospective validation of transient elastography for staging liver fibrosis in patients undergoing hepatectomy and liver transplantation. *J Hepatol*. 2017;**68**(1):199–200.
20. Llop E, Berzigotti A, Reig M, et al. Assessment of portal hypertension by transient elastography in patients with compensated cirrhosis and potentially resectable liver tumors. *J Hepatol*. 2012;**56**(1):103–108.
21. Teh SH, Christein J, Donohue J, et al. Hepatic resection of hepatocellular carcinoma in patients with cirrhosis: Model of End-Stage Liver Disease (MELD) score predicts perioperative mortality. *J Gastrointest Surg*. 2005;**9**(9):1207–1215.
22. Fromer MW, Aloia TA, Gaughan JP, Atabek UM, Spitz FR. The utility of the MELD score in predicting mortality following liver resection for metastasis. *Eur J Surg Oncol*. 2016;**42**(10):1568–1575.
23. Fan ST, Lai EC, Lo CM, Ng IO, Wong J. Hospital mortality of major hepatectomy for hepatocellular carcinoma associated with cirrhosis. *Arch Surg*. 1995;**130**(2):198–203.
24. Yokoyama Y, Ebata T, Igami T, Sugawara G, Mizuno T, Nagino M. The adverse effects of preoperative cholangitis on the outcome of portal vein embolization and subsequent major hepatectomies. *Surgery*. 2014;**156**(5):1190–1196.
25. Olthof PB, Wiggers JK, Groot Koerkamp B, et al. Postoperative liver failure risk score: identifying patients with resectable perihilar cholangiocarcinoma who can benefit from portal vein embolization. *J Am Coll Surg*. 2017;**225**(3):387–394.
26. Watanabe K, Yokoyama Y, Kokuryo T, et al. Segmental cholangitis impairs hepatic regeneration capacity after partial hepatectomy in rats. *HPB (Oxford)*. 2010;**12**(10):664–673.
27. Mansour JC, Aloia TA, Crane CH, Heimbach JK, Nagino M, Vauthey JN. Hilar cholangiocarcinoma: expert consensus statement. *HPB (Oxford)*. 2015;**17**(8):691–699.
28. Siniscalchi A, Aurini L, Spedicato S, et al. Hyperdynamic circulation in cirrhosis: predictive factors and outcome following liver transplantation. *Minerva Anestesiol*. 2013;**79**(1):15–23.
29. Villanueva C, Albillos A, Genesca J, et al. Development of hyperdynamic circulation and response to beta-blockers in compensated cirrhosis with portal hypertension. *Hepatology*. 2016;**63**(1):197–206.
30. Moller S, Hobolth L, Winkler C, Bendtsen F, Christensen E. Determinants of the hyperdynamic circulation and central hypovolaemia in cirrhosis. *Gut*. 2011;**60**(9):1254–1259.
31. Jimenez W, Rodes J. Impaired responsiveness to endogenous vasoconstrictors and endothelium-derived vasoactive factors in cirrhosis. *Gastroenterology*. 1994;**107**(4):1201–1203.
32. Moller S, Bendtsen F, Henriksen JH. Determinants of the renin-angiotensin-aldosterone system in cirrhosis with special emphasis on the central blood volume. *Scand J Gastroenterol*. 2006;**41**(4):451–458.

33. Moller S, Iversen JS, Krag A, Bie P, Kjaer A, Bendtsen F. Reduced baroreflex sensitivity and pulmonary dysfunction in alcoholic cirrhosis: effect of hyperoxia. *Am J Physiol Gastrointest Liver Physiol*. 2010;**299**(3):G784–G790.
34. Lenz K. Hepatorenal syndrome—is it central hypovolemia, a cardiac disease, or part of gradually developing multiorgan dysfunction? *Hepatology*. 2005;**42**(2):263–265.
35. Wiese S, Hove JD, Bendtsen F, Moller S. Cirrhotic cardiomyopathy: pathogenesis and clinical relevance. *Nat Rev Gastroenterol Hepatol*. 2014;**11**(3):177–186.
36. Desai MS, Mathur B, Eblimit Z, et al. Bile acid excess induces cardiomyopathy and metabolic dysfunctions in the heart. *Hepatology*. 2017;**65**(1):189–201.
37. Huffmyer JL, Nemergut EC. Respiratory dysfunction and pulmonary disease in cirrhosis and other hepatic disorders. *Respir Care*. 2007;**52**(8):1030–1036.
38. Gines P, Schrier RW. Renal failure in cirrhosis. *N Engl J Med*. 2009;**361**(13):1279–1290.
39. Arroyo V, Fernandez J. Management of hepatorenal syndrome in patients with cirrhosis. *Nat Rev Nephrol*. 2011;**7**(9):517–526.
40. Moller S, Krag A, Bendtsen F. Kidney injury in cirrhosis: pathophysiological and therapeutic aspects of hepatorenal syndromes. *Liver Int*. 2014;**34**(8):1153–1163.
41. Moller S, Henriksen JH, Bendtsen F. Central and noncentral blood volumes in cirrhosis: relationship to anthropometrics and gender. *Am J Physiol Gastrointest Liver Physiol*. 2003;**284**(6):G970–G979.
42. Mohanty A, Garcia-Tsao G. Hyponatremia and hepatorenal syndrome. *Gastroenterol Hepatol (N Y)*. 2015;**11**(4):220–229.
43. Ruiz-del-Arbol L, Serradilla R. Cirrhotic cardiomyopathy. *World J Gastroenterol*. 2015;**21**(41):11502–11521.
44. Gines P, Berl T, Bernardi M, et al. Hyponatremia in cirrhosis: from pathogenesis to treatment. *Hepatology*. 1998;**28**(3):851–864.
45. Kim G, Huh JH, Lee KJ, Kim MY, Shim KY, Baik SK. Relative adrenal insufficiency in patients with cirrhosis: a systematic review and meta-analysis. *Dig Dis Sci*. 2017;**62**(4):1067–1079.
46. Marik PE, Pastores SM, Annane D, et al. Recommendations for the diagnosis and management of corticosteroid insufficiency in critically ill adult patients: consensus statements from an international task force by the American College of Critical Care Medicine. *Crit Care Med*. 2008;**36**(6):1937–1949.
47. Marik PE, Zaloga GP. Adrenal insufficiency in the critically ill: a new look at an old problem. *Chest*. 2002;**122**(5):1784–1796.
48. Tripodi A, Mannucci PM. The coagulopathy of chronic liver disease. *N Engl J Med*. 2011;**365**(2):147–156.
49. Tripodi A, Salerno F, Chantarangkul V, et al. Evidence of normal thrombin generation in cirrhosis despite abnormal conventional coagulation tests. *Hepatology*. 2005;**41**(3):553–558.
50. Tripodi A, Primignani M, Lemma L, Chantarangkul V, Mannucci PM. Evidence that low protein C contributes to the procoagulant imbalance in cirrhosis. *J Hepatol*. 2013;**59**(2):265–270.
51. Intagliata NM, Argo CK, Stine JG, et al. Concepts and controversies in haemostasis and thrombosis associated with liver disease: proceedings of the 7th International Coagulation in Liver Disease Conference. *Thromb Haemost*. 2018;**118**(8):1491–1506.
52. Raparelli V, Basili S, Carnevale R, et al. Low-grade endotoxemia and platelet activation in cirrhosis. *Hepatology*. 2017;**65**(2):571–581.
53. Tripodi A, Chantarangkul V, Primignani M, et al. The international normalized ratio calibrated for cirrhosis (INR(liver)) normalizes prothrombin time results for model for end-stage liver disease calculation. *Hepatology*. 2007;**46**(2):520–527.
54. Muller MC, Straat M, Meijers JC, et al. Fresh frozen plasma transfusion fails to influence the hemostatic balance in critically ill patients with a coagulopathy. *J Thromb Haemost*. 2015;**13**(6):989–997.
55. Morgan DJ, McLean AJ. Therapeutic implications of impaired hepatic oxygen diffusion in chronic liver disease. *Hepatology*. 1991;**14**(6):1280–1282.
56. Morgan DJ, McLean AJ. Clinical pharmacokinetic and pharmacodynamic considerations in patients with liver disease. An update. *Clin Pharmacokinet*. 1995;**29**(5):370–391.
57. Tenhunen R, Marver HS, Schmid R. The enzymatic conversion of heme to bilirubin by microsomal heme oxygenase. *Proc Natl Acad Sci U S A*. 1968;**61**(2):748–755.
58. Gatecel C, Losser MR, Payen D. The postoperative effects of halothane versus isoflurane on hepatic artery and portal vein blood flow in humans. *Anesth Analg*. 2003;**96**(3):740–745.
59. Beck-Schimmer B, Breitenstein S, Urech S, et al. A randomized controlled trial on pharmacological preconditioning in liver surgery using a volatile anesthetic. *Ann Surg*. 2008;**248**(6):909–918.
60. Martin JL, Plevak DJ, Flannery KD, et al. Hepatotoxicity after desflurane anesthesia. *Anesthesiology*. 1995;**83**(5):1125–1129.
61. Cote G, Bouchard S. Hepatotoxicity after desflurane anesthesia in a 15-month-old child with Mobius syndrome after previous exposure to isoflurane. *Anesthesiology*. 2007;**107**(5):843–845.
62. van Miert MM, Eastwood NB, Boyd AH, Parker CJ, Hunter JM. The pharmacokinetics and pharmacodynamics of rocuronium in patients with hepatic cirrhosis. *Br J Clin Pharmacol*. 1997;**44**(2):139–144.
63. Khalil M, D'Honneur G, Duvaldestin P, Slavov V, De Hys C, Gomeni R. Pharmacokinetics and pharmacodynamics of rocuronium in patients with cirrhosis. *Anesthesiology*. 1994;**80**(6):1241–1247.
64. Lebrault C, Berger JL, D'Hollander AA, Gomeni R, Henzel D, Duvaldestin P. Pharmacokinetics and pharmacodynamics of vecuronium (ORG NC 45) in patients with cirrhosis. *Anesthesiology*. 1985;**62**(5):601–605.
65. Benson GD. Acetaminophen in chronic liver disease. *Clin Pharmacol Ther*. 1983;**33**(1):95–101.
66. Myers RP, Shaheen AA. Hepatitis C, alcohol abuse, and unintentional overdoses are risk factors for acetaminophen-related hepatotoxicity. *Hepatology*. 2009;**49**(4):1399–1400.
67. Prescott LF. Paracetamol, alcohol and the liver. *Br J Clin Pharmacol*. 2000;**49**(4):291–301.
68. Bosilkovska M, Walder B, Besson M, Daali Y, Desmeules J. Analgesics in patients with hepatic impairment: pharmacology and clinical implications. *Drugs*. 2012;**72**(12):1645–1669.
69. Bessone F. Non-steroidal anti-inflammatory drugs: what is the actual risk of liver damage? *World J Gastroenterol*. 2010;**16**(45):5651–5661.
70. Tegeder I, Lotsch J, Geisslinger G. Pharmacokinetics of opioids in liver disease. *Clin Pharmacokinet*. 1999;**37**(1):17–40.
71. O'Brien A, Williams R. Nutrition in end-stage liver disease: principles and practice. *Gastroenterology*. 2008;**134**(6):1729–1740.
72. Quigley EM. Gastrointestinal dysfunction in liver disease and portal hypertension. Gut-liver interactions revisited. *Dig Dis Sci*. 1996;**41**(3):557–561.

73. Madden AM, Bradbury W, Morgan MY. Taste perception in cirrhosis: its relationship to circulating micronutrients and food preferences. *Hepatology*. 1997;26(1):40–48.
74. Heiser C, Haller B, Sohn M, et al. Olfactory function is affected in patients with cirrhosis depending on the severity of hepatic encephalopathy. *Ann Hepatol*. 2018;17(5):822–829.
75. Bhonchal S, Nain CK, Prasad KK, et al. Functional and morphological alterations in small intestine mucosa of chronic alcoholics. *J Gastroenterol Hepatol*. 2008;23(7 Pt 2):e43–e48.
76. Muller MJ, Bottcher J, Selberg O, et al. Hypermetabolism in clinically stable patients with liver cirrhosis. *Am J Clin Nutr*. 1999;69(6):1194–1201.
77. Suttmann U, Ockenga J, Hoogestraat L, et al. Resting energy expenditure and weight loss in human immunodeficiency virus-infected patients. *Metabolism*. 1993;42(9):1173–1179.
78. Petrides AS, Stanley T, Matthews DE, Vogt C, Bush AJ, Lambeth H. Insulin resistance in cirrhosis: prolonged reduction of hyperinsulinemia normalizes insulin sensitivity. *Hepatology*. 1998;28(1):141–149.
79. McCullough AJ, Tavill AS. Disordered energy and protein metabolism in liver disease. *Semin Liver Dis*. 1991;11(4):265–277.
80. Owen OE, Reichle FA, Mozzoli MA, et al. Hepatic, gut, and renal substrate flux rates in patients with hepatic cirrhosis. *J Clin Invest*. 1981;68(1):240–252.
81. Selberg O, Burchert W, vd Hoff J, et al. Insulin resistance in liver cirrhosis. Positron-emission tomography scan analysis of skeletal muscle glucose metabolism. *J Clin Invest*. 1993;91(5):1897–1902.
82. Muller MJ, Willmann O, Rieger A, et al. Mechanism of insulin resistance associated with liver cirrhosis. *Gastroenterology*. 1992;102(6):2033–2041.
83. Rivera Irigoin R, Abiles J. [Nutritional support in patients with liver cirrhosis]. *Gastroenterol Hepatol*. 2012;35(8):594–601.
84. Italian Multicentre Cooperative Project on Nutrition in Liver Cirrhosis. Nutritional status in cirrhosis. *J Hepatol*. 1994;21(3):317–325.
85. Lautz HU, Selberg O, Korber J, Burger M, Muller MJ. Protein-calorie malnutrition in liver cirrhosis. *Clin Investig*. 1992;70(6):478–486.
86. Peng S, Plank LD, McCall JL, Gillanders LK, McIlroy K, Gane EJ. Body composition, muscle function, and energy expenditure in patients with liver cirrhosis: a comprehensive study. *Am J Clin Nutr*. 2007;85(5):1257–1266.
87. Lieber CS. Alcohol, liver, and nutrition. *J Am Coll Nutr*. 1991;10(6):602–632.
88. Manne V, Saab S. Impact of nutrition and obesity on chronic liver disease. *Clin Liver Dis*. 2014;18(1):205–218.
89. Prijatmoko D, Strauss BJ, Lambert JR, et al. Early detection of protein depletion in alcoholic cirrhosis: role of body composition analysis. *Gastroenterology*. 1993;105(6):1839–1845.
90. Cabre E, Nunez M, Gonzalez-Huix F, et al. Clinical and nutritional factors predictive of plasma lipid unsaturation deficiency in advanced liver cirrhosis: a logistic regression analysis. *Am J Gastroenterol*. 1993;88(10):1738–1743.
91. Amodio P, Bemeur C, Butterworth R, et al. The nutritional management of hepatic encephalopathy in patients with cirrhosis: International Society for Hepatic Encephalopathy and Nitrogen Metabolism Consensus. *Hepatology*. 2013;58(1):325–336.
92. Huisman EJ, Trip EJ, Siersema PD, van Hoek B, van Erpecum KJ. Protein energy malnutrition predicts complications in liver cirrhosis. *Eur J Gastroenterol Hepatol*. 2011;23(11):982–989.
93. Plauth M, Bernal W, Dasarathy S, et al. ESPEN guideline on clinical nutrition in liver disease. *Clin Nutr*. 2019;38(2):485–521.
94. Chin SE, Shepherd RW, Thomas BJ, et al. Nutritional support in children with end-stage liver disease: a randomized crossover trial of a branched-chain amino acid supplement. *Am J Clin Nutr*. 1992;56(1):158–163.
95. Plank LD, Gane EJ, Peng S, et al. Nocturnal nutritional supplementation improves total body protein status of patients with liver cirrhosis: a randomized 12-month trial. *Hepatology*. 2008;48(2):557–566.
96. Coolsen MM, Wong-Lun-Hing EM, van Dam RM, et al. A systematic review of outcomes in patients undergoing liver surgery in an enhanced recovery after surgery pathways. *HPB (Oxford)*. 2013;15(4):245–251.
97. Hughes MJ, McNally S, Wigmore SJ. Enhanced recovery following liver surgery: a systematic review and meta-analysis. *HPB (Oxford)*. 2014;16(8):699–706.
98. Hasse JM, Blue LS, Liepa GU, et al. Early enteral nutrition support in patients undergoing liver transplantation. *JPEN J Parenter Enteral Nutr*. 1995;19(6):437–443.
99. Plank LD, Metzger DJ, McCall JL, et al. Sequential changes in the metabolic response to orthotopic liver transplantation during the first year after surgery. *Ann Surg*. 2001;234(2):245–255.
100. Plank LD, Mathur S, Gane EJ, et al. Perioperative immunonutrition in patients undergoing liver transplantation: a randomized double-blind trial. *Hepatology*. 2015;61(2):639–647.
101. Fan ST, Lo CM, Lai EC, Chu KM, Liu CL, Wong J. Perioperative nutritional support in patients undergoing hepatectomy for hepatocellular carcinoma. *N Engl J Med*. 1994;331(23):1547–1552.
102. Hu QG, Zheng QC. The influence of enteral nutrition in postoperative patients with poor liver function. *World J Gastroenterol*. 2003;9(4):843–846.
103. Perseghin G, Mazzaferro V, Benedini S, et al. Resting energy expenditure in diabetic and nondiabetic patients with liver cirrhosis: relation with insulin sensitivity and effect of liver transplantation and immunosuppressive therapy. *Am J Clin Nutr*. 2002;76(3):541–548.
104. Mathur S, Peng S, Gane EJ, McCall JL, Plank LD. Hypermetabolism predicts reduced transplant-free survival independent of MELD and Child-Pugh scores in liver cirrhosis. *Nutrition*. 2007;23(5):398–403.
105. Selberg O, Bottcher J, Tusch G, Pichlmayr R, Henkel E, Muller MJ. Identification of high- and low-risk patients before liver transplantation: a prospective cohort study of nutritional and metabolic parameters in 150 patients. *Hepatology*. 1997;25(3):652–657.
106. European Association for the Study of the Liver. EASL Clinical Practice Guidelines for the management of patients with decompensated cirrhosis. *J Hepatol*. 2018;69(2):406–460.
107. Runyon BA, AASLD. Introduction to the revised American Association for the Study of Liver Diseases Practice Guideline management of adult patients with ascites due to cirrhosis 2012. *Hepatology*. 2013;57(4):1651–1653.
108. Afdhal NH, Giannini EG, Tayyab G, et al. Eltrombopag before procedures in patients with cirrhosis and thrombocytopenia. *N Engl J Med*. 2012;367(8):716–724.
109. Terrault N, Chen YC, Izumi N, et al. Avatrombopag before procedures reduces need for platelet transfusion in patients with chronic liver disease and thrombocytopenia. *Gastroenterology*. 2018;155(3):705–718.

110. Bedreli S, Sowa JP, Gerken G, Saner FH, Canbay A. Management of acute-on-chronic liver failure: rotational thromboelastometry may reduce substitution of coagulation factors in liver cirrhosis. *Gut*. 2016;**65**(2):357–358.
111. De Pietri L, Bianchini M, Montalti R, et al. Thrombelastography-guided blood product use before invasive procedures in cirrhosis with severe coagulopathy: a randomized, controlled trial. *Hepatology*. 2016;**63**(2):566–573.
112. Villanueva C, Colomo A, Bosch A, et al. Transfusion strategies for acute upper gastrointestinal bleeding. *N Engl J Med*. 2013;**368**(1):11–21.
113. Kopko PM, Popovsky MA, MacKenzie MR, Paglieroni TG, Muto KN, Holland PV. HLA class II antibodies in transfusion-related acute lung injury. *Transfusion*. 2001;**41**(10):1244–1248.
114. O'Leary JG, Demetris AJ, Friedman LS, et al. The role of donor-specific HLA alloantibodies in liver transplantation. *Am J Transplant*. 2014;**14**(4):779–787.
115. O'Leary JG, Kaneku H, Jennings LW, et al. Preformed class II donor-specific antibodies are associated with an increased risk of early rejection after liver transplantation. *Liver Transpl*. 2013;**19**(9):973–980.
116. Drolz A, Horvatits T, Roedl K, et al. Coagulation parameters and major bleeding in critically ill patients with cirrhosis. *Hepatology*. 2016;**64**(2):556–568.
117. Levy JH, Welsby I, Goodnough LT. Fibrinogen as a therapeutic target for bleeding: a review of critical levels and replacement therapy. *Transfusion*. 2014;**54**(5):1389–1405.
118. Thakrar SV, Mallett SV. Thrombocytopenia in cirrhosis: impact of fibrinogen on bleeding risk. *World J Hepatol*. 2017;**9**(6):318–325.
119. Drebes A, de Vos M, Gill S, Treckmann J, et al. Prothrombin complex concentrates for coagulopathy in liver disease: single-center, clinical experience in 105 patients. *Hepatol Commun*. 2019;**3**(4):513–524.
120. Abuelkasem E, Hasan S, Mazzeffi MA, Planinsic RM, Sakai T, Tanaka KA. Reduced requirement for prothrombin complex concentrate for the restoration of thrombin generation in plasma from liver transplant recipients. *Anesth Analg*. 2017;**125**(2):609–615.
121. Kirchner C, Dirkmann D, Treckmann JW, et al. Coagulation management with factor concentrates in liver transplantation: a single-center experience. *Transfusion*. 2014;**54**(10 Pt 2):2760–2768.
122. O'Leary JG, Greenberg CS, Patton HM, Caldwell SH. AGA clinical practice update: coagulation in cirrhosis. *Gastroenterology*. 2019;**157**(1):34–43.e1.
123. Siniscalchi A, Begliomini B, De Pietri L, et al. Increased prothrombin time and platelet counts in living donor right hepatectomy: implications for epidural anesthesia. *Liver Transpl*. 2004;**10**(9):1144–1149.
124. Tsui SL, Yong BH, Ng KF, Yuen TS, Li CC, Chui KY. Delayed epidural catheter removal: the impact of postoperative coagulopathy. *Anaesth Intensive Care*. 2004;**32**(5):630–636.

5

Liver function tests and assessment of liver function

Omar Y. Mousa and Patrick S. Kamath

Introduction

The liver has multiple functions, and results of serum biochemical tests of the liver are crucial in the evaluation and management of patients with liver diseases. It is recommended to use the term liver biochemical tests rather than liver function tests because the measured enzymes (aminotransferases and alkaline phosphatase (ALP)) do not reflect liver function. Aminotransferases and ALP are markers of hepatic dysfunction. Therefore, this chapter presents a review and assessment of liver 'biochemical' tests, in addition to hepatic synthetic function, global liver function, and dynamic tests of the liver.

History

Inspection of the liver (Greek term *hēpatoskōpia*) in antiquity among Babylonians, Etruscans, Greeks, and Romans to determine health was extraordinary prescient.[1] The liver was considered the site of the soul, and there are clay liver models from Mesopotamia that date back to 2000 BC which are held in the Middle East Department of the British Museum.[2] Leonardo da Vinci (1452–1519) studied the anatomy of the human liver thoroughly in the fourteenth century, and described different liver diseases including cirrhosis (Figure 5.1). Andreas Vesalius (1514–1564) described the anatomy of the hepatic vessels and biliary tracts. However, it was believed that the liver had no function other than bile production.[3]

In the following century, Francis Glisson (1597–1677) determined that the liver parenchyma had hepatic lobules and was responsible for liver function and production of bile. Cirrhosis was described in detail and ascites was tapped through the umbilicus in the seventeenth century. In the eighteenth and nineteenth centuries observations were made regarding gallstones, liver tumours, fatty liver, hepatic congestion, acute hepatic necrosis, and hepatic coma. The twentieth century was the beginning of the modern era of hepatology, as multiple scientists studied the lobules of the human liver, bile composition and function, glycogen and urea synthesis, as well as micro- and macro-vesicular fatty degeneration.[3] Different tests were developed, including the serum bilirubin test (1913), Bauer's galactose test (1906), hippuric acid synthesis, and dye tests.[3,4] However it was not until the 1950s that the value of serum transaminases was determined in the diagnosis of hepatitis.

Liver function 'biochemical' tests

The liver biochemical tests have many clinical applications, and include alanine aminotransferase (ALT), aspartate aminotransferase (AST), ALP, bilirubin, and gamma-glutamyl transferase (GGT).[5] The tests are essential non-invasive tools to screen for liver diseases, and are helpful when used as a combination to determine disease severity, monitor disease progression, and measure treatment efficacy. However, they can have poor sensitivity or specificity when used individually. Tests of global liver function, including the Child–Turcotte–Pugh (CTP) score and Model for End-Stage Liver Disease (MELD) score were developed using these liver biochemical tests, and will be discussed further in this chapter.

Serum bilirubin

Bilirubin is a potentially toxic product of haem metabolism, mediated by the catalytic degradation of haem using haem oxygenase and biliverdin reductase. Eighty per cent of the daily bilirubin production is derived from haemoglobin, and the rest is contributed by other haemoproteins and free haem.[6] Unconjugated bilirubin enters the hepatocytes for conjugation to glucuronic acid, where the enzyme uridine 5′-diphosphate (UDP) glucuronyl transferase in the endoplasmic reticulum solubilizes bilirubin. Conjugated bilirubin is then excreted into the bile canaliculi. Transport across the canalicular membrane requires ATP, the only step in bilirubin metabolism that is energy dependent. This explains why some patients with hepatic failure present with conjugated hyperbilirubinaemia. Conjugated bilirubin in the bile passes into the small intestine until it reaches the terminal ileum and colon, where it is hydrolysed by beta-glucuronidase-containing bacteria to unconjugated bilirubin and then reduced to colourless urobilinogen. Urobilinogen is absorbed passively by the intestine into the portal circulation, the

Liver function 'biochemical' tests 41

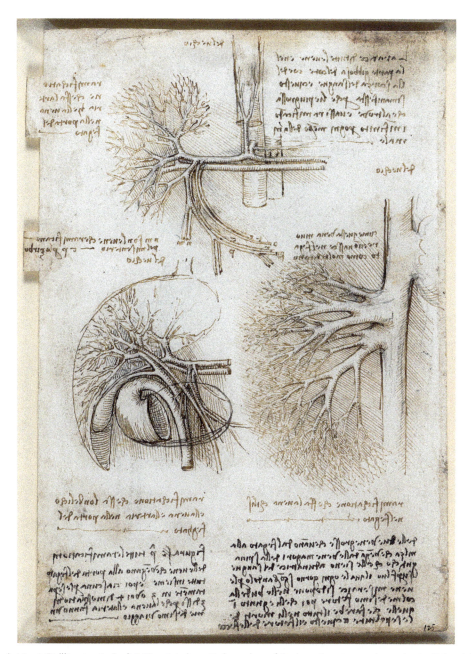

Figure 5.1 Leonardo da Vinci: *Dell'Anatomia Fogli B*. Top: intrahepatic branches of the hepatic artery and portal vein. Below left: branches of the umbilical vein, portal vein, hepatic artery, and bile duct. Gall bladder and bile duct. Below right: hepatic veins and their junction with the inferior vena cava.
Reproduced with permission from the Royal Collection Trust/© His Majesty King Charles III 2023. Available at: https://www.rct.uk/collection/919051/recto-the-vessels-and-nerves-of-the-neck-verso-the-vessels-of-the-liver

majority of which is eventually re-excreted by the liver and a small portion is excreted in the urine. A portion of urobilinogen is not absorbed, but is excreted unchanged or is oxidized and excreted as urobilin that has an orange colour.[7,8]

Measurement of conjugated and unconjugated bilirubin in patients with jaundice may not allow differentiation between the hepatocellular and cholestatic types of liver injury. When hyperbilirubinaemia is associated with elevated liver enzymes, the evaluation of a hepatocellular versus cholestatic process is possible. In addition, the degree and duration of elevation of bilirubin levels has not been assessed individually to estimate prognosis. However, bilirubin is a critical component of the MELD score, estimating patient survival in end-stage liver disease.

Conjugated and unconjugated bilirubin correspond to direct and indirect bilirubin. Table 5.1 summarizes the causes and mechanisms of isolated hyperbilirubinaemia in adults. Unconjugated hyperbilirubinaemia means that less than 15% of the total bilirubin is conjugated. It may result from overproduction of bilirubin through haemolytic disorders or ineffective erythropoiesis, impaired hepatocellular uptake of bilirubin by drugs like rifampin, impaired conjugation (Crigler–Najjar syndrome types I and II or Gilbert's syndrome), or overproduction of bilirubin from a

Table 5.1 Causes and mechanisms of isolated hyperbilirubinaemia in adults

Cause	Mechanism
Indirect hyperbilirubinaemia	
Haemolytic disorders	Overproduction of bilirubin
Inherited: • Red cell enzyme defects (e.g. glucose-6-phosphate dehydrogenase deficiency) • Sickle cell disease • Spherocytosis and elliptocytosis Acquired: • Drugs and toxins • Hypersplenism • Immune mediated • Paroxysmal nocturnal • Haemoglobinuria • Traumatic: macro- or microvascular injury	
Ineffective erythropoiesis	Overproduction of bilirubin
Cobalamin deficiency Folate deficiency Profound iron deficiency Thalassaemia	
Drugs Rifampin, probenecid	Impaired hepatocellular uptake
Inherited conditions	Impaired conjugation of bilirubin
Crigler–Najjar syndrome types I and II Gilbert's syndrome	
Other	
Haematoma and massive blood transfusion	Overproduction of bilirubin
Direct hyperbilirubinaemia	
Inherited conditions	
Dubin–Johnson syndrome Rotor syndrome	Impaired excretion of conjugated bilirubin

Reproduced with permission from Pratt, D.S. 'Liver Chemistry and Function Tests' in Feldman, M., Friedman, L.S., Brandt, L.J., *Sleisenger and Fordtran's Gastrointestinal and Liver Disease*, 10th edition, pp 1243–53, © Elsevier 2016.

Table 5.2 Causes of elevated serum aminotransferase levels

Chronic, mild elevations, ALT > AST (<150 U/L or 5× normal)
Hepatic causes α_1-Antitrypsin deficiency   Autoimmune hepatitis   Chronic viral hepatitis (B, C, and D)   Haemochromatosis   Medications and toxins   Steatosis and steatohepatitis   Wilson disease
Non-hepatic causes   Coeliac disease   Hyperthyroidism
Severe, acute elevations, ALT > AST (>1000 U/L or >20–25× normal)
Hepatic causes   Acute bile duct obstruction   Acute Budd–Chiari syndrome   Acute viral hepatitis   Drugs and toxins   Hepatic artery ligation   Ischaemic hepatitis   Wilson disease
Severe, acute elevations, AST > ALT (>1000 U/L or >20–25× normal)
Hepatic cause   Medications or toxins in a patient with underlying alcoholic liver injury   *Non-hepatic cause*   Acute rhabdomyolysis
Chronic, mild elevations, AST > ALT (<150 U/L, <5× normal)
Hepatic cause   Alcohol-related liver injury (AST/ALT > 2:1, AST nearly always <300 U/L)   *Non-hepatic causes*   Hypothyroidism   Macro-AST   Myopathy   Strenuous exercise

ALT, alanine aminotransferase; AST, aspartate aminotransferase.
Note: virtually any liver disease can cause moderate aminotransferase elevations (5–15× normal).
Reproduced with permission from Pratt, D.S. 'Liver Chemistry and Function Tests' in Feldman, M., Friedman, L.S., Brandt, L.J., *Sleisenger and Fordtran's Gastrointestinal and Liver Disease*, 10th edition, pp 1243–53, © Elsevier 2016.

haematoma or massive blood transfusion. Isolated conjugated hyperbilirubinaemia is caused by inherited diseases where excretion of conjugated bilirubin across the bile canaliculi is impaired (e.g. Dubin–Johnson syndrome and Rotor syndrome). Isolated conjugated hyperbilirubinaemia may also be seen when there is a fistula between the biliary tree and portal vein, sepsis, total parental nutrition, and systemic illnesses like lymphoma.

Clinically, scleral icterus is evident when the total serum bilirubin level is at least 3.0 mg/dL, though astute physicians may pick it up with a serum bilirubin level of 2 mg/dL. A patient with dark-coloured urine indicates hyperbilirubinaemia due to cholestasis.

Aminotransferases ('transaminases')

ALT and AST are serum aminotransferases that are increased in hepatocellular liver disease. ALT is more specific for liver injury than AST, given that the highest concentration of ALT is present in the liver. AST is also present in cardiac and skeletal muscle, kidney, brain, pancreas, lung, leucocytes, and erythrocytes. Similar to bilirubin, the degree of elevation of serum AST and ALT alone does not reflect the severity of liver injury. The increase in aminotransferase levels can be secondary to tissue damage or increased cell membrane permeability, and their half-lives are measured in days.[9] However, the degree and pattern of ALT and AST elevation is very helpful in guiding the diagnosis. For example, in patients with moderately elevated aminotransferase levels, a ratio of AST to ALT of more than 2 is quite suggestive of alcohol-related liver disease. By contrast, patients with viral hepatitis or non-alcoholic fatty liver disease typically have an AST to ALT ratio of less than 1. While the upper limit of normal (ULN) of AST and ALT varies between different laboratories, elevation in these tests above the ULN is associated with increased liver-related mortality. Among healthy controls, a normal ALT level ranges from 29 to 33 IU/L for males and 19 to 25 IU/L for females.[5] Table 5.2 summarizes the causes of elevated serum aminotransferase levels. A mild AST and/or ALT elevation is defined as 2–5× ULN, moderate AST and/or ALT elevation as 5–15× ULN, and severe AST and/or ALT elevation as >20× ULN.

Alkaline phosphatase

The major sources of serum ALP are the liver and bone. ALP is also present in the kidneys, small intestine, and placenta. ALP is ideally tested in the fasting state, and serum ALP elevations can be seen in

Table 5.3 Intrahepatic causes of cholestatic liver enzyme elevations in adults

Drugs[a]	**Other:**
Bland cholestasis:	• Crohn's disease
• Anabolic steroids	• Heavy metal exposure; beryllium, copper
• Oestrogens	• Hodgkin's disease
Cholestatic hepatitis:	**Viral hepatitis**
• Angiotensin-converting enzyme inhibitors: captopril, enalapril	HAV and HEV
• Antimicrobials: amoxicillin-clavulanic acid, ketoconazole	HBV and HCV, including fibrosing cholestatic hepatitis
• Azathioprine	EBV
• Chlorpromazine	Cytomegalovirus
• NSAIDs; sulindac, piroxicam	**Idiopathic adulthood ductopenia**
Granulomatous hepatitis:	**Genetic conditions**
• Allopurinol	Progressive familial intrahepatic cholestasis:
• Antibiotics: sulfonamides	• Type 1 (formerly Bylers's disease)
• Antiepileptics: carbamazepine, phenytoin	• Type 2
• Cardiovascular agents: hydralazine, procainamide, quinidine	• Type 3
• Phenylbutazone	Benign recurrent intrahepatic cholestasis:
Vanishing bile duct syndrome:	• Type 1
• Amoxicillin-clavulanic acid	• Type 2
• Chlorpromazine	CF
• Dicloxacillin	**Malignancy**
• Flucloxacillin	Hepatocellular carcinoma
• Macrolides	Metastatic disease
PBC	Paraneoplastic syndrome:
PSC	• Non-Hodgkin's lymphoma
Granulomatous liver disease	• Prostate cancer
Infections:	• Rental cell cancer
• Brucellosis	**Infiltrative liver disease**
• Fungal: histoplasmosis, coccidioidomycosis	Amyloidosis
• Leprosy	Lymphoma
• Q fever	**Intrahepatic cholestasis of pregnancy**
• Schistosomiasis	**TPN**
• TB, *Mycobacterium avium* complex, bacillus Calmette-Guérin	**Graft-versus-host disease**
Sarcoidosis	**Sepsis**
Idiopathic granulomatous hepatitis	

CF, cystic fibrosis; EBV, Epstein-Barr virus; HAV/HBV/HCV/HEV, hepatitis A, B, C, E virus; TB, tuberculosis; PBC, primary biliary cirrhosis; PSC, primary sclerosing cholangitis; TPN, total parental nutrition.
[a] Categorized by histological pattern. Drug lists are not meant to be comprehensive.
Reproduced with permission from Pratt, D.S. 'Liver Chemistry and Function Tests' in Feldman, M., Friedman, L.S., Brandt, L.J., *Sleisenger and Fordtran's Gastrointestinal and Liver Disease*, 10th edition, pp 1243-53, © Elsevier 2016.

patients with blood groups O and B following consumption of fatty food, due to release of intestinal ALP.[10] A benign increase in intestinal ALP can be familial, while adolescents can have higher levels of ALP (of bone origin) than adults due to bone growth. Adding GGT to the workup can help distinguish between liver and bone disease as a cause of elevated ALP. In addition, patients with Wilson disease, fulminant hepatitis, or haemolysis can have low serum levels of ALP, due to reduced enzyme activity and displacement of zinc by copper. Table 5.3 summarizes the intrahepatic causes of cholestatic liver enzyme elevations, and Box 5.1 shows the extrahepatic causes of cholestatic liver enzyme elevations in adults.

Gamma-glutamyl transferase

GGT is found in the liver, kidneys, pancreas, spleen, heart, brain, and seminal vesicles. It has a high sensitivity but low specificity for hepatobiliary disease. However, it is not increased in bone disease; therefore, it is helpful in the evaluation of an isolated increase in ALP. Elevated serum GGT levels can be caused by alcohol consumption, anti-HIV medications, or certain antiepileptics like phenytoin. Previous studies have suggested an association between ALP and the risk of hepatocellular carcinoma, choledocholithiasis, and increased mortality.[11-13]

5′-Nucleotidase

The 5′-nucleotidase level is mainly increased in hepatobiliary disease. It is associated with the canalicular and sinusoidal plasma membranes. It is also found in the intestine, brain, heart, blood vessels, and endocrine pancreas. This enzyme is seldom used in clinical practice, but elevation points to ALP elevations being of hepatic origin.

Tests of hepatic synthetic function

Albumin and prothrombin time

Albumin is synthesized by hepatocytes. The half-life for albumin is 2–3 weeks, and hypoalbuminaemia can occur secondary to chronic hepatic dysfunction or other non-hepatic causes including malnutrition, nephrotic syndrome, sepsis, and hormonal imbalance. Hypoalbuminaemia in the setting of liver disease suggests chronic liver injury. By contrast, an abnormal prothrombin time reflects acute hepatic dysfunction. Prothrombin time is a measure of the conversion time of prothrombin to thrombin, which involves coagulation factors that are synthesized in the liver (e.g. II, V, VII, and X). It is a measure of the time required for the plasma to clot.

> **Box 5.1** Extrahepatic causes of cholestatic liver enzyme elevations in adults
>
> **Intrinsic**
> *Choledocholithiasis*
> Immune-mediated duct injury:
> - Autoimmune pancreatitis
> - PSC
>
> *Malignancy:*
> - Ampullary cancer
> - Cholangiocarcinoma
>
> *Infections:*
> - AIDS cholangiopathy
> - Cytomegalovirus
> - Cryptosporidiosis
> - Microsporidiosis
> - Parasitic infections
> - Ascariasis
>
> **Extrinsic**
> *Malignancy:*
> - Gallbladder cancer
> - Metastases, including portal adenopathy from metastases
> - Pancreatic cancer
>
> *Mirizzi's syndrome*[a]
> *Pancreatitis*
> *Pancreatic pseudocyst*
>
> [a] Compression of the common hepatic duct by a stone in the neck of the gall bladder.
> Reproduced with permission from Pratt, D.S. 'Liver Chemistry and Function Tests' in Feldman, M., Friedman, L.S., Brandt, L.J., *Sleisenger and Fordtran's Gastrointestinal and Liver Disease*, 10th edition, pp 1243–53, © Elsevier 2016.

The international normalized ratio (INR) was introduced by the World Health Organization in 1983 to standardize the prothrombin time between different laboratories,[14] an important approach when managing patients with bleeding or clotting disorders, especially patients on warfarin therapy. Other causes of prothrombin time prolongation include impaired hepatic synthetic function, vitamin K deficiency (required for vitamin K-dependent factors II, VII, IX, and X), and disseminated intravascular coagulation (a decreased factor VIII level can distinguish disseminated intravascular coagulation from liver disease). Serum albumin level and prothrombin time have prognostic value in patients with liver disease, as they are components of the CTP (albumin and INR) and MELD scores (INR). These scores are described in further detail in the section 'Assessment of global liver function'.

Approach to a patient with abnormal liver biochemical tests

Evaluation of patients with abnormal liver biochemical tests should be initiated with a detailed medical history. A careful review of the possible risk factors for liver disease; medication history (including over-the-counter medications and herbal supplements); epidemiological history such as contact with other patients with hepatitis; associated medical conditions such as inflammatory bowel disease, cardiopulmonary disease, and haematological disorders; family history of hereditary forms of liver disease; and social history (alcohol use, substance abuse) is essential. Physical examination should assess the stigmata of chronic liver disease, including jaundice, ascites, hepatomegaly, splenomegaly, palmar erythema, Dupuytren's contractures, spider naevi, gynaecomastia, caput medusae, and hepatic encephalopathy. Decreased breath sounds in the setting of emphysema may suggest alpha-1-antitrypsin deficiency, bronze skin and arthritis can be seen in haemochromatosis, and Kayser–Fleischer rings seen by an expert ophthalmologist confirms a diagnosis of Wilson disease.

The pattern of liver biochemical test elevation is essential. The R ratio can help differentiate hepatocellular from cholestatic liver injury. It is calculated by the formula R = (ALT value ÷ ALT ULN) ÷ (ALP value ÷ ALP ULN). Hepatocellular injury is defined by an R ratio of greater than 5, and cholestatic injury is defined by an R ratio less than 2. A ratio of 2–5 suggests a mixed pattern of injury, where there is elevation of both ALP and AST and ALT levels.

Assessment of the temporal relationship between the elevation in AST, ALT, ALP, and bilirubin levels and the time of medication administration, for example, is important and very helpful in making a diagnosis of drug-induced liver injury. Repeating the liver biochemical tests is recommended to confirm that they are abnormal and the elevation is chronic. Assessment for the different causes of chronic liver disease through laboratory tests and radiological imaging should follow, before proceeding with a liver biopsy. Assessing causes of liver disease should include checking for viral hepatitis, fatty liver disease, autoimmune hepatitis, haemochromatosis, Wilson disease, and alpha-1-antitrypsin deficiency, as well as thyroid disease and coeliac disease.[5] Identifying drug-induced liver injury requires demonstrating a temporal relationship between use of the medication and elevation in the liver tests, and excluding other causes of liver disease. Often a diagnosis of drug-induced liver injury is based on expert opinion. The evaluation of asymptomatic elevation of serum aminotransferase levels is summarized in **Figure 5.2**. The evaluation of an isolated elevation of serum ALP level is shown in **Figure 5.3**.

Assessment of global liver function

Biochemical tests alone or combined with complications of portal hypertension like ascites and hepatic encephalopathy have been used to assess global hepatic function. Incorporation of both biochemical and clinical information to determine prognosis was the basis of the CTP score.[14,15] The CTP score utilized prothrombin time, serum albumin, serum bilirubin, ascites, and hepatic encephalopathy to evaluate patients for their suitability for portosystemic shunt surgery. Scores of 1–3 were assigned to the five individual variables, namely prothrombin time, bilirubin, albumin, ascites, and hepatic encephalopathy (**Table 5.5**). The sum of the scores from the five variables was then used to categorize the severity of liver disease. Patients with 5–6 points were classified as CTP class A, 7–9 points as CTP class B, and 10–15 points as CTP class C.

The MELD score was initially developed to identify patients at high risk of mortality following a transjugular intrahepatic portosystemic shunt procedure, and was later found to predict survival among patients with cirrhosis who did not require a transjugular intrahepatic portosystemic shunt. The variables in the model include serum total bilirubin, INR for prothrombin time, and serum creatinine. Before being widely accepted as a prognostic tool, the model was validated in hospitalized patients with cirrhosis; ambulatory patients with cirrhosis of varying aetiologies, including primary biliary cholangitis; and independently validated in an inception cohort of patients with cirrhosis

Practice guidelines and guidance

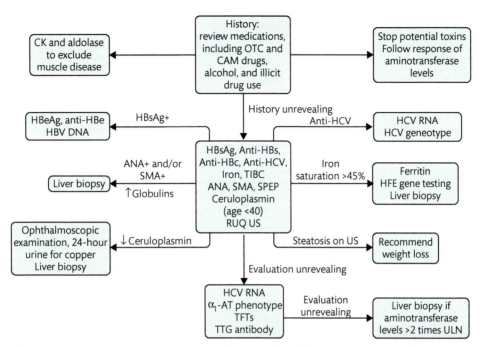

Figure 5.2 Evaluation of asymptomatic elevation of serum aminotransferase levels. α_1-AT, alpha-1-antitrypsin; ANA, antinuclear antibodies; Anti-HBc, antibody to hepatitis B core antigen; Anti-HBe, antibody to hepatitis B e antigen; Anti-HBs, antibody to hepatitis B surface antigen; Anti-HCV, antibody to hepatitis C virus; CAM, complementary and alternative medicines; CK, creatine kinase; HBeAg, hepatitis B e antigen; HBV DNA, hepatitis B virus deoxyribonucleic acid; HBsAg, hepatitis B surface antigen; HFE, haemochromatosis; OTC, over-the-counter; RNA, ribonucleic acid; RUQ US, right upper quadrant ultrasound; SMA, smooth muscle antibodies; SPEP, serum protein electrophoresis; TIBC, total iron binding capacity, TFTs, thyroid function tests; TTG, tissue transglutaminase; ULN, upper limit of normal.

Reproduced with permission from Pratt, D.S. 'Liver Chemistry and Function Tests' in Feldman, M., Friedman, L.S., Brandt, L.J., *Sleisenger and Fordtran's Gastrointestinal and Liver Disease*, 10th edition, pp 1243–53, © Elsevier 2016.

in Italy.[16] The MELD score also received a wide recognition as a prognostic tool to prioritize organ allocation among liver transplant candidates. The MELD score has subsequently been shown to be predictive of mortality in acute liver failure,[17] alcoholic hepatitis,[18] drug-induced liver injury,[19] and patients with cirrhosis undergoing surgery.[20] In January 2016, the 'Organ Procurement and Transplantation Network Policy 9.1 (MELD Score)' was updated to include serum sodium as a factor in the calculation of the MELD score, combined with the previously mentioned variables. Hyponatraemia is a common problem in patients with cirrhosis, and the severity of the hyponatraemia is a marker of the severity of the cirrhosis. The MELD-Sodium (MELD-NA) score is shown in Box 5.2.

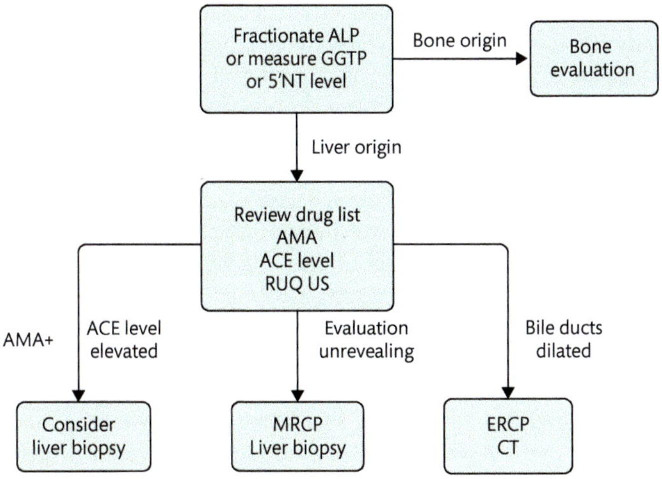

Practice guidelines and guidance

National and international medical societies have published guidelines for the evaluation of abnormal liver biochemical tests as

Figure 5.3 The evaluation of an isolated elevation of serum alkaline phosphatase level. ACE, angiotensin-converting enzyme; ALP, alkaline phosphatase; AMA, antimitochondrial antibodies; 5'NT, 5'-nucleotidase; RUQ, right upper quadrant.

Reproduced with permission from Pratt, D.S. 'Liver Chemistry and Function Tests' in Feldman, M., Friedman, L.S., Brandt, L.J., *Sleisenger and Fordtran's Gastrointestinal and Liver Disease*, 10th edition, pp 1243–53, © Elsevier 2016.

Table 5.5 Child–Turcotte–Pugh classification

CTP score—grading the severity of liver disease			
Biochemical and clinical variables			
Total bilirubin, mg/dL	1–2	2–3	>3
Serum albumin, g/dL	>3.5	2.8–3.5	<2.8
Prothrombin time, seconds	1–4	4–6	>6
Ascites	Absent	Slight	Moderate
Encephalopathy grade	None	1 and 2	3 and 4
Points	+1	+2	+3

Source: data from Child CG, Turcotte JG. Surgery and portal hypertension. In: Child CG, ed. *The Liver and Portal Hypertension*. Philadelphia, PA: Saunders; 1964: 50–64.

> **Box 5.2** MELD-Na Score
>
> - Biochemical variables:
>   - Total bilirubin.
>   - INR.
>   - Sodium.
>   - Creatinine.
> - Dialysis at least twice in the past week or continuous venovenous haemofiltration for more than 24 hours in the past week.
>
> Source: data from Kim WR, et al. Hyponatremia and mortality among patients on the liver-transplant waiting list. N Engl J Med. 2008;359(10):1018–26.

Table 5.6 Dynamic tests of liver performance

Clearance tests	• Sulfobromophthalein sodium (BSP) • Indocyanine green (ICG) • Caffeine test • Galactose • I^{131} Rose Bengal dye
Breath tests/$^{14}CO_2$ exhalation	• ^{14}C-aminopyrine • ^{3}C-methacetin • ^{14}C-diazepam • ^{14}C-phenacetin • ^{14}C- or ^{13}C-galactose
Metabolic capacity	• Lidocaine/monoethylglycinexylidide (MEGX) test

Sources: data from Sakka SG. Assessing liver function. *Curr Opin Crit Care*. 2007;13:207–214; Clavien P-A, Petrowsky H, DeOliveira ML, et al. Strategies for safe and liver surgery and partial liver transplantation. *N Engl J Med*. 2007;356:1545–1559; Burra P, Masier A. Dynamic tests to study liver function. *Eur Rev Med Pharmacol Sci*. 2004;8:19–21; Lewis AE. Investigation of hepatic function by clearance techniques. *Am J Physiol*. 1950;163:54–61; Stravitz RT, Ilan Y. Potential use of metabolic breath tests to assess liver disease and prognosis: has the time arrived for routine use in the clinic? *Liver Int*. 2017;37:328–336; Bosch J, Bureau C, Chalasani N, et al. ^{13}C-Methacetin breath test is a highly accurate non-invasive point of care test for detecting CSPH in patients with NASH. *J Hepatol*. 2018;68:S115.

follows: The American College of Gastroenterology (ACG) ('ACG Clinical Guideline: evaluation of abnormal liver chemistries', 2017),[5] the British Society of Gastroenterology ('Guidelines on the management of abnormal liver blood tests', 2017),[21] These references provide helpful guidance in the evaluation and management of patients with abnormal liver biochemical tests.

Dynamic tests of liver performance

There is a need in the field of hepatology for non-invasive assessment of dynamic liver performance. Liver performance tests should be able to assess early as well as late stages of liver disease. They should be well tolerated, reproducible, and operator independent. Previously, hepatic clearance tests, also called 'dynamic tests', were described but are rarely used in current clinical practice. Hepatic clearance tests reflect the ability of the liver to clear endogenous or exogenous substances from the circulation and depend on the circulation and organ perfusion, as well as on hepatocyte function.[22] The liver has to be the sole route of the removal of the compound from the plasma, and the compound should remain in the plasma in equilibrium with other fluid compartments before extraction by the liver for the test to accurately reflect hepatic function. Clearance from the plasma should be independent of its concentration.[23] These tests were initially used to assess the residual liver function in critically ill patients with shock or sepsis requiring vasopressors for haemodynamic support, and in patients undergoing liver resection or awaiting liver transplantation.[24] A list of the tests is shown in Table 5.6. A summary including a brief description of some dynamic liver tests is shown in Table 5.7. The disadvantages of these tests include a potential for inaccurate assessment of liver function, and limited availability and reproducibility. For example, when the compound is bound to plasma proteins until excretion by the liver, the test result can be influenced by changes in plasma albumin levels or by hepatic blood flow, as it is the case in the sulphobromophthalein (BSP) test. Indocyanine green (ICG) is a better test, as the compound is avidly bound to plasma proteins and has a more predictable distribution volume, its plasma level reflects hepatic uptake and it has excellent hepatic clearance.[22]

In addition, the liver's capacity to transport organic anions and metabolize exogenous compounds may allow assessment of the liver functionality and guide treatment response.[25] However, these tests are not helpful for screening purposes, are more difficult and expensive to perform, and therefore have fallen out of routine use.[22] Current research projects investigating liver function assessment include the HepQuant SHUNT test,[26] hepatobiliary scintigraphy,[27] and signal intensity on gadolinium-ethoxybenzyl-diethylenetriaminepentaacetic acid (Gd-EOB-DTPA)-enhanced magnetic resonance imaging during the interstitial and hepatobiliary phase.[28]

Artificial intelligence in hepatology

Over the past decade, the field of hepatology has witnessed substantial progress in the application of artificial intelligence (AI). AI encompasses statistical techniques ranging between advanced modelling and deep learning algorithms. Machine learning is the most exciting new application of AI in healthcare. In machine learning, the *machine* can *learn* complex relationships between variables and the outcomes of interest and develop prediction models.[29] It is powerful and can process many interactions between predictors. Multiple studies have focused on the detection of non-alcoholic fatty liver disease, liver fibrosis in patients with viral hepatitis, diagnosis of oesophageal varices, development of hepatocellular carcinoma, liver transplant prioritization, donor–recipient matching to predict survival following liver transplantation, and prediction of hepatic decompensation in primary sclerosing cholangitis. AI techniques may help determine the risk of liver fibrosis among patients with chronic liver disease, and help avoid invasive tests like liver biopsies.[30–32] Recently, AI has been used to develop an automated algorithm to help investigate and provide a cost-effective early diagnostic strategy for liver disease in the primary care setting. This is called intelligent liver function testing or 'iLFT'.[33] Future studies and applications of AI in liver disease are promising.

Table 5.7 Examples of dynamic tests of liver performance

Test	Description
Clearance tests	
Sulphobromophthalein (BSF)[13]	• First used in 1913 • Indication: assessment of dynamic liver function • Water soluble • Binds to plasma proteins • Conjugates with glutathione before excretion in bile Summary of the test: • IV injection of bromosulphthalein • Complete extraction by the liver • In normal individual: <10% remains in the serum by 30 min and less than 5% by 45 min • Extraction and removal by the liver is related to hepatic blood flow and canalicular bile transporter protein function Clinical application: • Slower rates of extraction are seen in liver disease • In patients undergoing liver resection, a negative prognosis can be predicted by increased retention after 15 minutes • Can differentiate between Dubin–Johnson syndrome and Rotor syndrome
Indocyanine green (ICG)[13,14]	• It was recommended to assess hepatic blood flow in 1957 • Indication: assessment of dynamic liver function • Excretion of ICG exclusively into bile • Does not undergo intrahepatic recirculation • Appears in bile acids within 8 min of intravenous infusion Summary of the test: • A transcutaneous system is used to assess the clearance rate and plasma disappearance rate non-invasively • In normal individuals: the clearance rate of ICG is >700 mL/min/m^2 and its plasma disappearance rate is >18%/min Clinical application: • Decreased rate of plasma disappearance in liver disease • Prognosticate patients undergoing liver resection • Evaluate potential liver donors for liver function
Caffeine test[13]	• Useful in severe liver lesions • Correlates with BSF and the $^{14}CO_2$ breath elimination test • Mechanism: quantifies hepatic microsomal activity Summary of test: • Caffeine is administered orally • Dose = 300 mg • Quantification of caffeine and caffeine metabolite levels in the blood Clinical application: • Caffeine elimination rates are increased in cirrhosis • Lower caffeine metabolite/caffeine ratio in cirrhosis
Breath tests	
^{14}C-Aminopyrine test[13]	• Most common • Correlates with the degree of liver damage • Radioactively labelled aminopyrine is ingested orally • Aminopyrine undergoes demethylation in the liver • Microsomal liver function can be assessed based on exhaled $^{14}CO_2$ Clinical application: • Prognostication of patients with chronic liver disease
Metabolic capacity	
MEGX test	• This test is based on the hepatic conversion of lidocaine to MEGX • Conversion is related to the cytochrome P450 (CYP) system • Use of this test is limited by the need for laboratory equipment/immunoassay • Can be influenced by patient-related factors, as well as hepatic metabolic capacity and blood flow • Consider interactions with substances or drugs that result from the cytochrome CYP3A/4A system Clinical application: • Quantitative assessing of pre- and post-transplant liver function
Tests rarely performed in clinical practice	
Amino acid clearance test[13]	• Evaluate periodic plasma clearance of amino acids after standardized infusion dose
Galactose elimination capacity[13]	• Used early in the clinical course of jaundice • Distinguishes between hepatocellular disease and biliary obstruction • Assesses the liver's capacity to convert galactose to its phosphorylated form: galalactose-1-phosphate • Clinical value is limited, especially due to galactose intolerance

Sources: data from Sakka SG. Assessing liver function. *Curr Opin Crit Care*. 2007;13:207–214; Clavien P-A, Petrowsky H, DeOliveira ML, et al. Strategies for safe and liver surgery and partial liver transplantation. *N Engl J Med*. 2007;356:1545–1559; Burra P, Masier A. Dynamic tests to study liver function. *Eur Rev Med Pharmacol Sci*. 2004;8:19–21; Lewis AE. Investigation of hepatic function by clearance techniques. *Am J Physiol*. 1950;163:54–61; Stravitz RT, Ilan Y. Potential use of metabolic breath tests to assess liver disease and prognosis: has the time arrived for routine use in the clinic? *Liver Int*. 2017;37:328–336; Bosch J, Bureau C, Chalasani N, et al. ^{13}C-Methacetin breath test is a highly accurate non-invasive point of care test for detecting CSPH in patients with NASH. *J Hepatol*. 2018;68:S115.

REFERENCES

1. Jastrow M. The liver in antiquity and the beginnings of anatomy. *Trans Stud Coll Physicians Phila*. 1907;**29**:117–139.
2. Cavalcanti de AMA, Martins C. History of liver anatomy: Mesopotamian liver clay models. *HPB (Oxford)*. 2013;**15**(4):322–323.
3. Franken FH. History of hepatology. In: Csomós G, Thaler H, eds. *Clinical Hepatology*. Berlin: Springer; 1983: 1–15.
4. McNee JW, Keefer CS. The clinical value of the Van Den Bergh reaction for bilirubin in blood: with notes on improvements in its technique. *Br Med J*. 1925;**2**(3367):52–54.
5. Kwo PY, Cohen SM, Lim JK. ACG Clinical Guideline: evaluation of abnormal liver chemistries. *Am J Gastroenterol*. 2017;**112**(1):18–35.
6. Berk PD, Howe RB, Bloomer JR, Berlin NI. Studies of bilirubin kinetics in normal adults. *J Clin Invest*. 1969;**48**(11):2176.
7. Poland R, Odell G. Physiologic jaundice: the enterohepatic circulation of bilirubin. *N Engl J Med*. 1971;**284**(1):1–6.
8. Lester R, Schmid R. Bilirubin metabolism. *N Engl J Med*. 1964;**270**:779–786.
9. Kallai L, Hahn A, Roeder V, et al. Correlation between histological findings and transaminase values in chronic diseases of the liver. *Acta Med Scand*. 1964;**175**:49–56.
10. Bamford K, Harris H, Luffman J, et al. Serum-alkaline phosphatase and the ABO blood groups. *Lancet* 1965;**1**(7384):530–531.
11. Hu G, Tuomilehto J, Pukkala E, et al. Joint effects of coffee consumption and serum gamma-glutamyltransferase on the risk of liver cancer. *Hepatology*. 2008;**48**(1):7–9.
12. Yang M, Chen T, Wang S, et al. Biochemical predictors for absence of common bile duct stones in patients undergoing laparoscopic cholecystectomy. *Surg Endosc*. 2008;**22**(7):1620–1624.
13. Pinkham CA, Krause KJ. Liver function tests and mortality in a cohort of life insurance applicants. *J Insur Med*. 2009;**41**(3):170–177.
14. Child CG, Turcotte JG. Surgery and portal hypertension. *Major Probl Clin Surg*. 1964;**1**:1–85.
15. Pugh RN, Murray-Lyon IM, Dawson JL, Pietroni MC, Williams R. Transection of the oesophagus for bleeding oesophageal varices. *Br J Surg*. 1973;**60**(8):646–649.
16. Kamath PS, Wiesner RH, Malinchoc M, et al. A model to predict survival in patients with end-stage liver disease. *Hepatology*. 2001;**33**(2):464–470.
17. Kremers WK, van IJperen M, Kim WR, et al. MELD score as a predictor of pretransplant and posttransplant survival in OPTN/UNOS status 1 patients. *Hepatology*. 2004;**39**(5):764–769.
18. Mayo Clinic. MELD score and 90-day mortality rate for alcoholic hepatitis. n.d. https://www.mayoclinic.org/medical-professionals/transplant-medicine/calculators/meld-score-and-90-day-mortality-rate-for-alcoholic-hepatitis/itt-20434719#
19. Hayashi PH, Rockey DC, Fontana RJ, et al. Death and liver transplantation within 2 years of onset of drug-induced liver injury. *Hepatology*. 2017;**66**(4):1275–1285.
20. Mayo Clinic. Post-operative mortality risk in patients with cirrhosis. n.d. http://www.mayoclinic.org/medical-professionals/model-end-stage-liver-disease/post-operative-mortality-risk-patients-cirrhosis
21. Newsome PN, Cramb R, Davison SM, et al. Guidelines on the management of abnormal liver blood tests. *Gut*. 2018;**67**(1):6–19.
22. Burra P, Masier A. Dynamic tests to study liver function. *Eur Rev Med Pharmacol Sci*. 2004;**8**(1):19–21.
23. Lewis AE. Investigation of hepatic function by clearance techniques. *Am J Physiol*. 1950;**163**(1):54–61.
24. Sakka SG. Assessing liver function. *Curr Opin Crit Care*. 2007;**13**(2):207–214.
25. Wagener G. *Liver Anesthesiology and Critical Care Medicine*. New York: Springer, 2018.
26. ClinicalTrials.gov. The HepQuant SHUNT test for monitoring liver disease and treatment effects by measuring liver function and physiology. 2021. https://clinicaltrials.gov/ct2/show/NCT03294941
27. Hoekstra LT, de Graaf W, Nibourg GA, et al. Physiological and biochemical basis of clinical liver function tests: a review. *Ann Surg*. 2013;**257**(1):27–36.
28. Ippolito D, Pecorelli A, Famularo S, et al. Assessing liver function: diagnostic efficacy of parenchymal enhancement and liver volume ratio of Gd-EOB-DTPA-enhanced MRI study during interstitial and hepatobiliary phase. *Abdom Radiol (NY)*. 2019;**44**(4):1340–1349.
29. Lovejoy CA, Keogh B, Maruthappu M. How will artificial intelligence affect diagnosis and treatment of liver disease? *Dig Liver Dis*. 2019;**51**(9):1350–1352.
30. Le Berre C, Sandborn WJ, Aridhi S, et al. Application of artificial intelligence to gastroenterology and hepatology. *Gastroenterology*. 2020;**158**(1):76–94.e2.
31. Spann A, Yasodhara A, Kang J, et al. Applying machine learning in liver disease & transplantation: a comprehensive review. *Hepatology*. 2020;**10**(3):1093–1105.
32. Eaton JE, Vesterhus M, McCauley BM, et al. Primary Sclerosing Cholangitis Risk Estimate Tool (PREsTo) predicts outcomes of the disease: a derivation and validation study using machine learning. *Hepatology*. 2020;**71**(1):214–224.
33. Dillon JF, Miller MH, Robinson EM, et al. Intelligent liver function testing (iLFT): a trial of automated diagnosis and staging of liver disease in primary care. *J Hepatol*. 2019;**71**(4):699–706.

6

Imaging

Ultrasound, computed tomography, magnetic resonance imaging, nuclear medicine, and angiography

Guido Costa, Ezio Lanza, Matteo Donadon, and Guido Torzilli

Introduction

Imaging studies represent a fundamental step both in the evaluation of liver anatomy, and in detecting and characterizing focal liver lesions and biliary tract disorders—especially in patients awaiting liver surgery. Moreover, from a surgical perspective, the role of imaging studies also includes the planning of the best surgical approach, meaning preoperative and intraoperative guidance in the operating room as well as monitoring of the postoperative course after surgery. This chapter will focus on the current roles of ultrasound, computed tomography (CT), magnetic resonance imaging (MRI), nuclear medicine, and angiography in the setting of patients awaiting liver surgery.

Ultrasound

Ultrasound represents a valid imaging modality for screening and first-level assessment, being a low-cost and safe technique, with no harmful effects on the patient and operator. It has some limitations mainly because it is not a reproducible study and its quality and reliability are heavily influenced by the skill and experience of the operator. Moreover, the presence of some structures, such as bone or air, may limit the field of the study due to the inability of the ultrasound wave to pass through these structures.

The physical phenomenon, that leads to the computation of the image, lies in the analysis of the intensity of the pulsatile waves emitted by the transducer of the probe after it has been reflected by different tissues. Different probes may emit ultrasound waves with different frequencies: high-frequency probes offer a better image resolution but with lower capability of tissue penetration and visualization of structures. By contrast, low-frequency probes allow for the study of deeper structures but with lower image definition. For the study of the vascular flow of the liver, Doppler ultrasound is a viable approach. It allows the study of vascular flow by computing the change in frequency of an ultrasound wave when reflected by a moving object, in this case circulating red blood cells.

The two acoustic windows mainly used for the study of the liver are subcostal and intercostal, with the patient lying in the supine or left lateral decubitus position. Usually the study of the liver is carried out following its segmental portal anatomy, in order to systematically visualize and study all the parenchyma of the organ and to assess the presence of anatomical variants. A normal liver is characterized by a uniform echogenicity, is usually hypoechoic compared to the spleen and iso-/hyperechoic to the renal cortex, and has a smooth contour. Some information regarding the liver parenchyma can be obtained by ultrasound: a diffusely hyperechoic parenchyma is typical in cases of hepatic steatosis, while a nodular contour of the organ may suggest the presence of liver cirrhosis. Moreover, ultrasound can show indirect features related to liver function, such as the presence of ascites or abdominal varices. However, the main role of liver ultrasound as a first-level imaging technique is in the detection and characterization of focal liver lesions. Such lesions are primarily characterized by their echogenicity in contrast to liver parenchyma and may be anechoic, hypoechoic, isoechoic, or hyperechoic. An anechoic focal liver lesion indicates the presence of a cystic lesion, which in most cases is benign. The inner structure, the presence of septa, and the content of a given cyst may suggest the presence of a complication, such previous bleeding, as well as its aetiology. Hypoechoic lesions are typical of many malignancies and are usually investigated with second-level studies such as CT or MRI. Hyperechogenicity includes both benign, such as focal fatty changes and hepatic haemangiomas, and malignant primary or secondary lesions. Even these latter lesions should be investigated by using second-level studies. In some cases, liver lesions have an appearance that does not markedly differ from the normal parenchyma: these lesions are called isoechoic lesions and are the most difficult to detect and characterize. In these situations, the use of ultrasound contrast agents, constituted by gas-filled hyperechogenic microbubbles administered intravenously, has proven to be useful in the detection and characterization of focal liver lesions.[1] Of note, these ultrasound contrast agents have not shown any nephrotoxicity so far and they can be used safely in patients with impaired renal function.

Ultrasound has an important role not only in the preoperative assessment but also in the surgical setting. During liver resection, the use of intraoperative ultrasound (IOUS) permits an accurate staging of hepatic disease and provides a fundamental guidance tool for resection. This is particularly important for the radical but conservative surgical policy that allows the parenchymal sacrifice to be minimized, thus reducing surgical risk, and offers a chance of cure to an increasing proportion of patients.[2,3] In fact, cases with a burden of disease and bi-lobar localization may not be considered surgically treatable using conventional dissection in the vertical planes because of an insufficient future remnant of liver.[4] With the aid of IOUS, the surgeon can adapt the dissection plane by following the tumour edges in real time, switching from the vertical to curved dissection planes that allow the removal of the tumour without sacrificing the vascular skeleton of the liver.[5] This approach results in potentially many surgical possibilities, with operations that are tailored to suit each patient.[6]

As a standard policy, the authors recommend liver explorations starting from the portal branches. The probe is placed along the midline that divides the liver into a lower and upper part and the portal bifurcation is the first structure to be seen. Then, with gentle tilting movements of the probe, the portal branches can be followed from their hilar origin to the periphery and all liver segments can be explored without extensive movements. This allows the surgeon to study the whole organ and to asses portal anatomical variations (Figure 6.1). After the exploration of the portal system, the probe is tilted upward to visualize the confluence of the hepatic veins.[7] After surgical exploration and staging of the disease, IOUS can provide the surgeon with important information during resection: with the aid of a gauze placed on the resection plane that leads to hyperechogenic air entrapment, the conducted dissection plane can be clearly visualized and corrected as needed. Moreover, IOUS-guided surgical manoeuvres[8,9] can provide an accurate and real-time *in vivo* assessment of the portal liver segmentation. This is particularly important for the treatment of primary liver tumours (i.e. hepatocellular carcinoma (HCC)) that could benefit oncologically from true anatomical resections.

The benefits of contrast-enhanced ultrasound for diagnosis and staging are also valid for the intraoperative setting (Figure 6.2).[10] Interestingly, the biliary tree may be investigated during IOUS by using injections of air and/or water into the cystic duct or a stump of a resected bile duct. This allows for a simple, and low-cost intraoperative cholangio-ultrasound. This may be very useful to confirm biliary tree integrity in case of suspected damage after surgical dissection or to define the amount of liver drained by a given resected bile duct.[11]

Finally, it is worth noting that the most modern ultrasound machines permit the integration and synchronization of the ultrasound image with CT or MRI. This type of application is very useful for localization of difficult lesions or IOUS-guided interventional procedures (i.e. biopsy or ablation). One of the main applications is the intraoperative identification of those lesions which have disappeared after chemotherapy: in such cases, the IOUS findings may be synchronized with pre-chemotherapy CT or MRI, where the lesions were still visible (see Figure 6.10d in 'Recent innovations').

Computed tomography

CT is frequently used in the study of liver masses and for follow-up after treatment. The basic principle that allows the computation of CT images relies on the different absorption capacities of X-rays by different tissues, and modified by the administration of contrast agents. High-density tissues, like bone, absorb most of the X-rays passing through, leading to a brighter image. The main difference and advantage from plain X-rays is that the X-ray source and multiple detectors are rotated around the patient (spiral CT). Many pieces of information are then acquired while the patient is moved through the rotating structure of the X-ray source and detectors while the image is reconstructed by a computer as a three-dimensional volume. This volume is then sliced in different planes, most commonly the axial, coronal, and sagittal planes. The main advantages of CT are that it is commonly available, and it has high spatial resolution compared to MRI; these characteristics have made CT the most commonly requested imaging modality in the study of the liver. It is important to note that CT is a modality that uses ionizing radiation and care should be taken as the patient population is being exposed increasingly to doses that are not trivial. Thus, CT should not be performed in pregnant patients and extra care should be taken in children and, when performing a contrast-enhanced examination, in patients with a history of reactions to contrast or impaired renal function.

An ideal and state-of-the-art CT examination for the study of the liver should combine a basal, pre-contrast scan, and different scans taken after the administration of an intravenous iodinated contrast agent. These scans include an early and arterial phase, a portal phase, and delayed phases. The evaluation of the liver is usually carried out using the standard abdomen soft tissue window. The evaluation of focal liver lesions is done considering the density of the lesion, its morphology, and enhancement after the administration of contrast agent.

Among the different benign focal lesions, hepatic haemangiomas have the characteristic peripheral nodular enhancement on arterial phase images while in the portal and late phases they show progressive centripetal enhancement that may not be complete in case

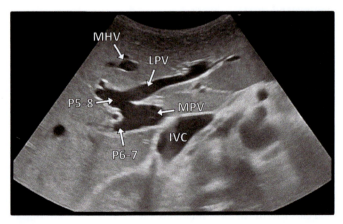

Figure 6.1 Portal bifurcation visualized with a conventional convex probe positioned in the midline, central position of the liver. The anterior (P5–8) and posterior (P6–7) right portal branches can be followed from their origin from the main portal vein (MPV). An anatomical variant, with the left portal vein (LPV) originating from the right anterior portal branch is easily detected. IVC, inferior vena cava; MHV, middle hepatic vein.

Computed tomography

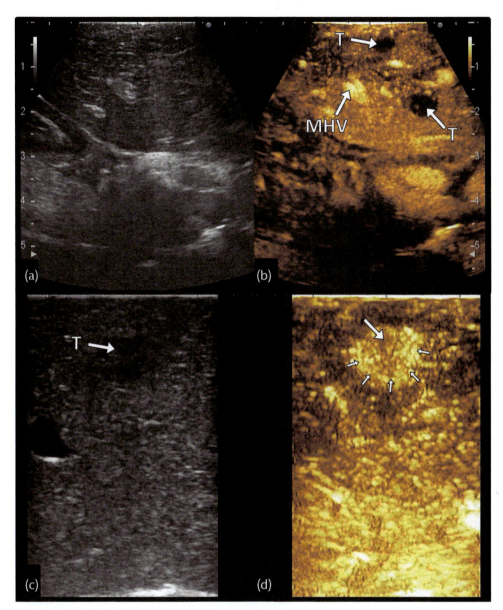

Figure 6.2 (a, b) After administration of intravenous ultrasound contrast (sulphur hexafluoride, SonoVue, Bracco Imaging) in a patient with multiple colorectal liver metastases, two lesions (T), located in segment 4, that were not detectable with the IOUS (a) became clearly detectable at parenchymatous phase of contrast-enhanced IOUS (b). In this case, the image was taken about 40 seconds after contrast administration. (c, d) Contrast-enhanced IOUS image of a patient with HCC. The lesion (T), mildly hypoechogenic at IOUS (c), after contrast administration (b) appears with a peripheral hypervascular rim (small arrow) and a less vascularized core (big arrow). The image was taken in an early vascular phase, about 25 seconds after contrast administration. MHV, middle hepatic vein.

of a giant haemangioma. Conversely, focal nodular hyperplasia is characterized by a diffuse homogeneous hyperenhancement in the arterial phase that progressively fades to the background hepatic parenchyma in the portal phase. A central scar, which progressively enhances on portal and delayed vascular phases, facilitates the diagnosis. This is, however, a sign that is present in only a minority of patients.[12]

Concerning liver malignancies, HCCs on CT show a typical hyperenhancement in the arterial phases and then become hypoattenuating to the liver parenchyma in the portal and late phases. This latter behaviour is termed 'wash-out' and reflects the pathological vascularization of the lesion (Figure 6.3a,b). A typical feature of HCCs is the presence of an enhancing tumoral capsule that has a different hyperattenuating behaviour from the lesion and the background parenchyma. Moreover, HCCs, especially in cirrhotic patients, show a peculiar tendency of invasion and thrombosis of portal and hepatic veins; in those cases, the visualization of a vascular tumour thrombus has the highest accuracy in the diagnosis of HCC. In larger lesions, the presence of multiple intralesional histological components is reflected in CT imaging by a peculiar mosaic pattern. The enhancing component represents the viable tumoral tissue, while the non-enhancing components are represented by fatty metamorphosis, necrosis, and haemorrhage.[13] Intrahepatic cholangiocarcinomas, on CT imaging, are typically focal lesions characterized by a lower attenuation and an enhanced peripheral rim. Of note, this type of tumour may have different,

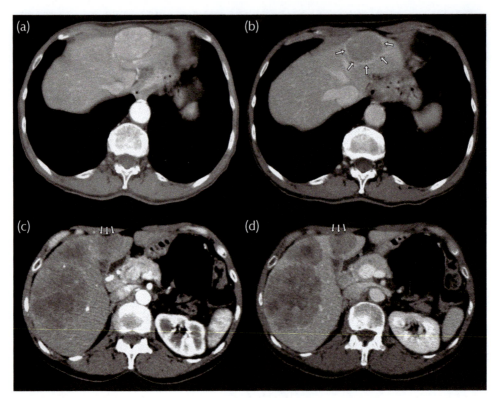

Figure 6.3 (a, b) CT scan of a patient with a HCC located in segment 3. The lesion shows typical behaviour after contrast administration. In the early arterial phase (a) it appears hyperenhanced while becoming hypoattenuated to liver parenchyma in portal phases (b). The tumoural capsule (small arrows) shows a different hyperattenuating behaviour from the lesion and the background parenchyma during wash-out. (c, d) Patient affected by multiple colorectal liver metastases. On contrast-enhanced CT scan, lesions appear mildly hypoattenuated in arterial phase with a mild peripheral hyperenhancement (c), while becoming clearly hypoattenuated in portal phase (d). Lesions have a cauliflower shape with a central, necrotic core that appear more hypoattenuating than the vital peripheral tissue. Moreover, retraction of the Glissonean sheath, another typical sign in colorectal liver metastases, is present (small arrows).

non-unique aspects on CT images, and expert hepatobiliary surgeons and radiologists are required for the differential diagnosis.[14] In perihilar cholangiocarcinoma, a ductal thickening is visible on CT as well as indirect signs of the presence of biliary obstruction, in particular, intrahepatic segmental or sectorial ductal dilatation in the biliary system above the obstruction as well as segmental or lobar atrophy (Figure 6.4). CT proved to be accurate in the detection of perihilar cholangiocarcinomas.[15] Besides diagnosis, a CT evaluation of perihilar cholangiocarcinoma should define the exact location and extent of disease in the biliary system, and the presence of any kind of vascular invasion and extrahepatic localization of disease. Moreover, a CT-based three-dimensional reconstruction and volumetric evaluation of the future liver remnant is often needed in order to define the best surgical strategy, considering that in this kind of disease a large parenchymal sacrifice is often necessary to achieve radical resection.

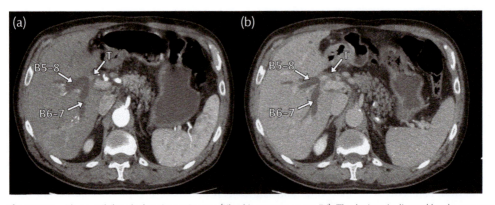

Figure 6.4 CT scan of a patient with a perihilar cholangiocarcinoma (Klatskin tumour, type IV). The lesion, indicated by the arrows, is visible and hyperattenuating in both arterial (a) and portal (b) phases. Biliary dilation in the upstream biliary system is present, with the right anterior and posterior biliary branches (B5–8 and B6–7) clearly visible.

Secondary liver malignancies have a heterogeneous appearance on CT. Usually they show lower attenuation compared to the surrounding parenchyma and their behaviour after contrast administration reflects their vascularization (Figure 6.3c,d). Hypervascular lesions show hyperattenuation during arterial phases and tend to be less visible during the portal phases. Hypovascular lesions are less attenuating than the background parenchyma during the portal phases.

From a surgical point of view, besides diagnosis, CT has an important role in the study of the vascular anatomy of the liver and in the definition of the vascular relationships of a given lesion in a patient awaiting hepatectomy. Moreover, the accurate definition of vascular structures after contrast administration allows proper visualization and characterization in cases of tumoral thrombi.

Magnetic resonance imaging

MRI is a technique that uses magnetic fields and radiofrequency pulses to generate and reconstruct images. The physical principle that allows the reconstruction of the images is the difference in moment and spin of certain atomic nuclei when exposed to different magnetic fields. When exposed to a static magnetic field, nuclei are aligned in the same or opposite parallel directions and have a spin or rotation with a fixed and stable frequency that depends on the nucleus and the intensity of the magnetic field. This static condition reaches an equilibrium with an almost equal number of nuclei aligned in the two opposite directions; the slight difference between the two unparallel groups generates a magnetic moment. Nuclei in the body are then excited after being exposed to a radiofrequency pulse, and when they return to their original state they generate a different measurable difference in the static magnetic moment. This process of returning to their original state is called relaxation and is the combination of two different processes, longitudinal (T1) and transverse (T2) relaxation, that can be separately analysed. In clinical practice, the most commonly analysed and imaged nucleus is the hydrogen (^{1}H) nucleus, as a surrogate of the water composition of the tissue. The acquired pieces of information are then reconstructed as multiplanar cross-sectional images that can be visualized and analysed by the operator. One of the main peculiarities of MRI is that the information provided is not only morphological, but also functional, because it reflects the atomic and molecular composition of the different tissues. In the evaluation of the liver pre-contrast T1, T2 and diffusion-weighted imaging sequences are commonly performed at first; contrast-enhanced T1-weighted sequences are then acquired with an additional hepatobiliary phase when liver-specific contrast agents are used. MRI contrast agents affect the T1 relaxation time in the tissue where they accumulate. In the hepatobiliary setting, two main categories of contrast agents are available, depending on their capability to be metabolized and excreted in the bile duct system by the hepatocellular tissue. New liver-specific agents (e.g. gadolinium ethoxybenzyl diethylenetriamine pentaacetic acid (Gd-EOB-DTPA), Primovist, or MultiHance) are metabolized and excreted into the biliary tree allowing acquisition of a late, pure parenchymal phase along with cholangiographic images. Of note is that the pure parenchymal phase after liver-specific agent injection correlates with the liver function.[16]

Focal liver lesions are characterized by low T1 signal intensity and variable intensity in T2-weighted sequences, cysts and hepatic haemangiomas are those with the higher signal intensity (Figure 6.5a–c). On contrast-enhanced MRI, the intensity signal in the different vascular phases reflects the vascularization of the lesion; the administration of hepato-specific contrast may be helpful in the detection of primary and secondary lesions.[17]

HCC is commonly characterized by a hypointense signal on T1-weighted phases and by an hyperintense signal on T2-weighted

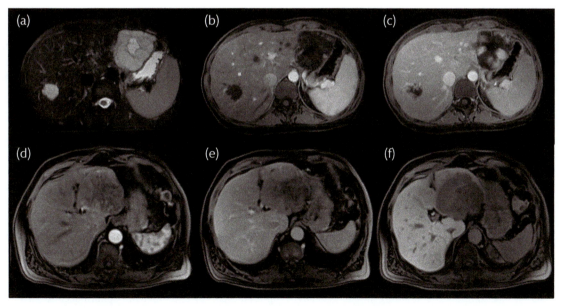

Figure 6.5 (a–c) MRI in a patient with hepatic haemangiomas in segments 2–3 and in segment 8. The lesions appear hyperintense in T2-weighted images (a) and show a typical progressively centripetal enhanced in T1-weighted contrast-enhanced arterial (b) and portal (c) phases. (d–f) MRI scan in a patient with a hepatocellular carcinoma located in the left lobe of the liver. The lesion is iso-hypointense in contrast-enhanced, T1-weighted, arterial phase (d) with the hyperenhanced tumoural capsule clearly visible. In portal phase (e), the lesion appears hypointense with a typical 'mosaic' pattern and in the late hepato-specific parenchymal phase (f), is clearly hypointense.

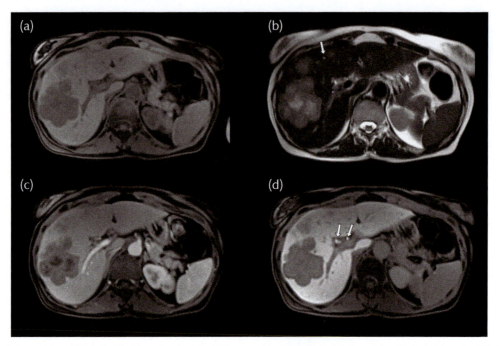

Figure 6.6 MRI study in a patient with colorectal liver metastases. Lesions appear hypodense in T1-weighted phase (a) and mildly hyperintense in T2-weighted images (b), where a tiny cyst lateral to the lesion in segment 4 is clearly visible (arrow). After contrast administration (c), the lesions appear hypointense with a mild peripheral contrast enhancement and a necrotic hypointense core. The late hepato-specific phase (d) allows the lesion to be visualized more clearly. The metabolized and biliary excreted contrast agent is clearly visible in the biliary tract (arrows).

phases. After contrast administration, it shows arterial hyperenhancement with a delayed dynamic phase washout; the signal intensity may be variable on contrast-enhanced MRI (Figure 6.5d–f). Intrahepatic cholangiocarcinomas are characterized by a high-intensity signal in T2-weighted phases and appear morphologically as lobulated lesions inducing capsular retraction when superficially located. After contrast administration, they show centripetal wash-in with peripheral enhancement. Concerning secondary liver malignancies, in general, liver metastases are characterized by a mild hypointense signal on T1-weighted images and a mild hyperintense signal on T2-weighted images. After contrast administration, their behaviour follows their vascularity as detailed in the previous section concerning CT (Figure 6.6).

Staging of colorectal liver metastases has improved after the introduction of Gd-EOB-DTPA and diffusion-weighted imaging. Indeed, higher sensitivity in detecting small lesions in the liver and particularly in confirming the disappearance of some metastases after systemic treatment has been shown for both MRI modalities.[18] Diffusion-weighted imaging adds the possibility of improving extrahepatic staging such as identifying lymph node involvement.[19]

Nuclear medicine

The main role of nuclear medicine imaging is in the detection of disease localization with the aid of a radiopharmaceutical agent. This agent is a radioactive compound containing an energetically unstable atom (radionuclide) that emits energy in the form of radiation when it reaches a lower-energy and more stable state. This emitted radiation can then be detected for diagnostic purposes or used for therapy.

Each radiopharmaceutical has its own peculiar pharmacokinetic properties that define its body distribution, in both normal and pathological tissues, and elimination. In the study and treatment of hepatobiliary diseases, radiopharmaceuticals and nuclear medicine application are typically used in the detection and staging of malignancies, in the evaluation of organ function, and in treatment by radioembolization. The two main techniques used in diagnostic nuclear medicine imaging are scintigraphy and positron emission tomography (PET). In scintigraphy, the radiation emitted by the radionuclide is captured by external detectors, the gamma cameras, and elaborated to form two-dimensional images with a process that resembles the acquisition of X-ray images. In PET studies, the information is acquired by multiple gamma cameras that detect pairs of emitted gamma rays and used to reconstruct three-dimensional images. These images are then linked and overlapped with a simultaneously performed unenhanced CT examination (PET-CT) in order to provide better tissue definition.

Concerning liver malignancies, PET-CT is usually performed using fluorodeoxyglucose marked with fluorine-18 as the radiopharmaceutical agent (^{18}F-FDG). Tumoral tissues tend to accumulate FDG more than non-neoplastic tissue and starting from this difference, PET-CT images are reconstructed (Figure 6.7a,b). One limitation of this agent is that brain tissue has a glucose-dependent metabolism, therefore limiting the capability of detection of tumoral localization. For the study of HCC, ^{18}F-FDG has demonstrated suboptimal accuracy and other radiopharmaceutical agents have been proposed and tested: ^{18}F-choline has shown a higher sensitivity in both newly diagnosed and recurrent HCC.[20–22] The biological rationale of the use of marked choline as a radiopharmaceutical agent is the reported higher activity of the key enzyme choline kinase

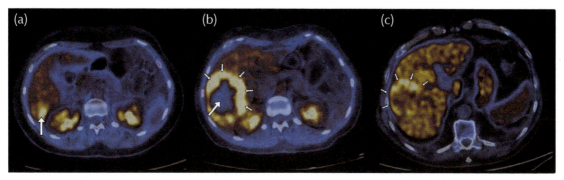

Figure 6.7 (a, b) ^{18}F-FDG PET-CT scan of a patient with multiple colorectal liver metastases. Two locations of pathological accumulation of the radiopharmaceutical agent are clearly visible: a smaller lesion is located in the inferior part of segment 6 (a), while a bigger one is visible cranially (b). The bigger lesion is characterized by a viable, metabolically active, peripheral tissue and a necrotic core that shows no sign of metabolic activity. The accumulation of the radiopharmaceutical agent visible in the urinary tract is due to the excretion of the radiopharmaceutical agent and is not pathological. (c) ^{11}C-Choline PET-CT scan of a patient with HCC. The lesion is located in the right hemiliver and presents a peripheral viable, metabolically active, tissue (arrows) and a central, metabolically inactive, necrotic core.

in HCC tumoral cells compared to background liver parenchyma (Figure 6.7c).[23]

The role of FDG-PET is not limited to initial diagnosis and staging and it may be useful in re-staging and in the evaluation of tumoral response after treatment. For this purpose, it is important to assess changes in tumour avidity for FDG or other radiopharmaceutical agents by the comparison of an examination performed before therapy with that performed after therapy.

Angiography

X-ray angiography is widely used as a diagnostic and interventional tool for procedures around and inside the liver.[24] Using iodinated contrast, angiography provides real-time visualization of vessels and bile ducts (percutaneous cholangiography[25]) and can be used to highlight tumours and biliary disease, as well as to advance guidewires, catheters, and different devices.

Biliary drainage

Obstructive jaundice can be caused by malignant biliary stenosis; it can also be due to biliary lithiasis or inflammatory disease. The role of interventional radiology is to restore biliary flow towards the duodenum, preferably using percutaneous transhepatic internal–external drainage (PTBD). PTBD has been used for jaundice relief since the 1970s and is considered a safe and effective approach.[26] Using a combined ultrasound and fluoroscopic approach, the operator is able to puncture a peripheral bile duct (e.g. in the sixth segment) with a small 18-gauge coaxial needle and to inject contrast to opacify the biliary tree (Figure 6.8). Then, access to the biliary bifurcation and to the duodenum is negotiated using a hydrophilic guidewire; an 8-French silicon multi-hole catheter with a pigtail tip is placed across the Vaterian sphincter. Similar procedures can be performed in the presence of a biliodigestive anastomosis.[27]

After biliary drainage, the patient should be hospitalized and monitored for sepsis and vital signs. Mild haemobilia can occur in up to 16% of cases and usually resolves within 24–48 hours.[28]

Venous bleeding occurs when the catheter crosses a branch of the hepatic or portal vein. Intermittent dark blood is often noted in the drainage bag; further cholangiography may be performed to confirm the diagnosis. Catheter repositioning is usually sufficient to move the catheter holes away from the parenchyma and inside the biliary tree. Some cases may require catheter upsizing.

Arterial bleeding occurs when fresh red blood is noted in the drain bag or around the catheter entry site. This is rarely a life-threatening situation and may frequently be caused by a pseudoaneurysm formed along the course of the catheter. Diagnostic angiography from the hepatic artery should be performed to evaluate any liver arterial bleeding, while the drainage catheter is still in place. If no active extravasation is seen, the catheter should be removed and the angiography repeated. Bleeding may be treated with embolization (see 'Emergency bleeding').

Transarterial embolization/chemoembolization

Liver tumours can be aggressively treated with transarterial embolization, with or without the addition of intra-arterial chemotherapy (transarterial chemoembolization).[29] Chemoembolization and bland embolization are the mainstays of treatment for multifocal, unresectable hepatocarcinomas,[30] but can also be performed for metastases of neuroendocrine and colorectal tumours.

Ultrasound-guided retrograde puncture of the right common femoral artery is the preferred access route. Then, under fluoroscopic guidance, a diagnostic catheter is placed in the coeliac trunk and diagnostic angiography is performed during injection of 20–25 mL of iodinated contrast to confirm the tumour's location and to plan the navigation route (Figure 6.9). In this setting, cone-beam CT and its derived three-dimensional reconstruction map can facilitate the understanding of vascular anatomy and reduce procedural time. A coaxial microcatheter is then advanced as close as possible to the tumour feeders. If transarterial embolization is the chosen approach, an embolizing agent such as small microspheres (e.g. polyvinyl alcohol, sodium polymethacrylate) is deployed to achieve the maximum ischaemic damage, relying on the tumour's almost exclusive arterial supply; when transarterial chemoembolization is performed, a chemotherapeutic drug (e.g. doxorubicin) is mixed with ethiodized oil or charged into small beads and then deployed in the target area, to induce cytotoxicity.

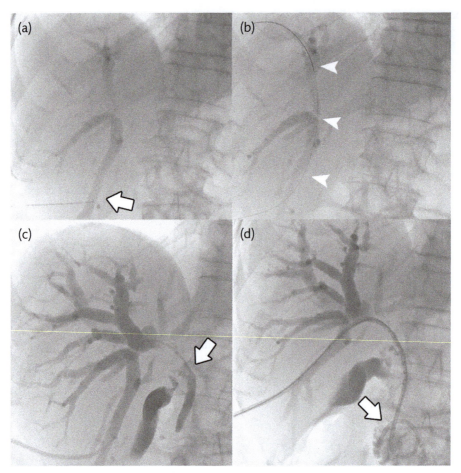

Figure 6.8 A 73-year-old man affected by hilar cholangiocarcinoma causing biliary obstruction. (a) After ultrasound-guided puncture, an 18-gauge Chiba needle is correctly positioned inside the biliary duct of the sixth liver segment (arrow). Contrast injection highlights the biliary ducts. (b) A 0.018-inch stiff guidewire (arrowheads) is advanced through the sixth and eighth segment biliary ducts to provide support for larger catheters. (c) After exchanging coaxial catheters, the main biliary duct is negotiated and an angiographic catheter is advanced in the choledocus (arrow) (d). A multi-hole 10-French pigtail catheter is finally positioned in the duodenum, restoring the normal biliary flow.

Emergency bleeding

X-ray angiography is an essential tool to perform emergency embolization in visceral bleeding, which in the liver may occur after a traumatic injury, or because of tumoral rupture. In both cases, the procedure is technically very similar to that previously detailed for transarterial embolization. It yields a very high success rate and is considered life-saving.[31]

Pre-procedural abdominal angio-CT is helpful to detect the exact site of bleeding and to speed up the procedure, thus reducing blood loss. Liquid embolic agents, such as *n*-butyl-cyanoacrylate or

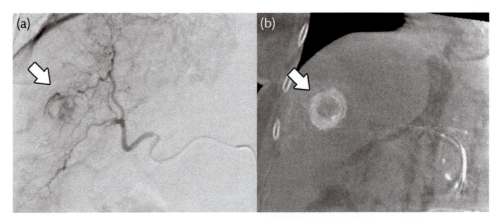

Figure 6.9 A 79-year-old woman undergoing transarterial embolization for HCC raised in a cirrhotic liver. Selective X-ray angiography of the right hepatic artery using a 1.8-French microcatheter shows an ill-defined hypervascular nodule in the eighth liver segment (a). The HCC nodule is better defined by cone-beam CT during intra-arterial contrast injection from the same stance (b).

ethylene vinyl alcohol, should be preferred in this setting because of the numerous arterial anastomoses typical of the liver architecture which are likely to reperfuse the bleeding site if proximal embolization (e.g. with metallic coils) is performed.

Complications include ischaemia and bilomas and have acceptable rates considering the quickness and minimal invasiveness of this intervention that allow stabilization of complex liver injuries.

Recent innovations

In the planning of a surgical strategy for patients undergoing liver resection, liver volumetric assessment and, more recently, liver three-dimensional reconstruction, represent a crucial step (Figure 6.10). In most cases the imaging modality used for the evaluation and reconstruction is CT, but reconstruction based on MRI is also possible. The most recent and advanced software available for three-dimensional reconstruction allows the surgeon to perform virtual preoperative reconstruction of the planned operation in order to assess the future remnant liver, even in complex surgical procedures. The 'virtual' resection can also be overlapped on the source imaging which, in turn, can be synchronized with the ultrasound machine in real time during the operation.

Another very recent application in the field of radiology worthy to be reported is represented by radiomics, a process that allows the extraction of large amounts quantitative features from medical images that can be subsequently elaborated and analysed. This process can be carried out starting from each of the different imaging modalities (US, CT, PET-CT, and MRI) and includes shape and volume characteristics and features of both the histogram of the image and the textural analysis of hepatic parenchyma, tumoral tissue, or tumour–parenchyma interface.[32] Radiomics has the potential to uncover disease features that cannot be appreciated by the naked eye which have diagnostic and prognostic significance.

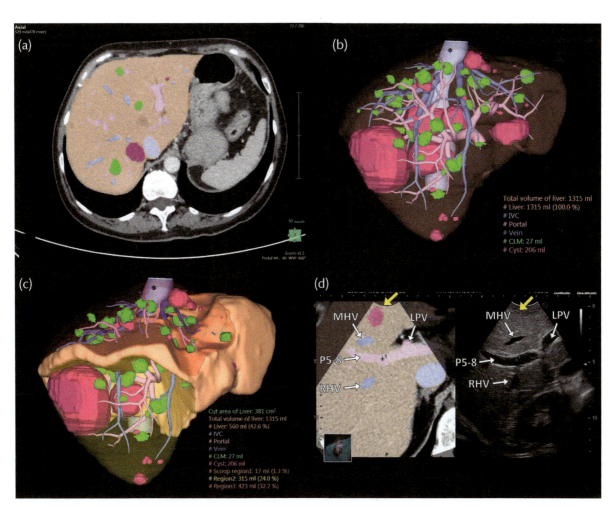

Figure 6.10 Three-dimensional reconstruction of the liver using Fujifilm SYNAPSE 3D software in a patient with multiple bi-lobar liver metastases and multiple liver cysts. Starting from the CT scan, liver parenchyma, portal system, hepatic veins, and focal lesion (both cysts, in purple, and metastases, in green) are recognized and highlighted (a). The software then provides a three-dimensional reconstruction of the liver parenchyma (b) and reports the volume of each of the reconstructed structures. The surgeon can then perform a virtual resection of the liver (c) with an estimation of the future liver remnant. The virtually planned operation can be then overlapped with the image of the CT scan, and subsequently synchronized with the IOUS image during the operation. Moreover, the three-dimensional reconstruction and synchronization with the IOUS can be performed on the pre-chemotherapy images in order to localize 'disappeared' lesions. In (d), a 'disappeared' lesion in S4 in a patient with multiple colorectal liver metastases, not visible with IOUS, is clearly localized (yellow arrow, lesion is marked in purple). LPV, left portal vein; MHV, middle hepatic vein; P5–8, right anterior portal branch; RHV, right hepatic vein.

REFERENCES

1. Brannigan M, Burns PN, Wilson SR. Blood flow patterns in focal liver lesions at microbubble-enhanced US. *Radiographics.* 2004;**24**(4):921–935.
2. Torzilli G, Montorsi M, Donadon M, et al. 'Radical but conservative' is the main goal for ultrasonography-guided liver resection: prospective validation of this approach. *J Am Coll Surg.* 2005;**201**(4):517–528.
3. Torzilli G, Vigano L, Gatti A, et al. Twelve-year experience of 'radical but conservative' liver surgery for colorectal metastases: impact on surgical practice and oncologic efficacy. *HPB (Oxford).* 2017;**19**(9):775–784.
4. Torzilli G, Procopio F, Botea F, et al. One-stage ultrasonographically guided hepatectomy for multiple bilobar colorectal metastases: a feasible and effective alternative to the 2-stage approach. *Surgery.* 2009;**146**(1):60–71.
5. Torzilli G, Procopio F, Costa G. Resection guidance. In: Torzilli G, ed. *Ultrasound-Guided Liver Surgery: An Atlas.* Milan: Springer-Verlag; 2014: 117–168.
6. Torzilli G. IOUS+R1vasc+CV=∞ A non-sense formula or a hepatectomies multiplier? *Surg Oncol.* 2020;**33**:193–195.
7. Torzilli G, Costa G, Botea F. Exploring the liver by ultrasound along its anatomy. In: Torzilli G, ed. *Ultrasound-Guided Liver Surgery: An Atlas.* Milan: Springer-Verlag; 2014: 25–42.
8. Makuuchi M, Hasegawa H, Yamazaki S. Ultrasonically guided subsegmentectomy. *Surg Gynecol Obstet.* 1985;**161**(4):346–350.
9. Torzilli G, Makuuchi M. Ultrasound-guided finger compression in liver subsegmentectomy for hepatocellular carcinoma. *Surg Endosc.* 2004;**18**(1):136–139.
10. Torzilli G, Del Fabbro D, Olivari N, et al. Contrast-enhanced ultrasonography during liver surgery. *Br J Surg.* 2004;**91**(9):1165–1167.
11. Torzilli G, Procopio F, Palmisano A. Intraoperative cholangio in the study of the biliary tree. In: Torzilli G, ed. *Ultrasound-Guided Liver Surgery: An Atlas.* Milano: Springer-Verlag; 2014: 169–182.
12. Shamsi K, De Schepper A, Degryse H, et al. Focal nodular hyperplasia of the liver: radiologic findings. *Abdom Imaging.* 1993;**18**(1):32–38.
13. Stevens WR, Gulino SP, Batts KP, et al. Mosaic pattern of hepatocellular carcinoma: histologic basis for a characteristic CT appearance. *J Comp Assist Tomogr.* 1996;**20**(3):337–342.
14. Kim SA, Lee JM, Lee KB, et al. Intrahepatic mass-forming cholangiocarcinomas: enhancement patterns at multiphasic CT, with special emphasis on arterial enhancement pattern—correlation with clinicopathologic findings. *Radiology.* 2011;**260**(1):148–157.
15. Feydy A, Vilgrain V, Denys A, et al. Helical CT assessment in hilar cholangiocarcinoma: correlation with surgical and pathologic findings. *AJR Am J Roentgenol.* 1999;**172**(1):73–77.
16. Zhang W, Wang X, Miao Y, et al. Liver function correlates with liver-to-portal vein contrast ratio during the hepatobiliary phase with Gd-EOB-DTPA-enhanced MR at 3 Tesla. *Abdom Radiol (N Y).* 2018;**43**(9):2262–2269.
17. Lafaro KJ, Roumanis P, Demirjian AN, et al. Gd-EOB-DTPA-enhanced MRI for detection of liver metastases from colorectal cancer: a surgeon's perspective! *Int J Hepatol.* 2013;**2013**:572307.
18. Macera A, Lario C, Petracchini M, et al. Staging of colorectal liver metastases after preoperative chemotherapy. Diffusion-weighted imaging in combination with Gd-EOB-DTPA MRI sequences increases sensitivity and diagnostic accuracy. *Eur Radiol.* 2013;**23**(3):739–747.
19. Bonifacio C, Viganò L, Felisaz P, et al. Diffusion-weighted imaging and loco-regional N staging of patients with colorectal liver metastases. *Eur J Surg Oncology.* 2019;**45**(3):347–352.
20. Lanza E, Donadon M, Felisaz P, et al. Refining the management of patients with hepatocellular carcinoma integrating 11C-choline PET/CT scan into the multidisciplinary team discussion. *Nucl Med Commun.* 2017;**38**(10):826–836.
21. Lopci E, Torzilli G, Poretti D, et al. Diagnostic accuracy of 11C-choline PET/CT in comparison with CT and/or MRI in patients with hepatocellular carcinoma. *Eur J Nucl Med Mol Imaging.* 2015;**42**(9):1399–1407.
22. Talbot JN, Gutman F, Fartoux L, et al. PET/CT in patients with hepatocellular carcinoma using [(18)F]fluorocholine: preliminary comparison with [(18)F]FDG PET/CT. *Eur Nucl J Med Mol Imaging.* 2006;**33**(11):1285–1289.
23. Kuang Y, Salem N, Tian H, et al. Imaging lipid synthesis in hepatocellular carcinoma with [methyl-11C]choline: correlation with in vivo metabolic studies. *J Nucl Med.* 2011;**52**(1):98–106.
24. Dittman W. Hepatic angiography. *Semin Liver Dis.* 1982;**2**(1):41–48.
25. Atkinson M, Happey MG, Smiddy FG. Percutaneous transhepatic cholangiography. *Gut.* 1960;**1**(4):357–365.
26. Covey AM, Brown KT. Percutaneous transhepatic biliary drainage. *Techn Vasc Interv Radiol.* 2008;**11**(1):14–20.
27. Okhotnikov OI, Yakovleva MV, Grigoriev SN. Interventional radiology in treatment of biliodigestive anastomoses strictures. *Khirurgiia.* 2016;**6**:37–42.
28. Kothaj P, Okapec S, Kúdelová A. Complications after percutaneous transhepatic drainage of the biliary tract. *Rozh Chir.* 2014;**93**(5):247–254.
29. Lanza E, Muglia R, Bolengo I, et al. Survival analysis of 230 patients with unresectable hepatocellular carcinoma treated with bland transarterial embolization. *PLoS One.* 2020;**15**(1):e0227711.
30. Lanza E, Donadon M, Poretti D, et al. Transarterial therapies for hepatocellular carcinoma. *Liver Cancer.* 2016;**6**(1):27–33.
31. Virdis F, Reccia I, Di Saverio S, et al. Clinical outcomes of primary arterial embolization in severe hepatic trauma: a systematic review. *Diagn Interv Imaging.* 2019;**100**(2):65–75.
32. Rizzo S, Botta F, Raimondi S, et al. Radiomics: the facts and the challenges of image analysis. *Eur Radiol Exp.* 2018;**2**(1):36.

7

Bacterial and parasitic infections of the liver

Chandan Kumar Kedarisetty, Mayank Jain, Thamarai S. Selvan, Varanasi Y. Bhargav, and Jayanthi Venkataraman

Introduction

The reticuloendothelial system plays an important defensive role against invasive organisms and the liver constitutes almost one-third of the mass of the reticuloendothelial system. It is therefore not uncommon to encounter bacterial and parasitic infections of the liver. Bacterial infections of the liver manifest as acute bacterial hepatitis, granulomatous liver disease, or liver abscess (pyogenic). Constitutional symptoms like malaise, fever, arthralgia, and anorexia are common in bacterial infections with elevations of aminotransferases. Some of the rare bacterial infections, such as Whipple's disease and *Bartonella* infection, which were not previously heard of in day-to-day clinical practice now seem to infect patients who are immunosuppressed, such as post-liver transplantation patients.

Several parasites have a predilection for the liver, with humans being incidental hosts on most occasions. Parasites residing in the biliary system often predispose patients to obstructive jaundice, secondary biliary cirrhosis, and cholangiocarcinoma. This chapter briefly outlines the clinical presentation, diagnosis, and impact of common and rare bacterial infections and parasitic infestations of the liver.

Bacterial infections

Pyogenic liver abscess

A liver abscess is the result of invasion and multiplication of microorganisms and occurs when microbes either enter directly from mucosal injury in the gastrointestinal tract through the blood vessels or via an infected biliary ductal system.[1] Other sources of infection that constitute less than 1% of cases are infections of hepatic cysts, post-traumatic injury, or post-transarterial chemoembolization for hepatocellular carcinoma. Most liver abscesses occur in the right lobe, in a ratio of 2:1, largely due to streamlining of blood to the right lobe of the liver via the relatively linear right portal vein, larger liver mass, and extensive biliary canalicular network.[2]

Patients present with right upper quadrant pain, fever with chills, pleuritic pain, cough, or in a state of shock due to septicaemia, leucocytosis, anaemia, and hypoalbuminaemia with abnormal liver biochemistry. Ultrasonographic examination of the abdomen is the initial screening modality. Computed tomography (CT) confirms the diagnosis, showing a typical rim enhancement (Figure 7.1). A pyogenic abscess is often polymicrobial in origin.[3,4] *Klebsiella pneumoniae* and *Escherichia coli* are the common pathogens. In biliary infection, Enterobacteriaceae are common; anaerobic species include *Bacteroides* spp., *Fusobacterium* spp., and microaerophilic and anaerobic streptococci.

Management is by ultrasound or CT-guided drainage of large abscesses, in conjunction with appropriate broad-spectrum antibiotics. An obstructed biliary system is drained by endoscopic retrograde cholangiopancreatography (ERCP) by placing internal biliary stents or a nasobiliary tube. The mortality is high in patients with jaundice, complicated/multiple abscesses leucocytosis, hypoalbuminaemia, and septic shock.

Brucellosis

This is a systemic febrile illness caused by *Brucella melitensis*. Its prevalence in India ranges between 3% and 8%. Exposure to domestic animals is the usual mode of transmission. The incubation period varies from few days to several months. Majority of patients have non-specific constitutional symptoms with hepatomegaly in 20–40%, elevations in aminotransferases in one-quarter, cholestatic jaundice in two-thirds, and liver abscesses. Histologically, granulomas are seen within the portal tract with cellular infiltration of the liver parenchyma and portal spaces, parenchymal damage, Kupffer cell hyperplasia, and, in the late stages, liver fibrosis and cirrhosis.[5–7] Blood culture is the gold standard for diagnosis with a higher yield in bone marrow culture. Enzyme-Linked Immunosorbent Assay (ELISA) and polymerase chain reaction (PCR) using blood and tissue are highly sensitive and specific. The bacteria respond to doxycycline 200 mg daily for 6 weeks in combination with either rifampin 600–900 mg daily for 6 weeks or intramuscular streptomycin 1 g daily for 2 weeks.

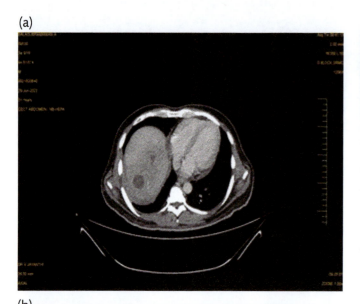
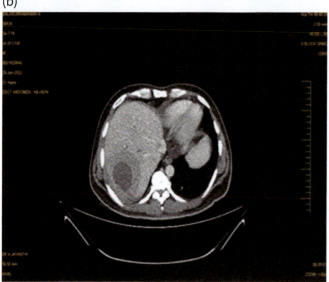

Figure 7.1 CECT scan of the abdomen showing a liver abscess with classical rim enhancement.

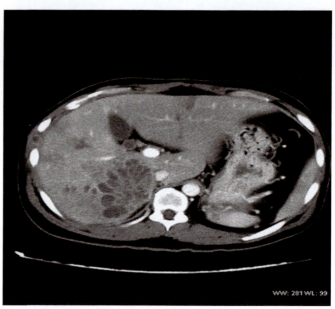

Figure 7.2 CECT scan showing hypodense, cavitary lesions with honeycomb pattern in liver and spleen in a patient with melioidosis. Reproduced with permission from Jain M, Patil V, Varghese J, et al. Meliodosis in cirrhosis of liver—a case series. *Gastroenterol Hepatol Int J.* 2016;1:000112.

Melioidosis

The bacterium *Burkholderia pseudomallei* is found in contaminated water and soil and causes a suppurative chronic multisystem infection with a predilection for the liver and spleen. Patients have a wide range of constitutional symptoms. A liver abscess is an important complication, which can be single, large with a honeycomb appearance or consist of several micro-abscesses (Figure 7.2). Gram staining and culture confirm the diagnosis.[8–10] An associated brain abscess, prostatic involvement, and septic arthritis is not uncommon.[10] Large abscesses require drainage along with intravenous ceftazidime 6- to 8-hourly for 10–14 days, followed by trimethoprim–sulfamethoxazole twice a day or amoxicillin/clavulanic acid, 8-hourly for 3–6 months.

Listeriosis

Listeriosis is caused by eating food contaminated with the bacterium *Listeria monocytogenes* and manifests in immunosuppressed individuals. Mild forms present as gastroenteritis and invasive forms manifest with neurological symptoms, or focal infections in the chest, abdomen, or arthritis. A liver abscess is common and may be solitary or multiple. Diffuse or granulomatous hepatitis has also been reported.[11] Diagnosis is by isolation of the bacterium in the tissue or body fluid. Invasive forms require parenteral antibiotics based on the sensitivity.

Hepatic actinomycosis

Hepatic actinomycosis is caused by the Gram-positive bacilli *Actinomyces israeli*. The liver is involved in 15% of cases and by contiguous haematogenous spread via the portal vein. The cause remains unknown in 80% and is polymicrobial in a third of cases.[12] Symptoms are often non-specific. Contrast-enhanced computed tomography (CECT) of the abdomen shows a typical solitary hypodense lesion (hyperintense on T2 magnetic resonance imaging) in two-thirds of patients, often in the right lobe of the liver (Figure 7.3). Documentation of basophilic filament aggregates and yellow 'sulphur' granules is confirmatory. Drainage of abscess in combination with any penicillin derivative—clindamycin or tetracycline for 3–6 months is the standard of care. The overall mortality is low.[13]

Acute bacterial hepatitis

Typhoid fever

Salmonella enterica serotype typhi is the causative agent of typhoid fever. Patients present with intermittent fever, headache, right lower quadrant abdominal pain and headache, relative bradycardia, rose spots on the chest and abdomen, erythematous papules (5–30%), and hepatosplenomegaly. Jaundice (0.4–26%)[14] and intestinal perforation are rare (1–3%). There is leucopenia and elevation of transaminases, serum bilirubin, and serum alkaline phosphatase (SAP). A positive blood culture is diagnostic (60–80%). Fluoroquinolones are the recommended treatment.

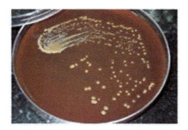
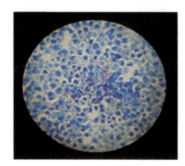
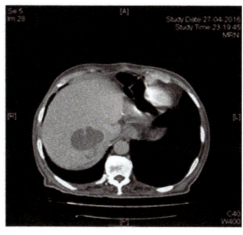

Figure 7.3 CECT image showing a 6.2 × 6 × 5.9 cm multiloculated hypodense collection with perilesional oedema; modified acid-fast stain was positive. Culture revealed *Nocardia*.
Reproduced with permission from Hanchnale P, Jain M, Varghese J, Venkataraman J, Rela M: Nocardia liver abscess post liver transplantation—a rare presentation. *Transplant Infectious Disease* 02/2017; doi:10.1111/tid.12670

Leptospirosis

Leptospirosis is caused by bacteria of the genus *Leptospira*. There is an initial acute phase followed by an immune phase. Liver dysfunction varies from mild to severe. *L icterohemorrhagica* is responsible for Weil's disease which occurs within a week of the clinical onset and lasts for more than a month.[15] It is characterized by deep jaundice, renal failure, and haemorrhage.[15,16] The liver is large and tender; the raised bilirubin and transaminase levels[17–19] are secondary to liver cell necrosis, intrahepatic cholestasis, and absorption of tissue haemorrhage. Death due to hepatic failure is rare.[16] One interesting study reported jaundice to be a predictor of severity in leptospirosis.[18] Penicillin is the drug of choice.

Granulomatous bacterial infection

There is a significant overlap of acute bacterial hepatitis (early stages) with granulomas in long-standing cases.[7]

Mycobacterium hepatic tuberculosis (TB)

Mycobacterium hepatic TB is an important extra-pulmonary manifestation of active TB. Pulmonary TB coexists with hepatic TB in 60–70% of cases. There has also been a sudden surge in hepatic TB with the increasing incidence of HIV/AIDS. There is essentially *miliary* and *localised* forms of hepatic TB.[20] The former accounts for 50–80% of cases[21] and is a result of haematogenous spread from the lung; the local variety is a consequence of spread from a focus in the gut and localizes around the portal tract, in the absence of a pulmonary focus.[22] There is a rise in SAP and gamma glutamyl transferase levels. CECT of the abdomen shows solitary or multiple lesions, mimicking a hepatoma or a liver abscess. Hepatic TB abscesses and tuberculomas occur in less than 1% of cases of TB; caseating granulomas are seen in 50–80%.[23] The detection rate of acid-fast bacilli on smear examination (0–45%) and culture are low (10–60%). Tissue PCR for *Mycobacterium* TB has a higher sensitivity and specificity.

The standard four-drug antituberculous treatment regimen is recommended for at least a year.

Syphilitic hepatitis

Syphilis is caused by the bacterium *Treponema pallidum*. In India, its prevalence along with other sexually transmitted infections like gonorrhoea, chlamydia, and trichomoniasis ranges from 0% to 3.9%. The three stages of syphilis are primary (chancre), a second stage of typical rash, and the third/tertiary stage (neurosyphilis, cardiovascular syphilis, or gummatous syphilis), which is the result of a cellular hypersensitivity reaction. The liver is rarely involved and is only suspected to be infected when there is an elevation of SAP levels. Syphilitic hepatitis occurs in the early stages of the disease, often in HIV-positive men.[24] Co-infection with hepatitis B and C has also been documented.[25]

Patients have hepatosplenomegaly with raised serum levels of SAP, gamma glutamyl transferase, and transaminases. Histology shows bile duct inflammatory changes, and at times granulomas.[26] Spirochaetes are seldom seen on liver histology. Parenteral penicillin is the treatment of choice for all stages of syphilis.

Whipple's disease

Whipple's disease is caused by the Gram-positive bacterium *Tropheryma whipplei*. The bacterium causes multisystem chronic disease (arthritis, diarrhoea) in an immunocompetent host. Liver involvement per se is uncommon. Three cases have been reported, following organ transplantation, with one case after a liver transplant.[27] Electron microscopy and *in situ* hybridization methods confirm the diagnosis. Girardin et al. diagnosed a case of hepatic epithelioid granuloma due to Whipple's disease in a 32-year-old male, with hepatomegaly after the patient presented with neurological symptoms.[28]

Cat scratch disease and peliosis (*Bartonella* infection)

Cat scratch disease is caused by *Bartonella henselae* (Gram negative), and is transmitted by the scratch or bite of a cat. Patients have a positive skin reaction, regional lymphadenopathy, and characteristic histology.[29] Hepatic bartonellosis occurs in 1–2% of cases and manifests with constitutional symptoms, tender hepatomegaly, necrotizing inflammatory granulomas on liver biopsy, and vascular tumours (peliosis).[30] *Bartonella* has been reported in a post-liver transplantation patient.[31] Immunohistochemical stains and molecular typing are confirmatory. Doxycycline and erythromycin are the recommended antibiotics.

Q fever

Q fever is a zoonotic infection caused by *Coxiella burnetii*, an intracellular Gram-negative coccobacillus. Cattle, goat, and sheep are the reservoirs. Cross-infection occurs by inhalation/ingestion or exposure to bacteria shed in the urine, faeces, or milk. Patients may be asymptomatic with mild elevations of transaminases (two to three times higher), or present with a flu-like illness, pneumonia, acute hepatitis,[32] or non-specific gastrointestinal tract symptoms. Lee et al.[33] reported typical fibrin ring, epithelioid, and necrotizing granulomas, with numerous eosinophils and multinucleated giant cells in liver specimens; hepatocyte necrosis is rare. Q fever has also been reported in the post-liver transplantation scenario.[34] A positive serology by indirect immunofluorescent assay confirms the diagnosis. Doxycycline is recommended for 14 days.

Parasitic liver diseases

The liver serves as a host organ for several parasites some of which are small and intracellular (e.g. *Plasmodium falciparum*) or extracellular (e.g. *Entamoeba histolytica*), or large (e.g. *Echinococcus*). Some have a reproductive capacity within the liver and others cause an injury to the host. Humans are incidental or accidental hosts. In an immunocompetent host, most parasitic infections adapt to the host and rarely cause severe symptoms. Some like schistosomiasis or echinococcosis are symptomatic and present with long-term sequelae.

Protozoal infections of the liver

Entamoeba histolytica and amoebic liver abscess (ALA)

There are two protozoal species, *Entamoeba dispar* (asymptomatic) and *E. histolytica*, that infect humans.[35] The latter is responsible for invasive disease. The clinical presentation includes amoebic dysentery (one-third) and extra-intestinal disease like an ALA and pulmonary, cardiac, and brain involvement.[36] ALA is seven to ten times more common in adult men, between 20 and 40 years of age.[37,38] Risk factors include low socioeconomic status and an immunosuppressed state.[39] It is rare in children.[40] ALA is a result of ascending infection via the portal venous system.[41] Clinical presentation is similar to a pyogenic liver abscess with leucocytosis, raised transaminases SAP. A large abscess can extend into the right lung or rupture into the peritoneal cavity (7%)[42]; a left liver lobe abscess can breach into the pericardium; rarely there is jaundice and a tender colonic mass (amoeboma).[43]

A chest X-ray shows an elevated right dome of diaphragm or a pleural effusion. On ultrasound examination the abscess is often single (70–80%), subcapsular, localized to the right lobe, isoechoic (solid abscess) in its early stage, and later hypoechoic. CECT and magnetic resonance imaging are confirmatory. Stool microscopy and PCR for amoebic antigen are rarely positive in patients with ALA.[44] Culture shows a polymicrobial profile.[39]

Definitive treatment includes tissue (metronidazole/tinidazole) and luminal (diloxanide furoate or paromomycin) agents with a cure rate of greater than 90%. When complicated, ultrasound or CT-guided drainage is recommended.[46,47] Resolution of ALA may take as long as 6–9 months on follow-up imaging.

Plasmodium falciparum and malarial hepatopathy

Malarial hepatopathy is characterized by high-grade fever (32–37 C), raised serum bilirubin (predominantly unconjugated), and transaminases (aspartate aminotransferase >alanine aminotransferase) in the absence of an inflammatory response within the liver. Most cases reported from Asian countries including India are due to *P. falciparum* infection.[48–50]

Pathologically, the maturing parasites induce formation of knobs on the surface of erythrocytes causing stickiness with adjacent red blood cells and endothelial cells resulting in occlusion of small blood vessels including portal venous radicles. The latter cause ischaemic injury to the hepatocytes and apoptosis.[51] Histologically, there is deposition of haemozoin, pigmentation in the Kupffer cells, reticuloendothelial hyperplasia, sinusoidal and portal infiltration, and cholestasis.[52] In the systemic circulation there is endotoxaemia and disseminated intravascular coagulopathy.

There has been a recent breakthrough in the understanding of the pathogenesis of malarial hepatopathy. *P. falciparum*, instead of infecting red blood cells after inoculation by the mosquito, reaches the liver and invades the hepatocytes and upregulates aquaporin3 (AQP3), resulting in rapid multiplication. These then invade the bloodstream to parasitize the red blood cells. Trials are ongoing with AQP3 inhibitors to treat the spread of falciparum infection.[53]

Clinically, patients are febrile with mild jaundice and hepatosplenomegaly.[54] There is also evidence of haemolysis. Severe infection results in altered sensorium and renal failure.[55] Treatment of malarial hepatopathy is essentially the management of the malarial infection.

Visceral leishmaniasis or black fever

Visceral leishmaniasis is caused by *Leishmania donovani* and transmitted by sandflies. The parasite after invasion, replicates within the host macrophages.[56] The incubation ranges from 2 to 6 months. The parasite has a predilection for the spleen, liver, and bone marrow. Patients present as fever of unknown origin, malaise, weight loss, moderate splenomegaly with or without a hepatomegaly, pancytopenia, and hypergammaglobulinaemia[57,58] with darkening of the skin.[59] In advanced cases, there can be signs of liver cell failure with jaundice and ascites. Bleeding gums or epistaxis is secondary to thrombocytopenia and liver cell failure. Rare presentations are chronic diarrhoea and malabsorption due to parasitosis of the small intestine.[60] Renal impairment is due to immune complex-mediated interstitial nephritis.[61] The diagnostic test is bone marrow culture and Giemsa-stained smear for intracellular (within macrophages) amastigotes (LD bodies).[62]

Molecular detection of parasite DNA using the PCR technique and serological testing (ELISA) for anti-leishmanial antibodies are confirmatory.

Drugs of choice include amphotericin B, pentavalent antimonial drugs, paromomycin, and miltefosine (the first oral drug for leishmaniasis).

Rare protozoal infections

Babesiois is a rare zoonotic tick-borne parasitic infection, common in certain regions of the USA. Its clinical presentation mimics falciform malarial fever. Symptoms begin a few weeks after exposure to a tick bite. Diagnosis is made on a peripheral blood smear examination. Classically an intra-erythrocytic organism is seen.[63] PCR is a sensitive test. Asymptomatic patients require no treatment. Intravenous clindamycin and quinine are reserved for severe infection.[64] Exchange transfusion is recommended for patients with severe parasitaemia (>10%), severe anaemia, and organ failure. Liver involvement is rare. Histology is similar to malarial infection.[65] Nassar et al. reported a case presenting as acute liver failure.[66]

Toxoplasmosis is caused by the protozoan *Toxoplasma gondii* and infects humans and animals. Typically, infection occurs after ingestion of raw or undercooked meat containing tissue cysts or from the environment. Most patients are asymptomatic; severity depends on immune status of the patient, parasite strain, and host species.[67–69] When acute, the course of the illness is usually benign and self-limited and consists of constitutional symptoms with maculopapular skin rash, hepatitis, and hepatosplenomegaly.[70] Granuloma and necrosis are seen on liver biopsy. An association with liver cirrhosis has also been reported.[71] Diagnosis is based on identification of immunoglobulin G or M antibodies to *T. gondii* (ELISA). The drug of choice is pyrimethamine in combination with sulphadiazine and leucovorin or clindamycin and leucovorin.

Echinococcosis

Echinococcosis is caused by a tapeworm *Echinococcus granulosus*. The definitive hosts are dogs, wolves, and foxes. Humans are intermediate hosts. The oncospheres in the small intestine enter the portal circulation to reach the liver where they mature to hydatid cysts. *E. granulosus* produces a single fluid-containing hepatic cyst with an expansive growth; *E. alveolaris* produces a multi-cystic form with an invasive property within the liver and to other organs. Patients may be asymptomatic or may complain of mild abdominal discomfort due to the size of the cyst.[72] Diagnosis is by serological tests (ELISA). Large cysts can rupture into the biliary tree when the pressure within the cyst exceeds 80 cmH$_2$O causing obstructive jaundice, cholangitis, and cholangitic liver abscess.[73,74] Ultrasound of the liver shows characteristic features (Gharbi classification).[74,75] On endoscopic ultrasound, floating cysts and membrane are typical.

Albendazole is given in combination with percutaneous aspiration and instillation of scolicidal agent ('PAIR'). Another alternative is surgery. ERCP is indicated for ruptured hydatid cysts in the biliary tree. The recommended dose of albendazole is 400 mg twice daily (≥60 kg body weight) or 15 mg/kg of body weight (for weight <60 kg) for 28 days with food.

Schistosomiasis

Schistosomiasis is caused by blood flukes of the genus *Schistosoma*. Acute forms present as a serum-like sickness (Katayama fever). Schistosomiasis may involve the liver early in the disease in about 30% of the patients (schistosomal hepatitis) or more commonly 5–10 years after the initial infection leading to periportal fibrosis and portal hypertension due to ova migration and development of hepatic granulomas followed by fibrosis.[76] Chronic forms present as non-cirrhotic portal fibrosis, characterized by massive splenomegaly and perisinusoidal portal hypertension; 20% of patients can progress to cirrhosis. Diagnosis is based on clinical findings and typical sonographic findings. Eosinophilia is present in 33–66% of patients. Serological assays, including ELISA, have a limited role. Praziquantel 40–60 mg/kg in divided doses for 1 day is the treatment of choice.

Toxocariasis (visceral larva migrans)

Human toxocariasis infection occurs by the accidental ingestion of embryonated eggs or larvae inhabiting dogs (*Toxocara canis*) or cats (*T. cati*). In humans it manifests as visceral and ocular larva migrans, neurotoxocariasis, and covert or common toxocariasis. Most infections are asymptomatic. Clinically overt infections are difficult to diagnose. Jain[77] reported a case of toxocariasis causing an eosinophilic abscess which resolved with albendazole (400 mg orally twice a day daily for 5 days) (Figure 7.4). Liver abscesses are often multiple, ill-defined, oval lesions that measure 1.0–1.5 cm in diameter and are best appreciated in the portal venous phase of contrast-enhanced CT and magnetic resonance imaging. Differential diagnoses include liver metastases, hepatocellular carcinoma, and granulomatous liver disease. Liver histology is diagnostic.[78]

Rare rodent-mediated hepatic parasitosis

Hepatic capillariasis is caused by the tissue-dwelling nematode *Capillaria hepatica*, essentially a zoonotic disease. Humans are incidental hosts and infection is acquired by ingesting food or water contaminated with infective eggs. The larva penetrates the intestinal wall and reaches the liver where it matures into an adult worm. It typically manifests as an acute hepatitis with hepatomegaly and fever with peripheral leucocytosis and eosinophilia. Rarely, there is a progression to liver failure as a result of heavy infestation. On histology, granulomas and hepatocyte necrosis are seen. Treatment is a combination of benzimidazoles and corticosteroids.[79]

Armillifer is an obligate parasite belonging to the Pentastomida subclass. Snakes are the definite hosts and humans are incidental hosts. The majority of infections occur after snake ingestion. Most patients are asymptomatic and incidentally suspected when there is a calcified parasite on imaging. In a systematic review of 40 patients, 50% had liver involvement.[80] Hepatic encephalopathy has also been reported. Other sites involved are the eyes, gut, peritoneum, and respiratory tract. An exact treatment protocol is yet to be reported.

The liver in biliary parasitosis

Several helminthic parasitic infestations in the biliary tract affect the liver during the parasite's life cycle.[81] These are more common in South East Asia and China and rarely seen in India. Humans

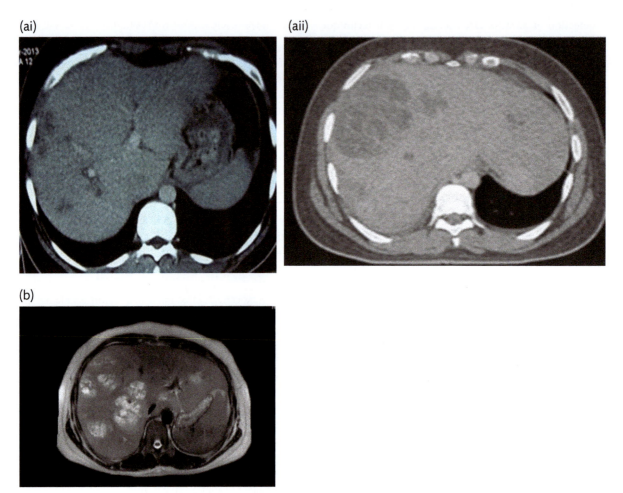

Figure 7.4 CECT (a) and MRI (b) showing an eosinophilic abscess in a patient with toxocariasis, and its response to albendazole.
Reproduced from Jain M. Liver involvement in visceral larva migrans. *Antiseptic*. 2018;115:37.

are invariably intermediate hosts. Parasites include adult worms of *Ascaris*, *Clonorchis sinensis*, *Opisthorchis felinues*, and *Fasciola hepatica* (Table 7.1). All these cause biliary obstruction and present with obstructive jaundice, recurrent pyogenic cholangitis, and occasionally liver abscess. Choledocholithiasis (brown pigment stones) and cholangiocarcinoma are two major complications. Diagnosis is usually by ultrasound, CECT of the abdomen, and endoscopic ultrasound. Therapeutic ERCP helps relieve symptoms in most patients.

Conclusion

The liver, with Kupffer cells in particular, is exposed to many systemic infectious pathogens and is either directly or indirectly (more often) involved in systemic viral, bacterial, parasitic, and fungal infections. While diagnosis is possible in most instances, a high index of suspicion is indicated for some of the less common pathogens. A good history and physical examination with appropriate diagnostic tests

Table 7.1 Hepatobiliary parasitosis: liver flukes and a rare protozoal infection

Parasite	Definite host	Intermediate host	Infective form	Liver pathology	Treatment	Dose
Ascaris	None	None	Embryonated eggs	Cholestatic jaundice	Albendazole	400 mg single dose
Clonorchis sinensis	Dog	Snail	Metacercaria	Portal and periportal fibrosis Secondary biliary cirrhosis	Praziquantel	25 mg/kg per day in three divided doses for 2–3 days
Opisthorchis felineus						
Fasciola hepatica	Sheep				Triclabendazole	10 mg/kg body weight in a single dose or repeated after 2weeks
Cryptosporidium				Secondary biliary cirrhosis due to sclerosing cholangitis	Nitazoxanide	500 mg twice a day for 3 days

like cultures and liver histology can confirm the diagnosis in most situations.

REFERENCES

1. Wong WM, Wong BCU, Hui CK, et al. Pyogenic liver abscess: retrospective analysis of 80 cases over a 10-year period. *J Gastroenterol Hepatol*. 2002;**17**(9):1001–1007.
2. Dutta A, Bandyopadhyay S. Management of liver abscess. *Med Update*. 2012;**22**:472–475.
3. Branum GD, Tyson GS, Branum MA, Meyers WC. Hepatic abscess. Changes in etiology, diagnosis, and management. *Ann Surg*. 1990;**212**(6):655–662.
4. Gyorffy EJ, Frey CF, SilvaJ Jr, McGahan J. Pyogenic liver abscess. Diagnostic and therapeutic strategies. *Ann Surg*. 1987;**206**:699–705.
5. Akritidis N, Tzivras M, Delladetsima I, et al. The liver in Brucellosis. *Clin Gastroenterol Hepatol*. 2007;**5**(9):1109–1112.
6. Ozturk-Engin D, Erdem H, Gencer S, et al. Liver involvement in patients with brucellosis: results of the Marmara study. *Eur J Clin Microbiol Infect Dis*. 2014;**33**:1253–1262.
7. Jain M, Varghese J, Venkataraman J. Hepatic granulomas: a clinician's perspective. *Indian J Clin Pract*. 2018;**28**:836–839.
8. Mukhopadhya A, Balaji V, Jesudason MV, et al. Isolated liver abscess in melioidosis. *Indian J Med Microbiol*. 2007;**25**(15):150–151.
9. Martin PF, TehCS, Casupang MA. Melioidosis: a rare cause of liver abscess. *Case Rep Hepatol*. 2016;**2016**:5910375.
10. Jain M, Patil V, Varghese J, et al. Melioidosis in cirrhosis of liver—a case series. *Gastroenterol Hepatol Int J*. 2016;**1**:000112.
11. Scholing M, Schneeberger PM, van den Dries P, et al. Clinical features of liver involvement in adult patients with listeriosis. Review of the literature. *Infection*. 2007;**35**(4):212–218.
12. Kanellopoulou T, Alexopoulou A, Tanouli MI, et al. Primary hepatic actinomycosis. *Am J Med Sci*. 2010;**339**(4):362–365.
13. Lakshmana Kumar YC, Javherani R, Malini A, Prasad SR. Primary hepatic actinomycosis. *Trans R Soc Trop Med Hyg*. 2005;**99**(11):868–870.
14. Ahmed A, Ahmed B. Jaundice in typhoid patients: differentiation from other common causes of fever and jaundice in the tropics. *Ann Afr Med*. 2010;**9**(3):135–140.
15. Levett P. Leptospirosis. *Clin Microbiol Rev*. 2001;**14**(2):296–326.
16. Vijayachari P, Sugunan AP, Shriram AN. Leptospirosis: an emerging global public health problem. *J Biosci*. 2008;**33**(4):557–569.
17. Deb Mandal M, Mandal S, Pal N. Is jaundice a prognosis of leptospirosis? *Asian Pacif J Trop Dis*. 2011;**1**:279–281.
18. Daher E, Lima R, Silva G Jr, et al. Clinical presentation of leptospirosis: a retrospective study of 201 patients in a metropolitan city of Brazil. *Braz J Infect Dis*. 2010;**14**(1):3–10.
19. Tailor P, Kapadia M, Modi K, Soni K. Study of routine biochemistry analytes in leptospirosis for evaluating organ and system specific involvement. Biochemistry analytes in leptospirosis for evaluating organ and system. *Natl J Integr Res Med*. 2014;**5**:45–47.
20. Chien RN, Lin PY, Liaw YF. Hepatic tuberculosis: comparison of miliary and local form. *Infection*. 1995;**23**(1):5–8.
21. Wang JY, Hsueh PR, Wang SK, et al. Disseminated tuberculosis: a 10-year experience in a medical center. *Medicine*. 2007;**86**:39–46.
22. Hersch C. Tuberculosis of the liver: a study of 200 cases. *S Afr Med J*. 1964;**38**:857–863.
23. Turhan N, Kurt M, Ozderin YO, Kurt OK. Hepatic granulomas: a clinicopathologic analysis of 86 cases. *Pathol Res Pract*. 2011;**207**(6):359–365.
24. Huang J, Lin S, Wan B, Zhu Y. A systematic literature review of syphilitic hepatitis in adults. *J Clin Transl Hepatol*. 2018;**6**(3):306–309.
25. Bhattar S, Aggarwal P, Sahani SK, Bhalla P. Co-infections and sero-prevalence of HIV, syphilis, hepatitis B and C infections in sexually transmitted infections clinic attendees of tertiary care hospital in north India. *J Res Health Sci*. 2016;**16**(3):162–165.
26. Young MF, Sanowski RA, Manne RA. Syphilitic hepatitis. *J Clin Gastroenterol*. 1992;**15**(2):174–176.
27. Vindigni SM, Taylor J, Quilter LAS, et al. Tropheryma whipplei infection (Whipple's disease) in a patient after liver transplantation. *Transpl Infect Dis*. 2016;**18**(4):617–624.
28. Girardin MFS, Zafrani ES, Chaumette MT, et al. Hepatic granulomas in Whipple's disease. *Gastroenterology*. 1984;**86**:753–756.
29. Hansmann Y, DeMartino S, Piemont Y, et al. Diagnosis of cat scratch disease with detection of Bartonella henselae by PCR: a study of patients with lymph node enlargement. *J Clin Microbiol*. 2005;**43**(8):3800–3806.
30. Kempf VA, Schaller M, Behrendt S, et al. Interaction of Bartonella henselae with endothelial cells results in rapid bacterial rRNA synthesis and replication. *Cell Microbiol*. 2000;**2**(5):431–441.
31. Bonatti H, Mendez J, Guerrero I, et al. Disseminated Bartonella infection following liver transplantation. *Transpl Int*. 2006;**19**(8):683–687.
32. Chang K, Yan JJ, Lee HC, et al. Acute hepatitis with or without jaundice: a predominant presentation of acute Q fever in southern Taiwan. *J Microbiol Immunol Infect*. 2004;**37**(2):103–108.
33. Lee M, Jang JJ, Kim YS, et al. Clinicopathologic features of Q fever patients with acute hepatitis. *Korean J Pathol*. 2012;**46**(1):10–14.
34. Petty LA, Te HS, Pursell K. A case of Q fever after liver transplantation. *Transpl Infect Dis*. 2017;**19**(5):e12737.
35. WHO/PAHO/UNESCO. A consultation of experts on amoebiasis. Mexico City, Mexico 28–29, 1997. *Epidemiol Bull*. 1997;**18**:13–14.
36. Haque R, Huston CD, Hughes M, et al. Amoebiasis. *N Engl J Med*. 2003;**348**(16):1565–1573.
37. Acuna-Soto R, Maguire JH, Wirth DF. Gender distribution in asymptomatic and invasive amebiasis. *Am J Gastroenterol*. 2000;**95**(5):1277–1283.
38. StanleySL Jr. Amoebiasis. *Lancet*. 2003;**361**(9362):1025–1034.
39. Singh A, Banerjee T, Kumar R, Shukla SK. Prevalence of cases of amebic liver abscess in a tertiary care centre in India: a study on risk factors, associated microflora and strain variation of Entamoeba histolytica. *PLoS One*. 2019;**14**:e0215774.
40. Jain M, Jain J, Gupta S. Amebic liver abscess in children—experience from Central India. *Indian J Gastroenterol*. 2016;**35**(3):248–249.
41. Aikat BK, Bhusnurmath SR, Pal AK, et al. The pathology and pathogenesis of fatal hepatic amebiasis-a study based on 79 autopsy cases. *Trans R Soc Trop Med Hyg*. 1979;**73**(2):188–192.
42. Adams EB, Macleod IN. I. Invasive amebiasis. Amebic dysentery and its complications. *Medicine (Baltimore)*. 1977;**56**(4):315–323.
43. Misra SP, Misra V, Dwivedi M. Ileocecal masses in patients with amoebic liver abscess: etiology and management. *World J Gastroenterol*. 2006;**12**(12):1933–1936.
44. Pritt BS, Clark CG. Amebiasis. *Mayo Clin Proc*. 2008;**83**(10):1154–1159.

45. Khanna S, Chaudhary D, Kumar A, Vij JC. Experience with aspiration in cases of amoebic liver abscess. *Eur J Clin Microbiol Infect Dis*. 2005;**24**(6):428–430.
46. Salata RA, Ravdin JI. The interaction of human neutrophils and Entamoeba histolytica increases cytopathogenicity for liver cell monolayers. *J Infect Dis*. 1986;**154**(1):19–26.
47. Ali WM, Ali I, Rizvi SAA, Rab AZ, Ahmed M. Recent trends in the epidemiology of liver abscess in western region of Uttar Pradesh: a retrospective study. *J Surg Anesth*. 2018;**2**:117.
48. Kochar DK, Singh P, Agarwal P, et al. Malarial hepatitis. *J Assoc Physicians India*. 2003;**51**:1069–1072.
49. Fazil A, Vernekar V, Gerian D, et al. Clinical profile and complication of malaria hepatopathy. *J Infect Public Health*. 2013;**6**(5):383–388.
50. Bhalla A, Suri V, Singh V. Malarial hepatopathy. *J Postgrad Med*. 2006;**52**(4):315–320.
51. Guha M, Kumar S, Dubey V, Maity P, Bandopadh U. Apoptosis in liver during malaria: role of oxidative stress and implication of mitochondrial pathway. *FASEB J*. 2006;**20**(8):1224–1226.
52. Chawla LS, Sidhu G, Sabharwal BD, Bhatia KL, Sood A. Jaundice in plasmodium falciparum. *J Assoc Physicians India*. 1989;**37**(6):390–391.
53. Posfai D, Sylvester K, Reddy A, et al. Plasmodium parasite exploits host aquaporin-3 during liver stage malaria infection. *PLoS Pathog*. 2018;**14**(5):e1007057.
54. Anand AC, Puri P. Jaundice in malaria. *J Gastroenterol Hepatol*. 2005;**20**(9):1322–1332.
55. Devarbhavi H, Alvares JF, Kumar KS. Severe falciparum malaria simulating fulminant hepatic failure. *Mayo Clin Proc*. 2005;**80**(3):355–358.
56. Bogdan C. Mechanisms and consequences of persistence of intracellular pathogens: leishmaniasis as an example. *Cell Microbiol*. 2008;**10**(6):1221–1234.
57. Jeronimo SMB, de QueirozSousa A, Pearson RD. Leishmaniasis. In: Guerrant RL, Walker DH, Weller PF, eds. *Tropical Infectious Diseases: Principles, Pathogens and Practice*, 3rd ed. Philadelphia, PA: Saunders Elsevier; 2011:696.
58. Sundar S, Rai M. Laboratory diagnosis of visceral leishmaniasis. *Clin Diagn Lab Immunol*. 2002;**9**(5):951–958.
59. Bern C, Joshi AB, Jha SN, et al. Factors associated with visceral leishmaniasis in Nepal: bed-net use is strongly protective. *Am J Trop Med Hyg*. 2000;**63**(3–4):184–188.
60. Baba CS, Makharia GK, Mathur P, et al. Chronic diarrhea and malabsorption caused by Leishmania donovani. *Indian J Gastroenterol*. 2006;**25**(6):309–310.
61. Verma N, Lal CS, Rabidas V, et al. Microalbuminuria and glomerular filtration rate in paediatric visceral leishmaniasis. *Biomed Res Int*. 2013;**2013**:498918.
62. Kager PA, Rees PH. Hematological investigations in visceral leishmaniasis. *Trop Geogr Med*. 1986;**38**(4):371–379.
63. Kjemtrup AM, Conrad PA. Human babesiosis: an emerging tick-borne disease. *Int J Parasitol*. 2000;**30**(12–13):1323–1337.
64. Sanchez E, Vannier E, Wormser GP, Hu LT. Diagnosis, treatment, and prevention of Lyme disease, human granulocytic anaplasmosis, and babesiosis: a review. *JAMA*. 2016;**315**(16):1767–1777.
65. Marathe A, Tripathi J, Handa V, Date V. Human babesiosis: a case report. *Indian J Med Microbial*. 2005;**23**(4):267–269.
66. Nassar Y, Richter S. Babesiosis presenting as acute liver failure. *Case Rep Gastroenterol*. 2017;**11**(3):769–773.
67. Montoya JG, Liesenfeld O. Toxoplasmosis. *Lancet*. 2004;**363**(9425):1965–1976.
68. Dawson D. Foodborne protozoan parasites. *Int J Food Microbiol*. 2005;**103**(2):207–227.
69. Dubey JP, Jones JL. Toxoplasma gondii infection in humans and animals in the United States. *Int J Parasitol*. 2008;**38**(11):1257–1278.
70. Demar M, Hommel D, Djossou F, et al. Acute toxoplasmoses in immunocompetent patients hospitalized in an intensive care unit in French Guiana. *Clin Microbiol Infect*. 2012;**18**(7):E221–E231.
71. Alvarado-Esquivel C, Torres-Berumen JL, Estrada-Martínez S, Liesenfeld O, Mercado-Suarez MF. Toxoplasma gondii infection and liver disease: a case–control study in a Northern Mexican Population. *Parasit Vectors*. 2011;**4**:75.
72. Amir Jahed AK, Fardin R, Farzad A, Bakshandeh K. Clinical echinococcosis. *Ann Surg*. 1975;**182**(5):541–546.
73. Dadoukis J, Gamvros O, Aletras H. Intrabiliary rupture of the hydatid cyst of the liver. *World J Surg*. 1984;**8**(5):786–790.
74. Al Karawi MA, Yasawy MI, Mohamed AE. Endoscopic management of biliary hydatid disease: report on six cases. *Endoscopy*. 1991;**23**(5):278–281.
75. Gharbi HA, Hassine W, Brauner MW. Ultrasound examination of the hydatid liver. *Radiology*. 1981;**139**(2):459–463.
76. Gryseels B, Polman K, Clerinx J, Kestens L. Human schistosomiasis. *Lancet*. 2006;**368**(9541):1106–1118.
77. Jain M. Liver involvement in visceral larva migrans. *Antiseptic*. 2018;**115**:37.
78. Jain M, Jain A, Bundiwal A, Ware S, Sircar S, Gupta A. A rare case of hepatic toxocariasis. *J Clin Expt Hepatol*. 2014;**4**:S66–S67.
79. Sawamura R, Fernandez MIM, Peres LC, et al. Hepatic capillariasis in children: report of 3 cases in Brazil. *Am J Trop Med Hyg*. 1999;**61**(4):642–647.
80. Ioannou P, Vamvoukaki R. Armillifer infections in humans: a systematic review. *Trop Med Infect Dis*. 2019;**4**(2):80.
81. Mas-Coma S, Bargues M. Human liver flukes: a review. *Res Rev Parasitol*. 1997:**57**(3–4):145–218.

8

Fatty liver in liver surgery

Nicolas Goldaracena and Lucas McCormack

Introduction

Liver surgery is the only curative treatment for patients with liver tumours.[1-3] Over the last two decades, new developments in surgical techniques and advances in the management of critical patients have increased the number of potential candidates for surgery.[4] Consequently, high-volume centres have reported a dramatic decrease in perioperative mortality after liver resection.[1,5,6]

As a result of significantly improved postoperative outcomes, indications for liver surgery and the extent of liver resections have expanded. Currently, major liver resections are performed routinely despite the presence of underlying liver disorders, such as steatosis.[6] While major hepatic resection (three or more liver segments) can be safely performed on healthy livers, the risk of such resection in patients with underlying hepatic disease remains challenging. Current data show wide variability with regard to postoperative mortality rates associated with liver failure following liver resections in either sick or healthy livers.[7,8] Moreover, the presence of numerous definitions of postoperative liver failure and the use of different classification systems to assess postoperative complications following liver resections make the interpretation of the literature difficult.[7,9,10]

A potentially increased risk of impaired postoperative recovery has been related to the presence of liver steatosis.[11] Data suggest that steatosis can have deleterious effects on ischaemic injury and regeneration. Moreover, it has been reported that it is liver steatosis per se that is the main preoperative risk factor for postoperative complications following major hepatectomy. Therefore, it is the presence of steatosis alone rather than the type (microsteatosis or macrosteatosis) that should be taken into account in the preoperative evaluation prior to extended liver resections.

It is the objective of this chapter to offer a comprehensive review and up-to-date management of the approach needed to perform safe liver surgery in patients with liver steatosis. In addition, a detailed description of the approach needed to safely utilize fatty livers for liver transplantation will be provided.

Fatty livers

Hepatic steatosis is characterized by an accumulation of lipids in the liver and it has been related to a spectrum of predisposing features such as obesity, diabetes, excessive use of alcohol, and a variety of drugs and toxins.[12,13] Fatty accumulation is considered pathological when the hepatic fat content, consisting mainly of triglycerides, exceeds 5% of the actual wet weight of the liver.[14]

In a retrospective study of a large series of hepatic resections, liver steatosis was found to be the most common underlying hepatic abnormality.[6] Although the global prevalence has yet to be evaluated, different studies have reported a prevalence of 10-20% in the lean population (body weight <110% of the ideal weight), 60-74% among obese individuals, and greater than 90% in morbidly obese individuals (body weight >200% of ideal weight).[15-17] Likewise, the incidence of steatohepatitis among lean, obese, and morbidly obese individuals is around 3%, 18%, and 50%, respectively. Moreover, the prevalence of steatosis and steatohepatitis has already increased dramatically in both Western and Eastern populations due to the concerning increase in obesity worldwide.

Steatosis is usually an incidental finding and hepatomegaly is often the only finding on physical examination. Despite widespread clinical use of imaging methods, ultrasound, computed tomography, or magnetic resonance imaging (MRI) can only, to some extent, detect the degree of steatosis. Saadeh et al. demonstrated the limitation of radiological modalities in a study where only steatosis greater than 25-30% could be reliably detected radiologically.[18] In addition, none of these modalities was able to distinguish either the grading or the type of liver fat or to detect the individual pathological features important to establish steatohepatitis, such as necro-inflammatory changes, hepatocyte ballooning, and fibrosis.[19] In 2017, a group at the University of Toronto evaluated in a cohort of 144 consecutive potential living liver donors the ability of magnetic resonance spectroscopy and MRI to distinguish between donors with and without clinically significant (>10%) hepatic steatosis. In their study they observed that a cut-off value of 5% for magnetic resonance spectroscopy and MRI improved the sensitivity for identifying steatosis greater than 10% correlated by liver biopsy. In this manner they established very high to perfect negative predictive values for MRI (95%) and magnetic resonance spectroscopy (100%) to exclude the presence of steatosis greater than 10% which is considered beyond the safe margin for living donation at the University of Toronto living donor liver transplant programme. Therefore, this resulted in the possibility to obviate the need for liver biopsy in this cohort when MRI-based hepatic quantification results imply absence or negligible hepatic steatosis (<5%).[20]

There is a consensus that the gold standard of diagnosis is at least two liver biopsies, as a single biopsy can result in substantial misdiagnosis and staging inaccuracies.[21] However, due to the risk of fatal bleeding after liver biopsy (0.4%), it is not routinely performed in patients without apparent complicated liver disease.[22] A uniform quantitative grading for steatosis and steatohepatitis has been suggested, combining the identified key pathological features.[23] Besides quantitative grading, steatosis can be classified qualitatively into microvesicular and macrovesicular forms (Figure 8.1). Most frequent is the macrovesicular one, and this is often associated with obesity, non-insulin-dependent diabetes, some dyslipidaemias, and alcohol abuse. Microvesicular steatosis is usually related to more acute conditions such as acute viral infections, metabolic disorders, and various toxins but also to acute fatty liver of pregnancy. The histopathological features of steatosis are evaluated in preoperative needle biopsies or operative wedge specimens that are frozen and/or deparaffinized. The staining methods currently used are haematoxylin and eosin with which the fatty changes are assessed by considering the non-stained regions. In addition, specific fat stains such as Oil Red O and Sudan III are used. However, there are several problems in the clinical application of these staining methods. The conventional techniques potentially underestimate the extent of fatty infiltration as they fail to identify microvesicular forms of steatosis.[24] In addition, the fat-specific stains have pitfalls, for example, in Oil Red O-stained liver tissue, the quality and quantity of the staining are highly operator dependent and false-positive results or overestimation of the severity are possible because of unspecific sinusoidal staining.[25]

Clinical conditions associated with hepatic steatosis

Patients with non-alcoholic fatty liver disease have an increased prevalence of non-insulin-dependent diabetes, but the actual role of diabetes in postoperative recovery is unclear as studies report contradictory results. Non-insulin-dependent diabetes was identified as an independent and significant variable predicting major postoperative complications in a cohort of 209 patients undergoing liver resection.[26] However, contrary to this study, a study including 525 diabetic and non-diabetic patients requiring hepatectomy reported no difference in perioperative morbidity or mortality and no effect was observed in long-term prognosis.[27] Although the impact of diabetes on postoperative complications remains unclear, an increased rate of wound infections was reported in an impressive cohort of over 20,000 patients.[28] From the analysis of a large database, it was concluded that a subset of diabetic patients having steatosis in the analysis of the liver specimens poorly tolerate major liver resection.[29] Thus, when contemplating major hepatectomy in patients with diabetes mellitus, surgeons should be aware that the presence of diabetes mellitus may lead to a higher incidence of hepatic failure postoperatively.

Obesity is crucially linked with steatosis as its prevalence among obese individuals is up to 75% and among morbidly obese individuals up to 100%.[13] In the past, obesity has been linked to increased perioperative technical complications leading to prolonged postoperative recovery. However, Dindo et al. prospectively investigated a cohort of 6336 patients undergoing elective surgery and found no increase in postoperative morbidity and mortality between obese and non-obese patients, not even in morbidly obese patients.[30] In contrast to general obesity, body fat accumulation (subcutaneous or intra-abdominal) has been reported to be independently associated with postoperative morbidity in a prospective study of 139 patients who underwent gastric or colorectal cancer surgery.[31]

Postoperative complications in patients with liver steatosis

Only a few studies have focused on liver steatosis as a risk factor for postoperative complications after liver resection. However, there are some general problems in the reporting of these studies. The histopathological methods for diagnosis of steatosis are not frequently, if ever, mentioned. So, the reliability of diagnosis of steatosis remains uncertain, rendering the comparison of the results difficult.

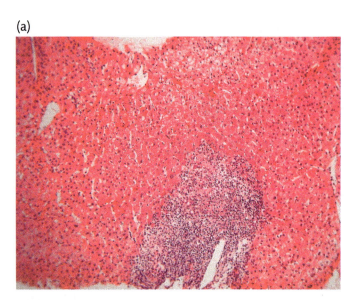

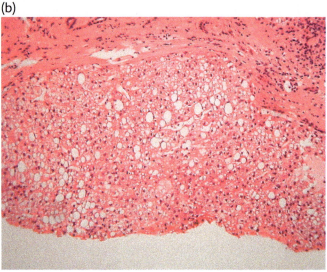

Figure 8.1 Haematoxylin and eosin-stained liver biopsies. (a) Non-fatty liver. (b) Severe steatotic liver containing macro- and microvesicular steatosis into the hepatocytes.

Uniform grading together with a more detailed description of the staining methods used and the number and sort of biopsies taken are important to compare different studies.[14] In the absence of a uniform classification system accepted by most to better stratify morbidity by severity, few data have been reported concerning the incidence of major complications after liver resection in steatotic patients. Finally, mortality is usually assessed as in-hospital mortality or 60-day mortality postoperatively, and there are no studies evaluating 5- or 10-year survival of steatotic patients after surgery.

In 1998, Behrns et al. evaluated, in a retrospective study of 135 patients, the safety of major resection in patients with hepatic steatosis.[32] They reported increased postoperative mortality, morbidity, and blood transfusion rates together with longer operative times in the presence of steatosis of 30% or higher. Belghiti et al., in a large database including 478 liver resections, detected the presence of hepatic steatosis (≥30%) in 37 (7.7%) patients, and they demonstrated that steatosis was an independent risk factor for postoperative complications but not for mortality.[5] In the analysis of a cohort of 1803 liver resections, the histological analysis demonstrated that only 55% of the liver specimens had normal parenchyma and 18% had liver steatosis.[6] In contrast, the presence of steatosis was not a risk factor for postoperative outcome after hepatectomy. Later, Kooby et al. reviewed the above-mentioned cohort to perform a case-matched study involving 325 steatotic patients compared with 160 with normal livers who were matched according to age, comorbidities, and the extent of resection.[33] Interestingly, they showed that steatosis was a predictor of postoperative complications, but mainly minor ones. Major postoperative complications, requiring major therapeutic intervention or mortality, were not affected by the presence of steatosis. To note, information regarding the presence of concomitant risk factors, such as nutritional parameters, kidney function, and cholestasis, were not included in this analysis. Furthermore, the histological analysis did not differentiate between the two types of liver steatosis or other histological features such as steatohepatitis or fibrosis. Therefore, we decided to investigate the influence of the quantitative and qualitative analysis of steatosis on the postoperative outcome after major liver resection.[11] In our study, each patient with liver steatosis was matched with a similar patient with a normal liver who required major hepatectomy according to the following variables: age, sex, American Society of Anesthesiologists score, diagnosis, extent of hepatectomy, and the need for a bilio-enteric bypass. We found that steatosis was the most significant preoperative risk factor for postoperative complications and should be considered for the planning of a major liver resection. Interestingly, neither the type nor the grading of liver steatosis influenced postoperative outcome after major hepatectomy. A novel finding in this study was that the presence of preoperative jaundice in a steatotic liver was an independent risk factor for mortality after surgery. Consequently, efforts should be made either to postpone surgery until normalization of bilirubin levels or to minimize the extent of liver resection in those patients (i.e. economic hepatectomy combined with ablation therapies, two-stage hepatectomy, etc.).

Liver steatosis in living donor hepatectomy

There is a worldwide discrepancy between the number of patients waiting for a liver transplant and the number of available liver grafts.[34] Living donor liver transplantation has emerged to mitigate this discrepancy and reduce mortality on the waiting list. However, as mentioned above, obesity has increased dramatically around the world and as a consequence the living donor pool is often populated with potential donors who are either overweight or obese and therefore have liver steatosis.[35]

It is well known that liver steatosis has potential impacts on liver regeneration, liver function, and postoperative complications for both donor and recipient. As donor safety is the highest priority in living donor liver transplantation, it is crucial that living donor hepatectomy is performed when liver steatosis in minimal. In the West, steatosis in living donor surgery is more restrictive and most centres will not consider performing a living donor hepatectomy in the presence of steatosis of greater than 10%. In this regard, in 2017 the Toronto group reported no difference in donor outcomes after right lobe living donor hepatectomy between patients with a body mass index greater than or less than 30 kg/m^2 but with macrosteatosis of up to 10%.[35] By contrast, some Asian centres have broader criteria and they have reported safely performing living donor liver surgery when liver steatosis does not exceed 30% of macrosteatosis. However, they would only consider such a degree of steatosis in living donor surgery if the donor age is less than 35 years old and the remnant liver volume is more than 35%.[36]

Use of steatotic grafts in liver transplantation

Liver transplantation is the treatment of choice for patients with end-stage liver disease. However, as mentioned above, in the past decades the number of patients waiting for a liver has increased substantially, far exceeding the number of available grafts. This has created a big discrepancy between supply and demand which has been impacted by increasing waiting list mortality.

Several strategies have been proposed to overcome this organ shortage, among them, the use of marginal liver grafts, such as the ones with steatosis (Figure 8.2).[37] Liver steatosis is found in up to 30% of cadaveric donors. Graft steatosis can be either macrovesicular or microvesicular, with microvesicular steatosis holding less of an influence on graft function following liver transplantation. The degree of steatosis has been proposed to be an independent risk factor for an adverse outcome after liver transplantation.[38] While those grafts with a mild degree of steatosis (<30%) are routinely used by most transplant centres, those livers with moderate (30–60%) and severe (60%) steatosis should be used with more caution, since they are more frequently associated with an increased risk of primary non-function of the graft. However, recent data suggest that under certain circumstances these organs can be safely used when other donor and recipient risk factors are minimized.[39]

Probably the main challenge when using steatotic grafts for liver transplantation is the ability to objectively predict or quantify the degree of steatosis. Liver biopsy is the gold standard to determine this but during the graft acceptance process this is not always possible and one has to rely on the donor surgeon's expertise.[40]

Therefore, the safest approach to achieve the best possible outcome following liver transplantation when using steatotic grafts is to minimize other donor and recipient risk factors. In this regard, if the liver graft has a steatosis of greater than 30%, the donor should be otherwise healthy and young, and the cold ischaemia time should

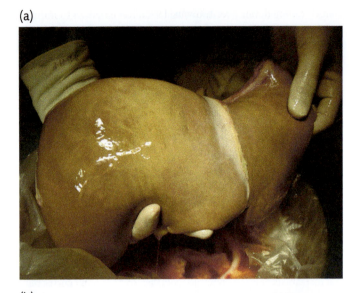
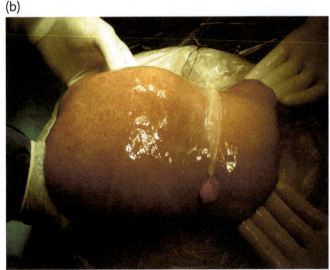

Figure 8.2 Macroscopic aspect of the liver graft before implantation. (a) Non-fatty liver. (b) Fatty liver.

be kept relatively short (<6 hours). Ideally, recipients of this type of graft should be patients in relatively good clinical condition, with low Model for End-Stage Liver Disease scores and without previous abdominal surgeries that would better tolerate transient graft dysfunction.[37–39]

Protective strategies in injured livers

Various approaches have been proposed to improve the poorer postoperative outcome of patients with steatosis after liver surgery. A positive correlation between preoperative liver function, operative time, blood transfusion requirement, and postoperative morbidity has been demonstrated.[41] In addition, the extent of blood loss by itself is responsible for short- and long-term complications.[42] Consequently, an intermittent Pringle manoeuvre (inflow occlusion by clamping of the portal triad) has been used to minimize blood loss during transection of the liver parenchyma in patients with liver disease or steatosis.[43] A randomized study confirmed the safety of using inflow occlusion during transection even in cirrhotic livers.[44] This strategy is particularly effective in preventing blood loss but only when associated with a low central venous pressure. Low central venous pressure anaesthesia, inflow and/or outflow vascular control, novel transection, or coagulation devices are all intended to reduce such losses.[45,46]

A randomized controlled trial showed that liver transection under inflow occlusion with the clamp crushing technique is associated with lower blood loss and reduced requirement for perioperative transfusions than resection performed with more sophisticated transection devices claimed to enable safe surgery without the need for inflow occlusion.[47] However, the Pringle manoeuvre induces ischaemic injury in the remnant liver, which is directly related to the duration of inflow occlusion and associated with increased morbidity and mortality.[48] The use of total vascular exclusion during hepatic resection greatly reduces blood loss, but liver regeneration is affected by the ischaemic organ injury suffered during this process.[5] Two protective strategies such as intermittent clamping and ischaemic preconditioning tend to reduce ischaemic injury and bleeding.[49–53]

There is growing evidence that liver steatosis is associated with a poorer outcome after hepatic resection.[11] Since in animal models it was observed that steatotic livers tolerate warm ischaemia during hepatectomy poorly, many surgeons have advocated developing protective strategies against ischaemic injury of these livers.[54] However, animal models applied in experimental studies on protective strategies have biases precluding the extrapolation of results to the clinical situation.[14,54] The development of clinically relevant experimental models is also hindered by the spectrum of patients with different aetiological factors. Different aetiological backgrounds lead to different forms of steatosis combined with a range of pathological features unique to some factors. Further, the clinical significance of the type and extent of steatosis is not clear as larger cohort studies applying uniform diagnostic criteria are missing. In two clinical randomized trials comparing ischaemic preconditioning or intermittent clamping versus continuous clamping the highly protective effect of both strategies in steatotic livers was clearly stated.[55,56] In another study, the protection conferred by intermittent clamping was fully preserved in steatotic livers, even if greater than 30% of steatosis was present, while this protective effect was weaker in the ischaemic preconditioning group.[49] These data may imply that intermittent clamping should be preferred in patients with severe steatosis and expected prolonged ischaemia times. However, more research is needed in this field of surgery as the prevalence of steatosis is dramatically increasing worldwide.

Conclusion

Liver steatosis is considered as a clinically important feature that influences patient morbidity and mortality after hepatic resection and liver transplantation. In the recent years, steatosis will become a major concern as the prevalence is closely linked to obesity, an epidemic disease in Western countries. There is an urgent need for reliable non-invasive methods to detect steatosis and related pathological features before an operation.

Surgeons should take the presence of injured livers into account when planning the extent and type of hepatic surgery. Preoperative and perioperative interventions should be considered to minimize the additional damage. The future goal should be to use by consensus a proper classification for morbidity and hepatic failure in liver surgery to compare results between centres. These centres should have a commitment to report all deaths related to hepatic failure after surgery.

Regarding choosing a standard of care and treatment for patients with chronic hepatic disease there are no fixed strategies. Each team should decide the best algorithm based on current evidence tailored to each patient to reach similar rates of morbidity and mortality compared to patients with healthy livers. Further randomized trials should focus on the evaluation of novel preoperative strategies, such as short-term intensive medical treatment of hepatic steatosis and preoperative portal vein embolization, to minimize risk in these patients.

REFERENCES

1. Fan ST, Lo CM, Liu CL, et al. Hepatectomy for hepatocellular carcinoma: toward zero hospital deaths. *Ann Surg*. 1999;**229**(3):322–330.
2. Jarnagin WR, Fong Y, DeMatteo RP, et al. Staging, resectability, and outcome in 225 patients with hilar cholangiocarcinoma. *Ann Surg*. 2001;**234**(4):507–517.
3. Tomlinson JS, Jarnagin WR, DeMatteo RP, et al. Actual 10-year survival after resection of colorectal liver metastases defines cure. *J Clin Oncol*. 2007;**25**(29):4575–4580.
4. Redaelli CA, Wagner M, Krahenbuhl L, et al. Liver surgery in the era of tissue-preserving resections: early and late outcome in patients with primary and secondary hepatic tumors. *World J Surg*. 2002;**26**(9):1126–1132.
5. Belghiti J, Hiramatsu K, Benoist S, Massault P, Sauvanet A, Farges O. Seven hundred forty-seven hepatectomies in the 1990s: an update to evaluate the actual risk of liver resection. *J Am Coll Surg*. 2000;**191**(1):38–46.
6. Jarnagin WR, Gonen M, Fong Y, et al. Improvement in perioperative outcome after hepatic resection: analysis of 1,803 consecutive cases over the past decade. *Ann Surg*. 2002;**236**(4):397–406.
7. Shirabe K, Shimada M, Gion T, et al. Postoperative liver failure after major hepatic resection for hepatocellular carcinoma in the modern era with special reference to remnant liver volume. *J Am Coll Surg*. 1999;**188**(3):304–309.
8. Schneider PD. Preoperative assessment of liver function. *Surg Clin North Am*. 2004;**84**(2):355–373.
9. Balzan S, Belghiti J, Farges O, et al. The '50-50 criteria' on postoperative day 5: an accurate predictor of liver failure and death after hepatectomy. *Ann Surg*. 2005;**242**(6):824–829.
10. Dindo D, Demartines N, Clavien PA. Classification of surgical complications: a new proposal with evaluation in a cohort of 6336 patients and results of a survey. *Ann Surg*. 2004;**240**(2):205–213.
11. McCormack L, Petrowsky H, Jochum W, Furrer K, Clavien PA. Hepatic steatosis is a risk factor for postoperative complications after major hepatectomy: a matched case-control study. *Ann Surg*. 2007;**245**(6):923–930.
12. Wanless IR, Lentz JS. Fatty liver hepatitis (steatohepatitis) and obesity: an autopsy study with analysis of risk factors. *Hepatology*. 1990;**12**(5):1106–1110.
13. Angulo P. Nonalcoholic fatty liver disease. *N Engl J Med*. 2002;**346**(16):1221–1231.
14. Vetelainen R, van Vliet A, Gouma DJ, van Gulik TM. Steatosis as a risk factor in liver surgery. *Ann Surg*. 2007;**245**(1):20–30.
15. Bellentani S, Saccoccio G, Masutti F, et al. Prevalence of and risk factors for hepatic steatosis in Northern Italy. *Ann Intern Med*. 2000;**132**(2):112–117.
16. Nomura H, Kashiwagi S, Hayashi J, Kajiyama W, Tani S, Goto M. Prevalence of fatty liver in a general population of Okinawa, Japan. *Jpn J Med*. 1988;**27**(2):142–149.
17. Luyckx FH, Desaive C, Thiry A, et al. Liver abnormalities in severely obese subjects: effect of drastic weight loss after gastroplasty. *Int J Obes Relat Metab Disord*. 1998;**22**(3):222–226.
18. Saadeh S, Younossi ZM, Remer EM, et al. The utility of radiological imaging in nonalcoholic fatty liver disease. *Gastroenterology*. 2002;**123**(3):745–750.
19. Rinella ME, Alonso E, Rao S, et al. Body mass index as a predictor of hepatic steatosis in living liver donors. *Liver Transpl*. 2001;**7**(5):409–414.
20. Satkunasingham J, Nik HH, Fischer S, et al. Can negligible hepatic steatosis determined by magnetic resonance imaging-proton density fat fraction obviate the need for liver biopsy in potential liver donors? *Liver Transpl*. 2018;**24**(4):470–477.
21. Ratziu V, Charlotte F, Heurtier A, et al. Sampling variability of liver biopsy in nonalcoholic fatty liver disease. *Gastroenterology*. 2005;**128**(7):1898–1906.
22. McGill DB, Rakela J, Zinsmeister AR, Ott BJ. A 21-year experience with major hemorrhage after percutaneous liver biopsy. *Gastroenterology*. 1990;**99**(5):1396–1400.
23. Brunt EM, Janney CG, Di Bisceglie AM, Neuschwander-Tetri BA, Bacon BR. Nonalcoholic steatohepatitis: a proposal for grading and staging the histological lesions. *Am J Gastroenterol*. 1999;**94**(9):2467–2474.
24. Urena M, Ruiz-Delgado F, Gonzales E, et al. Hepatic steatosis in liver transplant donors: common feature of donor population? *World J Surg*. 1998;**22**:837–844.
25. Markin RS, Wisecarver JL, Radio SJ, et al. Frozen section evaluation of donor livers before transplantation. *Transplantation*. 1993;**56**(6):1403–1409.
26. Shimada M, Matsumata T, Akazawa K, et al. Estimation of risk of major complications after hepatic resection. *Am J Surg*. 1994;**167**(4):399–403.
27. Poon RT, Fan ST, Wong J. Does diabetes mellitus influence the perioperative outcome or long term prognosis after resection of hepatocellular carcinoma? *Am J Gastroenterol*. 2002;**97**(6):1480–1488.
28. Cruse PJ, Foord R. The epidemiology of wound infection. A 10-year prospective study of 62,939 wounds. *Surg Clin North Am*. 1980;**60**(1):27–40.
29. Little SA, Jarnagin WR, DeMatteo RP, Blumgart LH, Fong Y. Diabetes is associated with increased perioperative mortality but equivalent long-term outcome after hepatic resection for colorectal cancer. *J Gastrointest Surg*. 2002;**6**(1):88–94.
30. Dindo D, Muller MK, Weber M, Clavien PA. Obesity in general elective surgery. *Lancet*. 2003;**361**(9374):2032–2035.
31. Tsukada K, Miyazaki T, Kato H, et al. Body fat accumulation and postoperative complications after abdominal surgery. *Am Surg*. 2004;**70**(4):347–351.
32. Behrns KE, Tsiotos GG, DeSouza NF, Krishna MK, Ludwig J, Nagorney DM. Hepatic steatosis as a potential risk factor for major hepatic resection. *J Gastrointest Surg*. 1998;**2**(3):292–298.
33. Kooby DA, Fong Y, Suriawinata A, et al. Impact of steatosis on perioperative outcome following hepatic resection. *J Gastrointest Surg*. 2003;**7**(8):1034–1044.

34. Goldaracena N, Barbas AS. Living donor liver transplantation. *Curr Opin Organ Transplant*. 2019;**24**(2):131–137.
35. Knaak M, Goldaracena N, Doyle A, et al. Donor BMI >30 is not a contraindication for live liver donation. *Am J Transplant*. 2017;**17**(3):754–760.
36. Lee SG. A complete treatment of adult living donor liver transplantation: a review of surgical technique and current challenges to expand indication of patients. *Am J Transplant*. 2015;**15**(1):17–38.
37. McCormack L, Petrowsky H, Jochum W, Mullhaupt B, Weber M, Clavien PA. Use of severely steatotic grafts in liver transplantation: a matched case-control study. *Ann Surg*. 2007;**246**(6):940–946.
38. McCormack L, Dutkowski P, El-Badry AM, Clavien PA. Liver transplantation using fatty livers: always feasible? *J Hepatol*. 2011;**54**(5):1055–1062.
39. Halazun KJ, Quillin RC, Rosenblatt R, et al. Expanding the margins: high volume utilization of marginal liver grafts among >200 liver transplants at a single institution. *Ann Surg*. 2017;**266**(3):441–449.
40. Yersiz H, Lee C, Kaldas FM, et al. Assessment of hepatic steatosis by transplant surgeon and expert pathologist: a prospective, double-blinded evaluation of 201 donor livers. *Liver Transpl*. 2013;**19**(4):437–449.
41. Wu CC, Yeh DC, Lin MC, Liu TJ, P'Eng FK. Improving operative safety for cirrhotic liver resection. *Br J Surg*. 2001;**88**(2):210–215.
42. Kooby DA, Stockman J, Ben-Porat L, et al. Influence of transfusions on perioperative and long-term outcome in patients following hepatic resection for colorectal metastases. *Ann Surg*. 2003;**237**(6):860–869.
43. Makuuchi M, Mori T, Gunven P, Yamazaki S, Hasegawa H. Safety of hemihepatic vascular occlusion during resection of the liver. *Surg Gynecol Obstet*. 1987;**164**(2):155–158.
44. Takayama T, Makuuchi M, Kubota K, et al. Randomized comparison of ultrasonic vs clamp transection of the liver. *Arch Surg*. 2001;**136**(8):922–928.
45. Emond JC, Samstein B, Renz JF. A critical evaluation of hepatic resection in cirrhosis: optimizing patient selection and outcomes. *World J Surg*. 2005;**29**(2):124–130.
46. Midorikawa Y, Kubota K, Takayama T, et al. A comparative study of postoperative complications after hepatectomy in patients with and without chronic liver disease. *Surgery*. 1999;**126**(3):484–491.
47. Lesurtel M, Selzner M, Petrowsky H, McCormack L, Clavien PA. How should transection of the liver be performed?: a prospective randomized study in 100 consecutive patients: comparing four different transection strategies. *Ann Surg*. 2005;**242**(6):814–822.
48. Wei AC, Tung-Ping Poon R, Fan ST, Wong J. Risk factors for perioperative morbidity and mortality after extended hepatectomy for hepatocellular carcinoma. *Br J Surg*. 2003;**90**(1):33–41.
49. Petrowsky H, McCormack L, Trujillo M, Selzner M, Jochum W, Clavien PA. A prospective, randomized, controlled trial comparing intermittent portal triad clamping versus ischemic preconditioning with continuous clamping for major liver resection. *Ann Surg*. 2006;**244**(6):921–928.
50. Belli G, Fantini C, D'Agostino A, Belli A, Russolillo N, Cioffi L. [Laparoscopic liver resection without a Pringle maneuver for HCC in cirrhotic patients]. *Chir Ital*. 2005;**57**(1):15–25.
51. Capussotti L, Nuzzo G, Polastri R, Giuliante F, Muratore A, Giovannini I. Continuous versus intermittent portal triad clamping during hepatectomy in cirrhosis. Results of a prospective, randomized clinical trial. *Hepatogastroenterology*. 2003;**50**(52):1073–1077.
52. Kim YI, Kitano S. Segment VIII resection of the cirrhotic liver under continuous pringle maneuver with in situ cooling followed by temporary portal decompression. *Am J Surg*. 1999;**177**(3):244–246.
53. Selzner N, Rudiger H, Graf R, Clavien PA. Protective strategies against ischemic injury of the liver. *Gastroenterology*. 2003;**125**(3):917–936.
54. Selzner M, Clavien P. Fatty liver in transplantation and surgery. *Sem Liver Dis*. 2001;**21**:105–113.
55. Belghiti J, Noun R, Malafosse R, et al. Continuous versus intermittent portal triad clamping for liver resection: a controlled study. *Ann Surg*. 1999;**229**(3):369–375.
56. Clavien PA, Selzner M, Rudiger HA, et al. A prospective randomized study in 100 consecutive patients undergoing major liver resection with versus without ischemic preconditioning. *Ann Surg*. 2003;**238**(6):843–850.

9
Cystic lesions of the liver

David Martin and Emmanuel Melloul

Introduction

Cystic lesions of the liver represent a heterogeneous group of fluid-filled lesions, benign or malignant, which differ in epidemiology, pathogenesis, and imaging findings. Most of these lesions are benign, discovered incidentally, and may be acquired, genetic, infectious, or parasitic. A minority can cause symptoms and may rarely be associated with complications. Hepatic cysts can be subdivided into simple and complex cysts, based on their characteristics. Differentiation is important because it can guide the need for further diagnostic procedures and treatment.[1]

In the workup, liver function tests may be performed but are usually normal unless the cyst is very large and compressing intra- or extrahepatic structures. In the case of an abscess or cyst infection, leucocytosis associated with elevation of inflammatory markers (C-reactive protein, procalcitonin) and positive blood cultures may occur. Radiological imaging assesses the size, characteristics, and location of cysts. Ultrasound (US) is typically the first-line imaging modality, as far as it is the most accessible, the least expensive, and it carries a sensitivity and specificity of about 90%.[2] The recent development of microbubble contrast-enhanced US enables the operator to visualize vascular flow within the septa or solid components of cysts.[2] Computed tomography (CT) scanning or magnetic resonance imaging (MRI) gives more detailed information about location, surrounding structures, nodularity, septations, and calcification within the cyst.[3,4] Aspiration of the cyst is generally not useful since the fluid analysis does not distinguish simple from neoplastic cysts, and no marker has been identified to determine malignant potential. Indeed, an elevated CA19-9 level in the cystic fluid does not correlate with malignant lesions.[1]

Nowadays, there are still controversies about the definition and classification of cysts. Furthermore, no consensus has been achieved on the optimal treatment of patients with symptoms, although several therapeutic approaches have been described.[5] This chapter provides an overview of the diagnosis and management of the most commonly observed hepatic cystic lesions.

Benign cystic lesion of the liver

Simple hepatic cyst

Epidemiology and pathogenesis

Hepatic cysts are the most commonly encountered hepatic lesions, occurring in 2.5–18% of the population, and have a predominance in females (ratio 1.5:1).[6–8] More than half of individuals older than 60 years are likely to have simple cysts, which are usually small, but can grow to more than 30 cm.[2] Large cysts may cause atrophy of the surrounding parenchyma. Their wall is lined by a biliary epithelium and the cavity contains clear fluid with a similar composition to serum.[8,9] Communication with the biliary ducts is very rare.[10] Hepatic cysts can rarely become complex as a result of rupture, haemorrhage, or infection.

Patients are usually asymptomatic, but cysts larger than 5 cm may cause symptoms, such as abdominal pain, early satiety, nausea, and vomiting.[9,11] Patients may have a palpable mass or hepatomegaly on clinical examination.

Imaging findings

Hepatic cysts are typically round structures that have an imperceptible wall and are usually multiple in number and vary in size.[8] US features include an anechoic fluid filled cavity, no septations, well-marginated borders, enhancement of the posterior wall, and posterior acoustic enhancement. CT and MRI show respectively attenuation and signal intensity (T1 hypointensity, T2 hyperintensity) like water (Figure 9.1).

Management

Cysts are generally asymptomatic and once the diagnosis is established, no further follow-up is required. Moreover, no treatment is needed unless they become large and symptomatic.[8] Treatment options include percutaneous aspiration with sclerotherapy, marsupialization, or surgical resection.[12,13] The choice between these modalities is made on the basis of the location of cysts, volume of the liver, and experience of the center.[14]

CHAPTER 9 Cystic lesions of the liver

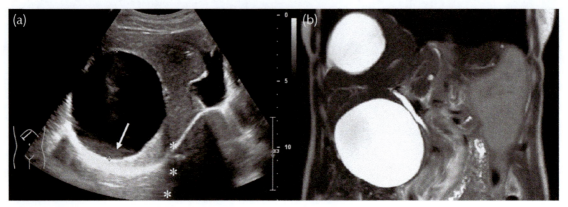

Figure 9.1 Simple hepatic cyst. (a) Classic sonographic features with well-marginated borders, no septations, enhancement of posterior wall (arrow), and posterior acoustic enhancement (asterisk). (b) MRI features on T2-weighted imaging (hyperintensity).

Aspiration-sclerotherapy is an effective method with few complications that has to be considered as first-line treatment.[14] US- or CT-guided aspiration is followed by contrast instillation that confirms the absence of communication with the biliary tree, which is a contraindication to therapy. The aspirated cavity is instilled with a sclerosing agent (alcohol) that is retained for 2 hours and then aspirated again. However, the recurrence rate is quite high, up to 20%.[15] Laparoscopic or open surgical fenestration techniques are similarly or even more effective in reducing cyst volume and symptoms, but have a significantly higher morbidity rate, such as bleeding or bile leaks.[16–18] Fenestration includes wide cystic wall deroofing (Figure 9.2). This wall should be sent for anatomopathological analysis to exclude malignancy. Intraoperative methylene blue cholangiography (through the cystic duct) is important to rule out communication with the bile duct. Hepatic parenchyma resection should be avoided because of the risk of postoperative bleeding or

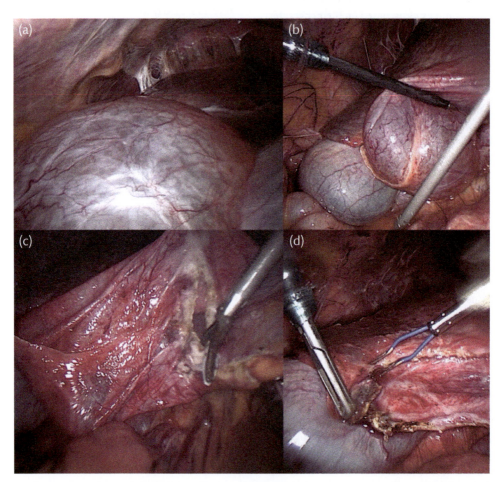

Figure 9.2 Laparoscopic fenestration of a simple hepatic cyst. (a) View of the cyst which appears as a protuberant bulge on the liver surface. (b) Volume reduction after cyst puncture. (c) Complete excision of the anterior wall of the cyst. (d) Inside view of the cyst and haemostasis using bipolar coagulation.

bile leaks. The recurrence rate after the deroofing technique ranges between 0% and 25%.[18-20]

Polycystic liver disease

Epidemiology and pathogenesis

Polycystic liver disease (PCLD) is an autosomal dominant genetic condition, which can occur concomitantly with polycystic kidney disease or may be confined to the liver, accounting for 10–20% of cases.[21] In isolated PCLD, inherited mutations of the protein C substrate *PRKCSH* gene or the *SEC36* gene are responsible.[2] It is a rare disease, with a prevalence rate ranging from 0.13% to 0.9%, and is predominantly discovered during the fourth or fifth decade of life.[21-23] PCLD has a slight predominance in females and hepatic cysts can emerge after the onset of puberty and dramatically increase in number and size through early and middle adult life.[24] The mechanism of cyst formation is not completely understood. One hypothesis is that small portions of the ductal system may become detached from the biliary tree and progressively dilate, forming cysts.[21] Cysts in PCLD are similar to simple hepatic cysts. They are lined by biliary epithelium and contain plasma-like serous fluid.[8]

Most patients are asymptomatic and pain is mainly caused by stretching of Glisson's capsule. Symptoms may also develop when PCLD progresses to advanced liver disease with complications, such as cyst haemorrhage, rupture, infection, biliary compression, venous outflow obstruction, and portal hypertension.

Imaging findings

Cysts seen in patients with PCLD are usually peripherally located and vary in size, ranging from a few millimetres to 80 mm.[8] The liver becomes enlarged and typically contains more than 20 cysts.[1,25] The diagnosis can also be made in case of a positive family history of PCLD and the presence of more than four liver cysts.[2,26] The cysts appear to be simple hepatic cysts on imaging (Figure 9.3).

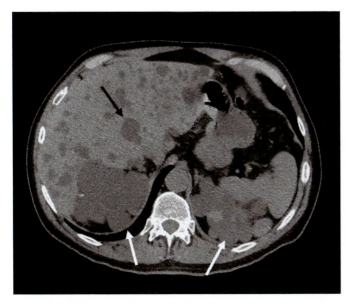

Figure 9.3 CT image: multiple cysts of varying sizes in liver (black arrow) and kidneys (white arrows), compatible with a polycystic liver and kidney disease.

Reproduced courtesy of Prof. Maurice Matter, Department of Visceral Surgery, University Hospital CHUV, University of Lausanne, Lausanne, Switzerland.

Management

The main objective of therapy is to reduce liver cyst volume to diminish the mass effect-related symptoms.[25] There is no effective medical therapy; however, there have been clinical trials, which have shown that it is possible to reduce liver volume and symptoms with somatostatin analogues octreotide or lanreotide.[27,28] Interventional and surgical options should be the last treatment option and include cyst aspiration and sclerosis, open or laparoscopic cyst fenestration, hepatic resection, and liver transplantation.[24] Aspiration-sclerotherapy and fenestration are indicated when PCLD consists of large cysts confined to a limited part of the liver.[2] It is important to select a dominant cyst that is likely to be responsible for the symptoms, usually the largest one. Most commonly, cysts with a diameter of more than 5 cm are good candidates for these therapies.[25] Surgical access has the advantage that multiple cysts can be treated at once during the procedure. In more extensive disease, segmental hepatic resection or even liver transplantation may be indicated.[25,29] Segmental hepatic resection may be considered in patients who harbour cyst-rich segments, but have predominantly normal liver parenchyma.[25] The extent of the resection depends on the distribution and location of cysts and ranges from a single-segment excision to an extended lobectomy. Liver transplantation is required when other therapies have failed and in patients with diffuse disease without enough healthy liver parenchyma sparing and concurrent hepatic dysfunction.[30]

Ciliated hepatic foregut duplication cyst

Epidemiology and pathogenesis

A ciliated hepatic foregut cyst is a rare congenital cystic lesion that is thought to arise from the embryonic foregut.[8] The cysts typically appear in the fifth decade with a slight male predominance.[31] Their histology is similar to those of bronchogenic cysts, lined by a ciliated pseudostratified columnar epithelial layer.[8,32] As this epithelium is able to secrete fluids of variable viscosity, the density may vary from a serous fluid to a viscous or mucous fluid.[8] Most patients are asymptomatic, and the cyst is discovered incidentally. However, malignant transformation into squamous cell carcinoma has been described in up to 5%.[31,33]

Imaging findings

A ciliated hepatic foregut cyst can be found in either of the major lobes of the liver but occurs most often in the medial segment of the left lobe (segment IV).[34] It typically measures less than 3 cm and is most commonly located in the subcapsular region.[32] With US imaging, cysts appear hypoechoic. On CT scans, the cysts are hyperattenuated to the surrounding liver parenchyma, and do not enhance with administration of contrast.[32] On MRI they are T2 hyperintense, however, usually not as hyperintense as a simple cyst, and have a variable appearance on T1-weighted images, including T1 hyper- or hypo-intensity.[35,36]

Management

Fine-needle aspiration biopsy can confirm the diagnosis.[37] Given the reported risk of malignant transformation, ciliated hepatic foregut cysts should be resected.[38] This resection can be done by laparoscopy.[39] Recurrent disease and malignant spread have not been described, and therefore, long-term follow-up after resection is not required.[33]

Pyogenic liver abscess

Epidemiology and pathogenesis

A pyogenic liver abscess is the development of an intrahepatic pus collection, secondary to a local inflammatory reaction by bacterial infection in the hepatic parenchyma.[40] It has an incidence varying from 1.1 to 2.3 for 100,000 habitants and has a slight preponderance in males.[41–43] The peak incidence is found in 50- to 65-year-old patients.[44] A pyogenic liver abscess can be of biliary, arterial (septicaemia), portal, or cryptogenic origin.[42] Those of biliary origin occur in patients with intrahepatic bile duct stones, extrahepatic bile duct stones, bilioenteric anastomoses, or biliary stents.[45] Other risk factors include diabetes, gastrointestinal tract cancers, diverticulitis, and cholecystitis.[46–48] The most commonly recorded bacterial infections are *Enterococcus* species, *Escherichia coli*, and *Klebsiella pneumonia*.[41] The infection may also be polymicrobial. Spreading of the infection is possible, with the main organs affected being the lungs, central nervous system, and eyes.[49]

Patients present with right upper quadrant pain, fever, chills, jaundice, weight loss, anorexia, and, occasionally from the outset, sepsis. Mortality is high, up to 6–14%.[40,41,48] Leucocytosis, an increase in C-reactive protein (average of 236 mg/L), hyperbilirubinaemia, and hypoalbuminaemia are common laboratory findings.[40,42]

Imaging

Pyogenic abscesses are mainly located in the right lobe of the liver. A high proportion manifests itself as a solitary abscess, but multiple bilateral abscesses are also possible.[44] On US, it may appear as an anechoic mass with well-defined or indistinct borders and may possibly contain echogenic debris or gas.[8] CT scanning has been reported to be more sensitive than US in the diagnosis of an abscess.[50] On CT, it is typically iso- or hypoattenuating compared with surrounding parenchyma in the unenhanced phase and has a peripheral rim of enhancement after intravenous administration of contrast (Figure 9.4).[51] On MRI, the central portion of the lesion will show low signal intensity on T1-weighted imaging and high signal intensity on T2-weighted imaging.[8] Moreover, a peripheral halo of hyperintensity indicating oedema may be seen on T2-weighted imaging.

Management

When the diagnosis of a pyogenic liver abscess is suspected, broad-spectrum intravenous antibiotics must be initiated after blood and abscess culture. Third- and fourth-generation cephalosporins, piperacillin/tazobactam, aminoglycosides, and carbapenems remain effective treatment options.[44,52] The optimal duration of intravenous antibiotics, as well as the duration of subsequent oral therapy, remain unclear and largely depend on the success of interventional treatments. For abscesses smaller than 5 cm, needle aspiration may be considered, but large abscesses should be drained percutaneously.[43,53] It has been shown that percutaneous drainage is more effective than percutaneous needle aspiration because it has a higher success rate, reduces the time required to achieve clinical relief, and supports a 50% reduction in abscess cavity size.[43] Percutaneous aspiration or drainage should be undertaken before surgery in terms of its lower morbidity and lower cost.[54] However, percutaneous treatment fails in approximately 10% of abscesses, and in those cases, surgical intervention is required.[8,41] The procedure involves incising the liver capsule, draining and irrigating the cavity, and disrupting the septa. The approach can be done by laparoscopy or laparotomy depending on the location of the abscess. In patients with recurrent abscesses as a result of multiple percutaneous drainage procedures or chronic biliary obstruction from multiple biliary drainages, a major hepatectomy may be considered as the last option.

Amoebic liver abscess

Epidemiology and pathogenesis

Amoebic abscesses are the result of *Entamoeba histolytica* infestation, and account for up to 10% of abscesses, and are more common in tropical areas as well as in tourists and in immigrants from developing countries.[44] Latin America, India, and Asia are endemic regions. Human contamination is by the faecal–oral route (contaminated food, water, or hands). Amoebic liver abscesses arise from haematogenous spread (probably via the portal circulation) of amoebic trophozoites that have breached the colonic mucosa.[55] Most patients have no bowel symptoms and stool microscopy is usually negative for *Entamoeba histolytica* trophozoites and cysts.[44] The diagnosis relies on imaging and positive amoebic serology, fluid aspiration from the lesion is therefore not necessary.[44] Amoebic serology is highly sensitive (>94%) and highly specific (>95%).[55]

The clinical presentation of patients with amoebic abscesses is similar to those with pyogenic abscesses. The mortality rate is between 1% and 3%.[44,55] Patients can present with an amoebic abscess months or even years after travel or residence in an endemic area.[44] Leucocytosis, mild anaemia, raised concentrations of alkaline phosphatase, and a high erythrocyte sedimentation rate are the most common laboratory observations.[55]

Imaging findings

US or CT scans are the radiological imaging of choice, insofar as both methods are very sensitive, but neither provides absolute specificity for amoebic liver abscesses.[55] US findings may vary, depending on the stage and evolution of the abscess. Initially, the

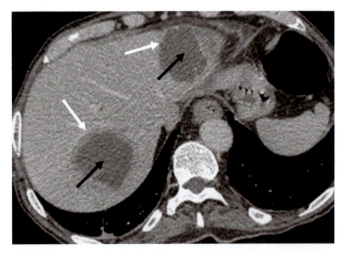

Figure 9.4 CT image of a pyogenic liver abscess (*Streptococcus milleri*) that is hypoattenuated compared with surrounding parenchyma (black arrows) and has a peripheral rim of enhancement (white arrows).
Reproduced courtesy of Dr Sabine Schmidt, Department of Radiology, University Hospital CHUV, University of Lausanne, Lausanne, Switzerland.

Benign cystic lesion of the liver

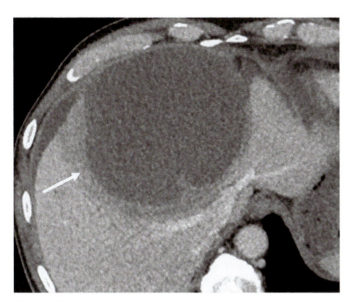

Figure 9.5 CT image of an amoebic liver abscess visible as an avascular hypodense liver mass with a thick wall and a ring of oedema (white arrow), forming a 'double-target' sign.
Reproduced courtesy of Dr Sabine Schmidt, Department of Radiology, University Hospital CHUV, University of Lausanne, Lausanne, Switzerland.

lesion has a greater echogenicity than the adjacent hepatic parenchyma and has a necrotic centre which is solid.[56] The necrotic solid component generates heterogeneous echogenicity. Later, liquefaction of the contents can occur, with debris in the bottom of the abscess. CT scans can detect small lesions and visualize detailed margins of the lesion and clues in the arterial and venous phases that allow differentiation between other common lesions, such as hepatic cysts, haemangiomas, or solid neoplasms. More precisely, a hypodense liver mass which is avascular with well-defined margins and has alternating hypervascular and hypovascular halos following contrast media enhancement can be viewed (Figure 9.5).[56] During the acute phase, MRI shows a homogeneous hypointense signal with clearly defined margins on a T1-weighted image, and a hyperintense and heterogeneous centre, depending on the fluidity and debris of the necrotic exudate.[56] After adequate treatment, follow-up imaging should be planned, as radiological resolution may take several months.

Management

Treatment includes an amoebicidal agent that targets hepatic infection (e.g. metronidazole). Interventional treatment is often not necessary. Most patients show a response to metronidazole (reduced fever and abdominal pain) within 72–96 hours.[44] Percutaneous treatment should be reserved for patients in whom the diagnosis is uncertain, in those who do not respond to metronidazole (persistent fever or abdominal pain) after 4 days of treatment, and if a large abscess is at the risk of rupture.[55] Surgical drainage is rarely required, and only in unusual cases such as haemorrhage, erosion into other organs, or sepsis not controlled by percutaneous drainage.

Cystic echinococcosis

Epidemiology and pathogenesis

A hydatid or echinococcal cyst (EC) is a widely endemic helminthic disease caused by accidental ingestion of eggs of *Echinococcus granulosus*. The parasite is ingested through contaminated food from the dog, the usual definitive host. Following ingestion, eggs hatch in the small intestine.[1] They then penetrate into the bloodstream, where they can migrate to their target organs, including the liver and lungs.[22] An EC is composed of three layers: the outer pericyst (compressed hepatic tissue), the endocyst (inner germinal layer), and the ectocyst (translucent thin interleaved membrane).[9] The maturation of a cyst is characterized by the development of daughter cysts in the periphery as a result of endocyst invagination. Cysts first appear in the liver 3–4 weeks after infection; however, they are very slow growing and may exist without developing symptoms for many years.[57] The highest prevalence of ECs is found in the temperate zones, including the Africa, the Middle East, Central Asia, South America, and parts of Europe.[58]

The clinical presentation includes abdominal pain, biliary obstruction, infection, and rarely cyst rupture, which can lead to an anaphylactic reaction.[8] The mortality rate of these lesions is higher than for simple cysts, estimated at 2–5%.[1,22] Aspiration should be avoided because of the anaphylaxis risk. Serodiagnostic tests to reveal *E. granulosus* antibodies have a sensitivity of 93.5% and specificity of 89.7%.[59]

Imaging findings

At an early stage of infection, an EC may appear as a simple cyst, but over time, it develops a thick and calcified wall with surrounding daughter cysts and several other complex features.[22] US typically demonstrates a cystic lesion with a hyperechogenic pattern combined with internal echoes such as snowflake-like inclusions or floating laminated membranes with multiple septa confined by a laminated border.[2] On CT, an EC appears as a well-defined lesion with distinguishable walls, calcified rims, intracystic septations, and peripheral daughter cysts (Figure 9.6).[60] MRI clearly demonstrates the pericyst, the matrix, and daughter cysts; however, it has not been proven to be cost-effective and has no added value compared to US and CT.[61]

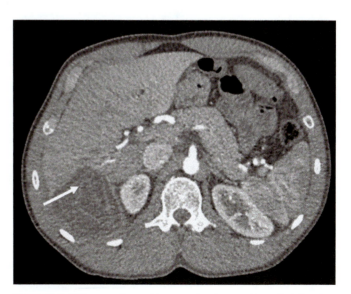

Figure 9.6 CT image of an echinococcal cyst: complex well-defined cystic lesion with distinguishable walls and intracystic septations (white arrow).

Management

For decades, surgical excision was the recommended approach for ECs. The availability of anthelminthic agents (albendazole) has made it possible to undertake US- or CT-guided transhepatic percutaneous drainage, termed puncture, aspiration, injection (scolicidal agents), and re-aspiration (PAIR).[62] The most frequently used scolicidal agents are hypertonic saline and ethanol. Patients with small and uncomplicated cysts can respond well to medical treatment alone. However, in larger or more complicated cysts, medical treatment should be used in combination with interventional procedures to minimize recurrence and achieve cure. PAIR appears to have lower rates of major and minor complications, mortality, and disease recurrence, and fewer days of hospitalization compared to patients treated surgically.[62] Patients undergoing PAIR typically receive oral albendazole for 7 days before and 1 month after drainage. This technique results in parasitological clearance in 95.8% of cases.[62] Surgery should be reserved for cystic echinococcosis refractory to PAIR because of difficult-to-manage cyst-biliary communication or obstruction. There are different surgical techniques, such as marsupialization (resection of the anterior wall and suture of the cut edges of the remaining cyst), capitonnage, cystectomy, pericystectomy, or liver resection (Figure 9.7). These interventions are either conservative or radical. In the conservative approach, removal of daughter cysts, resection of the active germinal lining, and removal of debris are essential. However, there is currently no universally accepted standard technique. Laparoscopic hepatic hydatid surgery has been described and seems to be a safe and effective method (Figure 9.8).[63,64] The surgical approach should be based on surgeon experience as well as on the location and size of the EC, and its proximity to biliary or vascular structures. Whatever the technique used, an anthelminthic agent should be used before surgery to sterilize the cyst and reduce the risk of dissemination and anaphylaxis.[65]

In terms of prevention, a new option for the control of *E. granulosus* in the intermediate host population is vaccination.[66]

Alveolar echinococcosis

Epidemiology and pathogenesis

Alveolar echinococcosis (AE) is caused by ingestion of the eggs of *Echinococcus multilocularis*, found in the excrement of foxes.[2] It is endemic in the Northern hemisphere, including North America and several Asian and European countries, such as France, Germany, Switzerland, and Austria.[67] The ingested eggs develop into an alveolar structure composed of small vesicles that grow slowly and are able to reach a diameter of 15–20 cm.[2,66] Each vesicle has the same wall structure as an EC.[2] Compared to the encapsulated growth of EC, AE presents an infiltrative neoplastic growth with potential metastasis to adjacent and distant organs (lungs, spleen, bone, and brain).[68] Serology tests (ELISA, Western blot) have a high diagnostic sensitivity of 90–100%, with a specificity of 95–100%.[69] Western blot allows us to distinguish between *E. granulosus*- and *E. multilocularis*-infected patients in 76% of cases.[70] However, serology does not allow the distinction between the active and inactive forms of both echinococcoses. AE usually has an asymptomatic phase of between 5 and 15 years prior to the development of symptoms, which are related to mass effect such as abdominal pain, weight loss, or fatigue.[71]

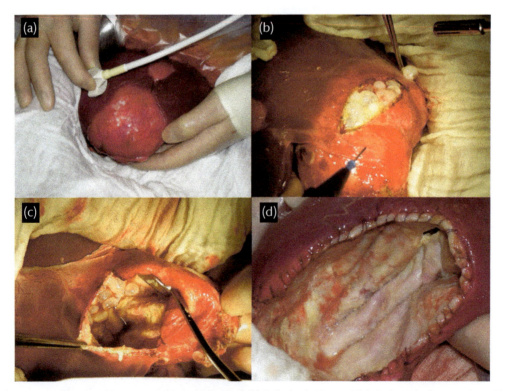

Figure 9.7 Surgical treatment of cystic echinococcosis (marsupialization). (a) Bulky hydatid cyst visible in the right liver, confirmed by intraoperative US. (b) Visible daughter cysts after capsule incision. (c) Removal of daughter cysts and resection of the active germinal lining. (d) Suture of the cut edges of the remaining cyst.

Reproduced courtesy of Prof. Nermin Halkic, Department of Visceral Surgery, University Hospital CHUV, University of Lausanne, Lausanne, Switzerland.

Benign cystic lesion of the liver

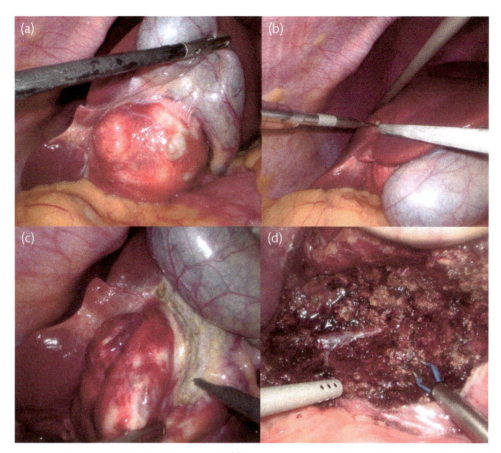

Figure 9.8 Laparoscopic surgical treatment of cystic echinococcosis. (a) Intraoperative view of the hydatic cyst near the gall bladder. (b) Puncture, aspiration, injection (scolicidal agents), and re-aspiration (PAIR procedure). (c) Pericystectomy. (d) Haemostasis of the operative field.
Reproduced courtesy of Prof. Nermin Halkic, Department of Visceral Surgery, University Hospital CHUV, University of Lausanne, Lausanne, Switzerland.

Imaging findings

US may show a mass with irregular limits and scattered calcification, surrounded by a hyperechogenic ring and a hypoechogenic centre with a multivesicular appearance.[66] Central necrosis may give the mass the appearance of a cystic-like structure.[72] On unenhanced CT, AE lesions appear as tumour-like masses with irregular borders, heterogeneous internal structures, and multiple distributed calcific foci (Figure 9.9). No significant intralesional enhancement is seen on contrast-enhanced CT, while mild enhancement can be seen in the peripheral tissue in the delayed phase.[73] On MRI, AE is visible in the form of small round cysts with a weak enhanced solid component.[74] The lesion can be large and irregular, which is clearly shown on T2-weighted imaging. T1-weighted images reveal more clearly the hepatic extension than CT, especially to hepatic veins, vena cava, and perihepatic spaces.[74]

Fluorodeoxyglucose positron emission tomography is useful for the detection of metabolic activity in AE.[75] It is therefore used for the assessment of lesion metabolism and the continuation or withdrawal of antiparasitic treatment. However, sophisticated equipment and high cost widely limit its use for routine evaluation.[75]

Management

The surgical management of AE is similar than that of a hepatic malignancy.[2] Radical resection is the only curative procedure, even though it is often difficult to achieve because of echinococcal dissemination.[67] It should be followed by a 2-year period of anthelminthic therapy (e.g. benzimidazole) and patients should be monitored for at least 10 years, because of the risk of recurrence.[67,76] Liver transplantation is indicated in advanced cases with liver failure and

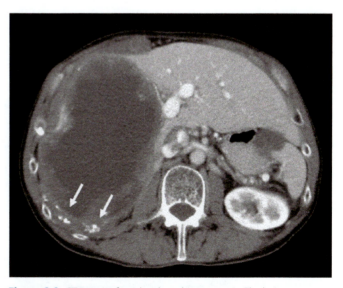

Figure 9.9 CT image of an alveolar echinococcosis. The lesion appears as a tumour-like masse with irregular borders, heterogeneous internal structures, and multiple distributed calcific foci (white arrows).

inability to achieve a radical resection.[77] The absence of extrahepatic localizations is mandatory for such cases.[69]

Biliary hamartoma (von Meyenburg complex)

Epidemiology and pathogenesis

Biliary hamartomas, also known as von Meyenburg complexes, are derived from embryonic bile ducts.[1] These benign congenital lesions consist of dilated small bile ducts surrounded by a fibrous stroma.[78] They are found in 5.6% of adults and in 0.9% of children.[79] No sex predilection has been reported.[8] Biliary hamartomas are the consequence of interrupted remodelling of the ductal plates during the late phase of embryological development of the small intrahepatic bile ducts.[80] Hamartomas may mimic metastases, and this diagnosis should be considered in patients with a primary malignant tumor.[78] Biopsy is necessary to confirm the diagnosis.

Biliary hamartomas are asymptomatic and are almost always discovered incidentally.[8]

Imaging findings

On imaging, biliary hamartomas present as multiple, small (<10–15 mm), round or irregular scattered cysts with a predilection for the subcapsular region.[8] On US, biliary hamartomas present as innumerable tiny hypoechoic or hyperechoic foci.[80] They also typically have a simple cystic appearance on CT (non-enhancing, hypoattenuation) and MRI (hypointense on T1-weighted and hyperintense on T2-weighted images).[8] The lack of communication with the biliary tree helps to differentiate biliary hamartomas from Caroli's disease.[8]

Management

Biliary hamartomas require no treatment.

Caroli's disease

Epidemiology and pathogenesis

Caroli's disease is a benign autosomal recessive disorder characterized by unilobular or bilobular segmental cystic dilatation of the intrahepatic biliary tract.[8,81] The incidence of the disease is estimated at 1/1,000,000 and more than 80% of patients are less than 30 years of age.[82] No sex predilection has been reported. The disease seems to be caused by the derangement in ductal plate remodelling of the large ducts.[8] The combination of Caroli's disease and hepatic fibrosis is designated as the Caroli syndrome, which is the more common variant.[8,83] Several renal disorders have been described in association with this liver disease, including autosomal polycystic kidney disease.[84]

Patients can present with recurrent attacks of fever, right upper quadrant pain, and rarely jaundice.[9] They may also develop liver abscesses, stones, and secondary biliary cirrhosis.[8] The incidence of cholangiocarcinoma varies from 5% to 10%.[81,85]

Imaging findings

Caroli's disease presents as a cystic dilatation of the intrahepatic ducts, as well as the 'central dot sign', which corresponds to a portal vein branch protruding into the lumen of a dilated bile duct.[86] The extrahepatic ducts remain intact and involvement can be diffuse or localized to one segment or one lobe, usually the left lobe (**Figure 9.10**).[8] These aspects can be observed with US, CT, or MRI.[81] Invasive exploration of the bile duct (endoscopic retrograde cholangiopancreatography, percutaneous cholangiography) is contraindicated because of the risk of developing severe cholangitis.

Management

Broad-spectrum antibiotic coverage is indicated in cases of cholangitis.[9] Thereafter, treatment relies on the location of the biliary abnormalities.[82] Hepatectomy is performed in patients with segmental or lobar disease and recurrent cholangitis. Liver transplantation may be required for patients with secondary biliary cirrhosis and portal hypertension.

Miscellaneous liver cysts: fungal abscesses, endometrial cysts, pseudocysts, traumatic cysts, bilomas, and haematomas

Invasive fungal infections are typically seen in the immunocompromised population, including diabetic patients, organ transplant recipients, postsplenectomy patients, and patients in the intensive care unit.[87] Pathogens most frequently found are *Candida* species, *Aspergillus* species, and *Cryptococcus*. On imaging, the lesions are usually small, less than 2 cm, and disseminated throughout the liver.[8] Management is the same as for pyogenic abscesses, including an intravenous antifungal agent (caspofungin) and drainage.

Endometrial cysts are rarely found in the liver and can mimic the appearance of mucinous cysts, as they are multiloculated with solid

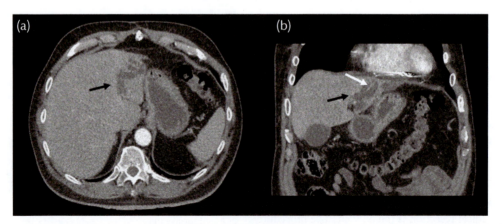

Figure 9.10 CT image of Caroli disease ((a) transverse plane, (b) coronal plane). Cystic intrahepatic ducts dilatation localized in the left lobe (black arrow). A portal vein branch protruding into the lumen of a dilated bile duct can be observed, which corresponds to the 'central dot sign' (white arrow).

and cystic components.[88] These cysts occur when endometrial tissue is implanted in the liver parenchyma, but the exact pathophysiology is not known.

An intrahepatic pseudocyst is an extremely rare condition that may occur in the setting of pancreatitis.[8] The spread of pancreatic enzymes along the hepatogastric and hepatoduodenal ligaments or along the portal triad into the liver parenchyma results in intrahepatic tissue damage and necrosis.[89] This fluid collection, like other collections in pancreatitis, can resolve or progress to become a pseudocyst with a fibrous capsule. It may require percutaneous or endoscopic drainage. On imaging, the lesion manifests as a simple fluid collection with an enhancing thin peripheral capsule, but will have a complex appearance if infected or in case of haemorrhage.[8,90]

The collection of bile, lymph, or blood products after injury to the liver parenchyma will result in the formation of a biloma, haematoma, or seroma, respectively.[8,91] These lesions may occur after blunt or penetrating trauma or iatrogenic injury, such as after cholecystectomy, liver surgery, liver transplantation, or other interventional procedures (percutaneous or endoscopic). A biloma is a collection of bile forming a cyst outside the biliary tract. It can present as either a simple or complex cyst.[85] Haematomas may appear cystic but are not true cysts because they are not surrounded by an epithelium. In the acute phase, they appear echogenic on US, hyperdense on CT and hyperintense on T1-weighted MRI. Afterwards, they can evolve and appear as cysts. Management depends on the type of collection, its size, and the patient's symptoms. Therapeutic approaches include conservative management, percutaneous or endoscopic drainage, and open or laparoscopic surgery.

Neoplastic cystic lesions of the liver

Biliary cystadenoma and cystadenocarcinoma

Epidemiology and pathogenesis

Biliary cystadenoma (BCA) and cystadenocarcinoma (BCAC) constitute cysts referred to as mucinous cystic neoplasms (MCNs) and account for 3–5% of all hepatic cysts.[22,92] More than 85% of BCAs are reported in women, and typically in the fifth decade of life (female:male ratio, 9:1).[81,93] These cysts are multilocular lesions that arise from ectopic rests of embryonic bile ducts or aberrant ducts.[2,94] Histologically, they are composed of three layers: a collagenous outer layer, a stromal layer, and, a mucin-secreting columnar epithelial layer.[1,22] The majority of the tumours contain ovarian-like stroma, grow slowly, and measure between 1.5 and 35 cm.[2,92] Malignant transformation of a BCA to a BCAC occurs in 20–30% of cases.[1,92] Imaging is not useful in distinguishing these two lesions, and the diagnosis is best done histologically. There is no significant difference in cystic fluid CA19-9 content between a benign biliary cystadenoma and a malignant biliary cystadenocarcinoma.[95]

Most patients are asymptomatic, but these lesions can cause jaundice from tumour invasion or compression at the porta hepatis, painful intracystic haemorrhage, rupture, fever due to secondary infection, ascites, and vena cava obstruction.[96,97]

Imaging findings

Most BCAs and BCACs are located in the central or left side of the liver, and are generally solitary.[98] By conventional US, these lesions are similar to complex cysts and, contain septa, wall, and mural nodules. On contrast-enhanced US, most of the MCNs (78%) have a typical honeycomb enhancement pattern of the cystic wall, septa, or mural nodules.[92] Hyperenhancement of the honeycomb septa during the arterial phase is more common in BCAs; however, hypoenhancement during the portal venous and late phases is more characteristic of BCACs. On CT scan, BCAs may be unilocular, multilocular, or may have septations.[81] MRI shows a well-defined lesion that does not enhance after the administration of intravenous contrast, and on T1-weighted imaging, the cyst shows a low signal, while in T2-weighted imaging, a very high-intensity signal is observed.[81] Wall nodularity, particularly nodules greater than 10 mm in diameter, is more suggestive of a BCAC.[1] However, despite the various diagnostic modalities, it remains difficult to differentiate BCAs from BCACs on preoperative imaging.

Management

Surgical removal of BCAs and BCACs by complete excision is the treatment of choice. It usually requires a central or left hepatectomy according to its more common location. Complete excision has a 5-year survival rate of 100% and a recurrence rate of only 13%.[99] Percutaneous fine-needle aspiration cytology is not recommended, especially because of the risk of peritoneal seeding.[100] BCAs are readily amenable to enucleation, but if there is any indication of malignancy, however, resection through normal tissue planes with negative margins is mandatory, in particular segmentectomy or hepatectomy.[98,100] Cholangiography is recommended to ensure an absence of communication with the biliary tree and to distinguish it from a cystic intraductal papillary mucinous neoplasm of the bile duct.

Cystic hepatocellular carcinoma

Epidemiology and pathogenesis

Cystic hepatocellular carcinomas (HCCs) may present as solid, cystic, or mixed lesions in the liver.[1] Areas of necrosis or haemorrhage within the tumour may create a cystic appearance on imaging.[81] This phenomenon can occur after interventional procedures, such as transarterial chemoembolization, cryoablation, or radiofrequency ablation. These interventional procedures may induce liquefactive necrosis that results in the cystic appearance of HCCs.[8] The incidence of cystic HCC following transarterial chemoembolization varies from 1% to 11%.[101,102] Cystic degradation may also rarely be spontaneous.

At pathological examination, the hypoattenuating central portion includes necrosis and the peripheral enhancing capsule contains malignant cells.[103]

Patients may present with acute fever and leucocytosis.[104]

Imaging findings

On contrast-enhanced US, a cystic HCC may present as a heterogeneous hypervascular mass during the arterial phase with rapid hypoenhancement during the portal venous phase (washout), and peripheral capsule enhancement.[81,105] On CT imaging, it may look like an abscess, with an irregular multilocular hypoattenuating lesion and a peripheral rim of enhancement.[104] Moreover, CT and MRI findings include underlying liver cirrhosis and intrinsic tumour characteristics of HCC as hypervascularity of solid components and tumour invasion of the portal and hepatic veins.[85]

Management

Spontaneous cystic HCC should be treated conventionally as a standard HCC. When the occurrence is post interventional, it may be treated conservatively. However, in cases of signs of infection or increase in size, percutaneous drainage, segmental hepatectomy, or internal drainage (metallic stent) combined with antibiotics should be considered.[101,102,106,107]

Embryonal hepatic sarcoma

Epidemiology and pathogenesis

Embryonal hepatic sarcoma (EHS) is a highly malignant hepatic neoplasm that is usually encountered in the paediatric population, most patients being between 6 and 10 years of age, with an equal female-to-male ratio.[108] It has the aspect of a very large and poorly differentiated tumour, and is of mesenchymal origin with sarcomatous features.[8]

Most patients present with non-specific symptoms, ranging from abdominal pain and fullness to nausea, fatigue, and weight loss.[109] Some report the occurrence of an abdominal mass. Tumour rupture is a potentially fatal complication and is due to rapid tumour growth.[110] The 20-year survival rate is 70%.[111]

Imaging findings

On US, an EHS appears as a solid lesion that is usually iso- to hyperechoic to the liver parenchyma and contains anechoic areas corresponding to necrosis or cystic degeneration.[8] On CT scan, the EHS appears cystic with near-water attenuation and contains septations and peripheral nodules.[112] On MRI, the lesion presents a low signal intensity on T1-weighted imaging and high signal intensity on T2-weighted imaging, but will show heterogeneous enhancement after contrast administration.[113]

Management

Treatment includes surgical resection, liver transplantation, and multiagent chemotherapy.[109] Patients with EHSs often present with large lesions that are not resectable at the time of diagnosis because of their proximity to major vascular structures.[109] Thereby, neoadjuvant chemotherapy can reduce the tumour size and can make it amenable to surgery.[114] Treatment regimens includes vincristine, actinomycin D, doxorubicin, cyclophosphamide, ifosfamide, and etoposide.[111,114,115] For lesions that remain unresectable despite neoadjuvant chemotherapy, and for those with recurrent disease after primary resection, liver transplantation can be considered.[109,111]

Cystic intraductal papillary mucinous neoplasm of the bile ducts

Epidemiology and pathogenesis

Cystic intraductal papillary mucinous neoplasms of the bile ducts (IPMN-Bs) are rare lesions formed by dilated intrahepatic ducts with intraluminal dysplastic biliary epithelium, which forms a polypoid mass and secretes mucus.[1,116] They occur commonly in the age group of 50–70 years, and there is a slight male predominance.[30] These tumours are highly differentiated and are considered as precursors to intrahepatic cholangiocarcinomas as they comprise 9–38% of all bile duct carcinomas.[116-118] They can develop throughout the biliary tree and cystic biliary dilatation is pathognomonic because of the mucin hypersecretion.[118] IPMN-B is classified into four epithelial subtypes: pancreatobiliary, intestinal, gastric, and oncocytic. They present a similar histology and pathology to cystadenoma, but they do not have an ovarian-like stroma and communication with the bile ducts.

Most patients are asymptomatic, but they can present with intermittent abdominal pain, acute cholangitis, or jaundice.[118]

Imaging findings

On US, diffuse bile duct ectasia, localized duct dilatation, and cystic dilatation are common findings. On CT scanning, the enhancement pattern is isodense or hyperdense during the late arterial phase and not hyperdense during the portal venous and delayed phase, as compared with the normal hepatic parenchyma.[119] On MRI, IPMN-Bs are iso- to hypointense masses on T1-weighted images and hyperintense masses on T2-weighted images.[120] Mucin cannot be detected on US, CT, and MRI.[118] Therefore, they are difficult to distinguish from cystadenomas or cystadenocarcinomas.

Management

To assess the extent of superficial spreading, biopsy might be essential, but it cannot always reflect the maximum degree of cytoarchitectural atypia.[118] IPMN-Bs should be considered for surgical resection as these lesions can cause recurrent cholangitis and obstructive jaundice even in the absence of malignant transformation.[30] The resection should be similar to that of cholangiocarcinoma.[121] This usually includes segmental resection and major hepatectomy with or without extrahepatic bile duct resection. The disease-free survival rate for patients who have undergone curative resection is 81% at 5 years.[122] As IPMN-B presents as a superficial spread along the bile duct lumen, intraoperative frozen section at the stumps of the bile duct is essential to confirm a cancer-free surgical margin.[118] Intraoperative cholangiography should be performed to assess the presence of a biliary communication. The indication for liver transplantation is very limited.

Cystic hepatic metastases

Epidemiology and pathogenesis

Hepatic metastatic disease is the most common malignant lesion of the liver, far more common than primary liver neoplasms.[123] Liver metastases can appear cystic in certain circumstances. Malignancies that lead to this cystic-appearing lesion are mainly neuroendocrine tumours, melanomas, and gastrointestinal stromal tumours.[81] Other malignancies that have been described to appear cystic include lung adenocarcinoma, colorectal carcinoma, transitional cell carcinoma, adenoid cystic carcinoma, ovarian carcinoma, choriocarcinoma, sarcoma, and lesions treated with chemotherapy.[8,124] These lesions may be due to rapid growth of the tumour with insufficient hepatic arterial supply, leading to central necrosis and cystic degeneration.[8,125] Approximately 11% of focal liver lesions in patients with a known primary carcinoma are found to be metastatic disease.[8,126]

Imaging findings

The radiological appearance of the cystic metastases depends on the primary cancer. A clinical history of primary and multiplicity of the lesions are classic features.[30] US provides only limited information for differentiation.[123] On CT scans, metastatic cystic lesions may be hypoattenuated against the background liver but will usually have an irregular peripheral rim of enhancement.[127] Liver abscess is an important differential diagnosis.[30] Calcifications are common with gastrointestinal, ovarian, breast, and renal metastases.[128]

Management

Treatment depends on the origin of the primary cancer, and includes different modalities, such as chemotherapy and surgical resection. Radiofrequency ablation, microwave ablation, and hepatic artery embolization are other treatment modalities that can normally be used in patients with unresectable disease or in those who cannot undergo surgical resection due to comorbidities.[81]

REFERENCES

1. Mavilia MG, Pakala T, Molina M, Wu GY. Differentiating cystic liver lesions: a review of imaging modalities, diagnosis and management. *J Clin Transl Hepatol.* 2018;**6**(2):208–216.
2. Lantinga MA, Gevers TJ, Drenth JP. Evaluation of hepatic cystic lesions. *World J Gastroenterol.* 2013;**19**(23):3543–3554.
3. Scherer K, Gupta N, Caine WP, Panda M. Differential diagnosis and management of a recurrent hepatic cyst: a case report and review of literature. *J Gen Intern Med.* 2009;**24**(10):1161–1165.
4. Suwan Z. Sonographic findings in hydatid disease of the liver: comparison with other imaging methods. *Ann Trop Med Parasitol.* 1995;**89**(3):261–269.
5. Taylor BR, Langer B. Current surgical management of hepatic cyst disease. *Adv Surg.* 1997;**31**:127–148.
6. Gaines PA, Sampson MA. The prevalence and characterization of simple hepatic cysts by ultrasound examination. *Br J Radiol.* 1989;**62**(736):335–337.
7. Carrim ZI, Murchison JT. The prevalence of simple renal and hepatic cysts detected by spiral computed tomography. *Clin Radiol.* 2003;**58**(8):626–629.
8. Borhani AA, Wiant A, Heller MT. Cystic hepatic lesions: a review and an algorithmic approach. *AJR Am J Roentgenol.* 2014;**203**(6):1192–1204.
9. Choi BY, Nguyen MH. The diagnosis and management of benign hepatic tumors. *J Clin Gastroenterol.* 2005;**39**(5):401–412.
10. Karavias DD, Tsamandas AC, Payatakes AH, et al. Simple (non-parasitic) liver cysts: clinical presentation and outcome. *Hepatogastroenterology.* 2000;**47**(35):1439–1443.
11. Bahirwani R, Reddy KR. Review article: the evaluation of solitary liver masses. *Aliment Pharmacol Ther.* 2008;**28**(8):953–965.
12. Moorthy K, Mihssin N, Houghton PW. The management of simple hepatic cysts: sclerotherapy or laparoscopic fenestration. *Ann R Coll Surg Engl.* 2001;**83**(6):409–414.
13. vanSonnenberg E, Wroblicka JT, D'Agostino HB, et al. Symptomatic hepatic cysts: percutaneous drainage and sclerosis. *Radiology.* 1994;**190**(2):387–392.
14. van Keimpema L, de Koning DB, Strijk SP, Drenth JP. Aspiration-sclerotherapy results in effective control of liver volume in patients with liver cysts. *Dig Dis Sci.* 2008;**53**(8):2251–2257.
15. Erdogan D, van Delden OM, Rauws EA, et al. Results of percutaneous sclerotherapy and surgical treatment in patients with symptomatic simple liver cysts and polycystic liver disease. *World J Gastroenterol.* 2007;**13**(22):3095–3100.
16. Fiamingo P, Tedeschi U, Veroux M, et al. Laparoscopic treatment of simple hepatic cysts and polycystic liver disease. *Surg Endosc.* 2003;**17**(4):623–626.
17. Hansman MF, Ryan JA Jr, Holmes JH 4th, et al. Management and long-term follow-up of hepatic cysts. *Am J Surg.* 2001;**181**(5):404–410.
18. Gigot JF, Legrand M, Hubens G, et al. Laparoscopic treatment of nonparasitic liver cysts: adequate selection of patients and surgical technique. *World J Surg.* 1996;**20**(5):556–561.
19. Zalaba Z, Tihanyi TF, Winternitz T, Nehez L, Flautner L. The laparoscopic treatment of non-parasitic liver cysts. Five years experience. *Acta Chir Hung.* 1999;**38**(2):221–223.
20. Gall TM, Oniscu GC, Madhavan K, Parks RW, Garden OJ. Surgical management and longterm follow-up of non-parasitic hepatic cysts. *HPB (Oxford).* 2009;**11**(3):235–241.
21. Abu-Wasel B, Walsh C, Keough V, Molinari M. Pathophysiology, epidemiology, classification and treatment options for polycystic liver diseases. *World J Gastroenterol.* 2013;**19**(35):5775–5786.
22. Marrero JA, Ahn J, Rajender Reddy K. ACG clinical guideline: the diagnosis and management of focal liver lesions. *Am J Gastroenterol.* 2014;**109**(9):1328–1347.
23. Van Keimpema L, De Koning DB, Van Hoek B, et al. Patients with isolated polycystic liver disease referred to liver centres: clinical characterization of 137 cases. *Liver Int.* 2011;**31**(1):92–98.
24. Everson GT, Taylor MR, Doctor RB. Polycystic disease of the liver. *Hepatology.* 2004;**40**(4):774–782.
25. Drenth JP, Chrispijn M, Nagorney DM, Kamath PS, Torres VE. Medical and surgical treatment options for polycystic liver disease. *Hepatology.* 2010;**52**(6):2223–2230.
26. Drenth JP, Chrispijn M, Bergmann C. Congenital fibrocystic liver diseases. *Best Pract Res Clin Gastroenterol.* 2010;**24**(5):573–584.
27. Hogan MC, Masyuk T, Bergstralh E, et al. Efficacy of 4 years of octreotide long-acting release therapy in patients with severe polycystic liver disease. *Mayo Clin Proc.* 2015;**90**(8):1030–1037.
28. van Keimpema L, Nevens F, Vanslembrouck R, et al. Lanreotide reduces the volume of polycystic liver: a randomized, double-blind, placebo-controlled trial. *Gastroenterology.* 2009;**137**(5):1661–1668.
29. Russell RT, Pinson CW. Surgical management of polycystic liver disease. *World J Gastroenterol.* 2007;**13**(38):5052–5059.
30. Rawla P, Sunkara T, Muralidharan P, Raj JP. An updated review of cystic hepatic lesions. *Clin Exp Hepatol.* 2019;**5**(1):22–29.
31. Bogner B, Hegedus G. Ciliated hepatic foregut cyst. *Pathol Oncol Res.* 2002;**8**(4):278–279.
32. Kadoya M, Matsui O, Nakanuma Y, et al. Ciliated hepatic foregut cyst: radiologic features. *Radiology.* 1990;**175**(2):475–477.
33. Ziogas IA, van der Windt DJ, Wilson GC, et al. Surgical management of ciliated hepatic foregut cyst. *Hepatology.* 2020;**71**(1):386–388.
34. Vick DJ, Goodman ZD, Deavers MT, Cain J, Ishak KG. Ciliated hepatic foregut cyst: a study of six cases and review of the literature. *Am J Surg Pathol.* 1999;**23**(6):671–677.
35. Ansari-Gilani K, Modaresi Esfeh J. Ciliated hepatic foregut cyst: report of three cases and review of imaging features. *Gastroenterol Rep.* 2017;**5**(1):75–78.
36. Fang SH, Dong DJ, Zhang SZ. Imaging features of ciliated hepatic foregut cyst. *World J Gastroenterol.* 2005;**11**(27):4287–4289.
37. Hornstein A, Batts KP, Linz LJ, Chang CD, Galvanek EG, Bardawil RG. Fine needle aspiration diagnosis of ciliated hepatic foregut cysts: a report of three cases. *Acta Cytol.* 1996;**40**(3):576–580.
38. Goodman MD, Mak GZ, Reynolds JP, Tevar AD, Pritts TA. Laparoscopic excision of a ciliated hepatic foregut cyst. *JSLS.* 2009;**13**(1):96–100.

39. Saravanan J, Manoharan G, Jeswanth S, Ravichandran P. Laparoscopic excision of large ciliated hepatic foregut cyst. *J Minim Access Surg.* 2014;**10**(3):151–153.
40. Lee KT, Wong SR, Sheen PC. Pyogenic liver abscess: an audit of 10 years' experience and analysis of risk factors. *Dig Surg.* 2001;**18**(6):459–465.
41. Meddings L, Myers RP, Hubbard J, et al. A population-based study of pyogenic liver abscesses in the United States: incidence, mortality, and temporal trends. *Am J Gastroenterol.* 2010;**105**(1):117–124.
42. Santos-Rosa OM, Lunardelli HS, Ribeiro-Junior MA. Pyogenic liver abscess: diagnostic and therapeutic management. *Arq Bra Cir Dig.* 2016;**29**(3):194–197.
43. Cai YL, Xiong XZ, Lu J, et al. Percutaneous needle aspiration versus catheter drainage in the management of liver abscess: a systematic review and meta-analysis. *HPB (Oxford).* 2015;**17**(3):195–201.
44. Lubbert C, Wiegand J, Karlas T. Therapy of liver abscesses. *Viszeralmedizin.* 2014;**30**(5):334–341.
45. Shi SH, Zhai ZL, Zheng SS. Pyogenic liver abscess of biliary origin: the existing problems and their strategies. *Semin Liver Dis.* 2018;**38**(3):270–283.
46. Thomsen RW, Jepsen P, Sorensen HT. Diabetes mellitus and pyogenic liver abscess: risk and prognosis. *Clin Infect Dis.* 2007;**44**(9):1194–1201.
47. Lai HC, Lin CC, Cheng KS, et al. Increased incidence of gastrointestinal cancers among patients with pyogenic liver abscess: a population-based cohort study. *Gastroenterology.* 2014;**146**(1):129–137.e1.
48. Alvarez Perez JA, Gonzalez JJ, Baldonedo RF, et al. Clinical course, treatment, and multivariate analysis of risk factors for pyogenic liver abscess. *Am J Surg.* 2001;**181**(2):177–186.
49. Lee SS, Chen YS, Tsai HC, et al. Predictors of septic metastatic infection and mortality among patients with Klebsiella pneumoniae liver abscess. *Clin Infect Dis.* 2008;**47**(5):642–650.
50. Lin AC, Yeh DY, Hsu YH, et al. Diagnosis of pyogenic liver abscess by abdominal ultrasonography in the emergency department. *Emerg Med J.* 2009;**26**(4):273–275.
51. Alsaif HS, Venkatesh SK, Chan DS, Archuleta S. CT appearance of pyogenic liver abscesses caused by Klebsiella pneumoniae. *Radiology.* 2011;**260**(1):129–138.
52. Siu LK, Yeh KM, Lin JC, Fung CP, Chang FY. Klebsiella pneumoniae liver abscess: a new invasive syndrome. *Lancet Infect Dis.* 2012;**12**(11):881–887.
53. Zerem E, Hadzic A. Sonographically guided percutaneous catheter drainage versus needle aspiration in the management of pyogenic liver abscess. *AJR Am J Roentgenol.* 2007;**189**(3):W138–W142.
54. Ferraioli G, Garlaschelli A, Zanaboni D, et al. Percutaneous and surgical treatment of pyogenic liver abscesses: observation over a 21-year period in 148 patients. *Dig Liver Dis.* 2008;**40**(8):690–696.
55. Stanley SL Jr. Amoebiasis. *Lancet.* 2003;**361**(9362):1025–1034.
56. Kimura K, Stoopen M, Reeder MM, Moncada R. Amebiasis: modern diagnostic imaging with pathological and clinical correlation. *Semin Roentgenol.* 1997;**32**(4):250–275.
57. Pakala T, Molina M, Wu GY. Hepatic echinococcal cysts: a review. *J Clin Transl Hepatol.* 2016;**4**(1):39–46.
58. Mandal S, Mandal MD. Human cystic echinococcosis: epidemiologic, zoonotic, clinical, diagnostic and therapeutic aspects. *Asian Pac J Trop Med.* 2012;**5**(4):253–260.
59. Sbihi Y, Rmiqui A, Rodriguez-Cabezas MN, Orduna A, Rodriguez-Torres A, Osuna A. Comparative sensitivity of six serological tests and diagnostic value of ELISA using purified antigen in hydatidosis. *J Clin Lab Anal.* 2001;**15**(1):14–18.
60. Haddad MC, Birjawi GA, Khouzami RA, Khoury NJ, El-Zein YR, Al-Kutoubi AO. Unilocular hepatic echinococcal cysts: sonography and computed tomography findings. *Clin Radiol.* 2001;**56**(9):746–750.
61. Sayek I, Onat D. Diagnosis and treatment of uncomplicated hydatid cyst of the liver. *World J Surg.* 2001;**25**(1):21–27.
62. Smego RA Jr, Sebanego P. Treatment options for hepatic cystic echinococcosis. *Int J Infect Dis.* 2005;**9**(2):69–76.
63. Ertem M, Karahasanoglu T, Yavuz N, Erguney S. Laparoscopically treated liver hydatid cysts. *Arch Surg.* 2002;**137**(10):1170–1173.
64. Seven R, Berber E, Mercan S, Eminoglu L, Budak D. Laparoscopic treatment of hepatic hydatid cysts. *Surgery.* 2000;**128**(1):36–40.
65. Smego DR, Smego RA Jr. Hydatid cyst: preoperative sterilization with mebendazole. *South Med J.* 1986;**79**(7):900–901.
66. Eckert J, Deplazes P. Biological, epidemiological, and clinical aspects of echinococcosis, a zoonosis of increasing concern. *Clin Microbiol Rev.* 2004;**17**(1):107–135.
67. Nunnari G, Pinzone MR, Gruttadauria S, et al. Hepatic echinococcosis: clinical and therapeutic aspects. *World J Gastroenterol.* 2012;**18**(13):1448–1458.
68. Kern P. Clinical features and treatment of alveolar echinococcosis. *Curr Opin Infect Dis.* 2010;**23**(5):505–512.
69. Brunetti E, Kern P, Vuitton DA. Expert consensus for the diagnosis and treatment of cystic and alveolar echinococcosis in humans. *Acta Trop.* 2010;**114**(1):1–16.
70. Liance M, Janin V, Bresson-Hadni S, Vuitton DA, Houin R, Piarroux R. Immunodiagnosis of Echinococcus infections: confirmatory testing and species differentiation by a new commercial Western blot. *J Clin Microbiol.* 2000;**38**(10):3718–3721.
71. Moro P, Schantz PM. Echinococcosis: a review. *Int J Infect Dis.* 2009;**13**(2):125–133.
72. Bresson-Hadni S, Delabrousse E, Blagosklonov O, et al. Imaging aspects and non-surgical interventional treatment in human alveolar echinococcosis. *Parasitol Int.* 2006;**55**(Suppl):S267–S272.
73. Bulakci M, Kartal MG, Yilmaz S, et al. Multimodality imaging in diagnosis and management of alveolar echinococcosis: an update. *Diagn Interv Radiol.* 2016;**22**(3):247–256.
74. Kodama Y, Fujita N, Shimizu T, et al. Alveolar echinococcosis: MR findings in the liver. *Radiology.* 2003;**228**(1):172–177.
75. Liu W, Delabrousse E, Blagosklonov O, et al. Innovation in hepatic alveolar echinococcosis imaging: best use of old tools, and necessary evaluation of new ones. *Parasite.* 2014;**21**:74.
76. Reuter S, Jensen B, Buttenschoen K, Kratzer W, Kern P. Benzimidazoles in the treatment of alveolar echinococcosis: a comparative study and review of the literature. *J Antimicrob Chemother.* 2000;**46**(3):451–456.
77. Koch S, Bresson-Hadni S, Miguet JP, et al. Experience of liver transplantation for incurable alveolar echinococcosis: a 45-case European collaborative report. *Transplantation.* 2003;**75**(6):856–863.
78. Lev-Toaff AS, Bach AM, Wechsler RJ, Hilpert PL, Gatalica Z, Rubin R. The radiologic and pathologic spectrum of biliary hamartomas. *AJR Am J Roentgenol.* 1995;**165**(2):309–313.
79. Redston MS, Wanless IR. The hepatic von Meyenburg complex: prevalence and association with hepatic and renal cysts among 2843 autopsies [corrected]. *Mod Pathol.* 1996;**9**(3):233–237.

80. Venkatanarasimha N, Thomas R, Armstrong EM, Shirley JF, Fox BM, Jackson SA. Imaging features of ductal plate malformations in adults. *Clin Radiol*. 2011;**66**(11):1086–1093.
81. Bakoyiannis A, Delis S, Triantopoulou C, Dervenis C. Rare cystic liver lesions: a diagnostic and managing challenge. *World J Gastroenterol*. 2013;**19**(43):7603–7619.
82. Yonem O, Bayraktar Y. Clinical characteristics of Caroli's disease. *World J Gastroenterol*. 2007;**13**(13):1930–1933.
83. Desmet VJ. What is congenital hepatic fibrosis? *Histopathology*. 1992;**20**(6):465–477.
84. Shedda S, Robertson A. Caroli's syndrome and adult polycystic kidney disease. *ANZ J Surg*. 2007;**77**(4):292–294.
85. Vachha B, Sun MR, Siewert B, Eisenberg RL. Cystic lesions of the liver. *AJR Am J Roentgenol*. 2011;**196**(4):W355–W366.
86. Brancatelli G, Federle MP, Vilgrain V, Vullierme MP, Marin D, Lagalla R. Fibropolycystic liver disease: CT and MR imaging findings. *Radiographics*. 2005;**25**(3):659–670.
87. De Rosa FG, Garazzino S, Pasero D, Di Perri G, Ranieri VM. Invasive candidiasis and candidemia: new guidelines. *Minerva Anestesiol*. 2009;**75**(7–8):453–458.
88. Hsu M, Terris B, Wu TT, et al. Endometrial cysts within the liver: a rare entity and its differential diagnosis with mucinous cystic neoplasms of the liver. *Hum Pathol*. 2014;**45**(4):761–767.
89. Scappaticci F, Markowitz SK. Intrahepatic pseudocyst complicating acute pancreatitis: imaging findings. *AJR Am J Roentgenol*. 1995;**165**(4):873–874.
90. Mofredj A, Cadranel JF, Dautreaux M, et al. Pancreatic pseudocyst located in the liver: a case report and literature review. *J Clin Gastroenterol*. 2000;**30**(1):81–83.
91. Yoon W, Jeong YY, Kim JK, et al. CT in blunt liver trauma. *Radiographics*. 2005;**25**(1):87–104.
92. Dong Y, Wang WP, Mao F, et al. Contrast enhanced ultrasound features of hepatic cystadenoma and hepatic cystadenocarcinoma. *Scand J Gastroenterol*. 2017;**52**(3):365–372.
93. Soares KC, Arnaoutakis DJ, Kamel I, et al. Cystic neoplasms of the liver: biliary cystadenoma and cystadenocarcinoma. *J Am Coll Surg*. 2014;**218**(1):119–128.
94. Wheeler DA, Edmondson HA. Cystadenoma with mesenchymal stroma (CMS) in the liver and bile ducts. A clinicopathologic study of 17 cases, 4 with malignant change. *Cancer*. 1985;**56**(6):1434–1445.
95. Wang C, Miao R, Liu H, et al. Intrahepatic biliary cystadenoma and cystadenocarcinoma: an experience of 30 cases. *Dig Liver Dis*. 2012;**44**(5):426–431.
96. Dixon E, Sutherland FR, Mitchell P, McKinnon G, Nayak V. Cystadenomas of the liver: a spectrum of disease. *Can J Surg*. 2001;**44**(5):371–376.
97. Ramacciato G, Nigri GR, D'Angelo F, et al. Emergency laparotomy for misdiagnosed biliary cystadenoma originating from caudate lobe. *World J Surg Oncol*. 2006;**4**:76.
98. Martel G, Alsharif J, Aubin JM, et al. The management of hepatobiliary cystadenomas: lessons learned. *HPB (Oxford)*. 2013;**15**(8):617–622.
99. Lauffer JM, Baer HU, Maurer CA, Stoupis C, Zimmerman A, Buchler MW. Biliary cystadenocarcinoma of the liver: the need for complete resection. *Eur J Cancer*. 1998;**34**(12):1845–1851.
100. Sang X, Sun Y, Mao Y, et al. Hepatobiliary cystadenomas and cystadenocarcinomas: a report of 33 cases. *Liver Int*. 2011;**31**(9):1337–1344.
101. Zhang B, Guo Y, Wu K, Shan H. Intrahepatic biloma following transcatheter arterial chemoembolization for hepatocellular carcinoma: incidence, imaging features and management. *Mol Clin Oncol*. 2017;**6**(6):937–943.
102. Yu JS, Kim KW, Jeong MG, Lee DH, Park MS, Yoon SW. Predisposing factors of bile duct injury after transcatheter arterial chemoembolization (TACE) for hepatic malignancy. *Cardiovasc Interven Radiol*. 2002;**25**(4):270–274.
103. Hagiwara S, Ogino T, Takahashi Y, et al. Hepatocellular carcinoma mimicking liver abscesses in a cirrhotic patient with severe septic shock as a result of salmonella O9 HG Infection. *Case Rep Gastroenterol*. 2009;**3**(1):56–60.
104. Falidas E, Pazidis A, Anyfantakis G, Vlachos K, Goudeli C, Villias C. Multicystic hepatocarcinoma mimicking liver abscess. *Case Rep Surg*. 2013;**2013**:374905.
105. Zech CJ, Reiser MF, Herrmann KA. Imaging of hepatocellular carcinoma by computed tomography and magnetic resonance imaging: state of the art. *Dig Dis*. 2009;**27**(2):114–124.
106. Sakamoto I, Iwanaga S, Nagaoki K, et al. Intrahepatic biloma formation (bile duct necrosis) after transcatheter arterial chemoembolization. *AJR Am J Roentgenol*. 2003;**181**(1):79–87.
107. Sun Z, Li G, Ai X, et al. Hepatic and biliary damage after transarterial chemoembolization for malignant hepatic tumors: incidence, diagnosis, treatment, outcome and mechanism. *Crit Rev Oncol Hematol*. 2011;**79**(2):164–174.
108. Stocker JT, Ishak KG. Undifferentiated (embryonal) sarcoma of the liver: report of 31 cases. *Cancer*. 1978;**42**(1):336–348.
109. Walther A, Geller J, Coots A, et al. Multimodal therapy including liver transplantation for hepatic undifferentiated embryonal sarcoma. *Liver Transpl*. 2014;**20**(2):191–199.
110. Hung TY, Lu D, Liu MC. Undifferentiated (embryonal) sarcoma of the liver complicated with rupture in a child. *J Pediatr Hematology Oncol*. 2007;**29**(1):63–65.
111. Bisogno G, Pilz T, Perilongo G, et al. Undifferentiated sarcoma of the liver in childhood: a curable disease. *Cancer*. 2002;**94**(1):252–257.
112. Crider MH, Hoggard E, Manivel JC. Undifferentiated (embryonal) sarcoma of the liver. *Radiographics*. 2009;**29**(6):1665–1668.
113. Chung EM, Lattin GE Jr, Cube R, et al. From the archives of the AFIP: Pediatric liver masses: radiologic-pathologic correlation. Part 2. Malignant tumors. *Radiographics*. 2011;**31**(2):483–507.
114. Kim DY, Kim KH, Jung SE, Lee SC, Park KW, Kim WK. Undifferentiated (embryonal) sarcoma of the liver: combination treatment by surgery and chemotherapy. *J Pediatr Surg*. 2002;**37**(10):1419–1423.
115. May LT, Wang M, Albano E, Garrington T, Dishop M, Macy ME. Undifferentiated sarcoma of the liver: a single institution experience using a uniform treatment approach. *J Pediatr Hematol Oncol*. 2012;**34**(3):e114–e116.
116. Watanabe A, Suzuki H, Kubo N, et al. An oncocytic variant of intraductal papillary neoplasm of the bile duct that formed a giant hepatic cyst. *Rare Tumors*. 2013;**5**(3):e30.
117. Barton JG, Barrett DA, Maricevich MA, et al. Intraductal papillary mucinous neoplasm of the biliary tract: a real disease? *HPB (Oxford)*. 2009;**11**(8):684–691.
118. Ohtsuka M, Shimizu H, Kato A, et al. Intraductal papillary neoplasms of the bile duct. *Int J Hepatol*. 2014;**2014**:459091.
119. Ogawa H, Itoh S, Nagasaka T, Suzuki K, Ota T, Naganawa S. CT findings of intraductal papillary neoplasm of the bile duct: assessment with multiphase contrast-enhanced examination using multi-detector CT. *Clin Radiol*. 2012;**67**(3):224–231.
120. Yoon HJ, Kim YK, Jang KT, et al. Intraductal papillary neoplasm of the bile ducts: description of MRI and added value of diffusion-weighted MRI. *Abdom Imaging*. 2013;**38**(5):1082–1090.

121. Pitchaimuthu M, Duxbury M. Cystic lesions of the liver—a review. *Curr Probl Surg*. 2017;**54**(10):514–542.
122. Lee SS, Kim MH, Lee SK, et al. Clinicopathologic review of 58 patients with biliary papillomatosis. *Cancer*. 2004;**100**(4):783–793.
123. Alobaidi M, Shirkhoda A. Malignant cystic and necrotic liver lesions: a pattern approach to discrimination. *Curr Probl Diagn Radiol*. 2004;**33**(6):254–268.
124. Federle MP, Filly RA, Moss AA. Cystic hepatic neoplasms: complementary roles of CT and sonography. *AJR Am J Roentgenol*. 1981;**136**(2):345–348.
125. Mortele KJ, Ros PR. Cystic focal liver lesions in the adult: differential CT and MR imaging features. *Radiographics*. 2001;**21**(4):895–910.
126. Schwartz LH, Gandras EJ, Colangelo SM, Ercolani MC, Panicek DM. Prevalence and importance of small hepatic lesions found at CT in patients with cancer. *Radiology*. 1999;**210**(1):71–74.
127. Robinson PJ. Imaging liver metastases: current limitations and future prospects. *Br J Radiol*. 2000;**73**(867):234–241.
128. Sica GT, Ji H, Ros PR. CT and MR imaging of hepatic metastases. *AJR Am J Roentgenol*. 2000;**174**(3):691–698.

10

Benign liver tumours

Sadhana Shankar, Evangelia Florou, and Parthi Srinivasan

Introduction

Benign liver tumours are a heterogeneous group of lesions which have various cellular origins. The extensive use of modern imaging techniques such as ultrasound (US), computed tomography (CT), and magnetic resonance imaging (MRI) has resulted in an increased detection of many asymptomatic benign liver lesions. Though often detected incidentally, benign tumours, owing to their sheer size, can often become symptomatic and demand medical or surgical intervention. Benign liver tumours are broadly classified into *epithelial* and *non-epithelial* tumours (Table 10.1).[1] These are further subclassified based on their cell of origin. The incidence of each of these tumours varies. It is important to recognize that some benign tumours have a malignant potential. The most frequently diagnosed benign liver lesions are cavernous haemangiomas and focal nodular hyperplasias (FNHs) which very rarely require treatment or long-term follow-up. Less frequently diagnosed lesions such as hepatic adenomas and angiomyolipomas may be associated with a high risk of complications such as bleeding or malignant transformation thereby necessitating surgical intervention. It is therefore crucial to have a comprehensive knowledge of the clinical, biological, radiological, and pathological characteristics of each of the benign liver tumours to ensure accurate diagnosis as well as appropriate management. This chapter aims to describe the aetiology, clinical features, pathological characteristics, diagnostic workup, and treatment strategy for many benign liver lesions. The focus has been placed on tumours occurring in the adult population. As radiological imaging plays a critical role in their diagnosis and management, special emphasis is placed on its role. The most recent guidelines in the management of these tumours have also been highlighted.

Epithelial tumours of hepatocellular origin

Hepatocellular adenoma

The hepatocellular adenoma (HCA) or hepatic adenoma is a rare benign tumour with a prevalence of less than 0.05% in the general population.[2] It has a strong predilection for women (female:male ratio of 9:1) and usually occurs in the reproductive age group (35–55 years). Though usually solitary, the presence of multiple adenomas (greater than ten in number) of varying sizes involving both lobes of the liver is termed hepatic adenomatosis and is found in up to one-third of patients. Adenomatosis is usually found associated with congenital syndromes like glycogen storage disorders (particularly type 1a glycogenosis) and familial adenomatosis. HCAs are of particular interest because of the extensive research into their aetiology and subtypes and their remarkable association with complications like malignant transformation.

Aetiology

HCA is of epithelial origin and is composed of hepatocytes. These tumours became widely recognized and reported after an association was found with use of the oral contraceptive pill (OCP), highlighting that hormonal influences may play a role in its pathogenesis. Oestrogen has been reported to be an independent risk factor for the development of HCA and use of the OCP increases the risk by 30 times.[2] Two-thirds of HCAs express oestrogen receptors

Table 10.1 Classification of benign liver tumours

Epithelial tumours	
Hepatocellular	Hepatocellular adenoma Focal nodular hyperplasia Nodular regenerative hyperplasia Arterialized nodular hyperplasia (FNH-like lesions) Dysplastic nodule
Cholangiocellular	Bile duct adenoma Biliary hamartoma (von Meyenburg complex) Biliary adenofibroma
Non-epithelial tumours	
Mesenchymal	Cavernous haemangioma Fatty lesions—angiomyolipoma, lipoma, myelolipoma, focal fatty change Lymphangioma Leiomyoma Mesenchymal hamartoma
Heterotopia	Splenic, pancreatic, adrenal, or endometriotic tissue
Miscellaneous	Peliosis hepatis Inflammatory pseudotumour Solitary fibrotic tumour

Source: data from Nagtegaal ID, Odze RD, Klimstra D, et al. The 2019 WHO classification of tumours of the digestive system. *Histopathology*. 2020;76(2):182–188.

and it is postulated that oestrogen may stimulate the development of HCA by promoting *HNF1A* gene mutations or germline mutations in *CYP1B1* involved in oestrogen metabolism.[3–5] The link between OCP and HCA is further strengthened by the demonstration of a dose-dependent relationship between the two. Conversely, spontaneous regression of HCA after cessation of OCP use has also been observed frequently.[6,7] Newer hormonal pills containing low-dose oestrogen or progesterone are associated with a lower risk suggesting that environmental factors may also play a role in the pathogenesis of HCA.

An increased risk of HCA has also been reported with the use of androgen preparations such as those used in patients with Fanconi's anaemia, paroxysmal nocturnal haemoglobinuria, hypogonadism, and hypopituitarism and in athletes who have abused anabolic steroids.[8,9] There have been sporadic reports of an increased incidence in patients with endogenous overproduction of androgens as in Klinefelter's syndrome and polycystic ovarian syndrome.[10,11] More recently, an increased incidence of HCA has been reported in obese patients (38–73% of patients with HCA) and in patients with non-alcoholic steatohepatitis, shifting the paradigm from modern oral contraceptives to obesity and metabolic syndrome as the major risk factors in the modern era.[12–14]

Several rare genetic syndromes have been associated with HCA, the most important being glycogen storage diseases (types I, III, and IV). The lifelong risk of developing HCA is significantly increased in these patients. Type 1a glycogenosis is particularly important as more than 50% of these patients have hepatic adenomatosis.[15] The tumours develop between the second and third decades of life with nearly half of them being subclassified as inflammatory hepatocellular adenomas (I-HCAs).[16] Reduction in their size and number has been observed after optimizing metabolic control. Other syndromes associated with HCA are the McCune–Albright syndrome, maturity-onset diabetes of the young type 3 (MODY 3), and iron-overload states such as hereditary haemochromatosis and beta thalassaemia.[17–19]

Pathology and molecular subtypes

Macroscopically, HCA appears as a solitary or as multiple well-defined lesions with large subcapsular vessels. On cut section, it appears as a fleshy, well-demarcated, sometimes encapsulated tumour ranging in colour from white to brown with heterogeneous areas of haemorrhage and necrosis (Figure 10.1). Microscopically, HCA is composed of benign hepatocytes with a low nuclear/cytoplasmic ratio and uniform nuclei, arranged in a trabecular pattern (Figure 10.2a). The hallmark is the absence of normal hepatic architecture including the portal structures and bile ducts. The hepatocytes may have increased intracellular fat or glycogen and there are numerous small vessels distributed throughout the tumour.

HCA is considered to be a heterogeneous disease with several molecular subtypes based on clonal hepatocellular proliferation, and each subtype is associated with distinct morphological characteristics and complications. Based on genomic analysis of mutation in specific genes, Bioulac-Sage et al., in a multicentric study, identified four subtypes of HCA and proposed the Bordeaux classification.[20] According to this classification, HCA is subdivided into HNF1α-mutated HCA (H-HCA), inflammatory (also called telangiectatic) HCA (I-HCA), β-catenin-mutated HCA (b-HCA), and an unclassified subtype. The main hallmarks of the different subtypes are summarized in Table 10.2. Molecular subtyping has

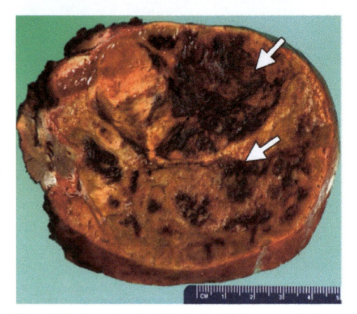

Figure 10.1 Cut section of an HCA showing a fleshy, encapsulated tumour with areas of haemorrhage (white arrows).

resulted in a better understanding of the tumorigenesis. While the size of HCA correlates well with complications of haemorrhage and malignant transformation, the molecular subtyping is essential to identify lesions which are highly associated with the risk of transformation into hepatocellular carcinoma (HCC). More recently, the Bordeaux classification has been further expanded into eight subtypes including HCA with β-catenin activation and IL6/JAK/STAT3 overexpression (b^{ex3} IHCA), HCA with weak β-catenin activation ($b^{ex7,8}$ HCA), Sonic hedgehog pathway-activated HCA (sh HCA), and argininosuccinate synthase-1-positive HCA (ASS+ HCA) in addition to the original four subtypes.[4]

Clinical features

Most HCAs are detected incidentally on US in patients with recognizable risk factors. Symptomatic patients usually present with abdominal pain. In patients with large tumours, the liver function tests may show a cholestatic pattern due to extrinsic compression of the biliary tree. I-HCA may present as a systemic inflammatory response syndrome with fever. Unlike other benign liver lesions, HCAs have a potential for haemorrhage and malignant transformation. Haemorrhage is the most common complication and has been reported in 25% of patients.[12] Risk factors for haemorrhage include size greater than 5 cm, I-HCA subtype, visualization of arteries within the tumour, location in the left lateral segment, and exophytic growth.[12,21] Pregnancy as a risk factor for tumour growth and rupture has been proposed, but several studies show that HCAs remain relatively stable during pregnancy.[21] The risk of malignant transformation is 4–5% and is associated with male sex (six- to ten-fold increased risk), androgen use, b-HCA subtype, and size greater than 5 cm (independent of subtype). I-HCAs can also contain β-catenin mutations and such a variety are at a risk of malignant transformation.[22–24] HCC that occurs in the setting of HCA is usually well differentiated without vascular invasion or satellite nodules and is usually found after histopathological examination of the resected adenoma specimen.[12,23] The serum alpha-fetoprotein level is usually normal in such a setting.

Epithelial tumours of hepatocellular origin

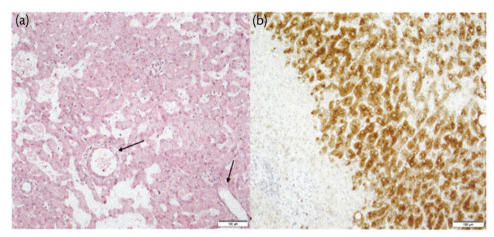

Figure 10.2 (a) High-power microscopy showing the inflammatory type of HCA with benign hepatocytes arranged in trabeculae with numerous unpaired vessels (black arrows) distributed throughout the tumour. (b) The tumour shows positive immunostaining with serum amyloid A.

Diagnosis

Most HCAs are incidentally picked up by US and may be hypo-, hyper-, or isoechoic and are generally well-defined, non-lobulated lesions which may appear heterogeneous due to intratumoural bleeding or necrosis (Figure 10.4a,b). On non-contrast CT scans, HCAs are typically iso- or hypoattenuating lesions when compared to the adjacent hepatic parenchyma. On contrast-enhanced CT scans they demonstrate moderate to intense enhancement

Table 10.2 Hepatocellular adenoma—Bordeaux classification for subtypes and features

Feature	HNF1α-mutated HCA (H-HCA)	Inflammatory HCA (I-HCA)	β-catenin mutated HCA (b-HCA)	Unclassified HCA
Incidence	30–40%	40–55%	10–20%	5–10%
Mutation involved	Inactivation of HNF1α protein involved in hepatocyte differentiation and metabolism control	Inactivation of JAK/STAT pathway by mutation of gp130 (*IL6ST*), *FRK*, *STAT3*, *GNAS*, and *JAK1*	Activation of β-catenin gene (*CTNNB1*) localized at hotspots in exons 3, 7, and 8. Some may be associated with additional mutations in the JAK/STAT pathway	No particular mutation identified
Clinical features	Tumours are found almost exclusively in women using the OCP (**Figure 10.3**). Germline mutations are found in familial adenomatosis and MODY 3. They never occur in glycogen storage diseases	Tumours are often found in patients with obesity, metabolic syndrome, and glycogen storage disorders. They produce a systemic inflammatory response with elevated C-reactive protein, erythrocyte sedimentation rate, alkaline phosphatase, and gamma glutamyl transaminase	This type has an association with male sex, androgen use, and has a younger age of onset	No specific clinical feature
Histological hallmark	Prominent steatosis	Clusters of small arteries surrounded by extracellular matrix and inflammatory infiltrates associated with foci of sinusoidal dilatation	Presence of cellular atypias, pseudoglandular formations, and cholestasis	No specific histological feature
Immunostaining	Absence of staining for liver fatty acid binding protein (LFABP) which is controlled by HNF1α, compared to strong positivity in the background liver	Staining with serum amyloid A (**Figure 10.2b**) and C-reactive protein (more sensitive, less specific)	Diffuse, strong glutamine synthetase positivity and positive β-catenin nuclear staining	None
Specific complication	None	Haemorrhage, systemic inflammatory response	Malignant transformation	Rarely malignant transformation
MRI features	Diffuse and homogeneous signal drop out on T1 out-of-phase sequences due to the presence of microscopic fat (sensitivity 86% and specificity 100%)	High signal intensity on T2-weighted images in the periphery which correlates with dilated sinusoids (Atoll sign). They demonstrate intense enhancement with gadolinium, which persists in the portal venous and delayed phase	Lack specific features on imaging and may show homogeneous or heterogeneous hyperintensity on T1- and T2-weighted images. They may also show strong arterial enhancement that may not persist on the delayed phase thereby mimicking HCC	Strong arterial enhancement and they do not show any delayed enhancement after gadolinium injection. Lack specific identifying features and may mimic HCC

Source: data from Zucman-Rossi J, Jeannot E, Van Nhieu JT, et al. Genotype–phenotype correlation in hepatocellular adenoma: new classification and relationship with HCC. *Hepatology*. 2006;43(3):515–524.

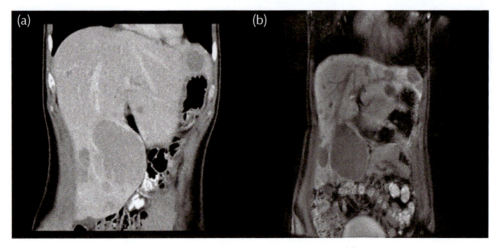

Figure 10.3 Multiple bilateral hepatic adenomas in a young woman taking oral contraceptives. (a) Coronal contrast-enhanced CT image. (b) Coronal T1-weighted MRI showing signal drop due to the presence of fat.

in the arterial phase and may remain hyperdense or washout in the portal venous phase (Figure 10.4c,d). Among all the imaging modalities available, MRI has the highest sensitivity (87–91%) and specificity (89–98%) to accurately diagnose HCA and to even classify the subtypes.[25,26] HCA is usually of moderate intensity on T2-weighted imaging and demonstrates enhancement in the arterial phase followed by a hyperintense appearance in the venous phase (Figures 4.5 and 4.6). Occasionally the lesions are hypointense in the venous phase and can be confused with HCC. When hepatobiliary-specific contrast agents such as gadolinium-EOB-DTPA (Primovist) and gadolinium-BOPTA (MultiHance) are used, they typically do not show uptake in the hepatobiliary phase due to a lack of functioning hepatocytes. The subtypes of HCA have noticeably different imaging features as summarized in Table 10.2 which can be used to differentiate them. Despite this, there may be considerable difficulty in differentiating them from

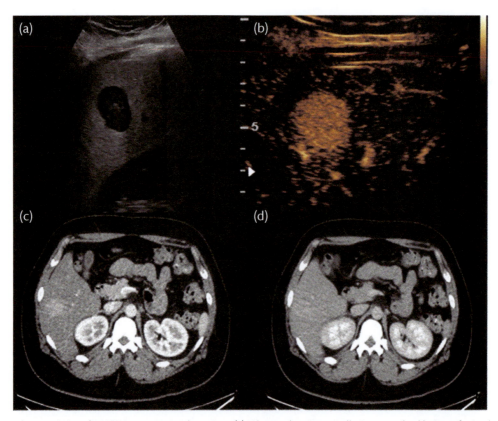

Figure 10.4 Imaging characteristics of a HCA in a young male patient. (a) US scan showing a well-circumscribed lesion of mixed echogenicity in the right lobe of the liver. (b) Contrast-enhanced US scan of the same lesion showing enhancement in the arterial phase. (c) Axial arterial phase contrast-enhanced CT scan showing enhancement of the lesion. The liver is mildly fatty but not cirrhotic. (d) Axial portal venous phase contrast-enhanced CT scan showing washout of the lesion which becomes iso-attenuating with the liver.

Epithelial tumours of hepatocellular origin

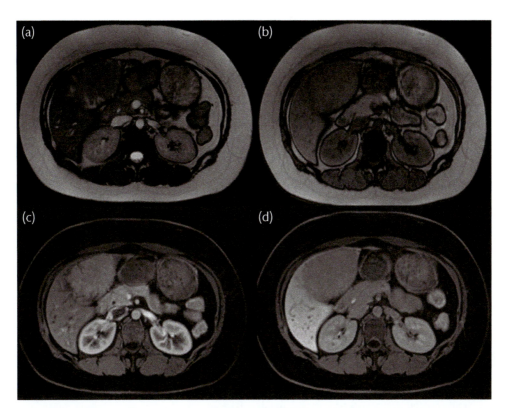

Figure 10.5 Axial phase MRI characteristics of I-HCA in a young female patient. (a) T2-weighted image with fat suppression shows a high intensity in the periphery corresponding to large sinusoids (Atoll sign). (b) In- and opposed-phase T1 image showing no signal drop out in the lesion. (c) Arterial phase T1 image demonstrating brisk enhancement of the lesion. (d) Portal venous phase T1 image showing washout from the lesion.

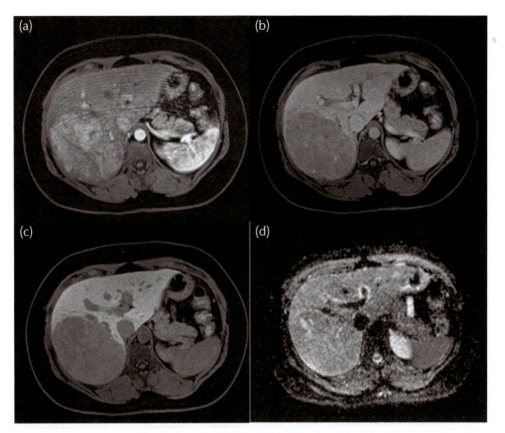

Figure 10.6 Axial MRI characteristics of a well-defined inflammatory HCA in a young male patient. (a) Arterial phase image showing intense enhancement. (b) Portal venous phase image showing washout. (c) A 20-minute delayed phase image with hepatobiliary-specific contrast agent Primovist demonstrating no uptake by the lesion. (d) Diffusion-weighted image showing no restriction of diffusion.

atypical FNHs or from HCCs in which case percutaneous biopsy may be necessary to establish the diagnosis.

Management

HCA has a potential for complications including malignant transformation. Once diagnosed, a thorough baseline assessment and a plan for further management including follow-up should be established. When risk factors are identified, lifestyle changes such as discontinuation of the OCP or anabolic steroids and weight control are recommended (Figure 10.7). In male patients, HCA should always be resected irrespective of size as it carries a higher risk of malignant transformation. In female patients, once imaging diagnosis is established, lifestyle changes are advised and a reassessment with contrast-enhanced MRI is recommended in 6 months (irrespective of the initial tumour size).[27] HCAs persistently greater than 5 cm or increasing in size (≥20% of tumour diameter as per RECIST criteria for solid malignant tumours) should be considered for resection irrespective of their molecular subtype.[28] A laparoscopic or open approach can be chosen for resecting these tumours depending upon the tumour location, number, and size. Regional lymphadenectomy is not indicated. HCAs less than 5 cm on reassessment or those showing a decrease in size require surveillance for a minimum period of 5 years. US is a cost-effective method of follow-up compared to MRI and is preferred for well-diagnosed lesions. Annual surveillance is recommended for all non-IHCA subtypes whereas biannual surveillance is recommended for the I-HCA subtype.[27] For lesions stable or decreasing in size after 5 years, biennial surveillance is recommended. Some centres have adopted a conservative approach with annual surveillance for tumours greater than 5 cm of the H-HCA subtype as the risk of complications is extremely low in them.[12]

In pregnant women with HCA, a closer surveillance with US every 6–12 weeks is recommended. Liaison with the obstetric team is essential if there is an increase in size during pregnancy as there is a risk of rupture. Prior to 24 weeks of gestation, surgery is the preferred treatment for tumours increasing in size to greater than 5 cm and after 24 weeks, transarterial embolization (TAE) can be an effective alternative treatment.[27,28] For smaller adenomas (<5 cm), not exophytic and not growing, a conservative approach is preferred and there are no data supporting elective Caesarean section over vaginal delivery.

In patients with adenomatosis, the risk of complications and the management depends on the size of the largest tumour rather than on the number of tumours.[12,20] In patients with unilobar disease with risk factors, hepatectomy is done as a one-staged or two-staged procedure. In bi-lobar disease, resection of lesions larger than 5 cm is advocated. In glycogen storage diseases, there is a lifelong risk of HCA recurrence and associated complications. Clinical guidelines suggest annual surveillance with US in such patients aged between 0 and 10 years and biannual surveillance after 10 years.

Though surgical resection remains the first-line treatment, non-surgical techniques such as TAE and radiofrequency ablation are being introduced for management of these tumours. TAE can be life-saving in patients presenting with acute haemorrhage and can help to manage the situation conservatively. It can even cause regression of the tumour. Under such circumstances, an MRI is repeated in 6 months, to look for residual tumour and if the tumour is less than 5 cm, it can be managed conservatively with regular surveillance. The same principle has been applied for the use of TAE to treat non-ruptured HCAs, especially for large and multiple tumours and also preoperatively to reduce the size to allow parenchymal-sparing surgery.[29] In patients with progression of residual tumours after resection, radiofrequency ablation can be considered as an alternative treatment option provided the size of the tumour is less than 4 cm for effective ablation.[30] Indications for liver transplantation in HCA have become limited and include multiple unresectable lesions in men, a large unresectable HCA with an intrahepatic venous shunt, and patients with glycogen storage disease unresponsive to medical treatment.[12,31,32]

Focal nodular hyperplasia

FNH is the second most common benign tumour of the liver with a prevalence of 0.2–3% in the population.[27] Like HCA, it shows a female preponderance with a female:male ratio of 9:1 and is usually found in the middle-aged group between 30 and 50 years.[33] FNH are usually solitary and less than 5 cm in size. About 20% are multiple and are found in association with vascular disorders like hereditary haemorrhagic telangiectasia, Budd–Chiari syndrome, and congenital absence of the portal vein. They may be found associated with hepatic adenomas in 20% of cases.

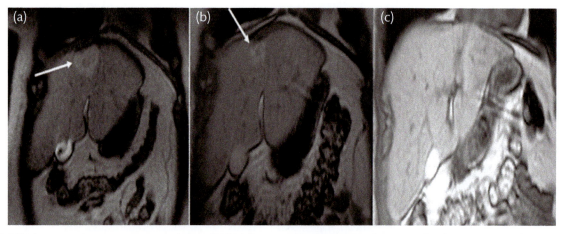

Figure 10.7 MRI demonstrating spontaneous resolution of HCA (white arrow) in a young female patient after discontinuation of oral contraceptives. (a) Image at diagnosis. (b) Image at 18 months of follow-up. (c) Image at 4 years of follow-up showing complete resolution.

Aetiopathogenesis

FNH is considered to be an aberrant regenerative response to an arterial malformation.[34] According to this hypothesis, arterial hyperperfusion of a localized area of liver parenchyma results in hyperplasia of the hepatocytes. This theory is supported by the fact that FNH is commonly found associated with vascular disorders of the liver like the Budd–Chiari syndrome, hereditary haemorrhagic telangiectasia, congenital absence of the portal vein, congenital portosystemic shunting (Abernethy syndrome), and portal vein thrombosis with subsequent arterialization. This hypothesis is further supported by molecular studies which demonstrate that FNH is a polyclonal regenerative process with deregulation of genes involved in vascular remodelling.[35] There is differential expression of angiopoietins resulting in an increased angiopoietin 1/angiopoietin 2 ratio resulting in arteriolar malformation. Molecular analysis also shows upregulation of extracellular matrix genes resulting in overexpression of transforming growth factor β (TGF-β) and Wnt/β-catenin target genes such as *GLUL* which encodes glutamine synthetase.[35] This results in a characteristic 'map-like' staining of glutamine synthetase typically at the periphery of the nodule on immunohistochemistry. This heterogeneous pattern of staining indicates that there is β-catenin activation without gene mutation supporting the polyclonal origin of FNH and, in turn, the vascular theory. Most FNHs remain stable in size which further supports that it is a regenerative response to an abnormal arterial blood supply. Another observation is that FNH and its surrounding tissue also expresses oestrogen receptors and is commonly found in middle-aged women taking oral contraceptives.[36] However, several studies have indicated that there is no hormonal influence on the growth of FNH and the lesion remains relatively stable in size even during pregnancy or after cessation of oral contraceptive use.[37]

Grossly, FNH is a well-circumscribed unencapsulated solitary lesion with a firm to rubbery consistency and a central stellate scar with radiating septa. Histologically, FNH is composed of benign-appearing hepatocytes arranged in liver plates of normal or slightly increased thickness separated by fibrous septa radiating from a central scar (Figure 10.8a). Kupffer cells and biliary ductules are found at the interface between the septa and the nodule and the septa may contain inflammatory infiltrates. The characteristic features which distinguish it from adenomas are the presence of large dystrophic arteries in the fibrous septa and positive immunostaining with glutamine synthetase in a map-like pattern (Figure 10.8b). Apart from the classical type, 'atypical FNH' has been described in 20% of cases. These atypical presentations include FNH without a central scar (see Figure 10.12 later in this section), steatotic FNH (containing fat), telangiectatic FNH, and mixed FNH (hyperplastic and adenomatous).[38]

Clinical features

FNH is usually asymptomatic and is incidentally detected during investigation for an unrelated cause. Very rarely, when large or subcapsular, they can cause symptoms such as abdominal discomfort due to compression of the adjacent structures or stretching of Glisson's capsule. Reports of pedunculated FNHs undergoing torsion and causing acute pain have also been documented. Nevertheless, complications are extremely rare and malignant transformation has never been described. Liver function tests are usually normal but a mild elevation of gamma glutamyl transferase and alkaline phosphatase has been observed in very large FNHs causing extrinsic compression of the bile ducts. Most FNHs remain stable in size over time and mild regression has also been reported in postmenopausal women.

Diagnosis

The radiological appearance of FNH is that of a lobulated, unencapsulated, homogeneous lesion with a central scar. FNH is generally hypo- or isoechoic on US and typically displaces the surrounding vessel, the very feature that makes it detectable on this modality (Figure 10.9a). Contrast-enhanced US demonstrates centrifugal filling from a central feeding artery with a 'spoke-wheel' pattern in the arterial phase which is a characteristic feature of FNH and helps to distinguish it from a hepatic adenoma (Figure 10.9b). On non-contrast CT, FNH appears as a hypoattenuating lesion and on arterial phase contrast, there is rapid enhancement which later becomes iso-attenuating to the surrounding liver in the portal and delayed venous phase (Figure 10.9c,d). The central hypoattenuating scar is seen only in one-third of the cases on contrast-enhanced CT.

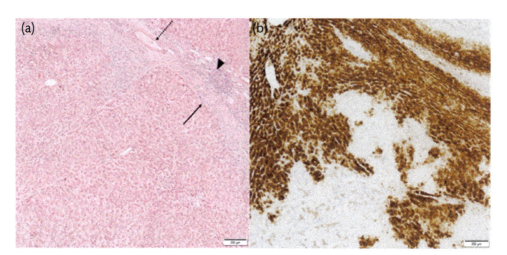

Figure 10.8 (a) High-power microscopic view of FNH showing sheets of benign hepatocytes separated by fibrous bands (solid arrow). Large dystrophic vessels (dotted arrow) and inflammatory infiltrates (arrowhead) are typically seen within the septa. (b) Immunostaining with glutamine synthetase shows the characteristic map-like pattern.

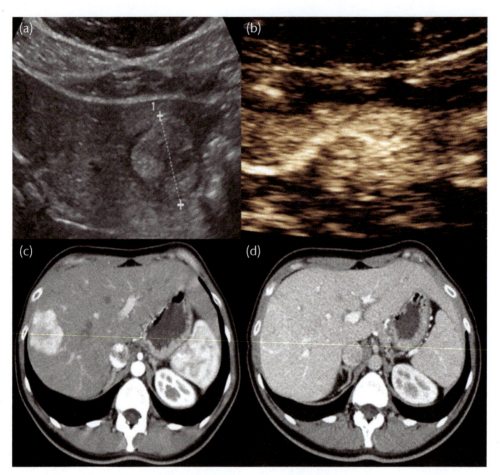

Figure 10.9 Imaging characteristics of FNH. (a) US scan demonstrating an isoechoic lesion. (b) Contrast-enhanced US scan of the same lesion shows a central feeding artery with a 'spoke-wheel' pattern. (c) Axial arterial phase contrast CT scan shows intense enhancement of FNH in segment 7 with a central scar. (d) Axial portal venous phase CT scan shows that the FNH becomes iso-attenuating with the liver.

MRI has the highest sensitivity (70–80%) and specificity (100%) for diagnosis of FNH and to differentiate it from other benign lesions. There are seven important MRI criteria to diagnose FNH and the presence of at least four is diagnostic of FNH (Figures 10.10 and 10.11).[26] They are as follows: a lesion that is homogeneous, lacks a capsule, lobulated, barely detectable on T1- and T2-weighted images, has a central scar which is hypointense on T1-weighted images and strongly hyperintense on T2-weighted images, shows intense arterial enhancement with no washout of contrast in the venous phase, and no prior history of cancer or chronic liver disease. A combination of contrast-enhanced US and MRI has the highest diagnostic accuracy for a small FNH and for an atypical FNH (Figure 10.12). Hepatobiliary-specific contrast (Primovist, MultiHance) has significantly improved accuracy in differentiating in FNH from hepatic adenoma. The presence of Kupffer cells results in uptake of technetium 99m-sulphur colloid and super para-magnetic iron oxide (SPIO) contrast agents which help to differentiate it from an adenoma. Hepatic angiography demonstrates a typical 'spoke-wheel' pattern but is not used routinely. Biopsy is generally not indicated unless all imaging modalities fail to establish an accurate diagnosis.

Management

Asymptomatic FNHs, irrespective of their size or number, do not require any treatment.[27] The patient should be reassured that there is no risk of malignant transformation and also educated about the natural history of the lesion. There is no justification for avoiding oral contraceptives and pregnancy nor is there a need for follow-up. Surgical resection is recommended for symptomatic patients and for patients with a pedunculated FNH with a risk of torsion. The presence of large surrounding veins supports formal liver resection over enucleation to reduce the risk of untoward bleeding. In some symptomatic patients, TAE and radiofrequency ablation have been tried with good results; however, these procedures are not routinely recommended.[39]

Nodular regenerative hyperplasia

Nodular regenerative hyperplasia (NRH), also known as nodular transformation or non-cirrhotic nodulation, is a benign condition characterized by diffuse involvement of the liver with micronodules 1–2 mm in size. It is recently being recognized as a clinical entity which is distinctly different in its biological behaviour from regenerative nodules found in cirrhosis and FNH.

Aetiopathogenesis

The prevalence of NRH is estimated to be around 2% and it is found equally in both sexes.[40] Several theories have been proposed for nodular transformation of the liver and they suggest that these nodules are basically hyperplastic hepatocytes triggered in

Epithelial tumours of hepatocellular origin | 95

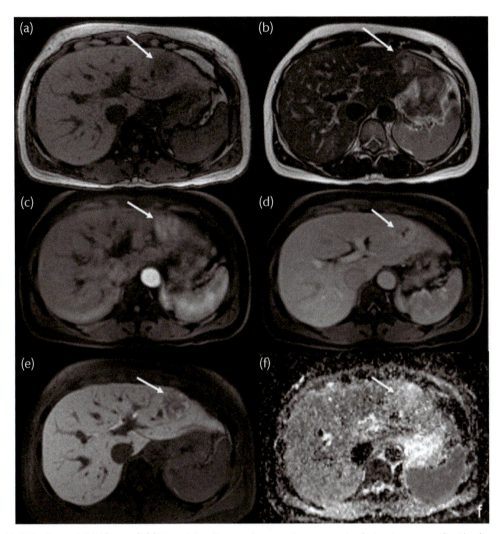

Figure 10.10 Axial MRI findings of FNH (arrows). (a) T1-weighted image shows an iso-attenuating lesion in segment 3 with a hypoattenuating central scar. (b) T2-weighted image shows a similar lesion with a hyperattenuating central scar. (c) Arterial phase MRI demonstrating intense enhancement of the lesion. (d) In the porto-venous phase, the lesion continues to enhance. (e) A 20-minute delayed image with Primovist demonstrates retention in the lesion. (f) Diffusion-weighted image shows restricted diffusion.

response to various causative factors. The vascular theory suggests that portal venulitis due to any insult results in obliteration of the portal veins and ischaemia of the central zone of hepatocytes which in turn triggers the hypertrophy of surrounding hepatocytes resulting in micronodular transformation.[41] Another theory suggests that NRH is a pre-neoplastic process based on the finding that some of these nodules harbour dysplasia (20–42%) and even HCC.[33,42] In support of the vascular theory, NRH is commonly found in association with a gamut of systemic diseases like myeloproliferative and lymphoproliferative disorders, chronic vascular disorders, rheumatological and collagen vascular diseases, solid organ transplantation, and portal venopathy.[43,44] Drugs such as steroids, azathioprine, and oxaliplatin have also been associated with it. The most notable association has been in patients taking oxaliplatin-based chemotherapy for colorectal liver metastasis. The prevalence of NRH in these patients is as high as 24%.[45] In such patients, NRH has been associated with high morbidity and mortality following major liver resection.[46]

Macroscopically, the liver is diffusely involved by nodules 1–2 mm in size. Histologically, the characteristic findings are those of hepatocyte hyperplasia, with plates more than one cell in thickness, occasional binucleation of hepatocytes, and coexistent compression of adjacent liver with condensation of reticulin around expanded nodules (**Figure 10.13**).[47] Kupffer cell hyperplasia is frequently present. There is, however, preservation of the basic architectural framework.

Clinical features

Clinically, NRH is usually asymptomatic and associated with normal liver function tests except with the occasional elevation of the serum alkaline phosphatase. However, 30% of patients may develop portal hypertension and subsequent varices, splenomegaly, and ascites.[48] In patients receiving oxaliplatin-based chemotherapy, an aspartate aminotransferase-to-platelet ratio index (APRI score) of greater than 0.36 and platelet count less than 100,000/mm³ is predictive of the presence of NRH and is a useful tool for preoperative risk assessment in these patients.[49]

Diagnosis

Imaging may often remain normal or show features of non-cirrhotic portal hypertension without nodules. Occasionally, livers with NRH

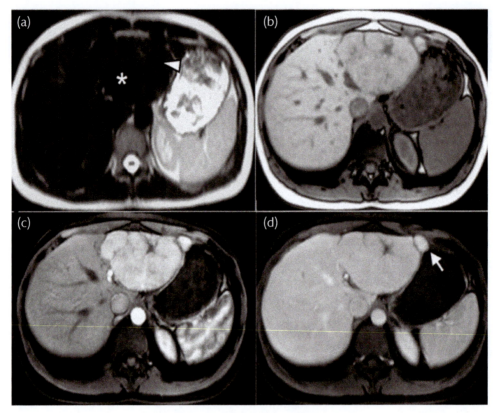

Figure 10.11 Axial MRI findings of FNH in a 66-year-old lady. (a, b) T2- and T1-weighted images show a barely detectable lesion with a central scar. (c) Arterial phase showing enhancement of FNH. (d) Porto-venous phase showing continued enhancement.

show diffuse nodules which are often hypodense on CT without significant enhancement. On MRI, these nodules appear hyperintense on T1-weighted images and hypo- or isointense on T2-weighted images (Figure 10.14). The nodules may take up technetium sulphur colloid and have variable echogenicity on sonography. They may fill from the periphery on angiography, are vascular, and sometimes contain small hypovascular areas due to haemorrhage. The absence of a central scar distinguishes it from FNH. Biopsy, either percutaneous or open to obtain an adequate tissue sample, remains the procedure of choice to establish accurate diagnosis and to rule out malignancy.

Management

In asymptomatic patients, no treatment is necessary. In patients with portal hypertension, appropriate management in the form of drug therapy, banding of oesophageal varices, and portocaval shunt procedures are recommended. In patients receiving oxaliplatin, addition of bevacizumab has been found to limit the development of NRH.[50] In the presence of NRH in such patients, the functional liver remnant must be carefully assessed and improved prior to undertaking any major liver resection as there is a high incidence of postoperative morbidity due to liver failure.

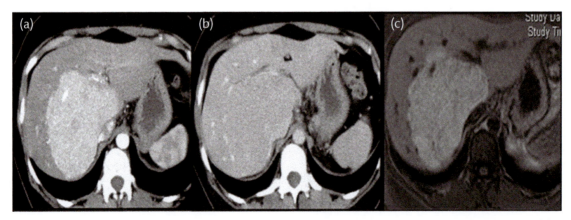

Figure 10.12 Atypical FNH without a central scar. (a) Arterial phase contrast-enhanced CT scan shows enhancement of the lesion. (b) Venous phase CT scan shows that the lesion becomes iso-attenuating. (c) Delayed phase MRI with Primovist demonstrates retention of contrast in the lesion.

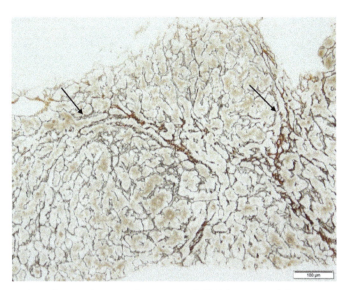

Figure 10.13 High-power microscopic view of a reticulin-stained specimen of NRH showing nodular arrangement (arrows) of benign-looking hepatocytes with no features of atypia surrounded by an intact reticulin framework.

Arterialized nodular hyperplasia

This category of lesions is called FNH-like lesions as they histologically resemble FNH but are seen in patients with underlying liver disease such as the Budd–Chiari syndrome, hereditary haemorrhagic telangiectasia, and congenital hepatic fibrosis or they may be found adjacent to a metastatic tumour (Figure 10.15). The exact aetiology is unknown but as all the above conditions are associated with decreased portal flow and increased arterial flow, these lesions may be considered as a hepatic response to vascular changes. Imaging with CT reveals nodules which strongly enhance on the arterial phase and may sometimes show a central scar. On MRI, they appear hyperintense on T1-weighted images and hypointense on T2-weighted images. Histologically, they are composed of benign hepatocytes which are CD34 positive with adjacent arterioles and portal tracts with an intact reticulin framework. Unlike FNH, these nodules may increase in size and number over time.

Dysplastic nodule

Dysplastic nodules are asymptomatic lesions usually found in cirrhotic livers and are considered to be precursors of HCC. They can be low grade or high grade and are usually less than 2 cm in size. They are incidentally detected during imaging or macroscopic examination of resected specimen. The alpha-feto protein level is normal or may be mildly elevated but never more than 200 ng/mL. Macroscopically,

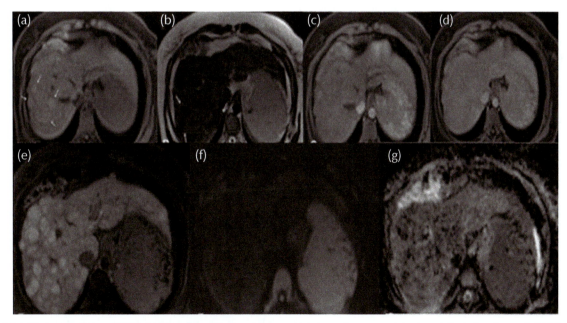

Figure 10.14 MRI characteristics of NRH. (a) T1-weighted image shows multiple hyperintense nodules in a cirrhotic liver (arrows). (b) T2-weighted image shows multiple hypodense nodular architecture of the liver. (c, d) Arterial and portal venous phase MRI demonstrate no enhancement. (e) A 20-minute delayed Primovist image shows no uptake or washout in the nodules. (f) Diffusion-weighted image and apparent diffusion coefficient (g) show no restriction of diffusion.

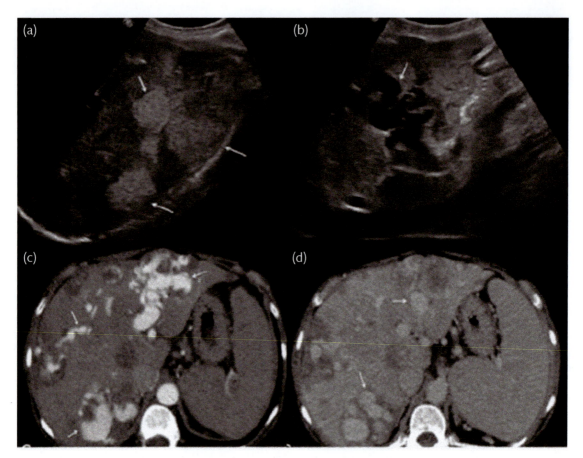

Figure 10.15 Hereditary haemorrhagic telangiectasis (Osler–Weber–Rendu syndrome) in a young female patient with associated arterialized nodular hyperplasia. (a) US scan shows multiple echogenic nodules (arrows) in a heterogeneous liver parenchyma. (b) US scan of the same patient showing hypertrophic hepatic arteries (arrow). (c, d) Arterial and portal venous phase contrast-enhanced CT scan demonstrating hypertrophic hepatic arteries forming arteriovenous shunts with the portal vein (arrows) with a heterogeneous hepatic parenchyma.

low-grade dysplastic nodules are well circumscribed and yellow to tan in colour whereas the high-grade dysplastic nodules may have irregular margins. Histologically, they show a spectrum of atypical features such as hyperchromatic nuclei, pseudoacinar pattern, focal reticulin loss, and unpaired arterioles. These changes may be present throughout the nodule or may be focal. An immunohistochemical profile is important to distinguish it from HCC. CK7(+) ductular reaction is present around more than 50% of the circumference of most high-grade dysplastic nodules, whereas this is focal or lost in most HCCs. Glypican-3 expression favours HCC rather than high-grade dysplasia especially if strong and diffuse. Imaging features that suggest malignant transformation of a high-grade dysplastic nodule include increasing size, hypervascularity, and nodule-in-nodule configuration. Nevertheless, biopsy is necessary to establish diagnosis and excision biopsy may be necessary to exclude focal malignancy. A biopsy confirmation of a high-grade dysplastic nodule warrants more frequent surveillance as the rate of malignant transformation is 32% per year.[51] Hence in some cases, ablation of the lesion has also been advocated.

Epithelial tumours of cholangiocellular origin

Bile duct adenoma

Bile duct adenoma, also called a cholangioma, is a benign epithelial lesion composed of peribiliary cystic structures resembling bile ducts. They are small and subcapsular in location and are often mistaken for metastatic deposits during surgery. The aetiology is unclear but BRAF V600E mutations are found in more than 50% of cases.[52] BRAF mutations are also commonly reported in intrahepatic cholangiocarcinoma suggesting that bile duct adenomas may be precursors of malignancy. However, this 'adenoma to carcinoma sequence' is not well established. Macroscopically, it appears as a single, small (<1 cm), whitish, subcapsular lesion which is firm in consistency. Microscopically, it contains uniformly sized tubules and acini with rounded outlines composed of a single layer of cuboidal to columnar cells that lack atypia, hyperchromasia, or mitoses against a background of fibrous stroma (Figure 10.16). Variant features include clear cell change, mucinous metaplasia, neuroendocrine differentiation, and α-1 antitrypsin globules. A circumscribed outline and lack of cytological atypia are the most important features to distinguish it from adenocarcinoma. Bile duct adenomas are considered to be indolent and hence resection is not justified.

Biliary hamartoma (von Meyenburg complex)

Biliary hamartoma or von Meyenburg complex is a developmental malformation caused by aberrant remodelling of the embryonic bile ducts. The prevalence is around 5% at autopsy.[53] They are generally sporadic but have also been found within the spectrum of numerous fibropolycystic diseases of liver including congenital hepatic fibrosis, Caroli's disease, and autosomal dominant polycystic

Epithelial tumours of cholangiocellular origin 99

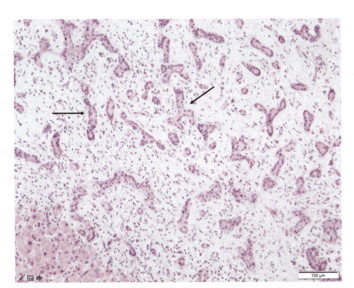

Figure 10.16 High-power microscopic view of bile duct adenoma showing simple non-cystic tubular glands (arrows) lined by cuboidal epithelium without atypia in a background of fibrous stroma. Note the absence of intraluminal bile within the glands.

liver disease. They are small (usually <0.5 cm), grey-white, multi-focal, subcapsular lesions with a whitish or greenish appearance. Microscopically, they are composed of angulated, branching, and irregular ducts embedded in dense fibrous stroma, found usually within or at the edge of portal tracts. The ducts are lined by cuboidal, often flattened epithelium and may contain eosinophilic protein-aceous debris or inspissated bile. Unlike bile duct adenoma they do not contain the BRAF V600E mutation. On US, they are classically very small hyperechoic cystic lesions associated with 'comet-tail' appearances (Figure 10.17). Contrast-enhanced CT demonstrates multiple, diffuse low-attenuation lesions with no perceptible enhancement. On MRI they appear as hypointense and hyperintense lesions on T1- and T2-weighted images respectively and may demonstrate mild mural enhancement. These are asymptomatic lesions found incidentally during imaging or surgery and do not require any treatment.

Biliary adenofibroma

Biliary adenofibroma is an extremely rare tumour which forms a large fibrous mass containing complex tubulo-cystic cavities lined by biliary epithelium. Only a few cases have been reported in the literature to date.[54] Biliary adenofibromas are found equally among men and women and vary in size from 5 to 20 cm. They may remain asymptomatic or cause abdominal discomfort due to compression of adjacent structures. Imaging reveals a well-circumscribed solid–cystic mass but the appearance is non-specific and the diagnosis is based on histological examination. Grossly, the tumour presents as an unencapsulated, well-circumscribed solid–cystic nodule.

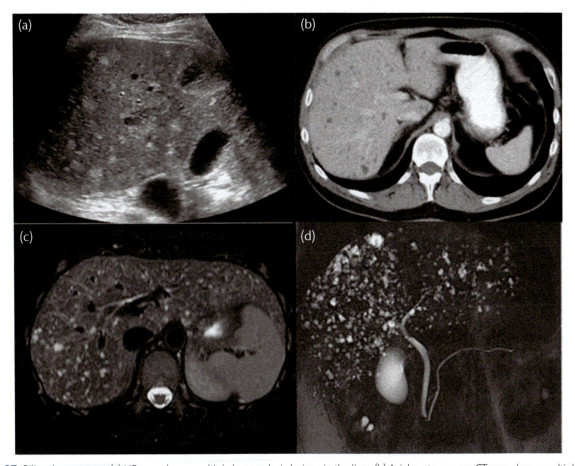

Figure 10.17 Biliary hamartoma. (a) US scan shows multiple hyperechoic lesions in the liver. (b) Axial porto-venous CT scan shows multiple well-defined low-attenuation lesions with faint peripheral enhancement. (c) Axial T2 weighted MRI shows multiple hyperintense nodules with central areas of low signal. (d) Coronal magnetic resonance cholangiopancreatography shows no communication with the biliary tree.

Histologically, it is composed of a tubulo-cystic proliferation of variable-sized bile ducts with an immunohistochemical profile suggestive of bile duct origin (CK7+, CK19+). The epithelial component is embedded in a moderately cellular fibrous stroma which is strongly immunoreactive for α-smooth muscle actin. Some tumours show amplifications of p53, CCND1, and ERBB2 which suggest that it may be a premalignant condition. Malignant transformation to cholangiocarcinoma has also been reported.[55] Hence complete surgical resection whenever possible is justified.

Non-epithelial tumours of the liver

Cavernous haemangioma

Cavernous haemangiomas are the most common benign tumours of the liver accounting for 70% of all benign lesions.[33] They can occur in any age group but due to significant differences in the histological features and presentation of haemangiomas between the paediatric and adult populations, only those occurring in adults are discussed in this chapter.

Aetiopathogenesis

The prevalence of hepatic haemangiomas varies between 0.4% and 20% based on autopsy studies.[27] It shows a preponderance for middle-aged females with a female:male ratio of 5:1.[56] Most haemangiomas are small, may be single or multiple (<10%), and are detected incidentally. Haemangiomas greater than 10 cm in size are called 'giant haemangiomas' and they may be associated with secondary changes. Diffuse hepatic haemangiomatosis is a condition characterized by multiple haemangiomas of varying sizes involving one or both lobes of the liver. It is usually found in the paediatric age group associated with other anomalies.

The pathogenesis of a haemangioma is unclear. It is thought to be a vascular malformation or a hamartoma of congenital origin. Some of these tumours express oestrogen receptors and show accelerated growth during puberty, pregnancy, oral contraceptive use, androgenic treatment, and even with drugs such as metoclopramide.[57–59] This theory advocates that hormonal influence may contribute to an increase in the size of these otherwise benign lesions. Though a large number of lesions remain stable, nearly 45% of them evolve by up to 5% in size over a protracted period of time.[60] Enlargement of these tumours occurs by ectasia rather than by hypertrophy or hyperplasia and is possibly caused by deactivation of endothelial cell proliferation inhibitors such as platelet factor 4, TGF-β, and interferon α.[61] It is worth remembering that these lesions do not undergo malignant transformation.

Macroscopically, haemangiomas appear as well-demarcated, purplish-blue, soft, and compressible lesions with blood-filled cavities and a thin capsule. Some degree of fibrosis, calcification, or thrombosis can be observed in larger lesions especially in giant haemangiomas. Microscopically, they appear as cavernous vascular spaces of varying sizes lined by flattened endothelium and supported by paucicellular fibrous septa (Figure 10.18). There is no endothelial atypia or mitotic activity. They derive their blood supply from the hepatic artery and show no portal or biliary structures. Larger and older lesions may show involutional changes such as calcification, hyalinization, thrombosis, and necrosis. A small haemangioma may become entirely fibrous and may present as a solitary fibrous nodule. Immunohistochemistry is strongly positive for CD34 showing a vascular differentiation.

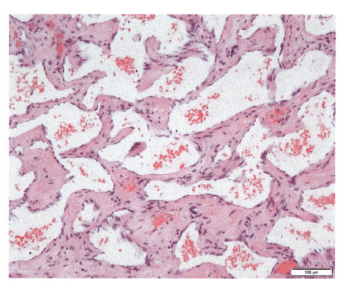

Figure 10.18 High-power microscopic view of a cavernous haemangioma composed of dilated vascular spaces containing blood with a flat endothelial lining. The intervening fibrous septa are paucicellular and of varying thickness.

Clinical features

Haemangiomas are typically asymptomatic lesions which are discovered incidentally at autopsy, radiological imaging, or laparotomy for unrelated reasons. The biochemical functions of the liver are unaffected. A large haemangioma can present as a palpable mass causing abdominal pain or can rarely cause jaundice due to compression of the biliary tree. Giant haemangiomas, in contrast, can become symptomatic due to three reasons: (1) alterations in internal architecture such as inflammation and necrosis secondary to thrombosis, (2) coagulation abnormalities which can lead to systemic complications like rupture and haemorrhage, and (3) compression of adjacent structures.[62] These complications are often associated with more widespread systemic manifestations.

Bornman et al.[62] described a syndrome of low-grade fever, weight loss, and abdominal pain in patients with a haemangioma. This clinical picture is accompanied by normal liver biochemistry and white blood cell count but high erythrocyte sedimentation rate, thrombocytosis, increased fibrinogen, and anaemia. Bornman et al. attributed this syndrome to intralesional thrombosis-induced systemic inflammatory response. Similarly, the Kasabach–Merritt syndrome is a unique complication of hepatic haemangiomas in adults characterized by consumptive coagulopathy presenting with thrombocytopenia, microangiopathic haemolysis, and disseminated intravascular coagulation.[63] It is associated with a high mortality of 30–40% due to bleeding. Both these syndromes are reversible after resection of the haemangioma. Diffuse hepatic haemangiomatosis usually presents in infancy and is associated with the Rendu–Osler–Weber syndrome or skeletal haemangiomatosis and results in high-output cardiac failure. Isolated diffuse hepatic haemangiomatosis without extrahepatic lesions is extremely rare in adults.[64,65]

Intratumoural haemorrhage can occur spontaneously or after abdominal trauma and anticoagulation therapy. Spontaneous rupture of giant subcapsular haemangiomas has also been reported during pregnancy or in association with the Kasabach–Merritt syndrome and carries a high mortality rate (30%). Nevertheless, the presence of these vascular liver tumours should not interfere with any form of therapy or advice given to patients taking into account their high prevalence and extremely low risk of complications.

Diagnosis

Haemangiomas are accurately diagnosed radiographically by their characteristic appearance. On US, the typical appearance is that of a well-defined hyperechoic mass with acoustic enhancement (Figure 10.19a). Contrast-enhanced US shows a well-defined mass with peripheral globular enhancement in the arterial and portal venous phases and an isoechoic pattern in the late phase.[66] Though rarely required, contrast-enhanced US is useful to diagnose atypical haemangiomas. The diagnostic criteria for haemangioma on CT include low attenuation in non-contrast CT (Figure 10.19b), peripheral nodular enhancement ('arterial puddles') in the arterial phase (sensitivity 67%, specificity 99%, positive predictive value 96%), followed by centripetal filling in the venous phase (Figure 10.19c,d).[67] MRI is the gold standard for the diagnosis of a haemangioma and has a high specificity and sensitivity of over 90%. The classic appearance is that of a hypointense lesion on T1-weighted sequences and hyperintense lesion on T2-weighted sequences with the characteristic 'light-bulb' appearance (Figure 10.20).[68] On diffusion-weighted sequences, haemangiomas show progressive decrease in intensity with increasing b-values (Figure 10.20).

Some haemangiomas may have atypical appearances in which case multiple imaging modalities in combination may be needed to establish the diagnosis. The most common atypical radiological lesions are giant haemangiomas and rapidly filling haemangiomas. Giant haemangiomas (>10 cm) may appear heterogeneous due to central thrombosis, fibrosis, or hyalinization (Figure 10.21). However, they show the characteristic early peripheral puddles in the arterial phase and strong peripheral hyperintensity on T2-weighted images. Progressive centripetal enhancement during the venous and delayed phases though present may not be complete. Rapidly filling haemangiomas are usually small (<2 cm) and show immediate homogeneous enhancement in the arterial phase (Figure 10.22). They can be differentiated from malignant lesions by strong hyperintensity on T2-weighted images with persistent enhancement during the delayed phase. Other uncommon atypical presentations include calcified haemangiomas, hyalinized haemangiomas, haemangioma with fluid–fluid levels (containing fluids with different intensities), pedunculated haemangiomas, and haemangiomas with capsular retraction.

The diagnosis of haemangioma against a background of an abnormal liver parenchyma is cumbersome but crucial to differentiate it from malignant lesions which are more common in such livers. In fatty livers, haemangiomas appear iso- or hypoechoic to the surrounding parenchyma on US and hyperintense on non-enhanced CT. Similarly, in cirrhotic livers, they may be compressed by the parenchyma and appear as fibrous nodules. MRI with T2 and fat-suppressed sequences are crucial in this setting to identify

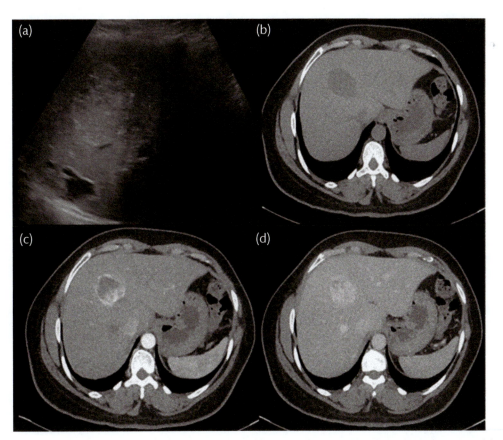

Figure 10.19 Radiological features of a hepatic cavernous haemangioma. (a) US scan shows a well-defined hypoechoic mass. (b) Axial non-contrast CT scan of the same patient shows a well-defined hypoattenuating lesion in segment 8. (c) Arterial phase contrast-enhanced CT scan shows the characteristic peripheral arterial puddles. (d) Venous phase CT scan shows progressive centripetal filling of the lesion.

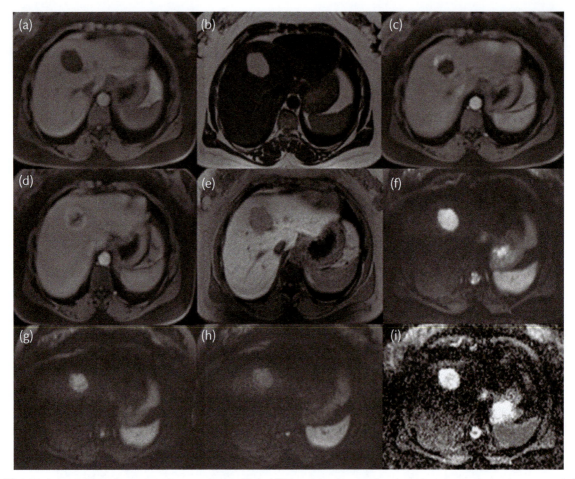

Figure 10.20 MRI characteristics of cavernous haemangioma of liver. (a) T1-weighted image showing a hypointense lesion in segment 8. (b) T2-weighted image shows characteristic strong hyperintensity (light bulb sign). (c) Arterial phase gadolinium-enhanced image shows peripheral puddles. (d) Venous phase gadolinium-enhanced image shows progressive centripetal filling. (e) A 20-minute delayed Primovist-enhanced image shows no uptake in the lesion. (f, g, h, i) Diffusion-weighted sequences showing progressive decrease in intensity of the lesion with increasing b-values with apparent restriction of diffusion.

haemangiomas which show persistent hyperintensity in contrast to underlying malignancy.

Less frequently used techniques for diagnosing haemangiomas are scintigraphy with technetium-99 pertechnetate-labelled erythrocytes, single-photon emission CT, and hepatic angiography which shows the characteristic 'cotton-wool' appearance. Percutaneous biopsy is not recommended for routine diagnosis as haemangiomas can be easily diagnosed radiologically and biopsy carries a high risk of bleeding. It is limited to exceptional cases when diagnosis remains uncertain despite multimodality imaging. Percutaneous biopsy can be done safely provided there is a cuff of hepatic parenchyma between the capsule and the haemangioma to provide adequate compression.

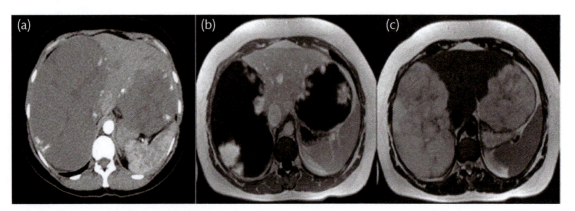

Figure 10.21 Multiple giant haemangiomata. Arterial phase contrast-enhanced CT scan (a) and arterial phase T2-weighted MRI (b) showing peripheral puddles. (c) Pre-contrast T2-weighted MRI showing hyperintense lesions.

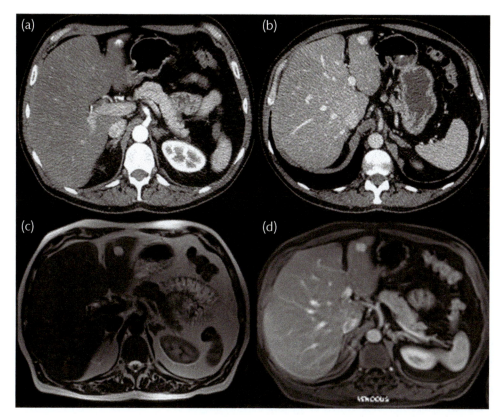

Figure 10.22 Rapidly filling haemangioma in segment 3 of liver. (a, b) Arterial and venous phase contrast-enhanced CT scans. (c) T2-weighted MRI showing hyperintense lesion. (d) T2-weighted delayed phase gadolinium-enhanced MRI showing continued uptake by the lesion.

Management

Asymptomatic haemangiomas of any size do not require treatment. Once the diagnosis is clearly established, there is no justification for serial monitoring or long-term follow-up except in a very few specific cases. It is important to reassure the patients about the rarity of growth and occurrence of complications in these otherwise benign lesions. They should also be reassured that it is not necessary to adopt any specific lifestyle and therapeutic measures such as avoiding pregnancy, sporting activity, or use of oral contraceptives.

Indications for treatment of haemangiomas include severe symptoms caused by extrinsic compression of adjacent structures, occurrence of complications, and inability to exclude malignancy. Giant haemangiomas are often symptomatic and require intervention. When indicated, the treatment of choice is surgical intervention by enucleation or formal resection through an open or laparoscopic approach. In Kasabach–Merritt syndrome, resection of the tumour becomes the gold standard of treatment to control consumptive coagulopathy. Other non-surgical options such as TAE or radiofrequency ablation can be used to reduce the size of the haemangioma and alleviate symptoms in unresectable cases.[69–71] TAE may be life-saving in case of rupture and acute haemorrhage, but is associated with complications like liver infarction, abscess formation, or failure of the procedure due to revascularization. Small case series have reported radiotherapy as an effective means to limit or regress growth as well as to decrease associated symptoms.[72] Rarely, liver transplantation has been successfully done in exceptional patients with complicated unresectable tumours or in patients with complicated diffuse haemangiomatosis.[73]

Fatty lesions of the liver

Angiomyolipoma

Hepatic angiomyolipoma (HAML) is a rare mesenchymal tumour belonging to a group of tumours derived from perivascular epithelioid cells (PECs) called PEComas. Morphologically, it is composed of proliferating blood vessels, smooth muscle cells, and adipose tissue in varying proportions.

Aetiopathogenesis

The prevalence of HAMLs is 0.3–2.1% and is less when compared to renal angiomyolipoma.[74] It is usually detected incidentally in non-cirrhotic livers and is not accompanied by serological abnormalities. The usual age of presentation is between 30 and 50 years and it has a predisposition for females (female:male ratio of 3:1). Most cases are sporadic and solitary. The pathogenesis remains unclear and there is no association with hormonal influence. Ten per cent of cases are associated with tuberous sclerosis in which case they are usually multiple. Most of these lesions are greater than 5 cm in size and may grow further. HAMLs are premalignant lesions and malignant transformation has been reported in 1% of cases.[74] Macroscopically, it appears as a solitary well-circumscribed lesion which is unencapsulated or partially encapsulated. The cut surface is soft and yellow or tan in colour and may contain areas of haemorrhage and necrosis. The background liver is typically

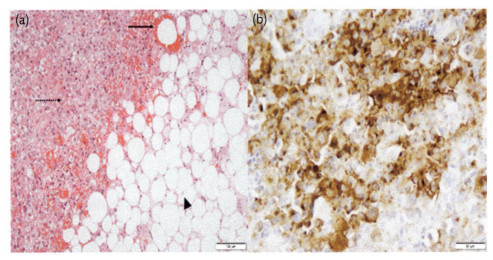

Figure 10.23 (a) High-power microscopic view of hepatic angiomyolipoma showing all the three characteristic elements, namely spindle-shaped myoid cells (dotted arrow), abnormal blood vessel (solid arrow), and adipose tissue (arrowhead). (b) The myoid component of the tumour showing positive immunostaining with HMB-45.

non-cirrhotic. Microscopically, it contains three elements: adipose tissue, smooth muscle (myoid) cells, and abnormal blood vessels in varying proportions (Figure 10.23a). The key diagnostic feature is the presence of myoid cells which may be of epithelioid type (large polygonal cells with fibrillar cytoplasm and eccentric eosinophilic nucleus) or spindle cell type (plump cells with thin rim of eosinophilic cytoplasm and a pale nucleus). The adipose component consists of mature adipose tissue and the vascular component consists of thick-walled and tortuous blood vessels. Histologically, HAML can be subdivided into the classic type with lipomatous, myomatous, or angiomatous predominance and an epithelioid variant with 10–100% of epithelioid cells. Immunohistochemical examination is necessary to differentiate it from other benign and malignant hepatic tumours and to increase the accuracy of diagnosis. The smooth muscle component of these tumours stains positively with human melanoma black 45 (HMB-45), actin, and MART-1 but is negative to cytokeratin (Figure 10.23b). In addition, they also stain positively with c-KIT (CD117).

Clinical features

HAML is often asymptomatic and is incidentally detected. Large tumours may become symptomatic due to a pressure effect. The majority of HAMLs are believed to be benign, although a number of cases have been reported with malignant behaviour including growth, recurrence after surgical resection, metastasis, and invasive growth patterns into the liver parenchyma and alongside the vessels.[75] Such malignant transformation is thought to occur mostly in the epithelioid type.

Diagnosis

HAMLs have a heterogeneous appearance on imaging due to their varying components. On contrast-enhanced imaging (US, CT, and MRI), they appear enhanced in the arterial phase without washout in the portal and delayed phases (Figure 10.24). On MRI, the adipose component appears hyperintense in T1-weighted images and a drop in intensity is seen in fat-supressed sequences but not in opposed-phase images which helps to differentiate it from other fat-containing hepatocellular tumours (Figure 10.25). The diagnostic accuracy of imaging modalities becomes low in the epithelioid variant which may resemble hepatic adenoma or HCC due to very little fat. In this case, percutaneous biopsy may help in establishing the diagnosis. Nevertheless, biopsy with HMB-45 staining might be superior compared to imaging with a diagnostic accuracy of 78.1% and becomes mandatory in most cases.[74]

Management

In asymptomatic patients, when the diagnosis of HAML is established and biopsy shows no atypical epithelioid pattern or high proliferative activity, a careful annual or biennial surveillance is necessary. In symptomatic patients and patients with uncertain diagnosis, atypical epithelioid pattern, and high proliferative activity, surgical resection of the tumour is necessary. Treatment with embolization, chemotherapy, sirolimus, and liver transplantation have also been reported but are less efficacious and surgical resection remains the treatment of choice whenever possible.[74]

Lipoma

Lipoma of the liver is a very rare benign lesion that is often diagnosed incidentally. Primary lipoma of the liver is extremely rare and was first described by Ramchand et al.[76] Since then there have been a few case reports describing their occurrence.[77] They are usually solitary lesions and can occur in any part of the liver. There is considerable debate about whether they are derived from lipomatous tissue within the parenchyma or from the capsule as they have been described in both locations. Macroscopically, they are well encapsulated and the cut surface appears homogeneous and yellowish in colour. Histologically, they are composed of mature adipose tissue. On non-contrast CT they appear as well-circumscribed, homogeneous lesions of fat attenuation without contrast enhancement. On MRI, they appear hyperintense on both T1- and T2-weighted images but the vital finding is the drop in intensity on fat-supressed images (Figure 10.26). Similarly, they do not drop signal intensity on opposed phase images which helps to differentiate them from other fat-containing hepatocellular tumours. The main differential

Non-epithelial tumours of the liver

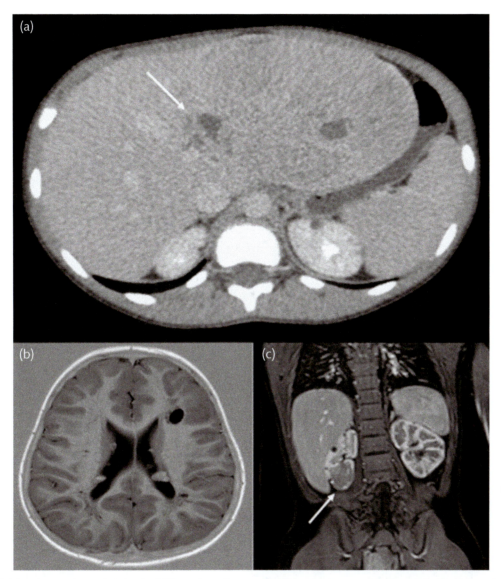

Figure 10.24 (a) Axial contrast-enhanced abdominal CT scan in an 8-year-old child with tuberous sclerosis showing hepatic angiomyolipoma (arrow) with heterogeneous enhancement. (b) Axial MRI of brain showing ependymal nodules. (c) Coronal MRI of abdomen showing angiomyolipoma in the lower pole of right kidney (arrow) in the same patient.

diagnosis includes angiomyolipoma from which it can be differentiated by HMB-45 staining as a true lipoma does not stain with HMB-45. Hepatic lipoma may also be confused with focal fatty change which shows a more geographic pattern of distribution and histologically is an abnormal accumulation of fat vesicles within the cytoplasm of hepatocytes. Nevertheless, true hepatic lipomas are harmless and do not require any treatment.

Myelolipoma

Hepatic myelolipoma is an extremely rare benign mesenchymal tumour containing mature adipose tissue and haematopoietic elements. It is usually found incidentally in patients over the age of 60 years and is more common in females than males (2:1).[78] It is often solitary and varies in size between 4 and 15 cm. Though the exact aetiology is not well understood, the most widely accepted theory is metaplasia of reticuloendothelial cells of blood capillaries. The other theories include translocation of differentiated bone marrow tissue or adrenal tissue during embryogenesis. Macroscopically, they appear as a well-defined yellowish mass with mature blood vessels. Microscopically, they are composed of irregularly mature fibrotic adipose tissue and some myeloid tissue with myeloid, erythroid, and megakaryocytic cells inside. Imaging can be helpful in diagnosing these tumours. US imaging shows hyperechoic lumps with clear boundaries. CT scanning demonstrates quasi-circular, sometimes lobulated masses with clear borders, partially or fully enveloped by a pseudo-capsule. These masses consist of variable low-density adipose tissue and medium density bone marrow tissue, and sometimes enhance with contrast due to calcification, infarction, or haemorrhage. MRI scans can detect hyperintense signals from fat tissue on the T1-weighted sequences while T2-weighted sequences may detect intermediate to hyperintense signals due to the different concentrations of myeloid components. Percutaneous biopsy remains the primary tool to confirm diagnosis and rule out malignancy. They usually remain asymptomatic but large lesions may cause

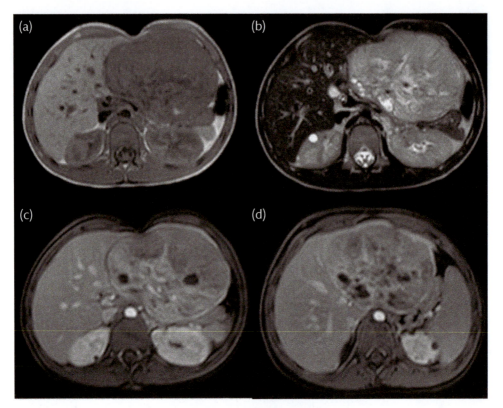

Figure 10.25 MRI characteristics of hepatic angiomyolipoma. (a) T1-weighted fat-supressed image showing a heterogeneously attenuating lesion with areas of hypoattenuation corresponding to the fat component. (b) T2-weighted image showing the same lesion with hyperattenuating fat-containing areas. (c) Arterial phase gadolinium-enhanced image showing enhancement of the vascular component. (d) Delayed phase gadolinium-enhanced image showing sustained enhancement.

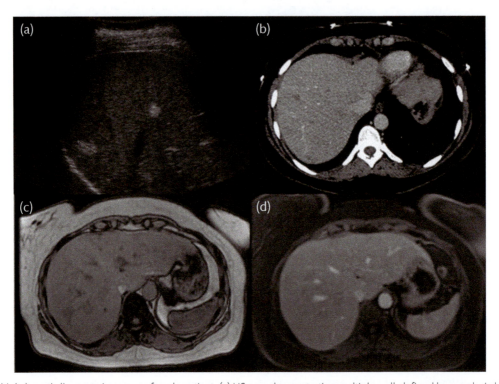

Figure 10.26 Multiple hepatic lipomata in a young female patient. (a) US scan demonstrating multiple well-defined hyperechoic lesions. (b) Contrast-enhanced CT scan showing multiple homogeneous round nodules of fat attenuation. (c) T1-weighted image showing multiple hyperintense lesions. (d) Gadolinium-enhanced T1-weighted image shows no significant arterial enhancement of the lesions.

symptoms due to pressure effects. Asymptomatic lesions require annual observation according to the guidelines published by American Association of Clinical Endocrinologists/American Association of Endocrine Surgeons (2009). Symptomatic lesions may require surgical resection. Intralesional haemorrhage, infarction, rupture, and suspicion of malignancy are also indications for surgery.

Focal fatty change

Hepatic steatosis is defined as intracellular accumulation of fat in more than 5% of hepatocytes and is usually a diffuse process. However, focal areas of steatosis or fat sparing (in steatotic livers) have also been described and become an important differential diagnosis while evaluating focal lesions for malignancy. Focal fatty lesions of the liver have a characteristic distribution in segment 4 just anterior to the porta hepatis or along the falciform ligament.[79] The pathogenesis has been attributed to regional hypoxia caused by the presence of abnormal vasculature in this region. These lesions frequently occur in patients with diabetes, obesity, hepatitis C infection, and non-alcoholic steatohepatitis. Hence, hormones and metabolic substances may also play a role in their pathogenesis.[80] On US, they appear hyperechoic with posterior shadowing due to attenuation of the US waves by fat. On CT, focal fatty lesions appear hypodense when compared to the surrounding parenchyma. Radiologically, the characteristic location, penetration by underlying vessels, and lack of mass effect can help to distinguish it from other focal lesions. MRI is the best modality for diagnosis and a focal fatty lesion appears as a well-defined or ill-defined hypointense lesion on opposed phase T1-weighted images, fat-suppressed T1- and T2-weighted images, and with hepatocyte-specific contrast agents such as gadobenate dimeglumine (Gd-BOPTA) and gadoxetic acid (Gd-EOB-DTPA). A ring of steatosis is often seen surrounding metastatic deposit from insulinoma. Segmental or patchy deposition of fat may also be found in patients with islet cell transplantation mimicking the distribution of the harvested islet cells following injection into the portal vein. Focal fat sparing has a similar distribution and appears hypoechoic on US, hyperdense on CT, and hyperintense on fat-suppressed MRI sequences mimicking hepatic adenoma or FNH. A knowledge of the existence and appearance of focal fatty change is important to distinguish it from other benign and malignant lesions of the liver.

Lymphangioma

Hepatic lymphangioma is an extremely rare benign lesion commonly found during childhood. It is formed by sequestration of lymphatic tissue within the hepatic parenchyma during embryogenesis. It is usually solitary, small (<4 cm), and asymptomatic. Multiple lymphangiomas have been reported rarely in literature. On imaging, it has a cystic appearance with some solid component and may contain peripheral calcification. Biopsy shows vascular lymphatic spaces lined by normal endothelium and immunostaining using D2-40, LYVE-1, and Prox-1 markers is helpful to discriminate the lymphatic from vascular endothelium and to establish the diagnosis.[81] Asymptomatic lesions require no treatment and surgical resection is reserved for giant symptomatic lymphangiomas.

Leiomyoma

Hepatic leiomyomas are extremely rare lesions that arise from smooth muscles of blood vessels or bile ducts. They are more common in females and occur in patients with immunodeficiency such as those with human immunodeficiency virus (HIV) or Epstein–Barr virus infection and post organ transplantation.[82] On imaging, they appear hypoechoic on US and hypoattenuating on CT scan with heterogeneous enhancement after injection of contrast material. On MRI, leiomyomas are hypointense on T1-weighted sequences and strongly hyperintense on T2-weighted sequences. Biopsy shows spindle cell proliferation without nuclear atypia, haemorrhage, or necrosis and immunostaining with mesenchymal markers such as vimentin and smooth muscle actin is positive. Liver resection with a good margin is usually recommended for these lesions.

Mesenchymal hamartoma

This is a developmental anomaly usually found in children less than 2 years of age. It is associated with balanced translocation involving chromosome band 19q13.4 or 19q13.3 found in association with uniparental disomy.[83] A vascular or toxic insult during fetal development of liver has also been hypothesized as the cause. It appears as a large, solid lesion with marked lymphoedema of portal tracts and cystic degeneration (Figure 10.27). Histologically, it is composed of a mixture of varying portions of mesenchymal cells, bile ducts, hepatocytes, blood vessels, and cystic spaces. Malignant transformation has been reported. Hence, surgical resection is advocated.[83]

Heterotopic tissue

Heterotopic tissue or choristoma is an abnormal location of normal tissue within the liver parenchyma. Ectopic splenic, pancreatic, adrenal, and endometriotic tissues within the liver have been previously reported in literature. The most common is hepatic splenosis caused by autotransplantation of splenic tissue following traumatic rupture. It is usually found in the left lobe of the liver and appears hypervascular on arterial phase imaging with washout on the venous phase. It is usually found incidentally and a high degree of suspicion is required to distinguish it from other benign or malignant liver lesions. Technetium 99m-labelled heat-denatured red blood cell scintigraphy can be used to differentiate it from other lesions and biopsy can establish a definite diagnosis.

Hepatic endometriosis is found in women of childbearing age and mostly associated with pelvic endometriosis. The pathogenesis is multifactorial and involves celomic metaplasia, retrograde menstruation, and lymphatic and iatrogenic dissemination. It is usually diagnosed incidentally during evaluation of abdominal symptoms and may require resection. Heterotopic pancreatic and adrenal tissues have also been reported within the liver.[84] They have been exclusively located in medium to large sized portal tracts and intermingled with peribiliary glands. Such tissue is often found communicating with bile duct lumina and empties its secretions into them. Biopsy and immunohistochemical staining can establish the diagnosis and it does not require any specific treatment.

Miscellaneous tumours

Peliosis hepatis

Peliosis hepatis is a rare condition diagnosed histologically by multiple cystic blood-filled cavities throughout the hepatic parenchyma. Peliosis hepatis was first described by Wagner in 1861 but the term

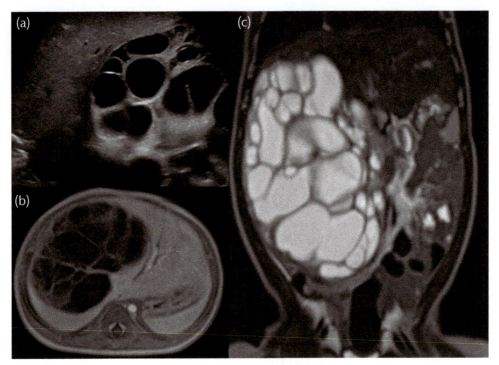

Figure 10.27 Hepatic mesenchymal hamartoma in a 14-month-old child presenting as a large well-defined solid-cystic lesion. (a) US appearance. (b) Axial T1-weighted gadolinium-enhanced MRI. (c) Coronal T2-weighted MRI.

was coined by Schoenlank in 1916.[85,86] It is derived from the Greek word '*Pelios*' meaning bluish. Though it is usually detected in the liver it may involve other organs of the lymphoreticular system and less commonly the lungs, kidneys, adrenals, pancreas, pituitary gland, stomach, and intestines.[87]

Aetiopathogenesis

The pathogenesis of peliosis remains unclear. While one theory favours congenital malformation of vessels or microcirculatory disturbances manifesting as peliosis under altered local intravascular pressure conditions, others favour an acquired vascular disorder triggered by toxic stimuli playing a key role in the pathogenesis.[87,88] However, none of them can satisfactorily explain the pathological findings in all cases. Several risk factors have been associated with peliosis hepatis.[89] These include drugs such as steroids, oral contraceptives, tamoxifen, methotrexate, thiopurine, azathioprine, and iron chelators in addition to toxins such as arsenic or thorium. It has also been associated with neoplastic conditions, especially myeloproliferative disease and Castleman's disease. There are some reported associations with arteritis, telangiectasia, cystic fibrosis, coeliac disease, and even with infections like HIV, tuberculosis, leprosy, syphilis, rickettsiosis, and bartonellosis.

On cut surface, multiple, randomly distributed, blood-filled cystic spaces can frequently be seen at gross inspection, giving the section a 'Swiss cheese' appearance. Microscopically, two different types of lesions have been described.[90] The first type is designated 'parenchymal peliosis' and consists of irregular cavities that are neither lined by sinusoidal cells nor by fibrous tissue with the adjacent hepatic tissue occasionally displaying liver cell necrosis. The second type is called 'phlebectatic peliosis' and is characterized by regular, spherical cavities lined by endothelium and/or fibrosis.

Immunohistochemical studies have revealed an increased deposition of collagen type III and type IV as well as laminin along the dilated liver sinusoids, thus suggesting a transformation of hepatic stellate cells into myofibroblasts in response to endothelial cell injury.

Clinical features

Patients with peliosis hepatis are usually asymptomatic and it is most commonly detected incidentally during autopsy or during evaluation for other conditions. The natural history of the disease is highly variable. In some cases, it may lead to progressive fibrosis and development of liver failure. In others, a regression has been observed after withdrawal of the inciting agent. Very rarely, rupture of the liver parenchyma and fatal haemorrhage has also been described.

Diagnosis

On imaging, there is diffuse involvement of the liver parenchyma with lesions which may vary in size from a few millimetres up to more than 4 cm (Figure 10.28). US may demonstrate multiple pseudocystic lesions with increased vascularity on colour Doppler but the appearance is highly variable. CT scans may show multiple hypodense lesions of varying sizes which enhance in the early arterial phase and then become isodense with the remaining parenchyma in the venous and delayed phases. Some degree of calcification and thrombosis can also be recognized. MRI is the gold standard for diagnosis especially when combined with a hepato-specific contrast agent. T1-weighted images show multiple heterogeneous lesions which show centrifugal enhancement with contrast administration. In T2-weighted sequences, they may appear as hyperintense lesions compared with the surrounding parenchyma with multiple high-signal-intensity spots that are attributable to haemorrhagic

Miscellaneous tumours

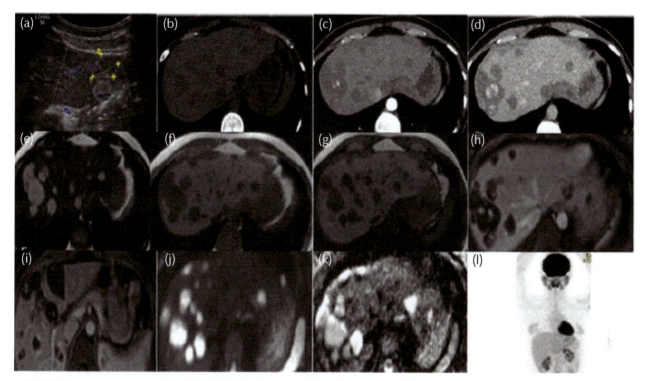

Figure 10.28 US, contrast-enhanced CT, Gd-EOB-DTPA-enhanced MRI, and fluorodeoxyglucose positron emission tomography images of a 34-year-old female with biopsy-confirmed peliosis hepatis. (a) Multiple hypo- and hyperechoic lesions in the liver on US (arrows). (b) Non-contrast CT scan showing multiple hypoattenuating lesions. (c, d) Arterial and porto-venous phase CT scan demonstrating multiple hypoattenuating lesions in the right lobe with central 'dot' enhancement. (e) T2-weighted image demonstrates multiple high-signal-intensity cystic lesions. (f, g) In- and out-of-phase MRI shows lack of intralesional fat. (h, i) Arterial and porto-venous MRI shows similar enhancement features as CT. (j, k) Diffusion-weighted image and apparent diffusion coefficient shows T2 shine through with no restriction of diffusion. (l) Fluorodeoxyglucose positron emission tomography scan confirms no uptake of the isotope tracer by the liver lesions.

necrosis. Biopsy is not indicated for diagnosis as there is a high risk of bleeding.

Management

Asymptomatic patients require no treatment. Interventions are required in the setting of rupture and acute haemorrhage. Surgical resection can be done in localized disease. TAE can be a life-saving procedure in such circumstances. Discontinuation of steroids and other incriminating drugs has also been advocated in progressive cases. In patients developing progressive liver failure, liver transplantation has also been performed with good outcomes.[91] In general, considering the atypical manifestations, variable imaging features, and serious complications, peliosis hepatis should be remembered in the differential diagnosis of hepatic nodules.

Inflammatory pseudotumours

An inflammatory pseudotumour of the liver (IPL), also known as an inflammatory myofibroblastic tumour and a plasma cell granuloma, is a rare benign tumour with an incidence of 0.2–0.7%.[92] Inflammatory pseudotumours can occur anywhere in the body but are most commonly found in the lungs. IPL accounts for 8% of extrapulmonary inflammatory pseudotumours. IPL is found between 35 and 65 years of age and is slightly more common in men. Their aetiology remains uncertain although infectious conditions, autoimmune phenomena, or the systemic inflammatory response syndrome have been suggested as possible triggers resulting in an exaggerated immune response. Recent studies hypothesize that IPL is of dendritic cell origin.[93]

IPL commonly occurs as a large solitary mass predominantly occurring in the right lobe of the liver but multicentricity has also been described. A perihilar variant has also been described which mimics hilar cholangiocarcinoma. Patients are usually symptomatic and present with low-grade fever, abdominal pain, weight loss, and fatigue. The perihilar variant may cause jaundice and cholangitis. Liver function tests are usually normal except for mild elevation of the alkaline phosphatase and gamma glutamyl transferase. In patients with perihilar IPL, an obstructive pattern of liver function test may be encountered. Inflammatory markers are usually elevated including immunoglobulin G4 when associated with immunoglobulin G-related sclerosing cholangitis. They are often mistaken for malignancy due to the clinical presentation but the tumour markers are normal on evaluation. The imaging findings are also not specific for diagnosis. IPL may appear as a large, heterogeneous, ill-defined lesion or a solitary encapsulated necrotic nodule or may appear as a perihilar inflammatory mass (Figure 10.29). On non-contrast CT, IPL appears as a low attenuation lesion and demonstrates inhomogeneous arterial enhancement on contrast. On MRI, it is hypointense on T1- and isointense on T2-weighted images. Gadolinium-enhanced MRI shows poorly defined peripheral rim-like enhancement at arterial phase. Diagnosis is established based on histological examination of a percutaneous needle biopsy or a surgically resected specimen which shows chronic infiltration of various inflammatory

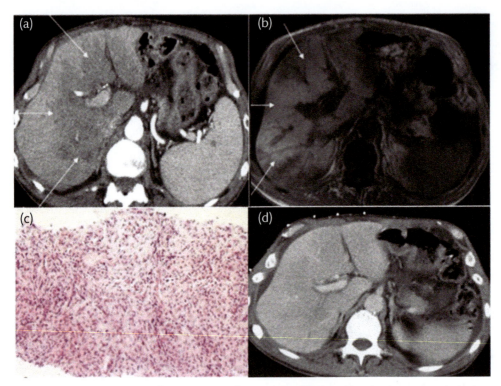

Figure 10.29 Imaging features of a biopsy-proven inflammatory pseudotumour in a 59-year-old male who presented with increased inflammatory markers and deranged liver function tests. (a) Arterial phase CT scan showing ill-defined low-attenuation areas involving both liver lobes (arrows). (b) Fat-suppressed T1-weighted MRI showing multiple areas of low intensities within the liver. (c) Histology of this abnormal area of liver demonstrating multiple inflammatory infiltrates. (d) Follow-up CT scan obtained after 8 weeks shows resolution of the lesion without any treatment.

cells (plasma cells, lymphocytes, neutrophils, and eosinophils) and a fibrous stroma. There may be associated thrombophlebitis of small portal venous branches and destruction of biliary ductules.

The diagnostic ambiguity of IPL often leads to misconception as malignancy and may result in major surgical resections carrying a high risk of complications. Hence, thorough investigation and, if necessary, repeat biopsy is advocated if the imaging findings are inconclusive and tumour markers are normal. IPL is a benign condition and when the diagnosis is certain, a conservative approach with antibiotics, steroids, and simple surveillance is recommended. A complete regression rate of greater than 90% has been observed with steroids which offer good symptom control as well.[92,93]

Solitary fibrotic tumour

A solitary fibrotic tumour or a solitary necrotic tumour is an uncommon benign entity that often mimics malignancy. The average age at presentation is 60 years and it is more common in males.[94] Most patients are asymptomatic and the lesion is picked up incidentally. It presents as a small (usually <2 cm), solitary, well-defined lesion. The aetiology is unclear but it may be associated with trauma or infection. On imaging, it appears as a well-defined heterogeneous lesion showing progressive enhancement in the delayed phase due to accumulation of contrast in the collagenous stroma. Diagnosis is established by biopsy and it shows central necrosis surrounded by a hyalinized capsule containing collagen and elastin with inflammatory infiltrates. Solitary fibrotic tumours are presumed to be benign and so a non-surgical management is advocated. In half the patients, there may be associated extrahepatic malignancy arising from the gastrointestinal tract and the lesion may show a focus of adenocarcinoma.[94] Hence, resection is justified if an absolute diagnosis cannot be established.

Conclusion

To conclude, benign liver tumours are often encountered in clinical practice, but rarely require surgical or radiological intervention. They can present with a wide array of clinical features, from remaining asymptomatic to producing pressure effects or even life-threatening haemorrhage, with some atypical variants undergoing malignant transformation. Due to this complex behaviour, it is important to understand their aetiopathogenesis to guide appropriate management and we hope this chapter has served the purpose.

Acknowledgements

We wish to thank Prof. Yoh Zen, Consultant Histopathologist, Institute of Liver Studies, King's College Hospital, London, UK and Dr Praveen Peddu, Consultant Radiologist and Clinical Lead for Liver Radiology, King's College Hospital, London UK for their contributions.

REFERENCES

1. Nagtegaal ID, Odze RD, Klimstra D, et al. The 2019 WHO classification of tumours of the digestive system. *Histopathology*. 2020;**76**(2):182–188.

2. Rooks JB, Ory HW, Ishak KG, et al. Epidemiology of hepatocellular adenoma: the role of oral contraceptive use. *JAMA*. 1979;**242**(7):644–648.
3. Torbenson M, Lee JH, Choti M, et al. Hepatic adenomas: analysis of sex steroid receptor status and the Wnt signaling pathway. *Mod Pathol*. 2002;**15**(3):189–196.
4. Nault JC, Bioulac-Sage P, Zucman-Rossi J. Hepatocellular benign tumors—from molecular classification to personalized clinical care. *Gastroenterology*. 2013;**144**(5):888–902.
5. Jeannot E, Poussin K, Chiche L, et al. Association of CYP1B1 germ line mutations with hepatocyte nuclear factor 1α-mutated hepatocellular adenoma. *Cancer Res*. 2007;**67**(6):2611–2616.
6. Gutiérrez SM, García IC, Nan ND, Hernández HJ. [Hepatic lesions and prolonged use of oral contraceptive]. *Rev Clin Esp*. 2007;**207**(5):257–258.
7. Edmondson HA, Reynolds TB, Henderson B, Benton B. Regression of liver cell adenomas associated with oral contraceptives. *Ann Intern Med*. 1977;**86**(2):180–182.
8. Nakao A, Sakagami K, Nakata Y, et al. Multiple hepatic adenomas caused by long-term administration of androgenic steroids for aplastic anemia in association with familial adenomatous polyposis. *J Gastroenterol*. 2000;**35**(7):557–562.
9. Socas L, Zumbado M, Perez-Luzardo O, et al. Hepatocellular adenomas associated with anabolic androgenic steroid abuse in bodybuilders: a report of two cases and a review of the literature. *Br J Sports Med*. 2005;**39**(5):e27.
10. Beuers U, Richter WO, Ritter MM, Wiebecke B, Schwandt P. Klinefelter's syndrome and liver adenoma. *J Clin Gastroenterol*. 1991;**13**:214–216.
11. Triantafyllopoulou M, Whitington PF, Melin-Aldana H, Benya EC, Brickman W. Hepatic adenoma in an adolescent with elevated androgen levels. *J Pediatr Gastroenterol Nutr*. 2007;**44**(5):640–642.
12. Dokmak S, Paradis V, Vilgrain V, et al. A single-center surgical experience of 122 patients with single and multiple hepatocellular adenomas. *Gastroenterology*. 2009;**137**(5):1698–1705.
13. Chang CY, Hernandez-Prera JC, Roayaie S, Schwartz M, Thung SN. Changing epidemiology of hepatocellular adenoma in the United States: review of the literature. *Int J Hepatol*. 2013;**2013**:604860.
14. Brunt EM, Wolverson MK, Di Bisceglie AM. Benign hepatocellular tumors (adenomatosis) in nonalcoholic steatohepatitis: a case report. *Semin Liver Dis*. 2005;**25**(2):230–236.
15. Lee P. Glycogen storage disease type I: pathophysiology of liver adenomas. *Eur J Pediatr*. 2002;**161**(1):S46–S49.
16. Sakellariou S, Al-Hussaini H, Scalori A, et al. Hepatocellular adenoma in glycogen storage disorder type I: a clinicopathological and molecular study. *Histopathology*. 2012;**60**(6B):E58–E65.
17. Nault JC, Fabre M, Couchy G, et al. GNAS-activating mutations define a rare subgroup of inflammatory liver tumors characterized by STAT3 activation. *J Hepatol*. 2012;**56**(1):184–191.
18. Shuangshoti S, Thaicharoen A. Hepatocellular adenoma in a beta-thalassemic woman having secondary iron overload. *J Med Assoc Thai*. 1994;**77**(2):108–112.
19. Radhi JM, Loewy J. Hepatocellular adenomatosis associated with hereditary haemochromatosis. *Postgrad Med J*. 2000;**76**(892):100–102.
20. Zucman-Rossi J, Jeannot E, Van Nhieu JT, et al. Genotype–phenotype correlation in hepatocellular adenoma: new classification and relationship with HCC. *Hepatology*. 2006;**43**(3):515–524.
21. Bieze M, Phoa SS, Verheij J, van Lienden KP, van Gulik TM. Risk factors for bleeding in hepatocellular adenoma. *Br J Surg*. 2014;**101**(7):847–855.
22. Khajornjiraphan N, Thu NA, Chow PK, et al. Malignant transformation of hepatocellular adenoma: how frequently does it happen? *Liver Cancer*. 2015;**4**(1):1–5.
23. Stoot JH, Coelen RJ, De Jong MC, Dejong CH. Malignant transformation of hepatocellular adenomas into hepatocellular carcinomas: a systematic review including more than 1600 adenoma cases. *HPB (Oxford)*. 2010;**12**(8):509–522.
24. Farges O, Ferreira N, Dokmak S, Belghiti J, Bedossa P, Paradis V. Changing trends in malignant transformation of hepatocellular adenoma. *Gut*. 2011;**60**(1):85–89.
25. Ronot M, Bahrami S, Calderaro J, et al. Hepatocellular adenomas: accuracy of magnetic resonance imaging and liver biopsy in subtype classification. *Hepatology*. 2011;**53**(4):1182–1191.
26. Husainy MA, Sayyed F, Peddu P. Typical and atypical benign liver lesions: a review. *Clin Imaging*. 2017;**44**:79–91.
27. European Association for the Study of the Liver (EASL). EASL Clinical Practice Guidelines on the management of benign liver tumours. *J Hepatol*. 2016;**65**(2):386–398.
28. Noels JE, van Aalten SM, van der Windt DJ, et al. Management of hepatocellular adenoma during pregnancy. *J Hepatol*. 2011;**54**(3):553–558.
29. Deodhar A, Brody LA, Covey AM, Brown KT, Getrajdman GI. Bland embolization in the treatment of hepatic adenomas: preliminary experience. *J Vasc Interv Radiol*. 2011;**22**(6):795–799.
30. van Vledder MG, van Aalten SM, Terkivatan T, Robert A, Leertouwer T, IJzermans JN. Safety and efficacy of radiofrequency ablation for hepatocellular adenoma. *J Vasc Interv Radiol*. 2011;**22**(6):787–793.
31. Visser G, Rake JP, Labrune P, et al. Consensus guidelines for management of glycogen storage disease type 1b—European study on glycogen storage disease type 1. *Eur J Pediatr*. 2002;**161**(1):S120–S123.
32. Lerut JP, Ciccarelli O, Sempoux C, et al. Glycogenosis storage type I diseases and evolutive adenomatosis: an indication for liver transplantation. *Transpl Int*. 2002;**16**(12):879–884.
33. Choi BY, Nguyen MH. The diagnosis and management of benign hepatic tumors. *J Clin Gastroenterol*. 2005;**39**(5):401–412.
34. Wanless IR, Mawdsley C, Adams R. On the pathogenesis of focal nodular hyperplasia of the liver. *Hepatology*. 1985;**5**(6):1194–1200.
35. Rebouissou S, Bioulac-Sage P, Zucman-Rossi J. Molecular pathogenesis of focal nodular hyperplasia and hepatocellular adenoma. *J Hepatol*. 2008;**48**(1):163–170.
36. Chandrasegaram MD, Shah A, Chen JW, et al. Oestrogen hormone receptors in focal nodular hyperplasia. *HPB (Oxford)*. 2015;**17**(6):502–507.
37. Rifai K, Mix H, Krusche S, Potthoff A, Manns MP, Gebel MJ. No evidence of substantial growth progression or complications of large focal nodular hyperplasia during pregnancy. *Scand J Gastroenterol*. 2013;**48**(1):88–92.
38. Nguyen BN, Fléjou JF, Terris B, Belghiti J, Degott C. Focal nodular hyperplasia of the liver: a comprehensive pathologic study of 305 lesions and recognition of new histologic forms. *Am J Surg Pathol*. 1999;**23**(12):1441–1454.
39. Hedayati P, Shamos R, Gillespie T, McMullen W. Treatment of symptomatic focal nodular hyperplasia with percutaneous radiofrequency ablation. *J Vasc Interv Radiol*. 2010;**21**(4):582–585.

40. Biecker E, Fischer HP, Strunk H, Sauerbruch T. Benign hepatic tumors. *J Gastroenterol*. 2003;**41**(2):191–200.
41. Al-Mukhaizeem KA, Rosenberg A, Sherker AH. Nodular regenerative hyperplasia of the liver: an under-recognized cause of portal hypertension in hematological disorders. *Am J Hematol*. 2004;**75**(4):225–230.
42. Ebrahimi DN, Ghaanati H, Haghpanah B, Bashashati M, Jahangiri NY, Shadman YA, Sayyah A. Nodular regenerative hyperplasia of the liver: report of a case. *Iranian J Radiol*. **3**(1):7–10.
43. Morris JM, Oien KA, McMahon M, et al. Nodular regenerative hyperplasia of the liver: survival and associated features in a UK case series. *Eur J Gastroenterol Hepatol*. 2010;**22**(8):1001–1005.
44. Hillaire S, Bonte E, Denninger MH, et al. Idiopathic non-cirrhotic intrahepatic portal hypertension in the West: a re-evaluation in 28 patients. *Gut*. 2002;**51**(2):275–280.
45. Hubert C, Sempoux C, Horsmans Y, et al. Nodular regenerative hyperplasia: a deleterious consequence of chemotherapy for colorectal liver metastases? *Liver Int*. 2007;**27**(7):938–943.
46. Wicherts DA, de Haas RJ, Sebagh M, et al. Regenerative nodular hyperplasia of the liver related to chemotherapy: impact on outcome of liver surgery for colorectal metastases. *Ann Surg Oncol*. 2011;**18**(3):659–669.
47. Forbes GM, Shilkin KB, Reed WD. Nodular regenerative hyperplasia of the liver: the importance of combined macroscopic and microscopic findings. *Med J Aust*. 1991;**154**(6):415–417.
48. Arvanitaki M, Adler M. Nodular regenerative hyperplasia of the liver. A review of 14 cases. *Hepatogastroenterology*. 2001;**48**(41):1425–1429.
49. Soubrane O, Brouquet A, Zalinski S, et al. Predicting high grade lesions of sinusoidal obstruction syndrome related to oxaliplatin-based chemotherapy for colorectal liver metastases: correlation with post-hepatectomy outcome. *Ann Surg*. 2010;**251**(3):454–460.
50. Rubbia-Brandt L, Lauwers GY, Wang H, et al. Sinusoidal obstruction syndrome and nodular regenerative hyperplasia are frequent oxaliplatin-associated liver lesions and partially prevented by bevacizumab in patients with hepatic colorectal metastasis. *Histopathology*. 2010;**56**(4):430–439.
51. Borzio M, Fargion S, Borzio F, et al. Impact of large regenerative, low grade and high grade dysplastic nodules in hepatocellular carcinoma development. *J Hepatol*. 2003;**39**(2):208–214.
52. Pujals A, Bioulac-Sage P, Castain C, Charpy C, Zafrani ES, Calderaro J. BRAF V600E mutational status in bile duct adenomas and hamartomas. *Histopathology*. 2015;**67**(4):562–567.
53. Redston MS, Wanless IR. The hepatic von Meyenburg complex: prevalence and association with hepatic and renal cysts among 2843 autopsies [corrected]. *Mod Pathol*. 1996;**9**(3):233–237.
54. Arnason T, Borger DR, Corless C, et al. Biliary adenofibroma of liver. *Am J Surg Pathol*. 2017;**41**(4):499–505.
55. Gurrera A, Alaggio R, Leone G, Aprile G, Magro G. Biliary adenofibroma of the liver: report of a case and review of the literature. *Pathol Res Int*. 2010;**2010**:504584.
56. Belghiti J, Cauchy F, Paradis V, Vilgrain V. Diagnosis and management of solid benign liver lesions. *Nat Rev Gastroenterol Hepatol*. 2014;**11**(12):737–749.
57. Conter RL, Longmire Jr WP. Recurrent hepatic hemangiomas. Possible association with estrogen therapy. *Ann Surg*. 1988;**207**(2):115–119.
58. Ozakyol A, Kebapci M. Enhanced growth of hepatic hemangiomatosis in two adults after postmenopausal estrogen replacement therapy. *Tohoku J Exp Med*. 2006;**210**(3):257–261.
59. Feurle GE. Arteriovenous shunting and cholestasis in hepatic hemangiomatosis associated with metoclopramide. *Gastroenterology*. 1990;**99**(1):258–262.
60. Hasan HY, Hinshaw JL, Borman EJ, Gegios A, Leverson G, Winslow ER. Assessing normal growth of hepatic hemangiomas during long-term follow-up. *JAMA Surg*. 2014;**149**(12):1266–1271.
61. Trotter JF, Everson GT. Benign focal lesions of the liver. *Clin Liver Dis*. 2001;**5**(1):17–42.
62. Bornman PC, Terblanche J, Blumgart RL, Jones EP, Pickard H, Kalvaria I. Giant hepatic hemangiomas: diagnostic and therapeutic dilemmas. *Surgery*. 1987;**101**(4):445–449.
63. Kasabach HH, Merritt KK. Capillary hemangioma with extensive purpura: report of a case. *Am J Dis Child*. 1940;**59**(5):1063–1070.
64. Moon WS, Yu HC, Lee JM, Kang MJ. Diffuse hepatic hemangiomatosis in an adult. *J Korean Med Sci*. 2000;**15**(4):471–474.
65. Kim EH, Park SY, Ihn YK, Hwang SS. Diffuse hepatic hemangiomatosis without extrahepatic involvement in an adult patient. *Korean J Radiol*. 2008;**9**(6):559–562.
66. Quaia E, Bertolotto M, Dalla Palma L. Characterization of liver hemangiomas with pulse inversion harmonic imaging. *Eur Radiol*. 2002;**12**(3):537–544.
67. Nino-Murcia M, Olcott EW, Jeffrey RB Jr, Lamm RL, Beaulieu CF, Jain KA. Focal liver lesions: pattern-based classification scheme for enhancement at arterial phase CT. *Radiology*. 2000;**215**(3):746–51.
68. Semelka RC, Brown ED, Ascher SM, et al. Hepatic hemangiomas: a multi-institutional study of appearance on T2-weighted and serial gadolinium-enhanced gradient-echo MR images. *Radiology*. 1994;**192**(2):401–406.
69. Zeng Q, Li Y, Chen Y, Ouyang Y, He X, Zhang H. Gigantic cavernous hemangioma of the liver treated by intra-arterial embolization with pingyangmycin-lipiodol emulsion: a multi-center study. *Cardiovasc Interv Radiol*. 2004;**27**(5):481–485.
70. Srivastava DN, Gandhi D, Seith A, Pande GK, Sahni P. Transcatheter arterial embolization in the treatment of symptomatic cavernous hemangiomas of the liver: a prospective study. *Abdom Imaging*. 2001;**26**(5):510–514.
71. Malagari K, Alexopoulou E, Dourakis S, et al. Transarterial embolization of giant liver hemangiomas associated with Kasabach-Merritt syndrome: a case report. *Acta Radiol*. 2007;**48**(6):608–612.
72. Biswal BM, Sandhu M, Lal P, Bal CS. Role of radiotherapy in cavernous hemangioma liver. *Indian J Gastroenterol*. 1995;**14**(3):95–98.
73. Ercolani G, Grazi GL, Pinna AD. Liver transplantation for benign hepatic tumors: a systematic review. *Dig Surg*. 2010;**27**(1):68–75.
74. Klompenhouwer AJ, Verver D, Janki S, et al. Management of hepatic angiomyolipoma: a systematic review. *Liver Int*. 2017;**37**(9):1272–1280.
75. Kamimura K, Nomoto M, Aoyagi Y. Hepatic angiomyolipoma: diagnostic findings and management. *Int J Hepatol*. 2012;**2012**:410781.
76. Ramchand S, Yusufuddin A, Baskerville L. Lipoma of the liver. *Arch Pathol*. 1970;**90**:331–333.
77. Nakamura N, Kudo A, Ito K, Tanaka S, Arii S. A hepatic lipoma mimicking angiomyolipoma of the liver: report of a case. *Surg Today*. 2009;**39**(9):825–828.
78. Li KY, Wei AL, Li A. Primary hepatic myelolipoma: a case report and review of the literature. *World J Clin Cases*. 2020;**8**(19):4615–4623.

79. Matsui O, Kadoya M, Takahashi S, et al. Focal sparing of segment IV in fatty livers shown by sonography and CT: correlation with aberrant gastric venous drainage. AJR. *Am J Roentgenol.* 1995;**164**(5):1137–1140.
80. Venkatesh SK, Hennedige T, Johnson GB, Hough DM, Fletcher JG. Imaging patterns and focal lesions in fatty liver: a pictorial review. *Abdom Radiol.* 2017;**42**(5):1374–1392.
81. Matsumoto T, Ojima H, Akishima-Fukasawa Y, et al. Solitary hepatic lymphangioma: report of a case. *Surg Today.* 2010;**40**(9):883–889.
82. Perini MV, Fink MA, Yeo DA, et al. Primary liver leiomyoma: a review of this unusual tumour. *ANZ J Surg.* 2013;**83**(4):230–233.
83. Stringer MD, Alizai NK. Mesenchymal hamartoma of the liver: a systematic review. *J Pediatr Surg.* 2005;**40**(11):1681–1690.
84. Terada T, Nakanuma Y, Kakita A. Pathologic observations of intrahepatic peribiliary glands in 1000 consecutive autopsy livers: heterotopic pancreas in the liver. *Gastroenterology.* 1990;**98**(5):1333–1337.
85. Wagner E. Fall von blutcysten der leber. *Arch Heilk.* 1861;**2**:369–370.
86. Schoenlank W. An instance of peliosis hepatis. *Virchows Arch Pathol Anat Physiol Clin Med.* 1916;**222**(3):358–364.
87. Tsokos M, Erbersdobler A. Pathology of peliosis. *Forensic Sci Int.* 2005;**149**(1):25–33.
88. Wanless IR, Huang WY. Vascular disorders. In: Burt AD, Portmann BC, Ferrell L, eds. *MacSween's Pathology of the Liver.* 6th ed. New York: Elsevier; 2012: 618–619.
89. Crocetti D, Palmieri A, Pedullà G, Pasta V, D'Orazi V, Grazi GL. Peliosis hepatis: personal experience and literature review. *World J Gastroenterol.* 2015;**21**(46):13188–13194.
90. Yanoff M. Peliosis hepatis. An anatomic study with demonstration of two varieties. *Arch Pathol.* 1964;**77**:159–165.
91. Hyodo M, Mogensen AM, Larsen PN, et al. Idiopathic extensive peliosis hepatis treated with liver transplantation. *J Hepatobiliary Pancreat Surg.* 2004;**11**(5):371–374.
92. Park JY, Choi MS, Lim YS, et al. Clinical features, image findings, and prognosis of inflammatory pseudotumor of the liver: a multicenter experience of 45 cases. *Gut Liver.* 2014;**8**(1):58–63.
93. Goldsmith PJ, Loganathan A, Jacob M, et al. Inflammatory pseudotumours of the liver: a spectrum of presentation and management options. *Eur J Surg Oncol.* 2009;**35**(12):1295–1298.
94. Deniz K, Çoban G. Solitary necrotic nodule of the liver: always benign? *J Gastrointest Surg.* 2010;**14**(3):536–540.

11

Modern management of liver trauma

Philip C. Müller, Valentin Neuhaus, Thomas Pfammatter, and Henrik Petrowsky

Introduction

Following trauma, the liver is one of the most often injured organs of the abdominal cavity. In Europe, hepatic trauma is frequently caused by blunt injury from traffic accidents, while in America and South Africa, up to one-fifth or even more are due to penetrating injures either from stab or gunshot wounds.[1–3]

Historically, liver trauma was associated with high morbidity and mortality rates from an aggressive surgical approach. During the past 25 years, a better understanding of the underlying pathophysiology, improved diagnostics, and additional therapies such as interventional embolization has led to a paradigm shift in management. The introduction of fast contrast-enhanced (CE) computed tomography (CT), has enabled a precise evaluation of injured solid abdominal organs.[4] In haemodynamically stable patients, nonoperative management (NOM) has become the standard of care for blunt liver trauma and in selected patients with penetrating trauma.[5,6] During the same time, there has been a paradigm shift away from aggressive surgical technique, such as formal hepatic resections, towards damage control surgery (DCS).[7] The main principles of DCS are the control of bleeding and contamination during the initial operation followed by planned reoperation for definitive repair and reconstruction after adequate resuscitation. Still, surgeons often face demanding challenges in the hostile environment of active bleeding livers, where resection techniques as in elective hepatic surgery are often not suitable. The time window for successful surgical treatment before the onset of the 'lethal triad' of coagulopathy, acidosis, and hypothermia is narrow and should not be missed.[8] However, the introduction of CECT, DCS, and percutaneous techniques such as angiography, embolization, or interventional drainages allow for an individualized approach with improved results. This chapter presents the current approach to hepatic trauma, describing the pathophysiology, classification, diagnostic workup, NOM, and surgical management.

Pathophysiology

Although the liver is protected by the ribcage, it is frequently involved in abdominal trauma. The large and anterior location makes the liver prone to penetrating abdominal injuries from gunshot (Figure 11.1) or stab wounds (Figure 11.2). Penetrating hepatic injuries often result in a sharp cut through the liver tissue and its vessels. Blunt hepatic injuries occur from direct compressive forces or shearing forces in the scenarios of acceleration and/or deceleration injuries (Figure 11.3).[9] While arterial blood vessels are less susceptible to tearing, the thin Glisson's capsule, the hepatic veins, and the liver parenchyma are less elastic and more susceptible to rupture. Due to its fixation to the diaphragm and the abdominal wall, injuries to the right hemiliver are much more frequent than to the left hemiliver.[10] Deceleration injuries are associated with tears between the right anterior and right posterior sectors at the junction between the triangular ligament and the Glisson's capsule. Deceleration is followed by rotation of the liver to the left, where the posterior ligamentous attachment to the diaphragm and the abdominal wall are especially sensitive to tension and shear or rotational forces will cause hepatic venous tears.[9,11] By contrast, direct blunt injuries lead to central, star-shaped injuries, and involve both the right and the left lobe due to compression between the ribcage and spine. Ongoing bleeding, multiple major bleeding sites, as well as coagulation disorders are potentially fatal combinations. In particular, liver cirrhosis and the deadly duo of pelvic fractures in combination with liver trauma are important additional factors that are associated with a poor outcome in liver trauma patients. Both hospital mortality (liver cirrhosis odds ratio 4.52) and complications (liver cirrhosis odds ratio 1.92) are significantly higher in this patient group (Box 11.1).[12–17]

Classification of liver injury

Liver trauma can range from a minor capsular tear without parenchymal injury to extensive disruption involving both hemilivers and injuries to major vascular structures such as the hepatic veins or vena cava. While the segmental anatomical classification by Couinaud is important in elective liver surgery, traumatic liver injuries often do not respect anatomical boundaries. The segmental anatomy is only used to describe the location of hepatic injuries. Therefore, the American Association for the Surgery of Trauma[18] developed a classification system particularly for liver trauma

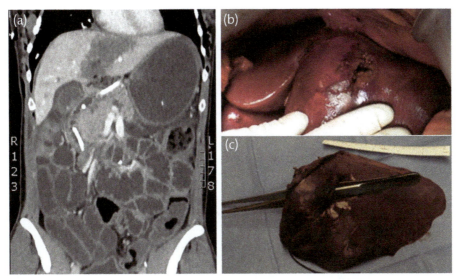

Figure 11.1 Clinical case of penetrating liver injury. A 27-year-old patient with gunshot injury arrived haemodynamically instable in the emergency department. Crush laparotomy was immediately performed in the trauma room. Due to massive bleeding, Pringle manoeuvre and exclusion of the infrahepatic vena cava was performed. The gunshot penetrated segment II/III through the left portal vein (a), pars 1 of the duodenum, and the right hemicolon. The laceration of segment II/III was approximated with sutures, while the left vena portae was oversewn in a first attempt to stop bleeding. Duodenum and right hemicolon were approximated and closed with sutures. According to the damage control surgery concept, definitive repair of the duodenum and the colon was postponed with the goal of correction of coagulopathy and haemodynamic stabilization achieved. Due to clinical deterioration and the suspicion of ongoing bleeding, the patient was taken to the operation room 12 hours later, where bisegmentectomy II/III was performed (b, c). The patient was discharged after 30 days.

that was recently updated[19] (Table 11.1). The initial system was based on intraoperative findings reflecting the rising mortality with increasing injury severity while the liver trauma grading in the 2018 updated liver injury scale relies on various features of imaging, intraoperative, or pathological criteria. Liver trauma is classified from grade I (e.g. subcapsular haematoma or parenchymal laceration) to grade V (e.g. injury to the vena cava, hepatic veins, or parenchymal disruption >75% of a hepatic lobe).

Diagnosis

The initial assessment of the patient with suspected hepatic trauma follows the principles of Advanced Trauma Life Support (ATLS).[20] First, the airway, breathing, and circulation are evaluated. Then, a thorough full-body examination is performed to detect additional injuries. Furthermore, the response to resuscitation is evaluated and serves as an important indicator for the further management

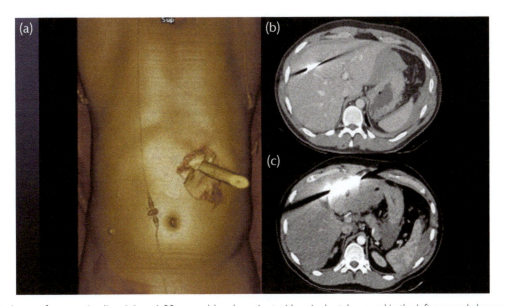

Figure 11.2 Clinical case of penetrating liver injury. A 32-year-old male patient with a single stab wound in the left upper abdomen was admitted to the trauma room. At admission, he presented with a knife in the left upper abdomen (a). A CECT scan shows the penetrating stitch channel through the entire liver (b, c). The patient underwent emergency laparotomy with removal of the knife, careful abdominal exploration, and local hepatic haemostasis.

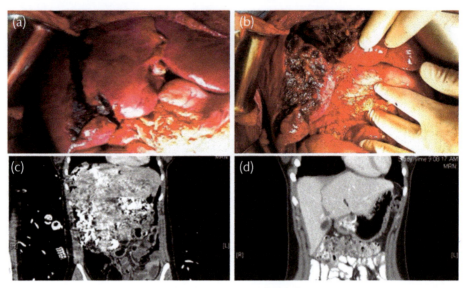

Figure 11.3 Clinical case of blunt liver injury. A 22-year-old female patient who fell from a second story balcony was admitted in the emergency room. Due to haemodynamic instability and positive FAST, emergent explorative laparotomy was performed. She had grade 5 liver injury with an almost complete split between the right and left lobe (a, b). There was massive bleeding with complete tear of the middle hepatic vein. The middle hepatic vein was sutured and the abdomen was packed with surgical sponges due to uncontrollable bleeding (c). After haemodynamic stability was achieved, the patient was taken to the operating room 2 days later in order to remove all surgical sponges. There was no bleeding from the parenchymal split surface and the abdomen was definitely closed (a, b). The patient was discharged after 10 days and fully recovered. A follow-up CT scan 2 months later showed a homogeneous-perfused liver with a split scar still apparent (d).

of the patient.[5] This depends on the pathophysiology of the trauma (blunt versus penetrating), the haemodynamic stability, and the clinical presentation (e.g. peritonitis or organ evisceration) of the patient. Patients with penetrating injuries, who are haemodynamically unstable (systolic blood pressure <90 mmHg after 1 L of fluids) irrespective of the trauma, and patients unresponsive to resuscitation should undergo emergent surgical exploration (Figure 11.4). Patients with blunt hepatic trauma and haemodynamic stability should undergo further diagnostic imaging. Abdominal ultrasound (US) often represents the first diagnostic modality in the evaluation of patients with blunt abdominal trauma.[5] Focused Assessment with Sonography for Trauma (FAST) is a sensitive and specific tool to detect free fluid in the perihepatic, perisplenic, and pelvic regions.[21,22] However, FAST is inappropriate for the identification of the intra-abdominal bleeding site and grading of the organ injury. Furthermore, FAST has drawbacks in terms of evaluation of hollow viscus and retroperitoneal injuries. Therefore, US is a valuable screening examination and, if positive, haemodynamically stable patients need a secondary and more definitive assessment preferably by CECT.[5] CECT has the highest sensitivity and specificity in detecting intra-abdominal injuries and has become the diagnostic technique of choice in abdominal trauma over the last 25 years (Figure 11.5).[4] In multitrauma patients, whole-body CT is increasingly used as the preferred imaging modality.[23] CECT allows the identification and comprehensive classification of parenchymal, vascular, and concomitant injuries while only 1.1% of associated abdominal injuries are missed by a CT scan.[24] In addition, CT is highly sensitive to detect vascular bleeding in patients with severe hepatic injuries. CECT detects arterial haemorrhage with an 85% specificity and 65% sensitivity.[23] The diagnostic importance of CT in trauma management becomes apparent by the fact that CT scanners are mandatory these days in trauma room planning and construction. Importantly, early whole-body CT reduces the time to decision-making while significantly reducing mortality rates.[4,24,27]

Non-operative management

NOM is the treatment of choice for blunt hepatic injury in haemodynamically stable patients without CT findings mandating surgery and amenable for clinical evaluation (Figure 11.4).[5,16] If there are no signs of a hollow viscus injury, NOM is the standard of care for blunt hepatic trauma, regardless of the grade or extent of the injury. However, for appropriate NOM, institutions need certain infrastructure and services:

1. A facility capable of continuous monitoring (intensive care unit (ICU), intermediate care unit (IMCU)).
2. The possibility to perform repeated CECT scans at any time.[25,28]
3. An operating room that is immediately available for emergency procedures.

Stable patients with blunt hepatic injury managed non-operatively are admitted to the ICU/IMCU for close haemodynamic monitoring

Box 11.1 Reported risk factors for increased mortality in liver trauma

- Liver cirrhosis.[12,14]
- Combined pelvic injury.[13]
- High injury severity score.[1,4,15]
- Associated severe head injury.[16]
- Multiorgan failure and sepsis.[16]
- Age.[17]

Non-operative management

Table 11.1 Classification of liver injury according to the 2018 revised Liver Injury Scale

AAST grade	AIS severity	Imaging criteria (CT findings)	Operative criteria	Pathologic criteria
I	2	• Subcapsular haematoma <10% surface area • Parenchymal laceration <1 cm in depth	• Subcapsular haematoma <10% surface area • Parenchymal laceration <1 cm in depth • Capsular tear	• Subcapsular haematoma <10% surface area • Parenchymal laceration <1 cm in depth • Capsular tear
II	2	• Subcapsular haematoma 10–50% surface area; intraparenchymal haematoma <10 cm in diameter • Laceration 1–3 cm in depth and ≤10 cm length	• Subcapsular haematoma 10–50% surface area; intraparenchymal haematoma <10 cm in diameter • Laceration 1–3 cm in depth and ≤10 cm length	• Subcapsular haematoma 10–50% surface area; intraparenchymal haematoma <10 cm in diameter • Laceration 1–3 cm depth and ≤10 cm length
III	3	• Subcapsular haematoma >50% surface area; ruptured subcapsular or parenchymal haematoma • Intraparenchymal haematoma >10 cm • Laceration >3 cm depth • Any injury in the presence of a liver vascular injury or active bleeding contained within liver parenchyma	• Subcapsular haematoma >50% surface area or expanding; ruptured subcapsular or parenchymal haematoma • Intraparenchymal haematoma >10 cm • Laceration >3 cm in depth	• Subcapsular haematoma >50% surface area; ruptured subcapsular or intraparenchymal haematoma • Intraparenchymal haematoma >10 cm • Laceration >3 cm in depth
IV	4	• Parenchymal disruption involving 25–75% of a hepatic lobe • Active bleeding extending beyond the liver parenchyma into the peritoneum	• Parenchymal disruption involving 25–75% of a hepatic lobe	• Parenchymal disruption involving 25–75% of a hepatic lobe
V	5	• Parenchymal disruption >75% of hepatic lobe • Juxtahepatic venous injury to include retrohepatic vena cava and central major hepatic veins	• Parenchymal disruption >75% of hepatic lobe • Juxtahepatic venous injury to include retrohepatic vena cava and central major hepatic veins	• Parenchymal disruption >75% of hepatic lobe • Juxtahepatic venous injury to include retrohepatic vena cava and central major hepatic veins

AAST, American Association for the Surgery of Trauma; AIS, Abbreviated Injury Scale.
Vascular injury is defined as a pseudoaneurysm or arteriovenous fistula and appears as a focal collection of vascular contrast that decreases in attenuation with delayed imaging.
Active bleeding from a vascular injury presents as vascular contrast, focal or diffuse, that increases in size or attenuation in delayed phase. Vascular thrombosis can lead to organ infarction.
Grade based on highest grade assessment made on imaging, at operation or on pathologic specimen.
More than one grade of liver injury may be present and should be classified by the higher grade of injury.
Advance one grade for multiple injuries up to a grade III.
Reproduced with permission from R.A. Kozar, M. Crandall, K. Shanmuganathan, B.L. Zarzaur, M. Coburn, C. Cribari, K. Kaups, K. Schuster, G.T. Tominaga, AAST Patient Assessment Committee, Organ injury scaling 2018 update: Spleen, liver, and kidney. J Trauma Acute Care Surg. 85 (2018) 1119-1122.

including serial abdominal examinations evaluating new or increased right upper quadrant tenderness. Initial NOM furthermore includes bed rest, nil by mouth, and repeated laboratory studies including blood counts, coagulation profile, and liver function tests. The length of surveillance stay in the ICU/IMCU depends on the severity of liver trauma and associated injures. Haemodynamically stable patients with isolated liver trauma are generally transferred to the ward after 36–48 hours. The start of a normal diet, deep vein thrombosis prophylaxis, and when to resume full activities varies between institutions.[29] It seems safe and important to start with deep vein thrombosis prophylaxis within the first 48 hours, especially in those at a high risk (e.g. spine/pelvic injuries).[30] Whether or not to perform routine follow-up imaging is another debatable question. While routine imaging is not indicated in mild cases, patients with high-grade injuries often undergo repeated CT scans in search of associated complications. In these scenarios, we in Zurich always recommend follow-up imaging before discharge. Typical indicators for NOM failure are drops in haematocrit, fever, increasing inflammation parameters, and new-onset haemodynamic instability. These indicators need further workup and management. Various studies have demonstrated a high success rate of NOM in the range of 85–96%.[1,4,16,31]

Non-operative interventions

Angiography and angioembolization

Angiographic embolization is an important and effective adjunct intervention in patients undergoing NOM (Figure 11.4).[32] An active extravasation on CECT scan most likely results from an injury to a branch of the hepatic artery and is an indication for hepatic arterial embolization preventing delayed haemorrhage and formation of pseudoaneurysms and arterio-venous fistulae (Figure 11.6). The embolization should be as selective as possible to minimize the risk of parenchymal ischaemia. The success rate of angiographic embolization is as high as 83%, however, no guidelines exist as to when and in which patients to perform angiography.[33] The most frequent complications after embolization are hepatic necrosis, abscess formation, and bile leaks.[34-36]

Image-guided percutaneous drainage

Bile collection and bile leakage due to biliary tree disruption is a frequent complication occurring in up to 20% of cases after liver injury.[37,38] In most cases, adequate external drainage using a CT- or US-guided approach is sufficient for closure of the bile leak. However, persistent high-output bile leaks may be diagnosed and

CHAPTER 11 Modern management of liver trauma

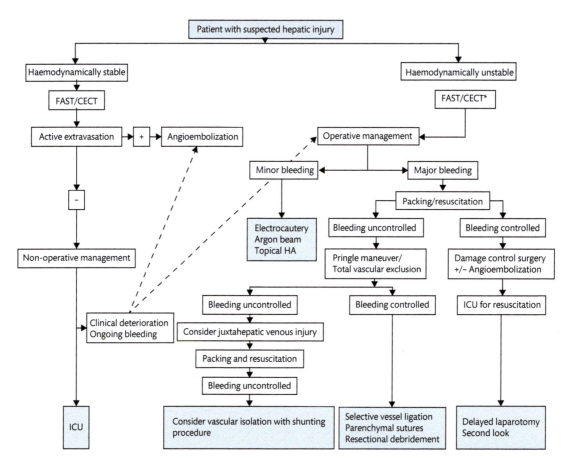

Figure 11.4 Treatment algorithm for the management of patients with suspected hepatic injury due to blunt trauma. CE-CT, contrast-enhanced computed tomography; FAST, Focused Assessment with Sonography for Trauma; HA, haemostatic agent; ICU, intensive care unit.

Adapted from Coccolini F et al. Liver trauma: WSES 2020 guidelines. *World J Emerg Surg*. 2020;15:24. https://doi.org/10.1186/s13017-020-00302-7 Under a Creative Commons Attribution 4.0 International License (http://creativecommons.org/licenses/by/4.0/).

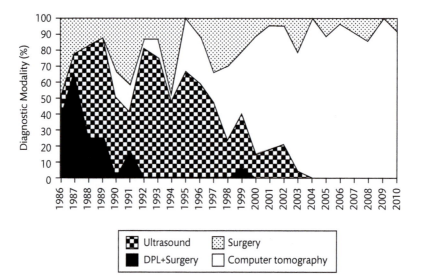

Figure 11.5 Distribution of initial diagnostic modality of liver trauma at admission for the period 1986–2010. CT has replaced US as the technique of choice to explore liver trauma over the last 25 years.

Reproduced with permission from H. Petrowsky, S. Raeder, L. Zuercher, A. Platz, H.P. Simmen, M.A. Puhan, M.J. Keel, P.-A. Clavien. A quarter century experience in liver trauma: a plea for early computed tomography and conservative management for all hemodynamically stable patients. *World J Surg*. 2012;36:247–254. https://doi.org/10.1007/s00268-011-1384-0

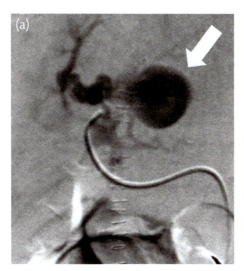 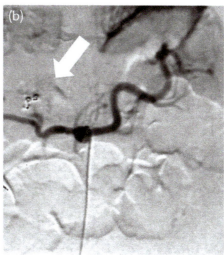

Figure 11.6 Following penetrating hepatic trauma, an arterio-biliary fistula (haemobilia) with formation of a pseudoaneurysm (arrow) of the left hepatic artery was managed by angioembolization (a). The left hepatic artery was coiled (arrow) resulting in complete elimination of the pseudoaneurysm (b).

treated by endoscopic retrograde cholangiopancreatography with stent placement to decompress the outflow of the biliary system.[39,40] Additionally, CT-guided percutaneous drainage is effective for the treatment of intrahepatic or perihepatic abscesses.[41]

Failure of non-operative management

Failure of NOM may or may not be liver related. It is more likely with higher grades of liver injury and generally due to ongoing haemorrhage (in 75% of the cases).[42,43] It is important that failure of NOM is recognized early and approached aggressively. In most cases, NOM failure becomes apparent by haemodynamic instability requiring blood transfusions and fluid resuscitation, often in combination with the onset of new or increased right upper quadrant pain. When stable, an angiography with embolization can be performed in carefully selected patients. However, a haemodynamically unstable patient should be taken to the operating room for surgical exploration immediately (Figure 11.4). Failure rates of NOM of hepatic trauma are generally below 10%; however, unsuccessful NOM is associated with increased mortality rates.[16,31]

Operative management

Haemodynamically unstable patients require immediate laparotomy to control bleeding (Figure 11.4). Exploratory laparotomy is performed through a midline incision, followed by evisceration of the small bowel and packing of the four abdominal quadrants. Using a retraction system facilitates the exposure of the liver; if the exposure is still inadequate, the incision should be extended. Packing the abdomen gives the anaesthetist time to resuscitate the patient. Then the abdominal cavity is systematically explored. In case of a suspected liver injury, the right upper quadrant should be explored last. According to the damage control concept, the major goal of the operation is to achieve physiological stability and haemostasis, rather than complete the immediate repair of the injuries. The idea behind this concept is to prevent the 'lethal triad' of coagulopathy, acidosis, and hypothermia, which are major contributors to early mortality.[44]

The 'open abdomen' treatment by vacuum-assisted closure is often used in DCS and has advantages related to shorter operation time, better abdominal decompression and minimizing the risk for abdominal compartment syndrome, and additional drainage.

Minor bleeding from superficial lacerations is controlled by local packing, electrocautery, and argon beam coagulation. For deeper lacerations, topical haemostatic agents or the greater omentum are placed into the laceration followed by packing. Approximating the laceration with liver sutures can also contribute to effective compression.

Bleeding from deeper liver lacerations, not manageable by local haemostatic techniques, should be stopped by compression through packing with surgical sponges. For effective haemostasis, it is of paramount importance that the injured parenchyma is compressed with packs placed above and below the laceration (Figure 11.7). However, overpacking can result in compression of the vena cava and subsequent hypotension or abdominal compartment syndrome. It is therefore advisable to wait a few minutes and observe the effect of the packing before finishing the operation.

If severe bleeding cannot be controlled by packing, inflow occlusion (Pringle manoeuvre) should be performed next (Figure 11.8). The index finger is passed through the foramen of Winslow (epiploic foramen) and a window is created in the pars flaccida of the gastrohepatic ligament. Then, a tape is passed through the opening between the gastrohepatic ligament and the foramen of Winslow thereby encircling the hepatoduodenal ligament. Both ends of the tape are then passed through a rubber tourniquet that is pushed down to the level of the hepatoduodenal ligament. For inflow occlusion, the tourniquet is tightened around the portal triad with a vascular clamp. It is important to keep the occlusion time to a minimum. In elective hepatic surgery, a 15-minute inflow occlusion time has been shown to be safe, while this time can be prolonged with intermittent clamping of 5 minutes. With this technique the total inflow occlusion time can be prolonged up to 120 minutes, although scientific evaluation in hepatic trauma patients is missing.[45]

In case of arterial injury, selective ligation of the bleeding hepatic artery may be necessary. If bleeding is localized to one of the hepatic

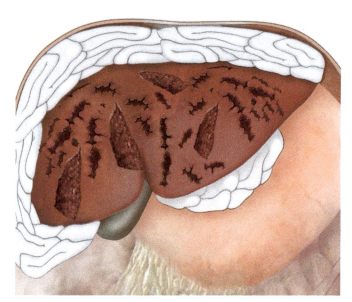

Figure 11.7 Circumferential packing of the liver with surgical sponges. For effective haemostasis, it is important that the injured parenchyma is compressed with packs placed above and below the laceration.
Reproduced courtesy of Carol De Simio, University Hospital Zurich, Zurich, Switzerland.

lobes, ligation of the right or left hepatic artery beyond the bifurcation of the proper hepatic artery can be used to manage bleeding. Alternatively, angiography with embolization can be used in stable patients (see 'Angiography and angioembolization').

When haemorrhage continues despite inflow occlusion, bleeding from injury to the retrohepatic veins, or the inferior vena cava is

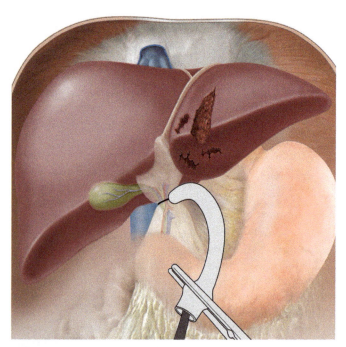

Figure 11.8 The Pringle manoeuvre for inflow occlusion. A tape is passed through the opening between the gastrohepatic ligament and the foramen of Winslow and the hepatoduodenal ligament is encircled. For inflow occlusion, the tourniquet is tightened around the portal triad with a vascular clamp.
Reproduced courtesy of Carol De Simio, University Hospital Zurich, Zurich, Switzerland.

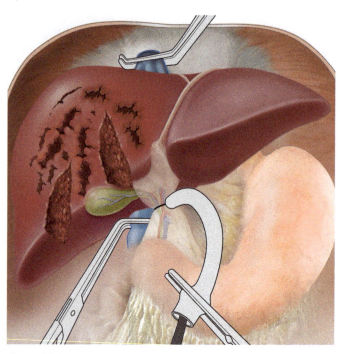

Figure 11.9 Total vascular exclusion includes clamping of the portal triad, and the infra- and suprahepatic vena cava. This type of clamping manoeuvre is often required for the surgical management of major vascular injuries including the hepatic veins and vena cava.
Reproduced courtesy of Carol De Simio, University Hospital Zurich, Zurich, Switzerland.

suspected. In the next step, packing and a quick decision on how to achieve outflow control is crucial. Any delay on the decision may worsen the prognosis of the patient and lead to massive blood loss. Total hepatic vascular occlusion is a major challenge in patients with ongoing haemorrhage as the clamping of the inferior vena cava is often poorly tolerated by the haemodynamically unstable patient (Figure 11.9). In addition, the surgical technique is more complex, especially outflow control of the surpahepatic vena cava. Despite the surgical feasibility of total hepatic vascular occlusion, patients with juxtahepatic vena caval injuries have a high mortality rate.

In extremely rare cases, liver transplantation may be an option for severe hepatic trauma where bleeding is controlled with total hepatectomy and a portocaval shunt. Analysing the outcomes of 73 recipients in the European Liver Transplant Registry, showed mortality and graft loss rates of 42.5% and 46.6%, respectively, at 90 days. Improved outcomes were observed for candidates with liver trauma not exceeding grade IV injuries and an injury severity score below 33.[46,47]

Extrahepatic biliary injury

The majority of extrahepatic biliary injuries result from penetrating trauma with the gallbladder as the most often involved structure.[48] While cholecystectomy can be attempted, the surgeon should keep in mind that cholecystectomy creates another source of haemorrhage in the liver bed. In case of massive haemorrhage and coagulopathy, simple closure with a stitch or drainage may be more suitable in the scenario of DCS. Minor injuries to the extrahepatic biliary tree can be managed by primary closure or external drainage. Major injuries require Roux-en-Y choledochojejunostomy or hepaticojejunostomy for definitive repair; however, haemodynamic stability and coagulopathy determine the management in these patients.[49] Drainage by T-tube insertion in the emergency setting and subsequent elective biliary reconstruction after resuscitation may often be a better option than direct repair.

Planned reoperation

Following DCS, we aim for a planned reoperation 24–48 hours after the initial procedure. However, this interval may be prolonged if severe medical conditions (e.g. pulmonary insufficiency, haemodynamic instability, coagulopathy) prevent reoperation.[7,8] For preoperative planning, CECT should be performed prior to the reoperation. After evacuation of the haemoperitoneum and exploration of the abdominal cavity, liver packing should be slowly removed with extreme care. Whenever bleeding is encountered, it should be stopped with local haemostatic techniques. If a bile leak is detected, it should be properly drained. If there is ongoing bleeding from the unpacked liver, consider repacking and early termination of the operation. When limited hepatic necrosis is present without signs of infection, local drainage or limited necrosectomy might be performed.

Postoperative complications

Abdominal compartment syndrome

Abdominal compartment syndrome after hepatic trauma may be due to various reasons including perihepatic packing, persistent bleeding, abdominal closure under tension, bile leakage, retroperitoneal bleeding due to a pelvic injury, or vigorous volume management. CT may be used to depict the intra- and retroperitoneal fluid. Patients with abdominal compartment syndrome are treated by urgent decompressive laparotomy while leaving the abdomen open using vacuum-assisted closure.

Biliary leak

Biliary tree disruption with formation of a biloma and/or persistent bile leak with or without biliary peritonitis is a frequent complication after both NOM and operative management of hepatic trauma. The incidence of biliary leakage ranges from 0.5% to 21%, while the majority are minor leaks that respond well to conservative treatment.[40,50] Risk factors for major bile leaks include high-grade liver injury, centrally located liver trauma, and the use of arterial embolization.[37,50] Magnetic resonance cholangiography is the diagnostic modality of choice to provide information on the source of the leak. Biliary leaks are often successfully managed by adequate percutaneous drainage and/or endoscopic retrograde cholangiopancreatography with sphincterotomy and biliary stent placement.[39,40]

Liver necrosis and hepatic abscess

The risk of hepatic necrosis increases with the severity of the liver trauma, following embolization or arterial injuries.[36] Small areas of hepatic necrosis do not require special treatment. However, major hepatic necrosis requires surgical treatment with surgical debridement or formal anatomical hepatic resection. Debridement of necrosis may be simpler but can lead to a prolonged postoperative course due to the need of repeated necrosectomy and the risk of biliary leaks. Hepatic abscesses have a low incidence in patients with hepatic trauma (0–7%).[36,41] They are usually due to infected hepatic parenchymal necrosis or infected bilomas. The majority of abscesses can be managed with CT- or US-guided percutaneous drainage.

Conclusion

In haemodynamically stable patients, NOM has become the standard of care for blunt liver trauma with a high success rate in the range of 85–96%. Angioembolization and image-guided percutaneous drainage are adjuncts of NOM leading to a less traumatic treatment of liver trauma. The paradigm shift away from aggressive surgical techniques with prolonged surgery such as shifting from formal hepatic resections towards DCS further results in improved outcomes of patients with liver trauma who require operation.

Acknowledgements

The authors thank Carol De Simio for creating the illustrations in Figures 11.7–11.9.

REFERENCES

1. Fodor M, Primavesi F, Morell-Hofert D, et al. Non-operative management of blunt hepatic and splenic injury: a time-trend and outcome analysis over a period of 17 years. *World J Emerg Surg.* 2019;**14**:29. https://doi.org/10.1186/s13017-019-0249-y
2. Zago TM, Pereira BM, Nascimento B, Alves MSC, Calderan TRA, Fraga GP. Hepatic trauma: a 21-year experience. *Rev Col Bras Cir.* 2013;**40**(4):318–322. https://doi.org/10.1590/s0100-69912013000400011
3. Clancy TV, Gary Maxwell JG, Covington DL, Brinker CC, Blackman D. A statewide analysis of level I and II trauma centers for patients with major injuries. *J Trauma.* 2001;**51**(2):346–351. https://doi.org/10.1097/00005373-200108000-00021
4. Petrowsky H, Raeder S, Zuercher L, et al. A quarter century experience in liver trauma: a plea for early computed tomography and conservative management for all hemodynamically stable patients. *World J Surg.* 2012;**36**(2):247–254. https://doi.org/10.1007/s00268-011-1384-0
5. Coccolini F, Coimbra R, Ordonez C, et al. Liver trauma: WSES 2020 guidelines. *World J Emerg Surg.* 2020;**15**:24. https://doi.org/10.1186/s13017-020-00302-7
6. Navsaria P, Nicol A, Krige J, Edu S, Chowdhury S. Selective nonoperative management of liver gunshot injuries. *Eur J Trauma Emerg Surg.* 2019;**45**(2):323–328. https://doi.org/10.1007/s00068-018-0913-z
7. Weber DG, Bendinelli C, Balogh ZJ. Damage control surgery for abdominal emergencies. *Br J Surg.* 2014;**101**(1):e109–e118. https://doi.org/10.1002/bjs.9360
8. Lamb CM, MacGoey P, Navarro AP, Brooks AJ. Damage control surgery in the era of damage control resuscitation. *Br J Anaesth.* 2014;**113**(2):242–249. https://doi.org/10.1093/bja/aeu233
9. Cheynel N, Serre T, Arnoux PJ, Ortega-Deballon P, Benoit L, Brunet C. Comparison of the biomechanical behavior of the liver during frontal and lateral deceleration. *J Trauma.* 2009;**67**(1):40–44. https://doi.org/10.1097/TA.0b013e31818cc429
10. Badger SA, Barclay R, Campbell P, Mole DJ, Diamond T. Management of liver trauma. *World J Surg.* 2009;**33**(12):2522–2537. https://doi.org/10.1007/s00268-009-0215-z
11. Cheynel N, Serre T, Arnoux PJ, et al. Biomechanic study of the human liver during a frontal deceleration. *J Trauma.* 2006;**61**(4):855–861. https://doi.org/10.1097/01.ta.0000196871.19566.92

12. Serrano E, Liu P, Nwabuo AI, Langness S, Juillard C. The effect of cirrhosis on trauma outcomes: a systematic review and meta-analysis. *J Trauma Acute Care Surg*. 2020;**88**(4):536–545. https://doi.org/10.1097/TA.0000000000002464
13. Grotz MRW, Gummerson NW, Gänsslen A, et al. Staged management and outcome of combined pelvic and liver trauma. An international experience of the deadly duo. *Injury*. 2006;**37**(7):642–651. https://doi.org/10.1016/j.injury.2005.11.009
14. Talving P, Lustenberger T, Okoye OT, et al. The impact of liver cirrhosis on outcomes in trauma patients: a prospective study. *J Trauma Acute Care Surg*. 2013;**75**(4):699–703. https://doi.org/10.1097/TA.0b013e31829a2c19
15. Schnüriger B, Inderbitzin D, Schafer M, Kickuth R, Exadaktylos A, Candinas D. Concomitant injuries are an important determinant of outcome of high-grade blunt hepatic trauma. *Br J Surg*. 2009;**96**(1):104–110. https://doi.org/10.1002/bjs.6439
16. Hommes M, Navsaria PH, Schipper IB, Krige JEJ, Kahn D, Nicol AJ. Management of blunt liver trauma in 134 severely injured patients. *Injury*. 2015;**46**(5):837–842. https://doi.org/10.1016/j.injury.2014.11.019
17. Chien LC, Lo SS, Yeh SY. Incidence of liver trauma and relative risk factors for mortality: a population-based study. *J Chin Med Assoc*. 2013;**76**(10):576–582. https://doi.org/10.1016/j.jcma.2013.06.004
18. Moore EE, Cogbill TH, Jurkovich GJ, Shackford SR, Malangoni MA, Champion HR. Organ injury scaling: spleen and liver (1994 revision). *J Trauma*. 1995;**38**(3):323–324. https://doi.org/10.1097/00005373-199503000-00001
19. Kozar RA, Crandall M, Shanmuganathan K, et al. Organ injury scaling 2018 update: spleen, liver, and kidney. *J Trauma Acute Care Surg*. 2018;**85**(6):1119–1122. https://doi.org/10.1097/TA.0000000000002058
20. Galvagno SM, Nahmias JT, Young DA. Advanced Trauma Life Support® update 2019: management and applications for adults and special populations. *Anesthesiol Clin*. 2019;**37**(1):13–32. https://doi.org/10.1016/j.anclin.2018.09.009
21. Stengel D, Leisterer J, Ferrada P, Ekkernkamp A, Mutze S, Hoenning A. Point-of-care ultrasonography for diagnosing thoracoabdominal injuries in patients with blunt trauma. *Cochrane Database Syst Rev*. 2018;**12**(12):CD012669. https://doi.org/10.1002/14651858.CD012669.pub2
22. Netherton S, Milenkovic V, Taylor M, Davis PJ. Diagnostic accuracy of eFAST in the trauma patient: a systematic review and meta-analysis. *CJEM*. 2019;**21**(6):727–738. https://doi.org/10.1017/cem.2019.381
23. Huber-Wagner S, Kanz KG, Hanschen M, van Griensven M, Biberthaler P, Lefering R. Whole-body computed tomography in severely injured patients. *Curr Opin Crit Care*. 2018;**24**(1):55–61. https://doi.org/10.1097/MCC.0000000000000474
24. Miller PR, Croce MA, Bee TK, Malhotra AK, Fabian TC. Associated injuries in blunt solid organ trauma: implications for missed injury in nonoperative management. *J Trauma*. 2002;**53**(2):238–242. https://doi.org/10.1097/00005373-200208000-00008
25. Poletti PA, Mirvis SE, Shanmuganathan K, Killeen KL, Coldwell D. CT criteria for management of blunt liver trauma: correlation with angiographic and surgical findings. *Radiology*. 2000;**216**(2):418–427. https://doi.org/10.1148/radiology.216.2.r00au44418
26. Furugori S, Kato M, Abe T, Iwashita M, Morimura N. Treating patients in a trauma room equipped with computed tomography and patients' mortality: a non-controlled comparison study. *World J Emerg Surg*. 2018;**13**:16. https://doi.org/10.1186/s13017-018-0176-3
27. Huber-Wagner S, Lefering R, Qvick LM, et al. Effect of whole-body CT during trauma resuscitation on survival: a retrospective, multicentre study. *Lancet*. 2009;**373**(9673):1455–1461. https://doi.org/10.1016/S0140-6736(09)60232-4
28. Fang JF, Wong YC, Lin BC, Hsu YP, Chen MF. The CT risk factors for the need of operative treatment in initially hemodynamically stable patients after blunt hepatic trauma. *J Trauma*. 2006;**61**(3):547–553. https://doi.org/10.1097/01.ta.0000196571.12389.ee
29. Rostas JW, Manley J, Gonzalez RP, et al. The safety of low molecular-weight heparin after blunt liver and spleen injuries. *Am J Surg*. 2015;**210**(1):31–34. https://doi.org/10.1016/j.amjsurg.2014.08.023
30. Schellenberg M, Inaba K, Biswas S, et al. When is it safe to start VTE prophylaxis after blunt solid organ injury? A prospective study from a level I trauma center. *World J Surg*. 2019;**43**(11):2797–2803. https://doi.org/10.1007/s00268-019-05096-7
31. van der Wilden GM, Velmahos GC, Emhoff T, et al. Successful nonoperative management of the most severe blunt liver injuries: a multicenter study of the research consortium of New England centers for trauma. *Arch Surg*. 2012;**147**(5):423–428. https://doi.org/10.1001/archsurg.2012.147
32. Letoublon C, Morra I, Chen Y, Monnin V, Voirin D, Arvieux C. Hepatic arterial embolization in the management of blunt hepatic trauma: indications and complications. *J Trauma*. 2011;**70**(5):1032–1036. https://doi.org/10.1097/TA.0b013e31820e7ca1
33. Virdis F, Reccia I, Di Saverio S, et al. Clinical outcomes of primary arterial embolization in severe hepatic trauma: a systematic review. *Diagn Interv Imaging*. 2019;**100**(2):65–75. https://doi.org/10.1016/j.diii.2018.10.004
34. Green CS, Bulger EM, Kwan SW. Outcomes and complications of angioembolization for hepatic trauma: a systematic review of the literature. *J Trauma Acute Care Surg*. 2016;**80**(3):529–537. https://doi.org/10.1097/TA.0000000000000942
35. Hagiwara A, Murata A, Matsuda T, Matsuda H, Shimazaki S. The efficacy and limitations of transarterial embolization for severe hepatic injury. *J Trauma*. 2002;**52**(6):1091–1096. https://doi.org/10.1097/00005373-200206000-00011
36. Dabbs DN, Stein DM, Scalea TM. Major hepatic necrosis: a common complication after angioembolization for treatment of high-grade liver injuries. *J Trauma*. 2009;**66**(3):621–627. https://doi.org/10.1097/TA.0b013e31819919f2
37. Wahl WL, Brandt MM, Hemmila MR, Arbabi S. Diagnosis and management of bile leaks after blunt liver injury. *Surgery*. 2005;**138**(4):742–747. https://doi.org/10.1016/j.surg.2005.07.021
38. Asensio JA, Roldán G, Petrone P, et al. Operative management and outcomes in 103 AAST-OIS grades IV and V complex hepatic injuries: trauma surgeons still need to operate, but angioembolization helps. *J Trauma*. 2003;**54**(4):647–653. https://doi.org/10.1097/01.TA.0000054647.59217.BB
39. Lubezky N, Konikoff FM, Rosin D, Carmon E, Kluger Y, Ben-Haim M. Endoscopic sphincterotomy and temporary internal stenting for bile leaks following complex hepatic trauma. *Br J Surg*. 2006;**93**(1):78–81. https://doi.org/10.1002/bjs.5195
40. Anand RJ, Ferrada PA, Darwin PE, Bochicchio GV, Scalea TM. Endoscopic retrograde cholangiopancreatography is an effective treatment for bile leak after severe liver trauma. *J Trauma*. 2011;**71**(2):480–485. https://doi.org/10.1097/TA.0b013e3181efc270

41. Bala M, Gazalla SA, Faroja M, et al. Complications of high grade liver injuries: management and outcome with focus on bile leaks. *Scan J Trauma Resusc Emerg Med*. 2012;**20**:20. https://doi.org/10.1186/1757-7241-20-20
42. Kozar RA, Moore FA, Cothren CC, et al. Risk factors for hepatic morbidity following nonoperative management: multicenter study. *Arch Surg*. 2006;**141**(5):451–458. https://doi.org/10.1001/archsurg.141.5.451
43. Leppäniemi AK, Mentula PJ, Streng MH, Koivikko MP, Handolin LE. Severe hepatic trauma: nonoperative management, definitive repair, or damage control surgery? *World J Surg*. 2011;**35**(12):2643–2649. https://doi.org/10.1007/s00268-011-1309-y
44. Sherren PB, Hussey J, Martin R, Kundishora T, Parker M, Emerson B. Lethal triad in severe burns. *Burns J Int Soc Burn Inj*. 2014;**40**(8):1492–1496. https://doi.org/10.1016/j.burns.2014.04.011
45. Rüdiger HA, Kang KJ, Sindram D, Riehle HM, Clavien PA. Comparison of ischemic preconditioning and intermittent and continuous inflow occlusion in the murine liver, *Ann Surg*. 2002;**235**(3):400–407. https://doi.org/10.1097/00000658-200203000-00012
46. Krawczyk M, Grąt M, Adam R, et al. Liver transplantation for hepatic trauma: a study from the European Liver Transplant Registry. *Transplantation*. 2016;**100**(11):2372–2381. https://doi.org/10.1097/TP.0000000000001398
47. Kaltenborn A, Reichert B, Bourg CM, et al. Long-term outcome analysis of liver transplantation for severe hepatic trauma. *J Trauma Acute Care Surg*. 2013;**75**(5):864–869. https://doi.org/10.1097/TA.0b013e3182a8fe8a
48. Thomson BNJ, Nardino B, Gumm K, et al. Management of blunt and penetrating biliary tract trauma. *J Trauma Acute Care Surg*. 2012;**72**(6):1620–1625. https://doi.org/10.1097/TA.0b013e318248ed65
49. Kaptanoglu L, Kurt N, Sikar HE. Current approach to liver traumas. *Int J Surg Lond Engl*. 2017;**39**:255–259. https://doi.org/10.1016/j.ijsu.2017.02.015
50. Yuan KC, Wong YC, Fu CY, Chang CJ, Kang SC, Hsu YP. Screening and management of major bile leak after blunt liver trauma: a retrospective single center study. *Scand J Trauma Resusc Emerg Med*. 2014;**22**:26. https://doi.org/10.1186/1757-7241-22-26

12

Extrahepatic portal venous obstruction, idiopathic non-cirrhotic portal fibrosis, and hepatic venous outflow tract obstruction

Mohammad Qasim Khan and Patrick S. Kamath

Introduction

Disorders of the hepatic and portal venous systems of the liver constitute a group of uncommon conditions which collectively represent a significant health problem within the realm of liver diseases. With the exception of the upper oesophagus and distal rectum, the entire gastrointestinal tract drains into the liver via the portal venous system, accompanied by venous drainage from the spleen, pancreas, and gallbladder (Figure 12.1). The portal vein is formed by the union of the superior mesenteric vein and splenic vein behind the neck of the pancreas.[1] The left gastric vein drains into the portal vein at or near the confluence of the superior mesenteric vein and splenic vein. The inferior mesenteric vein is a tributary of the splenic vein. The portal vein divides into the left and right portal vein branches in the hilum of the liver. The umbilical vein drains into the left portal vein. Blood from the portal vein and the hepatic artery drain into hepatic sinusoids, which drain into the inferior vena cava (IVC) via the hepatic veins: right, middle, and left. The right hepatic vein drains separately into the IVC. The left and middle hepatic veins usually form a common trunk that drains into the IVC separately but adjacent to the confluence of the right hepatic vein with the IVC. The caudate lobe has independent drainage into the IVC. Disorders of the portal venous and hepatic venous systems can result in portal hypertension, idiopathic portal hypertension, Budd–Chiari syndrome (BCS) which results from hepatic venous outflow obstruction and may be complicated by cirrhosis, hepatocellular carcinoma, and rarely acute liver failure.

In this chapter we discuss the epidemiology, aetiology, clinical features, diagnosis, and management of extrahepatic portal venous obstruction, idiopathic non-cirrhotic portal hypertension (INCPH), and hepatic venous outflow obstruction,

Extrahepatic portal venous obstruction

Definition

Extrahepatic portal venous obstruction (EHPVO) as a cause of portal hypertension refers to the obstruction of the extrahepatic portal vein (portal vein thrombosis (PVT)), with or without involvement of the intrahepatic portal veins or other segments of the splanchnic venous system. Isolated thrombosis of the splenic or superior mesenteric veins is also a cause of portal hypertension.

Epidemiology

Due to the lack of a standardized classification system and heterogeneity of risk factors, the incidence and prevalence of EHPVO has been difficult to ascertain and is highly variable in the literature. An autopsy study of almost 24,000 patients from Sweden revealed a prevalence of EHPVO of 1%.[2] Another autopsy study out of Japan revealed a prevalence of 0.05% in patients without cirrhosis and 6.59% in patients with cirrhosis.[3] Recent reports utilizing national hospital discharge data and liver transplant registries have illustrated prevalence rates in patients with cirrhosis between 1.3% and 9.8%.[2,4–8] While there are few prospective studies evaluating incidence of PVT in patients with cirrhosis, this generally ranges between 3.2% and 4.1% at 1 year after diagnosis.[9–12]

Aetiology and risk factors

Multiple aetiologies and risk factors for PVT have been identified (Box 12.1). According to one study, in patients with acute PVT, one risk factor was identified in 67% of patients and in 18% of patients, two risk factors were identified.[13] As such, it is not rare for a patient with PVT to have multiple contributory risk factors.

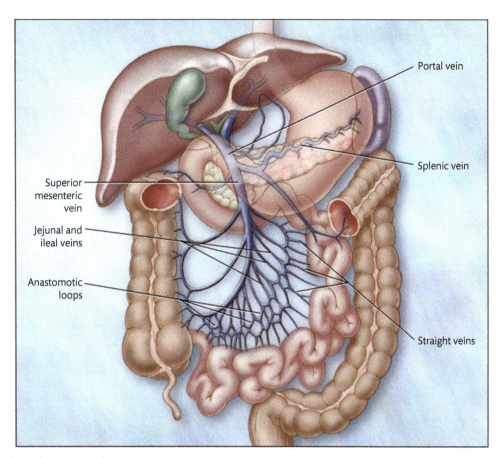

Figure 12.1 Normal portal venous circulation.
Reproduced with permission from Kumar S, Sarr MG, Kamath PS. Mesenteric venous thrombosis. *N Engl J Med.* 2001;345:1683–1688.

Thrombophilia represents the most common cause of PVT in patients without cirrhosis.[11,13] Notably, myeloproliferative neoplasms account for one-quarter of the cases of PVT.[4,14,15] Of the inherited causes of thrombophilia, factor V Leiden, and prothrombin G20210A gene mutations are the most common in the United States, with others including deficiencies of protein C, protein S, antithrombin, as well as the antiphospholipid syndrome.[16] Oestrogen-based oral contraceptives also pose increased risk for the development of PVT.[17]

Endothelial injury secondary to intra-abdominal surgeries, trauma, and intra-abdominal inflammatory processes such as pancreatitis, inflammatory bowel disease, diverticulitis, appendicitis, or cholecystitis can also increase the risk for the development of PVT.[17,18]

Cirrhosis and congestive heart failure promote stasis of flow in the portal venous system. The severity of liver disease and portal hypertension are important predictors of PVT development in patients with cirrhosis.[11,12,19–21] Additionally, obesity, metabolic syndrome, and cirrhosis secondary to non-alcoholic steatohepatitis have been identified as independent risk factors for PVT.[22–24] It is pertinent to note that hepatocellular carcinomas can invade the portal vein and cause PVT in patients with cirrhosis. As a result, contrast-enhanced imaging should be considered to differentiate bland from tumour thrombus in these patients.[25] Tumour thrombosis is characterized by arterial streaks within the portal vein, commonly referred to as the 'threads and streaks' sign. PVT may also be classified based on the extent of thrombosis, aetiology, and duration.[26]

Clinical features

In patients without cirrhosis, upper abdominal pain, which may be severe, is a prominent feature of PVT.[27] The presence of spiking fevers associated with chills, septic shock, and tender hepatomegaly raises the suspicion for septic thrombosis or pylephlebitis.[27] Other clinical features associated with PVT include ascites and nausea; splenomegaly suggests either chronicity or a myeloproliferative neoplasm as a cause of the PVT.[28,29] A sizable number of patients with cirrhosis who develop PVT may, however, be asymptomatic with thrombosis being incidentally detected during imaging studies.[30] In contrast, PVT may be associated with worsening portal hypertension and/or hepatic decompensation, that is, ascites, variceal bleeding, encephalopathy, and worsening jaundice.[27,30] If the obstruction to the portal vein extends to the superior mesenteric vein, features of intestinal ischaemia may develop.[30] Infrequently, patients may present with biliary-type pain, pancreatitis, and cholecystitis owing to the development of portal hypertensive cholangiopathy, that is, compression of the intra- and extrahepatic bile ducts by collateral veins of a cavernoma.[31,32] In the developing world, EHPVO is a major cause of paediatric portal hypertension (54% of cases) and paediatric upper gastrointestinal bleeding (68–84% of cases).[33] There is a bimodal distribution of cases with patients affected by omphalitis and umbilical sepsis presenting in the first few years of life, whereas those with intra-abdominal infections, prothrombotic conditions, and other contributing factors present in late childhood and adolescence. Forty-six to ninety per cent of paediatric cases of

> **Box 12.1** Causes of extrahepatic portal vein obstruction
>
> **Thrombophilia**
>
> *Acquired*
> - Myeloproliferative neoplasm.
> - Intra-abdominal malignancy.
> - Paroxysmal nocturnal haemoglobinuria.
> - Nephrotic syndrome.
> - Pregnancy.
> - Oral contraceptive use.
>
> *Inherited*
> - Inherited thrombophilic conditions: factor V Leiden mutation, prothrombin gene mutation, protein C/S deficiency, antithrombin deficiency, antiphospholipid syndrome, and methylenetetrahydrofolate reductase TT677 polymorphism.
> - Sickle cell disease.
>
> **Injury to the portal venous endothelium**
> - Intra-abdominal inflammation: pancreatitis, inflammatory bowel disease, diverticulitis, appendicitis, and cholecystitis.
> - Local surgery or procedure: cholecystectomy, colectomy, splenectomy, TIPS, surgical portosystemic shunt creation, liver transplantation, and locoregional therapy for hepatic tumours.
> - Abdominal trauma.
>
> **Sluggish portal venous flow**
> - Cirrhosis.
> - Congestive heart failure.
> - Hepatocellular carcinoma.
> - Cholangiocarcinoma.
> - Nodular regenerative hyperplasia.
> - Sinusoidal obstruction syndrome.

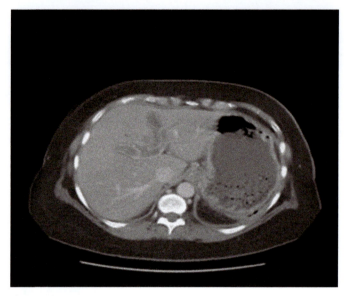

Figure 12.2 CT appearance of acute portal vein thrombosis revealing central lucency in an expanded, well-defined vein with rim-enhanced walls.

EHPVO present with gastrointestinal bleeding and approximately 25% of patients have splenomegaly.[34] Splenomegaly may be massive, associated with dragging left upper quadrant abdominal pain, sharp pleuritic-type pain with splenic infarction, malnutrition, and growth retardation. Patients may also present with hypersplenism, portal biliopathy, and minimal hepatic encephalopathy. While liver synthetic function is generally preserved in children with EHPVO, with prolonged duration of disease, liver dysfunction characterized by hypoalbuminemia and ascites may develop.[34]

Diagnosis

PVT is suspected on Doppler ultrasound and confirmed via contrast-enhanced computed tomography (CT) scanning or magnetic resonance imaging (MRI) of the abdomen.[29] Broadly, these studies reveal evidence of portal vein obstruction, presence of solid intraluminal material, or portal vein cavernoma, that is, serpiginous collaterals in the area of the portal vein with non-visualization of the main portal vein.[29,32,35,36] The lower cost, wider availability, and lack of radiation exposure make Doppler ultrasound a favourable first-line investigative test.[28] For the diagnosis of PVT, Doppler ultrasound in one report had a sensitivity of 93%, specificity of 99%, positive predictive value of 97%, and negative predictive value of 98% when compared with angiography.[28] However, CT imaging or MRI confer the additional advantage of higher resolution for evaluation of thrombosis extension, presence of hepatocellular carcinoma, local factors that cause PVT such as tumours or inflammatory bowel disease, and bowel ischaemia.[27,29]

An acute PVT appears as a central lucency with an expanded and well-defined vein on contrast-enhanced cross-sectional imaging (Figure 12.2).[27] A tumour thrombus secondary to hepatocellular carcinoma will reveal arterialization of the clot.[27] In addition to imaging studies, investigations to identify risk factors for development PVT should be concurrently initiated, especially in patients without cirrhosis.

Management

Treatment considerations

Anticoagulation is the mainstay of treatment in patients with acute PVT.[37] Early initiation of anticoagulation is associated with favourable clinical outcomes[29] and is initiated with either infusions of unfractionated heparin or subcutaneous low-molecular-weight heparin (LMWH).[27,29,37] Anticoagulation is generally maintained with either oral vitamin K antagonists (VKA) or LMWH.[27,37] Whereas the recently developed direct-acting oral anticoagulants (DOACs) are promising agents, there is limited data on their use in patients with PVT. If there are concerns for pylephlebitis, either piperacillin-tazobactam or a combination of metronidazole with either ceftazidime or cefepime should be administered.[38]

Management of PVT in patients with and without cirrhosis is considered separately given (1) different treatment goals; (2) alterations to the haemostatic, coagulation, anticoagulation, and fibrinolytic pathways specific to cirrhosis; and (3) varied clinical presentations in the setting of pre-existing portal hypertension. In patients without cirrhosis, the goals of treatment of recent PVT are to (1) promote recanalization of the portal vein and prevent the development of portal hypertension and (2) prevent extension of the obstruction to the mesenteric veins and subsequent development of intestinal ischaemia. The additional goals of treatment of PVT in cirrhotic patients are to (1) prevent worsening of portal hypertension and its downstream sequelae and (2) prevent progression of portal venous obstruction that may hinder a future liver transplant. The presence of venous collaterals in patients with cirrhosis make the risk of intestinal ischaemia less likely.[37]

Management in non-cirrhotic patients

Anticoagulation

A large prospective trial of 95 consecutive non-cirrhotic patients with recent PVT revealed complete recanalization of the portal vein in 38% of patients after early initiation of anticoagulation (LMWH, VKAs).[13] Two patients developed intestinal infarction secondary to thrombus progression and nine patients developed bleeding complications while on anticoagulation.[11] Large database analyses evaluating the safety and efficacy of traditional anticoagulants suggest that morbidity and mortality in non-cirrhotic patients with portal venous thrombosis is higher and that overall bleeding risk from anticoagulation is low.[39,40]

DOACs are quickly becoming popular choices for anticoagulation in non-cirrhotic patients with portal vein obstruction given promising data from several small retrospective studies.[41,42] A large retrospective single-centre cohort study evaluating non-cirrhotic patients with PVT treated with VKAs, LMWH, and DOACs found DOACs to have higher rates of thrombus resolution and less major bleeding when compared to warfarin.[43] However, this was a heterogeneous group of patients with varied aetiologies and extents of PVT. Therefore, prospective studies are required, stratifying patients according to the aetiology and extent of PVT.

In patients with reversible causes of PVT, anticoagulation is recommended for about 6 months,[27,44] whereas in patients with thrombophilia, long-term anticoagulation should be considered.[27,44] While on anticoagulation, cross-sectional imaging should be considered after 2–3 months of therapy to assess treatment response.[37]

Alternative therapies—thrombolysis, transjugular intrahepatic portosystemic shunt, and surgical thrombectomy

Thrombolytic therapy is generally considered as adjunctive therapy or salvage therapy after failure of anticoagulation in cases where PVT is extending to the superior mesenteric vein, risking bowel ischaemia. Recanalization rates have been found to be similar to those for anticoagulation alone.[45–47] Furthermore, rates of procedure-related morbidity and mortality are particularly high and therefore thrombolytic therapy in patients with acute PVT should be considered only very selectively.[45–47]

Transjugular intrahepatic portosystemic shunts (TIPSs) have been used in patients with PVT with or without cirrhosis. A recent meta-analysis revealed 12-month recanalization rates with TIPSs of 79% in patients with PVT.[48] Recanalization rates post-TIPS were comparable in patients with and without cirrhosis.[48] The reduction of portal venous pressures post-procedure makes TIPS a promising option for patients with chronic PVT complicated by refractory ascites or recurrent bleeding.[19]

Surgical thrombectomy achieves portal vein recanalization in 30% of patients with PVT. Recurrence rates are particularly high if performed more than 30 days after onset.[49] Given its invasive nature, the procedure is typically reserved for patients undergoing surgery for intestinal infarction and is carried out at the time of laparotomy.

Prevention of complications of extrahepatic portal venous thrombosis

Portal hypertension and its sequelae (e.g. variceal bleeding, ascites, encephalopathy, and portal hypertensive cholangiopathy) represent the major complications of chronic PVT. Ascites and hepatic encephalopathy are more common in patients with cirrhosis and PVT, whereas portal hypertensive cholangiopathy is more common in patients without cirrhosis.

Since variceal bleeding is the most common portal hypertensive complication in patients with PVT without cirrhosis, endoscopic evaluation should be considered in all patients to assess for the presence of high-risk varices.[27,37] Beta-blockers have been shown to reduce the risk of bleeding from large varices and improve survival in studies with small numbers of patients with non-cirrhotic PVT.[32,50] Head-to-head comparisons of endoscopic band ligation versus beta-blockers among patients with chronic PVT and varices are lacking in the literature. However, based on data from patients with cirrhosis and oesophageal and/or gastric varices, beta-blockers are considered the first choice for primary prophylaxis against variceal bleeding and band ligation is considered in patients intolerant to or with contraindications to beta-blocker therapy.[29] For patients with recurrent bleeding that fails to respond to beta-blocker therapy and band ligation, a TIPS procedure should be carried out when technically feasible. The role of portosystemic shunt surgery in preventing variceal rebleeding is discussed in Chapter 13.

Extrahepatic biliary ductal obstruction from stones or strictures secondary to portal hypertensive cholangiopathy warrants endoscopic retrograde cholangiopancreatography for stone removal and stent placement, respectively. Caution must be taken during these manoeuvres as rupture of intrabiliary varices can lead to massive haemobilia. Surgical portosystemic shunts may reverse the biliary changes.

Management in cirrhotic patients

Anticoagulation

There is often reluctance to prescribe anticoagulation in patients with cirrhosis given their impaired haemostatic and coagulation pathways. However, in cirrhotic patients with PVT, the benefits of anticoagulation include delaying progression to hepatic decompensation. In a meta-analysis of eight studies with patients with cirrhosis and PVT, patients treated with LMWH or warfarin had higher rates of partial or complete recanalization (71% vs 42%; odds ratio (OR) 4.8, 95% confidence interval (CI) 2.7–8.7), compared with untreated patients. Major and minor bleeding rates were equal (11%) between anticoagulated and untreated patients. Specifically, variceal bleeding rates were *lower* in anticoagulated patients compared with untreated patients (2% vs 12%; OR 0.23, 95% CI 0.06–0.94).[51] The target international normalized ratio range on warfarin is 2–3.

The initial trials evaluating DOACs for the prophylaxis and treatment of venous thromboembolism and atrial fibrillation excluded patients with cirrhosis. Knowledge of the pharmacodynamics of DOACs in patients with cirrhosis is also limited. Having said that, there is growing clinical experience with the use of DOACs in highly selected cohorts of patients with compensated cirrhosis.[52–56] This is likely secondary to their ease of use, comparable safety profile in compensated cirrhotic patients and patients without cirrhosis, as well as recent development of direct reversal agents.[57,58] In a recent study evaluating patients with cirrhosis undergoing anticoagulation for atrial fibrillation, both warfarin and DOACs were associated with reduced all-cause mortality. Warfarin was associated with more bleeding compared to no anticoagulation. DOACs were associated with a lower incidence of bleeding when compared to warfarin.[54]

While the use of DOACs is expanding in patients with all indications for anticoagulation, prospective studies are needed to delineate the safety and efficacy of these agents in patients with cirrhosis and PVT.

The recommended duration of anticoagulation for patients with cirrhosis and acute PVT, without an additional thrombophilia, is long term or until liver transplantation.[27] Of note, patients with tumour thrombosis secondary to hepatocellular carcinoma do not benefit from anticoagulation.[59]

Given that complete recanalization may be seen in 13% of cirrhotic patients with main PVT who do not receive anticoagulation, watchful waiting with surveillance imaging may be considered in asymptomatic patients who are not candidates for liver transplantation.[51] This would allow for anticoagulation to be considered in select patients with progression of obstruction, involvement of mesenteric veins, or evidence of bowel ischaemia. However, it is pertinent to note that early initiation of anticoagulation therapy, within 6 months of onset, has been shown to provide greater benefit with respect to portal vein recanalization.[60,61] Anticoagulation is not required for patients with PVT restricted to the branches of the portal vein since spontaneous recanalization is common.

Transjugular intrahepatic portosystemic shunt

TIPS is a particularly favourable option in patients with PVT who have sequelae of portal hypertension. A meta-analysis of 13 studies evaluating TIPS for PVT revealed a 12-month recanalization rate of 81% in patients with cirrhosis. The 12-month TIPS patency rate was 84%. Major complications such as bleeding or death were seen in 1% of patients when evaluating studies that looked at TIPS alone. Cavernous transformation of the portal vein was identified as a major contributor to technical failure; however, employment of trans-splenic and transhepatic routes resulted in greater success.[48]

Liver transplant considerations

Anticoagulation in patients listed for liver transplantation yields complete recanalization in 42–75% of patients.[10,30] While obstruction of the extrahepatic portal vein does not increase waitlist mortality in patients listed for liver transplantation, it may pose technical difficulties during the transplant procedure and is associated with increased post-transplant mortality in the transplant recipient.[62,63] It is unknown whether regression of portal vein obstruction prior to transplantation improves post-transplant survival as there are currently no randomized controlled trials that have studied this question. As a result, depending on centre experience and available expertise, extensive obstruction of the portal vein may lead to removal from the transplant waitlist due to anticipated challenges.

Prognosis

In patients with acute uncomplicated extrahepatic portal venous thrombosis, long-term survival is good and depends on the underlying aetiology of PVT. In the absence of cirrhosis, 5-year survival is generally greater than 70%.[31,32,50,64,65] However, in patients presenting with acute intestinal ischaemia, in-hospital mortality rates may be as high as 44%.[66] With appropriate therapy, recanalization of the portal vein should occur within 6 months.[13] Furthermore, approximately 55% of patients not achieving recanalization will develop gastro-oesophageal varices. The 2-year probability of variceal bleeding and development of ascites in patients with failure of recanalization is 12% and 16%, respectively.[67]

Idiopathic non-cirrhotic portal hypertension

Background

INCPH is a syndrome characterized by portal hypertension without biopsy-proven cirrhosis and in the absence of obstruction in the extrahepatic portal vein or hepatic venous outflow tract.[68] Exclusion of other causes of liver disease and other aetiologies of non-cirrhotic portal hypertension (e.g. sinusoidal obstruction syndrome, sarcoidosis, schistosomiasis, and congenital hepatic fibrosis) are key prerequisites to diagnosis.[68] Earlier literature from across the globe illustrated ambiguity with regard to the nomenclature of this condition. In the Western world, the terms hepatoportal sclerosis, idiopathic portal hypertension, incomplete septal cirrhosis, and nodular regenerative hyperplasia have been used. In the Indian subcontinent, the condition has been termed non-cirrhotic portal fibrosis, whereas in Japan and other Asian countries, it has been termed idiopathic portal hypertension. As all these entities share a very similar clinical and histopathologic profile, 'idiopathic non-cirrhotic portal hypertension' has been proposed as the preferred terminology, describing a singular, distinct entity with various pathological features, as opposed to numerous distinct clinicopathological entities.[68]

Epidemiology

INCPH has a greater incidence and prevalence in developing countries compared to developed countries. These differences are thought to be secondary to differences in socioeconomic status, living conditions, hygiene, and ethnic background.[69] In the Indian subcontinent, prevalence estimates among patients with portal hypertension as high as 23.3% have been reported,[69,70] although these figures have not been updated since the 1980s. In contrast, in the Western world, INCPH is thought to be responsible for only 3–5% of all cases of portal hypertension.[71] Slight sex differences have been noted in studies across the globe, although the disease tends to affect younger individuals around the fourth decade of life.[68,69]

Pathophysiology and aetiology

While it remains to be proven, it is theorized that INCPH arises secondary to (1) increased splenic blood flow and (2) increased intrahepatic resistance secondary to obliteration of the portal venous microcirculation.[68,72]

The aetiology of INCPH remains unknown; however, multiple triggers have been implicated in the development of this disease state. These include (1) exposures to drugs or toxins, (2) chronic or recurrent infections, (3) immunological disorders, (4) genetic anomalies, and (5) hypercoagulable states[68,73] (Box 12.2). Since hypercoagulable states are associated with both extrahepatic PVT and INCPH and given the approximately 20–40% prevalence of PVT in patients with INCPH, these two conditions are postulated to be the ends of the same disease spectrum.

Clinical presentation and diagnosis

Variceal bleeding represents the most common clinical presentation of INCPH.[44,69] Hypersplenism is common but rarely symptomatic. In late stages of the disease, patients can develop other features of portal hypertension. Ascites may be associated with poor survival.[74] Hepatic encephalopathy can develop in the setting of massive

> **Box 12.2** Conditions associated with idiopathic non-cirrhotic portal hypertension
>
> **Haematological diseases**
> - Aplastic anaemia.
> - Myeloproliferative disorders.
> - Hodgkin's lymphoma.
> - Multiple myeloma.
>
> **Prothrombotic conditions**
> - Protein C or S deficiency.
> - Prothrombin G20210A gene mutation.
> - Factor V Leiden mutation.
> - Antiphospholipid syndrome.
> - ADAMTS13 deficiency.
>
> **Immunological and inflammatory disorders**
> - Common variable immune deficiency.
> - Systemic lupus erythematosus.
> - Scleroderma.
> - Rheumatoid arthritis.
> - HIV.
> - Coeliac disease.
> - Repeated gastrointestinal infections.
>
> **Drugs**
> - Didanosine.
> - Azathioprine.
> - Thioguanine.
> - Oxaliplatin.
>
> **Genetic conditions**
> - Hereditary haemorrhagic telangiectasia.
> - Turner syndrome.
> - Adams–Oliver syndrome.
> - TERT mutations.
> - Cystic fibrosis.

> **Box 12.3** Diagnostic criteria of idiopathic non-cirrhotic portal hypertension
>
> 1. Clinical signs of portal hypertension (any one of the following):
>   - Splenomegaly/hypersplenism.
>   - Oesophageal varices.
>   - Non-malignant ascites.
>   - Increased hepatic venous pressure gradient.
>   - Porto-venous collaterals.
> 2. Exclusion of cirrhosis on liver biopsy.
> 3. Exclusion of chronic liver disease causing cirrhosis or non-cirrhotic portal hypertension:
>   - Chronic viral hepatitis B and/or C.
>   - Non-alcoholic steatohepatitis/alcoholic steatohepatitis.
>   - Autoimmune hepatitis.
>   - Hereditary haemochromatosis.
>   - Wilson's disease.
>   - Primary biliary cirrhosis.
> 4. Exclusion of conditions causing non-cirrhotic portal hypertension:
>   - Congenital liver fibrosis.
>   - Sarcoidosis.
>   - Schistosomiasis.
> 5. Patent portal and hepatic veins (Doppler ultrasound or CT scanning).
>
> Adapted with permission from Schouten JN, Garcia-Pagan JC, Valla DC, Janssen HL. Idiopathic noncirrhotic portal hypertension. Hepatology. 2011;54:1071–1081.

portosystemic shunting.[75] Hepatopulmonary syndrome has also been described in association with INCPH.[76]

More often than in patients with cirrhosis, INCPH has been associated with a conspicuously enlarged spleen.[70,77] Massive splenomegaly, as in children with PVT, may be associated with dragging left upper quadrant abdominal pain, sharp pleuritic type pain with splenic infarction, and malnutrition.

Liver biochemical tests are usually normal or near-normal with mild elevations of alkaline phosphatase.[68,73,77]

Abdominal ultrasonography in patients with INCPH demonstrates nodularity of the liver surface and thickening of the portal vein walls in combination with features of portal hypertension. While this can often lead to a misdiagnosis of cirrhosis in these patients, liver–spleen stiffness ratios can help differentiate INCPH from cirrhosis. Liver stiffness higher than spleen stiffness favours cirrhosis, whereas spleen stiffness greater than liver stiffness favours INCPH.[78] Mean liver stiffness alone in a large cohort of patients with INCPH was 9.2 kPa, significantly lower than those observed in patients with cirrhosis (>12–12.5 kPa).[79]

The most common histological features of INCPH are phlebosclerosis, nodular regeneration, sinusoidal dilatation, paraportal shunt vessels, and perisinusoidal fibrosis.[74,77,80]

A diagnosis of INCPH requires that all of the following criteria be met, in keeping with expert recommendations: (1) clinical evidence of portal hypertension, (2) exclusion of cirrhosis on liver biopsy, (3) exclusion of other chronic liver disease that may cause cirrhosis, (4) exclusion of other conditions that may cause non-cirrhotic portal hypertension, and (5) imaging showing patent portal and hepatic veins (Box 12.3).

Management

The primary focus of management in patients with INCPH is prevention and treatment of portal hypertension and its complications, particularly variceal haemorrhage. These patients are typically managed in a manner similar to those with portal hypertension secondary to cirrhosis.[37,44] In addition, any contributory, underlying medical conditions should be concurrently treated and offending drugs should be removed (Box 12.2). Patients with variceal bleeding are candidates for portosystemic shunts especially if variceal bleeding recurs despite a combination of endoscopic variceal ligation and non-selective beta-blockers used as secondary prophylaxis. Liver transplantation may be required in some patients. INCPH may rarely occur post liver transplantation.[81]

Prognosis

There are limited data available regarding overall outcomes and prognoses of patients with INCPH. Generally, as a result of preserved liver synthetic function, most patients with INCPH have a better prognosis compared to patients with cirrhosis with a similar degree of portal hypertension. However, a subgroup of patients with nodular transformation of the liver and extensive portal fibrosis may progress to hepatic insufficiency, necessitating liver transplantation.[82,83] *De novo* PVT can develop in 20–40% of patients within 5 years of follow-up, with early anticoagulation leading to recanalization in 54% of patients.[73,84] A few case reports and series have suggested an association of INCPH with hepatocellular carcinoma and intrahepatic cholangiocarcinoma.[85–87]

CHAPTER 12 Non-cirrhotic portal hypertension

Hepatic venous outflow obstruction

Introduction

Diffuse impairment of venous outflow from the liver can occur secondary to lesions at the level of the sinusoids (sinusoidal obstruction syndrome), the hepatic veins, suprahepatic IVC (BCS), and the heart. At the microscopic level, these entities can cause sinusoidal dilatation, congestion, oedema, as well as hepatic cord compression and atrophy.[88] For the purposes of this discussion, we will focus herein on BCS.

Budd–Chiari syndrome

Background and classification

BCS is the obstruction of the hepatic venous outflow tract, anywhere from the small intrahepatic venules, up to the junction of the IVC and the right atrium, in the absence of intracardiac or pericardial obstruction.[89] Primary BCS is characterized by thrombotic obstruction of the hepatic venous outflow tract, whereas secondary BCS refers to extrinsic compression of the hepatic veins or obstruction of the hepatic venous outflow tract, for example, by malignant tumors.[27] Secondary BCS will not be discussed here.

Epidemiology

Primary BCS is a rare disorder that primarily affects individuals in the third to fourth decade of life, with a reported incidence in Western countries between 0.5 and 2 per million population per year.[27] The global prevalence of primary BCS ranges from 1.40 to 7.69 per million, with the highest prevalence in Asian countries, such as South Korea and China.[90–92] In non-Asian countries, BCS is more common in women and the obstruction may predominantly involve the hepatic veins. Conversely, in Asian countries, BCS shows a slight male predominance and the obstruction frequently occurs either purely in the suprahepatic IVC or a combination of the IVC and hepatic veins.[93,94]

Aetiology

An underlying prothrombotic condition can be identified in most patients with primary BCS. At least one prothrombotic disorder can be identified in 79–84% of patients, whereas two or more risk factors can be identified in up to 46% of patients.[89,90] There is considerable overlap in the prothrombotic risk factors for BCS and those for EHPVO (Box 12.4), with myeloproliferative disorders accounting for about half of the cases of primary BCS.

Pathogenesis

Thrombosis of the hepatic veins leads to increased hepatic venous and sinusoidal pressures. This leads to marked sinusoidal distension with congestion and oedema. Raised hepatic venous and sinusoidal pressures lead to ascites formation and slow portal venous inflow, increasing the risk for intra- and extrahepatic PVT (Figure 12.3). The decrease in hepatic blood flow causes pericentral ischaemic coagulative necrosis, apoptosis with eventual loss of hepatocytes, and fibrosis (Figure 12.4).

Clinical presentation and diagnosis

The clinical presentation of BCS varies widely, ranging from complete absence of symptoms to acute liver failure.[44] Fifteen to twenty percent of patients are asymptomatic, with the diagnosis being made incidentally on imaging studies obtained for other indications.[89,95] In acute cases, the most common signs and symptoms at the time of initial diagnosis are acute-onset abdominal pain with ascites, hepatomegaly, and elevated liver chemistries. Other complications of portal hypertension such as gastro-oesophageal variceal bleeding and hepatic encephalopathy may follow.[89] Acute liver failure may arise if the thrombosis is extensive and develops rapidly, but is uncommon. Laboratory studies reveal variable alterations of serum aminotransferases and alkaline phosphatase (usually three to five times the upper limit of normal), bilirubin, albumin, and prothrombin time depending on the acuity and extent of thrombosis.[89,96] The diagnosis of BCS is generally suspected on non-invasive testing with Doppler ultrasonography. CT- and MRI-based tests can be performed to confirm the diagnosis and facilitate treatment planning. Typical features of BCS on Doppler ultrasonography include presence of thrombus within or non-visualization of the hepatic vein, presence of collateral veins, transformation of the hepatic vein into a fibrous cord with lack of flow signals, and caudate lobe hypertrophy. CT imaging and MRI can show rapid clearance of contrast from the caudate lobe and patchy hepatic enhancement due to uneven portal perfusion (Figure 12.5).[37] Other non-specific imaging findings include hepatomegaly, splenomegaly, ascites, atrophy of hepatic lobes, and compression or narrowing of the IVC (Figures 12.6 and 12.7).

Management

The goals of therapy in BCS include restoration of hepatic venous outflow, management of portal hypertension, and management of the underlying causative factor. The recommended management of BCS comprises a stepwise approach, including anticoagulation, interventional vascular therapies (e.g. thrombolysis, percutaneous angioplasty and stenting, TIPS), and orthotopic liver transplantation (Figure 12.8).[29] Surgical procedures may be effective but are seldom carried out nowadays because of the widespread availability of TIPS.

Anticoagulation

Long-term anticoagulation should be initiated in all patients with BCS in order to reduce the risk of clot extension and prevent new

---

Box 12.4 Risk factors and causes of primary Budd–Chiari syndrome

Thrombophilia
- Myeloproliferative neoplasms.
- Paroxysmal nocturnal haemoglobinuria.
- Inherited thrombophilic conditions: factor V Leiden mutation, prothrombin gene mutation, protein C/S deficiency, antithrombin deficiency, antiphospholipid syndrome, and methylenetetrahydrofolate reductase TT677 polymorphism.
- Hyperhomocysteinaemia.
- Pregnancy.
- Oral contraceptive use.

Systemic conditions
- Sarcoidosis.
- Vasculitis.
- Behçet's disease.
- Connective tissue disease.
- Inflammatory bowel disease.

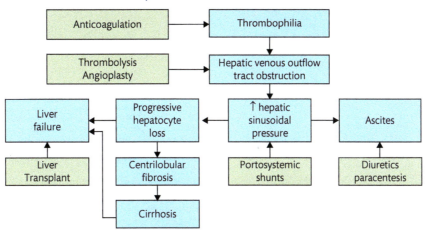

Figure 12.3 Pathophysiology of Budd–Chiari syndrome and rationale for treatment.
Reproduced with permission of Mayo Foundation for Medical Education and Research, all rights reserved.

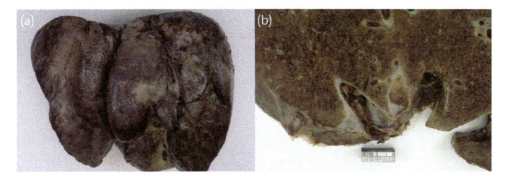

Figure 12.4 Gross pathological appearance of Budd–Chiari syndrome. (a) Swollen and congested liver with a tense, reddish-purple capsule. (b) Classic nutmeg appearance of the liver with evidence of a clot in the hepatic vein.

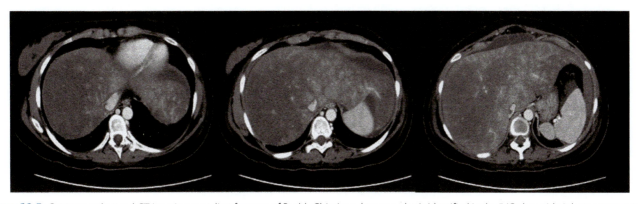

Figure 12.5 Contrast-enhanced CT imaging revealing features of Budd–Chiari syndrome: a clot is identified in the IVC alongside inhomogeneous enhancement of the liver parenchyma.

CHAPTER 12 Non-cirrhotic portal hypertension

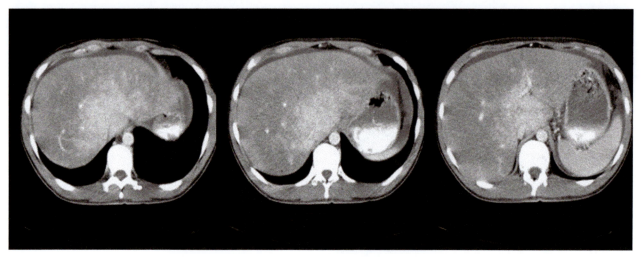

Figure 12.6 Contrast-enhanced CT imaging revealing features of Budd–Chiari syndrome: enlargement of the caudate lobe. Greater enhancement of the caudate lobe and central liver parenchyma is also seen, relative to the periphery.

thrombotic episodes. In the acute setting, either unfractionated heparin or LMWH can be initiated, followed by oral VKAs.[27,29,37,44] The target international normalized ratio on warfarin is 2–3 as in patients with PVT. While the DOACs are an attractive and promising alternative, there are very limited data on their use in BCS.[55] While major bleeding frequently occurs in patients with BCS, anticoagulation is not contraindicated in patients with previous portal hypertensive bleeding provided that appropriate prophylactic interventions to prevent rebleeding have been initiated.[29] Anticoagulation alone may suffice in over 80% of patients.

Interventional vascular therapies

Systemic or arterially delivered thrombolytic agents are ineffective in BCS.[27] However, in select cases of acute and incomplete thrombosis, local infusion of recombinant tissue plasminogen activator, streptokinase or urokinase, in combination with balloon angioplasty may be effective in re-establishing vascular patency.[97] Thrombolysis may also have a role in re-establishing patency of hepatic vein stents and TIPSs.[97]

Hepatic vein angioplasty with or without stenting has been shown to be particularly successful in a select group of BCS patients who have short-segment hepatic vein stenosis.

Transjugular intrahepatic portosystemic shunt and surgical management

Surgical shunt procedures such as mesocaval, side-to-side portocaval, and mesoatrial shunts have been previously carried out to decompress the liver in the setting of hepatic venous outflow obstruction. However, owing to significant perioperative mortality risk, up to 10–20%, these surgical shunt procedures have been largely replaced by TIPS.[98,99]

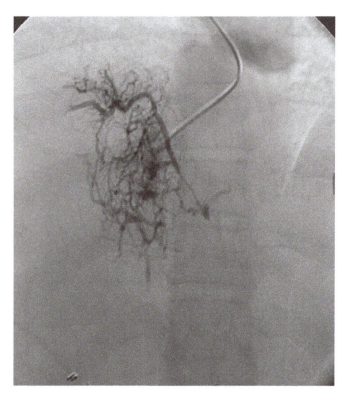

Figure 12.7 Hepatic venogram revealing 'spider venogram'—the presence of multiple tiny, thread-like collateral vessels forming a dense network, analogous to a spider's web.

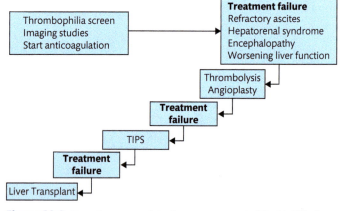

Figure 12.8 Stepwise approach to the management of Budd–Chiari syndrome.

Reproduced with permission of Mayo Foundation for Medical Education and Research, all rights reserved.

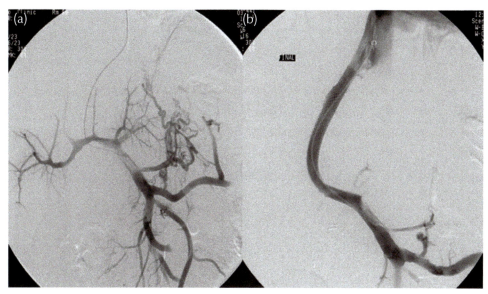

Figure 12.9 TIPS in Budd–Chiari syndrome. Through the right jugular vein, the TIPS needle is advanced to the level of the liver at which point the needle is punctured through the caval wall inside the liver tissue to reach the right portal vein after which the catheter is advanced to access the main portal vein (a). Shunts are then deployed, with portography revealing adequate intrashunt flow between the portal vein and inferior vena cava (b).

TIPS procedures offer a less invasive alternative to surgical shunts with excellent long-term outcomes (Figure 12.9). If the obstruction of the hepatic vein is extensive, the TIPS procedure can become more challenging and often a portocaval approach, involving direct puncture from the IVC to the right portal vein, may be required.[100] A large cohort of patients with BCS unresponsive to medical therapy and treated with TIPS had a 5-year transplant-free survival of 72%.[95] The BCS-TIPS prognostic index score is a useful tool that uses age, bilirubin, and international normalized ratio to help predict transplant-free survival in patients receiving a TIPS. Patients with a score of 7 or greater are likely to have a poor outcome following TIPS and thus orthotopic liver transplantation should be considered.[29,95]

Liver transplantation

Liver transplantation is required in the less than 10% of patients who fail anticoagulation and interventional radiological techniques. Patients selected for transplantation should not have an underlying thrombophilia that is associated with poor prognosis.

REFERENCES

1. Kumar S, Sarr MG, Kamath PS. Mesenteric venous thrombosis. *N Engl J Med*. 2001;**345**(23):1683–1688.
2. Ogren M, Bergqvist D, Bjorck M, Acosta S, Eriksson H, Sternby NH. Portal vein thrombosis: prevalence, patient characteristics and lifetime risk: a population study based on 23,796 consecutive autopsies. *World J Gastroenterol*. 2006;**12**(13):2115–2119.
3. Okuda K, Ohnishi K, Kimura K, et al. Incidence of portal vein thrombosis in liver cirrhosis. An angiographic study in 708 patients. *Gastroenterology*. 1985;**89**(2):279–286.
4. Yerdel MA, Gunson B, Mirza D, et al. Portal vein thrombosis in adults undergoing liver transplantation: risk factors, screening, management, and outcome. *Transplantation*. 2000;**69**(9):1873–1881.
5. Cagin YF, Atayan Y, Erdogan MA, Dagtekin F, Colak C. Incidence and clinical presentation of portal vein thrombosis in cirrhotic patients. *Hepatobiliary Pancreat Dis Int*. 2016;**15**(5):499–503.
6. Cool J, Rosenblatt R, Kumar S, et al. Portal vein thrombosis prevalence and associated mortality in cirrhosis in a nationally representative inpatient cohort. *J Gastroenterol Hepatol*. 2019;**34**(6):1088–11092.
7. Fan X, Huang X, Hershman M, et al. Portal vein thrombosis prevalence and mortality among alcoholic cirrhosis in a nationwide inpatient cohort. *Eur J Gastroenterol Hepatol*. 2020;**32**(9):1160–1167.
8. Violi F, Corazza GR, Caldwell SH, et al. Portal vein thrombosis relevance on liver cirrhosis: Italian Venous Thrombotic Events Registry. *Intern Emerg Med*. 2016;**11**(8):1059–1066.
9. Violi F, Corazza GR, Caldwell SH, et al. Incidence and recurrence of portal vein thrombosis in cirrhotic patients. *Thromb Haemost*. 2019;**119**(3):496–499.
10. Francoz C, Belghiti J, Vilgrain V, et al. Splanchnic vein thrombosis in candidates for liver transplantation: usefulness of screening and anticoagulation. *Gut*. 2005;**54**(5):691–697.
11. Nery F, Chevret S, Condat B, et al. Causes and consequences of portal vein thrombosis in 1,243 patients with cirrhosis: results of a longitudinal study. *Hepatology*. 2015;**61**(2):660–667.
12. Noronha Ferreira C, Marinho RT, Cortez-Pinto H, et al. Incidence, predictive factors and clinical significance of development of portal vein thrombosis in cirrhosis: a prospective study. *Liver Int*. 2019;**39**(8):1459–1467.
13. Plessier A, Darwish-Murad S, Hernandez-Guerra M, et al. Acute portal vein thrombosis unrelated to cirrhosis: a prospective multicenter follow-up study. *Hepatology*. 2010;**51**(1):210–218.
14. Singal AK, Kamath PS, Tefferi A. Mesenteric venous thrombosis. *Mayo Clin Proc*. 2013;**88**(3):285–294.
15. De Stefano V, Qi X, Betti S, Rossi E. Splanchnic vein thrombosis and myeloproliferative neoplasms: molecular-driven diagnosis and long-term treatment. *Thromb Haemost*. 2016;**115**(2):240–249.

16. Crowther MA, Kelton JG. Congenital thrombophilic states associated with venous thrombosis: a qualitative overview and proposed classification system. *Ann Intern Med*. 2003;**138**(2):128–134.
17. Janssen HL, Wijnhoud A, Haagsma EB, et al. Extrahepatic portal vein thrombosis: aetiology and determinants of survival. *Gut*. 2001;**49**(5):720–724.
18. Rebours V, Boudaoud L, Vullierme MP, et al. Extrahepatic portal venous system thrombosis in recurrent acute and chronic alcoholic pancreatitis is caused by local inflammation and not thrombophilia. *Am J Gastroenterol*. 2012;**107**(10):1579–1585.
19. Gaballa D, Bezinover D, Kadry Z, et al. Development of a model to predict portal vein thrombosis in liver transplant candidates: the Portal Vein Thrombosis Risk Index. *Liver Transpl*. 2019;**25**(12):1747–1755.
20. Stine JG, Wang J, Shah PM, et al. Decreased portal vein velocity is predictive of the development of portal vein thrombosis: a matched case-control study. *Liver Int*. 2018;**38**(1):94–101.
21. Abdel-Razik A, Mousa N, Elhelaly R, Tawfik A. De-novo portal vein thrombosis in liver cirrhosis: risk factors and correlation with the Model for End-stage Liver Disease scoring system. *Eur J Gastroenterol Hepatol*. 2015;**27**(5):585–592.
22. Stine JG, Argo CK, Pelletier SJ, Maluf DG, Caldwell SH, Northup PG. Advanced non-alcoholic steatohepatitis cirrhosis: a high-risk population for pre-liver transplant portal vein thrombosis. *World J Hepatol*. 2017;**9**(3):139–146.
23. Ayala R, Grande S, Bustelos R, et al. Obesity is an independent risk factor for pre-transplant portal vein thrombosis in liver recipients. *BMC Gastroenterol*. 2012;**12**:114.
24. Hernandez-Conde M, Llop E, Fernandez-Carrillo C, et al. Visceral fat is associated with cirrhotic portal vein thrombosis. *Expert Rev Gastroenterol Hepatol*. 2019;**13**(10):1017–1022.
25. Danila M, Sporea I, Popescu A, Sirli R. Portal vein thrombosis in liver cirrhosis—the added value of contrast enhanced ultrasonography. *Med Ultrason*. 2016;**18**(2):218–233.
26. Sarin SK, Philips CA, Kamath PS, et al. Toward a comprehensive new classification of portal vein thrombosis in patients with cirrhosis. *Gastroenterology*. 2016;**151**(4):574–577.
27. Simonetto DA, Singal AK, Garcia-Tsao G, Caldwell SH, Ahn J, Kamath PS. ACG clinical guideline: disorders of the hepatic and mesenteric circulation. *Am J Gastroenterol*. 2020;**115**(1):18–40.
28. Bach AM, Hann LE, Brown KT, et al. Portal vein evaluation with US: comparison to angiography combined with CT arterial portography. *Radiology*. 1996;**201**(1):149–154.
29. de Franchis R, Baveno VIF. Expanding consensus in portal hypertension: report of the Baveno VI Consensus Workshop: stratifying risk and individualizing care for portal hypertension. *J Hepatol*. 2015;**63**(74):3–52.
30. Amitrano L, Guardascione MA, Brancaccio V, et al. Risk factors and clinical presentation of portal vein thrombosis in patients with liver cirrhosis. *J Hepatol*. 2004;**40**(5):736–741.
31. Rajani R, Bjornsson E, Bergquist A, et al. The epidemiology and clinical features of portal vein thrombosis: a multicentre study. *Aliment Pharmacol Ther*. 2010;**32**(9):1154–1162.
32. Orr DW, Harrison PM, Devlin J, et al. Chronic mesenteric venous thrombosis: evaluation and determinants of survival during long-term follow-up. *Clin Gastroenterol Hepatol*. 2007;**5**(1):80–86.
33. Khanna R, Sarin SK. Non-cirrhotic portal hypertension—diagnosis and management. *J Hepatol*. 2014;**60**(2):421–441.
34. Feldman AG, Sokol RJ. Noncirrhotic portal hypertension in the pediatric population. *Clin Liver Dis (Hoboken)*. 2015;**5**(5):116–119.
35. Kalra N, Shankar S, Khandelwal N. Imaging of portal cavernoma cholangiopathy. *J Clin Exp Hepatol*. 2014;**4**(Suppl 1):44–52.
36. Sassoon C, Douillet P, Cronfalt AM, Odievre M, Chaumont P, Doyon D. Ultrasonographic diagnosis of portal cavernoma in children: a study of twelve cases. *Br J Radiol*. 1980;**53**(635):1047–1051.
37. Northup PG, Garcia-Pagan JC, Garcia-Tsao G, et al. Vascular liver disorders, portal vein thrombosis, and procedural bleeding in patients with liver disease: 2020 practice guidance by the American Association for the Study of Liver Diseases. *Hepatology*. 2021;**73**(1):366–413.
38. Chirinos JA, Garcia J, Alcaide ML, Toledo G, Baracco GJ, Lichtstein DM. Septic thrombophlebitis: diagnosis and management. *Am J Cardiovasc Drugs*. 2006;**6**(1):9–14.
39. Ageno W, Riva N, Schulman S, et al. Long-term clinical outcomes of splanchnic vein thrombosis: results of an international registry. *JAMA Intern Med*. 2015;**175**(9):1474–1480.
40. Riva N, Ageno W, Poli D, et al. Safety of vitamin K antagonist treatment for splanchnic vein thrombosis: a multicenter cohort study. *J Thromb Haemost*. 2015;**13**(6):1019–1027.
41. Janczak DT, Mimier MK, McBane RD, et al. Rivaroxaban and apixaban for initial treatment of acute venous thromboembolism of atypical location. *Mayo Clin Proc*. 2018;**93**(1):40–47.
42. Nery F, Valadares D, Morais S, Gomes MT, De Gottardi A. Efficacy and safety of direct-acting oral anticoagulants use in acute portal vein thrombosis unrelated to cirrhosis. *Gastroenterol Res*. 2017;**10**(2):141–143.
43. Naymagon L, Tremblay D, Zubizarreta N, et al. The efficacy and safety of direct oral anticoagulants in noncirrhotic portal vein thrombosis. *Blood Adv*. 2020;**4**(4):655–666.
44. European Association for the Study of the Liver. EASL Clinical Practice Guidelines: vascular diseases of the liver. *J Hepatol*. 2016;**64**:179–202.
45. Hollingshead M, Burke CT, Mauro MA, Weeks SM, Dixon RG, Jaques PF. Transcatheter thrombolytic therapy for acute mesenteric and portal vein thrombosis. *J Vasc Interv Radiol*. 2005;**16**(5):651–661.
46. Liu K, Li WD, Du XL, Li CL, Li XQ. Comparison of systemic thrombolysis versus indirect thrombolysis via the superior mesenteric artery in patients with acute portal vein thrombosis. *Ann Vasc Surg*. 2017;**39**:264–269.
47. Smalberg JH, Spaander MV, Jie KS, et al. Risks and benefits of transcatheter thrombolytic therapy in patients with splanchnic venous thrombosis. *Thromb Haemost*. 2008;**100**(6):1084–1088.
48. Rodrigues SG, Sixt S, Abraldes JG, et al. Systematic review with meta-analysis: portal vein recanalisation and transjugular intrahepatic portosystemic shunt for portal vein thrombosis. *Aliment Pharmacol Ther*. 2019;**49**(1):20–30.
49. Malkowski P, Pawlak J, Michalowicz B, et al. Thrombolytic treatment of portal thrombosis. *Hepatogastroenterology*. 2003;**50**(54):2098–2100.
50. Condat B, Pessione F, Hillaire S, et al. Current outcome of portal vein thrombosis in adults: risk and benefit of anticoagulant therapy. *Gastroenterology*. 2001;**120**(2):490–497.
51. Loffredo L, Pastori D, Farcomeni A, Violi F. Effects of anticoagulants in patients with cirrhosis and portal vein thrombosis: a systematic review and meta-analysis. *Gastroenterology*. 2017;**153**(2):480–487.
52. Intagliata NM, Henry ZH, Maitland H, et al. Direct oral anticoagulants in cirrhosis patients pose similar risks of bleeding when compared to traditional anticoagulation. *Dig Dis Sci*. 2016;**61**(6):1721–1727.

53. Intagliata NM, Maitland H, Northup PG, Caldwell SH. Treating thrombosis in cirrhosis patients with new oral agents: ready or not? *Hepatology.* 2015;**61**(2):738–739.
54. Serper M, Weinberg EM, Cohen JB, Reese PP, Taddei TH, Kaplan DE. Mortality and hepatic decompensation in patients with cirrhosis and atrial fibrillation treated with anticoagulation. *Hepatology.* 2021;**73**(1):219–232.
55. De Gottardi A, Trebicka J, Klinger C, et al. Antithrombotic treatment with direct-acting oral anticoagulants in patients with splanchnic vein thrombosis and cirrhosis. *Liver Int.* 2017;**37**(5):694–699.
56. Hum J, Shatzel JJ, Jou JH, Deloughery TG. The efficacy and safety of direct oral anticoagulants vs traditional anticoagulants in cirrhosis. *Eur J Haematol.* 2017;**98**(4):393–397.
57. Lee HF, Chan YH, Chang SH, et al. Effectiveness and safety of non-vitamin K antagonist oral anticoagulant and warfarin in cirrhotic patients with nonvalvular atrial fibrillation. *J Am Heart Assoc.* 2019;**8**(5):e011112.
58. Lee SR, Lee HJ, Choi EK, et al. Direct oral anticoagulants in patients with atrial fibrillation and liver disease. *J Am Coll Cardiol.* 2019;**73**(25):3295–3308.
59. Garcia-Tsao G, Bosch J. Management of varices and variceal hemorrhage in cirrhosis. *N Engl J Med.* 2010;**362**(9):823–832.
60. Delgado MG, Seijo S, Yepes I, et al. Efficacy and safety of anticoagulation on patients with cirrhosis and portal vein thrombosis. *Clin Gastroenterol Hepatol.* 2012;**10**(7):776–783.
61. Senzolo M, Sartori TM, Rossetto V, et al. Prospective evaluation of anticoagulation and transjugular intrahepatic portosystemic shunt for the management of portal vein thrombosis in cirrhosis. *Liver Int.* 2012;**32**(6):919–927.
62. Englesbe MJ, Kubus J, Muhammad W, et al. Portal vein thrombosis and survival in patients with cirrhosis. *Liver Transpl.* 2010;**16**(1):83–90.
63. Englesbe MJ, Schaubel DE, Cai S, Guidinger MK, Merion RM. Portal vein thrombosis and liver transplant survival benefit. *Liver Transpl.* 2010;**16**(8):999–1005.
64. Amitrano L, Guardascione MA, Scaglione M, et al. Prognostic factors in noncirrhotic patients with splanchnic vein thromboses. *Am J Gastroenterol.* 2007;**102**(11):2464–2470.
65. Spaander MC, Hoekstra J, Hansen BE, Van Buuren HR, Leebeek FW, Janssen HL. Anticoagulant therapy in patients with non-cirrhotic portal vein thrombosis: effect on new thrombotic events and gastrointestinal bleeding. *J Thromb Haemost.* 2013;**11**(3):452–459.
66. Schoots IG, Koffeman GI, Legemate DA, Levi M, van Gulik TM. Systematic review of survival after acute mesenteric ischaemia according to disease aetiology. *Br J Surg.* 2004;**91**(1):17–27.
67. Turnes J, Garcia-Pagan JC, Gonzalez M, et al. Portal hypertension-related complications after acute portal vein thrombosis: impact of early anticoagulation. *Clin Gastroenterol Hepatol.* 2008;**6**(12):1412–1417.
68. Schouten JN, Garcia-Pagan JC, Valla DC, Janssen HL. Idiopathic noncirrhotic portal hypertension. *Hepatology.* 2011;**54**(3):1071–1081.
69. Sarin SK, Kumar A, Chawla YK, et al. Noncirrhotic portal fibrosis/idiopathic portal hypertension: APASL recommendations for diagnosis and treatment. *Hepatol Int.* 2007;**1**(3):398–413.
70. Dhiman RK, Chawla Y, Vasishta RK, et al. Non-cirrhotic portal fibrosis (idiopathic portal hypertension): experience with 151 patients and a review of the literature. *J Gastroenterol Hepatol.* 2002;**17**(1):6–16.
71. Iber FL. Obliterative portal venopathy of the liver and 'idiopathic portal hypertension'. *Ann Intern Med.* 1969;**71**(3):660–661.
72. Sato Y, Sawada S, Kozaka K, et al. Significance of enhanced expression of nitric oxide syntheses in splenic sinus lining cells in altered portal hemodynamics of idiopathic portal hypertension. *Dig Dis Sci.* 2007;**52**(8):1987–1994.
73. Cazals-Hatem D, Hillaire S, Rudler M, et al. Obliterative portal venopathy: portal hypertension is not always present at diagnosis. *J Hepatol.* 2011;**54**(3):455–461.
74. Schouten JN, Nevens F, Hansen B, et al. Idiopathic noncirrhotic portal hypertension is associated with poor survival: results of a long-term cohort study. *Aliment Pharmacol. Ther* 2012;**35**(12):1424–1433.
75. Krasinskas AM, Eghtesad B, Kamath PS, Demetris AJ, Abraham SC. Liver transplantation for severe intrahepatic noncirrhotic portal hypertension. *Liver Transpl.* 2005;**11**(6):627–634.
76. Babbs C, Warnes TW, Haboubi NY. Non-cirrhotic portal hypertension with hypoxaemia. *Gut.* 1988;**29**(1):129–131.
77. Hillaire S, Bonte E, Denninger MH, et al. Idiopathic non-cirrhotic intrahepatic portal hypertension in the West: a re-evaluation in 28 patients. *Gut.* 2002;**51**(2):275–280.
78. Navin PJ, Hilscher MB, Welle CL, et al. The utility of MR elastography to differentiate nodular regenerative hyperplasia from cirrhosis. *Hepatology.* 2019;**69**(1):452–454.
79. Ziol M, Handra-Luca A, Kettaneh A, et al. Noninvasive assessment of liver fibrosis by measurement of stiffness in patients with chronic hepatitis C. *Hepatology.* 2005;**41**(1):48–54.
80. Verheij J, Schouten JN, Komuta M, et al. Histological features in western patients with idiopathic non-cirrhotic portal hypertension. *Histopathology.* 2013;**62**(7):1083–1091.
81. Devarbhavi H, Abraham S, Kamath PS. Significance of nodular regenerative hyperplasia occurring de novo following liver transplantation. *Liver Transpl.* 2007;**13**(11):1552–1556.
82. Isabel Fiel M, Thung SN, Hytiroglou P, Emre S, Schiano TD. Liver failure and need for liver transplantation in patients with advanced hepatoportal sclerosis. *Am J Surg Pathol.* 2007;**31**(4):607–614.
83. Bernard PH, Le Bail B, Cransac M, et al. Progression from idiopathic portal hypertension to incomplete septal cirrhosis with liver failure requiring liver transplantation. *J Hepatol.* 1995;**22**(4):495–499.
84. Siramolpiwat S, Seijo S, Miquel R, et al. Idiopathic portal hypertension: natural history and long-term outcome. *Hepatology.* 2014;**59**(6):2276–2285.
85. Isobe Y, Yamasaki T, Yokoyama Y, Kurokawa F, Hino K, Sakaida I. Hepatocellular carcinoma developing six and a half years after a diagnosis of idiopathic portal hypertension. *J Gastroenterol.* 2007;**42**(5):407–409.
86. Hidaka H, Ohbu M, Kokubu S, Shibuya A, Saigenji K, Okayasu I. Hepatocellular carcinoma associated with idiopathic portal hypertension: review of large nodules in seven non-cirrhotic portal hypertensive livers. *J Gastroenterol Hepatol.* 2005;**20**(3):493–494.
87. Penrice D, Simonetto DA. Nodular regenerative hyperplasia associated with primary liver malignancies. *Hepatology.* 2020;**71**(2):760–761.
88. Nakhleh RE. Pathology and differential diagnosis of hepatic venous outflow impairment. *Clin Liver Dis (Hoboken).* 2017;**10**:49–52.
89. Darwish Murad S, Plessier A, Hernandez-Guerra M, et al. Etiology, management, and outcome of the Budd-Chiari syndrome. *Ann Intern Med.* 2009;**151**(2):167–175.

90. Ollivier-Hourmand I, Allaire M, Goutte N, et al. The epidemiology of Budd-Chiari syndrome in France. *Dig Liver Dis*. 2018;**50**(9):931–937.
91. Ki M, Choi HY, Kim KA, Kim BH, Jang ES, Jeong SH. Incidence, prevalence and complications of Budd-Chiari syndrome in South Korea: a nationwide, population-based study. *Liver Int*. 2016;**36**(7):1067–1073.
92. Zhang W, Qi X, Zhang X, et al. Budd-Chiari syndrome in China: a systematic analysis of epidemiological features based on the Chinese literature survey. *Gastroenterol Res Pract*. 2015;**2015**:738548.
93. Plessier A, Valla DC. Budd-Chiari syndrome. *Semin Liver Dis*. 2008;**28**(3):259–269.
94. Darwish Murad S, Valla DC, de Groen PC, et al. Determinants of survival and the effect of portosystemic shunting in patients with Budd-Chiari syndrome. *Hepatology*. 2004;**39**(2):500–508.
95. Seijo S, Plessier A, Hoekstra J, et al. Good long-term outcome of Budd-Chiari syndrome with a step-wise management. *Hepatology*. 2013;**57**(5):1962–1968.
96. Dilawari JB, Bambery P, Chawla Y, et al. Hepatic outflow obstruction (Budd-Chiari syndrome). Experience with 177 patients and a review of the literature. *Medicine (Baltimore)*. 1994;**73**(1):21–36.
97. Sharma S, Texeira A, Texeira P, Elias E, Wilde J, Olliff SP. Pharmacological thrombolysis in Budd Chiari syndrome: a single centre experience and review of the literature. *J Hepatol*. 2004;**40**(1):172–180.
98. Panis Y, Belghiti J, Valla D, Benhamou JP, Fekete F. Portosystemic shunt in Budd-Chiari syndrome: long-term survival and factors affecting shunt patency in 25 patients in Western countries. *Surgery*. 1994;**115**(3):276–281.
99. Zeitoun G, Escolano S, Hadengue A, et al. Outcome of Budd-Chiari syndrome: a multivariate analysis of factors related to survival including surgical portosystemic shunting. *Hepatology*. 1999;**30**(1):84–89.
100. Garcia-Pagan JC, Heydtmann M, Raffa S, et al. TIPS for Budd-Chiari syndrome: long-term results and prognostics factors in 124 patients. *Gastroenterology*. 2008;**135**(3):808–815.

13 Medical management of portal hypertension and its complications

Mohammad Qasim Khan and Patrick S. Kamath

Natural history of portal hypertension

Portal hypertension can arise in the setting of many conditions, making it challenging to outline the course of disease in such a heterogeneous population. The natural history of portal hypertension is typically described in the setting of cirrhosis, the main cause of portal hypertension in Western countries. Compensated cirrhosis is generally an asymptomatic phase with a median survival of over 12 years; however, once decompensating events such as variceal haemorrhage, ascites or hepatic encephalopathy (HE) occur, the median survival decreases to 1.8 years.[1] Approximately 35% of individuals with cirrhosis decompensate over a 5-year period. Ascites is the most common decompensating event.[2] Once refractory ascites has developed, the probability of survival at 1 year is 52%.[3] Compensated cirrhosis with oesophageal varices portends a worse prognosis than compensated cirrhosis without varices, with a 5-year mortality of 10% and 1.5%, respectively.[2] Variceal haemorrhage in the absence of other decompensations has a 5-year mortality rate of 20%. However, when more than two decompensating events are present, the 5-year mortality is nearly 90%.[2]

Pathophysiology of portal hypertension

The portal venous circulation normally delivers blood to the liver from the capillaries of the oesophagus, stomach, intestines, spleen, pancreas, and gallbladder. The portal vein is formed by the union of the superior mesenteric and splenic veins behind the neck of the pancreas, and ultimately divides into the right and left portal vein branches in the hilum of the liver, feeding the right and left sides of the liver, respectively. Portal venules drain into hepatic sinusoids, and the flow then generally follows to the right, middle, and left hepatic veins to the inferior vena cava. An exception is the caudate lobe, which drains directly into the inferior vena cava.

Portal hypertension, defined as an increase in hepatic sinusoidal pressure to 6 mmHg or greater, can be measured via direct cannulation of the portal vein, or via indirect assessment utilizing the gradient between the portal vein and the inferior vena cava, defined as the hepatic venous pressure gradient (HVPG). Indirect assessment is the most common method, performed using a balloon catheter. Under fluoroscopic guidance, a branch of the hepatic vein is balloon-occluded or wedged, measuring the wedged hepatic venous pressure (WHVP). The WHVP measures the pressure within upstream sinusoids, a surrogate for portal venule pressure. Upon deflation of the balloon, the free hepatic venous pressure (FHVP) is measured. The FHVP reflects inferior vena cava pressure and serves as the reference for measurement of portal pressure. The HVPG is therefore calculated as the difference between the WHVP and FHVP.[4] Although HVPG values of 6 mmHg or greater are diagnostic of portal hypertension, clinically significant portal hypertension with its associated complications develops at values greater than 10 mmHg.[5]

In most circumstances, portal hypertension is driven by both increased portal resistance and increased portal inflow. Ohm's law ($\Delta P = \times R$) can be used to describe the interplay of these factors, with blood flow (Q) and vascular resistance (R) affecting portal pressure (ΔP). Increased vascular resistance can occur at any point within the portal venous system. In cirrhosis, for example, increased vascular resistance occurs due to both architectural distortion from fibrosis and regenerative nodule formation, as well as from increased endogenous vasoconstrictors within the sinusoids. Reduced nitric oxide and increased endothelin and other vasoconstrictors are released by sinusoidal endothelial cells in the hepatic microcirculation.[6] In contrast, there is an increase in nitric oxide production in the systemic and splanchnic circulation, resulting in primarily splanchnic vasodilation and higher volume portal venous flow. These changes are a manifestation of the hyperdynamic circulation in portal hypertension which also include a decreased mean arterial pressure and increased cardiac output.[6]

In response to the elevated portal pressure, a collateral circulation develops and varices are formed. Collateral formation is driven by increased flow and angiogenesis.[7,8]

In the collateral vessels, the normal flow in the portal circulation is reversed and shifts towards the systemic venous circulation. Collateral formation takes place at sites where the portal circulation is in close proximity to the systemic circulation, such as at the gastro-oesophageal junction and in the rectum.

Causes of portal hypertension

The causes of portal hypertension are commonly classified by sites of increased resistance to portal flow, that is, prehepatic, intrahepatic and posthepatic (Table 13.1). Such a classification is useful in interpreting portal pressure measurements (Table 13.2); however, there are several conditions that can cause increased resistance at more than one site, often depending on the stage of the disease. The HVPG is not elevated in prehepatic and presinusoidal causes of portal hypertension.

Prehepatic portal hypertension

The primary cause of prehepatic portal hypertension is portal vein thrombosis. Similar to venous thrombosis elsewhere in the body, portal vein thrombosis develops in the presence of factors in Virchow's triad: hypercoagulability, slow blood flow, and endothelial injury. Cirrhosis is the most common cause of portal vein thrombosis in the West. The high-volume, but slow-flow portal vein haemodynamics in cirrhosis provide a favourable environment for the development of thrombosis, and decreased portal venous velocity has been found to be a significant risk factor for portal vein thrombosis.[9] The fine balance between pro- and anticoagulant factors is also tipped towards the hypercoagulable state in decompensated cirrhosis.[10] A systemic hypercoagulable state is the most common risk factor for the development of portal vein thrombosis in the absence of cirrhosis. A myeloproliferative disorder is identified in approximately 30% of patients. Often, several predisposing factors are present within one individual, including inherited prothrombotic conditions, localized inflammation, or other malignancies.[11,12]

Intrahepatic portal hypertension

Intrahepatic portal hypertension can be further divided into the site of increased vascular resistance within the liver, namely within presinusoidal, sinusoidal, or postsinusoidal capillaries (Table 13.1).

Schistosomiasis represents one of the most common causes of portal hypertension worldwide. Schistosome eggs embolize to the liver via the portal vein, causing granulomatous presinusoidal inflammation and associated periportal fibrosis.[13] Portal granulomas in sarcoidosis also cause increased presinusoidal resistance. Nodular regenerative hyperplasia is defined by nodular transformation in the absence of fibrosis. The pathological changes appear to be driven by changes in the hepatic microvasculature, particularly embolization of portal venules, leading to areas of focal hypertrophy and atrophy. Nodular regenerative hyperplasia is associated with several conditions, such as autoimmune diseases, malignancy, human immunodeficiency virus infection, pulmonary hypertension, and portal vein thrombosis, as well as immunosuppressive medications.[14,15]

Cirrhosis causes more than 90% of portal hypertension in Western countries. Although cirrhosis is broadly considered a cause of sinusoidal portal hypertension, there are often alternative sites of increased resistance that appear early in the disease course, depending on the background cause of liver disease. For example, portal hypertension first develops in primary biliary cholangitis due to presinusoidal changes prior to the development of cirrhosis.[16] Screening for varices in individuals with primary biliary cholangitis, therefore, is not only recommended in cirrhosis, but also in the presence of a transient elastography value of greater than 7 kPa.[17] In addition to cirrhosis, sinusoidal portal hypertension can be caused by infiltrative conditions, such as amyloidosis and systemic mastocytosis. Postsinusoidal portal hypertension is primarily seen in the sinusoidal obstruction syndrome. Small hepatic veins become occluded and the sinusoidal endothelium in zone 3 is damaged in the setting of haematopoietic stem cell transplantation or exposure to other drugs and toxins, such as oxaliplatin-based chemotherapy.[18]

Posthepatic portal hypertension

Hepatic venous outflow tract obstruction and cardiac disease are the primary causes of posthepatic portal hypertension, which is characterized by venous outflow impairment. Budd–Chiari syndrome is eponymous for hepatic venous outflow tract obstruction, and can occur anywhere along the course of the small hepatic veins to the inferior vena cava. Even more so than portal vein thrombosis, myeloproliferative disorders are strongly associated with the development of the Budd–Chiari syndrome. Other causes include solid organ malignancies, infection, inflammatory disorders, trauma, and polycystic liver disease. Inherited prothrombotic conditions are often also present, particularly factor V Leiden mutation.[19]

Table 13.1 Aetiologies of portal hypertension

Prehepatic	Intrahepatic			Posthepatic
	Presinusoidal	Sinusoidal	Postsinusoidal	
Portal vein thrombosis	Schistosomiasis	Cirrhosis	Sinusoidal obstruction syndrome	Budd–Chiari syndrome
Splenic vein thrombosis	Sarcoidosis	Alcoholic hepatitis		Severe tricuspid regurgitation
Splanchnic arteriovenous fistula	Polycystic liver disease	Acute fatty liver of pregnancy		Right-sided heart failure
Extrinsic compression of portal/splenic vein	Amyloidosis	Amyloidosis		Constrictive pericarditis
	Idiopathic non-cirrhotic portal hypertension, including nodular regenerative hyperplasia	Gaucher disease		
		Mastocytosis		
	Liver metastasis	Viral hepatitis		
	Cholangiopathy	Acute hepatic injury		
	Congenital hepatic fibrosis			

Table 13.2 Hepatic venous pressure gradient changes by type of portal hypertension

Catheter measurement	Portal hypertension				
	Prehepatic	Presinusoidal	Sinusoidal	Postsinusoidal	Posthepatic
WHVP	Normal	Normal	Increased	Increased	Increased
FHVP	Normal	Normal	Normal	Normal	Increased
HVPG	Normal	Normal	Increased	Increased	Normal

Complications of portal hypertension

Variceal haemorrhage

Prophylaxis

Screening for gastro-oesophageal varices by upper gastrointestinal endoscopy is recommended in individuals diagnosed with cirrhosis. An exception might be individuals with a platelet count greater than 150 × 10⁹/L and mean liver stiffness of less than 20 kPa, as these factors are associated with a low risk of clinically significant varices.[20,21]

Oesophageal varices in the palisade zone around the gastro-oesophageal junction are at particular risk of haemorrhage as there are no associated perforating veins to help decompress flow to periesophageal veins.[22] On endoscopy, they are classified to be small (<5 mm) or large (≥5 mm). The risk of bleeding increases as varices enlarge, with an annual risk of haemorrhage of 5% and 15% for small and large varices, respectively.[23] Hence, prophylactic therapy is recommended to prevent the first haemorrhage in those with large varices and in those with small varices and red wale signs or advanced hepatic dysfunction (Child–Pugh class C). Primary prophylaxis can be achieved with repeat endoscopic band ligation every few weeks until obliteration of the varices is achieved or via pharmacological therapy with non-selective beta-blockers (NSBBs). Nadolol or propranolol are the NSBBs recommended, titrated up to achieve a resting heart rate of 55–60 beats per minute. Alternatively, carvedilol can be used, starting at 3.125 mg twice daily, and increased to 6.25 mg twice daily as tolerated with no need to achieve a target heart rate. Beta-blockade should be withheld in individuals with ascites if systolic blood pressure decreases to less than 90 mmHg, or if hyponatraemia (sodium <130 mEq/L) or acute kidney injury develops.[20] There is no need for repeat endoscopy after the initiation of beta-blockade; however, the recurrence rate of oesophageal varices after ligation approximates 90%, and therefore ongoing surveillance is required if endoscopy is the management approach selected, generally at 3–6 months after eradication and then annually thereafter. A recent network meta-analysis suggests that NSBB monotherapy may decrease all-cause mortality and the risk of first variceal bleeding while carrying a lower risk of serious complications compared with variceal band ligation.[24] Therefore, NSBB may be the preferred therapy for primary prophylaxis against oesophageal variceal bleeding.

Gastric varices occur more commonly in continuity with oesophageal varices than in other areas of the stomach, partly due to less collateral flow through the short gastric veins that drain the fundus to the splenic vein.[22] However, isolated gastric varices can occur. Gastric varices are typically described using Sarin's classification.[25] Isolated gastric varices type 1 are at the highest risk of bleeding and are more likely to be seen in cirrhosis and with thrombosis of the portal or splenic vein; hence their discovery should prompt cross-sectional imaging.[25,26] Primary prophylaxis with NSBBs can be considered for fundal-type varices based on limited evidence.[27]

Management of acute variceal haemorrhage

Gastro-oesophageal variceal bleeding presents with haematemesis and melena. After assessing and managing the acute haemodynamic instability, additional supportive care can be initiated, including transfusion of blood products if needed, vasoactive agents, and antimicrobial prophylaxis, followed by endoscopic assessment.

A restrictive transfusion strategy is now considered the best approach in acute gastrointestinal haemorrhage based on a large randomized controlled trial.[28] Limiting the transfusion threshold to 7 g/dL showed improved survival in patients with Child–Pugh class A and B cirrhosis, but not class C. Despite somatostatin administration, patients randomized to a liberalized transfusion strategy with a transfusion threshold of 9 g/dL had increased portal pressures and rebleeding.[28]

There is good evidence to support the use of vasoactive agents in acute variceal haemorrhage. Somatostatin is a 14-amino acid peptide that reduces portal hypertension via splanchnic vasoconstriction by both direct vasoconstriction and inhibition of vasodilatory peptides, such as glucagon. Octreotide is a longer-acting synthetic analogue of somatostatin.[29,30] Terlipressin is a synthetic analogue of vasopressin that allows a more sustained reduction in portal pressure. Although terlipressin decreases portal pressure via a decreased cardiac output and increased splanchnic vasoconstriction and systemic vascular resistance, it is a safer alternative to vasopressin, which is associated with more haemodynamic side effects, including bradycardia.[31] Compared to placebo, terlipressin is associated with increased haemostasis and decreased mortality as shown in a meta-analysis.[32] However, increased complications and decreased haemostasis were seen compared to octreotide. Another meta-analysis comparing 30 randomized controlled trials has found that all vasoactive agents were associated with decreased transfusion requirements and decreased 7-day mortality at a moderate level of evidence, with no differences in haemostasis or mortality when comparing vasoactive agents, although a very low quality of evidence was noted.[33] Vasoactive agents are generally recommended for up to 5 days.

Patients who present with cirrhosis and gastrointestinal haemorrhage are at a high risk of bacterial infection. Randomized controlled trial evidence supports the use of antibiotic prophylaxis to decrease infection, rebleeding, and mortality.[34,35] Early administration of antibiotic prophylaxis, either before or within 8 hours of endoscopy, is associated with decreased mortality in comparison to a delayed approach.[36] A 7-day course of intravenous ceftriaxone 1 g every 24 hours has demonstrated increased efficacy compared to oral norfloxacin, although high local resistance to quinolones may have accounted for the differences seen.[37]

Oesophagogastroduodenoscopy is recommended after stabilization of the haemodynamic parameters and within 12 hours of presentation.[38] Endoscopic variceal ligation should be completed in the setting of ongoing oesophageal variceal bleeding; evidence of recent haemorrhage, such as a clot or 'white nipple' sign; and in the presence of oesophageal varices without another identifiable cause for bleeding. If band ligation is not technically feasible, sclerotherapy or topical haemostatic powder are alternative options, although repeat endoscopy for definitive ligation within 12-24 hours is required after topical powder administration.[39] Balloon tamponade or endoscopically placed expandable metal stents can be used as a temporizing measure for less than 24 hours, or up to 7 days, respectively.[40,41] Rescue transjugular intrahepatic portosystemic shunt (TIPS) placement provides more definitive therapy by connecting the portal vein to the lower-pressure inferior vena cava, allowing rapid reduction in portal pressures.[20,42]

Bleeding gastro-oesophageal varices type 1 (GOV1), which are in continuity with oesophageal varices and extend along the lesser curvature of the stomach, can be treated similarly to oesophageal varices with band ligation, or alternatively with cyanoacrylate injection.[43] Use of TIPS also effectively controls haemorrhage from gastric varices, and can be considered first-line therapy in managing bleeding gastric fundal varices.[42]

Prevention of rebleeding

Early or pre-emptive TIPS should be performed within 24-72 hours of admission and considered in patients at high risk of oesophageal variceal haemorrhage recurrence. High risk patients are considered Child-Pugh class C (10-13 points) and/or those with an HVPG of greater than 20 mmHg. In one study, those with Child-Pugh class B and active bleeding were also included.[44] Compared to standard medical treatment after endoscopic variceal ligation, early TIPS in this high-risk population has demonstrated decreased rebleeding and improved patient survival.[44,45] Many patients are ineligible for early TIPS, including those with very advanced liver disease (Child-Pugh score >13), age over 75, advanced hepatocellular carcinoma, recurrent HE, and pulmonary hypertension, among others.[44,46]

For those who do not undergo early TIPS, combination therapy with NSBB and ongoing endoscopic variceal ligation is recommended as first-line management and is more beneficial than monotherapy with either approach.[47] However, it appears most of the effect is driven by pharmacological therapy. In patients who experience rebleeding despite first-line combination therapy, TIPS is the most effective approach to prevent recurrent haemorrhage.[48]

There are limited data to support NSBB use in gastric variceal rebleeding. Although NSBBs are recommended to prevent GOV1 rebleeding, repeat cyanoacrylate injection has been shown to be superior to NSBBs in managing cardiofundal varices.[49] Balloon-occluded retrograde transvenous obliteration (BRTO) or TIPS can also be considered for secondary prophylaxis of cardiofundal variceal haemorrhage. BRTO involves applying sclerosant throughout the fundal varices and associated collaterals by cannulation of the left renal vein via a femoral or jugular vein approach. The procedure requires the presence of a portosystemic shunt between the renal vein and the splenic vein. By obliterating shunts, BRTO can also reduce the risk of HE, but may increase portal hypertension and the risk of bleeding from oesophageal varices.[50-52] Decreased rebleeding has been demonstrated with TIPS; although no randomized trials have been conducted with BRTO, rebleeding rates range from 0% to 15%, lower than rebleeding rates of up to 30% seen with TIPS.[41,51,53,54]

Ascites

Pathogenesis and diagnosis of ascites

The splanchnic vasodilatation in portal hypertension results in a decrease in the effective arterial blood volume. These altered haemodynamics activate the renin–angiotensin–aldosterone system, antidiuretic hormone, and sympathetic nervous system. The activation of these systems results in sodium and water retention, as well as renal vasoconstriction and the development of ascites. The fluid retained is compartmentalized to the peritoneal space as a result of portal hypertension. An HVPG of 10 mmHg is necessary for ascites to occur. Ascites can be recognized on physical examination by the presence of a fluid wave and shifting dullness, and may coincide with peripheral oedema.[55] Ultrasonography can confirm the presence of ascites with as little as 100 mL of fluid.[56]

A diagnostic paracentesis should be performed once ascites develops to elucidate its underlying aetiology. It should also be performed to rule out infection (spontaneous bacterial peritonitis (SBP)) in individuals with cirrhosis and ascites who present to hospital or have a change in their clinical status, such as worsening HE or a deterioration in kidney function. Ascitic fluid analysis should include cell counts, with both total nucleated cell counts and polymorphonuclear neutrophil (PMN) counts, albumin level, total protein, and bacterial culture sent in blood culture bottles. A concomitant serum albumin level should be measured to calculate the serum–ascites albumin gradient (SAAG). A SAAG value of 1.1 g/dL or more can generally confirm the diagnosis of portal hypertensive-related ascites.[57] The other primary aetiology for a high SAAG is ascites related to hepatic venous outflow impairment (e.g. cardiac ascites), for which the ascitic fluid total protein concentration is typically 2.5 g/dL or higher (Table 13.3). Cirrhosis with portal hypertension is the cause of approximately 85% of ascites, and clinical suspicion of other underlying diagnoses determines the need for further ascitic fluid testing, such as cytology and mycobacterial culture.[58]

Management of ascites

Management of ascites in the setting of cirrhosis and portal hypertension is centred on achieving a negative sodium balance and is described here. The management of other causes of ascites centres on the treatment of the underlying disorder. First-line treatment in cirrhosis and ascites focuses on dietary sodium restriction to less than 2000 mg/day.[59] Additionally, medications should be reviewed to ensure those which are nephrotoxic, non-steroidal

Table 13.3 Causes of ascites by serum-ascites albumin gradient (SAAG)

SAAG (g/dL)	
≥1.1	<1.1
Cirrhosis	Nephrotic syndrome
Acute liver failure	Peritoneal carcinomatosis
Cardiac ascites	Tuberculous peritonitis
Budd–Chiari syndrome	Pancreatitis
	Myxoedema

anti-inflammatories, high-dose beta-blockers, or other inappropriate drugs are not being administered.

Dietary restriction alone may not result in resolution of ascites, and diuretic therapy is typically initiated shortly thereafter. A ratio of spironolactone to furosemide at 100:40 is best to maintain normal serum potassium levels and achieve rapid natriuresis.[59] Diuretic therapy is titrated to achieve mobilization of fluid, targeting approximately 0.5 kg of daily weight loss in those without lower limb oedema.[60] If ascites is non-responsive to diuretics or increases at any point, the diet should be carefully re-evaluated to ensure appropriate sodium restriction. The patient should also be evaluated for SBP, malignancy, and portal or hepatic vein thrombosis. Urine sodium can be measured to determine if the patient is achieving a net sodium deficit. A low-sodium diet of less than 2000 mg/day equates to less than 88 mmol of sodium per day. With approximately 10 mmol of non-urinary sodium excretion daily, individuals will be expected to excrete 78 mmol of urinary sodium per day to maintain their weight. Therefore, an excess of 78 mmol in urine per day (whether through spontaneous natriuresis or diuretic therapy) should result in fluid loss in the setting of dietary adherence.[59,61]

If individuals are intolerant to diuretic therapy due to orthostasis, renal injury, or hyponatraemia, or have fluid overload unresponsive to therapy, a diagnosis of diuretic-intolerant or refractory ascites is made. Such individuals are initially managed with intermittent therapeutic large-volume paracentesis. When large-volume paracentesis (>5 L) is performed, post-paracentesis circulatory dysfunction can occur, characterized by hypotension and renal dysfunction, with a high risk of mortality.[62] Intravenous infusion of 25% albumin is an important preventative measure, as up to 80% of individuals can experience post-paracentesis circulatory dysfunction in the absence of plasma expansion. Generally, 6–8 g of albumin is infused for every 1 L of ascitic fluid removed.

Alternatives to large-volume paracentesis in refractory ascites are TIPS, automated pumps connecting the peritoneal cavity with the bladder, and liver transplantation. Refractory ascites resolves in 50–75% of patients after TIPS placement.[63–65] Subcutaneous automated pump devices are effective in mobilizing peritoneal fluid to the bladder; however, they are associated with numerous complications without improvement in survival and are currently not recommended as a part of routine clinical practice.[66,67] In individuals near the end of life, percutaneous externally draining catheters may be placed in the setting of palliation; however, these may be problematic in other circumstances due to the high risk of infection.[68,69]

Spontaneous bacterial peritonitis

The clinical presentation of SBP can be variable, ranging from an asymptomatic increase in serum creatinine to marked encephalopathy. A diagnosis can be easily missed if a paracentesis is not performed. Diagnosis of SBP is confirmed by the presence of greater than 250 PMNs/mL in a patient with cirrhosis and ascites without a secondary source of infection, and should be differentiated from other variants (Table 13.4).[70]

Management of SBP and culture-negative neutrocytic ascites are similar and include prompt antimicrobial therapy and albumin administration. Empiric intravenous cefotaxime 2 g every 8 hours should be given as first-line antibiotic therapy as it targets the typical flora involved and has excellent penetration into the ascitic fluid.[71,72]

Table 13.4 Spontaneous bacterial peritonitis variants

Variant	PMN/mL	Bacterial culture
SBP	≥250	Positive
Culture negative neutrocytic ascites	≥250	Negative
Monomicrobial non-neutrocytic bacteriascites	<250	Positive
Polymicrobial bacteriascites	<250	Positive

Source: data from Runyon BA. Spontaneous bacterial peritonitis variants. In: *UpToDate*, Post TW (Ed), UpToDate, Waltham, MA. Available at: https://www.uptodate.com/contents/spontaneous-bacterial-peritonitis-in-adults-treatment-and-prophylaxis (Accessed 19 December 2022).

The addition of albumin 1.5 g/kg of body weight at diagnosis and albumin 1.0 g/kg on day 3 has been shown to reduce mortality.[73]

Hepatic encephalopathy

Pathogenesis and classification of hepatic encephalopathy

HE represents a constellation of neuropsychiatric symptoms ranging from marginal alterations in concentration to coma. The underlying mechanisms that cause HE remain under investigation. Hepatic dysfunction and portosystemic shunting allow ammonia, other nitrogenous compounds, and other harmful products normally metabolized by the liver to be transported to the brain.[74] The role of ammonia, inflammatory cytokines, oxidative stress, intestinal microbiota, sarcopenia, and other factors on the development of abnormal neurotransmission and brain oedema continues to be examined.[75] Symptomatic HE is a decompensating event and is common in patients with cirrhosis, occurring in approximately 30% throughout the disease course.[76,77]

Each episode of HE should be classified by aetiology, severity, time course, and precipitating factors to guide workup and management.[78] Aetiology refers to the type of underlying hepatic abnormality, and is subclassified to HE associated with acute liver failure (type A), portosystemic shunting (type B), and cirrhosis (type C). Disease severity is generally by the West Haven criteria (Table 13.5); however, covert HE is now also recognized, generally defined as a neurological abnormality identified on psychometric testing without overt clinical symptoms.[78] The International Society for Hepatic Encephalopathy and Nitrogen Metabolism consensus statement divides HE into covert (minimal and grade 1) and overt (grades 2–4) for standardization in clinical trials.[79] Its time course is divided into episodic, recurrent, and persistent HE, and the disease

Table 13.5 West Haven criteria for grading of hepatic encephalopathy

Grade	Symptoms
1	Altered mood or behaviour, decreased concentration
2	Drowsy, inappropriate behaviour, minimal disorientation
3	Marked confusion, somnolence
4	Coma

Source: data from Vilstrup H, Amodio P, Bajaj J, et al. Hepatic encephalopathy in chronic liver disease: 2014 practice guideline by the American Association for the Study of Liver Diseases and the European Association for the Study of the Liver. *Hepatology*. 2014;60:715.

is also subclassified into spontaneous or precipitated HE. Infection is one of the most common precipitating factors for HE, although medications, gastrointestinal haemorrhage, dehydration, electrolyte disturbance, and constipation, among others, can be implicated.[80]

The diagnosis of covert HE is based on psychometric and neurophysiological testing; however, no superior method of assessment has been identified. Some available tests include the Stroop test (computerized psychomotor speed testing), Portosystemic Encephalopathy Syndrome test (paper–pencil testing), and the Continuous Reaction Time test (reaction time measurement to auditory stimuli).[81–83] Such a diagnosis of covert HE can be valuable in providing patients with an explanation for their symptoms and signify prognosis for future overt HE events.[76] Overt HE is diagnosed clinically using a detailed history and physical examination, West Haven criteria, and the Glasgow Coma Scale.[84] The spectrum of neuropsychiatric symptoms seen in HE are non-specific, and alternative causes that may explain patient presentation must be ruled out (e.g. uraemia, intracranial haemorrhage, diabetes mellitus, medications, and neurological complications of alcohol, such as Wernicke's encephalopathy and Korsakoff syndrome).

Management of hepatic encephalopathy

Targeted therapy is typically initiated upon the development of overt HE; however, covert symptoms may be treated if affecting the patient's function or quality of life. Management is directed at correcting the underlying cause, and administering drug therapy to reduce ammonia levels. Once an episode of overt HE has occurred, patients should be generally continued on prophylactic therapy indefinitely thereafter, unless a clear isolated precipitant is identified and eliminated.

Lactulose is a non-absorbable disaccharide that reduces ammonia via increased frequency of bowel movements and acidification of the colon, allowing conversion of ammonia to ammonium, and modifying the gut flora to non-urease-producing species. It is considered first-line therapy for overt HE based on decades of clinical experience and should be titrated to achieve two to three semi-formed bowel movements per day. The impact of lactulose on HE has been variable in studies, confounded by inclusion criteria, heterogeneity of precipitants, and subjectivity of assessment tools, among other issues. However, a recent meta-analysis has now demonstrated that non-absorbable disaccharide use is associated with reduced mortality, and can also prevent HE development and other liver-related adverse events.[85]

Rifaximin is a non-absorbable antibiotic that works to lower blood ammonia by decreasing bacterial load in the gut, modifying bacterial metabolism, and inhibiting bacterial translocation. Rifaximin was first positioned as an adjunct to lactulose in the prevention of overt HE recurrence, and it has also been shown to reduce HE-related hospitalization in this setting.[86] Adding rifaximin to lactulose is also more effective than lactulose alone in reversing overt HE.[87] Rifaximin monotherapy can improve cognitive function in cirrhosis and minimal HE, likely through modulation of bacterial metabolism.[88]

There is emerging evidence for the use of other agents in the management and prevention of HE. L-ornithine-L-aspartate (LOLA) lowers ammonia concentrations by increasing its metabolism to glutamine and urea by activating key enzymes in glutamine and urea synthesis within the liver and skeletal muscle. There is evidence for the beneficial effect of LOLA in the treatment of minimal and overt HE and secondary prophylaxis of overt HE, but the agent is not widely available.[89,90] Oral branched-chain amino acids (BCAAs) are thought to be beneficial in HE by rebalancing the BCAA to aromatic amino acid ratio that is usually decreased in cirrhosis, thereby altering central nervous system neurotransmitter synthesis. Although BCAAs have not been shown to reduce mortality, they were associated with improvement of the manifestations of HE on meta-analysis.[91] Probiotics have also been studied in HE; however, recommendations on probiotic use in HE cannot be made at this time given the very low quality of evidence available.[92] Low serum zinc levels are common in cirrhosis and associated with HE. Limited data suggest mild HE can be improved when zinc is added to lactulose.[93] Zinc administration was also beneficial in some individuals with refractory HE in one study, and is generally well tolerated.[94]

In addition to pharmacological strategies, cross-sectional imaging to identify large portosystemic shunts should be considered in individuals with overt HE, particularly in the setting of adequate liver function. Embolization of shunts can successfully treat overt HE.[95]

Conclusion

In conclusion, heightened vigilance is necessary for the early identification and management of clinically significant portal hypertension and its sequelae in patients with cirrhosis. Specifically, identifying patients who may benefit from beta-blockade, antibiotic prophylaxis, or TIPS is imperative to prevent or mitigate decompensation, and improve overall survival.

REFERENCES

1. D'Amico G, Pasta L, Morabito A, et al. Competing risks and prognostic stages of cirrhosis: a 25-year inception cohort study of 494 patients. *Aliment Pharmacol Ther.* 2014;**39**(10):1180–1193.
2. D'Amico G, Garcia-Tsao G, Pagliaro L. Natural history and prognostic indicators of survival in cirrhosis: a systematic review of 118 studies. *J Hepatol.* 2006;**44**(1):217–231.
3. Moreau R, Delègue P, Pessione F, et al. Clinical characteristics and outcome of patients with cirrhosis and refractory ascites. *Liver Int.* 2004;**24**(5):457–464.
4. Groszmann RJ, Wongcharatrawee S. The hepatic venous pressure gradient: anything worth doing should be done right. *Hepatology.* 2004;**39**(2):280–283.
5. Ripoll C, Groszmann R, Garcia-Tsao G, et al. Hepatic venous pressure gradient predicts clinical decompensation in patients with compensated cirrhosis. *Gastroenterology.* 2007;**133**(2):481–488.
6. Iwakiri Y, Groszmann RJ. Vascular endothelial dysfunction in cirrhosis. *J Hepatol.* 2007;**46**(5):927–934.
7. Fernandez M, Vizzutti F, Garcia-Pagan JC, Rodes J, Bosch J. Anti-VEGF receptor-2 monoclonal antibody prevents portal-systemic collateral vessel formation in portal hypertensive mice. *Gastroenterology.* 2004;**126**(3):886–894.
8. Sumanovski LT, Battegay E, Stumm M, van der Kooij M, Sieber CC. Increased angiogenesis in portal hypertensive rats: role of nitric oxide. *Hepatology.* 1999;**29**(4):1044–1049.
9. Stine JG, Wang J, Shah PM, et al. Decreased portal vein velocity is predictive of the development of portal vein thrombosis: a matched case-control study. *Liver Int.* 2018;**38**(1):94–101.

10. Tripodi A, Primignani M, Lemma L, et al. Detection of the imbalance of procoagulant versus anticoagulant factors in cirrhosis by a simple laboratory method. *Hepatology*. 2010;**52**(1):249–255.
11. Denniger MH, Chaït Y, Casadevall N, et al. Cause of portal or hepatic venous thrombosis in adults: the role of multiple concurrent factors. *Hepatology*. 2000;**31**(3):587–591.
12. Valla D, Casadevall N, Huisse MG, et al. Etiology of portal vein thrombosis in adults. A prospective evaluation of primary myeloproliferative disorders. *Gastroenterology*. 1988;**94**(4):1063–1069.
13. Ross AG, Bartley PB, Sleigh AC, et al. Schistosomiasis. *N Engl J Med*. 2002;**346**(16):1212–1220.
14. Wanless I. Micronodular transformation (nodular regenerative hyperplasia) of the liver: a report of 64 cases among 2500 autopsies and a new classification of benign hepatocellular nodules. *Hepatology*. 1990;**11**(5):787–797.
15. Hartleb M, Gutkowski K, Milkiewicz P. Nodular regenerative hyperplasia: evolving concepts on underdiagnosed cause of portal hypertension. *World J Gastroenterol*. 2011;**17**(11):1400–1409.
16. Gores GJ, Wiesner RH, Dickson ER, Zinsmeister AR, Jorgensen RA, Langworthy A. Prospective evaluation of esophageal varices in primary biliary cirrhosis: development, natural history, and influence on survival. *Gastroenterology*. 1989;**96**(5):1552–1559.
17. Lindor KD, Bowlus CL, Boyer J, Levy C, Mayo M. Primary biliary cholangitis: 2018 practice guidance from the American Association for the Study of Liver Diseases. *Hepatology*. 2019;**69**(1):394–419.
18. Valla DC, Cazals-Hatem D. Sinusoidal obstruction syndrome. *Clin Res Hepatol Gastroenterol*. 2016;**40**(4):378–385.
19. Khan F, Armstrong MJ, Mehrzad H, et al. Review article: a multidisciplinary approach to the diagnosis and management of Budd-Chiari syndrome. *Aliment Pharmacol Ther*. 2019;**49**(7):840–863.
20. de Franchis R; Baveno VI Faculty. Expanding consensus in portal hypertension: report of the Baveno VI Consensus Workshop: stratifying risk and individualizing care for portal hypertension. *J Hepatol*. 2015;**63**(3):743–752.
21. Maurice JB, Brodkin E, Arnold F, et al. Validation of the Baveno VI criteria to identify low risk cirrhotic patients not requiring endoscopic surveillance for varices. *J Hepatol*. 2016;**65**(5):899–905.
22. Vianna A, Hayes P, Moscoso G, et al. Normal venous circulation of the gastroesophageal junction. A route to understanding varices. *Gastroenterology*. 1987;**93**(4):876–889.
23. D'Amico G, Luca A. Natural history: clinical-haemodynamic correlations: prediction of the risk of bleeding. *Baillieres Clin Gastroenterol*. 1997;**11**(2):243–256.
24. Sharma M, Singh S, Desai V, et al. Comparison of therapies for primary prevention of esophageal variceal bleeding: a systematic review and network meta-analysis. *Hepatology*. 2019;**64**(4):1657–1675.
25. Sarin SK, Lahoti D, Saxena SP, Murthy NS, Makwana UK. Prevalence, classification and natural history of gastric varices: a long term follow-up study in 568 portal hypertension patients. *Hepatology*. 1992;**16**(6):1343–1349.
26. Kim T, Shijo H, Kokawa H, et al. Risk factors for hemorrhage from gastric fundal varices. *Hepatology*. 1997;**25**(2):307–312.
27. Mishra SR, Sharma BC, Kumar A, Sarin SK. Primary prophylaxis of gastric variceal bleeding comparing cyanoacrylate injection and beta-blockers: a randomized controlled trial. *J Hepatol*. 2011;**54**(6):1161–1167.
28. Villanueva C, Colomo A, Bosch A, et al. Transfusion strategies for acute upper gastrointestinal bleeding. *N Engl J Med*. 2013;**368**(1):11–21.
29. Abraldes JG, Bosch J. Somatostatin and analogues in portal hypertension. *Hepatology*. 2002;**35**(6):1305–1312.
30. Ludwig D, Schadel S, Bruning A, et al. 48-hour hemodynamic effects of octreotide on postprandial splanchic hyperemia in patients with liver cirrhosis and portal hypertension: double-blind, placebo-controlled study. *Dig Dis Sci*. 2000;**45**(5):1019–1027.
31. Moller S, Hansen EF, Becker U, et al. Central and systemic haemodynamic effects of terlipressin in portal hypertensive patients. *Liver*. 2000;**20**(1):51–59.
32. Zhou X, Tripathi D, Song T, et al. Terlipressin for the treatment of acute variceal bleeding: a systematic review and meta-analysis of randomized controlled trials. *Medicine*. 2019;**97**:e13437.
33. Wells M, Chande N, Adams P, et al. Meta-analysis: vasoactive medications for the management of acute variceal bleeds. *Aliment Pharmacol Ther*. 2012;**35**(11):1267–1278.
34. Bernard B, Grangé JD, Khac EN, Amiot X, Opolon P, Poynard T. Antibiotic prophylaxis for the prevention of bacterial infections in cirrhotic patients with gastrointestinal bleeding: a meta-analysis. *Hepatology*. 1999;**29**(6):1655–1661.
35. Chavez-Tapia NC, Barrientos-Gutierrez T, Tellez-Avila F, et al. Meta-analysis: antibiotic prophylaxis for cirrhotic patients with upper gastrointestinal bleeding—an updated Cochrane review. *Aliment Pharmacol Ther*. 2011;**34**(5):509–518.
36. Brown MR, Jones G, Nash KL, Wright M, Guha IN. Antibiotic prophylaxis in variceal hemorrhage: timing, effectiveness and Clostridium difficile rate. *World J Gastroenterol*. 2010;**16**(42):5317–5323.
37. Fernández J, Ruiz del Arbol L, Gómez C, et al. Norfloxacin vs ceftriaxone in the prophylaxis of infections in patients with advanced cirrhosis and hemorrhage. *Gastroenterology*. 2006;**131**(4):1049–1056.
38. Hsu YC, Chung CS, Tseng CH, et al. Delayed endoscopy as a risk factor for in-hospital mortality in cirrhotic patients with acute variceal hemorrhage. *J Gastroenterol Hepatol*. 2009;**24**(7):1294–1299.
39. Ibrahim M, El-Mikkawy A, Abdel Hamid M, et al. Early application of haemostatic powder added to standard management for oesophagogastric variceal bleeding: a randomized trial. *Gut*. 2019;**68**(5):844–853.
40. Garcia-Tsao G, Sanyal AJ, Grace ND, Carey W. Prevention and management of gastroesophageal varices and variceal hemorrhage in cirrhosis. *Hepatology*. 2007;**46**(3):922–938.
41. Escorsell A, Pavel O, Cardenas A, et al. Esophageal balloon tamponade versus esophageal stent in controlling acute refractory variceal bleeding: a multicenter randomized, controlled trial. *Hepatology*. 2016;**63**(6):1957–1967.
42. Chau TN, Patch D, Chan YW, Nagral A, Dick R, Burroughs AK. Salvage transjugular intrahepatic portosystemic shunts—gastric fundal compared with esophageal variceal bleeding. *Gastroenterology*. 1998;**114**(5):981–987.
43. El Amin H, AAbdel BL, Sayed Z, et al. A randomized trial of endoscopic variceal ligation versus cyanoacrylate injection for treatment of bleeding junctional varices. *Trop Gastroenterol*. 2010;**31**(4):279–284.
44. García-Pagán JC, Caca K, Bureau C, et al. Early use of TIPS in patients with cirrhosis and variceal bleeding. *N Engl J Med*. 2010;**362**(25):2370–2379.

45. Monescillo A, Martínez-Lagares F, Ruiz-del-Arbol L, et al. Influence of portal hypertension and its early decompression by TIPS placement on the outcome of variceal bleeding. *Hepatology*. 2004;**40**(4):793–801.
46. Maimone S, Saffioti F, Filomia R, et al. Predictors of re-bleeding and mortality among patients with refractory variceal bleeding undergoing salvage transjugular intrahepatic portosystemic shunt (TIPS). *Dig Dis Sci*. 2019;**64**(5):1335–1345.
47. Puente A, Hernandez-Gea V, Graupera I, et al. Drugs plus ligation to prevent rebleeding in cirrhosis: an updated systematic review. *Liver Int*. 2014;**34**(6):823–833.
48. Holster IL, Tjwa ET, Moelker A, et al. Covered transjugular intrahepatic portosystemic shunt versus endoscopic therapy + beta-blocker for prevention of variceal rebleeding. *Hepatology*. 2016;**63**(2):581–589.
49. Mishra SR, Chander SB, Kumar A, Sarin SK. Endoscopic cyanoacrylate injection versus beta-blocker for secondary prophylaxis of gastric variceal bleed: a randomised controlled trial. *Gut*. 2010;**59**(6):729–735.
50. Trudeau W, Prindiville T. Endoscopic injection sclerosis in bleeding gastric varices. *Gastrointest Endosc*. 1986;**32**(4):264–268.
51. Saad WE, Sabri SS. Balloon-occluded retrograde transvenous obliteration (BRTO): technical results and outcomes. *Semin Intervent Radiol*. 2011;**28**(3):333–338.
52. Park JK, Saab S, Kee ST, et al. Balloon-occluded retrograde transvenous obliteration (BRTO) for treatment of gastric varices: review and meta-analysis. *Dig Dis Sci*. 2015;**60**(6):1543–1553.
53. Lo GH, Liang HL, Chen WC, et al. A prospective, randomized controlled trial of transjugular intrahepatic portosystemic shunt versus cyanoacrylate injection in the prevention of gastric variceal rebleeding. *Endoscopy*. 2007;**39**(8):679–685.
54. Jang SY, Kim GH, Park SY, et al. Clinical outcomes of balloon-occluded retrograde transvenous obliteration for the treatment of gastric variceal hemorrhage in Korean patients with liver cirrhosis: a retrospective multicenter study. *Clin Mol Hepatol*. 2012;**18**(4):368–374.
55. Williams JW, Simel DL. Does this patient have ascites? *J Amer Med Assoc*. 1992;**267**(19):2645–2648.
56. Goldberg BB, Goodman GA, Clearfield HR. Evaluation of ascites by ultrasound. *Radiology*. 1970;**96**(1):15–22.
57. Runyon BA, Montano AA, Akriviadis EA, Antillon MR, Irving MA, McHutchison JG. The serum-ascites albumin gradient is superior to the exudate-transudate concept in the differential diagnosis of ascites. *Ann Intern Med*. 1992;**117**(3):215–220.
58. Akriviadis EA, Runyon BA. The value of an algorithm in differentiating spontaneous from secondary bacterial peritonitis. *Gastroenterology*. 1990;**98**(1):127–133.
59. Runyon BA. Care of patients with ascites. *N Engl J Med*. 1994;**330**(5):337–342.
60. Pockros PJ, Reynolds TB. Rapid diuresis in patients with ascites from chronic liver disease: the importance of peripheral edema. *Gastroenterology*. 1986;**90**(6):1827–1833.
61. Eisenmenger WJ, Blondheim SH, Bongiovanni AM, Kunkel HG. Electrolyte studies on patients with cirrhosis of the liver. *J Clin Invest*. 1950;**29**(11):1491–1499.
62. Alessandria C, Elia C, Mezzabotta L, et al. Prevention of paracentesis-induced circulatory dysfunction in cirrhosis: standard vs half albumin doses. A prospective, randomized, unblinded pilot study. *Dig Liver Dis*. 2011;**43**(11):881–886.
63. Bureau C, Thabut D, Oberti F, et al. Transjugular intrahepatic portosystemic shunts with covered stents increase transplant-free survival of patients with cirrhosis and recurrent ascites. *Gastroenterology*. 2017;**151**(1):157–163.
64. Albillos A, Banares R, Gonzalez M, Catalina MV, Molinero LM. A meta-analysis of transjugular intrahepatic portosystemic shunt versus paracentesis for refractory ascites. *J Hepatol*. 2005;**43**(6):990–996.
65. Ochs A, Rossle M, Haag K, et al. The transjugular intrahepatic portosystemic stent-shunt procedure for refractory ascites. *N Engl J Med*. 1995;**332**(18):1192–1197.
66. Bellot P, Welker MW, Soriano G, et al. Automated low flow pump system for the treatment of refractory ascites: a multicenter safety and efficacy study. *J Hepatol*. 2013;**58**(5):922–927.
67. Bureau C, Adebayo D, Chalret de Rieu M, et al. Alfapump® system vs. large volume paracentesis for refractory ascites: a multicenter randomized controlled study. *J Hepatol*. 2017;**67**(5):940–949.
68. Knight JA, Thompson SM, Fleming CJ, et al. Safety and effectiveness of palliative tunneled peritoneal drainage catheters in the management of refractory malignant and non-malignant ascites. *Cardiovasc Intervent Radiol*. 2018;**41**(5):753–761.
69. Reinglas J, Amjadi K, Petrcich B, Momoli F, Shaw-Stiffel T. The palliative management of refractory cirrhotic ascites using the PleurX (©) catheter. *Can J Gastroenterol Hepatol*. 2016;**2016**:4680543.
70. Runyon BA, Antillon MR. Ascitic fluid pH and lactate: insensitive and nonspecific tests in detecting ascitic fluid infection. *Hepatology*. 1991;**13**(5):929–935.
71. Felisart J, Rimola A, Arroyo V, et al. Randomized comparative study of efficacy and nephrotoxicity of ampicillin plus tobramycin versus cefotaxime in cirrhotics with severe infections. *Hepatology*. 1985;**5**(3):457–462.
72. Runyon BA, Akriviadis EA, Sattler FR, Cohen J. Ascitic fluid and serum cefotaxime and desacetyl cefotaxime levels in patients treated for bacterial peritonitis. *Dig Dis Sci*. 1991;**36**(12):1782–1786.
73. Sort P, Navasa M, Arroyo V, et al. Effect of intravenous albumin on renal impairment and mortality in patients with cirrhosis and spontaneous bacterial peritonitis. *N Engl J Med*. 1999;**341**(6):403–409.
74. Wijdicks EF. Hepatic encephalopathy. *N Engl J Med*. 2016;**375**(17):1660–1670.
75. Swaminathan M, Ellul MA, Cross TJS. Hepatic encephalopathy: current challenges and future prospects. *Hepat Med*. 2018;**10**:1–11.
76. Romero-Gómez M, Boza F, García-Valdecasas MS, García E, Aguilar-Reina J. Subclinical hepatic encephalopathy predicts the development of over hepatic encephalopathy. *Am J Gastroenterol*. 2001;**96**(9):2718–2723.
77. Das A, Dhiman RK, Saraswat VA, Verma M, Naik SR. Prevalence and natural history of subclinical hepatic encephalopathy in cirrhosis. *J Gastroenterol Hepatol*. 2001;**16**(5):531–535.
78. Ferenci P, Lockwood A, Mullen K, Tarter R, Weissenborn K, Blei AT. Hepatic encephalopathy—definition, nomenclature, diagnosis, and quantification: final report of the working party at the 11th World Congresses of Gastroenterology, Vienna, 1998. *Hepatology*. 2002;**35**(3):716–721.
79. Bajaj JS, Cordoba J, Mullen KD. Review article: the design of clinical trials in hepatic encephalopathy—an International Society for Hepatic Encephalopathy and Nitrogen Metabolism (ISHEN) consensus statement. *Aliment Pharmacol Ther*. 2011;**33**(7):739–747.

80. Cordoba J, Ventura-Cots M, Simón-Talero M, et al. Characteristics, risk factors, and mortality of cirrhotic patients hospitalized for hepatic encephalopathy with and without acute-on-chronic liver failure (ACLF). *J Hepatol*. 2014;**60**(2):275–281.
81. Bajaj JS, Thacker LR, Heumann DM, et al. The Stroop smartphone application is a short and valid method to screen for minimal hepatic encephalopathy. *Hepatology*. 2013;**58**(3):1122–1132.
82. Weissenborn K, Ennen JC, Schomerus H, Ruckert N, Hecker H. Neuropsychological characterization of hepatic encephalopathy. *J Hepatol*. 2001;**34**(5):768–773.
83. Lauridsen MM, Thiele M, Kimer N, Vilstrup H. The continuous reaction times method for diagnosing, grading, and monitoring minimal/covert hepatic encephalopathy. *Metab Brain Dis*. 2013;**28**(2):231–234.
84. Montagnese S, Amodio P, Moran MY. Methods for diagnosing hepatic encephalopathy in patients with cirrhosis: a multidimensional approach. *Metab Brain Dis*. 2004;**19**(3–4):281–312.
85. Gluud LL, Vilstrup H, Morgan MY. Non-absorbable disaccharides for hepatic encephalopathy: a systematic review and meta-analysis. *Hepatology*. 2016;**64**(3):908–922.
86. Hudson M, Schuchmann M. Long-term management of hepatic encephalopathy with lactulose and/or rifaximin: a review of the evidence. *Eur J Gastroenterol Hepatol*. 2019;**31**(4):434–450.
87. Sharma BC, Sharma P, Lunia MK, et al. A randomized, double-blind, controlled trial comparing rifaximin plus lactulose with lactulose alone in treatment of overt hepatic encephalopathy. *Am J Gastroenterol*. 2013;**108**(9):1458–1463.
88. Bajaj JS, Heuman DM, Sanyal AJ, et al. Modulation of the metabiome by rifaximin in patients with cirrhosis and minimal hepatic encephalopathy. *PLoS One*. 2013;**8**(4):e60042.
89. Butterworth RF, Kircheis G, Hilger N, McPhail MJW. Efficacy of L-ornithine L-aspartate for the treatment of hepatic encephalopathy and hyperammonemia in cirrhosis: systematic review and meta-analysis of randomized controlled trials. *J Clin Exp Hepatol*. 2018;**8**(3):301–313.
90. Butterworth RF. Beneficial effects of L-ornithine L-aspartate for prevention of overt hepatic encephalopathy in patients with cirrhosis: a systematic review with meta-analysis. *Metab Brain Dis*. 2020;**35**(1):75–81.
91. Gluud LL, Dam G, Les I, et al. Branched-chain amino acids for people with hepatic encephalopathy. *Cochrane Database Syst Rev*. 2017;**5**(5):CD001939.
92. Dalal R, McGee RG, Riordan SM, Webster AC. Probiotics for people with hepatic encephalopathy. *Cochrane Database Syst Rev*. 2017;**2**(2):CD008716.
93. Shen YC, Chang YH, Fang CJ, Lin YS. Zinc supplementation in patients with cirrhosis and hepatic encephalopathy: a systematic review and meta-analysis. *Nutr J*. 2019;**18**(1):34.
94. Takuma Y, Nouso K, Makino Y, Hayashi M, Takahashi H. Clinical trial: oral zinc in hepatic encephalopathy. *Aliment Pharmacol Ther*. 2010;**32**(9):1080–1090.
95. Laleman W, Simon-Talero M, Maleux G, et al. Embolization of large spontaneous portosystemic shunts for refractory hepatic encephalopathy: a multi-center survey on safety and efficacy. *Hepatology*. 2013;**57**(6):2448–2457.

14

Interventional radiological and surgical treatment of portal hypertension

Mohammad Qasim Khan and Patrick S. Kamath

Introduction

In patients with portal hypertension, portosystemic shunts decompress the high-pressure portal venous system into the lower pressure systemic venous system, reducing the risk of variceal bleeding. Portosystemic shunts may occur spontaneously, typically as splenorenal shunts. Spontaneous portosystemic shunts are associated with a higher risk of hepatic encephalopathy[1] and portopulmonary hypertension.[2] Portosystemic shunts can also be created to treat portal hypertension, either by interventional radiologists via a transjugular route (transjugular intrahepatic portosystemic shunts (TIPS) or surgically. Both TIPS and surgical shunts decrease the risk of portal hypertension-related bleeding but are associated with an increased risk of hepatic encephalopathy and reduced patency of the shunt in the long term. There are other interventions, both surgical and interventional radiological, that are used to treat complications of portal hypertension without creating a portosystemic shunt.

Interventional radiological procedures to treat complications of portal hypertension

Transjugular intrahepatic portosystemic shunts

By creating a tract between the hepatic vein and an intrahepatic branch of the portal vein, TIPS reduce elevated portal pressures. A TIPS is functionally a side-to-side portacaval shunt which decreases hepatic sinusoidal pressure and has been used in the treatment of variceal bleeding, refractory ascites, Budd–Chiari syndrome, and hepatic hydrothorax. TIPS can be placed by an interventional radiologist via a percutaneous route with a mortality rate of less than 1–2%. The procedure is carried out with the patient under sedation; platelet count greater than 60,000/mm³ and an international normalized ratio less than 1.5 are desirable but are not essential in an emergency. Broad-spectrum antibiotic coverage is recommended if the TIPS procedure is carried out in a patient with variceal bleeding as an emergency procedure and in the presence of biliary obstruction, as in patients with primary sclerosing cholangitis. The hepatic vein is cannulated through a transjugular approach, and using a Rosch needle, the portal vein is punctured. A guidewire connects the hepatic vein and a branch of the portal vein. Following dilation of the tract, a stent is placed, bridging usually the right hepatic vein and the right portal vein (Figure 14.1). The stent is dilated as required to reduce the portacaval pressure gradient (the pressure difference between the portal vein and the hepatic vein at the confluence of the inferior vena cava) to less than 12 mmHg. A coated stent with the polytetrafluoroethylene-coated portion lining the tract in the liver parenchyma and an uncoated portion anchoring the stent to the portal vein and the draining hepatic vein is preferred to a bare-metal stent. Shunt stenosis is less likely with coated stents as compared with bare-metal stents.

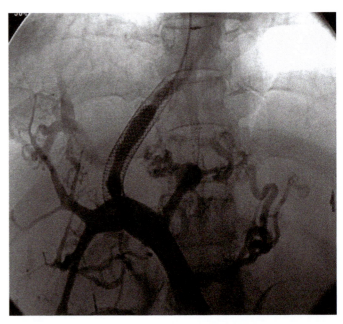

Figure 14.1 Radiographic image demonstrating stent deployment and subsequent successful creation of an intrahepatic portosystemic shunt.

Indications for TIPS

Portal hypertension-related bleeding

The most common indication for TIPS is refractory variceal bleeding, either for control of acute variceal bleeding or to prevent recurrent variceal rebleeding following failure of pharmacological and endoscopic therapies. Early TIPS within 72 hours of control of variceal bleeding may also be indicated in patients at high risk of rebleeding (Child–Pugh class C, class B with active bleeding, or a Model for End-stage Liver Disease (MELD) score ≥18 and a transfusion requirement of ≥4 units of red blood cells). This early use of TIPS is associated with lower mortality and a reduced rate of variceal rebleeding compared with a combination of pharmacological and endoscopic therapy.[3] In acute variceal bleeding that cannot be controlled after two sessions of endoscopic therapy within a 24-hour period, TIPS is used as rescue therapy. In such situations, TIPS is effective in controlling oesophageal variceal bleeding in more than 90% of patients with decompensated cirrhosis, but the mortality rate is greater than 60% within 90 days. TIPS may also be used to control bleeding and prevent rebleeding from isolated gastric fundal varices.

In a meta-analysis of 12 randomized controlled trials that compared TIPS with endoscopic therapy in the prevention of bleeding from oesophageal varices, the rebleeding rate was lower with TIPS, but the frequency of encephalopathy was higher.[4] There was no survival difference between the groups. Covered TIPS is superior to a combination of variceal ligation and beta-blockers to prevent variceal rebleeding but does not improve survival and is associated with higher rates of early hepatic encephalopathy. Indeed, there is considerable uncertainty regarding the survival benefit of any treatment used for prevention of variceal rebleeding.[5]

TIPS-related complications and outcomes

Complications following the procedure are classified as (1) procedure related, (2) early (occurring within 30 days), or (3) late (occurring after 30 days) (Table 14.1). Shunt stenosis, hepatic encephalopathy, and mortality risk require further discussion.

Table 14.1 Complications post transjugular intrahepatic portosystemic shunt placement

Timing of complication	Complication
Procedure related: major	Carotid artery puncture injury Intraperitoneal haemorrhage Sepsis Contrast nephropathy Cardiopulmonary failure Radiation skin burns/ulcers
Procedure related: minor	Haematoma at puncture site Contrast-induced reactions Fever
Early post-procedure (1–30 days)	*Shunt related:* Shunt thrombosis Stent migration Portobiliary fistula *Systemic:* Hepatic encephalopathy Progressive hepatic failure Cardiac arrhythmia Pulmonary arterial hypertension Haemolytic anaemia

Adapted with permission from Kamath PS, McKusick MA. Transjugular intrahepatic portosystemic shunts. *Gastroenterology*. 1996;111:1700–1705.

The frequency of stenosis of non-covered TIPS ranges from 20% to 78% depending on the surveillance technique used. The risk of shunt stenosis has been reduced to about 15% with the use of a covered stent. Doppler ultrasound evaluation every 6 months is generally used as the surveillance tool to identify TIPS stenosis, but with low negative predictive value and only fair positive predictive value. TIPS stenosis is strongly suspected when there is recurrence of the problem that necessitated the TIPS, irrespective of Doppler ultrasound findings. Shunt patency is best demonstrated by means of a TIPS venogram and measurement of the portacaval pressure gradient; a portocaval gradient greater than 12 mmHg indicates shunt stenosis and requires either dilation of the stent or placement of an additional stent to reduce the gradient.

TIPS may worsen liver function by diverting portal blood flow away from the liver. The shunting of portal blood away from the liver increases the risk of hepatic encephalopathy and may decrease survival in some patients. Hepatic encephalopathy is more common in older patients and with wider diameter shunts; therefore, if TIPS is used at all in patients older than 60 years, care should be taken to use as narrow a shunt diameter as possible to reduce portal pressure. Emergency TIPS is clearly associated with a higher mortality rate, especially in centres which perform less than 20 procedures a year.[6] Child–Turcotte–Pugh (CTP) class C patients have lower survival post TIPS (Table 14.2). The MELD score (http://www.mayoclinic.org/gi-rst/mayomodel6.html) is a mathematical model that may be used to accurately determine survival following the procedure.[7] The MELD score is calculated using the serum creatinine level, international normalized ratio, serum bilirubin level, and aetiology of liver disease as variables. The probability of mortality following TIPS placement can be calculated with use of an online formula (https://www.mayoclinic.org/medical-professionals/model-end-stage-liver-disease/probability-mortality-following-transjugular-intrahepatic-portosystemic-shunts). In general, patients with a MELD score of 14 or less have excellent survival after TIPS placement and the procedure may be carried out routinely in such patients when indicated. Patients with a MELD score greater than 24 have a mortality rate approaching 30% at 3 months post-TIPS placement; the high risk should be discussed with the patient before carrying out the procedure, especially if patients are not candidates for liver transplantation. In the intermediate group with MELD scores ranging between 15 and 24, TIPS placement

Table 14.2 Child–Turcotte–Pugh scoring system and Child–Pugh classification

Parameter	CTP numerical score		
	1	2	3
Ascites	None	Slight	Moderate/severe
Encephalopathy	None	Slight/moderate	Moderate/severe
Bilirubin (mg/dL)	<2	2–3	>3
Albumin (g/dL)	>3.5	2.8–3.5	<2.8
Prothrombin time (seconds)	1–3	4–6	>6

Note: class A: 5–6 points; class B: 7–9 points; class C: 10–15 points.
Source: data from: Pugh RN, Murray-Lyon IM, Dawson JL, Pietroni MC, Williams R. Transection of the oesophagus for bleeding oesophageal varices. *Br J Surg*. 1973;60(8):646–649.

may be carried out following shared decision-making between the physician and the patient.

Other interventional radiological procedures

Balloon-occluded retrograde transvenous obliteration (BRTO)

BRTO of gastric varices may be used to occlude gastric varices that are bleeding or at risk for bleeding. Such a technique is possible when a large splenorenal shunt is identified on abdominal cross-sectional imaging. The splenorenal shunt is catheterized via the left renal vein using a femoral vein approach or via an existing TIPS or via a transjugular approach. The gastric varices are embolized with coils following occlusion of the shunt with a balloon. The long-term durability of the variceal obliteration is uncertain, but BRTO has been used for both the prevention and control of gastric variceal bleeding increasingly because of its safety and efficacy in treating gastric varices.[8]

Surgical procedures to treat complications of portal hypertension

Surgical treatment of portal hypertension includes three groups of procedures: (1) non-shunt interventions, (2) portosystemic shunts, and (3) liver transplantation. Liver transplantation is a definitive procedure for portal hypertension and is reliably associated with increased survival as compared with all other interventions in patients with cirrhosis. Liver transplantation which should be considered in all patients with cirrhosis who have a variceal bleed is discussed in Chapter 13. Surgical procedures (other than liver transplantation) are rescue therapies when a combination of pharmacological and endoscopic procedures is unable to control variceal bleed or prevent recurrent bleeding. Patients with non-cirrhotic causes of portal hypertension (portal vein thrombosis and idiopathic non-cirrhotic portal hypertension or non-cirrhotic portal fibrosis) and the rare patient with CTP class A cirrhosis when the expertise to carry out TIPS is not available are candidates for surgical procedures. Surgical treatment in patients with non-cirrhotic portal hypertension after even a single bleeding episode may be considered when patients live at a great distance from centres with the expertise to treat variceal bleeding or in patients with rare blood types. Failure of standard therapy is not well defined and is best individualized depending on the patient's circumstances and available resources.

Non-shunt surgical procedures

Non-shunt procedures, which include oesophageal transection and gastro-oesophageal devascularization, are performed infrequently nowadays. Oesophageal transection which involves transecting and stapling the oesophagus used to be highly effective in controlling variceal bleeding and was associated with a lower risk of encephalopathy than portosystemic shunts. It was considered when endoscopic therapy could not control variceal bleeding but was not found to be superior to endoscopic therapy. Oesophageal transection for variceal bleeding, thus, may be an obsolete procedure.

Devascularization procedures are carried out to prevent recurrent variceal bleeding in patients with portal vein thrombosis when a portal vein branch at least 8 mm in diameter is not available for creation of a portosystemic shunt. Gastro-oesophageal devascularization is combined with a splenectomy and is carried out via an abdominal approach or laparoscopically. The operation requires total devascularization of the greater curve of the stomach, the upper two-thirds of the lesser curve of the stomach, and circumferential devascularization of the lower 7.5 cm of the oesophagus. The rate of recurrent bleeding following this procedure may be as high as 40%.[9]

Mesenterico–left portal venous bypass ('Rex shunt')

The mesenterico–left portal venous bypass, or Rex shunt, is carried out in patients with extrahepatic portal vein thrombosis when the intrahepatic portion of the left portal vein is patent.[10] The operation is called a Rex shunt since the anastomosis to the left portal vein is in the recessus of Rex which is where the left portal vein divides to supply segments III and IV of the liver. A jugular vein graft may be used to bridge the superior mesenteric vein to the intrahepatic portion of the left portal vein in the Rex recessus. The Rex shunt is not a true portosystemic shunt since the procedure involves restoring portal blood flow by bypassing the occluded extrahepatic portal vein segment; no portal blood is shunted into the systemic venous system. Children who undergo a mesenterico–left portal vein bypass have a reduction in the risk of hepatic encephalopathy and long-term learning disability. Therefore, the Rex shunt is the preferred surgical procedure when feasible in children with extrahepatic portal venous obstruction. Because of limited data on the efficacy of endoscopic or pharmacological therapy in children, the Rex bypass is recommended for secondary prophylaxis of variceal bleeding in patients with extrahepatic portal vein obstruction whenever surgical expertise is available. The procedure is also carried out in adults in whom portal vein thrombosis develops following liver transplantation.[11]

Portosystemic shunts

Surgical shunts are seldom carried out for refractory variceal bleeding in patients with cirrhosis since TIPS is widely available. Surgical shunts are carried out almost exclusively for refractory bleeding due to non-cirrhotic portal hypertension, such as in patients with idiopathic portal hypertension, congenital hepatic fibrosis, and portal vein thrombosis. Portosystemic shunts are carried out even in the absence of variceal bleeding in some patients with portal cavernomas where cholangiopathy results in biliary obstruction (portal cavernoma cholangiopathy).[12]

Depending on the degree of portal blood shunted into the systemic circulation, surgical portosystemic shunts are classified as *selective shunts*, such as a distal splenorenal shunt; *partial shunts*, such as a side-to-side calibrated portacaval shunt; and *total shunts*. Total shunts completely divert portal flow and include, among other shunts, the portacaval shunt.

Selective portosystemic shunts

The most widely used selective shunt is the distal splenorenal shunt (DSRS) originally described by Dr W. Dean Warren.[13] With the DSRS shunt, only varices at the gastro-oesophageal junction and spleen are decompressed. Portal hypertension in the superior mesenteric vein and portal vein is not corrected. Thus, variceal bleeding is controlled whereas the risk of ascites remains. In carrying out the DSRS shunt a portoazygos disconnection is required followed by an

Surgical procedures to treat complications of portal hypertension

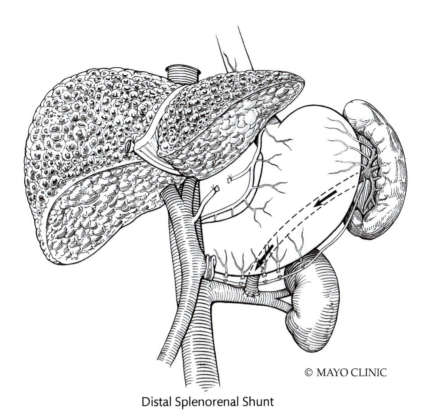

Distal Splenorenal Shunt

Figure 14.2 Distal splenorenal shunt. The distal end of the splenic vein is anastomosed to the side of the left renal vein. The right gastric, left gastric, and right gastroepiploic veins and all branches to the gastroepiploic vein are ligated. However, the short gastric veins are preserved, to decompress the gastro-oesophageal junction through the shunt. Portal hypertension persists in the superior mesenteric and portal veins and ascites does not improve.
Reproduced with permission of Mayo Foundation for Medical Education and Research, all rights reserved.

end-to-side anastomosis between the splenic vein and left renal vein (Figure 14.2). The splenic vein is disconnected from the superior mesenteric vein and is separated from the pancreas with ligation of all its collaterals. The entire length of the pancreas requires mobilization and the left adrenal vein is ligated. The portal system is thus disconnected from the azygos system to allow flow from the gastro-oesophageal junction through the short gastric veins into the splenic vein. The splenic vein is then anastomosed to the left renal vein, end to side. Following a DSRS, variceal bleeding is prevented in approximately 90% of patients with a lower rate of hepatic encephalopathy than with total shunts.

Partial portosystemic shunts

Any shunt with a diameter less than 12 mm using an interposition graft or a direct vein-to-vein anastomosis results in partially diverting portal blood flow.

The typical partial portosystemic shunt requires using a synthetic interposition graft between the portal vein or superior mesenteric vein and the inferior vena cava (Figure 14.3). Antegrade flow in the portal vein is maintained by using an 8 mm diameter graft which usually results in reducing portal pressure to less than 12 mmHg. Rates of preventing variceal rebleeding and encephalopathy following this shunt are comparable to DSRS. Like patients who have undergone a DSRS, ascites occurs in approximately 20% of patients with partial portosystemic shunts since hepatic sinusoidal pressure is not reduced.[14]

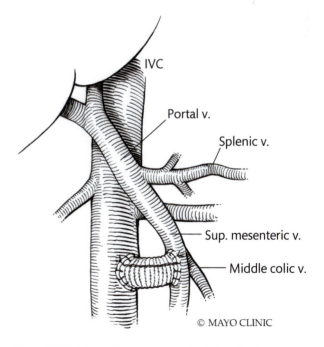

Figure 14.3 Interposition mesocaval shunt. A synthetic graft is interposed between the superior mesenteric vein and the inferior vena cava (IVC). A graft 8 mm in diameter reduces portal hypertension while maintaining some antegrade portal blood flow.
Reproduced with permission of Mayo Foundation for Medical Education and Research, all rights reserved.

Total portosystemic shunts

Total shunts include the end-to-side portacaval shunt (Eck fistula) (Figure 14.4), side-to-side portacaval shunt, large-diameter interposition shunts, and the conventional splenorenal shunt (Figure 14.5). Hepatic sinusoidal pressure is reduced with total shunts, thus reducing the risk of ascites.

Only the side-to-side portacaval shunt is in current use. Any interpositional shunt greater than 12 mm in diameter functions as a total shunt. Variceal bleeding and ascites are well controlled because the hepatic sinusoids are decompressed. Side-to-side portacaval shunts may be carried out occasionally in patients with Budd–Chiari syndrome. Surgical side-to-side portacaval shunts were previously also carried out in a small number of centres as an emergency procedure to control oesophageal variceal haemorrhage. Given that TIPS may be carried out with a lower risk of mortality and morbidity, surgical portosystemic shunts are not used any longer in patients with cirrhosis. In patients with non-cirrhotic portal hypertension where a markedly enlarged spleen is associated with abdominal discomfort and hypersplenism, a splenectomy with a splenorenal shunt may be indicated (Figure 14.5). Results of splenectomy with splenorenal shunt in children with extrahepatic portal vein thrombosis causing portal hypertension are particularly encouraging.[15]

Though hepatic encephalopathy occurs in 30–40% of patients following a total shunt, variceal rebleeding occurs in less than 10% of patients. Patients who have had a portacaval shunt previously may have an increased risk of operative morbidity and intraoperative transfusion requirements when undergoing liver transplantation. However, the long-term outcomes of transplant are not significantly different from patients who have not had a portacaval shunt. Nevertheless, it is recommended that surgical portacaval shunts be avoided in patients who are potential candidates for liver transplantation.

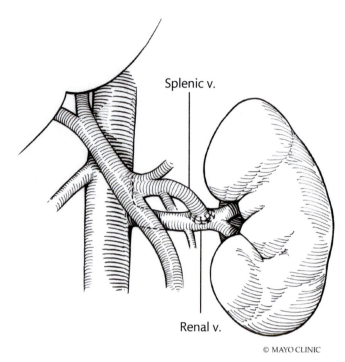

Figure 14.5 Splenectomy with splenorenal shunt. An end-to-side anastomosis is performed between the splenic vein and the left renal vein following splenectomy.

Reproduced with permission of Mayo Foundation for Medical Education and Research, all rights reserved.

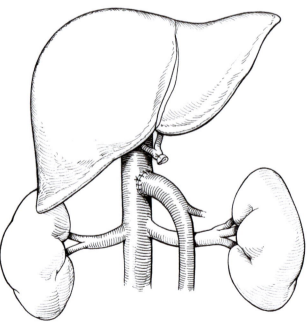

Figure 14.4 End-to-side portacaval shunt. The portal vein is ligated into the hilum of the liver and the distal portion of the portal vein is anastomosed to the infrahepatic inferior vena cava. An end-to-side portacaval shunt does not reduce hepatic sinusoidal pressure and ascites persists. This shunt is no longer performed.

Reproduced with permission of Mayo Foundation for Medical Education and Research, all rights reserved.

Transjugular intrahepatic portosystemic shunts versus surgical portosystemic shunts

A surgical portosystemic shunt may be preferred over TIPS in selected patients with non-cirrhotic portal hypertension when expertise is available. Meta-analyses suggest the benefit of surgical shunting over TIPS for treatment of refractory or recurrent variceal haemorrhage even in patients with CTP class A cirrhosis because of improved survival and less frequent shunt failure.[16] However, the studies included mostly patients undergoing TIPS with bare-metal stents which are associated with a higher risk of shunt stenosis. Given the very low certainty of the available evidence and risks of random errors in the analyses, firm conclusions cannot be drawn.[17] Thus, surgical portosystemic shunts are best reserved for patients with non-cirrhotic portal hypertension.

REFERENCES

1. Nardelli S, Riggio O, Turco L, et al. Relevance of spontaneous portosystemic shunts detected with CT in patients with cirrhosis. *Radiology.* 2021;**299**(1):133–140.
2. Talwalkar JA, Swanson KL, Krowka MJ, Andrews JC, Kamath PS. Prevalence of spontaneous portosystemic shunts in patients with portopulmonary hypertension and effect on treatment. *Gastroenterology.* 2011;**141**(5):1673–1679.

3. Nicoara-Farcau O, Han G, Rudler M, et al. Effects of early placement of transjugular portosystemic shunts in patients with high-risk acute variceal bleeding: a meta-analysis of individual patient data. *Gastroenterology*. 2021;**160**(1):193–205.
4. Halabi SA, Sawas T, Sadat B, et al. Early TIPS versus endoscopic therapy for secondary prophylaxis after management of acute esophageal variceal bleeding in cirrhotic patients: a meta-analysis of randomized controlled trials. *J Gastroenterol Hepatol*. 2016;**31**(9):1519–1526.
5. Plaz Torres MC, Best LM, Freeman SC, et al. Secondary prevention of variceal bleeding in adults with previous oesophageal variceal bleeding due to decompensated liver cirrhosis: a network meta-analysis. *Cochrane Database Syst Rev*. 2021;**3**(3):CD013122.
6. Sarwar A, Zhou L, Novack V, Tapper EB, Curry M, Malik R, Ahmed M. Hospital volume and mortality after transjugular intrahepatic portosystemic shunt creation in the United States. *Hepatology*. 2018;**67**(2):690–699.
7. Malinchoc M, Kamath PS, Gordon FD, Peine CJ, Rank J, ter Borg PC. A model to predict poor survival in patients undergoing transjugular intrahepatic portosystemic shunts. *Hepatology*. 2000;**31**(4):864–871.
8. Lee EW, Shahrouki P, Alanis L, Ding P, Kee ST. Management options for gastric variceal hemorrhage. *JAMA Surg*. 2019;**154**(6):540–548.
9. Caps MT, Helton WS, Johansen K. Left-upper-quadrant devascularization for 'unshuntable' portal hypertension. *Arch Surg*. 1996;**131**(8):834–838.
10. di Francesco F, Grimaldi C, de Ville de Goyet J. Meso-Rex bypass—a procedure to cure prehepatic portal hypertension: the insight and the inside. *J Am Coll Surg*. 2014;**218**(2):e23–e36.
11. Han D, Tang R, Wang L, Li A, Huang X, Shen S, Dong J. Case report of a modified Meso-Rex bypass as a treatment technique for late-onset portal vein cavernous transformation with portal hypertension after adult deceased-donor liver transplantation. *Medicine (Baltimore)*. 2017;**96**(25):e7208.
12. Dhiman RK, Saraswat VA, Valla DC, et al. Portal cavernoma cholangiopathy: consensus statement of a working party of the Indian national association for study of the liver. *J Clin Exp Hepatol*. 2014;**4**(Suppl 1):S2–S14.
13. Richards WO. W. Dean Warren, MD, FACS, Father of selective shunts for variceal hemorrhage: lessons learned. *Am Surg*. 2020;**86**(9):1049–1055.
14. Henderson JM. The distal splenorenal shunt. *Surg Clin North Am*. 1990;**70**(2):405–423.
15. Prasad AS, Gupta S, Kohli V, Pande GK, Sahni P, Nundy S. Proximal splenorenal shunts for extrahepatic portal venous obstruction in children. *Ann Surg*. 1994;**219**(2):193–196.
16. Clark W, Hernandez J, McKeon B, et al. Surgical shunting versus transjugular intrahepatic portasystemic shunting for bleeding varices resulting from portal hypertension and cirrhosis: a meta-analysis. *Am Surg*. 2010;**76**(8):857–864.
17. Brand M, Prodehl L, Ede CJ. Surgical portosystemic shunts versus transjugular intrahepatic portosystemic shunt for variceal haemorrhage in people with cirrhosis. *Cochrane Database Syst Rev*. 2018;**10**(10):CD001023.

15

Budd–Chiari syndrome, veno-occlusive disease, and secondary vascular diseases of the liver

Patricia Sánchez-Velázquez and Fernando Burdío

Budd–Chiari syndrome

Budd–Chiari syndrome (BCS) is a clinical disorder resulting from the obstruction of the hepatic venous outflow, whatever the cause of its obstruction, which can be traced back to the small hepatic venules at the entrance to the inferior vein cava[1] (**Figure 15.1**). However, the syndrome has a variable clinical presentation, depending on the number of hepatic veins involved, the degree of venous obstruction, and the speed at which the thrombosis occurs. Since Chiari recorded the first ten cases in 1899, more than 8000 cases of BCS have been described in the medical literature.[2] Even though BCS remains a relatively uncommon condition, its incidence has now increased

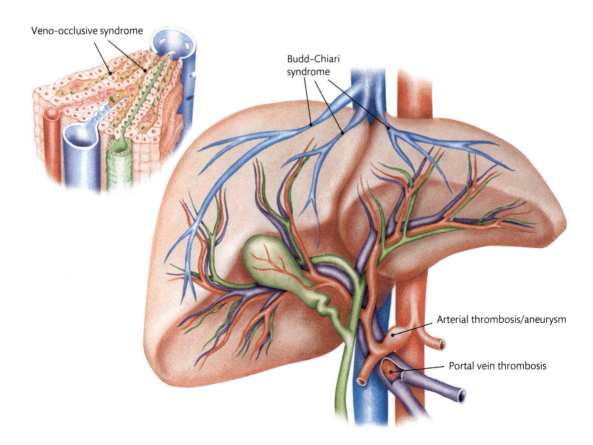

Figure 15.1 Representative picture of the vascular disorders of the liver, which affect the liver inflow and outflow.

substantially (to around 1 per million per year) probably as a result of more accurate diagnostic imaging and the widespread use of thrombogenic agents, such as oral contraceptives.[1,2] BCS may progress to death from liver failure in weeks, months, or even years, according to the rapidity and extent of the outflow obstruction, usually from bleeding from oesophageal varices. However, this dismal prognosis has improved in recent years with the adoption of a stepwise approach that includes less invasive measures, such as the transjugular intrahepatic portosystemic shunt (TIPS), while liver transplantation remains a good option when conservative measures fail.[1-5]

Aetiology

In Parker's classical description of 1959, the predisposing conditions for BCS were unknown in 70% of the patients while in recent studies (Table 15.1), this figure has dropped to less than 30%. In three recent wide-ranging European studies, a number of factors or predisposing conditions have been described in most patients[6-8] (Table 15.1). Multiple prothrombotic conditions are found in 15–20% of patients, suggesting that when one of the causal factors is identified, additional factors should be investigated. Conversely, no risk factor was found in some patients.[1] In studies with large patient populations in the United States, the most frequent predisposing conditions are myeloproliferative neoplasms such as polycythaemia vera, essential thrombocythaemia and primary myelofibrosis.[9] In these populations the JAK2 mutation is especially frequent,[10] although this mutation may also be an independent risk factor for BCS itself (Table 15.1). Other causes include paroxysmal nocturnal haemoglobinuria, antiphospholipid syndrome, and inherited protein C or S and antithrombin III deficiencies. In a number of patients with BCS, protein C deficiency has also been associated with a myeloproliferative disorder.[9]

BCS may also develop during pregnancy or in the postpartum state within a few weeks or months after delivery, while many cases occur in women taking oral contraceptives. Although a definitive causative link is lacking, a multicentre case–control study suggested that the relative risk of hepatic vein thrombosis is 2.37, which is similar to the relative risk of stroke, myocardial infarction, and venous thromboembolism in women taking oral contraceptives.[11] A number of infectious diseases may also be associated with BCS, including amoebic abscess, aspergillosis, or hydatid disease. Rare causes or predisposing factors are systemic diseases (e.g. connective disease disorders), abdominal surgery, or trauma. However, regional variations between East and West must be taken into account, as some conditions that are rare in the West are frequent in the East. For example, membranous obstruction of the vena cava, which is almost unknown in the West is one of the most frequent conditions seen in the East, as are infections such as amoebiasis.[1,12]

Clinical manifestations and diagnosis

Clinical manifestations of BCS are extremely heterogeneous and may vary from severe forms of acute liver failure to asymptomatic forms accidentally diagnosed when studying mild alterations of the liver enzymes.[1,9] The diagnosis is generally made after complications related to portal hypertension, mainly ascites, occur. Ascites (83%), hepatomegaly (67%), and abdominal pain (61%) were the most frequent clinical manifestations in a European cohort of 163 BCS patients,[13] in which 58% of the patients had oesophageal varices at diagnosis. Although less common, acute liver failure may be the initial presentation in around 5% of cases. This wide range of clinical presentations probably correlates with both time to establishment and extension of the hepatic vein thrombosis. Obstruction of a hepatic vein can promote the development of collateral circulation and the patient remains asymptomatic. Typical laboratory findings are aminotransferase elevation reflecting subjacent necrosis and a decrease in prothrombin time in severe cases. Another clinical finding in these patients is the presence of benign regenerative nodules in around 60–70% of pathology studies[14] but in only 36% in an imaging study.[15] Less frequently, patients with BCS may also develop hepatocellular carcinoma. A systematic review of 16 studies that reported hepatocellular carcinoma prevalence in BCS highlights huge differences in the reported rates, ranging from 2.0% to 46.2%. This is probably due, at least in part, to the heterogeneity of the studies included: geographical differences, dissimilar follow-up times, diverse enrolment periods, different diagnostic tools and treatments, and different survivals rates.[16] Hepatocellular carcinoma surveillance is recommended in all cases of patients with chronic BCS; while 6-monthly ultrasound (US) is the most widely endorsed strategy.[1]

BCS should be suspected in any patient with acute or chronic liver disease, especially when its aetiology is unknown and/or if there is

Table 15.1 Risk factors for Budd–Chiari syndrome in three recent European cohort studies

	N tested (% positive)
Acquired conditions	
Myeloproliferative neoplasms	168 (41%)
JAK2^{V617F} mutation	168 (35%)
Antiphospholipid syndrome	165 (10%)
Paroxysmal nocturnal haemoglobinuria	152 (7%)
Inherited hypercoagulable conditions	
Factor V Leyden	165 (8%)
Factor II gene mutation	168 (3%)
Protein C deficiency	150 (5%)
Protein S deficiency	147 (4%)
Antithrombin deficiency	153 (1%)
External factors	
Recent pregnancy	168 (1%)
Recent oral contraceptive use	168 (22%)
Systemic diseases	168 (6%)
Connective tissue disease	
Coelic disease	
Behçet's disease	
Mastocytosis	
Inflammatory bowel disease	
Human immunodeficiency virus infection	
Sarcoidosis	
Myeloma	
Inflammatory intrabdominal lesions	168 (2%)
Acute pancreatitis	
Biliary infection	
Intestinal infection	
Intrabdominal surgery	168 (1%)
Abdominal trauma	168 (1%)
>1 risk factor	168 (19%)
No cause	168 (24%)

Reproduced with permission from Hernández et al. Current knowledge in pathophysiology and management of Budd-Chiari syndrome and non-cirrhotic non-tumoral splanchnic vein thrombosis. J Hepatol. 2019;71(1):175–199.

an underlying prothrombotic condition. The key feature is to demonstrate obstruction of the hepatic venous outflow. Non-invasive imaging techniques (Doppler US, computed tomography, or magnetic resonance imaging) are the mainstays of an adequate diagnosis. Direct signs include visualization of the occluded veins, presence of endoluminal thrombi in the hepatic vein, non-visualization of the hepatic vein, stagnant or inverted venous flow, and collateral networks, all of which are most frequently found in acute BCS. Chronic forms are usually associated with indirect signs such as hypertrophy of the caudate lobe, a caudate vein larger than 3 mm and concomitant atrophic lobes, a dysmorphic liver, parenchymal heterogeneity, heterogeneous enhancement, and benign regenerative nodules. Hepatic venography is only recommended if the diagnosis remains uncertain, even though the above-cited investigations classically reveal a spider's web pattern, formed by a rich collateral circulation[1,9] (Figure 15.2).

Prognosis and management

The prognosis of BCS has dramatically changed in the last decade, with an improvement in survival rates as a consequence of better management based on anticoagulation, TIPS, and liver transplantations.[4,5] Several parameters or combinations of parameters can be used to predict BCS prognosis. Liver function tests such as the Child–Pugh[17] and Model for End-stage Liver Disease scores are able to predict BCS outcomes[18] but BCS-specific prognostic scores such as BCS-TIPS can also identify patients with poor outcomes, despite TIPS[19] or BCS-specific scores for predicting transplant-free survival.[20]

BCS management is based on recommendations from clinical experience, retrospective studies, and expert consensus, since randomized clinical studies are still lacking. The current BCS treatment strategy thus relies on progressively escalating invasiveness[4,5,13] (Figure 15.3):

1. Anticoagulation should be administered to all patients, even those without an underlying prothrombotic disorder or those who are initially asymptomatic, to attempt to reduce the risk of clot extension and new thrombotic episodes.[1,4] Either low-molecular-weight heparin or vitamin antagonists are the treatment of choice to initiate anticoagulation.

2. Reports of thrombolysis in BCS are limited. Recombinant tissue plasminogen activator, streptokinase, or urokinase have been used through a peripheral vein or locally after catheterization of the thrombosed vein. These agents may be useful in patients with recent and incomplete thrombosis, usually combined with angioplasty stenting to restore venous outflow,[21] but as bleeding complications with these techniques may be fatal,[22] thrombolysis should only be attempted in selected cases with acute or subacute BCS at experienced centres.[1,4]

3. Percutaneous angioplasty is an effective and safe approach for restoring the physiological hepatic outflow, with or without stenting, in segmental stenosis in the cranial part of a hepatic vein or the suprahepatic inferior vein cava.[1,4] However, as this is only found in a small percentage of patients, this technique would only benefit a small proportions of BCS patients.[5] While stenting may reduce restenosis, stent misplacement may make future TIPS or liver transplantation more challenging.[1]

4. Derivative techniques are to be used when the aforementioned treatments are not possible or fail to solve the obstruction. Before the 1990s, surgical shunts (mesocaval, portocaval, or mesocaval–atrial shunts) were the mainstay treatments in this setting[23,24] but were generally associated with significant

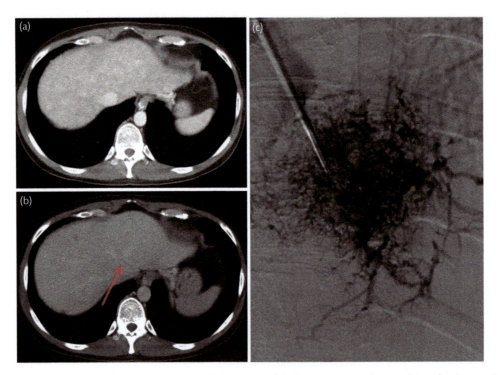

Figure 15.2 (a) Computed tomography scan shows absence of enhancement of the hepatic veins in the portal specific phase; only in the late phase (b) can the suprahepatic veins (arrow) just be distinguished. (c) Spider's web pattern after vein opacification in venography.
Reproduced courtesy of Dr Marta Solá, Parc Taulí Hospital, Sabadell.

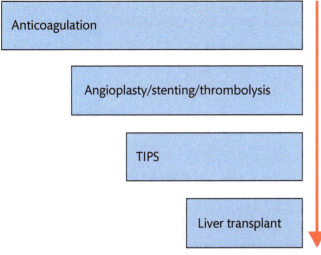

Figure 15.3 Recommend stepwise therapeutic algorithm of BCS.[4,5]
Adapted with permission from Garcia-Pagán JC, Buscarini E, Janssen HLA, et al. EASL Clinical Practice Guidelines: vascular diseases of the liver. *J Hepatol*. 2016;64(1):179-202. doi:10.1016/j.jhep.2015.07.040

morbidity and mortality. However, in patients surviving surgery in whom the shunt remains patent, the outcome was excellent.[25] In any case, since the 1990s surgical shunts have mostly been replaced by less invasive techniques like TIPS, which has been shown to be more effective in maintaining patency and is associated with lower mortality and morbidity in patients with failed medical treatment or when recanalization has failed.[4]

5. Liver transplants in patients with BCS may represent a technical challenge because of the presence of retroperitoneal fibrosis related to hepatic vein thrombosis, liver enlargement or adhesions, while the classic 'piggyback' technique becomes more challenging due to the larger caudate lobe and occlusion of the hepatic vein ostia.[1,26] A large European study showed good actuarial survival rates of 76%, 71%, and 68% at 1, 5, and 10 years, respectively.[27]

Veno-occlusive disease/sinusoidal obstruction syndrome

As a rare cause of posthepatic portal hypertension, veno-occlusive disease (VOD) is characterized by primary damage to the sublobular venules in the absence of thrombosis of the major hepatic veins, unlike the BCS, which leads to postsinusoidal obstruction and can seriously jeopardize patients' lives.

Aetiology

Despite the many situations that can lead to VOD, the illness was first recognized in Jamaica in the mid 1950s by Bras et al.[28] and soon after in Africa[29] in children who ingested comfrey herb tea, which is now known to be rich in pyrrolizidine alkaloids. The patients presented with jaundice and abdominal tenderness, followed by either acute or subacute liver failure. At that time an occlusive process involving the terminal branches of the venous tree had already been recognized as a common feature in biopsies.

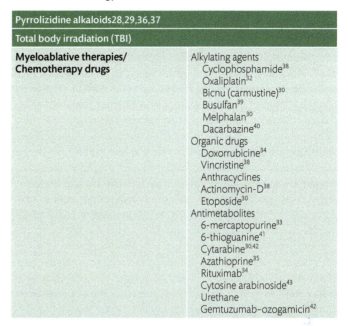

Table 15.2 Aetiology of veno-occlusive disease

Pyrrolizidine alkaloids[28,29,36,37]	
Total body irradiation (TBI)	
Myeloablative therapies/ Chemotherapy drugs	Alkylating agents 　Cyclophosphamide[38] 　Oxaliplatin[32] 　Bicnu (carmustine)[30] 　Busulfan[39] 　Melphalan[30] 　Dacarbazine[40] Organic drugs 　Doxorrubicine[34] 　Vincristine[38] 　Anthracyclines 　Actinomycin-D[38] 　Etoposide[30] Antimetabolites 　6-mercaptopurine[33] 　6-thioguanine[41] 　Cytarabine[30,42] 　Azathioprine[35] 　Rituximab[34] 　Cytosine arabinoside[43] 　Urethane 　Gemtuzumab–ozogamicin[42]

Nowadays, VOD, also known as the sinusoidal obstruction syndrome (SOS), occurs most frequently as a consequence of myeloablative regimens before haematopoietic stem cell transplantation (HSCT).[30] These 'conditioning' regimens include high-dose cytotoxic drugs together with or without total body irradiation. BEAM schema (bicnu, etoposide, cytarabine, and melphalan)[30] or busulfan and cyclophosphamide in combination are the most commonly used therapies which are known to present the highest incidence of VOD.[31] Prolonged exposure to other conventional chemotherapeutic agents such as oxaliplatin,[32] 6-mercaptopurine,[33] R-CHOP regimen as treatment of non-Hodgkin lymphoma,[34] or immunosuppressive drugs after an organ transplant,[35] are also linked to VOD to a lesser extent. Table 15.2 summarizes the reported causes related to VOD.

Incidence

The VOD incidence varies widely according to the intensity of the conditioning regimen, the clinical diagnostic criteria applied, and most importantly the presence or absence of risk factors. Some well-known individual risk factors favour its appearance, such as pre-existent liver disease (hepatitis C virus, hepatic cirrhosis), use of norethisterone in women, or individual carriers of the haemochromatosis C282Y allele mutation,[44] but there are also even more important hepatic-related and transplant-related factors, which have an enormous impact on VOD development.[31] Historically, VOD/SOS was reported to occur in up to 60% of patients undergoing HSCT; however, it seems that the real incidence is lower than believed, around 14%,[45] but it is still burdened with a high mortality rate due to multiorgan failure in severe cases.

Clinical manifestations and diagnosis

Due to sinusoidal occlusion, VOD usually presents initially with signs of portal hypertension, that is, weight gain with or without ascites, right upper quadrant pain, hepatomegaly, and jaundice. The problem is, however, that as the chronology of the disease is somewhat dynamic, these clinical features vary widely in severity from mild VOD/SOS to multiorgan failure and death, which makes diagnosis challenging. After ruling out other potential causes and in the absence of serological diagnostic markers, diagnosis has to be by consensus criteria, classically the Baltimore[46] and Seattle criteria,[47] which have in common serum bilirubin greater than 2 mg/dL, tender hepatomegaly, and weight gain due to fluid accumulation. The European Society for Blood and Marrow Transplantation updated criteria[31] now include a compendium of both with a timing differentiation in terms of early/late onset within 21 days after HSCT.

Imaging techniques such as US were claimed in the 1990s to be the gold standard for VOD diagnosis; however, over time, no strong correlation has been found between the US findings and the presence of VOD, as US does not identify specific abnormalities, but simply signs of portal hypertension, which preclude accurate diagnosis in the early onset of symptoms. An attempt has been made to standardize criteria, so that they can now be summarized as seven items: hepatomegaly, splenomegaly, ascites and portal venous flow alterations, portal vein (PV) diameter greater than 12 mm, gallbladder wall thickening greater than 6 mm, hepatic veins less than 3 mm, and visualization of the paraumbilical veins.[48]

Nevertheless, the gold standard for confirming the diagnosis is hepatic venous gradient measurement together with transjugular biopsy,[49] but this technique is not available in all centres and is potentially burdened with complications in the case of severe coagulopathy. Liver biopsy shows similar results in all scenarios (Figure 15.4): centrilobular bands of sinusoidal congestion secondary to the swollen endothelial cells, which all together obstruct the sinusoidal blood flow. No hepatocytes necrosis is usually revealed, but rather a high rate of centrilobular fibrosis, whereby the small hepatic veins will be partially occluded.[50]

Treatment and prevention

Treatment of VOD/SOD depends largely on the severity of the clinical manifestations. Up to 85% of the patients will recover spontaneously with only supportive treatment such as diuretics, sodium restriction, and paracentesis, as they suffer only a mild variant. In some exceptional cases a TIPS could be useful to decompress the portal circulation and control the ascites. Few cases have been reported of VOD treated by liver transplantation,[51-53] which is only possible in cases of benign disease and because most HSCT causes have an underlying malignancy in their background, liver transplantation for VOD is practically anecdotal.

Portal vein thrombosis/extrahepatic portal vein obstruction

Acute or chronic, portal vein thrombosis (PVT) involves the closure of the main PV and can in some cases seriously jeopardize the patient's life. This condition is present more often than is thought, as has been shown in a Swedish study that demonstrated the prevalence of PVT in autopsies in nearly 1% of the population.[54,55] However, the time of the onset, either acute or chronic, together with the location and completeness of the PVT are fundamental in its clinical implications, management, and prognosis. Despite these differences in treatment and severity, the aetiology of both entities is quite similar. The first cause of PVT is hepatic cirrhosis,[56,57] followed by abdominal

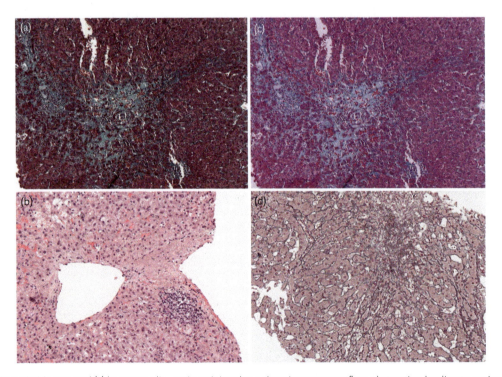

Figure 15.4 (a) Tricromic Masson and (c) haematoxylin–eosin staining show chronic venous outflow obstruction leading to perivenular fibrosis, pericellular fibrosis, and central fibrous bridges characteristic from the SOS. In detail (b) medium power imaging haematoxylin–eosin staining shows occlusion of terminal hepatic veins by cellular debris and retained erythrocytes, with partial fibrotic organization. (d) Perisinusoidal fibrosis and occlusion of the lumen of the venule is easily identified by using special stains for connective tissue (reticuline).
Reproduced courtesy of Dr Alba Díaz Lorca, Hospital Clinic, Barcelona.

cancer or an inflammatory focus in the abdomen.[53] When these frequent causes can be ruled out, most of the non-cirrhotic, non-oncological patients suffer from prothrombotic conditions, with factor V Leiden mutation,[58,59] antiphospholipid syndrome, and protein C and S deficiency[60] being the most common.

There are, however, special situations which have to be considered separately, such as direct injury to the portal venous system after surgery (i.e. splenectomy,[61] liver transplantation,[62,63] and hepatectomy) because these will require a particular treatment approach and thus will have a special mention in this chapter.

Below we focus on the details of acute compared to chronic PVT in non-cirrhotic patients, while having the same aetiological background requires a different approach.

Acute portal vein thrombosis

This is defined as the sudden obstruction of the PV, which can vary in length and completeness and extend downstream to the right/left portal branches[64] or upstream to the superior mesenteric vein (SMV) and splenic vein.[64]

The clinical manifestations are mid-abdominal and colicky pain in about 90% of cases and in most instances accompanied by ascites, while the liver enzymes are rarely increased.[65] Up to 50% of patients can develop fever and elevation of inflammatory parameters such as C-reactive protein. Abdominal symptomatology can sometimes be subclinical, so that in some cases PVT is first diagnosed when signs of gastrointestinal bleeding due to portal hypertension appear.[66] The most severe and life-threatening complication of acute PVT is small bowel infarction, as impairment of the visceral outflow can easily lead to bowel wall infarction and peritonitis.[67]

The first-line approach for PVT diagnosis is usually US,[68] which has a high sensitivity, ranging between 88% and 98%.[69] Several classifications have been proposed to stratify PVT, the most extensive perhaps being that described by Yerdel et al.,[70] initially conceived to assess PVT before liver transplantation and thus perhaps the most accurate. It grades the PVT from grade 1 to 4, which varies from minimal or partial thrombosis of the PV (thrombosis <50% of the lumen), with or without minimal extension into the SMV, to a complete thrombosis of the PV and SMV (proximal and distal).

In the absence of an experienced operator, the alternative to diagnosis is contrast-enhanced abdominal computed tomography[68] in the portal phase (Figure 15.5), which also gives an excellent insight into the small bowel situation and other intra-abdominal pitfalls.

Overall, anticoagulation therapy is the first treatment option for acute PVT, with the double aim of achieving recanalization of the PV and avoiding extension of the thrombosis. A prospective trial[65] demonstrated the benefit of early treatment with heparin-based anticoagulation therapies in terms of thrombus extension and achieving a partial recanalization rate of 30% in the main PV and up to 60% in the SMV/splenic vein at 6-month follow-up. However, the treatment length and the onset of heparin-based therapies are still controversial, even though most studies agree on starting the anticoagulation early in the clinical course and maintaining it for at least 3–6 months, according to the radiological development of the thrombus.[4,63,71] Bleeding complications derived from anticoagulation have been described as less than 5%.[64]

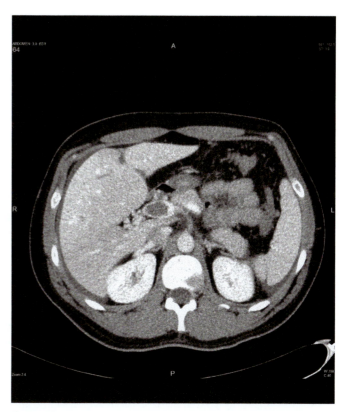

Figure 15.5 Computed tomography scan in portal specific phase shows a subtotal thrombosis of the portal vein without signs of hepatic damage.
Reproduced courtesy of Dr A. Radosevic, Hospital del Mar, Barcelona.

Other interventional approaches (surgical thrombectomy, systemic or *in situ* thrombolysis, or TIPS) are emerging alternatives in this setting, but are still not widespread. All these techniques are applied mostly in cases of bowel infarction or clinical impairment because their effectiveness has not yet been shown to be superior to the classic medical approach, although they are burdened with a high complication rate.

Mechanical thrombectomy involves percutaneous access to the PV system (i.e. normally by the transhepatic approach), and restoring the flow within the PV by balloon thrombectomy, rheolytic thrombectomy, or suction thrombectomy.[72,73] The latter consists of inflating the balloon past the clot in order to pull it away, followed by an angioplasty,[74] while rheolytic thrombectomy applies a device to fragment the clot, allowing passive thrombus evacuation.[72] Thrombolysis by the jugular route has shown an encouraging success rate of 53% complete recanalization, but only in small patient cohorts,[75,76] therefore the results have to be handled with caution.

Surgical exploration with or without surgical thrombolysis[77] is reserved for patients with suspected peritonitis secondary to small bowel infarction, in which bowel resection could be extensive with a large necrotic delimited area. However, this necrosis can be overestimated, leading to a massive bowel resection, which will seriously jeopardize the patient's life.

Acute PVT is a special situation after a liver transplantation operation, since its clinical implications are much more severe than those described so far, and therefore in many cases can lead to retransplantation.[73]

Chronic portal vein thrombosis

From a theoretical point of view, the main difference between acute and chronic PVT is the timing of onset, which means that in the absence of re-permeabilization of the PV it is replaced by multiple collaterals, defined as a cavernomatous transformation.[4,63] This is usually associated with the development of collateral circulation in the splanchnic territory and leads to portal hypertension. Although the most common aetiology of chronic PVT is hepatic cirrhosis, which is not within the scope of this chapter, there are also cases of non-cirrhotic portal hypertension, such as prothrombotic conditions, which can follow a slightly different course.[78]

The main clinical manifestation involves upper gastrointestinal bleeding due to rupture of the oesophageal varices; however, this clinical scenario is now rare in developed countries.[79] Diagnosis is thus normally accidental during investigating other causes of hypersplenism or portal hypertension such as thrombocytopenia, splenomegaly, collateral varices on imaging, or gastropathy. Interestingly, patients with non-cirrhotic portal hypertension develop variceal bleeding earlier than cirrhotic patients.[78]

Treatment fundamentally involves two aspects: prevention of gastrointestinal bleeding and recurrent thrombosis through anticoagulation.[63] Screening for oesophageal varices and prophylactic endoscopic sclerosis[80] seems to reduce the risk of upper gastrointestinal bleeding, while very few data are available concerning TIPS, splenectomy, or surgical devascularization procedures, such as the Sugiura operation.[81]

Anticoagulation is recommended in patients with non-cirrhotic PVT due to the risk of recurrent thrombosis and also because they mostly have an underlying prothrombotic disease.[82]

Hepatic vascular malformations by hereditary haemorrhagic telangiectasia

Hereditary haemorrhagic telangiectasia, also known as Rendu–Osler–Weber syndrome, is an autosomal dominant congenital disorder, which involves vascular malformations mainly in the skin, lung, brain, and liver. Its incidence is very rare, affecting 1–2/8000,[83] although about 75% of the patients remain asymptomatic. When focusing on the liver effects of the disease it is important to perform US screening to assess vascular malformations, which will impact patient management. In its advanced state it is common to find complex changes in the hepatic artery and its branches, such as dilatation or aneurysms, with marked flow abnormalities.[4]

No treatment has been recommended for asymptomatic patients; however, those with symptomatic liver vascular malformations require intensive medical treatment either for high-output cardiac failure or for portal hypertension complications and encephalopathy. Liver transplant is the treatment of choice if the symptoms fail to respond to medical treatment.[83]

REFERENCES

1. Hernández-Gea V, De Gottardi A, Leebeek FWG, Rautou PE, Salem R, Garcia-Pagan JC. Current knowledge in pathophysiology and management of Budd-Chiari syndrome and non-cirrhotic non-tumoral splanchnic vein thrombosis. *J Hepatol.* 2019;**71**(1):175–199. doi:10.1016/j.jhep.2019.02.015
2. William R. Jarnagin MD. *Blumgart's Surgery of the Liver, Biliary Tract and Pancreas.* 6th ed. Philadelphia, PA: Elsevier; 2016. doi:0.1016/C2011-1-00123-6
3. Molmenti EP, Segev DL, Arepally A, et al. The utility of TIPS in the management of Budd-Chiari syndrome. *Ann Surg.* 2005;**241**(6):978–983. doi:10.1097/01.sla.0000164180.77824.12
4. Garcia-Pagán JC, Buscarini E, Janssen HLA, et al. EASL clinical practice guidelines: vascular diseases of the liver. *J Hepatol.* 2016;**64**(1):179–202. doi:10.1016/j.jhep.2015.07.040
5. Seijo S, Plessier A, Hoekstra J, et al. Good long-term outcome of Budd-Chiari syndrome with a step-wise management. *Hepatology.* 2013;**57**(5):1962–1968. doi:10.1002/hep.26306
6. Turon F, Cervantes F, Colomer D, Baiges A, Hernández-Gea V, Garcia-Pagán JC. Role of calreticulin mutations in the aetiological diagnosis of splanchnic vein thrombosis. *J Hepatol.* 2015;**62**(1):72–74. doi:10.1016/j.jhep.2014.08.032
7. Poisson J, Plessier A, Kiladjian J-J, et al. Selective testing for calreticulin gene mutations in patients with splanchnic vein thrombosis: a prospective cohort study. *J Hepatol.* 2017;**67**(3):501–507. doi:10.1016/j.jhep.2017.04.021
8. Bureau C, Laurent J, Robic MA, et al. Central obesity is associated with non-cirrhotic portal vein thrombosis. *J Hepatol.* 2016;**64**(2):427–432. doi:10.1016/j.jhep.2015.08.024
9. Menon KVN, Shah V, Kamath PS. The Budd–Chiari syndrome. *N Engl J Med.* 2004;**350**(6):578–585.
10. Smalberg JH, Murad SD, Braakman E, Valk PJ, Janssen HLA, Leebeek FWG. Myeloproliferative disease in the pathogenesis and survival of Budd-Chiari syndrome. *Haematologica.* 2006;**91**(12):1712–1713.
11. Valla D, Le MG, Poynard T, Zucman N, Rueff B, Benhamou JP. Risk of hepatic vein thrombosis in relation to recent use of oral contraceptives. A case-control study. *Gastroenterology.* 1986;**90**(4):807–811. doi:10.1016/0016-5085(86)90855-3
12. Jarnagin WR, Gonen M, Fong Y, et al. Improvement in perioperative outcome after hepatic resection: analysis of 1,803 consecutive cases over the past decade. *Ann Surg.* 2002;**236**(4):397–406. doi:10.1097/01.SLA.0000029003.66466.B3
13. Murad SD, Plessier A, Hernandez-Guerra M, et al. Etiology, management, and outcome of the Budd-Chiari syndrome. *Ann Intern Med.* 2009;**151**(3):167–175. doi:10.7326/0003-4819-151-3-200908040-00004
14. Tanaka M, Wanless IR. Pathology of the liver in Budd-Chiari syndrome: portal vein thrombosis and the histogenesis of venocentric cirrhosis, veno-portal cirrhosis, and large regenerative nodules. *Hepatology.* 1998;**27**(2):488–496. doi:10.1002/hep.510270224
15. Vilgrain V, Lewin M, Vons C, et al. Hepatic nodules in Budd-Chiari syndrome: imaging features. *Radiology.* 1999;**210**(2):443–450. doi:10.1148/radiology.210.2.r99fe13443
16. Ren W, Qi X, Yang Z, Han G, Fan D. Prevalence and risk factors of hepatocellular carcinoma in Budd–Chiari syndrome: a systematic review. *Eur J Gastroenterol Hepatol.* 2013;**25**(7):830–841. doi:10.1097/MEG.0b013e32835eb8d4
17. Tang TJ, Batts KP, de Groen PC, et al. The prognostic value of histology in the assessment of patients with Budd–Chiari syndrome. *J Hepatol.* 2001;**35**(3):338–343. doi:10.1016/S0168-8278(01)00131-3
18. Murad SD, Kim WR, de Groen PC, et al. Can the model for end-stage liver disease be used to predict the prognosis in patients with Budd-Chiari syndrome? *Liver Transplant.* 2007;**13**(6):867–874. doi:10.1002/lt.21171
19. Garcia–Pagán JC, Heydtmann M, Raffa S, et al. TIPS for Budd-Chiari syndrome: long-term results and prognostics

factors in 124 patients. *Gastroenterology*. 2008;**135**(3):808–815. doi:10.1053/j.gastro.2008.05.051
20. Rautou PE, Moucari R, Escolano S, et al. Prognostic indices for Budd-Chiari syndrome: valid for clinical studies but insufficient for individual management. *Am J Gastroenterol*. 2009;**104**(5):1140–1146. doi:10.1038/ajg.2009.63
21. Sharma S, Texeira A, Texeira P, Elias E, Wilde J, Olliff S. Pharmacological thrombolysis in Budd Chiari syndrome: a single centre experience and review of the literature. *J Hepatol*. 2004;**40**(1):172–180. doi:10.1016/J.JHEP.2003.09.028
22. Smalberg JH, Spaander MVMCW, Jie K-SG, et al. Risks and benefits of transcatheter thrombolytic therapy in patients with splanchnic venous thrombosis. *Thromb Haemost*. 2008;**100**(6):1084–1088.
23. Bismuth H, Sherlock DJ. Portasystemic shunting versus liver transplantation for the Budd-Chiari syndrome. *Ann Surg*. 1991;**214**(5):581–589. doi:10.1097/00000658-199111000-00008
24. Orloff MJ, Daily PO, Orloff SL, Girard B, Orloff MS. A 27-year experience with surgical treatment of Budd-Chiari syndrome. *Ann Surg*. 2000;**232**(3):340–352. doi:10.1097/00000658-200009000-00006
25. Bachet J-B, Condat B, Hagège H, et al. Long-term portosystemic shunt patency as a determinant of outcome in Budd–Chiari syndrome. *J Hepatol*. 2007;**46**(1):60–68. doi:10.1016/j.jhep.2006.08.016
26. Yoon YI, Lee SG, Moon DB, et al. Surgical techniques and long-term outcomes of living-donor liver transplantation with inferior vena cava replacement using atriocaval synthetic interposition graft for Budd-Chiari syndrome. *Ann Surg*. 2019;**269**(4):e43–e45. doi:10.1097/SLA.0000000000002847
27. Mentha G, Giostra E, Majno PE, et al. Liver transplantation for Budd–Chiari syndrome: a European study on 248 patients from 51 centres. *J Hepatol*. 2006;**44**(3):520–528. doi:10.1016/j.jhep.2005.12.002
28. Bras G, Jellife D, Stuart KL. Veno-occlusive disease of liver with nonportal type of cirrhosis. *AMA Arch Pathol*. 1954;**57**(4):285–300.
29. Stein H. Veno-occlusive disease of liver in African children. *Br Med J*. 1957;**1**(5034):1496. doi:10.1136/bmj.1.5034.1496
30. Tavernier E, Chalayer E, Cornillon J, et al. Fulminant hepatitis due to very severe sinusoidal obstruction syndrome (SOS/VOD) after autologous peripheral stem cell transplantation: a case report. *BMC Res Notes*. 2018;**11**(1):436. doi:10.1186/s13104-018-3533-0
31. Mohty M, Malard F, Abecassis M, et al. Revised diagnosis and severity criteria for sinusoidal obstruction syndrome/veno-occlusive disease in adult patients: a new classification from the European Society for Blood and Marrow Transplantation. *Bone Marrow Transplant*. 2016;**51**(7):906–912. doi:10.1038/bmt.2016.130
32. Tominaga K, Kurumiya Y, Sekoguchi E, Kobayashi S, Kawai K, Kiriyama M. Severe liver injury due to sinusoidal obstruction syndrome induced by oxaliplatin in a patient with resectable colorectal liver metastases. *Japanese J Cancer Chemother*. 2018;**45**(6):989–992.
33. McNerney KO, Vasquez JC, Kent MW, McNamara JM. Sinusoidal obstruction syndrome during maintenance therapy for acute lymphoblastic leukemia with 6-mercaptopurine and methotrexate: a pediatric case report. *J Pediatr Hematol Oncol*. 2017;**39**(8):e454–e455. doi:10.1097/MPH.0000000000000776
34. Sakumura M, Tajiri K, Miwa S, et al. Hepatic sinusoidal obstruction syndrome induced by non-transplant chemotherapy for non-Hodgkin lymphoma. *Intern Med*. 2017;**56**(4):395–400. doi:10.2169/internalmedicine.56.7669
35. Galeano Valle F, Muñoz Roldán I, Donis Sevillano E. Azathioprine-induced hepatic sinusoidal obstruction syndrome. *Med Clin (Barc)*. 2018;**151**(3):127–128. doi:10.1016/j.medcli.2017.12.012
36. Ridker PM, Mcdermott WV. Comfrey herb tea and hepatic veno-occlusive disease. *Lancet*. 1989;**333**(8639):657–658. doi:10.1016/S0140-6736(89)92154-5
37. Jelliffe DB, Bras G, Stuart KL. The clinical picture of veno-occlusive disease of the liver in Jamaican children. *Ann Trop Med Parasitol*. 1954;**48**(4):386–396. doi:10.1080/00034983.1954.11685639
38. Choi A, Kang YK, Lim S, Kim DH, Lim JS, Lee JA. Severe hepatic sinusoidal obstruction syndrome in a child receiving vincristine, actinomycin-D, and cyclophosphamide for rhabdomyosarcoma: successful treatment with defibrotide. *Cancer Res Treat*. 2016;**48**(4):1443–1447. doi:10.4143/crt.2016.096
39. Chen S, Osborn JD, Chen X, Boyer MW, McDonald GB, Hildebrandt GC. Subacute hepatic necrosis mimicking veno-occlusive disease in a patient with HFE H63D homozygosity after allogeneic hematopoietic cell transplantation with busulfan conditioning. *Int J Hematol*. 2015;**102**(6):729–731. doi:10.1007/s12185-015-1878-x
40. Houghton AN, Shafi N, Rickles FR. Acute hepatic vein thrombosis occurring during therapy for Hodgkin's disease. A case report. *Cancer*. 1979;**44**(6):2324–2329. doi:10.1002/1097-0142(197912)44:6<2324::AID-CNCR2820440648>3.0.CO;2-8
41. Toksvang LN, Schmidt MS, Arup S, et al. Hepatotoxicity during 6-thioguanine treatment in inflammatory bowel disease and childhood acute lymphoblastic leukaemia: a systematic review. *PLoS One*. 2019;**14**(5):e0212157. doi:10.1371/journal.pone.0212157
42. Stone RM, Moser B, Sanford B, et al. High dose cytarabine plus gemtuzumab ozogamicin for patients with relapsed or refractory acute myeloid leukemia: Cancer and Leukemia Group B study 19902. *Leuk Res*. 2011;**35**(3):329–333. doi:10.1016/j.leukres.2010.07.017
43. Cortes J, Tsimberidou AM, Alvarez R, et al. Mylotarg combined with topotecan and cytarabine in patients with refractory acute myelogenous leukemia. *Cancer Chemother Pharmacol*. 2002;**50**(6):497–500. doi:10.1007/s00280-002-0539-y
44. Helmy A. Review article: updates in the pathogenesis and therapy of hepatic sinusoidal obstruction syndrome. *Aliment Pharmacol Ther*. 2006;**23**(1):11–25. doi:10.1111/j.1365-2036.2006.02742.x
45. Coppell JA, Richardson PG, Soiffer R, et al. Hepatic veno-occlusive disease following stem cell transplantation: incidence, clinical course, and outcome. *Biol Blood Marrow Transplant*. 2010;**16**(2):157–168. doi:10.1016/j.bbmt.2009.08.024
46. Mcdonald GB, Sharma P, Matthews DE, Shulman HM, Thomas ED. Venocclusive disease of the liver after bone marrow transplantation: diagnosis, incidence, and predisposing factors. *Hepatology*. 1984;**4**(1):116–122. doi:10.1002/hep.1840040121
47. Jones RJ, Lee KSK, Beschorner WE, et al. Venoocclusive disease of the liver following bone marrow transplantation. *Transplantation*. 1987;**44**(6):778–783. doi:10.1097/00007890-198712000-00011
48. Ravaioli F, Colecchia A, Alemanni LV, et al. Role of imaging techniques in liver veno-occlusive disease diagnosis: recent advances and literature review. *Expert Rev Gastroenterol Hepatol*. 2019;**13**(5):463–484. doi:10.1080/17474124.2019.1588111

49. Jones RJ, Lee KSK, Beschorner WE, et al. Venoocclusive disease of the liver following bone marrow transplantation. *Transplantation*. 1987;**44**(6):778–783.
50. Rubbia-Brandt L, Lauwers GY, Wang H, et al. Sinusoidal obstruction syndrome and nodular regenerative hyperplasia are frequent oxaliplatin-associated liver lesions and partially prevented by bevacizumab in patients with hepatic colorectal metastasis. *Histopathology*. 2010;**56**(4):430–439. doi:10.1111/j.1365-2559.2010.03511.x
51. Kim I-D, Egawa H, Marui Y, et al. A successful liver transplantation for refractory hepatic veno-occlusive disease originating from cord blood transplantation. *Am J Transplant*. 2002;**2**(8):796–800.
52. Rapoport AP, Doyle HR, Starzl T, Rowe JM, Doeblin T, DiPersio JF. Orthotopic liver transplantation for life-threatening veno-occlusive disease of the liver after allogeneic bone marrow transplant. *Bone Marrow Transplant*. 1991;**8**(5):421–424.
53. Nimer SD, Milewicz AL, Champlin RE, Busuttil RW. Successful treatment of hepatic venoocclusive disease in a bone marrow transplant patient with orthotopic liver transplantation. *Transplantation*. 1990;**49**(4):819–821.
54. Ögren M, Bergqvist D, Björck M, Acosta S, Eriksson H, Sternby NH. Portal vein thrombosis: prevalence, patient characteristics and lifetime risk: a population study based on 23796 consecutive autopsies. *World J Gastroenterol*. 2006;**12**(13):2115–2119. doi:10.3748/wjg.v12.i13.2115
55. Qi X. Portal vein thrombosis: recent advance. *Advs Exp Med Adv Intern Med*. 2017;**906**:229–239. doi:10.1007/5584_2016_118
56. Harding DJ, Perera MTPR, Chen F, Olliff S, Tripathi D. Portal vein thrombosis in cirrhosis: controversies and latest developments. *World J Gastroenterol*. 2015;**21**(22):6769–6784. doi:10.3748/wjg.v21.i22.6769
57. Amitrano L, Guardascione MA, Brancaccio V, et al. Risk factors and clinical presentation of portal vein thrombosis in patients with liver cirrhosis. *J Hepatol*. 2004;**40**(5):736–741. doi:10.1016/j.jhep.2004.01.001
58. Bhattacharyya M, Makharia G, Kannan M, Ahmed RPH, Gupta PK, Saxena R. Inherited prothrombotic defects in Budd-Chiari syndrome and portal vein thrombosis: a study from North India. *Am J Clin Pathol*. 2004;**121**(6):844–847. doi:10.1309/F2U1-XBV4-RXYU-AYG0
59. Janssen HL, Meinardi JR, Vleggaar FP, et al. Factor V Leiden mutation, prothrombin gene mutation, and deficiencies in coagulation inhibitors associated with Budd-Chiari syndrome and portal vein thrombosis: results of a case-control study. *Blood*. 2000;**96**(7):2364–2368.
60. Qi X, De Stefano V, Wang J, et al. Prevalence of inherited antithrombin, protein C, and protein S deficiencies in portal vein system thrombosis and Budd-Chiari syndrome: a systematic review and meta-analysis of observational studies. *J Gastroenterol Hepatol*. 2013;**28**(3):432–442. doi:10.1111/jgh.12085
61. Dong F, Luo S-H, Zheng L-J, et al. Incidence of portal vein thrombosis after splenectomy and its influence on transjugular intrahepatic portosystemic shunt stent patency. *World J Clin Cases*. 2019;**7**(17):2450–2462. doi:10.12998/wjcc.v7.i17.2450
62. Ding L, Deng F, Yu C, et al. Portosplenomesenteric vein thrombosis in patients with early-stage severe acute pancreatitis. *World J Gastroenterol*. 2018;**24**(35):4054–4060. doi:10.3748/wjg.v24.i35.4054
63. Deleve LD, Valla D-C, Garcia-Tsao G; American Association for the Study Liver Diseases. Vascular disorders of the liver. *Hepatology*. 2009;**49**(5):1729–1764. doi:10.1002/hep.22772
64. Senzolo M, Riggio O, Primignani M. Vascular disorders of the liver: recommendations from the Italian Association for the Study of the Liver (AISF) ad hoc committee. *Dig Liver Dis*. 2011;**43**(7):503–514. doi:10.1016/j.dld.2010.11.006
65. Plessier A, Darwish-Murad S, Hernandez-Guerra M, et al. Acute portal vein thrombosis unrelated to cirrhosis: a prospective multicenter follow-up study. *Hepatology*. 2010;**51**(1):210–218. doi:10.1002/hep.23259
66. Altun E, El-Azzazi M, Semelka RC. Vascular disorders of the liver. In: Altun E, El-Azzazi M, Semelka RC, eds. *Liver Imaging MRI with CT Correlation*. Oxford: Wiley; 2015: 267–284. doi:10.1002/9781118484852.ch14
67. Shaji K, Sarr MG, Patrick K. Mesenteric venous thrombosis. *N Engl J Med*. 2001;**345**(23):1683–1688. doi:10.1056/NEJMra010076
68. Hall TC, Garcea G, Metcalfe M, Bilku D, Dennison AR. Management of acute non-cirrhotic and non-malignant portal vein thrombosis: a systematic review. *World J Surg*. 2011;**35**(11):2510–2520. doi:10.1007/s00268-011-1198-0
69. Berzigotti A, García-Criado Á, Darnell A, García-Pagán JC. Imaging in clinical decision-making for portal vein thrombosis. *Nat Rev Gastroenterol Hepatol*. 2014;**11**(5):308–316. doi:10.1038/nrgastro.2013.258
70. Yerdel MA, Gunson B, Mirza D, et al. Portal vein thrombosis in adults undergoing liver transplantation: risk factors, screening, management, and outcome. *Transplantation*. 2000;**69**(9):1873–1881. doi:10.1097/00007890-200005150-00023
71. de Franchis R. Evolving consensus in portal hypertension. Report of the Baveno IV consensus workshop on methodology of diagnosis and therapy in portal hypertension. *J Hepatol*. 2005;**43**(1):167–176. doi:10.1016/j.jhep.2005.05.009
72. Song JH, He X, Lou WS, et al. Application of percutaneous AngioJet thrombectomy in patients with acute symptomatic portal and superior mesenteric venous thrombosis. *Zhonghua Yi Xue Za Zhi*. 2017;**97**(13):991–995. doi:10.3760/cma.j.issn.0376-2491.2017.13.006
73. Hollingshead M, Burke CT, Mauro MA, Weeks SM, Dixon RG, Jaques PF. Transcatheter thrombolytic therapy for acute mesenteric and portal vein thrombosis. *J Vasc Interv Radiol*. 2005;**16**(5):651–661. doi:10.1097/01.RVI.0000156265.79960.86
74. Seedial SM, Mouli SK, Desai KR. Acute portal vein thrombosis: current trends in medical and endovascular management. *Semin Intervent Radiol*. 2018;**35**(3):198–202. doi:10.1055/s-0038-1660798
75. Klinger C, Riecken B, Schmidt A, et al. Transjugular local thrombolysis with/without TIPS in patients with acute non-cirrhotic, non-malignant portal vein thrombosis. *Dig Liver Dis*. 2017;**49**(12):1345–1352. doi:10.1016/j.dld.2017.05.020
76. Rosenqvist K, Ebeling Barbier C, Rorsman F, Sangfelt P, Nyman R. Treatment of acute portomesenteric venous thrombosis with thrombectomy through a transjugular intrahepatic portosystemic shunt: a single-center experience. *Acta Radiol*. 2018;**59**(8):953–958. doi:10.1177/0284185117742683
77. Jung HJ, Lee SS. Combination of surgical thrombectomy and direct thrombolysis in acute abdomen with portal and superior mesenteric vein thrombosis. *Vasc Spec Int*. 2014;**30**(4):155–158. doi:10.5758/vsi.2014.30.4.155
78. Gioia S, Nardelli S, Pasquale C, et al. Natural history of patients with non cirrhotic portal hypertension: comparison with patients with compensated cirrhosis. *Dig Liver Dis*. 2018;**50**(8):839–844. doi:10.1016/j.dld.2018.01.132

79. Condat B, Pessione F, Helene Denninger M, Hillaire S, Valla D. Recent portal or mesenteric venous thrombosis: increased recognition and frequent recanalization on anticoagulant therapy. *Hepatology*. 2000;**32**(3):466–470. doi:10.1053/jhep.2000.16597
80. Zargar SA, Javid G, Khan BA, et al. Endoscopic ligation compared with sclerotherapy for bleeding esophageal varices in children with extrahepatic portal venous obstruction. *Hepatology*. 2002;**36**(3):666–672. doi:10.1053/jhep.2002.35278
81. Selzner M, Tuttle-Newhall JE, Dahm F, Suhocki P, Clavien PA. Current indication of a modified Sugiura procedure in the management of variceal bleeding. *J Am Coll Surg*. 2001;**193**(2):166–173. doi:10.1016/S1072-7515(01)00937-1
82. Spaander MCW, Hoekstra J, Hansen BE, Van Buuren HR, Leebeek FWG, Janssen HLA. Anticoagulant therapy in patients with non-cirrhotic portal vein thrombosis: effect on new thrombotic events and gastrointestinal bleeding. *J Thromb Haemost*. 2013;**11**(3):452–459. doi:10.1111/jth.12121
83. Govani FS, Shovlin CL. Hereditary haemorrhagic telangiectasia: a clinical and scientific review. *Eur J Hum Genet*. 2009;**17**(7):860–871. doi:10.1038/ejhg.2009.35

16

Treatment of hepatocellular carcinoma
A surgical perspective

Vincenzo Mazzaferro, Michele Droz dit Busset, and Matteo Virdis

'Operable hepatocellular carcinoma' is still a definition that counts

Management of hepatocellular carcinoma (HCC) has markedly improved since the early 2010s when new molecular classes of systemic treatments entered clinical practice, after having demonstrated a significant survival benefit in randomized control trials conducted in patients with advanced, non-operable tumours. Since then, an extraordinary research effort has been performed on HCC. Thus, a tumour that used to be an orphan in medical oncology due to its resistance to conventional chemotherapeutic agents and to its frequent coexistence with chronic liver diseases—a major limiting factor for any kind of treatment—gained the attention of the oncology community.

Current systemic therapies, including immune-checkpoint inhibitors, tyrosine kinase inhibitors (TKIs), and monoclonal antibodies, have challenged the use of conventional therapies, mainly locoregional and surgically oriented. While 50–60% of patients with HCC are estimated to be exposed to systemic therapies in their lifespan, surgical interventions still represent the cornerstone of treatment and the sole ones with curative potential.[1,2]

As research proceeds in investigating molecular mechanisms to be targeted with new drugs for 'unresectable HCC', attention should remain on the large group of patients with 'operable HCC', either at the time of diagnosis or when various combinations of systemic and locoregional treatments maintain and downstage the tumour to conditions eligible for curative surgical removal. After all, the surgical operability of HCC—either by liver resection (LR) or liver transplantation (LT)—is still the main prognostic factor, as removal of the tumour can lead to the consideration of the patient as 'tumour free' and even 'cured', according to the presenting stage of the disease and the interval from surgical resection. As the majority of non-surgical treatments for HCC are proposed for 'unresectable' or 'non-transplantable' patients, any condition favouring surgical intervention is hierarchically predominant over other options. Determination of surgical operability of any HCC should be pursued at any stage of intrahepatic HCC development.

This chapter is focused on the current perspectives offered by surgical interventions in the general debate on the best treatment for HCC according to its various stages.[2–4]

Perspectives of surgical interest in the epidemiology of hepatocellular carcinoma

HCC is the fifth most common cancer globally and the second most frequent cause of cancer-related death in the world. The disease has a higher incidence with advancing age and has a strong preponderance for the male sex. The incidence of HCC in the last 20 years has increased in parallel with the greater longevity of the population. In recent years, there has been a reduction in the areas at high incidence (Southeast Asia and sub-Saharan Africa) to the detriment of Western continents such as Europe and North America; this shift is mainly linked to the change in the aetiology of chronic liver disease or cirrhosis that precedes tumour genesis.

According to all sources, HCC is a global problem. Differently from other 'big killers', such as lung, breast, colorectal, ovarian, and prostate cancers, the incidence and mortality rates for HCC remain very similar—over 850,000 new cases are registered each year with over 800,000 deaths—with homogeneous trends observed in high versus low human development index regions in the world, both in men and women (**Figure 16.1**).

Projections of incidence and deaths in the Western world estimate that, over the next 10 years, HCC will be the third leading cause of cancer-related death, preceding colorectal, breast, and prostate cancers. Chronic hepatitis C virus (HCV) and hepatitis B virus (HBV) infection continue to represent significant factors related to HCC development, particularly among immigrants from countries with endemic hepatotropic infections; however, the increasing incidence of metabolic syndrome, non-alcoholic fatty liver disease (NAFLD), and non-alcoholic steatohepatitis (NASH) means they are likely to become the main aetiological factors of HCC in the years to come (**Figure 16.2**). Metabolic imbalances are becoming a major concern due to the chronic inflammatory conditions that they generate both systemically and in the hepatic microenvironment. Chronic metabolic conditions such as the metabolic syndrome, diabetes, uncontrolled hypertension, and high body mass index increase the risk of HCC, with an additive effect in patients with concomitant virus-related chronic hepatitis. Overall, NAFLD is becoming the most relevant cause of HCC in Western countries, being that the reported HCC incidence in this context is between 0.25% and 7.6%. NASH

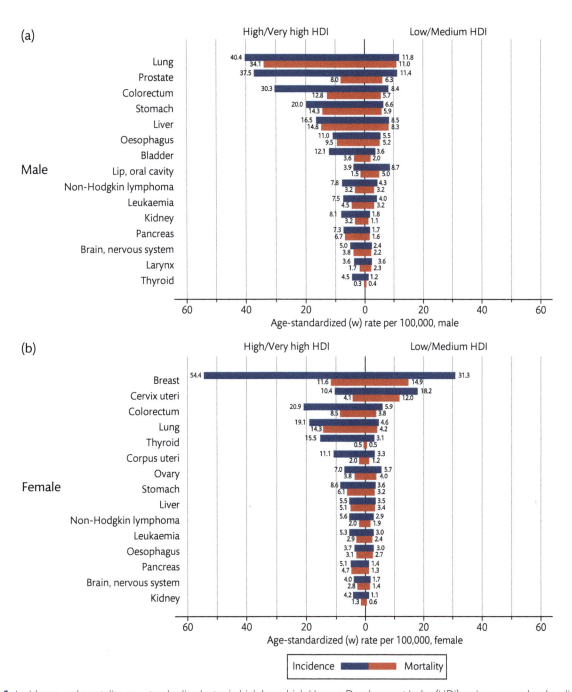

Figure 16.1 Incidence and mortality age-standardized rates in high/very-high Human Development Index (HDI) regions versus low/medium HDI regions among (a) men and (b) women in 2018.
Reproduced with permission from Bray, F., Ferlay, J., Soerjomataram, I., Siegel, R.L., Torre, L.A. and Jemal, A. (2018), Global cancer statistics 2018: GLOBOCAN estimates of incidence and mortality worldwide for 36 cancers in 185 countries. *CA: A Cancer Journal for Clinicians*, 68: 394–424. Original data from: World Health Organization, Global Health Observatory, Geneva 2018. https://www.who.int/data/gho

is the precursor step in the development of HCC in patients with diabetes mellitus or obesity. Owing to the present epidemic condition of obesity, NASH has become the most common cause of cirrhosis. Since 2010, the proportion of HCC attributed to NASH has rapidly increased, currently representing 15–20% of cases in the West. Furthermore, the role for HCC development attributable to metabolic syndrome and NASH in the general population is likely to be above 20%, owing to its coexistence in patients with other liver diseases.

Differently from NASH/NAFLD-related HCC, HBV-related HCC could be significantly reduced in the near future and even eliminated in many endemic countries. Due to the extensive vaccination of youth against HBV infection and neonatal transmission, the rate of HBV and HBV-related HCC has decreased. In addition, suppression of viraemia with oral therapies such as tenofovir and entecavir is now routinely practised, resulting in a significant 5-year reduction of the HCC incidence from 14% to 4%, particularly in cirrhotic patients.

CHAPTER 16 Treatment of hepatocellular carcinoma

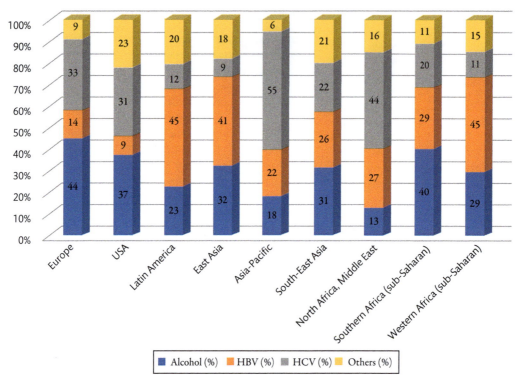

Figure 16.2 Geographical distribution of risk factors contributing to HCC development.
Source: data from Global Burden of Disease Liver Cancer Collaboration, Akinyemiju T, Abera S, et al. The burden of primary liver cancer and underlying etiologies from 1990 to 2015 at the global, regional, and national level: results from the Global Burden of Disease Study 2015. *JAMA Oncol.* 2017;3(12):1683–1691. doi:10.1001/jamaoncol.2017.3055

In addition, HCV-related HCC decreases significantly in patients who achieve sustained virological response by means of combination therapies with direct-acting antivirals, with a predicted 50% reduction of all-cause HCV-related mortality and of the risk of HCC occurrence in the following 5 years. In the particular context of surgical therapy of HCC, the new generation of direct-acting antivirals have proved effective in reducing the risk of postoperative liver failure and late recurrence from '*de novo*' HCC in patients undergoing LR or local ablation. In addition, direct-acting antivirals are recommended for prevention and treatment of HCV recurrence after LT, a condition that used to significantly affect the rate of post-transplant graft failure and the non-cancer-related mortality following LT in HCV-positive patients.

With respect to alcohol-related liver cirrhosis and cancer, the progression of chronic liver disease to cirrhosis is proportional to the lifetime alcohol intake. It should be noted that about 40% of new cases of HCC in Europe occur in alcohol abusers also frequently carrying concomitant conditions affecting liver function (e.g. viral infection, metabolic syndrome, etc.).

The incidence of HCC is also increased in patients with HIV infection compared to the general population, with several reports describing an accelerated course of cancer evolution and multifocality in HIV-positive patients.[1,3,5,6]

Influence of individual components and local conditions in the composition of guidelines for hepatocellular carcinoma

Surgical intervention is the mainstay of treatment in all major guidelines on clinical management of HCC. It is well accepted that surgery for HCC can be proposed as LR or LT. In general, surgical procedures should be proposed when curative-intent tumour removal can be pursued—namely, when the removal of all visible disease with clear margins is possible, according to tumour presentation, liver functional reserve, and patient status. If these conditions are satisfied, a 5-year overall survival as high as 60–80% can be achieved.

In current guidelines, the inherent locoregional nature of surgical intervention limits the use of surgery to patients with HCC at its early phases of development, even though more advanced tumour stages can be treated with either LR or LT. While consistent progress has been made in defining objective conditions with an independent impact on postoperative survival of HCC patients, the definition of the best candidate for LR and/or liver LT is still a matter of debate, making the eligibility for LR or LT very difficult to homogenize within the hepato-oncology and surgical communities.

In daily practice, quite often the heterogeneity of HCC presentation may lead to conditions in which the patient does not exactly fulfil all the characteristics for being allocated to one treatment slot or another. This is typically observed in the intermediate stage (i.e. Barcelona Clinic Liver Cancer (BCLC) B stage) in which patients with good (i.e. Child–Pugh class A) or suboptimal (i.e. Child–Pugh class B, ≥7) liver function and limited (just above the Milan criteria) or extensive tumour burden (large/multifocal disease) can be comprised.

As medical decisions on the best treatment are based not only on tumour characteristics but also on the patient's general condition and liver function, the management pattern in the various evolutionary stages of HCC may differ quite significantly from one centre to another, according to different expertise and local conditions. However, in a comprehensive perspective, surgical aggressiveness and pure technical considerations should be hierarchically organized within a multidisciplinary team decision, since a single surgical

Influence of individual components and local conditions in the composition of guidelines for hepatocellular carcinoma

Table 16.1 Differences in HCC staging systems in major international guidelines

	EASL	AASLD	APASL	NCCN	JSH	KLCSG
Performance status	Yes	Yes	No	No	No	No (ECOG 0–1)
Liver function	Yes	Yes	Yes	No	Yes	No (Child–Pugh A)
Tumour factors	Yes	Yes	Yes	Yes (AJCC TNM 8)	Yes	Yes (mUICC)

AJCC, American Joint Committee on Cancer; ECOG, Eastern Cooperative Oncology Group; mUICC, modified Union for International Cancer Control staging system; TNM, tumour, node, metastasis.

Source: data from Jogi S, Varanai R, Bantu SS, et al. Selecting the first line treatment in non-metastatic hepatocellular carcinoma—comparing clinical practice guidelines. Oncol Rev. 2020;14(2):515. doi:10.4081/oncol.2020.515

treatment cannot fit all patients and tumour presentations; moreover, the differential impact in terms of treatment benefit that surgery may offer to the individual patient with respect to non-surgical alternatives has to be considered.

The complexity of selecting the best candidate for various available treatments in HCC is appreciable when considering the heterogeneity of criteria informing the major guidelines (Table 16.1).

Comparing guidelines from different geographical and cultural areas of the world can be a complex exercise. As highlighted in Figure 16.3 and Table 16.1, Western guidelines (European Association for the Study of the Liver (EASL) and American Association for the Study of Liver Diseases (AASLD)) use a series of factors derived from the BCLC staging system such as performance status, liver function, Child–Pugh score, and tumour parameters obtained from radiology

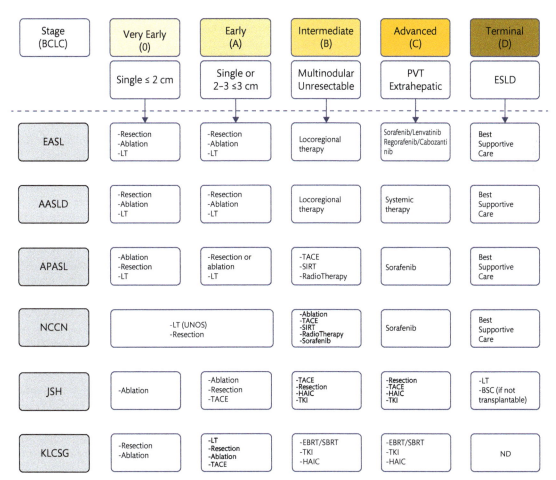

Figure 16.3 Comparison of various criteria and therapeutic alternatives informing major national and international guidelines on clinical management of HCC. AASLD, American Association for the Study of Liver Disease; APASL, Asian Pacific Association for the Study of the Liver; BCLC, Barcelona Clinic Liver Cancer; EASL, European Association for the Study of the Liver; EBRT, external beam radiation therapy; HAIC, hepatic artery infusion chemotherapy; JSH, Japanese Society for Hepatology; KLCSG, Korean Liver Cancer Association-National Cancer Center Korea Practice Guidelines; LT, liver transplantation; NCCN, National Comprehensive Cancer Network; PVT, portal vein thrombosis; TACE, trans-arterial chemoembolization; TARE, trans-arterial radioembolization; SBRT, stereotactic body radiation therapy; TKI, tyrosine-kinase inhibitors.

Adapted with permission from Foerster F, Galle PR. Comparison of the current international guidelines on the management of HCC. JHEP Rep. 2019;1(2):114–119. doi:10.1016/j.jhepr.2019.04.005

and pathology staging (i.e. number of tumour nodules, dimensions of the largest lesions and presence of tumour macrovascular invasion). Other guidelines especially from the East (the Asian Pacific (APASL), Korean (KLCSG), and Japanese (JSH) guidelines) but also the US National Comprehensive Cancer Network (NCCN) guidelines have a more liberal approach in terms of potential therapeutic alternatives to be offered at various stages of disease.

Guidelines are based on different grades of scientific evidence. However, the proliferation of various recommendations for patients carrying the same tumour in different contexts denotes that any judgements on efficacy, toxicity, and impact on the outcome of a given therapy within the frame of a guideline may vary according to specific populations, different aetiologies, various resources, and local expertise. A good example of how much individual components not considered in guidelines influence final recommendations (e.g. tumour responsiveness, tumour location within the liver, patient age, expected benefit with respect to alternatives, centre expertise, etc.) is the variability in indications for locoregional therapies. Similar to pharmacological-driven regimens for HCC depending on the availability of active clinical trials, locoregional treatments such as ablation and intra-arterial therapies are influenced by local expertise as well as LR and LT, whose results are related not only to sound technical procedures but also to external conditions such as access to intensive care facilities, organ donation rate, and waitlist dynamics.

The process behind the construction of guidelines has influenced the way surgeons approach the multidisciplinary discussion of HCC patients. In fact, the definition of the optimal surgical candidate has evolved, incorporating factors that are accessible to either surgical or non-surgical specialists. For instance, in the EASL guidelines, LR is recommended after a multiparametric, composite evaluation that has to consider an appropriate balance of liver function (i.e. compensated Child–Pugh class A liver function and Model for End-Stage Liver Disease (MELD) score <9), grade of portal hypertension, and predicted remnant liver volume. Laparoscopic, robotic, and other minimally invasive approaches are advocated whenever possible, with an expected perioperative mortality and morbidity that should not exceed 3% and 20%, respectively, also including a post-surgical severe liver failure rate of less than 5%.

The heterogeneity of guidelines reiterates the fact that surgery (LR and LT) could maintain a central role in the treatment algorithm of HCC, provided that non-surgical treatments are part of the surgical strategy. In fact, non-surgical alternatives should be considered instrumental to facilitate curative surgical removal of HCC and eventually improve patients' outcomes.[3-7]

Innovations in liver resection for hepatocellular carcinoma

When applied to very early and early stages of HCC in patients with compensated cirrhosis (Child–Pugh class A) with no portal hypertension, LR is associated with survival rates approaching 70% at 5 years. Advances in surgical technique and postoperative care have led to perioperative mortality rates in referral centres of below 1%, with a blood transfusion requirement below 10%.

In the last decade, several innovative perspectives have renovated the surgical approach to HCC. However, despite significant advances, LR remains a technically demanding procedure with outcomes largely dependent on a number of variables related to tumour presentation, surgical expertise, patient comorbidities, and underlying liver conditions. As a result, LR performed in non-referral centres is still burdened by consistent morbidity, with liver decompensation the most fearful complication and the leading cause of prolonged hospitalization, increased costs, and poor long-term outcomes. Two main perspectives have innovated LR for HCC in recent years: minimally invasive liver surgery (MILS) and prevention/management of postoperative liver malfunction and failure.[3,6,8]

Laparoscopic liver resection is a model of minimization of surgical morbidity for hepatocellular carcinoma

A large burden of scientific evidence has confirmed laparoscopic LR in cirrhotic patients to be equivalent to the conventional open approach in terms of tumour-negative margins of resection and long-term patient outcomes, with virtually no mortality and a morbidity rate around 25%, mostly related to manageable grade I complications according to the Clavien–Dindo classification. The strength of evidence in favour of laparoscopic LR has increased in the last decade up to the point that minimally invasive resection is recommended whenever possible, since it is associated with clear benefits in term of complication rate, blood loss, and duration of hospital stay.

Laparoscopic resections in cirrhotic patients offer a protective effect against postoperative liver decompensation and ascites, also in mildly decompensated liver disease (Child–Pugh class B). Such an effect may be even more prominent in major resections, as collateral blood vessels and lymphatic circulation in cirrhotic patients are disrupted in the case of a large abdominal incision, while they are preserved in the case of a laparoscopic approach.

In addition, laparoscopic resections reduce intraoperative blood loss and transfusion requirements due to minimization of bleeding from hepatic vein branches and to the positive intra-abdominal pressure generated by the pneumo-peritoneum. Finally, the field magnification, part of the video-assisted surgical procedures, allows more precise control of small intrahepatic vessels with the contribution of advanced haemostatic instruments and stapling devices.

A large number of studies agree on the benefits of laparoscopy in terms of reduction of postoperative pain, rapid patient mobilization, lower rates of wound infection, dehiscence, and incisional hernias, and fewer pulmonary complications as opposed to conventional laparotomy, usually conducted through large subcostal incisions and rib retraction. All these characteristics of laparoscopic LR—also applicable to robotic MILS approaches—translate into shorter hospital stay with respect to conventional surgery in patients undergoing LR according to the extent (minor or major) of parenchyma removal.

From the technical standpoint, laparoscopic resections should be the standard of care in case of minor resections, left lateral lobectomy (segment II and III), and anteroinferior segmentectomies (i.e. segments II–VI). In major hepatectomies and in case of 'difficult segments' (i.e. posterior-superior segments, namely segment VII and VIII, and also for the caudate lobe, segment I) the evidence is less robust, even though several results show that in experienced centres MILS of HCC in unfavourable locations can be performed safely, while maintaining the short-term advantages. In **Figure 16.4**,

Innovations in liver resection for hepatocellular carcinoma

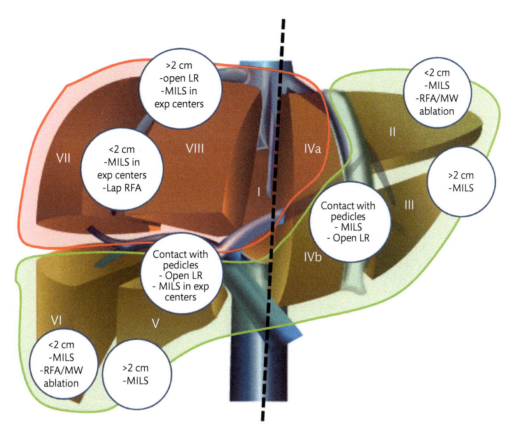

Figure 16.4 Indications for laparoscopic and open liver resections according to HCC size and location. Tumours in unfavourable locations (posterosuperior segments in the red area: segment I, IVa, VII, and VIII) can be removed through laparoscopic (Lap) approach (minimally invasive liver surgery (MILS)) only in high-experienced (exp) centres. HCCs <2 cm centrally located in the red area may be treated with laparoscopic radiofrequency (RFA) or microwave (MW) ablation, as an alternative to conventional open liver resection (LR), usually requiring significant amounts of parenchyma removal. HCCs >2 cm located in the anteroinferior locations (green area: segments II, III, IVb, V, and VI) can safely be approached laparoscopically with less technical issues. HCC <2 cm in the green favourable area can benefit from ablation if patients are unfit for surgery. Centrally located HCCs close to main portal pedicle containing major vascular and biliary branches may require an open approach, even though MILS is possible in a significant number of cases, especially when vascular and biliary structures of the left liver is considered. Tumour proximity to hilar structures usually contraindicates ablation.

an example of a decision-making algorithm for laparoscopic and open LRs is shown, based on the available scientific evidence and on tumour size and location.[6–10]

Postoperative liver failure in patients with hepatocellular carcinoma and with chronic liver diseases can be minimized if the risk is calculated on objective preoperative parameters

As described above, the decision to proceed with LR in patients with chronic liver diseases and cirrhosis should be based on a multiparametric assessment, aimed at objectively quantifying the associated risks, to be balanced against the expected outcomes of non-surgical options.

Among the many factors considered in the decision process, relevant portal hypertension and abnormal bilirubin are the most frequently described predictors of postoperative decompensation and early mortality. According to guidelines, portal hypertension is defined as a hepatic vein–portal vein pressure gradient of at least 10 mmHg; when such measurement is not available, evidence of oesophageal varices at gastroscopy associated with splenomegaly and platelet count less than 100,000/mL are considered indirect signs of portal hypertension.

Even if a large number of surgical studies demonstrated that LR in selected patients with portal hypertension and abnormal bilirubin is possible, LR should not be the standard for all patients carrying such high-risk indicators of poor surgical outcome. However, the grade of portal hypertension and liver function measured through bilirubin, indocyanine green clearance test, or other comprehensive scores such as the Child–Pugh, ALBI (albumin–bilirubin), and MELD scores are privileged prognostic factors accessible preoperatively for discussion in multidisciplinary meetings before surgery.

Another key element to be considered preoperatively is the predicted extent of LR, a pure technical factor that the surgeon in charge of the operation can determine, according to HCC presentation at computed tomography or magnetic resonance imaging scan.

The risk of postoperative liver failure in HCC patients with chronic liver disease can be predicted by the hierarchic combination of the three preoperative indicators listed above and summarized in **Figure 16.5**. In the presence of portal hypertension, major resections are contraindicated due to high risks of liver decompensation and mortality, while major hepatectomies in well-compensated livers or minor resections in patients with portal hypertension are associated with an intermediate risk of postoperative liver failure. In patients with no portal hypertension undergoing minor resections, a MELD

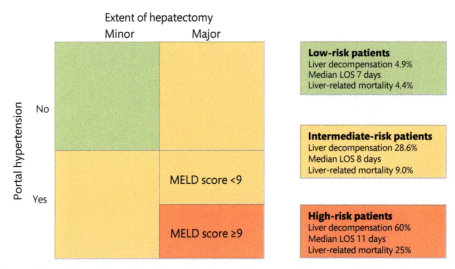

Figure 16.5 Prognostic interaction and possible combinations of the three main preoperative prognostic factors for postoperative liver failure (presence of portal hypertension, MELD score, and extent of liver resection). Three risk classes can be identified, associated with increased rate of liver decompensation, length of hospital stay (LOS), and liver-related mortality.
Adapted with permission from Citterio D, Facciorusso A, Sposito C, et al. Hierarchic Interaction of Factors Associated With Liver Decompensation After Resection for Hepatocellular Carcinoma. JAMA Surg. 2016;151(9):846–853. doi:10.1001/jamasurg.2016.1121

score less than 9 can sub-stratify a subset of patients who will have a particularly favourable postoperative outcome.[7]

Borderline presentations of hepatocellular carcinoma are not recommended for upfront resection, although neoadjuvant non-surgical therapies may convert a proportion of them to surgically sound options, to be offered on an individual basis after multidisciplinary discussion

As described above, LR in patients with chronic liver disease and HCC is an option to be considered in all cases but in need of confirmation, after the many factors influencing short- and long-term results are carefully scrutinized and compared with those related to alternative non-surgical options. Therefore, it is not surprising that 'borderline' indications for surgical interventions may emerge after multidisciplinary discussion on individual patients, whose complexities are not fully captured by HCC clinical management guidelines. Among several borderline HCCs worth a mention, the following are the most relevant.[2,3]

LR for HCC after induction of lobar hypertrophy

Several techniques for inducing slow versus rapid lobar hypertrophy in case of an anticipated insufficient liver remnant are part of the surgical knowledge and are described in detail in other parts of this book. A simplified scheme of the alternatives in place, also in case of HCC, is presented in Figure 16.6.

Apart from technical and functional considerations, the underlying condition limiting the application of these techniques in the context of patients with HCC is the presence of advanced fibrosis and cirrhosis that impair regeneration and cause low rates of future liver remnant volume increase. Such reduced growth of the future liver remnant in the case of chronically injured liver parenchyma have been described after both portal vein embolization or ligation and after the so-called associating liver partition and portal vein ligation. Kinetic growth and hypertrophy after associating liver partition and portal vein ligation decrease with progressive degrees of fibrosis, and are reduced by up to 50% in cirrhosis, although they remain higher than portal vein embolization. Preoperative assessment of the degree of liver fibrosis (through FibroScan or liver biopsy) may be helpful in predicting the regenerative outcome.

When considering these techniques, the issue of tumour growth while awaiting hypertrophy has to be considered, which may even preclude resection for tumours close to major biliary or vascular structures. In order to overcome these concerns and improve tumour control, a sequential approach combining transarterial chemoembolization (TACE) followed by hypertrophy-inducing techniques has been advocated. More recently, the role of transarterial radioembolization has been evaluated in patients with insufficient future liver remnant, due to its ability to induce atrophy of the treated lobe with contralateral hypertrophy (radiation lobectomy) while simultaneously providing local tumour control of the diseased hemi-liver.

Finally, a drawback to be considered about resections of regenerated livers affected by liver cirrhosis is the impaired function related to less mature hepatocytes. Due to accelerated hypertrophy—as liver volume is not equal to liver function—those HCC patients who may complete the process are at increased risk of morbidity and mortality related to post-hepatectomy liver failure, an outcome that should be avoided through very careful patient selection.[2,11–13]

LR for multinodular HCC

In patients with multifocal HCC, the standard of care in most guidelines is locoregional treatment, mainly TACE. However, a limited number of nodules within the Milan criteria (i.e. ≤3 nodules ≤3 cm each) still belong to the category of early HCC, in which curative surgical intervention has a proven efficacy in prolonging survival. For multinodular HCC beyond the Milan criteria, LR may be offered in patients with preserved hepatic function and potentially curative interventions, particularly in tumours responding to locoregional or combined non-surgical treatments. Such migration in the eligibility

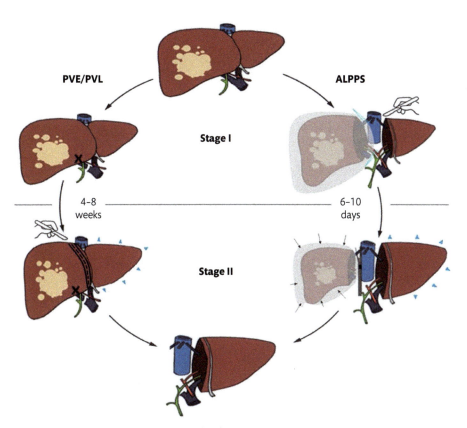

Figure 16.6 Regenerative techniques of the future liver remnant (FLR) to increase resectability. Slow (PVE: portal vein embolization; PVL: portal vein ligation) versus rapid techniques (ALPPS: associating liver partition and portal vein ligation for staged hepatectomy) have different indications and outcomes. Time of liver transection (stage II) after partial portal inflow interruption (stage I) is also indicated. Arrowheads indicate hypertrophy of the left lobe.
Adapted with permission from Mazzaferro V, Gorgen A, Roayaie S, et al. Liver resection and transplantation for intrahepatic cholangiocarcinoma. J Hepatol. 2020;72(2):364-377. doi:10.1016/j.jhep.2019.11.020

for curative resection at different times during the medical history of a patient with HCC undergoing multiple treatment is in agreement with the reverse 'stage migration' concept described in recent guidelines, aimed at offering the best available treatment to HCC patients, regardless of their previous medical history.

Of course, survival after LR in multinodular HCC is suboptimal if compared to tumour removal performed in its earlier stages; however, several studies showed that LR, when feasible, outperforms TACE. Patient selection is once again the key to success in proposing surgical interventions for non-optimal candidates.[2]

LR in combination with ablation

For many years, LR and ablation competed for the same group of HCC patients at their initial stage of development and, although a definitive study confirming the equivalence of these treatment options has never been produced, it is widely accepted that the results of ablative treatments for HCC smaller than 3 cm are similar to those achieved with LR. Differently from the past, liver surgeons therefore should include tumour ablation (by means of radiofrequency ablation, microwave ablation, or percutaneous ethanol injection) within the operation room armamentarium, especially for centrally located lesions and in patients with borderline liver function and comorbidities. Thus, on top of being considered the standard of care for patients with early HCC not amenable to surgical treatment, ablative techniques can become a very efficient companion of resection in multifocal HCC, even though such a combination has never been assessed in rigorous prospective randomized trials.

In addition, ablation is part of the current standard of HCC downstaging for subsequent tumour resection and transplantation and modern techniques of MILS may include ultrasound-guided ablation of small central HCC lesions. This reduces invasiveness of resection, complication rate, hospital stay, and costs.

In multinodular HCC, multimodal treatment with a combination of resection and ablative therapies achieves better results than locoregional treatments alone. Due to the inherent heterogeneity of HCC presentation, a patient-tailored approach is strongly advocated in this context and several studies are underway to evaluate different combinations and sequential treatments including ablation, TACE, transarterial radioembolization, and also systemic therapy.[2,14]

Resection of recurrent HCC

The main outcome issue related to LR for HCC is the high rate of tumour recurrence, as high as 50–70% at 5 years. Early relapses (occurring ≤2 years after tumour resection) carry a significantly worse prognosis and are thought to be the consequence of residual microscopic tumour foci left at the time of primary resection. Late recurrences (>2 years from resection) are mainly related to the development of new tumour sites and behave quite similarly to primary tumours. Multinodular disease, tumour size greater than 5 cm, satellite nodules, microvascular invasion, and persistence of high alpha-fetoprotein (AFP) levels increase the risk of recurrence. There is no recognized adjuvant treatment able to significantly reduce the recurrence rate as none of the many options proposed in this area has entered clinical practice. In this respect, promising results are expected from trials currently testing checkpoint inhibitors and other immunotherapies, alone or in combination with TKIs.

Prophylactic (pre-emptive) LT has been advocated for transplantable patients exhibiting high-risk features following LR for HCC, such as microvascular invasion, poor differentiation, presence of microsatellites, multiple tumours, and gene-expressing signatures associated with aggressive behaviour. Also, salvage transplantation at the time of recurrence can offer a therapeutic chance if within-acceptable selection criteria in the recurring tumour are met.

However, due to several limitations in the access to LT, repeated LR along the lines described above is a sound option in about 15–30% of patients with recurrent HCC, with recent studies showing improved outcomes when laparoscopic procedures are employed, as these patients are at significant risk of postoperative morbidity.

For patients with recurring multifocal HCC or in case of macrovascular portal invasion limited at the segmental level, locoregional and systemic treatment are proposed as first option, with surgery to be considered at a later time if the tumour is downstaged and eligibility for resection is maintained. Several studies showed improved outcomes for a combination or sequential treatments of different locoregional therapies, TKIs, and immunotherapy. In all these instances, surgical removal could be beneficial in controlled/downstaged HCC, if curative procedures aimed at complete tumour removal are thought to be feasible.[15]

Innovations in liver transplantation for the treatment of hepatocellular carcinoma

LT is the best treatment option currently available for HCC, as it extends the conventional margins of surgical oncology by eliminating both the visible tumour and those concurrent conditions favouring cancer origin and progression (i.e. cirrhosis, chronic liver damage, and inflammation). The use of LT for the treatment of certain forms of cancer remains a unique example of innovation that generated an entire field of interest defined as 'transplant oncology'. However, the most relevant limitation to the expanded use of LT in such contexts largely depends on the availability of donated organs.

Due to the persistent gap between the number of transplant candidates and the available grafts, a priori determination of 'selection criteria' is necessary for indicating the best candidates to be offered the limited resource of transplantation. In support of the need for patient and tumour selection are the unequivocal data showing that the strongest predictor of post-transplant mortality in patients with HCC remains HCC recurrence.

Furthermore, as LT is a salvage therapy for other forms of non-cancer-related liver diseases, the competition among cancer and non-cancer indications has increased and has been paralleled by the need to balance various indications within a common waiting list, according to the general principles of organ transplant allocation, which are the following:

- Urgency: focused on the mortality risk derived by the missing opportunity to receive a LT while on the waiting list.
- Utility: focused on maximization of post-transplant outcome.
- Benefit: measuring the survival gain achieved by liver transplant as compared to the available non-transplant options for the same disease conditions.[16,17]

Liver transplantation has different metrics with respect to any other treatment options against hepatocellular carcinoma

With respect to surgical resection and to other locoregional and systemic options considered in the clinical management of HCC, LT demands specific and adjunctive metrics. Similar to a lens decomposing the light spectrum, the multifaceted prism of LT is able to open new perspectives and give new interpretations of the results of other non-transplant therapies (Figure 16.7).

Non-transplant therapies acting through surgical and non-surgical interventions against HCC can be scrutinized under the eye of transplantation and revisited in perspective. For instance, a partial response to systemic or locoregional therapies can be reconsidered

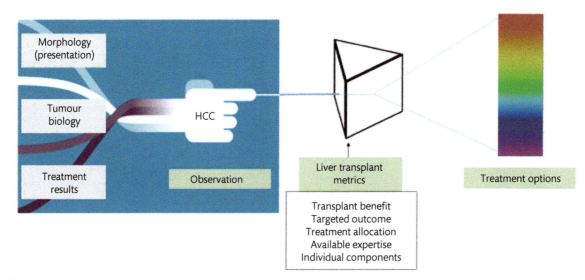

Figure 16.7 The multiple metrics of transplantation for HCC revisit the principles derived from observations and expand their therapeutic applications.

using the transplant benefit principle and the available access to LT and used to target or not the unprecedented outcome achievable with transplantation, providing that selection criteria are satisfied. In general, the spectrum of characteristics that are considered in each active therapy against HCC can be expanded if LT is considered among the options. In fact, the large majority of 'conventional' and 'borderline' indications for total hepatectomy and consequent liver replacement emerge after multidisciplinary discussion on individual patients, whose complexities are not fully captured by guidelines but deemed sufficient for considering transplant eligibility.[17]

Transplant criteria and the importance of a flexible approach to transplant eligibility

After decades of systematic use of LT as the standard of care in eligible patients with HCC, some interesting conclusions emerged from meta-analyses on thousands of patients receiving transplants with the aim to cure liver cancer:

- A promising decrease in HCC recurrence and improvement of survival after LT have been observed over the last 35 years. This may be due to the implementation of neoadjuvant cancer-limiting therapies preceding LT and to progressive reduction of non-cancer-related adverse prognostic factors in chronically immunosuppressed recipients, such as recurrent hepatitis, chronic immunological events, and comorbidities causing non-cancer-related deaths.
- Milan criteria (single HCC <5 cm in size, or up to three HCC nodules, each ≤3 cm) still determines a significant difference in predicting recurrence and patient outcomes. In fact, the Milan criteria represents the benchmark for any attempt to expand transplantation indications. A large sample of the proposed 'expanded criteria' are summarized in Table 16.2.
- HCC recurrences are observed more frequently in Asian series with respect to Western countries. This may be the consequence of less stringent selection criteria in living-donor liver transplantation (LDLT), more frequently applied in the East, possibly exceeding Milan criteria, as well as differences in viral aetiology, as HBV infection is the primary underlying cause of HCC in Asia compared to HCV in Western countries.

Regardless of the criteria adopted in different contexts, in which different general and local conditions play a role, the wider the expansion of tumour burden thought to be eligible for LT, the higher the HCC recurrence rate after transplantation, and consequently the lower the expected patient survival.

As reported in Table 16.3, several factors acting as surrogates of tumour biology are considered in modern selection criteria to complement the conventional morphological ones. Among others, the best surrogate of tumour biology in clinical practice remains the serum level of AFP, which is more valuable in this context than in the HCC screening of cirrhotic patients.

The interaction between tumour morphology as assessed at radiology (size and number of nodules) and AFP levels is systematically deducible with the 'Metroticket' model, a web-based calculator (freely available at http://www.hcc-olt-metroticket.org) able to accurately predict the post-transplant survival in any HCC

Table 16.2 Expanded selection criteria for liver transplantation in HCC patients, with the associated survival outcomes

Centre	Morphological criteria	Biomarker criteria	Survival
Milan	1 lesion ≤6.5 cm, 2–3 lesions ≤4.5 cm each	None	4 yr OS: 85%
UCSF	1 lesion ≤6.5 cm, 2–3 lesions ≤4.5 cm each Total tumour diameter ≤8 cm	None	5 yr OS: 72.4%
Pamplona	1 lesion ≤6 cm, 2–3 lesions ≤5 cm each	None	5 yr OS: 79%
Edmonton	1 lesion <7.5 cm, multiple lesions <5 cm each	None	4 yr OS: 82.9% 4 yr RFS: 76.8%
Dallas	1 lesion ≤6 cm, 2–4 lesions ≤5 cm each	None	5 yr RFS: 1 lesion ≤6 cm: 63.9% 2–4 lesions 3–5 cm: 64.6%
Valencia	1–3 lesions ≤5 cm each Total tumour diameter ≤10 cm	None	5 yr OS: 67%
Up-to-Seven	The sum of the size and number of tumours not exceeding 7 in the absence of microvascular invasion	None	5 yr OS: 71.2%
Hangzhou	Total tumour diameter ≤8 cm Total tumour diameter >8 cm with histopathological grade I or II	If total tumour diameter >8 cm: AFP ≤400 ng/mL	5 yr OS: 70.7% 5 yr DFS: 62.4%
Rome	Total tumour diameter ≤8 cm	AFP ≤400 ng/mL	5 yr DFS: 74.4%
Warsaw	UCSF or Up-to-Seven criteria	AFP <100 ng/mL	5 yr OS: 100%
Geneva	Total tumour volume ≤115 cm³	AFP ≤400 ng/mL	4 yr OS: 74.6%
Toronto	Milan criteria Any size and number + G1–2 + no cancer-related symptoms	AFP ≤500 ng/mL AFP ≤500 ng/mL	5 yr OS: 78% 5 yr OS: 68%
Metroticket 2.0	Up-to-Seven Up-to-Five Up-to-Four	AFP ≤200 ng/mL AFP ≤400 ng/mL AFP ≤1000 ng/mL	5 yr cancer-specific survival: 75%

DFS, disease-free survival; OS, overall survival; RFS, recurrence-free survival.

Table 16.3 Composite criteria aimed at individualization of prognosis to be used for different priority within the transplant waitlist

Prognostic composite criteria	Time to assess	Variables	Formula—ranges categories or calculator	Endpoint of prediction
MORAL	Pre LT At LT	NLR ≥5 (6 point); AFP ≥200 (4 points) Maximum diameter >3 cm (3 points) Grade 4 (6 points), vascular invasion (2 points) Maximum diameter >3 cm (3 points) Number >3 (2 points)	0–2 Low risk 3–6 Medium risk 7–10 High risk >10 Very high risk	RFS
HALT-HCC	Pre LT	TBS, AFP, MELD-Na (TBS = √number of lesions + maximum diameter)	(1.27 × TBS) + (1.85 × lnAFP) +(0.26 × MELD-Na)	OS
French Model		Number of lesions: 1–3 (0 points), ≥4 (1 point) Maximum diameter (cm): ≤3 (0 points), 3–6 (1 point), >6 (4 points) AFP: ≤100 (0 points), 100–1000 (2 points), >1000 (3 points)	0–2 Low risk >2 High risk	RFS OS
Metroticket 2.0	Pre LT	Number of lesions (active) + maximum diameter (active) AFP	http://www.hcc-olt-metroticket.org/ (individual prognostication calculator)	OS and HCC-specific survival

NLR, neutrophil-to-lymphocyte ratio; OS, overall survival; RFS, recurrence-free survival; TBS, Tumour Burden Score.

patient considered for listing and while on the waitlist. Notably, the Metroticket calculator is a versatile instrument to monitor the HCC 'vital' part of the tumour in case of pretransplant neoadjuvant treatments. Through multiple predictions made at each interval after tumour downstaging, variation of prognosis during the course of disease can be determined as a consequence of various treatments. This translates into a flexible approach to listing and priority according to the measured chances of success of LT at different time intervals during the treatment history of the patient (Figure 16.8).[17-19]

Hepatocellular carcinoma response to pretransplant therapies is the most effective driver for criteria expansion

As in the Metroticket model, any a priori defined flexible approach to transplant eligibility criteria for HCC—to be challenged with local conditions and waitlist dynamics—creates a differential scale of transplant priority that depends on tumour presentation and response to neoadjuvant, pretransplant therapies.

The inherent heterogeneity of HCC presentations is paralleled by a wide range of downstaging efficacy, particularly when combination treatments are attempted at different time intervals. It has been demonstrated that not only the initial response of HCC to available treatments but also the tumour tendency to regrowth after treatment varies quite significantly. This speaks in favour of a variable time-related propensity to tumour progression after radiological response, also confirming the common clinical observation that clinical evolution and response to therapy in HCC may be different in different patients (Figure 16.9).

The spectrum of end-treatment presentations of HCC is granular and goes from complete response, to sustained response beyond Milan criteria, to various degrees of partial responses in or beyond Milan criteria, to no response at all. This is worth a differential offer

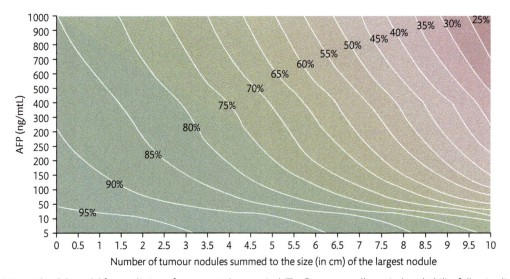

Figure 16.8 The Metroticket 2.0 model for prediction of post-transplant survival. The 5-year overall-survival probability following liver transplantation according to HCC presentation (i.e. number of nodules summed to the size of the largest tumour) and serum level of AFP is presented in a contour plot scheme. Multiple measurements can be taken at various times of the medical history and according to the response to neoadjuvant treatments.
Reproduced with permission from Mazzaferro V, Sposito C, Zhou J, et al. Metroticket 2.0 Model for Analysis of Competing Risks of Death After Liver Transplantation for Hepatocellular Carcinoma. *Gastroenterology.* 2018;154(1):128–139. doi:10.1053/j.gastro.2017.09.025

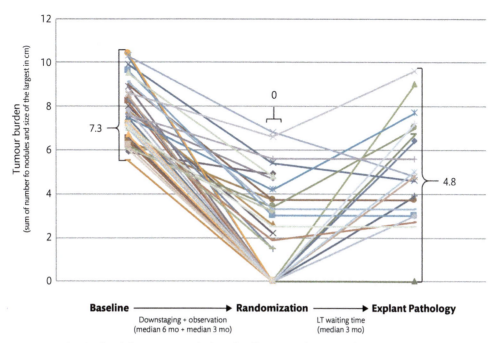

Figure 16.9 In a prospective randomized trial demonstrating the benefit of liver transplantation after HCC downstaging, tumour burden assessment over time shows how both the grade of tumour response to treatment and tumour progression after treatment undergo significant variations in different patients.

Reproduced with permission from Mazzaferro V, Citterio D, Bhoori S, et al. Liver transplantation in hepatocellular carcinoma after tumour downstaging (XXL): a randomised, controlled, phase 2b/3 trial. Lancet Oncol. 2020;21(7):947–956. doi:10.1016/S1470-2045(20)30224-2

of LT, reflecting a stratification of stages of responses and tumour progressions that ultimately defines a scale of priority to receive organs procured from deceased donors.

The search for the best allocation of donated organs and priority for HCC patients is a persistently unsolved issue, ever since the MELD system—unable to capture presentation, biology, and evolution of cancer—was introduced as the driver for prioritizing LT candidates on the basis of acuity of the candidate's medical conditions.

Balancing priority across different indications is in fact an unfinished project. For instance, the system currently applied in the United States assigns exception points to patients within Milan criteria and to those beyond criteria successfully downstaged to Milan criteria, although HCC patients with compensated cirrhosis have persistently very low MELD scores and difficult access to deceased donor LT. The current systems do not satisfy the increasing request to adopt versatile models for HCC (such as the Metroticket model) for expanding the transplant offer with reasonable success in patients with HCC beyond Milan criteria.

In Figure 16.10, a systematic scale of priority in the transplant offer for HCC undergoing neoadjuvant therapies is presented. This kind of model is likely to be introduced into clinical practice because predetermined cancer conditions are not required upfront, while eligibility for transplantation and priority are defined at the end of the therapeutic neoadjuvant process, namely after the best available therapy has been completed. A further advantage in following such a strategy is that preliminary tumour response to treatments could become the most flexible and defined criteria for expanding the indication for LT in HCC beyond the Milan criteria, without compromising the post-transplant outcome and therefore fully justifying the use of donated organs for cancer patients.

To complement this line of reasoning, several studies and meta-analyses correlate favourable tumour biology with response to neoadjuvant treatments, also showing that LT efficacy is increased in tumours beyond the Milan criteria, achieving an objective response to locoregional treatments. Providing the exclusion of patients with severe comorbidities, advanced age, or other reasons impeding surgical consideration, any intrahepatic presentation of HCC could be considered for LT, with the decision on eligibility and priority to be taken after tumour downstaging. Finally, the evolution of neoadjuvant treatments is able to change allocation and prioritization issues, as the degree of tumour response is the main driver of access to LT. Due to recent advancements in targeted therapies, both TKIs and immunotherapy may improve the current results of tumour downstaging obtained with locoregional treatments, converting more advanced patients to curative perspectives.

Definitive confirmation of this flexible strategy emerged in a randomized control trial (XXL trial) demonstrating with good evidence that, after sustained and successful downstaging of HCC beyond Milan criteria, LT achieves a significant survival benefit with respect to any other non-transplant therapy.[16–21]

The donor pool for patients with hepatocellular carcinoma should be expanded

Expansion of the donor pool in cancer patients through living donation is analysed in detail in other parts of this book. General indications for LDLT in case of HCC should not differ from those employing deceased donors; however, tumour extension considered suitable for LDLT is usually less restrictive, since the reduction of expected survival in LDLT is felt acceptable in the context of organ donation as a personal gift rather than a resource to be distributed in the community. In a European perspective in which living donation

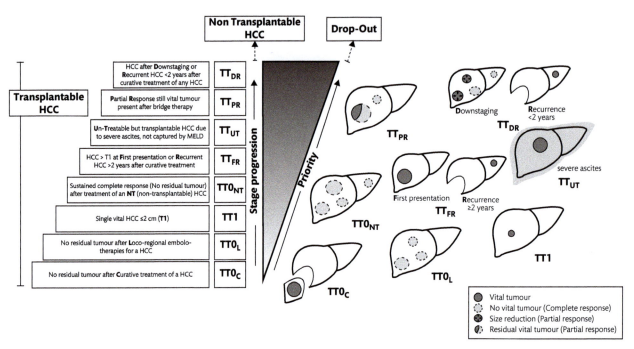

Figure 16.10 Staging and priority allocation for HCC according to definition of end-treatment tumour presentation. Several levels of priority can be identified at the end of neoadjuvant therapy, according to tumour response and to the risk of waitlist drop-out because of tumour progression beyond predefined criteria.
Reproduced with permission from: Mazzaferro V. Squaring the circle of selection and allocation in liver transplantation for HCC: an adaptive approach. *Hepatology*. 2016;63(5):1707–1717. doi:10.1002/hep.28420

still represents a marginal component of LT activity, in addition to optimization of graft allocation through prioritization, several strategies have been implemented aimed at expanding the limited resource of available grafts.

A modern area of interest is represented by expanded criteria donors with use of marginal grafts and donors after cardiac death (DCD). Recent advances in organ preservation and reconditioning by means of perfusion machines reduce the risk of failure related to the ischaemia-reperfusion injury in marginal grafts and also allow for a real-time assessment of graft quality before implantation in low MELD score recipients, a common condition in HCC patients. The inhibition of inflammatory reaction associated with ischaemia-reperfusion injury may even lower the risk of tumour recurrence in livers from donors after cardiac death reconditioned with hypothermic oxygenated perfusion, as compared to conventional brain-dead donors. This may be due to an impact of perfusion on the early immune response of the recipient, with reduction of metastatic tumour cells engraftment in the transplanted liver.[22]

Conclusion

In conclusion, LR and LT are the mainstay of treatment of HCC with a strong prognostic impact as compared to locoregional and systemic therapies. Although current guidelines only capture a segment of the potentials of surgical therapies, resectability should be pursued—if not applied—at any stage of intrahepatic HCC, either at presentation or after non-surgical treatments have reduced or controlled the tumour. Minimally invasive approaches, neoadjuvant treatments, technical improvements, and models for accurate prediction of postoperative liver failure in cirrhotic patients allow the expansion of resection to borderline indications. Tumour response to non-surgical therapies is the most effective tool to select patients for surgical interventions, especially for LT in HCCs beyond conventional criteria. Despite new advancements in medical therapies, surgical interventions will continue to play a central role in the curative treatment of HCC.

REFERENCES

1. Llovet JM, Kelley RK, Villanueva A, et al. Hepatocellular carcinoma. *Nat Rev Dis Prim*. 2021;**7**(1):6.
2. Galle PR, Tovoli F, Foerster F, et al. The treatment of intermediate stage tumours beyond TACE: from surgery to systemic therapy. *J Hepatol*. 2017;**67**(1):173–183.
3. Jogi S, Varanai R, Bantu SS, et al. Selecting the first line treatment in non-metastatic hepatocellular carcinoma—comparing clinical practice guidelines. *Oncol Rev*. 2020;**14**(2):158–163.
4. Foerster F, Galle PR. Comparison of the current international guidelines on the management of HCC. *JHEP Rep*. 2019;**1**(2):114–119.
5. Galle PR, Forner A, Llovet JM, et al. EASL Clinical Practice Guidelines: management of hepatocellular carcinoma. *J Hepatol*. 2018;**69**(1):182–236.
6. Chin KM, Prieto M, Cheong CK, et al. Outcomes after curative therapy for hepatocellular carcinoma in patients with non-alcoholic fatty liver disease: a meta-analysis and review of current literature. *HPB (Oxford)*. 2021;**23**(8):1164–1174.
7. Citterio D, Facciorusso A, Sposito C, et al. Hierarchic interaction of factors associated with liver decompensation after resection for hepatocellular carcinoma. *JAMA Surg*. 2016;**151**(9):846–853.

8. Sun Z, Li Z, Shi XL, et al. Anatomic versus non-anatomic resection of hepatocellular carcinoma with microvascular invasion: a systematic review and meta-analysis. *Asian J Surg*. 2021;**44**(9):1143–1150.
9. Swaid F, Geller DA. Minimally invasive primary liver cancer surgery. *Surg Oncol Clin N Am*. 2019;**28**(3):215–227.
10. Di Sandro S, Danieli M, Ferla F, et al. The current role of laparoscopic resection for HCC: a systematic review of past ten years. *Transl Gastroenterol Hepatol*. 2018;**3**:68.
11. Loveday BPT, Jaberi A, Moulton CA, et al. Effect of portal vein embolization on treatment plan prior to major hepatectomy for hepatocellular carcinoma. *HPB (Oxford)*. 2019;**21**(8):1072–1078.
12. Glantzounis GK, Tokidis E, Basourakos SP, et al. The role of portal vein embolization in the surgical management of primary hepatobiliary cancers. A systematic review. *Eur J Surg Oncol*. 2017;**43**(1):32–41.
13. Zhang J, Huang H, Bian J, et al. Safety, feasibility, and efficacy of associating liver partition and portal vein ligation for staged hepatectomy in treating hepatocellular carcinoma: a systematic review. *Ann Transl Med*. 2020;**8**(19):1246.
14. Teo JY, Allen JC, Ng DC, et al. A systematic review of contralateral liver lobe hypertrophy after unilobar selective internal radiation therapy with Y90. *HPB (Oxford)*. 2016;**18**(1):7–12.
15. Tampaki M, Papatheodoridis GV, Cholongitas E. Intrahepatic recurrence of hepatocellular carcinoma after resection: an update. *Clin J Gastroenterol*. 2021;**14**(3):699–713.
16. Mehta N, Bhangui P, Yao FY, et al. Liver transplantation for hepatocellular carcinoma. Working Group report from the ILTS Transplant Oncology Consensus Conference. *Transplantation*. 2020;**104**(6):1136–1142.
17. Mazzaferro V. Squaring the circle of selection and allocation in liver transplantation for HCC: an adaptive approach. *Hepatology*. 2016;**63**(5):1707–1717.
18. Mazzaferro V, Sposito C, Zhou J, et al. Metroticket 2.0 model for analysis of competing risks of death after liver transplantation for hepatocellular carcinoma. *Gastroenterology*. 2018;**154**(1):128–139.
19. Mazzaferro V, Citterio D, Bhoori S, et al. Liver transplantation in hepatocellular carcinoma after tumour downstaging (XXL): a randomised, controlled, phase 2b/3 trial. *Lancet Oncol*. 2020;**21**(7):947–956.
20. Younossi Z, Stepanova M, Ong JP, et al. Nonalcoholic steatohepatitis is the fastest growing cause of hepatocellular carcinoma in liver transplant candidates. *Clin Gastroenterol Hepatol*. 2019;**17**(4):748–755.
21. Tan DJH, Wong C, Ng CH, et al. A meta-analysis on the rate of hepatocellular carcinoma recurrence after liver transplant and associations to etiology, alpha-fetoprotein, income and ethnicity. *J Clin Med*. 2021;**10**(2):238.
22. Kubal C, Mihaylov P, Holden J. Oncologic indications of liver transplantation and deceased donor liver allocation in the United States. *Curr Opin Organ Transplant*. 2021;**26**(2):168–175.

17
Cholangiocarcinoma

Mohamed Rela and Mettu Srinivas Reddy

Overview of cholangiocarcinoma

Cholangiocarcinomas (CCs) are a group of cancers originating in the biliary tract. The cell of origin is the cholangiocyte lining the entire biliary tract and these tumours are classified depending on their location of origin from the intrahepatic biliary ductules to the distal bile duct entering the ampulla of Vater. They are uncommon, slow-growing tumours and seen after the sixth decade of life. They usually present late in their natural history and curative options are limited.

Anatomical classification

Tumours arising from the intrahepatic biliary tract proximal to the second-order bile ducts are usually classified as intrahepatic cholangiocarcinomas (IHCCs) constituting 20% of all CCs. Perihilar cholangiocarcinomas (PHCCs) include all cancers developing in the biliary tract from the second-order bile ducts up to the cystic duct origin. Tumours distal to the cystic duct are classified as distal cholangiocarcinomas (dCCs) (Figure 17.1). Cancers developing in the gall bladder have a distinct pathology and natural history and are not included in the CC group. This chapter will cover IHCCs and PHCCs; dCCs and cancers of the gall bladder are dealt with elsewhere in this book.

Epidemiology, risk factors, and natural history

CCs are uncommon, constituting approximately 3% of all abdominal malignancies. Multiple longitudinal studies have shown that their incidence has been increasing worldwide. The disease has distinct geographical variations in incidence and is more common in Eastern countries, probably related to the higher prevalence of parasitic infections in this region. It is usually seen in the sixth decade of life and has a slight male preponderance.

There are several well-defined risk factors for CC, though the majority of tumours develop in the absence of any of these predisposing factors. Primary sclerosing cholangitis (PSC) is a strong risk factor

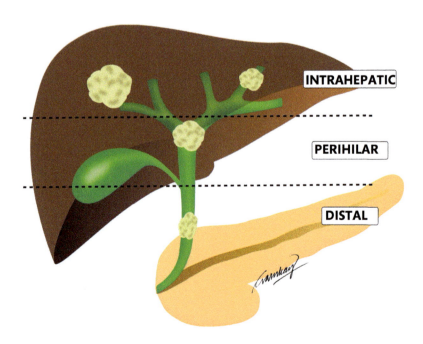

Figure 17.1 Types of CC.
Reproduced courtesy of Dr Ramkiran Reddy Cherukuru, Consultant Surgeon, Dr Rela Institute & Medical Center, Chennai, India.

for CC. Inflammatory bowel disease, particularly long-standing ulcerative colitis (UC), is another risk factor. Chronic parasitic infections of the biliary tract (e.g. *Clonorchis sinensis*),[1] congenital diseases of the biliary tract (e.g. choledochal cyst), and Caroli's disease[2] are also associated with an increased risk. Occupational exposure to chemicals and solvents and asbestos has been associated with CC.[3]

Most CCs present late and hence do not have curative options. The potential for curative treatment is higher for dCC due to earlier presentation with jaundice, while it is lowest for IHCC. Once diagnosed, the median survival in patients who are unsuitable for any treatment options is 3.9 months, ranging from 3.0 months for IHCC to 5.9 months for PHCC.[4] In another study of patients who received palliative treatments such as biliary drainage and chemotherapy, the survival after clinical presentation was 19% at 2 years and 9% at 3 years.[5]

Pathology

Ninety per cent of CCs are adenocarcinomas with biliary differentiation. The remaining tumours present with papillary, squamous, adenosquamous, or mucinous differentiation. Histologically, these tumours have malignant cells with desmoplastic stroma. Multifocality is common and several precursors or premalignant lesions have been recognized. These include intra-epithelial biliary neoplasms, intraductal papillary neoplasms, and intraductal tubular neoplasms.[6]

Perihilar cholangiocarcinoma

Morphologically, these are classified as papillary, nodular, nodular infiltrating, or diffuse infiltrating types. Papillary types are better differentiated and more likely to be resectable.

Tumours may be classified into well-, moderately, and poorly differentiated forms based on the percentage of gland formation (Figure 17.2a,b).

Intrahepatic cholangiocarcinoma

Morphologically, these have been classified into four pathological variants: mass-forming type, periductal infiltrating type, intraductal growth type, and mixed variant.[6] Histologically, IHCC can be classified into a cholangiolar type and a bile duct type[7] (Figure 17.2c). The cholangiolar type is composed of cuboidal to low columnar tumour cells that contain scanty cytoplasm while the bile duct type is composed of tall columnar tumour cells arranged in a large glandular pattern. The cholangiolar-type IHCC is frequently associated with viral hepatitis, whereas the bile duct type is associated with hepatolithiasis. Precancerous lesions such as biliary intraepithelial neoplasms or intraductal papillary neoplasms of the bile duct are frequently associated with the bile duct-type IHCC. Prognostically, the cholangiolar variants have a better long-term survival.

Tumour staging

The eighth edition of the Union for International Cancer Control (UICC) staging for PHCC and IHCC is presented in Tables 17.1 and 17.2.[8] Prognostic factors for CC are tumour size, number of lesions, locoregional spread and presence of vascular invasion, lymph nodal involvement, and distant metastases.

Therapeutic options

The clinical management of PHCC and IHCC are distinct and will be dealt with separately in the following sections. Surgical resection

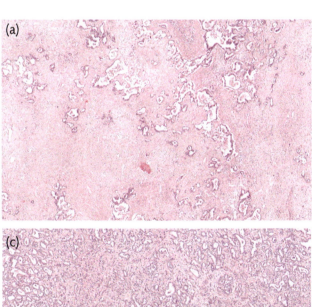
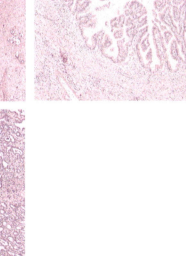
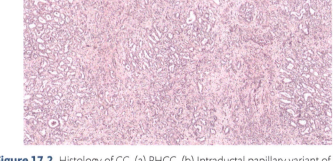

Figure 17.2 Histology of CC. (a) PHCC. (b) Intraductal papillary variant of PHCC. (c) IHCC (bile duct type).
Reproduced courtesy of Dr Mukul Vij, Department of Pathology, Dr Rela Institute & Medical Center, Chennai, India.

Table 17.1 UICC staging (eighth edition) for perihilar cholangiocarcinoma

T–primary tumour	
TX	Primary tumour cannot be assessed
T0	No evidence of primary tumour
Tis	Carcinoma *in situ*
T1	Tumour confined to the bile duct, with extension up to the muscle layer or fibrous tissue
T2a	Tumour invades beyond the wall of the bile duct to surrounding adipose tissue
T2b	Tumour invades adjacent hepatic parenchyma
T3	Tumour invades unilateral branches of the portal vein or hepatic artery
T4	Tumour invades the main portal vein or its branches bilaterally; or the common hepatic artery; or unilateral second-order biliary radicals with contralateral portal vein or hepatic artery involvement
N–regional lymph nodes	
NX	Regional lymph nodes cannot be assessed
N0	No regional lymph node metastasis
N1	Metastases to 1–3 regional lymph nodes
N2	Metastases to 4 or more regional nodes
M–distant metastasis	
M0	No distant metastasis
M1	Distant metastasis

Stage–perihilar bile ducts			
Stage 0	Tis	N0	M0
Stage I	T1	N0	M0
Stage II	T2a, T2b	N0	M0
Stage IIIA	T3	N0	M0
Stage IIIB	T4	N0	M0
Stage IIIC	Any T	N1	M0
Stage IVA	Any T	N2	M0
Stage IVB	Any T	Any N	M1

Reproduced with permission from Brierley, JD, Gospodarowicz MK, and Wittekind C, *TNM Classification of Malignant Tumours*, 8th edition, UICC/Wiley-Blackwell, 2017, pp. 87–88.

Table 17.2 UICC staging (eighth edition) for intrahepatic cholangiocarcinoma

T–primary tumour	
T0	No evidence of primary tumour
Tis	Carcinoma *in situ* (intraductal tumour)
T1a	Solitary tumour 5 cm or less in greatest dimension without vascular invasion
T1b	Solitary tumour more than 5 cm in greatest dimension without vascular invasion
T2	Solitary tumour with intrahepatic vascular invasion *or* multiple tumours, with or without vascular invasion
T3	Tumour perforating the visceral peritoneum
T4	Tumour involving local extrahepatic structures by direct hepatic invasion
N–regional lymph nodes	
NX	Regional lymph nodes cannot be assessed
N0	No regional lymph node metastasis
N1	Regional lymph node metastasis
M–distant metastasis	
M0	No distant metastasis
M1	Distant metastasis

Stage–intrahepatic bile ducts			
Stage I	T1	N0	M0
Stage IA	T1a	N0	M0
Stage IB	T1b	N0	M0
Stage II	T2	N0	M0
Stage IIIA	T3	N0	M0
Stage IIIB	T4	N0	M0
	Any T	N1	M0
Stage IV	Any T	Any N	M1

Reproduced with permission from Brierley, JD, Gospodarowicz MK, and Wittekind C, *TNM Classification of Malignant Tumours*, 8th edition, UICC/Wiley-Blackwell, 2017, pp. 83–84.

is the only treatment option with a chance of long-term survival in these patients. The aim of surgery is an R0 resection leaving sufficient volume of healthy liver to support the patient's recovery.

The feasibility of surgery depends on multiple interrelated factors. These include tumour factors including the stage and location, baseline liver function including the size of the future liver remnant (FLR), performance status, and the cardiopulmonary fitness of these patients to undergo a major surgical resection. Ideally, all patients should be discussed in a multidisciplinary tumour board setting before proceeding to surgery. Many of these patients may need preoperative interventions to optimize their condition and improve the safety of the operation.

Non-surgical options are primarily palliative and can improve symptoms and extend survival. These include interventions to treat jaundice, locoregional therapies such as chemo- or radioembolization, radiotherapy, and photodynamic therapy, or palliative chemotherapy.

Perihilar cholangiocarcinoma

PHCCs constitute 50% of all CCs and include all CCs arising between the second-order division of right and left hepatic ducts and the origin of the cystic duct. Based on the location of the main tumour and laterality of the ducts involved these tumours are further classified into five types (Figure 17.3).

Clinical presentation and diagnostic workup

Obstructive jaundice is the most common symptom at presentation in PHCC and occurs when biliary drainage from both sides of the liver is obstructed. Early lesions are also identified during routine imaging for other medical conditions. Surveillance in conditions such as PSC or UC can detect these tumours at an early stage.

Diagnostic imaging

The first line of investigation in patients presenting with jaundice is an ultrasound scan to look for biliary obstruction. Ultrasound can

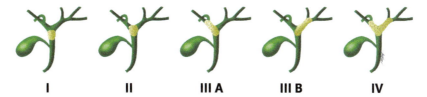

Figure 17.3 Bismuth Corlette classification of PHCC.
Reproduced courtesy of Dr Ramkiran Reddy Cherukuru, Consultant Surgeon, Dr Rela Institute & Medical Center, Chennai, India.

reveal dilated intrahepatic bile ducts and occasionally a hilar mass. Cross-sectional imaging with a contrast computed tomography (CT) scan or magnetic resonance imaging (MRI) is necessary to evaluate these tumours in greater detail. This may show a dilated intrahepatic biliary tract with an abrupt cut-off at the hilum. The tumour itself may be evident as thickening of the biliary tract, a hilar mass lesion, or an intraluminal papillary lesion. Imaging can also reveal intrahepatic metastases, cholangitic abscesses, and lymphadenopathy. A triple-phase contrast CT scan is the best modality for assessing arterial and portal vein involvement. Ideally, cross-sectional imaging should be performed prior to biliary drainage procedures to avoid the artefactual issues due to indwelling catheters and stents (Figure 17.4).

Histological diagnosis

Endoscopic retrograde cholangiopancreatography (ERCP) and percutaneous transhepatic cholangiography are primarily indicated for therapeutic procedures such as biliary drainage or for biopsy/brushing cytology of suspicious lesions. Preoperative histological diagnosis of PHCC is difficult due to the high false negativity rates of standard endo-biliary biopsy and cytology techniques. The use of newer techniques such as SpyGlass imaging to guide intraluminal biopsies and endoscopic ultrasound-guided fine-needle aspiration cytology of hilar lesions and use of genomic and proteomic studies for evaluating biopsies have the potential to improve the diagnostic yield.[9] However, in the presence of a potentially resectable lesion, lack of histological diagnosis of PHCC should not delay definitive surgical treatment.

Tumour marker carbohydrate antigen 19-9 (CA19-9)

CA19-9 is a commonly used tumour marker for pancreaticobiliary malignancies. While mild elevations are non-specific and could be related to cholangitis or obstructive jaundice, a level greater than 1000 U/mL is likely to be due to CC. High levels of CA19-9 also correlate with advanced disease and the presence of metastases. Elevated CA19-9 levels secondary to obstructive jaundice or cholangitis fall significantly after biliary drainage procedures. CA19-9 has also been used clinically to assess response to chemotherapy and to monitor for tumour recurrence though the evidence is not robust.[8]

Differential diagnosis

A variety of benign and malignant processes can mimic PHCC. Benign biliary strictures secondary to bile duct injury, inflammatory bile duct tumours, immunoglobulin G4-related cholangitis, and infections such as tuberculosis may mimic PHCC. Malignancies such as lymphomas can masquerade as PHCC. Dominant biliary strictures in the setting of PSC may be difficult to characterize even after repeated brush biopsy or SpyGlass examinations.

Surgery for perihilar cholangiocarcinoma: considerations

Resection of the primary tumour with clear margins is the only treatment modality with the potential for long-term cure in PHCC. These patients will usually need a major liver resection as part of the surgery. Only a third of patients with CC are amenable for resection.[11] Patients are unresectable usually due to extensive local disease rather than metastases. Intensive preoperative optimization strategies and

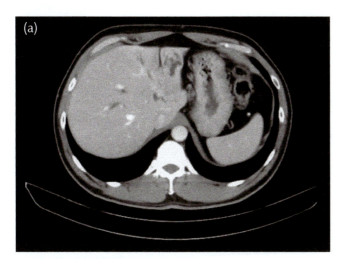 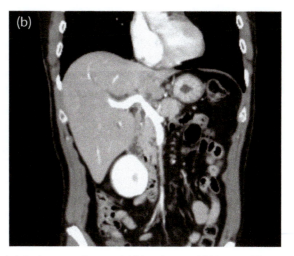

Figure 17.4 PHCC (contrast CT) showing the reciprocal left lobe atrophy and right lobe hypertrophy on axial (a) and coronal (b) images. The coronal image shows the abrupt cut-off of the left portal vein at its origin, which is responsible for the left lobe atrophy.

aggressive surgery can improve resectability. Management of these patients should preferably be undertaken in high-volume centres, with expertise in major liver resection, liver transplantation (LT), and interventional endoscopy and radiology for best outcomes, both in terms of resectability and survival after resection. Multiple factors have an impact in deciding whether a patient with PHCC is suitable for surgical resection. Many staging systems do not include important considerations such as remnant liver volume and underlying liver disease and are hence impractical for clinical use or intercentre comparison. The International Cholangiocarcinoma Group has developed a staging system taking into consideration many of these factors which dictate the feasibility of surgical resection in these patients[12] (Table 17.3).

Extent of tumour and vascular involvement

Assessment of the true extent of PHCC is complicated by the fact that a mass lesion is not always present. PHCC has the tendency to spread both radially into surrounding structures and longitudinally along the bile ducts. Bile duct resection thus has to be generous beyond the visible tumour margins to ensure complete clearance. The nature and extent of liver resection depends on the location and laterality of the tumour and associated vascular involvement. Unilateral biliary obstruction or vascular involvement can lead to a significant atrophy–hypertrophy response which should be taken into consideration during surgical planning (Figure 17.4).

Vascular involvement is common in PHCC due to the close proximity of the tumour to the hepatic inflow structures (Figure 17.5). The bile duct with its bifurcation lies dorsal to the main portal vein bifurcation. Posterior extension of the tumour can infiltrate the portal bifurcation early. Similarly, the right hepatic artery after originating from the common hepatic artery to the left of bile duct reaches the right side by crossing the common hepatic duct—usually posteriorly—where it can be involved by the tumour. While actual tumour infiltration of the arterial wall is uncommon due to its innate resistance to tumour infiltration, the artery can get encased by tumour tissue. The left hepatic artery remains to the left of the bile duct before entering the Rex recess and is usually away from the tumour.[13] In advanced cases, both the main portal vein and the common hepatic artery can be encased by the tumour.

Lymph nodal involvement

Lymph nodal involvement is common in PHCC. The commonly involved nodes are in the hepatoduodenal ligament, the hepatic artery, and the retropancreatic lymph nodes and these should be included in the field of resection. Lymph nodal involvement beyond these fields (i.e. coeliac and para-aortic) indicates systemic disease and curative surgery may not be possible.

Locoregional spread and metastases

Locally advanced PHCC can infiltrate the duodenum, pyloro-antral region, and the lesser curvature of the stomach. Involvement of the surrounding organs is a late event in these tumours and usually portends a poor prognosis. However, occasionally localized duodenal involvement may be present and if there are no other contraindications, curative resection is feasible. Distant metastases indicate advanced disease and surgery should be avoided.

Underlying liver disease

PHCCs cause progressive biliary obstruction due to their indolent nature. Obstructive jaundice leads to cholestatic liver injury

Table 17.3 Staging classification of the International Cholangiocarcinoma Group

Label	Side/location	Description
Bile duct (B)		
B1		Common bile duct
B2		Hepatic duct confluence
B3	Right	Right hepatic duct
B3	Left	Left hepatic duct
B4		Right and left hepatic duct
Tumour size (T)		
T1		<1 cm
T2		1–3 cm
T3		>3 cm
Tumour form (F)		
Sclerosing		Sclerosing (or periductal)
Mass		Mass-forming (or nodular)
Mixed		Sclerosing and mass-forming
Polypoid		Polypoid (or intraductal)
Portal vein involvement (180*)		
PV0		No portal involvement
PV1		Main portal vein
PV2		Portal vein bifurcation
PV3	Right	Right portal vein
PV3	Left	Left portal vein
PV4		Right and left portal veins
Hepatic artery involvement (180*)		
HA0		No arterial involvement
HA1		Proper hepatic artery
HA2		Hepatic artery bifurcation
HA3	Right	Right hepatic artery
HA3	Left	Left hepatic artery
HA4		Right and left hepatic artery
Liver remnant volume (V)		
V0		No information on the volume needed (liver resection not foreseen)
V%	Indicate segments	Percentage of the total volume of a putative remnant liver after resection
Underlying liver disease (D)		
		Fibrosis
		Non-alcoholic steatohepatitis
		Primary sclerosing cholangitis
Lymph nodes (N)		
N0		No lymph node involvement
N1		Hilar and/or hepatic artery lymph node involvement
N2		Peri-aortic lymph node involvement
Metastases (M)		
M0		No distant metastases
M1		Distant metastases (including liver and peritoneal metastases)

Reproduced with permission from Deoliveira ML, Schulick RD, Nimura Y, Rosen C, Gores G, Neuhaus P, et al. New staging system and a registry for perihilar cholangiocarcinoma. *Hepatology*. 2011 Apr;53(4):1363–71.

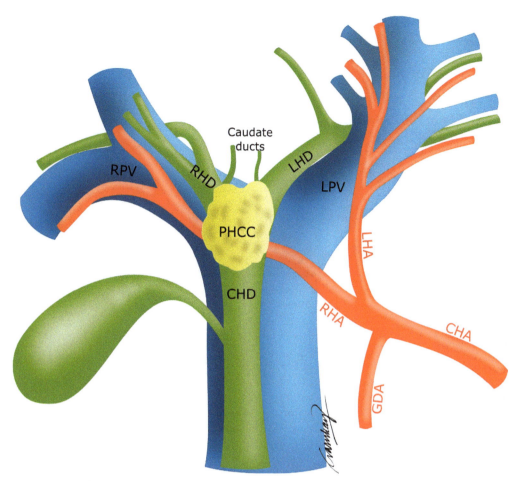

Figure 17.5 Anatomical relation of a PHCC to adjacent vascular structures. CHA, common hepatic artery; CHD, common hepatic duct; GDA, gastroduodenal artery; LHA, left hepatic artery; LHD, left hepatic duct; LPV, left portal vein; RHA, right hepatic artery; RHD, right hepatic duct; RPV, right portal vein.
Reproduced courtesy of Dr Ramkiran Reddy Cherukuru, Consultant Surgeon, Dr Rela Institute & Medical Center, Chennai, India.

impacting the regenerative potential of the remnant liver. If the obstruction is unilateral, as in the case of type III PHCC, prolonged biliary obstruction leads to hemi-atrophy of the involved segments with contralateral hypertrophy. This can increase the safety of liver resection due to an increased FLR. Background PSC may also lead to significant background liver disease and can contraindicate major resection.

Preoperative optimization

Careful utilization of preoperative optimization strategies has led to better resection rates and postoperative outcomes of PHCC. These measures are primarily aimed at improving the preoperative fitness of the patient, treating sepsis and malnutrition, and enhancing the safety of major liver resection.

Preoperative biliary drainage (POBD)

POBD is necessary in patients with high levels of jaundice and cholangitis. POBD improves the symptoms of itching and loss of appetite and helps in reduction of cholestatic liver injury. The choice of procedure depends on the level and anatomy of the biliary obstruction and the expertise available. While nasobiliary drainage or ERCP stenting is preferred by many centres, percutaneous transhepatic biliary drainage may be required in patients with high levels of obstruction. The future remnant liver should preferably be drained unless contralateral cholangitis mandates drainage of both sides. Preferential drainage of the FLR provides an opportunity for the hemiliver to recover and regenerate rapidly prior to surgery (Figure 17.6).

Preoperative biliary drainage has associated risks such as bleeding for percutaneous transhepatic biliary drainage and pancreatitis for ERCP. In addition, instrumentation of an obstructed biliary system has the potential to introduce infection. The overall impact of POBD on outcomes for PHCC is unclear. A recent meta-analysis suggested increased morbidity in patients undergoing routine POBD especially when the POBD to surgery interval was longer than 2 weeks.[14] It is unclear whether the poorer outcomes are a direct result of POBD or simply indicate advanced disease. The bilirubin cut-off at which POBD should be considered varies between centres. Our protocol is to perform biliary drainage if the patient needs a major hepatectomy and the bilirubin level is greater than 10 mg/dL and/or has ongoing cholangitis. Once a biliary drainage procedure is performed, bilirubin levels should reduce to less than 3 mg/dL prior to surgery. Failure of bilirubin levels to decrease after POBD is an indication of ongoing sepsis or inadequate function in the remnant liver and would contraindicate surgery.

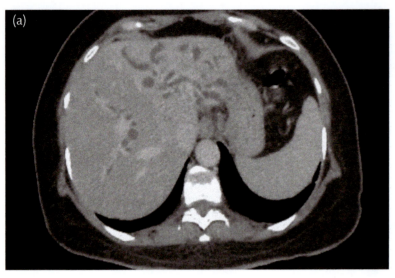
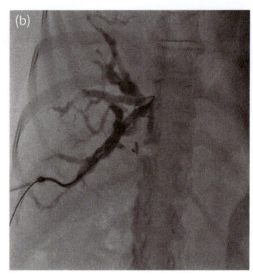

Figure 17.6 (a) PHCC with left lobe atrophy and bilateral bile duct dilatation. (b) Percutaneous biliary drainage of the right ductal system is being performed.

Portal vein embolization (PVE)

This technique is used to induce rapid hypertrophy of the FLR by preferentially diverting the entire portal blood flow to it, leading to a classic atrophy–hypertrophy response. A 20–25% increase in the FLR volume can be expected over 4–6 weeks with this approach, significantly improving the safety of major resection. Indications for PVE vary between centres but PVE is usually considered when the calculated FLR is less than 30% in healthy livers and less than 40% in patients with some underlying liver disease.[15] In cholestatic livers planned for a major resection, a combination of biliary drainage of the FLR and PVE of the contralateral liver lobe, performed either simultaneously or sequentially, can be considered. The percutaneous access for PVE should be through the unobstructed side. If the portal vein access is through the ipsilateral obstructed side, a biliary drainage should be carried out first to avoid severe life-threatening bacteraemia during the procedure. The extent of hypertrophy is an indirect marker of the quality of the underlying liver and a poor response to PVE or incomplete resolution of jaundice by drainage of the FLR predicts a higher risk of post-hepatectomy liver failure. This 4–6-week interval also provides an opportunity to optimize nutrition and improve muscle strength and deconditioning (Figure 17.7).

Surgical resection for perihilar cholangiocarcinoma

Staging laparoscopy is selectively utilized in patients with locally advanced PHCC and can avoid a laparotomy in the presence of peritoneal disease or hepatic metastases.

Curative surgery in PHCC usually involves a hemi- or extended hepatectomy, caudate lobe resection, and bile duct excision. Caudate bile ducts arise at the hepatic duct bifurcation and are involved early by PHCC.[16] En bloc resection of the caudate lobe improves clearance and has been shown to improve outcomes in these patients.[17] Frozen section examination of proximal and distal bile duct margins is usually performed in most centres to confirm an absence of tumour involvement.

The nature and extent of hepatectomy is guided by the laterality of the hilar tumour and presence and extent of vascular involvement. Bile duct excision alone is not recommended for PHCC as the risk of residual disease is very high. Limited liver resection of segments

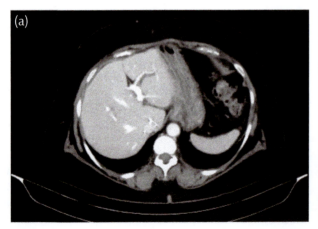
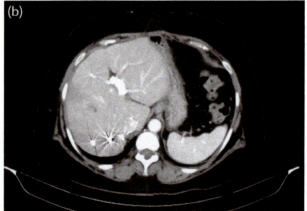

Figure 17.7 PVE to induce hypertrophy of FLR in PHCC. (a) This patient needed a right trisectionectomy for complete resection of the tumour. The patient underwent PVE of the right portal vein and segment IV portal veins as the left lateral segment (FLR) was deemed small. (b) Note the increase in size of the left lateral segment in the post-PVE scan.

4b and the caudate lobe along with bile duct excision may be feasible for type I and type II tumours. In patients with a type IIIA tumour, a right trisectionectomy or a right hepatectomy with excision of segment 4b and caudate lobe is usually required. The left hepatic duct is transected left of the hilum, so that any periductal spread of the tumour is included in the resection, while still obtaining one or two ducts for anastomosis. Post-hepatectomy liver failure due to a low FLR is the primary risk with this approach and hence they are the best candidates for preoperative left-sided POBD and PVE of the right and segment 4 portal veins. Type IIIB tumours will need a left hemihepatectomy or a left trisectionectomy along with caudate lobe excision. Low FLR is not usually a concern in this instance but there is a high chance of multiple bile ducts. In patients with type IV PHCC, the choice of resection should be tailored to the presence of atrophy–hypertrophy of the liver and the presence and laterality of vascular involvement.

Vascular resection for perihilar cholangiocarcinoma

The close relationship of the biliary bifurcation to the hepatic vascular inflow and improvements in surgical expertise have made vascular resection for treating locally advanced PHCC increasingly accepted as a valid option. Clear preoperative planning is necessary to decide on the nature of vascular resection and the options for reconstruction. A contrast CT scan with arterial and portal phase imaging is the best modality currently available for assessing vascular involvement.

Portal vein resection

The extent of portal vein involvement can range from simple extrinsic compression and adherence of the tumour to the dorsal aspect of the portal bifurcation, through cicatricial involvement of a first-order branch, to the whole portal vein being encircled or infiltrated by the tumour. Usually, when a first-order branch is completely encased by the tumour, there is associated ipsilateral atrophy of the hemiliver and the main portal vein and the contralateral hemiportal veins are uninvolved. In such cases, resection of the involved segment at the level of the bifurcation along with an end-to-end anastomosis or a vein patch repair is usually possible. More extensive involvement will need a wider resection of the portal vein and an interposition vein graft for a tension-free anastomosis. Routine vascular resection to achieve wide clearance and improve local control rates has been proposed by some authors.[18,19]

Arterial resection

Arterial resection and reconstruction in locally advanced PHCC with arterial involvement is increasingly being utilized in experienced centres to increase resectability.[20,21] Right hepatic artery involvement is common in PHCC due to the usual retro-choledochal course of the right hepatic artery from left to right. Involvement of the right hepatic artery in a right-sided resection is of no consequence. But in a left-sided resection, involvement of the right hepatic artery requires arterial excision and reconstruction of the arterial supply to the right lobe. Confirmation of a sufficient segment of uninvolved right hepatic artery or right posterior hepatic artery to the right of the tumour is important prior to any irreversible steps during the operation. Mobilization of the common hepatic artery after division of the gastroduodenal artery usually provides sufficient length for direct anastomosis after resection though an interposition graft may be rarely necessary. It is recommended that vascular resection and reconstruction is delayed until completion of the parenchymal transection. This will shorten the ischaemia time to the FLR and the vascular anastomoses are not stretched during transection and specimen removal. Though early reports suggested high morbidity and mortality after arterial resections, recent publications from large-volume centres have been more promising with low perioperative complication rates and long-term outcomes similar to patients who have not needed arterial resection.[20,21]

Associating liver partition and portal vein ligation for staged hepatectomy procedure in perihilar cholangiocarcinoma

The technique of associating liver partition and portal vein ligation for staged hepatectomy (ALPPS) has been utilized in the surgical treatment of PHCC to mitigate the risk of a small liver remnant. ALPPS is a two-staged procedure initially developed for bi-lobar colorectal metastases. Here, the first procedure involves parenchymal transection and ligation of the portal branch to the hemiliver planned for resection. This induces a strong regenerative response in the FLR. The second stage, usually after a gap of 1–2 weeks, involves completion of the transection, hilar division, and removal of the specimen. While the technique is theoretically sound, the procedure is associated with increased morbidity, prolonged hospital stay and cost of treatment, and inability to complete the second phase of the procedure due to septic complications. It is unclear whether ALPPS provides an additional benefit over traditional optimization techniques such as PVE.[22,23]

Perioperative outcomes

Perioperative morbidity is primarily in the form of bile leaks, sepsis, and post-hepatectomy liver failure. Postoperative care should prioritize nutritional support, early mobilization, and good chest physiotherapy and treating any foci of sepsis. The reported mortality after resection has ranged from 5% to 25%. However, recent reports have shown improvements in complication rates and survival particularly in those needing vascular resection. A 2016 review of over 4000 resections for PHCC reported an overall perioperative morbidity and mortality of 42% (6–70%) and 5% (0–12%) respectively.[24]

Liver transplantation for perihilar cholangiocarcinoma

Early results of LT for PHCC were associated with poor outcomes. In 2000, De Vreede et al reported their initial results of 11 patients with early PHCC who underwent LT after a period of neoadjuvant chemoradiotherapy with excellent long-term results.[25] A multicentre study confirmed the efficacy of the 'Mayo Clinic protocol' in a cohort with a 5-year survival of 65%.[26] LT in this setting is primarily indicated for locally advanced tumours without metastatic disease but are unresectable either due to major vascular invasion or due to poor liver function as in the case of PSC. In fact, a recent study reported better outcomes with LT even for patients with resectable PHCC.[27] Clarity is still awaited on the diagnostic criteria for listing for LT, need for neoadjuvant therapy, and the role of early living donor LT in these patients.[28]

Role of adjuvant therapy

Adjuvant therapy for PHCC after a potentially curative resection is controversial. While early studies had shown limited or no benefit, there is increasing evidence that adjuvant chemotherapy alone or in combination with radiotherapy may be beneficial, especially in patients at high risk of recurrence such as node-positive disease or margin-positive resections.[29,30] For an individual patient, the performance status, postoperative condition and the histology of the resected tumour should be taken into consideration when deciding on adjuvant therapy.

Outcomes after resection for perihilar cholangiocarcinoma

Long-term survival for PHCC primarily depends on the feasibility of complete resection. Five-year survival in excess of 50% has been reported in patients undergoing R0 resection. Hartog et al. reported a R0 resection rate of 78% in 4251 cases of PHCC undergoing surgery with a median survival of 38 months.[24] Survival is worse after R1 resection but may still be better than patients not suitable for surgery. The majority of early recurrences are local near the hilum and can present with jaundice or gastric outlet obstruction. Palliative stenting is the primary means of managing this complication, though successful resection of recurrence has been reported.[31]

Intrahepatic cholangiocarcinoma

IHCCs are intrahepatic tumours and constitute 20% of all CCs. They are the second most common primary hepatic malignancy after hepatocellular carcinoma.

Clinical presentation and diagnostic workup

These are indolent tumours and present late usually with abdominal pain and weight loss. Early lesions are usually identified during routine imaging for other medical conditions. The presence of risk factors such as UC and PSC or viral hepatitis-related chronic liver disease indicate the need for regular surveillance to help early detection. The main differential diagnosis for an IHCC are hepatocellular carcinoma (HCC), fibrolamellar HCC, liver metastases, or benign tumours such as atypical haemangiomas.

Diagnostic workup

The initial diagnosis is usually through ultrasound imaging or abnormal liver function tests. Investigations for IHCC are the same as those for evaluating a liver mass. All patients will need liver function tests, viral serology, and tumour markers. Most patients will need a contrast-enhanced CT scan or an MRI to evaluate the lesion. IHCCs are hypodense lesions on CT while on MRI they show a high signal intensity on T2-weighted images and low signal intensity on T1-weighted imaging. Other characteristic findings of mass-forming IHCC are peripheral enhancement, late central enhancement, liver capsular retraction, dilatation of peripheral bile ducts, and presence of satellite lesions.[32]

If the imaging suggests a potentially resectable tumour, investigations to rule out distant metastases are necessary. Depending on the clinical scenario this could be a chest CT scan or a whole-body positron emission tomography (PET)-CT scan. PET-CT has a sensitivity of over 90% for the primary tumour and for metastases. High standardized uptake values on PET-CT have been associated with poor differentiation and worse survival in IHCC.[33]

Percutaneous biopsy of IHCC is not recommended if curative options are being considered due to the risk of tumour seeding. Biopsy is only indicated in case of planned palliative chemotherapy, or in case of unclear differentiation with HCC in the setting of a planned LT, as LT for unselected IHCC has a poorer survival compared to HCC.

Surgery for intrahepatic cholangiocarcinoma: considerations

Only 10% of patients with IHCC are amenable for resection at presentation. Assessment of suitability for surgery depends on the actual extent of the tumour, the quality of the underlying liver parenchyma, and the patient's performance status. There is now sufficient evidence to suggest that management of these patients should preferably be undertaken in high-volume centres with liver resection and LT services, for best outcomes in terms of resectability and the survival after resection.[34]

Extent of tumour

The extent of tumour needs to be carefully assessed on cross-sectional imaging especially for the presence of satellite nodules around the primary tumour and any metastatic lesions away from the planned resection volume. Multiple tumours especially in the contralateral lobe of the liver indicate advanced disease and such patients are not suitable candidates for curative resection. Involvement of surrounding structures, such as the diaphragm, duodenum, and colon, indicates advanced disease and benefits of resection should be carefully evaluated. Patients planned for major resection should ideally have CT volumetry to confirm sufficient remnant liver volume.

Vascular and lymph nodal involvement

Vascular involvement in IHCC is primarily related to extrinsic compression of major vascular structures by the tumour. Actual infiltration of vessels is uncommon and occurs in the late stages of the disease. Local vascular involvement is not a contraindication for resection if R0 resection can be achieved with sufficient FLR. Lymph nodal involvement is seen in around 40% of IHCCs at presentation. Involvement is usually restricted to the regional lymph nodes—those in the hepatoduodenal ligament and around the hepatic artery. For right-sided lesions, the retropancreatic nodes and for left-sided lesions, the nodes along the lesser curvature of stomach and the cardia are also considered as regional lymph nodes. Involvement of the coeliac, para-aortic, and mediastinal lymph nodes may be seen in advanced tumours and suggests extensive spread.

Underlying liver condition

Any pre-existing liver disease is a major factor in deciding treatment options. While IHCCs may develop in the absence of any liver disease, these tumours mostly occur in the older age group and many of these patients may have an element of fatty liver, fibrosis, or even cirrhosis secondary to non-alcoholic steatohepatitis which can complicate postoperative recovery after major resection. If the tumour involves the hilar bile ducts, it can cause cholestatic liver injury and impact recovery after resection. While routine preoperative biopsy of the healthy liver is not recommended, it should be considered preoperatively in patients with other associated features of chronic liver disease and an expected marginal remnant.

Preoperative optimization

Preoperative biliary drainage may be necessary in patients who are jaundiced at presentation. Similarly, unilateral preoperative PVE of the planned resected hemiliver may be necessary to increase the volume of future remnant.

Surgical resection for intrahepatic cholangiocarcinoma

Staging laparoscopy with frozen section biopsy is useful in selected patients with doubtful lesions in the contralateral liver and peritoneal disease on cross-sectional imaging. Surgery for IHCC involves resection of the tumour containing liver with clear margins. A resection margin of 1 cm is recommended to reduce the risk of recurrence, though this may not always be feasible in large tumours close to major vascular structures.[35]

In tumours involving the biliary confluence, bile duct excision with a hepaticojejunostomy may be required to achieve clearance. The survival benefit of lymphadenectomy during resection for IHCC is unclear though the presence of lymph nodes positive for tumour indicates a worse prognosis.[36] We recommend limited lymphadenectomy of the hepatoduodenal ligament and the retropancreatic and hepatic artery lymph nodes. Aggressive surgical techniques including *ex vivo* resection and autotransplantation and the ALPPS procedure have also been reported for IHCC.[37,38]

Liver transplantation for intrahepatic cholangiocarcinoma

The role of LT for IHCC was initially suggested from retrospective data of incidental IHCC in explants of patients transplanted for HCC. Five-year survival rates of 65% and 45% were reported in patients with very early tumours (single tumour <2 cm).[39] In a small single-centre study, six patients with stable unresectable IHCC received LT after neoadjuvant chemotherapy with a 50% recurrence-free survival at 36 months.[40] A recent consensus recommendation states that the role of LT for IHCC is unclear and should only be considered in the setting of clinical trials.[28]

Locoregional therapies

Locoregional therapies such as transarterial chemoembolization, transarterial radioembolization, and stereotactic body radiation therapy have been used for local control of tumours in patients not suitable for resection. Overall survival of 12–18 months has been reported with these procedures which is superior to palliative care or even palliative chemotherapy. The choice of technique depends on the patient's performance status and availability of these treatment options.[41,42]

Adjuvant and palliative chemotherapy

There is limited evidence for routine adjuvant chemotherapy after resection for IHCC. However, it may be considered in patients with good performance status in case of node-positive disease or when resection margins are positive. Gemcitabine plus cisplatin is the current recommendation for adjuvant therapy.

Outcomes and survival

Resection offers the best chance of cure in patients with IHCC. A median overall survival ranging from 20 to 30 months with a 5-year survival ranging from 15% to 40% have been reported in resected patients. Recurrent disease, primarily intrahepatic recurrence, is the main cause of death. The majority of recurrences occur within 24 months and are predominantly within the remnant liver. Recurrences after 24 months are usually extrahepatic. Median survival of up to 80 months has been reported in patients who undergo R0 resection and have node-negative disease.

REFERENCES

1. Prueksapanich P, Piyachaturawat P, Aumpansub P, Ridtitid W, Chaiteerakij R, Rerknimitr R. Liver fluke-associated biliary tract cancer. *Gut Liver*. 2018;**12**(3):236–245.
2. Madadi-Sanjani O, Wirth TC, Kuebler JF, Petersen C, Ure BM. Choledochal cyst and malignancy: a plea for lifelong follow-up. *Eur J Pediatr Surg*. 2019;**29**(2):143–149.
3. Kubo S, Kinoshita M, Takemura S, et al. Characteristics of printing company workers newly diagnosed with occupational cholangiocarcinoma. *J Hepatobiliary Pancreat Sci*. 2014;**21**(11):809–817.
4. Park J, Kim M-H, Kim K, et al. Natural history and prognostic factors of advanced cholangiocarcinoma without surgery, chemotherapy, or radiotherapy: a large-scale observational study. *Gut Liver*. 2009;**3**(4):298–305.
5. Farley DR, Weaver AL, Nagorney DM. 'Natural history' of unresected cholangiocarcinoma: patient outcome after noncurative intervention. *Mayo Clin Proc*. 1995;**70**(5):425–429.
6. Vijgen S, Terris B, Rubbia-Brandt L. Pathology of intrahepatic cholangiocarcinoma. *Hepatobiliary Surg Nutr*. 2017;**6**(1):22–34.
7. Liau J-Y, Tsai J-H, Yuan R-H, Chang C-N, Lee H-J, Jeng Y-M. Morphological subclassification of intrahepatic cholangiocarcinoma: etiological, clinicopathological, and molecular features. *Mod Pathol*. 2014;**27**(8):1163–1173.
8. Brierley JD, Gospodarowicz MK, Wittekind C. *TNM Classification of Malignant Tumours*. 8th ed. Chichester: UICC/Wiley-Blackwell; 2017.
9. Yachimski P, Pratt DS. Cholangiocarcinoma: natural history, treatment, and strategies for surveillance in high-risk patients. *J Clin Gastroenterol*. 2008;**42**(2):178–190.
10. Grunnet M, Mau-Sørensen M. Serum tumor markers in bile duct cancer—a review. *Biomarkers*. 2014;**19**(6):437–443.
11. Rassam F, Roos E, van Lienden KP, et al. Modern work-up and extended resection in perihilar cholangiocarcinoma: the AMC experience. *Langenbecks Arch Surg*. 2018;**403**(3):289–307.
12. Deoliveira ML, Schulick RD, Nimura Y, et al. New staging system and a registry for perihilar cholangiocarcinoma. *Hepatology*. 2011;**53**(4):1363–1371.
13. Govil S, Reddy MS, Rela M. Surgical resection techniques for locally advanced hilar cholangiocarcinoma. *Langenbecks Arch Surg*. 2014;**399**(6):707–716.
14. Mehrabi A, Khajeh E, Ghamarnejad O, et al. Meta-analysis of the efficacy of preoperative biliary drainage in patients undergoing liver resection for perihilar cholangiocarcinoma. *Eur J Radiol*. 2020;**125**:108897.
15. Chaudhary RJ, Higuchi R, Nagino M, et al. Survey of preoperative management protocol for perihilar cholangiocarcinoma at 10 Japanese high-volume centers with a combined experience of 2,778 cases. *J Hepatobiliary Pancreat Sci*. 2019;**26**(11):490–502.
16. Nimura Y, Hayakawa N, Kamiya J, Kondo S, Shionoya S. Hepatic segmentectomy with caudate lobe resection for bile duct carcinoma of the hepatic hilus. *World J Surg*. 1990;**14**(4):535–543.
17. Dinant S, Gerhards MF, Busch ORC, Obertop H, Gouma DJ, Van Gulik TM. The importance of complete excision of the caudate

lobe in resection of hilar cholangiocarcinoma. *HPB (Oxford)*. 2005;**7**(4):263–267.
18. Neuhaus P, Thelen A. Radical surgery for right-sided klatskin tumor. *HPB (Oxford)*. 2008;**10**(3):171–173.
19. Rela M, Rajalingam R, Shanmugam V, O' Sullivan A, Reddy MS, Heaton N. Novel en-bloc resection of locally advanced hilar cholangiocarcinoma: the Rex recess approach. *Hepatobiliary Pancreat Dis Int*. 2014;**13**(1):93–97.
20. Nagino M, Nimura Y, Nishio H, et al. Hepatectomy with simultaneous resection of the portal vein and hepatic artery for advanced perihilar cholangiocarcinoma: an audit of 50 consecutive cases. *Ann Surg*. 2010;**252**(1):115–123.
21. Govil S, Bharatan A, Rammohan A, et al. Liver resection for perihilar cholangiocarcinoma—why left is sometimes right. *HPB (Oxford)*. 2016;**18**(7):575–579.
22. Olthof PB, Coelen RJS, Wiggers JK, et al. High mortality after ALPPS for perihilar cholangiocarcinoma: case-control analysis including the first series from the international ALPPS registry. *HPB (Oxford)*. 2017;**19**(5):381–387.
23. Lang H, de Santibanes E, Clavien PA. Outcome of ALPPS for perihilar cholangiocarcinoma: case-control analysis including the first series from the international ALPPS registry. *HPB (Oxford)*. 2017;**19**(5):379–380.
24. Hartog H, Ijzermans JNM, van Gulik TM, Groot Koerkamp B. Resection of perihilar cholangiocarcinoma. *Surg Clin North Am*. 2016;**96**(2):247–267.
25. De Vreede I, Steers JL, Burch PA, et al. Prolonged disease-free survival after orthotopic liver transplantation plus adjuvant chemoirradiation for cholangiocarcinoma. *Liver Transplant*. 2000;**6**(3):309–316.
26. Darwish Murad S, Kim WR, Harnois DM, et al. Efficacy of neoadjuvant chemoradiation, followed by liver transplantation, for perihilar cholangiocarcinoma at 12 US centers. *Gastroenterology*. 2012;**143**(1):88–98.
27. Ethun CG, Lopez-Aguiar AG, Anderson DJ, et al. Transplantation versus resection for hilar cholangiocarcinoma: an argument for shifting treatment paradigms for resectable disease. *Ann Surg*. 2018;**267**(5):797–805.
28. Sapisochin G, Javle M, Lerut J, et al. Liver transplantation for cholangiocarcinoma and mixed hepatocellular cholangiocarcinoma: working group report from the ILTS Transplant Oncology Consensus Conference. *Transplantation*. 2020;**104**(6):1125–1130.
29. Wang G, Wang Q, Fan X, Ding L, Dong L. The significance of adjuvant therapy for extrahepatic cholangiocarcinoma after surgery. *Cancer Manag Res*. 2019;**11**:10871–10882.
30. Nassour I, Mokdad AA, Porembka MR, et al. Adjuvant therapy is associated with improved survival in resected perihilar cholangiocarcinoma: a propensity matched study. *Ann Surg Oncol*. 2018;**25**(5):1193–1201.
31. Kitano Y, Yamashita Y, Nakagawa S, et al. Effectiveness of surgery for recurrent cholangiocarcinoma: a single center experience and brief literature review. *Am J Surg*. 2020;**219**(1):175–180.
32. Seo N, Kim DY, Choi J-Y. Cross-sectional imaging of intrahepatic cholangiocarcinoma: development, growth, spread, and prognosis. *Am J Roentgenol*. 2017;**209**(2):W64–W75.
33. Breitenstein S, Apestegui C, Clavien P-A. Positron emission tomography (PET) for cholangiocarcinoma. *HPB (Oxford)*. 2008;**10**(2):120–121.
34. Kommalapati A, Tella SH, Goyal G, et al. Association between treatment facility volume, therapy types and overall survival in patients with intrahepatic cholangiocarcinoma. *HPB (Oxford)*. 2019;**21**(3):379–386.
35. Tang H, Lu W, Li B, Meng X, Dong J. Influence of surgical margins on overall survival after resection of intrahepatic cholangiocarcinoma. *Medicine (Baltimore)*. 2016;**95**(35):e4621.
36. Weber SM, Ribero D, O'Reilly EM, Kokudo N, Miyazaki M, Pawlik TM. Intrahepatic cholangiocarcinoma: expert consensus statement. *HPB (Oxford)*. 2015;**17**(8):669–680.
37. Vicente E, Quijano Y, Ielpo B, et al. Ex situ hepatectomy and liver autotransplantation for cholangiocarcinoma. *Ann Surg Oncol*. 2017;**24**(13):3990.
38. Li J, Moustafa M, Linecker M, et al. ALPPS for locally advanced intrahepatic cholangiocarcinoma: did aggressive surgery lead to the oncological benefit? An international multi-center study. *Ann Surg Oncol*. 2020;**27**(5):1372–1384.
39. Sapisochin G, Facciuto M, Rubbia-Brandt L, et al. Liver transplantation for 'very early' intrahepatic cholangiocarcinoma: international retrospective study supporting a prospective assessment. *Hepatology*. 2016;**64**(4):1178–1188.
40. Lunsford KE, Javle M, Heyne K, et al. Liver transplantation for locally advanced intrahepatic cholangiocarcinoma treated with neoadjuvant therapy: a prospective case-series. *Lancet Gastroenterol Hepatol*. 2018;**3**(5):337–348.
41. Al-Adra DP, Gill RS, Axford SJ, Shi X, Kneteman N, Liau S-S. Treatment of unresectable intrahepatic cholangiocarcinoma with yttrium-90 radioembolization: a systematic review and pooled analysis. *Eur J Surg Oncol*. 2015;**41**(1):120–127.
42. Tao R, Krishnan S, Bhosale PR, et al. Ablative radiotherapy doses lead to a substantial prolongation of survival in patients with inoperable intrahepatic cholangiocarcinoma: a retrospective dose response analysis. *J Clin Oncol*. 2016;**34**(3):219–226.

18

Primary neoplasms of the liver
Hepatoblastoma

Paolo Muiesan,† Andrea Schlegel, Chiara Grimaldi, and Kejd Bici

Introduction

Primary malignant tumours of the liver are extremely rare and account for only 1% of all paediatric malignancies.[1] Hepatoblastoma (HB) is the most prevalent liver tumour in childhood, accounting for up to 80% of all paediatric liver tumour cases, and is the third most common abdominal solid tumour in very young children after neuroblastoma and nephroblastoma.[2,3] The incidence of HB is low, with approximately 1.5 new cases per million per year and its peak is within the first 3 years of life.[4]

This embryonic tumour arises from abnormal differentiation of hepatocyte precursors from primitive epithelial cells of the fetal liver and, typically, has a rapid rate of growth. HB is usually associated with prematurity, low birth weight, and a number of inherited conditions.[5] Moreover, parental tobacco use, loss of heterozygosity at 11p15, and mutations in genes have been reported to increase the risk of HB in some studies, despite inconsistent reports.[6-10] Though there is a clear syndromic association, the underlying liver is typically normal.

Most children with HB present with an enlarging abdominal mass, non-specific symptoms such as anorexia and weight loss, and in 70% of cases are in an advanced stage at diagnosis.[4] HB is more frequent in boys and presents with abdominal distension, a mass, pain, and failure to thrive. It can also present as intra-abdominal haemorrhage secondary to rupture. Serum alpha-fetoprotein (AFP) levels are raised in at least 70% of children with HB: when elevated at presentation, this tumour marker is an excellent aid in the diagnosis, monitoring response to therapy, and, crucially, in the early detection of disease recurrence. Low serum AFP level (<100 ng/mL) at presentation is a poor prognostic factor. HB spreads by vascular invasion, typically to the lungs. Abdominal lymph node involvement is very infrequent. Histologically, most HBs have an epithelial and mesenchymal component. The epithelial component can be of a fetal or embryonal subtype. Pure fetal histology seems to be more favourable. Macrotrabecular and undifferentiated anaplastic subtypes are uncommon. Whether a diagnostic biopsy is obtained, via surgical or percutaneous sampling, can be misleading and limits the prognostic value of the initial histology.

Overview of classification and staging

In the last decade, the classification of HB has significantly evolved. However, numerous different study groups and trials overlap and, sometimes, differ in definition and recommendation, leading to possible confusion.

Historically, four separate multicentre study groups worldwide have systematically reviewed and defined the treatment of HB in children: the International Childhood Liver Tumor Study Group (SIOPEL), the Children's Oncology Group (COG), the German Society of Pediatric Oncology and Hematology (GPOH), and the Japanese Study Group for Pediatric Liver Tumors (JPLT).

Although every single group contributed to improving treatments and outcomes of HB, they have developed different staging systems and prognostic factors, making comparison challenging.

As a great example of a cooperative attitude, all the above-mentioned groups created the Children's Hepatic tumours International Collaboration (CHIC) consortium, with the main goal of developing a common and global risk stratification system for HB.[11]

The CHIC pooled data from 1605 HB patients treated in eight different clinical trials (SIOPEL-2, SIOPEL-3, COG-INT0098, COG-P9645, GPOH-HB89, GPOH-HB99, JPLT-1, JPLT-2) from COG, SIOPEL, Germany, and Japan over two decades, to harmonize clinical, radiological, and pathological prognostic factors. CINECA, an Italian supercomputing centre run by an interuniversity consortium, was contracted to host and manage access to the dataset (**Figure 18.1**).[11]

The CHIC Steering Committee selected the data variables and set the database up. The dataset is constantly updated, in particular with the data from the currently recruiting trials.

This was instrumental to develop the Children's Hepatic tumor International Collaboration–Hepatoblastoma Stratification (CHIC-HS), a new, simplified risk staging system that levelled the differences between the four study groups.[12]

The Pediatric Liver Tumor Consensus Classification (PLTCC) was introduced in 2011, during the first International Pathology Symposium. This classification includes the most relevant histological types of HB.[13]

† It is with regret that we report the passing of Paolo Muiesan during the writing of this volume.

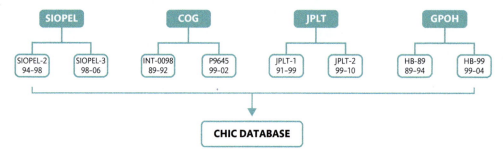

Figure 18.1 Children's Hepatic tumor International Collaboration (CHIC) database.

Both PLTCC and CHIC-HS are the backbones of the Pediatric Hepatic International Tumor Trial (PHITT), the largest clinical trial undertaken in paediatric liver cancer patients, opened in the US and Europe in 2017 and due to be completed in 2022. Its primary objective is to validate a new global risk stratification, defined by CHIC, and also to allow straightforward comparisons of biological material and molecular markers.

Differential diagnosis with hepatocellular carcinoma

Hepatocellular carcinoma (HCC) inevitably comes into the differential diagnosis. However, HCC is more frequently seen in older children and adolescents, either in a non-cirrhotic liver or in association with a variety of fibrosing diseases or cirrhosis of different aetiologies. In the Western world, HCC is much less frequent than HB. This is because HCC is usually associated with background liver disease including hepatitis B virus, which is less frequent in the West, and tyrosinaemia, which is treated with 2-(2-nitro-4-trifluoromethylbenzoyl)-1,3-cyclohexanedione (NTBC), an enzyme inhibitor, which confers some protection.

HCC also presents with abdominal distension and a mass, however abdominal pain and vomiting are also common. The serum AFP is raised in the majority of patients but to a lesser extent than in HB. HCC spreads by both lymphatic involvement of the hilar, para-aortic, and mediastinal lymph nodes and vascular invasion in the form of pulmonary metastases.

Histology is essential for the appropriate planning of the therapeutic strategies of HB given its high chemosensitivity. HCC, on the other hand, is poorly responsive to chemotherapy, is mainly diagnosed with imaging, and needs an upfront surgical approach, including primary resection or liver transplantation (LT). Childhood HCC is known to be more aggressive than HB and is associated with a higher risk of recurrence and worse overall survival, reflecting differences in the underlying tumour biology.[14] Biopsy of liver masses in children with a liver lesion suspicious for HB is useful to exclude benign tumours or HCC. Information on pathological subtypes of HB helps to define prognosis and therapeutic management.[15]

Biology and genetics

HB develops in the absence of liver disease and has a relatively stable genome. Cytogenetic or cytogenomic analysis of the tumour demonstrates only a limited number of chromosomal structural and numerical abnormalities.[16] Several genetic syndromes have been associated with an increased risk of HB, including the Beckwith–Wiedemann syndrome, familial adenomatous polyposis coli, Simpson–Golabi–Behmel syndrome, Sotos, syndrome and constitutional trisomy.[15,17–19] Several studies investigated the role of genetic mutations in the development of HB and there is growing support that the WNT signalling pathway and its molecular targets play a significant role in HB tumorigenesis.[20,21] The mutation of the *CTNNB1* gene encoding beta-catenin (β-catenin), the main transducer in the canonical WNT pathway, was first reported by Koch et al. in 1999 in sporadic HB.[22] It is the most frequent mutation observed and can occur in up to 80% of tumours that have tested positive for mutations.[23,24]

The JPLT-2 trial demonstrated that a large deletion of *CTNNB1* was detected in 107 cases among 212 HBs collected in the period 2000–2010, and that mutation of *CTNNB1* exon 3 was detected in 56 cases.[25]

The WNT/β-catenin cascade plays an important modulatory role in liver development and regeneration. The degradation of β-catenin is inhibited, and this protein accumulates in the cytoplasm and nucleus. Next, the β-catenin interacts with the T-cell factor/lymphoid enhancement factor (TCF/LEF) to control transcription, resulting in the expression of different genes and functions, including c-*MYC*, *CCND1*, *EGFR*, and glutamine synthetase.[26,27]

The second most common gene mutation in HB, accounting for 5–10% of HB tested, is in *NFE2L2*, which plays a key role in the antioxidant response and is associated with poor prognosis.[28]

The histological specimens obtained from HBs exhibit nuclear accumulation of both β-catenin and YAP proto-oncogene. Of note, the expression of only one of the two oncogenes does not induce tumour development, but the simultaneous overexpression of both, β-catenin and YAP, leads invariably to the rapid growth of HB in murine experimental models.[29]

The mammalian target of rapamycin complex 1 (mTORC1) signalling, involved in many functions of normal and neoplastic cells, was activated both in human and YAP/β-catenin mice.[30] A further study confirmed the importance of these associations, showing that rapamycin fat-diet mice significantly decreased the HB burden when compared to controls, indicating a possible relevant therapeutic role of mTORC inhibitors.[27,31]

Histology

Willis first described the term 'hepatoblastoma' referring to a tumour mass composed of hepatic epithelial parenchyma resembling fetal or embryonal liver.[32] HB is an embryonal tumour that originates from the hepatoblast, the precursor of the hepatocytes. It resembles the stages of liver development with a combination of different histological patterns.[33]

The modern classification proposed by CHIC is based on Ishak and Glunz's first description of two distinctive histological patterns of HB: the epithelial tumour, further subclassified into fetal and embryonal, and a mixed epithelial and mesenchymal type.[34]

In the last two decades, the correlation between histology and prognosis has been described by different studies.[35] In order to validate this relationship, an International Pathology Symposium was sponsored by the COG Liver Tumor Committee in 2011. Twenty-two pathologists and experts in paediatric liver tumours from each of the four study groups reviewed 50 paediatric HB cases and developed the histological classification PLTTC (Table 18.1).[13] On this occasion, new prognostic morphological categories were identified: the favourable, well-differentiated fetal (WDF) HB, the aggressive, small cell undifferentiated (SCU) HB, and the hepatocellular neoplasm not otherwise classified (HCN-NOS).

Epithelial tumours are composed of uniformly polygonal small cells measuring 10–20 micrometres in diameter. Cells have a central nucleus without nucleoli and abundant eosinophilic cytoplasm. They usually grow in sheets or have one- to two-cell-thick trabeculae.[36] Two types of epithelial HB are recognized: the *crowded fetal HB* and the *WDF HB* or 'pure fetal' HB. The former is mitotically active, while the latter has low mitotic activity and complete surgical excision has been shown to be curative.[37,38] In the COG trials INT-0098 and P9645, patients with WDF histology who had undergone primary surgery without any neoadjuvant or adjuvant chemotherapy showed a 100% recurrence-free survival. Thus, in contrast to SIOPEL, who recommend chemotherapy for all patients, COG proposed surgery alone as the curative option for patients with WDF histology.[39] This statement has been adopted by the new guidelines proposed by the PHITT trial, but two considerations are necessary: post-chemotherapy histology cannot be classified as 'pure fetal' and the diagnosis of WDF HB must be made only on primarily resected tumours composed entirely by fetal cells.[25]

SCU HB is the second most clinically relevant histological type. It is defined by cells measuring 7–8 micrometres in size that usually form clusters mixed with other epithelial cells or nests in a near-organoid pattern but may also grow in a diffuse pattern.[2] The SCU HB is associated with an aggressive biological behaviour and has been related to a worse prognosis even in tumours showing only a small SCU component.[40–43] Of note, only 5% of analysed specimens are shown to be entirely composed of small undifferentiated cells.

Anti-INI1 (an integrase interactor 1 gene) antibody is an important immunohistochemical staining, used to determine SCU HB. A small subset of INI1-negative SCU HBs shows morphological and biological features of malignant rhabdoid tumours but whether these SCU have further aggressive behaviour remains to be determined.[2]

The *embryonal HB* is an epithelial tumour with a better prognosis compared to SCU. It displays a common histological pattern: it is composed of cells resembling the embryonic stage of the liver, at 6–8 weeks of gestational age. The cells measure approximately 10–15 micrometres and have a high nuclear/cytoplasm ratio.[2,28] This is the most common histological pattern as 67% of HBs are epithelial with a combination of mixed embryonal and fetal patterns.[25]

Another epithelial type, often seen in post-chemotherapy specimens, is the *pleomorphic* epithelial HB. This is characterized by bizarre pleomorphic cells including giant cells.[2] Sometimes, if seen as the only component in a pre-chemotherapy specimen, it may mimic an HCC. Immunohistochemistry and the absence of both anaplasia and atypical mitoses can help to differentiate between the two tumour types.[13]

Rarer epithelial HB subtypes include *macrotrabecular* HB and *cholangioblastic* HB. The former accounts for approximately 5% of all cases and represents a morphological pattern rather than a histotype. The cholangioblastic HB is mainly composed of cells that show a prominent ductular differentiation. This needs to be distinguished from a ductular reaction, often noted at the periphery of the tumour itself, or from the very rare cholangioblastic tumours found in children.[28,44]

The *mixed epithelial and mesenchymal* HB comprises both epithelial and mesenchymal elements. Osteoid is the most common mesenchymal element noted, followed by cartilage and skeletal muscle.[45] The mesenchymal component represents an integral part of the tumour and should be distinguished from the result of chemotherapy or metaplastic change.

Table 18.1 Histological classification—Pediatric Liver Tumor Consensus Classification (PLTCC)

Epithelial			Mixed	HCN-NOS
Fetal	Well-differentiated (WDF)/pure fetal	Low mitotic activity	Mixed epithelia and mesenchymal	
	Crowded fetal	High mitotic activity		
Small cell undifferentiated (SCU)	INI1 positive			
	INI1 negative			
Embryonal				
Pleomorphic				
Cholangioblastic				
Macrotrabecular				

Source: data from López-Terrada D et al. Towards an international pediatric liver tumor consensus classification: proceedings of the Los Angeles COG liver tumors symposium. *Mod Pathol.* 2014;27(3):472–491.

The *teratoid* HB is a tumour displaying an overlap of different histological components such as endoderm, neuroectoderm, or melanin-containing cells.[46]

Poorly differentiated, clinically aggressive epithelial tumours, typical of older children have been identified as *transitional liver tumours*.[47] This histological type shows HCC-like features that are challenging to interpret. In recent years, this hybrid tumour showing genetic characteristics between HB and HCC has been defined as a *HCN-NOS*. The PHITT trial might help in improving our knowledge of the clinical and prognostic significance of HCN-NOS.[28]

Imaging

Progressive improvements in high-definition cross-sectional imaging have been crucial to better diagnose and stage HB.[48]

Ultrasound (US) remains the modality of choice for primary assessment of abdominal masses in children as it does not require the use of harmful ionizing radiation and of general anaesthesia. The main goal is to identify the origin of the tumour, thus allowing the radiologist to appropriately protocol the subsequent cross-sectional imaging study. US studies can also identify the intrahepatic extent, and the relationship of the mass to major venous structures, which is essential for staging and assessment of resectability. HB usually appears as a hyperechoic mass in the US image. Further cross-sectional and high-quality images are then necessary to evaluate the involvement of the liver segments and the precise relationship to portal pedicles and vascular structures including the inferior vena cava, hepatic veins, and their branches.[49,50] Cross-sectional imaging is therefore essential to correctly characterize and stage the tumours and for a more reproducible follow-up of the response to chemotherapy.

US studies may occasionally become useful again as a 'second-look' tool to complement the cross-sectional images, to better define subtle vascular invasion, and to support the follow-up after chemotherapy or surgical treatment.

Magnetic resonance (MRI) has quickly become the modality of choice for the evaluation of liver lesions in children. The lack of ionizing radiations and superior soft tissue contrast resolution are the main advantages over computed tomography (CT).[50,51] Axial and coronal images are acquired, with at least two pulse sequences, including T1 and either fat-suppressed T2, short-TI inversion recovery, or fat-suppressed fast/turbo. And images may be non-breath-hold or breath-hold depending on the patient's age.

Hepatocyte-specific contrast agents added not only the ability to identify the liver mass but also to detect vascular invasion.[51] These contrast agents are gadolinium based, and are taken up by hepatocytes and then excreted. This is an important feature to identify a multifocal disease.[52]

The CT scan, though penalized by ionizing radiations, still plays a key role in the diagnosis of lung metastasis, as recommended by both the previous and current research trials. Given its speed and multiple reconstructing algorithms, CT may be occasionally indicated for a complete evaluation of the child to minimize the duration of anaesthesia/sedation and to avoid multiple contrast agent administrations.[50]

PRETEXT and annotation factors

The 'Risk Group Stratification' is the milestone of the current management of HB. It is based on the PRE-Treatment EXTent of the tumour (PRETEXT) system that most cooperative group trials worldwide have adopted as the main system of risk stratification for HB and paediatric HCC.

The SIOPEL study group first introduced the PRETEXT system in 1992 and defined it as a method to stratify the imaging evaluation of children suffering from HB before any kind of treatment was attempted.[53]

Initially, this risk stratification system was not adopted by all the study groups. For example, the trials COG-INT0098 and P9645 recommended to attempt surgical resection of the tumour in every case and handed the decision to operate to the individual surgeon.[25] The classification used by the COG group, named Evan's stages I, II, III, was therefore based on the surgeon's decision whether to resect or not. Operable lesions were allocated to hepatectomy and postoperative chemotherapy, based on the histological findings. Patients with non-resectable tumours underwent biopsy, followed by chemotherapy and delayed surgery.[54]

In the 2000s, PRETEXT, the adult tumour, node, and metastasis (TNM) system, and Evan's surgical stages were introduced by the German GOPH and by JPLT following the improvements of high-quality cross-sectional images.[39] Their studies confirmed the reproducibility and reliability of the PRETEXT groups and their ability to predict the overall survival of patients affected by HB.[35,55–62] The GOC moved away from its original classification and adopted the PRETEXT staging system.[25]

The PRETEXT system represents the extent of the tumour through the four liver sectors/sections and its main purpose is to predict resectability. It is determined by calculating the number of contiguous sections to be resected to completely remove the tumour or, conversely, by calculating the number of contiguous tumour-free sections (Figure 18.2).

Given the above, four different stages have been defined:

- PRETEXT 1, three contiguous sections must be tumour free; therefore, the mass can involve only either the left lateral or right posterior section. Usually, these are small lesions.
- PRETEXT 2, two adjacent sections must be tumour free; the mass can involve one or two sections but is limited either to the right lobe or to the left lobe of the liver. Of note, tumours, involving left medial or right anterior sections are staged as PRETEXT 2.
- PRETEXT 3, the tumour extends both, into the left and right hemiliver. It may involve either two or three sections, resulting in only one adjacent section free from the tumour. Usually, central tumours, involving right anterior and left medial sections are considered PRETEXT 3: only one contiguous section (left lateral or right posterior) is tumour free.
- PRETEXT 4, no tumour-free sections. These tumours are mostly multifocal or infiltrative, and, in some cases, are large enough to compromise all four liver sections.[49,50]

Although anatomical delimitation of HB, defined by PRETEXT, can itself predict the tumour's resectability, there are some limitations related to vascular anomalies/variants, tumour shapes, and

PRETEXT and annotation factors | 191

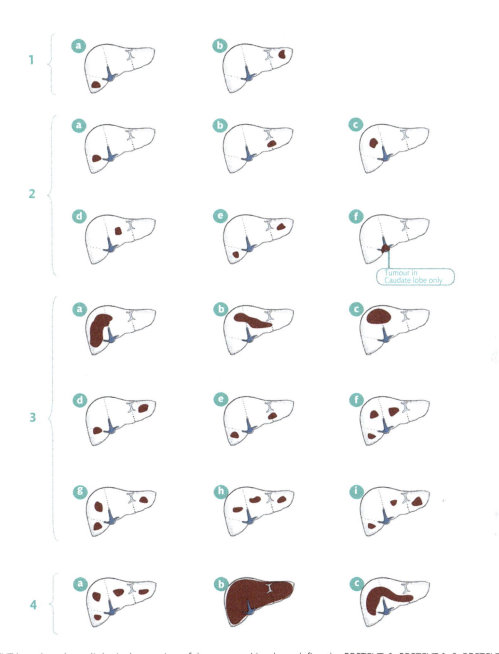

Figure 18.2 PRETEXT based on the radiological extension of the tumour. Numbers define the PRETEXT. 1, PRETEXT 1; 2, PRETEXT 2; 3, PRETEXT 3; 4, PRETEXT 4. See text for further explanation.

the distinction between invasion/displacement of a given hepatic section.[55,62,63]

In case of hepatic vein variants, such as duplicated right hepatic veins, the closest vessel to the middle hepatic vein insertion to the inferior vena cava (IVC) should be considered to be the right hepatic vein; when the middle hepatic vein is duplicated, the one that best aligns with the gall bladder should be considered the middle hepatic vein. In cases of left hepatic vein duplications, it may be difficult to select the correct PRETEXT group, and it may be useful to identify the segmental anatomy first.

Similarly, it is frequently challenging to allocate a pedunculated tumour to a PRETEXT group. In general, the hepatic section, where the tumour arises from, is considered to be the involved section.

Finally, another challenge consists in assessing the infiltration by large tumours or displacement of the adjacent segments. A close examination of the vessels may help to define the tumour's characteristics; however, in case of uncertainty, it is appropriate to presume tumour invasion and allocate the patient to a higher PRETEXT class.[50]

In addition to a pre-treatment staging, a POST-Treatment EXTent of the disease (POSTEXT) is assigned with the same modalities, usually following every two cycles of chemotherapy. POSTEXT is therefore used to customize either further chemotherapy cycles or surgical options.[64]

The annotation factors V, P, E, M, C, F, N, and R, together with the PRETEXT group, complete the PRETEXT system.

Annotation factors

Although PRETEXT was adopted as the main staging system used in the trials by all study groups, the same cannot be said with regard to the annotation factors which are known to affect patients' outcomes and survivals. These annotation factors have received different definitions from the various study groups.[29,50]

For this reason, PHITT tried to overcome the discrepancies in defining the annotation factors and has outlined a new consensus classification (Table 18.2).

For example, the involvement/invasion of the hepatic veins and/or the IVC widely differed between the groups. SIOPEL considered hepatic veins and IVC to be involved where the tumour completely obstructed or circumferentially encased the vessels or there were findings of neoplastic thrombosis; further annotations, such as V1, V2, or V3 were used to determine the number of hepatic veins involved.[65]

COG's AHEP-0731 trial used different criteria. Tumours were defined as V+ if IVC or all of the three hepatic veins met one of the following criteria: V0—tumour within 1 cm of the vessel, V1—tumour abutting the vessel, V2—tumour compressing the vessel, and V3—intravascular tumour thrombus.[48]

To eliminate these differences, the PHITT trial assigned a simpler V+ or V− status, *de facto* eliminating the degree of the vessel's invasion. HBs are therefore categorized as V+ when the following parameters are met, including:

- Obliteration (lumen not visible) of all three first-order (confluence between the IVC and most central hepatic vein branch) hepatic veins or ICV.
- Encasement (>50% of the lumen or >180° of circumference) of all three first-order hepatic veins or intrahepatic IVC.
- Tumour thrombus within one or more first-order hepatic vein or intrahepatic IVC.[50]

SIOPEL and COG defined PV involvement (P), another important prognostic annotation factor, using similar criteria used to define hepatic venous involvement. However, the annotation number among SIOPEL could only be extended to two (main portal vein and its two main branches).[48,65] Again, the PHITT assigned a simpler P+ or P− status relying on the same principles used to determine V+.

The prognostic role of distant metastasis (M) in determining a patient's survival has been identified during the early stages of the trials. The lungs are the most common site of metastasis but less than 20% of children with HB present with lung metastasis at diagnosis.[11] Metastatic disease strongly affects surgical management and clinical outcomes, and it is considered a relative contraindication for LT.[48]

The PHITT definition of pulmonary metastases (M+) includes at least one non-calcified nodule greater than 5 mm in diameter, or two or more non-calcified nodules, each greater or equal to 3 mm in diameter.[50]

Although the lungs are the most common site of metastasis, brain and bone disease have both been described, mostly as case reports.[66] However, in contrast to the previous SIOPEL and COG recommendations, a bone scan or brain MRI are not routinely indicated, unless the child is symptomatic.[50]

Three annotation factors that display a strong influence on surgical strategy and outcomes include multifocality (F), extrahepatic disease (E) and tumour rupture (R).

Twenty per cent of HB are multifocal at diagnosis and their outcome is worse when compared to solitary lesions.[67,68]

Multifocality significantly limits the surgical options and represents a real challenge for most surgeons.[48] It is also demanding for radiologists to detect small multifocal tumour residues on cross-sectional studies, particularly following effective chemotherapy.[63,69] MRI with hepatocyte-specific contrasts is more effective than conventional MRI or CT scans in identifying very small metastatic deposits in the liver.[70]

There are no significant differences between the study groups regarding multifocality. The PHITT system defines HB F+ when the tumour is composed of two or more hepatic masses with normal intervening liver tissue.[50]

In contrast, the assessment of the extrahepatic disease has been one of the most confusing aspects of the original PRETEXT classification. PHITT slightly changed the definition of extrahepatic disease proposed in the 2005 revision.[65,71,72] An HB is considered E+ if it is seen to cross boundaries/tissue planes (i.e. above and below the diaphragm) or to be surrounded by normal tissue by greater than 180°, or, finally, if there is at least one peritoneal nodule greater than 10 cm or two peritoneal nodules greater than 5 cm. However, E+ HB is uncommon and represents only 5% of cases.[50]

In general, it is rare, that a HB presents with tumour rupture as the first clinical sign. A recent CHIC analysis confirmed that this portends towards a worse prognosis.[11] It is important to note that ascites and subcapsular fluids are common findings in children with HB, therefore they should not be considered as tumour rupture in the PRETEXT staging. Haemorrhage following liver biopsy and surgical rupture (not present at diagnosis), should also not be considered to be PRETEXT R+. In contrast, a rupture following chemotherapy could be identified as R+ in the POSTEXT assessment.

Caudate lobe involvement is defined by the C annotation factor. C+ tumours are assigned conventionally to at least PRETEXT 2 and should be carefully evaluated in surgical planning. Lymph node metastases, in contrast to HCC, are an uncommon feature with HB. The different study groups have used variable and multivariate

Table 18.2 Annotation factors

V+	Tumour obliterates all three HVs or IVC
	Tumour encases (>50% or 80%) all three HVs or IVC
P+	Tumour obliterates all two portal branches or main PV
	Tumour encases (>50% or 80%) all two portal branches or main PV
	Tumour thrombus in anyone (or both) portal branches or main PV
E+	Tumour crosses boundaries/tissue plans
	Tumour surrounded by normal tissue by >180°
	At least one peritoneal nodule >10 cm or two peritoneal nodules >5 cm
F+	Two or more hepatic mass with normal intervening liver tissue
R+	Internal complexity/septation within fluid
	High-density fluid on CT
	Imaging of blood or blood degradation products on MRI
	Heterogeneous fluid on US with echogenic debris
	Visible rupture/hepatic capsular defect on imaging

HV, hepatic vein; IVC, inferior vena cava; PV: portal vein.
Source: data from Towbin AJ, et al. 2017 PRETEXT: radiologic staging system for primary hepatic malignancies of childhood revised for the Paediatric Hepatic International Tumour Trial (PHITT). *Pediatr Radiol.* 2018;48(4):536–554.

morphological criteria to assess their involvement. Unfortunately, data for C and N were not collected by all studies, therefore CHIC decided to exclude them from the retrospective analysis conducted to validate the CHIC-HS and they are not currently used to risk stratify the patients.[38]

Risk stratification

PRETEXT and its annotation factors has been a useful tool to evaluate a patient's prognosis. Each of the study groups has recently used PRETEXT, defining, based on its own experience, non-standard risk groups that would further guide patients' treatment.

So, for example, SIOPEL and GPOH stratified patients in standard- and high-risk groups, based on PRETEXT with its annotation factors, histology, and AFP levels (SIOPEL). JLPT stratified patients into three different groups: low/standard, intermediate and high risk. COG, instead, introduced an additional category to the three reported by JLPT, the very low-risk group. Patients belonging to this category were affected by HB, usually PRETEXT 1 or 2, that was immediately resectable at diagnosis and had a pure fetal histology. In such cases, upfront surgery is considered curative without the need for neoadjuvant or adjuvant chemotherapy.[48]

Nevertheless, every trial has reported specific negative or positive prognostic factors. For example, AFP less than 100 ng/mL, SCU histology, tumour rupture, and PRETEXT 4 were considered negative prognostic factors in SIOPEL, while other variables such as multifocality (GPOH), lymph node involvement (JPLT), age at diagnosis, very high levels of AFP (>1.2 million ng/mL) were proposed prognostic risk factors from other study groups. Given the rarity of HB and the small number of patients included in each trial, it remained demanding to assess an accurate prognostic significance for each factor.[68]

For that reason, Czauderna et al. initially retrospectively analysed the CHIC database of 1605 HB patients and reached several conclusions.[11] First, they confirmed the relationship between PRETEXT and its annotation factors with outcomes: survival decreased proportionally to higher PRETEXT stages. Second, metastatic tumours, consisting of less than 20% of all HBs, were confirmed to be strongly associated with a poor prognosis. Third, an AFP serum level less than 100 ng/mL and more than 1 million ng/mL was also associated with poor outcome. Patient age was found to affect clinical results as well, with a worse prognosis for older children (>2 years old).[11]

Other potential risk factors previously identified by smaller series, including prematurity, low birth weight, sex, and the Beckwith–Wiedemann syndrome, were not found to be associated with adverse prognosis.[11]

PRETEXT group (I, II, III, IV, V), AFP of 100 ng/ml or less, and presence of metastases have been proved to significantly affect the outcome in children with HB also by preceding studies.[35,55,68,73]

In a multivariate analysis performed on the 1263 patients appertaining to the CHIC database, Meyers et al. called these components 'traditional risk factors'.[38] Hence, they introduced a classification based on five different 'backbones':

- Backbone 1: PRETEXT 1 and 2.
- Backbone 2: PRETEXT 3.
- Backbone 3: PRETEXT 4.
- Backbone 4: metastatic tumour.
- Backbone 5: AFP less than 100 ng/mL.

Each backbone was then investigated in a multivariate analysis with the additional factors thought to be more likely related to the worse outcome: AFP between 100 and 1000 ng/mL; AFP greater than 1 million ng/mL; age less than 1 year, 1–2 years, 3–7 years and more than 8 years; and the presence/absence of the annotation factors V, P, E, F, and R. The latter were considered as a single factor to simplify the analysis and considered positive if at least one of the annotation factors was found at diagnosis.[38]

The event-free survival (EFS) at 5 years, defined as the time interval from enrolment in the protocol and the time of the first occurrence of tumour progression, relapse, diagnosis of second malignancy, or death for any cause, was used as the main outcome and guided the conception of four risk groups (Figure 18.3):

- Very low and low risk for an EFS greater than 89%.
- The intermediate risk for an EFS between 50% and 88%.
- High risk for a EFS less than 50%

Finally, they created the CHIC-HS, the current risk stratification tree that, starting from the established PRETEXT groups, guides to four risk categories (Figure 18.4):

- Very low risk.
- Low risk.

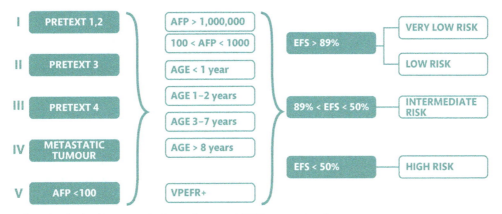

Figure 18.3 Evolution from the five backbones to the four risk groups. VPEFR, annotation factors, see text.

CHAPTER 18 Primary neoplasms of the liver

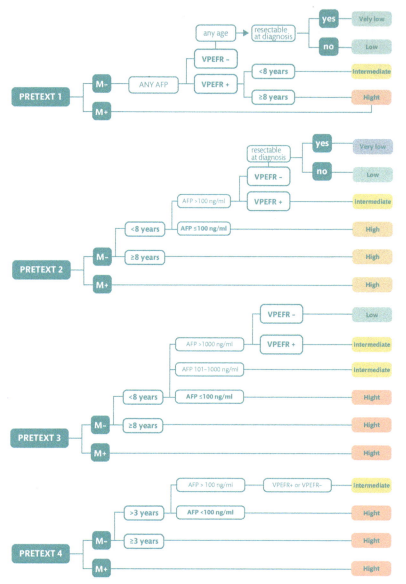

Figure 18.4 Children's Hepatic Tumor International Collaboration-Hepatoblastoma Stratification (CHIC-HS). M, metastasis; VPEFR, annotation factors, see text.

- Intermediate risk.
- High risk.

PRETEXT 1 and 2 were split to highlight the importance of tumour resectability at diagnosis which differentiates the very low-risk from the low-risk category.

Only a few patients who presented with low PRETEXT (1 or 2) and positive annotation factors (VPEFR+) showed a moderate to high risk, therefore they have been considered intermediate risk.

AFP less than 100 ng/mL did not affect EFS in the subgroup of PRETEXT 1 tumours; it was therefore not considered as an additional variable in this stratification group.

AFP less than 100 ng/mL confers a worse outcome in children with PRETEXT 3 tumour and below 8 years of age, so these patients were considered high risk.[38]

Ultimately, age at diagnosis may be considered a novel risk factor, but its relevance across the risk groups is variable. Only two subgroups of age (<8 and >8 years) were identified in all PRETEXT groups except for PRETEXT 4, where patients between 3 and 7 years old showed a worse prognosis, like older patients.[38]

Variability of the influence of age on outcome was further confirmed by Haeberle et al.[74] They stratified all patients from the CHIC dataset in 13 age groups (from 1 year to >13 years old) to evaluate how age could affect the prognosis. They concluded that the risk of an event in a patient suffering from HB increases uniformly in elder children. In contrast, older age at diagnosis seemed to attenuate the prognostic relevance of the other adverse risk factors: that is, in older children, metastatic disease conferred a lower risk.[74]

The histology classification PLTCC was not included in this stratification as it has been only recently developed. One of the PHITT clinical trial's goals is to merge clinical findings with biological parameters. A separate analysis to reassign a PTLCC-based histological subtype to patients included in the CHIC database is in progress.

Biopsy

The biopsy is usually performed percutaneously. The aim is to obtain sufficient material, not less than ten cores of the tumour, where two should contain an interface between the normal liver and tumour, one core normal liver, and at least two cores should be frozen. The material obtained from the normal liver is important for genetic testing. To decrease the risk of tumour seeding, the needle should pass through a short portion of the non-lesional liver and should not cross and contaminate segments of the liver that will not be resected during a later surgery. Moreover, US guidance will help to avoid large hepatic vessels or soft and necrotic parts of the tumour, thus reducing the risks of haemorrhage and rupture, respectively. The interventional radiologist and the surgeon should discuss these issues before the biopsy. If an unsafe biopsy path or inadequate tissue is expected with a percutaneous approach, then a laparoscopic or even open biopsy is recommended.

Chemotherapy

Chemotherapy has been a critical step in the management of paediatric malignant liver tumours.

Before the introduction of chemotherapy, the only chance of cure for children suffering from HB was, if feasible, surgical resection. In the 1980s, new chemotherapeutic regimens drastically changed the management and survival of these patients.[75] Cisplatin has become the main chemotherapeutic agent for HB. Even nowadays, most HB tumours, considered not resectable at initial presentation due to their extension and/or vascular involvement, benefit from chemotherapeutic regimens. Neoadjuvant chemotherapy has proven to effectively reduce the volume of initially non-resectable tumours to a size suitable for radical surgical removal. The involvement of vascular structures may also recede, allowing a better excision.[2]

The effort of all study groups led to the development of new therapeutic regimens, which improved overall patient survival up to 80%.[39,57,76–78] For example, the SIOPEL 4 regimen showed an impressive survival improvement in patients with metastatic disease at diagnosis, using a scheme of weekly dose-dense cisplatin chemotherapy, with a 98% response rate.[79] However, given different risk stratification systems, every group used different treatments.

The CHIC-HS prognostic stratification allowed children with HB to be uniformly treated according to their risk group. One of the main purposes of the PHITT trial is to validate the effectiveness of novel treatments in high-risk patients and the feasibility of reducing the intensification of chemotherapy in low-risk patients, thus avoiding excessive drug toxicity.[38]

To evaluate different treatments previously proposed by the trial groups, PHITT will, in some cases, randomize patients belonging to the same risk categories into different chemotherapeutic regimens to define which treatment would lead to a better outcome.[80] For instance, children affected by HB will be distributed into four groups (A, B, C, and D), which reflect the four risk categories of the CHIC-HS (very low risk, low risk, intermediate risk, and high risk) (Figure 18.5).

In group A, the reduced exposure to chemotherapy toxicity for patients, whose tumour shows a favourable histological pattern and low PRETEXT, is an important innovation introduced by the PHITT trial. It overcomes the SIOPEL theory of extending chemotherapy to all children suffering from HB. However, the histological pattern must be centrally reviewed to consider patients suitable for this treatment group.[80]

By contrast, patients belonging to the low-risk category (group B), suffering from a non-resectable mass, and absence of negative prognostic factors, receive two cycles of cisplatin monotherapy. It has been shown that most of the chemotherapeutic response occurs following the first two cycles, hence, resectability would be reconsidered after this initial treatment.[64]

Patients who are accounted for surgery are further randomized, following the resection, into two different treatment groups: two versus four additional cycles of cisplatin. Children still suffering from unresectable tumours, have two further cycles of cisplatin before being reconsidered for surgery. The PHITT trial will evaluate if a less toxic post-surgery chemotherapy would achieve a similar benefit, compared to more aggressive adjuvant treatment.

Patients with an extended HB, stage PRETEXT 4, or lower PRETEXT with positive annotation factors (VPEFR+), are considered to belong to risk group C. Such participants are randomized into three different chemotherapeutic strategies: (1) the one proposed by SIOPEL, based on a cocktail of cisplatin, carboplatin, and doxorubicin (SIOPEL 3HR) given for a total of five cycles; (2) the COG therapeutic scheme (C5VD), consisting of five cycles of cisplatin, 5-fluorouracil, vincristine, and doxorubicin; and (3) six cycles of cisplatin monotherapy (CDDP–M).

For each treatment scheme, surgery, when indicated, is performed at least before the last two cycles of chemotherapy.[80]

Children affected by metastatic HB belong to group D. They usually have a challenging primary disease and are eligible for a liver transplant. For these patients, PHITT recommends three blocks of cisplatin-intensive induction, the SIOPEL-4 regimen, alternating cisplatin and doxorubicin. Patients are then assessed to evaluate the metastatic response to chemotherapy alone or associated with thoracic surgery. In case metastases are cleared, children will follow a standard consolidation therapy of a further three cycles of cisplatin and doxorubicin. If metastases are not cleared, patients are randomized into two different groups of additional treatment:

- Carboplatin and doxorubicin, alternated with carboplatin and etoposide.
- Carboplatin and doxorubicin, alternated with vincristine and irinotecan.[80]

Outcomes in patients with metastatic HB have been historically poor. As previously mentioned, the novel SIOPEL 4 regimen, based on weekly dose-dense cisplatin chemotherapy, has shown a 98% partial response. Patients who had a complete or partial pulmonary response following induction experienced 95% and 53% EFS at 3 years, respectively. However, the great majority of patients experienced a grade 3–4 haematological toxicity.[54]

The PHITT trial will also assess the toxicity in those patients who cleared the metastases following the induction treatment and compare two different chemotherapy regimens, based on agents that have been proven effective in relapse and refractory disease.

CHAPTER 18 Primary neoplasms of the liver

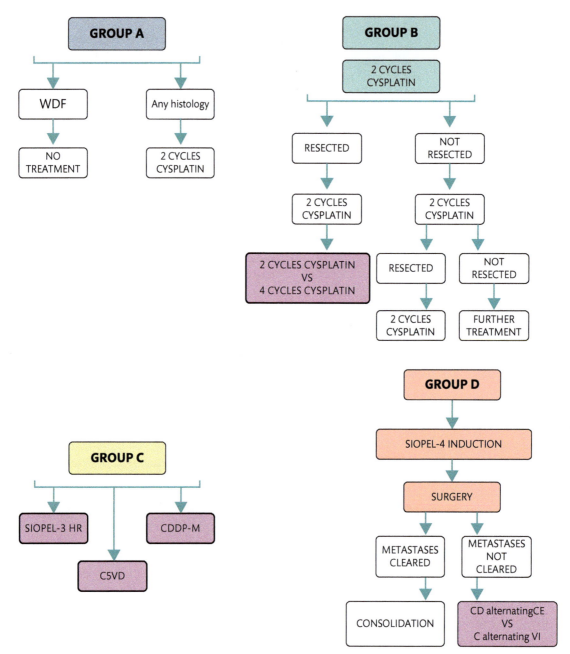

Figure 18.5 Diagram of chemotherapeutic treatment. CDDP-M, six cycles of cisplatin monotherapy; C5VD, five cycles of cisplatin, 5-fluorouracil, vincristine, doxorubicin; SIOPEL 3HR, five cycles based on a cocktail of cisplatin, carboplatin, and doxorubicin; SIOPEL-4 Induction, See text.

Surgical resection

The aim of surgery for a malignant tumour is complete excision, a requirement for cure.

The cisplatin-based chemotherapy used in the 1980s was the critical step that improved the overall survival of patients operated for HB from 35% to 70%.[3] Recent trials reported survival rates close to 80%.[4,5] Chemotherapy has been less successful in HCC, and surgical resection continues to offer the only real chance for cure in these children.

Advances in surgical technique have taken place in the past few years, but their significance has been relatively small compared to the efficacy of chemotherapy. The surgical strategy for HB should be based on a deep understanding of liver anatomy and surgical skills with different types of liver resections, including the most extreme ones (*ante situ* and *ex situ* resections). Surgery is best performed along anatomical planes, determined by segmental hepatic anatomy, while non-anatomical, atypical resections are mostly avoided except in particular cases. In fact, young children without any background liver disease, given the ability of their livers to regenerate rapidly, can tolerate very extensive liver resections, up to 80% of the whole liver.

The size and position of the lesion dictate the amount of parenchyma which will need to be removed. Although the main goal is to radically excise the tumour, the width of resection margins does not need to be greater than 1 cm.[81] However, in case of a good response to preoperative chemotherapy, the presence of microscopic residual disease at the resection margin is not a major adverse determinant of survival.[82-84]

Based on Coinaud's intrahepatic anatomical classification, the main types of liver resection include left lateral segmentectomy (segments 2–3), left hemihepatectomy (segments 1–4), left trisectionectomy (segments 1–4 plus 5 and 8), right hemihepatectomy (segments 5–8), and right trisectionectomy (segments 4–8). The surgical strategy and the extent of resection should be planned based on the preoperative imaging results.

The corresponding software for surgical planning, mostly used for living donation procedures, can provide a three-dimensional model that helps the surgeon's understanding of the position of the tumour in relation to vascular and biliary structures. It also has the ability to calculate volumes of every single liver segment and their relative function in the percentage of the whole liver, thus providing an estimate of the residual liver volume post-resection. In modern liver surgery, this has become a useful tool to plan accurate surgical strategies, perform resections along the correct anatomical planes, and avoid post-hepatectomy liver failure. At laparotomy, intraoperative US is used to confirm the tumour extent, the proximity of major intrahepatic vascular structures, and to assist the surgeon in choosing the best line of resection.

HB holds a similar physiological behaviour to HCC in the uptake of indocyanine green (ICG); therefore fluorescence-guided surgery can be a valuable option. The major advantages of ICG fluorescence imaging are clinical safety and feasibility. It has been reported that HB visualization can be greatly enhanced by near-infrared reflectance light.[85,86] Given that HB occasionally develops lymph node metastasis and dissemination in the abdominal cavity, it is best to administer ICG 72–96 hours before surgery to allow the background non-specific fluorescence in the intestinal loops to dissipate. An important technical limitation lies in the fact that the fluorescence emitted from ICG penetrates only 5–10 mm into the tissues, so that deep lesions display limited visibility. It remains somehow unclear whether ICG-guided surgery does improve the postoperative prognosis. While a tendency towards reduction of early recurrence rates of HCC has been reported after the introduction of ICG fluorography, no true survival benefits have yet been observed.[87] Based on the lower incidence of HBs in general, any benefit will need prolonged time to be demonstrated.[88]

The equipment required in the operating room usually includes an intraoperative US machine, energy devices, ultrasonic surgical aspirator, and bipolar forceps or argon beam.

Intraoperative US was introduced in the 1980s and has been a very useful tool to define the extent of the mass and its relation to the significant intrahepatic vascular and biliary structures.[89] It can detect new lesions, not diagnosed preoperatively, or reveal new information about the tumour and, therefore, it may alter the surgical strategy in approximately 20% of cases.[90]

Appropriate surgical strategy and technique allow for meticulous control of intraoperative bleeding which is required to reduce the need for blood transfusions, a factor linked with tumour recurrence, and perioperative morbidity. For this purpose, it is necessary to start with adequate surgical exposure. This can be achieved through a bilateral subcostal or hockey-stick incision and by mobilizing the liver from its ligaments and the retro-hepatic vena cava. Further steps include control of the hepatoduodenal ligament and of the vena cava above and below the liver. Hepatic tumours growing towards the porta hepatis or involving the hepato-caval confluence and inferior vena cava are at particular risk for copious haemorrhage, air embolism, and consequently increased postoperative morbidity and mortality.

In special cases requiring very extensive resection and vascular reconstruction, including *ante situm* procedures, the patient may require cold perfusion of the portal vein *in situ*. In rare, challenging circumstances, *ex situ* resections can be performed on the back table, after total hepatectomy, vena cava replacement, and temporary portocaval shunting, followed by reimplantation of the residual liver segments. These extreme techniques have been utilized in selected paediatric cases of borderline resectability.[91,92] In case of doubt about the possibility of resection, it has been suggested to proceed to surgery with a liver graft available for potential transplantation in standby. A backup transplant recipient should also be brought in hospital, in case a radical resection can be safely completed in the HB patient.[93,94] The determination of resectability of some tumours may vary between surgeons. Given the widespread availability of LT, the risks of a heroic resection must be carefully weighed against those of transplantation. Some authors even suggest primary transplantation for most children with PRETEXT 3 or 4.[95,96]

In more recent times, minimally invasive liver resection has been made available for paediatric patients affected by benign and malignant lesions. Laparoscopic liver resection has been reported for HB with excellent results in children as small as 9 months of age and 7 kg of weight.[97] However patient selection is essential to ensure that the resection is carried out with radical intent, safely, and with minimal bleeding. As with open surgery, a thorough preoperative CT assessment of the hilar anatomy, resection plane, and major vascular structures is necessary. Also, if patient safety or a clear resection margin becomes uncertain during the procedure, it is important to convert to open surgery without hesitation.

Postoperative complications

Surgical mortality rates have dropped to 4%,[98] though the postoperative morbidity still reaches 15–30%.[99] The main surgical complications include bleeding, tumour rupture, cholestasis, and bile leak.[99-101]

Postoperative complications have been shown to be more frequent in the high-risk HBs and bear a negative impact on survival and outcome after liver resection in the high-risk group with a decline of 5-year overall survival from 72% to 50%.[102] In the high-risk HB group, postoperative complications and vessel involvement by the tumour were both reported as independent negative prognostic factors. Surgical complications may also delay the start of adjuvant chemotherapy thus potentially compromising the prognosis.[102]

Haemorrhage

Intraoperative or postoperative haemorrhage is the most life-threatening complication during liver resections.[103] Unlike adults, children have small blood volumes and can become cardiovascularly unstable even from limited haemorrhages. Additionally, the liver parenchyma damaged by preoperative chemotherapy is more likely to be susceptible to bleeding. Therefore, meticulous surgical techniques and maintaining a low central venous pressure (2–4 mmHg) can help decrease the blood loss.[104]

When a difficult resection is anticipated, a Pringle's manoeuvre, a temporary clamping of the hepatoduodenal ligament, can be intermittently used to minimize intraoperative bleeding. Short-term complete hepatic vascular exclusion by clamping all three hepatic veins or even the IVC may help in avoiding a catastrophic haemorrhage or air embolism in case of accidental injury to the vena cava or the main hepatic veins. A normal liver texture is remarkably tolerant for ischaemia of up to 60 minutes. However, a planned intermittent clamping is usually utilized, and it involves 10–15 minutes of ischaemia followed by 5 minutes of reperfusion.

Bile leak

Bile leak occurs in approximately 7–10% of cases and its frequency has remained stable over the years.[102] The bile ducts, particularly at the level of the hilum, are more easily disrupted at the emergence of smaller branches. If a leak is recognized intraoperatively by retrograde cholangiogram of saline injection in the bile duct, it can be directly repaired with fine polydioxanone sutures. In case of injury or division of major ducts during the resection, drainage with a Roux loop should be considered.

Liver failure

Causes of post-hepatectomy liver failure include a functional small liver remnant, arterial or portal devascularization, venous congestion, and long warm ischaemia time due to a prolonged Pringle manoeuvre. This may manifest with early signs of cardiovascular instability such as lactic acidaemia or coagulopathy and later with jaundice, ascites, susceptibility to infections, and multiorgan failure. In the absence of improvement, an early assessment for LT is indicated.

Cardiac arrest

Intraoperative cardiac arrest occurs in 1–2% of major liver resections. The main causes include massive intraoperative bleeding, air emboli from caval or hepatic vein injuries, tumour emboli, and cardiac dysfunction from doxorubicin-related cardiotoxicity.

Liver transplantation

The management of HB has significantly evolved during the past three decades. The disease-free survival for HB has increased considerably from 30% in the pre-chemotherapy era to 70–80% in most recent studies.[48] Despite this increase, disease-free survival depends on complete surgical removal of the tumour. The role of LT as a treatment for unresectable HB has grown over time and is an important pillar of the multidisciplinary modern treatment concept of HB. The management of children affected by HB should be centralized in paediatric centres with expertise in radiology, oncology, liver surgery, and transplantation. Patients who respond to chemotherapy but whose tumour continues to be unresectable should be assessed for LT as primary surgery. The following HB types will qualify for LT: tumours invading all four sectors of the liver (HB classified into PRETEXT IV) or for those where the surgical excision may be incomplete due to close contact with either a hepatic vein or portal vein (some PRETEXT III or centrally located tumours). In PRETEXT IV multifocal HB, one sector may apparently clear during chemotherapy. Although it is tempting to consider radiological clearance as freedom from disease, partial hepatectomy in this setting has been shown to potentially leave viable microscopic residues leading to recurrence[100,105] (Table 18.3).

Absolute contraindications to LT for unresectable HB include persistent active metastatic disease (i.e. pulmonary metastases) and viable extrahepatic deposits not amenable to surgical excision after neoadjuvant chemotherapy. However, LT is a viable option with good long-term results for children who present with lung metastases which clear with chemotherapy. An additional thoracotomy may be indicated for surgical excision of residual pulmonary metastatic disease. If a radical excision is possible, even macroscopic venous invasion of the portal or hepatic veins is not an absolute contraindication to transplantation.

Patients generally receive additional cycles of chemotherapy following LT.

Outcomes of liver transplantation

Overall patient survival after adult and paediatric LT has improved in the past 30 years. Disease-free survival for HB has increased significantly from 30% in the prechemotherapy era to 70–80% in recent years. Overall, 5-year survival after LT in the SIOPEL-1 study, which included 154 children with HB, was 75%.[56] The presence of distant metastatic disease and PRETEXT staging were significant prognostic variables in this study. The 5-year survival of children with metastatic disease was 57% compared to 81% in those without. Regarding the extent of the tumour, the 5-year survival of patients with PRETEXT IV HBs was 57% compared to 100% of those with PRETEXT I lesions.[56] A SIOPEL group study has shown that the wider use of LT for HB has led to improved outcomes in patients with locally advanced disease.[106] Recent single-centre experiences have shown a disease-free survival of greater than 80% at 5 and 10 years post LT and superior results compared to outcomes of LT for children with HCC.[107,108] The survival for children with HB after resection or LT is essentially equivalent, despite the higher rate of advanced disease, vascular invasion, and satellite lesions among transplant patients.[109]

Similar excellent outcomes have also been reported in developing countries with limited resources when these children are managed by a multidisciplinary team with expertise in both complex liver

Table 18.3 Indications for liver transplantation

1	Multifocal PRETEXT IV	Except responders well downgraded to PRETEXT III, who may do as well with partial hepatectomy
2	Unifocal PRETEXT IV	If no clear margin for resection after neoadjuvant chemotherapy
3	PRETEXT III	If proximity to major vessels and doubtful tumour clearance
4	IVC and HVs	Tumour extension to IVC and all three HVs
5	PV	Invasion of main or both right and left PV
6	Intrahepatic recurrence or residual tumour after resection	'Salvage' transplantation

HV, hepatic vein; IVC, inferior vena cava; PRETEXT, Pre-treatment extension of tumor; PV, portal vein.
Source: data from Czauderna P, et al. Guidelines for surgical treatment of hepatoblastoma in the modern era—recommendations from the Childhood Liver Tumour Strategy Group of the International Society of Paediatric Oncology (SIOPEL). *Eur J Cancer*. 2005;41(7):1031–1036; and Otte JB, de Ville de Goyet J, Reding R. Liver transplantation for hepatoblastoma: indications and contraindications in the modern era. *Pediatr Transplant*. 2005;9(5):557–565.

surgery and LT, consisting of a paediatric oncologist, paediatric hepatologist, and an experienced paediatric hepatobiliary/pancreatic and liver transplant surgeon.[110]

Specific complications after liver transplantation

LT is associated with several complications, including surgical, vascular, and biliary complications, opportunistic infections exacerbated by immunosuppressive anti-rejection therapy, and vulnerability of the transplanted liver by chemotherapy. Hepatic artery thrombosis is a significant cause of graft loss and morbidity after paediatric LT.[111,112] Children affected by HB may be at higher risk for thrombosis because of technical challenges associated with anastomoses of smaller vessels, the use of whole paediatric grafts, and the prothrombotic state associated with hepatic malignant neoplasms. At King's College Hospital (London, UK) using a selective policy of retransplantation, revascularization, and conservative treatment, 83% of children survived the occurrence of hepatic artery thrombosis after LT. Approximately 40% of children with hepatic artery thrombosis survived without retransplantation.[112]

Prognostic factors in the context of liver transplantation

Histological vascular invasion, response to chemotherapy, and salvage LT have been reported as prognostic factors for HB recurrence after LT.[96,113–115] Other reported indicators for tumour recurrence and decreased survival after transplantation include the SIOPEL high-risk status and PRETEXT stage IV disease, tumour rupture, older age at the time of the LT, the presence of metastatic HB at initial presentation, persistently elevated AFP levels after neoadjuvant chemotherapy, and prolonged time spent on the transplant waiting list. In this context, United Network for Organ Sharing and NHS Blood and Transplant policies in the US and UK, respectively, grant a higher status particularly in the time window after chemotherapy, thus reducing waiting times.

The general response to chemotherapy at LT, evaluated by the dynamic change of serum AFP levels, could become a useful tool to predict post-LT recurrence for patients receiving both primary and rescue LT. Given that a significant proportion of patients receive salvage chemotherapy, recently established intensified first-line chemotherapy should contribute to an increase in the response rate and therefore the cure rate of patients receiving primary LT.[116,117] Novel salvage chemotherapy incorporating molecular targeting drugs, such as mTOR inhibitors, could be an alternative option for patients who are unable to tolerate high-dose chemotherapy.[118]

Salvage transplantation

In 2004, Otte et al. reviewed the world experience of transplantation for HB.[96] They reported an overall 6-year post LT survival of 82% in 106 children who received a primary transplant. In contrast, the survival was only 30% in 41 patients who had undergone a salvage transplant after hepatic recurrence or incomplete resection following partial hepatectomy.[96] Salvage transplantation remains a controversial concept within the transplant community. The hypothesis is that extrahepatic micrometastases, which cannot be eradicated by neoadjuvant chemotherapy, may lead to post-LT relapse. However, a SIOPEL review in 2012 showed that microscopic residue in HB was not associated with a decreased survival.[119] Additionally, Umeda et al. found no significant differences in overall survival rates between patients receiving primary and salvage LT and demonstrated a recurrence rate of 27% and 5-year overall survival of 72% following salvage transplantation in 11 patients.[117] Similarly, Ramos-Gonzalez et al. reported acceptable results of 66% survival with salvage transplantation for recurrent disease following liver resection. Although these outcomes might be inferior to primary transplantation, it can be argued that in particular cases it is the only option for a potential cure.[107] The development of better prognostic markers based on the molecular biology of HB will be crucial for the risk stratification and selection of patients for salvage transplantation and when deciding between extreme resections versus LT.

Metastatic disease

Lung metastases showing complete response to chemotherapy with or without surgical resection do not pose a contraindication to LT. Early involvement of the portal or hepatic veins and vena cava is not a contraindication, although the outcome is likely inferior with long-term survival ranging from 54% to 77%.[71,96]

Absolute contraindications for LT for HB include viable extrahepatic disease and persistent pulmonary metastases not suitable for surgical resection.

Candidates for LT not only require careful evaluation of their tumour but also their fitness for transplantation. The child's nutritional status should be optimized prior to transplantation. A detailed echocardiogram and assessment of renal function are essential before transplantation. This is due to the known side effects of adjuvant chemotherapy; for example, doxorubicin is cardiotoxic and cisplatin is both nephrotoxic and ototoxic. Such effects will add up to those of post-transplant immunosuppression. Liver transplant recipients are at an increased lifelong risk of malignancy regardless of the initial underlying disease or indication for the transplant. The immunosuppression may further increase the risk of a metastatic spread of existing malignancies.

The potential benefits of LT should therefore be weighed against the risks of complications and life-long immunosuppression. Ruth et al. reported a 50% rejection activity index in 20 children transplanted for HB, compared to 75% of 60 children transplanted for extrahepatic biliary atresia. Children transplanted for HB, when compared to the overall paediatric transplant population, showed a lower rate of rejection, a higher mortality secondary to sepsis/malignant progression, and renal function compromised by chemotherapy.[57,120] These findings would suggest that that LT for HB may require less immunosuppression.

Timing of liver transplantation

Chemotherapy must be continued until the time of transplantation to maintain control of the tumour. However, continuous administration of chemotherapy after four cycles does not increase the likelihood of conventional resectability of the tumour.[121] In such patients, where LT is required, the ideal timing of LT is after four cycles of neoadjuvant chemotherapy.[48] The interval between the last course of chemotherapy and LT should not exceed 4 weeks. A delayed resection or transplantation after the completion of four cycles will increase the risk of tumour resistance and poor outcomes.[122] Given the unpredictable nature of deceased donor availability, transplantation for HB is particularly suited for primary living donor liver transplantation (LDLT) as it is possible to plan the transplant at the desired timing. Similarly, LDLT can be used as a backup, in case there are no deceased donor offers within the window of opportunity. Several countries have also prioritized the allocation of cadaveric livers to a national HB list which, in the UK scheme, is positioned just below the tier of super-urgent indications. Although this leads to a high number of inappropriate offers, it also increases the likelihood that children will be transplanted within the post-chemotherapy window. Should the child not get an offer in time, chemotherapy is commenced again to provide a new window of transplantability to the patient.

Surgical technique and type of donors

LDLT has shown similar survival rates when compared with cadaveric donation for HB. However, potential advantages of LDLT include shorter waiting times, better graft quality, and, as mentioned earlier, improved timing of transplantation in combination with pre-transplant chemotherapy.[113] The latter is particularly relevant given the reported increased recurrence rate for those children who waited longer for a liver on the cadaveric transplant list.[108] Conversely, the advantages of cadaveric donation include the avoidance of a major operative procedure to a healthy donor and the availability of longer blood vessels from cadaveric donor grafts that allow for simpler vascular reconstructions.

Depending on the size of the donor and recipient, the most frequently transplanted liver grafts include a left lateral segment, a left lobe, or a whole liver. The transplantation of an entire liver is less likely due to the scarcity of paediatric donors, with implantation using the vena cava replacement technique to increase the radicality of the hepatectomy. Left-sided grafts (segments 2–3 and 2–4), given the absence of donor vena cava, are usually implanted with the piggyback technique and preservation of the IVC. However, when HB is the indication for LT, a replacement of the native IVC with an iliac vein from a cadaveric donor or with a jugular vein, in case of living donation, is recommended before implantation.[123]

Management of recurrence

The recurrence of HB after LT is observed in approximately 20–30% of children, and the outcomes for such patients are extremely poor.[96,108] The most frequently reported organs of recurrence include the lung and the transplanted liver, or both.

In patients with initial normal AFP levels, which increase again during the follow-up, the identification of the exact site of recurrence may be challenging. A total body ^{18}F fluorodeoxyglucose positron emission tomography may be useful.

However, when recurrence is confined to the liver, or to very few extrahepatic sites only, and especially when the tumour remains chemosensitive, the possibility of repeating chemotherapy and surgery should be contemplated. In recurrent, refractory disease, phase I and II clinical trials should be considered.[78] Alternative agents including irinotecan, oxaliplatin, targeted agents, gene-directed therapy, immunotherapy, and combinations of these are new potential strategies. A combination treatment of oxaliplatin, vincristine, and topotecan paired with radiofrequency ablation in patients with multiple refractory/recurrent pulmonary HB lesions has shown to yield a 2-year EFS rate of 33%.[124]

Conclusion

The potential for cure with combined surgical resection and modern chemotherapy is greater for HB when compared to children with HCC. Although some centres have reported their overall experience with HB while others have reported their experience with transplanted patients only, it is clear that most children with a diagnosis of HB will survive long term.

Although individual centres treat relatively small numbers of patients, the best overall survival rates are obtained in experienced units that offer all therapeutic options, including LT.

REFERENCES

1. Stiller CA, Pritchard J, Steliarova-Foucher E. Liver cancer in European children: incidence and survival, 1978–1997. Report from the Automated Childhood Cancer Information System project. *Eur J Cancer*. 2006;**42**(13):2115–2123.
2. Sharma D, Subbarao G, Saxena R. Hepatoblastoma. *Semin Diagn Pathol*. 2017;**34**(2):192–200.
3. Haas JE, Muczynski KA, Krailo M, et al. Histopathology and prognosis in childhood hepatoblastoma and hepatocarcinoma. *Cancer*. 1989;**64**(5):1082–1095.
4. Herzog CE, Andrassy RJ Eftekhari F. Childhood cancers: hepatoblastoma. *Oncologist*. 2000;**5**(6):445–453.
5. Stocker JT. Hepatoblastoma. *Semin Diagn Pathol*. 1994;**11**(2):136–143.
6. Chitragar S, Iyer VK, Agarwala S, Gupta SD, Sharma A, Wari MN. Loss of heterozygosity on chromosome 11p15.5 and relapse in hepatoblastomas. *Eur J Pediatr Surg*. 2011;**21**(1):50–53.
7. Sorahan T, Lancashire RJ. Parental cigarette smoking and childhood risks of hepatoblastoma: OSCC data. *Br J Cancer*. 2004;**90**(5):1016–1018.
8. Yang A, Sisson R, Gupta A, Tiao G, Geller JI. Germline APC mutations in hepatoblastoma. *Pediatr Blood Cancer*. 2018;**65**(4):10.1002/pbc.26892.
9. Zhang W, Meyfeldt J, Wang H, et al. Beta-catenin mutations as determinants of hepatoblastoma phenotypes in mice. *J Biol Chem*. 2019;**294**(46):17524–17542.
10. Heck JE, Meyers TJ, Lombardi C, et al. Case-control study of birth characteristics and the risk of hepatoblastoma. *Cancer Epidemiol*. 2013;**37**(4):390–395.
11. Czauderna P, Haeberle B, Hiyama E, et al. The Children's Hepatic tumors International Collaboration (CHIC): novel global rare tumor database yields new prognostic factors in hepatoblastoma and becomes a research model. *Eur J Cancer*. 2016;**52**:92–101.
12. Meyers RL, Maibach R, Hiyama E, et al. Risk-stratified staging in paediatric hepatoblastoma: a unified analysis from the Children's Hepatic tumors International Collaboration. *Lancet Oncol*. 2017;**18**(1):122–131.
13. López-Terrada D, Alaggio R, de Dávila MT, et al. Towards an international pediatric liver tumor consensus classification: proceedings of the Los Angeles COG liver tumors symposium. *Mod Pathol*. 2014;**27**(3):472–491.
14. Gupta AA, Gerstle JT, Ng V, et al. Critical review of controversial issues in the management of advanced pediatric liver tumors. *Pediatr Blood Cancer*. 2011;**56**(7):1013–1018.
15. Trobaugh-Lotrario AD, López-Terrada D, Li P, Feusner JH. Hepatoblastoma in patients with molecularly proven familial adenomatous polyposis: clinical characteristics and rationale for surveillance screening. *Pediatr Blood Cancer*. 2018;**65**(8):e27103.
16. Tomlinson GE, Douglass EC, Pollock BH, Finegold MJ, Schneider NR. Cytogenetic evaluation of a large series of hepatoblastomas: numerical abnormalities with recurring

aberrations involving 1q12-q21. *Genes Chromosomes Cancer.* 2005;**44**(2):177–184.

17. Mussa A, Molinatto C, Baldassarre G, et al. Cancer risk in Beckwith-Wiedemann syndrome: a systematic review and meta-analysis outlining a novel (epi)genotype specific histotype targeted screening protocol. *J Pediatr.* 2016;**176**:142–149.

18. Oue T, Kubota A, Okuyama H, et al. Hepatoblastoma in children of extremely low birth weight: a report from a single perinatal center. *J Pediatr Surg.* 2003;**38**(1):134–137.

19. Valentin LI, Perez L, Masand P. Hepatoblastoma associated with trisomy 18. *J Pediatr Genet.* 2015;**4**(4):204–206.

20. Koch A, Waha A, Hartmann W, et al. Elevated expression of Wnt antagonists is a common event in hepatoblastomas. *Clin Cancer Res.* 2005;**11**(12):4295–4304.

21. Tan X, Apte U, Micsenyi A, et al. Epidermal growth factor receptor: a novel target of the Wnt/beta-catenin pathway in liver. *Gastroenterology.* 2005;**129**(1):285–302.

22. Koch A, Denkhaus D, Albrecht S, Leuschner I, von Schweinitz D, Pietsch T. Childhood hepatoblastomas frequently carry a mutated degradation targeting box of the beta-catenin gene. *Cancer Res.* 1999;**59**(2):269–273.

23. Lee H, El Jabbour T, Ainechi S, et al. General paucity of genomic alteration and low tumor mutation burden in refractory and metastatic hepatoblastoma: comprehensive genomic profiling study. *Hum Pathol.* 2017;**70**:84–91.

24. Buendia MA. Genetic alterations in hepatoblastoma and hepatocellular carcinoma: common and distinctive aspects. *Med Pediatr Oncol.* 2002;**39**(5):530–535.

25. Czauderna P, Lopez-Terrada D, Hiyama E, Häberle B, Malogolowkin MH, Meyers RL. Hepatoblastoma state of the art: pathology, genetics, risk stratification, and chemotherapy. *Curr Opin Pediatr.* 2014;**26**(1):19–28.

26. Monga SP. β-catenin signaling and roles in liver homeostasis, injury, and tumorigenesis. *Gastroenterology.* 2015;**148**(7):1294–1310.

27. Calvisi DF, Solinas A. Hepatoblastoma: current knowledge and promises from preclinical studies. *Transl Gastroenterol Hepatol.* 2020;**5**:42.

28. Ranganathan S, Lopez-Terrada D, Alaggio R. Hepatoblastoma and pediatric hepatocellular carcinoma: an update. *Pediatr Dev Pathol.* 2020;**23**(2):79–95.

29. Tao J, Calvisi DF, Ranganathan S, et al. Activation of β-catenin and Yap1 in human hepatoblastoma and induction of hepatocarcinogenesis in mice. *Gastroenterology.* 2014;**147**(3):690–701.

30. Harada N, Oshima H, Katoh M, Tamai Y, Oshima M, Taketo MM. Hepatocarcinogenesis in mice with beta-catenin and Ha-ras gene mutations. *Cancer Res.* 2004;**64**(1):48–54.

31. Molina L, Yang H, Adebayo Michael AO, et al. mTOR inhibition affects Yap1-β-catenin-induced hepatoblastoma growth and development. *Oncotarget.* 2019;**10**(15):1475–1490.

32. Willis RA. Some uncommon and recenty identified tmours. In: Cameron R, Payling Wright G, eds. *The Pathology of the Tumours of Children.* Springfield, IL: Charles C. Thomas; 1962: 57–61.

33. Finegold MJ, Lopez-Terrada DH, Bowen J, Washington MK, Qualman SJ, College of American Pathologists. Protocol for the examination of specimens from pediatric patients with hepatoblastoma. *Arch Pathol Lab Med.* 2007;**131**(4):520–529.

34. Ishak KG, Glunz PR. Hepatoblastoma and hepatocarcinoma in infancy and childhood. Report of 47 cases. *Cancer.* 1967;**20**(3):396–422.

35. Meyers RL, Rowland JR, Krailo M, Chen Z, Katzenstein HM, Malogolowkin MH. Predictive power of pretreatment prognostic factors in children with hepatoblastoma: a report from the Children's Oncology Group. *Pediatr Blood Cancer.* 2009;**53**(6):1016–1022.

36. Weinberg AG, Finegold MJ. Primary hepatic tumors of childhood. *Hum Pathol.* 1983;**14**(6):512–537.

37. Malogolowkin MH, Katzenstein HM, Meyers RL, et al. Complete surgical resection is curative for children with hepatoblastoma with pure fetal histology: a report from the Children's Oncology Group. *J Clin Oncol.* 2011;**29**(24):3301–3306.

38. Meyers RL, Maibach R, Hiyama E, et al. Risk-stratified staging in paediatric hepatoblastoma: a unified analysis from the Children's Hepatic tumors International Collaboration. *Lancet Oncol.* 2017;**18**(1):122–131.

39. Perilongo G, Malogolowkin M, Feusner J. Hepatoblastoma clinical research: lessons learned and future challenges. *Pediatr Blood Cancer.* 2012;**59**(5):818–821.

40. Kasai M, Watanabe I. Histologic classification of liver-cell carcinoma in infancy and childhood and its clinical evaluation. A study of 70 cases collected in Japan. *Cancer.* 1970;**25**(3):551–563.

41. Gonzalez-Crussi F. Undifferentiated small cell ('anaplastic') hepatoblastoma. *Pediatr Pathol.* 1991;**11**(1):155–161.

42. Conran RM, Hitchcock CL, Waclawiw MA, Stocker JT, Ishak KG. Hepatoblastoma: the prognostic significance of histologic type. *Pediatr Pathol.* 1992;**12**(2):167–183.

43. Haas JE, Feusner JH, Finegold MJ. Small cell undifferentiated histology in hepatoblastoma may be unfavorable. *Cancer.* 2001;**92**(12):3130–3134.

44. Zimmermann A, Perilongo, G. eds. *Pediatric Liver Tumors.* Berlin: Springer Science & Business Media; 2011.

45. Saxena R, Leake JL, Shafford EA, et al. Chemotherapy effects on hepatoblastoma. A histological study. *Am J Surg Pathol.* 1993;**17**(12):1266–1271.

46. Manivel C, Wick MR, Abenoza P, Dehner LP. Teratoid hepatoblastoma. The nosologic dilemma of solid embryonic neoplasms of childhood. *Cancer.* 1986;**57**(11):2168–2174.

47. Prokurat A, Kluge P, Kościesza A, Perek D, Kappeler A, Zimmermann A. Transitional liver cell tumors (TLCT) in older children and adolescents: a novel group of aggressive hepatic tumors expressing beta-catenin. *Med Pediatr Oncol.* 2002;**39**(5):510–518.

48. Meyers RL, Tiao G, de Ville de Goyet J, Superina R, Aronson DC. Hepatoblastoma state of the art: pre-treatment extent of disease, surgical resection guidelines and the role of liver transplantation. *Curr Opin Pediatr.* 2014;**26**(1):29–36.

49. Coran AG, Adzick NS. *Pediatric Surgery.* Philadelphia, PA: Elsevier Mosby; 2012.

50. Towbin AJ, Meyers RL, Woodley H, et al. 2017 PRETEXT: radiologic staging system for primary hepatic malignancies of childhood revised for the Paediatric Hepatic International Tumour Trial (PHITT). *Pediatr Radiol.* 2018;**48**(4):536–554.

51. Pugmire BS, Towbin AJ. Magnetic resonance imaging of primary pediatric liver tumors. *Pediatr Radiol.* 2016;**46**(6):764–777.

52. Meyers AB, Towbin AJ, Geller JI, Podberesky DJ. Hepatoblastoma imaging with gadoxetate disodium-enhanced MRI—typical, atypical, pre- and post-treatment evaluation. *Pediatr Radiol.* 2012;**42**(7):859–866.

53. MacKinlay G, Pritchard J. A common language for childhood liver tumours. *Pediatr Surg Int.* 1992;**7**(4):325–326.

54. Ortega JA, Douglass EC, Feusner JH, et al. Randomized comparison of cisplatin/vincristine/fluorouracil and cisplatin/continuous infusion doxorubicin for treatment of pediatric hepatoblastoma: a report from the Children's Cancer Group and the Pediatric Oncology Group. *J Clin Oncol.* 2000;**18**(14):2665–2675.

55. Aronson DC, Schnater JM, Staalman CR, et al. Predictive value of the pretreatment extent of disease system in hepatoblastoma: results from the International Society of Pediatric Oncology Liver Tumor Study Group SIOPEL-1 study. *J Clin Oncol.* 2005;**23**(6):1245–1252.

56. Brown J, Perilongo G, Shafford E, et al. Pretreatment prognostic factors for children with hepatoblastoma—results from the International Society of Paediatric Oncology (SIOP) study SIOPEL 1. *Eur J Cancer.* 2000;**36**(11):1418–1425.

57. Pritchard J, Brown J, Shafford E, et al. Cisplatin, doxorubicin, and delayed surgery for childhood hepatoblastoma: a successful approach—results of the first prospective study of the International Society of Pediatric Oncology. *J Clin Oncol.* 2000;**18**(22):3819–3828.

58. Perilongo G, Shafford E, Maibach R, et al. Risk-adapted treatment for childhood hepatoblastoma. Final report of the second study of the International Society of Paediatric Oncology—SIOPEL 2. *Eur J Cancer.* 2004;**40**(3):411–421.

59. Darcy DG, Malek MM, Kobos R, Klimstra DS, DeMatteo R, La Quaglia MP. Prognostic factors in fibrolamellar hepatocellular carcinoma in young people. *J Pediatr Surg.* 2015;**50**(1):153–156.

60. Qiao G, Cucchetti A, Li J, et al. Applying of pretreatment extent of disease system in patients with hepatocellular carcinoma after curative partial hepatectomy. *Oncotarget.* 2016;**7**(21):30408–30419.

61. Weeda VB, Murawski M, McCabe AJ, et al. Fibrolamellar variant of hepatocellular carcinoma does not have a better survival than conventional hepatocellular carcinoma—results and treatment recommendations from the Childhood Liver Tumour Strategy Group (SIOPEL) experience. *Eur J Cancer.* 2013;**49**(12):2698–2704.

62. Meyers RL. Tumors of the liver in children. *Surg Oncol.* 2007;**16**(3):195–203.

63. Meyers RL, Czauderna P, Otte JB. Surgical treatment of hepatoblastoma. *Pediatr Blood Cancer.* 2012;**59**(5):800–808.

64. Lovvorn HN 3rd, Ayers D, Zhao Z, et al. Defining hepatoblastoma responsiveness to induction therapy as measured by tumor volume and serum alpha-fetoprotein kinetics. *J Pediatr Surg.* 2010;**45**(1):121–128.

65. Roebuck DJ, Aronson D, Clapuyt P, et al. 2005 PRETEXT: a revised staging system for primary malignant liver tumours of childhood developed by the SIOPEL group. *Pediatr Radiol.* 2007;**37**(2):123–132.

66. Yadav SS, Lawande MA, Patkar DA, Pungavkar SP. Rare case of hemorrhagic brain metastasis from hepatoblastoma. *J Pediatr Neurosci.* 2012;**7**(1):73–74.

67. Saettini F, Conter V, Provenzi M, et al. Is multifocality a prognostic factor in childhood hepatoblastoma? *Pediatr Blood Cancer.* 2014;**61**(9):1593–1597.

68. Maibach R, Roebuck D, Brugieres L, et al. Prognostic stratification for children with hepatoblastoma: the SIOPEL experience. *Eur J Cancer.* 2012;**48**(10):1543–1549.

69. Dall'Igna P, Cecchetto G, Toffolutti T, et al. Multifocal hepatoblastoma: is there a place for partial hepatectomy? *Med Pediatr Oncol.* 2003;**40**(2):113–116.

70. Kolbe AB, Podberesky DJ, Zhang B, Towbin AJ. The impact of hepatocyte phase imaging from infancy to young adulthood in patients with a known or suspected liver lesion. *Pediatr Radiol.* 2015;**45**(3):354–365.

71. Reyes JD, Carr B, Dvorchik I, et al. Liver transplantation and chemotherapy for hepatoblastoma and hepatocellular cancer in childhood and adolescence. *J Pediatr.* 2000;**136**(6):795–804.

72. Roebuck DJ, Sebire NJ, Pariente D. Assessment of extrahepatic abdominal extension in primary malignant liver tumours of childhood. *Pediatr Radiol.* 2007;**37**(11):1096–1100.

73. Fuchs J, Rydzynski J, Von Schweinitz D, et al. Pretreatment prognostic factors and treatment results in children with hepatoblastoma: a report from the German Cooperative Pediatric Liver Tumor Study HB 94. *Cancer.* 2002;**95**(1):172–182.

74. Haeberle B, Rangaswami A, Krailo M, et al. The importance of age as prognostic factor for the outcome of patients with hepatoblastoma: analysis from the Children's Hepatic tumors International Collaboration (CHIC) database. *Pediatr Blood Cancer.* 2020;**67**(8):e28350.

75. Hiyama E. Pediatric hepatoblastoma: diagnosis and treatment. *Transl Pediatr.* 2014;**3**(4):293–299.

76. Hishiki T, Matsunaga T, Sasaki F, et al. Outcome of hepatoblastomas treated using the Japanese Study Group for Pediatric Liver Tumor (JPLT) protocol-2: report from the JPLT. *Pediatr Surg Int.* 2011;**27**(1):1–8.

77. Haeberle B, Schweinitz D. Treatment of hepatoblastoma in the German cooperative pediatric liver tumor studies. *Front Biosci (Elite Ed).* 2012;**4**:493–498.

78. Zsiros J, Brugieres L, Brock P, et al. Dose-dense cisplatin-based chemotherapy and surgery for children with high-risk hepatoblastoma (SIOPEL-4): a prospective, single-arm, feasibility study. *Lancet Oncol.* 2013;**14**(9):834–842.

79. Qayed M, Katzenstein HM. Dose-intensive cisplatin for hepatoblastoma: have you heard? *Lancet Oncol.* 2013;**14**(9):791–792.

80. Morland B. Paediatric Hepatic International Tumour Trial. University of Birmingham. 2018. https://www.birmingham.ac.uk/Documents/college-mds/trials/crctu/phitt/Protocol/Current/PHITT-Protocol-version-3-0-17Oct2018.pdf

81. Dicken BJ, Bigam DL, Lees GM. Association between surgical margins and long-term outcome in advanced hepatoblastoma. *J Pediatr Surg.* 2004;**39**(5):721–725.

82. Perilongo G, Shafford E, Maibach R, et al. Risk-adapted treatment for childhood hepatoblastoma. Final report of the second study of the International Society of Paediatric Oncology—SIOPEL 2. *Eur J Cancer.* 2004;**40**(3):411–421.

83. Stringer MD, Hennayake S, Howard ER, et al. Improved outcome for children with hepatoblastoma. *Br J Surg.* 1995;**82**(3):386–391.

84. Schnater JM, Aronson DC, Plaschkes J, et al. Surgical view of the treatment of patients with hepatoblastoma: results from the first prospective trial of the International Society of Pediatric Oncology Liver Tumor Study Group. *Cancer.* 2002;**94**(4):1111–1120.

85. Kitagawa N, Shinkai M, Mochizuki K, et al. Navigation using indocyanine green fluorescence imaging for hepatoblastoma pulmonary metastases surgery. *Pediatr Surg Int.* 2015;**31**(4):407–411.

86. Yamamichi T, Oue T, Yonekura T, et al. Clinical application of indocyanine green (ICG) fluorescent imaging of hepatoblastoma. *J Pediatr Surg.* 2015;**50**(5):833–836.

87. Morita Y, Sakaguchi T, Unno N, et al. Detection of hepatocellular carcinomas with near-infrared fluorescence imaging using indocyanine green: its usefulness and limitation. *Int J Clin Oncol.* 2013;**18**(2):232–241.

88. Yamada Y, Ohno M, Fujino A, et al. Fluorescence-guided surgery for hepatoblastoma with indocyanine green. *Cancers (Basel)*. 2019;**11**(8):1215.
89. Makuuchi M, Hasegawa H, Yamazaki S, Takayasu K, Moriyama N. The use of operative ultrasound as an aid to liver resection in patients with hepatocellular carcinoma. *World J Surg*. 1987;**11**(5):615–621.
90. van Vledder MG, Pawlik TM, Munireddy S, Hamper U, de Jong MC, Choti MA. Factors determining the sensitivity of intraoperative ultrasonography in detecting colorectal liver metastases in the modern era. *Ann Surg Oncol*. 2010;**17**(10):2756–2763.
91. Fusai G, Steinberg R, Prachalias A, Heaton ND, Spitz L, Rela M. Ex vivo liver surgery for extraadrenal pheochromocytoma. *Pediatr Surg Int*. 2006;**22**(3):282–285.
92. Schlegel A, Sakuraoka Y, Motwani K, et al. Outcome after ex situ or ante situm liver resection with hypothermic perfusion and auto-transplantation: a single-centre experience in adult and paediatric patients. *J Surg Oncol*. 2020;**122**(6):1122–1131.
93. Millar AJ, Hartley P, Khan D, Spearman W, Andronikou S, Rode H. Extended hepatic resection with transplantation back-up for an 'unresectable' tumour. *Pediatr Surg Int*. 2001;**17**(5–6):378–381.
94. Srinivasan P, McCall J, Pritchard J, et al. Orthotopic liver transplantation for unresectable hepatoblastoma. *Transplantation*. 2002;**74**(5):652–655.
95. Pimpalwar AP, Sharif K, Ramani P, et al. Strategy for hepatoblastoma management: transplant versus nontransplant surgery. *J Pediatr Surg*. 2002;**37**(2):240–245.
96. Otte JB, Pritchard J, Aronson DC, et al. Liver transplantation for hepatoblastoma: results from the International Society of Pediatric Oncology (SIOP) study SIOPEL-1 and review of the world experience. *Pediatr Blood Cancer*. 2004;**42**(1):74–83.
97. Kwon H, Lee JY, Cho YJ, Kim DY, Kim SC, Namgoong JM. et al. How to safely perform laparoscopic liver resection for children: a case series of 19 patients. *J Pediatr Surg*. 2019;**54**(12):2579–2584.
98. Tannuri AC, Tannuri U, Gibelli NE, Romão RL. Surgical treatment of hepatic tumors in children: lessons learned from liver transplantation. *J Pediatr Surg*. 2009;**44**(11):2083–2087.
99. Pham TH, Iqbal CW, Grams JM, et al. Outcomes of primary liver cancer in children: an appraisal of experience. *J Pediatr Surg*. 2007;**42**(5):834–839.
100. Czauderna P, Otte JB, Aronson DC, et al. Guidelines for surgical treatment of hepatoblastoma in the modern era—recommendations from the Childhood Liver Tumour Strategy Group of the International Society of Paediatric Oncology (SIOPEL). *Eur J Cancer*. 2005;**41**(7):1031–1036.
101. Fuchs J, Rydzynski J, Hecker H, et al. The influence of preoperative chemotherapy and surgical technique in the treatment of hepatoblastoma—a report from the German Cooperative Liver Tumour Studies HB 89 and HB 94. *Eur J Pediatr Surg*. 2002;**12**(4):255–261.
102. Becker K, Furch C, Schmid I, von Schweinitz D, Häberle B. Impact of postoperative complications on overall survival of patients with hepatoblastoma. *Pediatr Blood Cancer*. 2015;**62**(1):24–28.
103. Lin CC, Chen CL, Cheng YF, Chiu KW, Jawan B, Hsaio CC. Major hepatectomy in children: approaching blood transfusion-free. *World J Surg*. 2006;**30**(6):1115–1119.
104. Wang WD, Liang LJ, Huang XQ, Yin XY. Low central venous pressure reduces blood loss in hepatectomy. *World J Gastroenterol*. 2006;**12**(6):935–939.
105. Otte JB, de Ville de Goyet J, Reding R. Liver transplantation for hepatoblastoma: indications and contraindications in the modern era. *Pediatr Transplant*. 2005;**9**(5):557–565.
106. Zsiros J, Maibach R, Shafford E, et al. Successful treatment of childhood high-risk hepatoblastoma with dose-intensive multiagent chemotherapy and surgery: final results of the SIOPEL-3HR study. *J Clin Oncol*. 2010;**28**(15):2584–2590.
107. Ramos-Gonzalez G, LaQuaglia M, O'Neill AF, et al. Long-term outcomes of liver transplantation for hepatoblastoma: a single-center 14-year experience. *Pediatr Transplant*. 2018;**22**(6):e13250.
108. Pham TA, Gallo AM, Concepcion W, Esquivel CO, Bonham CA. Effect of liver transplant on long-term disease-free survival in children with hepatoblastoma and hepatocellular cancer. *JAMA Surg*. 2015;**150**(12):1150–1158.
109. McAteer JP, Goldin AB, Healey PJ, Gow KW. Surgical treatment of primary liver tumors in children: outcomes analysis of resection and transplantation in the SEER database. *Pediatr Transplant*. 2013;**17**(8):744–750.
110. Shanmugam N, Scott JX, Kumar V, et al. Multidisciplinary management of hepatoblastoma in children: experience from a developing country. *Pediatr Blood Cancer*. 2017;**64**(3):e26249.
111. Rela M, Muiesan P, Bhatnagar V, et al. Hepatic artery thrombosis after liver transplantation in children under 5 years of age. *Transplantation*. 1996;**61**(9):1355–1357.
112. Stringer MD, Marshall MM, Muiesan P, et al. Survival and outcome after hepatic artery thrombosis complicating pediatric liver transplantation. *J Pediatr Surg*. 2001;**36**(6):888–891.
113. Faraj W, Dar F, Marangoni G, et al. Liver transplantation for hepatoblastoma. *Liver Transpl*. 2008;**14**(11):1614–1619.
114. Kasahara M, Ueda M, Haga H, et al. Living-donor liver transplantation for hepatoblastoma. *Am J Transplant*. 2005;**5**(9):2229–2235.
115. Browne M, Sher D, Grant D, et al. Survival after liver transplantation for hepatoblastoma: a 2-center experience. *J Pediatr Surg*. 2008;**43**(11):1973–1981.
116. Zsiros J, Brugieres L, Brock P, et al. Dose-dense cisplatin-based chemotherapy and surgery for children with high-risk hepatoblastoma (SIOPEL-4): a prospective, single-arm, feasibility study. *Lancet Oncol*. 2013;**14**(9):834–842.
117. Umeda K, Okajima H, Kawaguchi K, et al. Prognostic and therapeutic factors influencing the clinical outcome of hepatoblastoma after liver transplantation: a single-institute experience. *Pediatr Transplant*. 2018;**22**(2):e13113.
118. Bagatell R, Norris R, Ingle AM, et al. Phase 1 trial of temsirolimus in combination with irinotecan and temozolomide in children, adolescents and young adults with relapsed or refractory solid tumors: a Children's Oncology Group Study. *Pediatr Blood Cancer*. 2014;**61**(5):833–839.
119. Czauderna P. Hepatoblastoma throughout SIOPEL trials—clinical lessons learnt. *Front Biosci (Elite Ed)*. 2012;**4**:470–479.
120. Lee WS, Grundy R, Milford DV, et al. Renal function following liver transplantation for unresectable hepatoblastoma. *Pediatr Transplant*. 2003;**7**(4):270–276.
121. Warmann SW, Fuchs J. Drug resistance in hepatoblastoma. *Curr Pharm Biotechnol*. 2007;**8**(2):93–97.
122. Kremer N., Walther AE, Tiao GM. Management of hepatoblastoma: an update. *Curr Opin Pediatr*. 2014;**26**(3):362–369.
123. Chardot C, Saint Martin C, Gilles A, et al. Living-related liver transplantation and vena cava reconstruction after total hepatectomy including the vena cava for hepatoblastoma. *Transplantation*. 2002;**73**(1):90–92.
124. Zhang YT, Chang J, Yao YM, Li YN, Zhong XD, Liu ZL. Novel treatment of refractory/recurrent pulmonary hepatoblastoma. *Pediatr Int*. 2020;**62**(3):324–329.

19

Primary neoplasms of the liver
Other neoplasms

Jan Lerut and Quirino Lai

Introduction

Liver tumours arise, in decreasing order of frequency, from epithelial (hepatocytes, cholangiocytes) and mesenchymal (endothelial) cells. Unlike hepatocellular (HCC) and cholangiocellular carcinomas, diagnostic and therapeutic algorithms of other, rare primary neoplasms are far from being standardized.[1,2] This is not only explained by their protean clinical, morphological, and histopathological presentation but also by the limited awareness of the medical community for these 'orphan' diseases (defined as a disease occurring in less than six people per million).[3–9] Not surprisingly, many debates concerning their optimal management are still ongoing. This chapter aims to give, based on data both from recent literature and the European Liver Transplant Registry (ELTR), an up-to-date overview of these particular groups of liver tumours, looking thereby in particular to the possible value of liver transplantation (LT) in the therapeutic algorithm.[10–13] The larger panel of vascular liver tumours will first be discussed, followed by an overview of different types of liver sarcoma.

Vascular liver neoplasms

Vascular tumours were seen for a long time as a continuum going from the most benign lesion, the haemangioma, via the less aggressive hepatic epithelioid haemangioendothelioma (HEHE) to the most aggressive tumour, the hepatic haemangiosarcoma (HHS). Molecular biology recently showed that this concept was incorrect, as the different tumours result from very different mutations. HHS presents HRAS, KRAS, NRAS, and PTPRB mutations; the t(1; 3) (p36; q25) translocation leads to the EHE-specific fusion oncogene *WWTR1–CAMTA1*, and a small group (6%) of HEHE patients bear the *YAP1–TFE3* fusion oncogene.[14,15]

Hepatic epithelioid haemangioendothelioma

The epithelioid haemangioendothelioma (EHE) is a rare vascular tumour with an epithelioid and histiocytoid appearance, originating from vascular endothelial or pre-endothelial cells. EHE represents less than 1% of all vascular tumours. The HEHE is a rare (<1 person per million), low-grade malignancy.[3,16,17] Dail and Liebow first recognized this tumour as a lung tumour; later on, EHE was found in soft tissues, head and neck region, pleura, bones, and many other organs. The first case series, of 32 patients, published in 1984, was expanded by Makhlouf to 137 patients.[16,18] The Haemangioendothelioma, Epithelioid haemangioendothelioma And Related vascular Disorders (HEARD) Support Group internet database showed that EHE is most common in the liver, alone (21%) or combination with lung (18%) lesions, followed by bone alone (14%) and lung alone lesions (12%).[19] Pulmonary and hepatic lesions behave similarly.[17] HEHE is more frequent in middle-aged women (female:male ratio of 4:1) but exceptional in children.[20] Although a causal relationship between chronic *Bartonella* infection and the development of HEHE has been suggested through the induction of vasoproliferation, no definitive aetiological factor has been identified.[21]

The clinical manifestation is highly variable and non-specific, ranging from an asymptomatic status (25% of patients) to (the rare) hepatic failure. Upper abdominal discomfort or pain (60%), weight loss (20%), impaired general condition, due to weakness and fatigue (20%), and dyspnoea (5%) are the most frequent symptoms. Hepatosplenomegaly (30%) is frequent; jaundice, portal hypertension, and Budd–Chiari syndrome caused by tumour compression or venous infiltration are rare (5%). One-third of patients present with cholestasis and cytolysis. Kasabach–Merritt syndrome is exceptional. and serum tumour markers are always normal in the absence of underlying liver disease.

Two typical imaging features linked to tumour progression are seen: initially peripheral, nodular, usually bi-lobar, and subcapsular lesions ('peripheral pattern') are present, later on these lesions ('diffuse pattern') become confluent; eventually, macrovascular invasion and remodelling of the non-tumourous parenchyma appears. Most frequently, larger HEHE lesions present on contrast magnetic resonance imaging (MRI) a late, peripheral, ring arterial enhancement with progressive enhancement towards the centre (targetoid appearance) (**Figure 19.1**).[22] Capsular retraction and focal calcifications (due to central tumour necrosis) can develop. Angiography (if done) reveals a moderate vascularization only with displacement

Vascular liver neoplasms

(60%) contain bilateral multiple or solitary pulmonary nodules (measuring up to 5 cm in 10–20% of cases) or multiple pulmonary reticulonodular opacities; the (less favourable) pleural invasion presents as a diffuse infiltrative thickening. Bone metastases appear as osteolytic lesions.[24,25]

The diagnosis of HEHE is based on a high index of suspicion, integrating the following clinical and radiological findings: the presence of numerous intrahepatic tumours in young, mostly female, adults presenting in a good condition despite (a usually) long-lasting clinical history.[9,10,12] Histopathology, including haematoxylin and eosin and immunohistochemical (IHC) staining completed with molecular biology, will confirm the diagnosis. Cytology may contribute to the right diagnosis, but histology on larger (laparoscopically procured) samples is usually needed to differentiate HEHE from HHS, secondary malignancies and other rare tumours.[9,26,27] Macroscopic examination reveals several fibrous masses with characteristic, necrosis-related, central zoning; microscopic examination shows pleomorphic, medium and large-sized epithelioid cells spreading within sinusoids and small veins but, importantly, preserved portal tract landmarks. Lymph nodes can be negative on haematoxylin and eosin staining, but positive on IHC. Cellular atypia, nuclear fission, the presence of spindle cells, necrotic tumour changes and Ki-67 index greater than 10–15% indicate more aggressive tumours.[17,26,28,29] The observation made in a European cohort that HEHE was more aggressive in paediatric patients was not confirmed in the United Network for Organ Sharing (UNOS) survey.[30] IHC of the vascular endothelial markers, factor VIII-related antigen, Fli-1 (a protein expressed by the endothelium), and CD31, CD34, and ERG (a ETS family transcription factor expressed on endothelial cells) confirms the diagnosis.[14,31] Concordant clinical, radiological, histopathological, cytological, IHC, and molecular biology findings will confirm the diagnosis.

Four findings are important to differentiate HHS from HEHE: the higher incidence in men; the eventual involvement of environmental, toxic factors (see further); the higher aggressivity (frequently linked to a compromised liver function); and the destruction of lobular and portal landmarks on histology.[11,13,26,32]

The treatment algorithm of HEHE is complicated because of its rarity and unpredictable behaviour. The role of surgery has been questioned for a long time due to, some, well-documented 'spontaneous, long-term' (up to 28 years) survivals, the frequent absence of symptoms (25%), the presence of extrahepatic lesions at the moment of diagnosis (45%), the lack of prognostic clinical or histological criteria, the high recurrence rate after surgery (33%) and the lack of detailed long-term outcome reporting.[10,12,17,18,30] The Pittsburgh (USA; 16 patients), Canadian multicentre (11 patients), and UNOS (110 patients) experiences reported 5-year patient (PS) and disease-free survival (DFS) rates after LT ranging from 64% to 82% and 60% to 69%.[30,32,33] The 2006 Mehrabi review (286 patients) favoured partial and total liver resection as the treatment of choice.[34–36] Five-year PS rates after partial resection, LT, chemo-/radiotherapy, and therapeutic abstention were 75%, 55%, 30%, and 4.5%, respectively. Unfortunately, partial resection is only possible in less than 10% of patients harbouring single or few (four or fewer) lesions. The Mayo experience reported a 62% 5-year PS after partial resection in such 11 selected patients.[36]

The value of non-surgical approaches, such as radiotherapy, tumour ablation, transarterial (chemo-)embolization, hormone

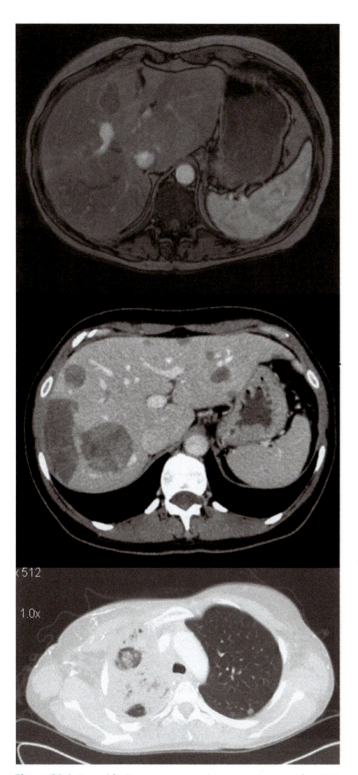

Figure 19.1 Typical findings on computed tomography scan of multiple confluent lesions in both liver lobes. This young female patient also presented with an extensive invasion of the right lung and pleura.

of the intrahepatic vascular tree by the tumour masses; liver biopsy is therefore not per se contraindicated. Thoracic computed tomography scan, scintigraphy, and fluorodeoxyglucose positron emission tomography scanning are necessary to stage the disease.[23] Chest lesions can be pulmonary, pleural, and mediastinal. There are three major different thoracic patterns. The lungs most frequently treatment, systemic or locoregional radiochemotherapy, and antiangiogenic or antitumour pharmacotherapy is still difficult to judge because of the lack of uniformity and, especially, of long-term follow-up. Radiotherapy is useful for local pain control.

The 2007 and 2017 ELTR– European Liver and Intestine Transplant Association (ELITA) HEHE reports, including 149 HEHE patients with a long-term follow-up, modified the outlook of these patients worldwide.[10,12,13] Both publications changed the 'medical awareness' towards these patients, as shown by the steep rise in patients reported to the registry and the high number of (personal) online consults. The ELTR–ELITA studies validated the place of LT as an even curative treatment with 5- and 10-year post-transplant PS rates of 81% and 77% and, most importantly, DFS rates of 79% and 73%, respectively. Pre-LT treatment (28%), lymph node invasion (27%), and limited extrahepatic disease (26.8%) did not significantly influence the outcome in these series, whereas micro- and macrovascular invasion (13% and 48%) did. The Leuven group even reported successful sequential (lung after liver, with 10- and 8-year post-transplant survival despite pleural and diaphragmatic invasion at transplantation) and simultaneous liver–lung transplantation (with 7 and 1 years of post-transplant survival, without signs of disease progression despite bone metastases at the moment of transplantation) in cases of multifocal chest and liver disease.[37] Recurrent disease, observed in and outside the graft in 25% of patients, remains of concern. If it occurs, an aggressive approach is warranted, as prolonged (disease-free) survival can be regained. The value of re-LT remains to be determined.[26] The ELTR–ELITA study clearly confirmed that long-term DFS can also be obtained for multifocal disease; these results should even incite to consider pre-emptive LT in asymptomatic patients.

Development of prognostic scores and efficacious neo- and adjuvant oncological therapies are needed to progress. Lau et al. identified the presence of pulmonary lesions, multiorgan involvement, disease progression, presence of ascites, age 55 years or older, and male sex as poor prognostic factors.[19] After the ELITA–ELTR HEHE study a prognostic score based on macrovascular and hilar lymph node invasion and waiting time was developed. Based on the 5-year DFS rates of 94%, 77%, and 38.5% in case of low (0–2), intermediate (3–5), and high (6–10) scores, respectively, a therapeutic HEHE algorithm has been proposed (**Figure 19.2**).[13] The waiting time on the LT list of some months is a useful 'tool' to differentiate HEHE from HHS as the latter invariably progresses rapidly within some months after diagnosis.

Several drugs have been administered to (small numbers) of EHE, HHS, and liver sarcoma patients aiming at counteracting the angiogenic pathways (bevacizumab, oral tyrosine-kinase inhibitors (sorafenib, sunitinib, pazopanib, and paclitaxel)) or non-VEGF angiogenic pathways (angiopoietin peptibody, PDGFR, and endoglin inhibitors). Other vascular target agents (thalidomide, lenalidomide, interferon, and beta-blockers), chemotherapies (cyclophosphamide, doxorubicin, and carboplatin–etoposide), and beta-blockers have also been tried. As these tumours contain VEGF receptors, treatments based on anti-VEGF antibodies seem logical. The higher content of such receptors and of beta-adrenergic receptors might improve outcome.[38–45] The phase II trials of the French sarcoma group (sorafenib; 15 HEHE patients) and the Eastern Cooperative Oncology Group (bevacizumab; seven HEHE patients) including advanced, non-resectable, metastatic diseases showed a stabilization of the disease up to 10 months in 20–40% and a 6-month partial response in 10% of patients.[46,47]

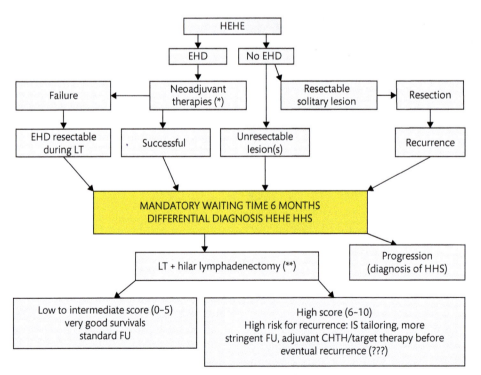

Figure 19.2 Therapeutic algorithm for hepatic epithelioid haemangioendothelioma. (*) non-standardized neo-adjuvant approach; (**) histological examination combining immunohistochemistry and haematoxylin and eosin staining. CHTH, chemotherapy; EHD, extrahepatic disease; FU, follow-up; IS, immunosuppression; HHS, hepatic haemangiosarcoma; LT, liver transplantation.

Better understanding of the biochemical, histological (mitotic index and pleomorphism), and molecular behaviour of this little-understood disease is required to monitor the efficacy of emerging neo- and adjuvant treatments and to identify aggressive tumour subtypes.[34,48,49] The confirmation of the monoclonal nature of all different lesions of a multifocal HEHE in the same patient is important. This allows us to suppose that multifocality and extrahepatic spread are metastatic implants of the same neoplastic clone rather than (as thought for a long time), the synchronous occurrence of multiple different clones. The Leuven group is extending this clonal research to simultaneous hepatic and extrahepatic lesions in order to confirm this hypothesis. If so, (neo-)adjuvant medical treatment will be equally effective for both hepatic and extrahepatic lesions.[50]

Hepatic infantile haemangioendothelioma

Hepatic infantile haemangioendothelioma (HIHE), the most common hepatic tumour in infants (<3 years), is usually diagnosed during the first 6 months of life. HIHE is more frequent in females and presents with (a)symptomatic hepatosplenomegaly, failure to thrive, congestive cardiac failure (15%), due to intra-tumour arteriovenous shunting, and cutaneous haemangiomas (20–40%). It appears as a histologically benign tumour. Histology identifies two types of HIHE: the 'benign' type I and the more pleomorphic type II. Tumours with type II features remain difficult to diagnose and to differentiate from angiosarcoma. Due to their more aggressive morphology and behaviour, they are nowadays considered by many to be childhood HHS.[51] The differentiation between HEHE and (type I) HIHE is important because the latter does not metastasize. Several lesions, present simultaneously in different organs such as the spleen, lungs, and bone, are probably separate lesions. HEHE can be differentiated from HIHE based on different age-related, clinical, and pathological features. The natural history of HIHE is variable; up to two-thirds of symptomatic patients die of complications such as heart failure.[19,34] In several cases, also in the ELTR–ELITA vascular tumour study, HHS foci have been reported. These patients have an extremely poor outcome. Treatment modalities include antiangiogenic drugs (using or combined with high-dose steroids, interferon, chemo- or radiotherapy), interventional radiological, and surgical interventions.[19,52,53] The Boston group developed an algorithm for the treatment of these children.[19] Partial hepatectomy is indicated in case of a solitary lesion or of lesions confined to one liver lobe; LT is required in diffuse lesions and a lack of response to steroid therapy. In case of rapid tumour growth, HHS should be suspected and a futile LT avoided.[54]

Hepatic haemangiosarcoma

HHS is the most common primary liver sarcoma, accounting for up to 2% of all primary liver tumours. It occurs mostly during the sixth and seventh decades of life and is more frequent in males (M:F ratio of 3:1). It is rarely seen in children.[34,55–57] HHS has been linked to many environmental carcinogens such as thorium dioxide, vinyl chloride monomers, radium, pesticides, external radiation, cyclophosphamide, arsenical compounds, use of androgenic/anabolic steroids, and iron, but most cases are sporadic.[9,16,58,59] The delay between toxic exposure and tumour development may be extremely long (up 65 years!).[58,59] The diagnosis can be challenging, even using modern imaging and pathology.[6,32,60–63] Macroscopically, HHS presents as an ill-defined spongy haemorrhagic nodule(s) involving the whole liver. Different growth patterns have been described: multiple nodules and/or a sizeable dominant mass and, more rarely, diffusely infiltrating macro-nodular tumours.[3,16] At diagnosis, 40% of patients already exhibit extrahepatic disease mostly in the lungs, spleen, bones, and adrenal glands. HHS patients are sicker than those with HEHE; they frequently present with signs of portal hypertension and liver failure. Hepatosplenomegaly, thrombocytopenia, pain, jaundice, ascites, peripheral oedema, and acute abdomen, related to the frequent tumour rupture, can also be present.[11,55]

The ELTR–ELITA HHS study, including 20 liver recipients, gave a better insight into the differential diagnosis with HEHE and the non-value of LT in its treatment. All but one patients were symptomatic. Weakness and fatigue (75%), upper abdominal pain and discomfort (60%), anorexia and nausea (50%), hepatomegaly (80%), weight loss (60%), and jaundice and ascites (45%) are the most frequent symptoms and signs. Portal hypertension (25%) and acute liver failure (10%) can be part of the disease presentation. On MRI, progressive, heterogeneous, nodular enhancement towards the centre and haemorrhage are commonly seen.[64] Pathology shows diffuse bi-lobar involvement in nearly all cases. The outcome after partial or total hepatectomy (LT) is very poor. All patients die after a median interval of 6 months due to recurrent disease.[11,55,56,65–84] LT is thus an absolute contraindication for HHS[11,76] (Table 19.1).

The combination of surgery and adjuvant chemotherapy seems to extend survival, reaching 84 months in the exceedingly rare case of a resectable solitary or the multinodular confined form. Encouraging results of chemotherapy have been reported in some cases of multinodular, metastasized HHS.[85] Transarterial embolization is useful in the case of bleeding after tumour rupture.[86] Radiotherapy is not helpful due to the radioresistant character of the tumour.[87] Similar to HEHE, the search for adequate medical therapy, based on the expression of angiogenic growth factor receptors and vascular-targeted agents, are needed to improve the outcome. Some drug combinations and immunotherapy (anti-PD1), occasionally combined with standard chemotherapy, led to a sporadic (partial) response.[55,88,89]

Haemangiopericytoma

Haemangiopericytoma (HPC), an uncommon vascular tumour comprising less than 2% of soft tissue sarcomas, arises from the pericytes of Zimmermann, the small oval cells that surround the capillaries. HPC is usually seen in adults of both sexes as a painless mass. The lower limbs, abdomen, retroperitoneal space, head, neck, and central nervous system are most commonly affected, while liver involvement is rare. They can present as solitary and multiple lesions. HPC presents as a hypervascular, well-circumscribed lesion(s) containing spindle-shaped cells. Half of them are malignant. Large tumour size (>20 cm), more than four mitoses per ten high-power fields, the presence of pleomorphic cells with chromatin pattern, and central necrosis or intratumour haemorrhage indicate malignant transformation. Histology, molecular biology, and IHC allow its differentiation from other sarcomas.[90–92]

The clinical presentation is very variable ranging from an absence of symptoms to paraneoplastic syndromes at diagnosis or at the time of development of metastases. Hypoglycaemia, secondary to the release of the insulin-like growth factors, appears in the later stage of the disease. Although aggressive surgery is the treatment of choice for both primary and metastatic lesions, in two-thirds of patients

Table 19.1 Literature review of liver transplantation for hepatic haemangiosarcoma

First author	Year	Ref.	Country	Article type	Age	N	Donor type	Death	Post-LT FU (mo)	Recurrence
Ringe	1989	65	Germany	Case series	Adult	1	DDLT	Yes	5	Yes
Penn	1991	66	Penn ITTS	Registry	–	14	DDLT	n = 14 (100%)	<27.5	9/14 (64.3%)
Von Schönfeld	1992	67	Germany	Case report	65	1	DDLT	Yes	14	No
Moreno-González	1993	68	Spain	Case series	–	1	LT	Yes	5	Yes
Rojter	1995	69	US	Case series	59	1	DDLT	Yes	6	Yes
Awan	1996	70	UK	Case series	Paediatric	1	DDLT	Yes	4	No
Vennarecci	1997	71	UK	Case series	–	2	DDLT	n = 2	3 and 5	n = 2
Pichlmayr	1997	72	Germany	Case series	Adult	1	DDLT	Yes	0	No
Pimentel Cauduro	2002	73	USA	Case report	70	1	DDLT	Yes	0.5	No
Dimashkieh	2004	74	USA	Case report	5	1	LT	No	14	Yes
Walsh	2004	75	USA	Case report	3 months	1	Split	No	17	No
Maluf	2005	56	USA	Case report	61	1	DDLT	No	12	Yes
			UNOS, USA	Registry	–	7	LT	–	8.7 (mean)	–
Husted	2006	76	Penn ITTS, USA	Registry	53.3 (med) (35–66.8)	6	DDLT	n = 6	5.7 (med) 2.6–15.4	n = 6
Bismuth	2009	77	France	Case report	44	1	DDLT	Yes	30	Yes
Matthaei	2009	78	Germany	Case series	19	2	DDLT	Yes	73	Yes
					51		DDLT	No	141	Yes
Geramizadeh	2011	79	Iran	Case report	Paediatric	7	LDLT	Yes	3	No
Orlando	2013	11	ELTR, Europe	Registry	N = 6 <15 yr 35.3 ± 22.6 yr (med: 41) (range:1–65)	22	DDLT	n = 22	7.2 (med)	n = 17 (77.3%)
Terzi	2014	80	Turkey	Case series	–	2	LT	n = 1 n = 1 Lost FU	18 –	n = 1 n = 1 Lost FU
Xue	2014	81	USA	Case report	5	1		No	27	No
Huerta-Orozco	2015	82	Mexico	Case report	41	1	LDLT	Yes	6	Yes
Pilbeam	2018	83	USA	Case report	2	1	DDLT	No	24	No
Konstantinidis	2018	84	National Cancer Database, USA	Registry	–	24	LT	–	6 (med)	–

DD/LDLT, deceased donor/living donor liver transplantation; FU, follow-up; ITTR, International Transplant Tumor Registry; mo, months; N, number; Ref., reference number.

the lesion recurs even after an R0 resection. The role of chemo- and radiotherapy is uncertain. The detection of recurrence is difficult because of the diversity of the tumour size and the lack of specific markers. Positron emission tomography scanning is very useful for diagnosis and follow-up if the initial tumour had tracer uptake. After R0 resection, 5-year DFS reaches 50%. Long-term follow-up is necessary as 10% of tumours recur after 5 years. Repeated surgery may be useful in case of paraneoplastic syndromes, in particular to counter hypoglycaemia.[92] Four patients were identified in the ELTR–ELITA vascular tumour study, two each had primary or metastatic HPC. One (metastatic) patient had a DFS of 12 years after LT and multiple abdominal, thoracic, and orthopaedic reinterventions.[93] Radio- and chemotherapy have been shown to be unsuccessful. Some partial responses have been obtained using combination therapies such as temozolomide and bevacizumab. Again, as for other soft tissue sarcomas, the search for specific molecular tumour markers will be necessary to improve outlook.[94]

Hepatic small vessel neoplasm

Recently, hepatic small vessel neoplasm (HSVN) has been described as an infiltrative hepatic neoplasm. Despite this infiltrative nature (mimicking HHS) and share of GNAQ and GNA14 mutations (which are also seen in some types of HHS and Kaposiform haemangioendothelioma), HSVN is considered to be a benign or low-grade tumour because of the lack of cellular atypia and increased proliferation.[95,96] The diagnosis needs detailed histological and molecular biology examination. Resection is the best treatment. Given its rarity, infiltrative nature, and insufficient follow-up data, the benign versus the potential, low-grade, malignant nature of this tumour type is questioned.[97]

Conclusion

Vascular tumours represent a diagnostic and therapeutic challenge for clinicians, mainly because of their rarity and their protean clinical, morphological, and histopathological manifestations. The complex and many times difficult differential diagnosis between these tumour types has been refined using immunohistochemistry and molecular biology. Surgery is the mainstay in the therapeutic algorithm. As partial hepatectomy is possible only in a minority of patients due to tumour multifocality, total hepatectomy (or LT) frequently remains the only therapeutic option. In the case of HEHE, pre-emptive or therapeutic LT may result in an excellent 5-year DFS even if the limited extrahepatic disease is present. Conversely, HHS patients have an unfortunate outcome; partial resection is rarely possible and LT is absolutely contraindicated due to the universal, rapid recurrence and short-term survival. LT is also futile in case of rapidly evolving (type II) HIHE. Despite the high recurrence rate, surgery, including LT, can offer a good palliation in HPC especially when a paraneoplastic syndrome is present. For all vascular tumours, effective medical (neo-)adjuvant treatment targeting the 'diseased' vessels is needed to improve outcome.[98]

Sarcomatous hepatocellular carcinoma or carcinosarcoma

Sarcomatous hepatocellular carcinoma (SaHCC), a rare variant of HCC, combines both HCC and spindle cell components.[99] SaHCC is also known as spindle cell carcinoma, sarcomatoid carcinoma, pseudo-sarcoma, and carcinosarcoma.[100] This tumour represents a mosaic of components with distinct histogenesis and carcinogenic pathways. Similar to the vascular neoplasms, SaHCC is very rare, behaviour and natural history are poorly understood and the management remains empirical. The diagnosis of this increasingly seen cancer is difficult as serological tumour markers are normal and typical imaging findings are missing. The sarcomatous component of HCC is probably derived from dedifferentiated anaplastic cells. The frequently present intra- and/or extrahepatic metastases and the aggressive tumour biology explain the dismal prognosis. Response to locoregional treatment (e.g. transarterial chemoembolization) is poor. Early (metastatic) recurrence is the rule after partial resection and LT.[101,102] Similar to mixed hepatocellular–cholangiocellular carcinomas, the prognosis is steered by the most aggressive (thus sarcomatous) tumour component.[101-106] In order to avoid futile LT, percutaneous biopsy should be, despite its poor sensitivity, more frequently used in case of unspecific liver tumour findings.[101,107] The Asan Medical Centre (Seoul, Korea) experience showed that liver biopsy is the only method to make the distinction between sarcomatous and ordinary HCC.[101] Again detailed pathological examination including extensive IHC and molecular biology is the key for making the diagnosis and predicting the outcome. Only seven (six in Eastern countries) SaHCC LT cases have been reported[101,108-110] (Table 19.2). In all, the tumour was seen in adults (age range from 40 to 65 years); four of them had a living donor LT. Early recurrence and extrahepatic metastases were the rule: one patient was disease free at 58 months, five died after 3–27 months, and one was alive at 22 months with recurrent disease.

Conclusion

SaHCC is challenging to diagnose. Clinical awareness and recognition are critical to dictate the treatment strategy which relies on the aggressiveness of the respective tumour components. Because of the poor outcome, LT should not be performed.

Undifferentiated embryonal liver sarcoma

Undifferentiated embryonal liver sarcoma (UELS) is a rare tumour accounting for 9–15% of paediatric liver malignancies.[111] It represents the third most common malignant liver tumour in children, following hepatoblastoma and HCC.[112] The peak incidence is between 6 and 10 years of age, but such a tumour has also been reported in, predominantly female, young adults.[113,114] UELS arises more commonly in the right liver lobe and merely presents as a large (10–30 cm) mass.[115] This mass formation explains the clinical presentation with non-specific symptoms of abdominal pain, (high) fever (due to tumour necrosis), weight loss, nausea, and anorexia (Figure 19.3).[111,113,115] Occasionally, patients present with abdominal pain after trauma leading to an erroneous diagnosis of a haematoma. MRI typically shows cystic and solid components.[116,117] Tumour markers are usually normal. UELS has a mesenchymal origin with sarcomatous features. Histologically, the tumour cells appear variable with spindle-, oval-, and stellate-shaped cells in a myxoid background; mitotic indices are usually high and anisonucleosis with hyperchromasia is often marked.[115] Chromosomal aberrations, such as the common breakpoint at 19q13.4, suggest that UESL may result from a malignant transformation of a mesenchymal hamartoma (precursor lesion).[118]

Historically, the treatment was mainly surgical with limited use of chemo- and radiotherapy. The outcome was very poor with less than 1 year PS linked to a high metastatic recurrence rate.[111] As this tumour is chemosensitive, successful multimodal treatments, combining aggressive adjuvant chemotherapy and R0 resection, were developed.

Table 19.2 Literature review of liver transplantation for sarcomatous hepatocellular cancer

First author	Year	Ref.	Country	Article type	Adult/paediatric	DD/LDLT	N	Death	FU (mo)	Recurrence
Garcez-Silva	2006	108	Brazil	Case report	40	DDLT	1	Yes	5	Yes
Hwang	2008	101	South Korea	Case series	54	LDLT	4	Yes	3	Yes
					59	LDLT		No	58	No
					46	LDLT		Yes	27	Yes
					56	DDLT		No	22	Yes
Kaneko	2010	109	Japan	Case report	53	LDLT	1	Yes	12	Yes
Orlando	2020	110	Belgium	Case report	65	DDLT	1	Yes	7	Yes

DD/LDLT, deceased donor/living donor; FU, follow-up; mo, months; N, number; Ref., reference number.

CHAPTER 19 Primary neoplasms of the liver

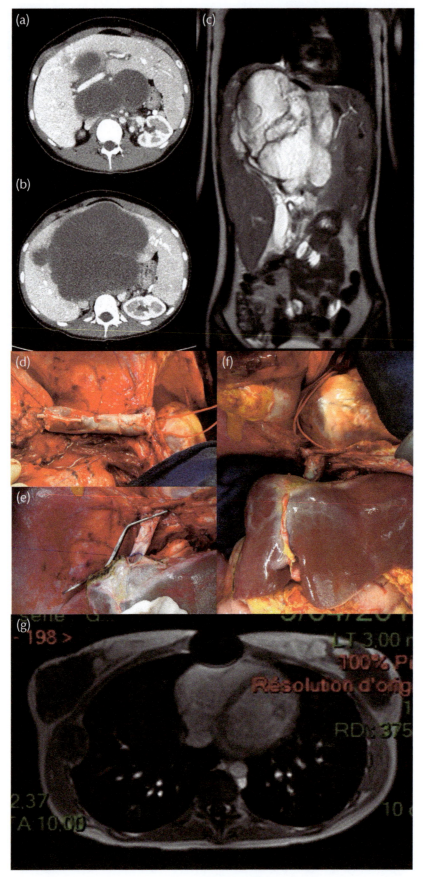

Figure 19.3 (a–c) Computed tomography scan showing a massive central hepatic tumour englobing the hilar structures as well as the inferior vena cava. This young female adult had high-grade fever until the day of LT due to extensive tumour necrosis. (d–f) Living donor LT, with the replacement of the entire inferior vena cava, was done using the small-sized left liver allograft from the patient's mother. The inferior vena cava was replaced with a free iliac vessel graft from a postmortem donor. (g) Thirty months post LT there was development of rib metastasis needing extensive thoracic wall reconstruction. The patient died of disease recurrence 9 months later.

Such a combination not only prolongs survival but also cures some adult patients.[119,120] The role of neoadjuvant chemotherapy is under investigation.[121] When a tumour remains unresectable despite aggressive chemotherapy, LT can be of value. Most LT literature regarding UELS concerns small case series or case reports (Table 19.3).[114, 22–134] The literature survey comprises 19 liver recipients and three US registry-series, including 17, 12, and 10 patients.[131,132,134] Most patients were paediatric; only four patients were aged over 20 years. The recurrence rate in 36 monitored cases was 13.9% (5/36 patients); five out of 31 (16.1%) patients died after a mean follow-up of 37 months (range from 4 to 123). Results of the (largest) US Scientific Registry of Transplant Recipients series (n = 17) are very encouraging with 5- and 10-year PS rates of 67.2%; DFS was 88%.[134]

Conclusion

The combination of both aggressive adjuvant chemotherapy and surgery markedly improves the outlook of UELS patients. The role of neoadjuvant chemotherapy is under evaluation. Surgery is the gold standard whenever it is possible or when the tumour is made resectable after chemotherapy. LT may play a valuable role in case of unresectable tumours after efficacious medical therapy or in case of post-resection recurrence.

Other sarcomas

Reports of LT for other, very uncommon, sarcomas are anecdotal.[134–140] Eighteen cases have been reported: leiomyosarcoma (LMS) (ten patients), biliary embryonal rhabdomyosarcoma (BERS) (seven patients), and Kupffer cell sarcoma (one patient) (Table 19.4).[134–142] All but five (age range 18–68 years) patients were children. Ten patients died after a follow-up of 0.5–141 months and recurrence was reported five times.

Six children and four adults were transplanted because of LMS. Three adults presented a recurrence several years after LT (Table 19.4). The US Scientific Registry of Transplant Recipients data (n = 6) reported only one recurrence in children; satisfactory results were observed with 5- and 10-year PS rates of 62.5%.[134]

BERS is the most common biliary tumour in children. Therapeutic modalities have been well studied by the European, German, and Italian soft tissue sarcoma consortia.[141–143] Results have again been markedly improved (50–85% long-term survival) by combining neoadjuvant radiochemotherapy and radical surgery. Age over 10 years, botryoid histology, large tumour, primary, and R1 surgery are all unfavourable prognostic factors.[142–143] The role of external beam radiotherapy has not been fully proven. In case of complete remission, surgery should be advocated due to a high recurrence rate.[143] Six of seven observed BERS cases were observed in children (Table 19.4). The 5-year PS can now reach 57%.[141–144]

Similar to UELS, the results of BERS treatment have been markedly improved by the combination of R0 surgery and chemotherapy.

Conclusion

LT may gain a place in the treatment of sarcoma patients when adhering to a multimodal treatment scheme. Because only a handful 'other sarcoma' patients have been reported in the transplant literature,

Table 19.3 Literature review of liver transplantation for undifferentiated embryonal liver sarcoma

First author	Year	Ref.	Country	Article type	Adult/paediatric	DD/LDLT	N	Death	FU (mo)	Recurrence
Otte	1996	122	Belgium	Case series	Paediatric	DDLT	2	Yes	<6	Yes
						LDLT		Yes	<6	No
Chen	2006	123	USA	Case series	6	DDLT	2	No	45	No
					7	DDLT		No	29	No
Okajima	2009	124	Japan	Case series	15	LDLT	1	No	18	No
Kelly	2009	125	USA	Case report	9	DDLT	1	No	60	No
Dhanasekaran	2012	126	USA	Case report	54	DDLT	1	No	123	No
Plant	2013	127	USA	Case series	<20 yr	DDLT	1	No	61	Yes
Ismail	2013	128	Poland	Case series	4	DDLT	1	Yes	4	No
Walther	2014	129	USA	Case series	13	DDLT	3	No	24	No
					11	DDLT		No	24	No
					7	DDLT		No	84	No
Schluckebier	2016	130	Switzerland	Case report	10	DDLT	1	No	36	No
Techavichit	2016	131	USA	Case series	22	DDLT	1	No	28	No
			UNOS US	Registry	Paediatric	DDLT	12	n = 1 (8.3%)	–	–
Shi	2017	132	USA	Registry	Paediatric	LT	10	n = 0	>60	–
Khan	2017	114	Pakistan	Case report	21	LT	1	No	18	No
Lerut	2019	133	Belgium	Case	Adult	LDLT and IVC replacement	1	Yes	39	Yes
Vinayak	2017	134	UNOS US	Registry	Paediatric	LT	17	5 yr: 67%	–	2/17
			USA	Case series	3.6 (1–7)	3 DDLT	3	No	>60	No

DD/LDLT, deceased donor/living donor liver transplantation; FU, follow-up; IVC, inferior vena cava; mo, months; N, number; Ref., reference number.

Table 19.4 Literature review of liver transplantation for leiomyosarcoma and biliary embryonal rhabdomyosarcoma

Author	Year	Ref.	Country	Article type	Age	N	DD/LDLT	Death	Post-LT FU (mo)	Recurrence
Calne	1977	135	UK	Case series	Paediatric	Kupffer cell sarcoma	DDLT	–	–	–
Saint-Paul	1993	136	France	Case series	68	LMS	DDLT	Yes	0.5	No
Matthaei	2009	137	Germany	Case series	19	LMS	DDLT	Yes	73	Yes
					51	LMS	DDLT	Yes	141	Yes
Liang	2010	138	China	Case report	44	LMS	DDLT	Yes	34	Yes
Paganelli	2014	139	Canada	Case report	2	BERS	DDLT	No	48	No
Shen	2016	140	China	Case report	10	BERS	DDLT	No	6	No
Perruccio	2017	142	Italy	Case series	Paediatric	BERS: 2	LT	n = 2	2 and 9	n = 1
Vinayak	2017	134	UNOS US	Registry	Paediatric	LMS: 6	LT	5 yr: 63%	–	n = 1
			USA	Case series	Paediatric	BERS	LT	No	60	No
Guerin	2019	141	Europe	Registry	Paediatric	BERS	LT	Yes	Early death	No
Lerut	2020	–	Belgium	Personal communication	18	BERS	LDLT	Yes (suicide)	60	No

DD/LDLT, deceased-donor/living donor liver transplantation; FU, follow-up; mo, months; N, number; Ref., reference number.

conclusions are difficult to draw. Extension of these exceptional experiences is needed to define clearly the role of LT in this setting.

General conclusion

Rare liver neoplasms should gain greater attention in the hepatological, oncological, surgical, and transplantation communities. Their rarity and protean presentations compromise diagnostic and therapeutic algorithms. Multimodal therapies, including LT (a better R0 therapy), will allow the future development of this, largely underrated, part of hepatobiliary and transplant oncology.

REFERENCES

1. Bridgewater J, Galle PR, Khan SA, et al. Guidelines for the diagnosis and management of intrahepatic cholangiocarcinoma. *J Hepatol*. 2014;**60**(6):1268–1289.
2. European Association for the Study of the Liver. EASL Clinical Practice Guidelines: management of hepatocellular carcinoma. *J Hepatol*. 2018;**69**(1):182–236.
3. Ishak K, Goodman Z, Stocker J. *Tumors of the Liver and Intrahepatic Bile Ducts* (Atlas of Tumour Pathology, Third series, fascicle 31). Washington, DC: Armed Forces Institute of Pathology; 1999.
4. Sempoux C, Balabaud C, Paradis V, et al. Hepatocellular nodules in vascular liver diseases. *Virchows Arch*. 2018;**473**(1):33–44.
5. Valla DC, Cazals-Hatem D. Vascular liver diseases on the clinical side: definitions and diagnosis, new concepts. *Virchows Arch*. 2018;**473**(1):3–13.
6. Thampy R, Elsayes KM, Menias CO, et al. Imaging features of rare mesenchymal liver tumours: beyond haemangiomas. *Br J Radiol*. 2017;**90**(1079):20170373.
7. Semelka RC, Nimojan N, Chandana S, et al. MRI features of primary rare malignancies of the liver: a report from four university centres. *Eur Radiol*. 2018;**28**(4):1529–1539.
8. Ehman EC, Torbenson MS, Wells ML, et al. Hepatic tumours of vascular origin: imaging appearances. *Abdom Radiol (NY)*. 2018;**43**(8):1978–1990.
9. Studer LL, Selby DM. Hepatic epithelioid hemangioendothelioma. *Arch Pathol Lab Med*. 2018;**142**(2):263–267.
10. Lerut JP, Orlando G, Adam R, et al. The place of liver transplantation in the treatment of hepatic epithelioid hemangioendothelioma: report of the European liver transplant registry. *Ann Surg*. 2007;**246**(6):949–957.
11. Orlando G, Adam R, Mirza D, et al. Hepatic hemangiosarcoma: an absolute contraindication to liver transplantation—the European Liver Transplant Registry experience. *Transplantation*. 2013;**95**(6):872–877.
12. Lerut JP, Weber M, Orlando G, et al. Vascular and rare liver tumours: a good indication for liver transplantation? *J Hepatol*. 2007;**47**(4):466–475.
13. Lai Q, Feys E, Karam V, et al. Hepatic epithelioid hemangioendothelioma and adult liver transplantation: proposal for a prognostic score based on the analysis of the ELTR-ELITA Registry. *Transplantation*. 2017;**101**(3):555–564.
14. Flucke U, Vogels RJ, de Saint Aubain Somerhausen N, et al. Epithelioid Hemangioendothelioma: clinicopathologic, immunhistochemical, and molecular genetic analysis of 39 cases. *Diagn Pathol*. 2014;**9**:131.
15. Antonescu CR, Le Loarer F, Mosquera JM, et al. Novel YAP1-TFE3 fusion defines a distinct subset of epithelioid hemangioendothelioma. *Genes Chromosomes Cancer*. 2013;**52**(8):775–784.
16. Ishak KG, Sesterhenn IA, Goodman ZD, et al. Epithelioid hemangioendothelioma of the liver: a clinicopathologic and follow-up study of 32 cases. *Hum Pathol*. 1984;**15**(9):839–852.
17. Sardaro A, Bardoscia L, Petruzzelli MF, et al. Epithelioid hemangioendothelioma: an overview and update on a rare vascular tumour. *Oncol Rev*. 2014;**8**(2):259.
18. Makhlouf HR, Ishak KG, Goodman ZD. Epithelioid hemangioendothelioma of the liver: a clinicopathologic study of 137 cases. *Cancer*. 1999;**85**(3):562–582.

19. Lau K, Massad M, Pollak C, et al. Clinical patterns and outcome in epithelioid hemangioendothelioma with or without pulmonary involvement: insights from an internet registry in the study of a rare cancer. *Chest*. 2011;**140**(5):1312–1318.
20. Sharif K, English M, Ramani P, et al. Management of hepatic epithelioid haemangio-endothelioma in children: what option? *Br J Cancer*. 2004;**90**(8):1498–1501.
21. Mascarelli PE, Iredell JR, Maggi RG, et al. Bartonella species bacteremia in two patients with epithelioid hemangioendothelioma. *J Clin Microbiol*. 2011;**49**(11):4006–4012.
22. Lee JH, Jeong WK. Magnetic resonance findings of hepatic epithelioid hemangioendothelioma: emphasis on hepatobiliary phase using Gd-EOB-DTPA. *Abdom Radiol (NY)*. 2017;**42**(9):2261–2271.
23. Nguyen BD. Epithelioid hemangioendothelioma of the liver with F-18 FDG PET imaging. *Clin Nucl Med*. 2004;**29**(12):828–830.
24. Bagan P, Hassan M, Le Pimpec Barthes F, et al. Prognostic factors and surgical indications of pulmonary epithelioid hemangioendothelioma: a review of the literature. *Ann Thorac Surg*. 2006;**82**(6):2010–2013.
25. Duarte Mesquita R, Sousa M, Trinidad C, et al. New insights about pulmonary epithelioid hemangioendothelioma: review of the literature and two case reports. *Case Rep Radiol*. 2017;**2017**:5972940.
26. Demetris AJ, Minervini M, Raikow RB, et al. Hepatic epithelioid hemangioendothelioma: biological questions based on pattern of recurrence in an allograft and tumour immunophenotype. *Am J Surg Pathol*. 1997;**21**(3):263–270.
27. Campione S, Cozzolino I, Mainenti P, et al. Hepatic epithelioid hemangioendothelioma: pitfalls in the diagnosis on fine needle cytology and 'small biopsy' and review of the literature. *Pathol Res Pract*. 2015;**211**(9):702–705.
28. Dong K, Wang XX, Feng JL, et al. Pathological characteristics of liver biopsies in eight patients with hepatic epithelioid hemangioendothelioma. *Int J Clin Exp Pathol*. 2015;**8**(9):11015–11023.
29. Kitaichi M, Nagai S, Nishimura K, et al. Pulmonary epithelioid haemangioendothelioma in 21 patients, including three with partial spontaneous regression. *Eur Respir J*. 1998;**12**(1):89–96.
30. Rodriguez JA, Becker NS, O'Mahony CA, et al. Long-term outcomes following liver transplantation for hepatic hemangioendothelioma: the UNOS experience from 1987 to 2005. *J Gastrointest Surg*. 2008;**12**(1):110–116.
31. Miettinen M, Wang ZF, Paetau A, et al. ERG transcription factor as an immunohistochemical marker for vascular endothelial tumours and prostatic carcinoma. *Am J Surg Pathol*. 2011;**35**(3):432–441.
32. Madariaga JR, Marino IR, Karavias DD, et al. Long-term results after liver transplantation for primary hepatic epithelioid hemangioendothelioma. *Ann Surg Oncol*. 1995;**2**(6):483–487.
33. Nudo CG, Yoshida EM, Bain VG, et al. Liver transplantation for hepatic epithelioid hemangioendothelioma: the Canadian multicentre experience. *Can J Gastroenterol*. 2008;**22**(10):821–824.
34. Mehrabi A, Kashfi A, Fonouni H, et al. Primary malignant hepatic epithelioid hemangioendothelioma: a comprehensive review of the literature with emphasis on the surgical therapy. *Cancer*. 2006;**107**(9):2108–2121.
35. Jung DH, Hwang S, Hong SM, et al. Clinicopathological features and prognosis of hepatic epithelioid hemangioendothelioma after liver resection and transplantation. *Ann Transplant*. 2016;**21**:784–790.
36. Grotz TE, Nagorney D, Donohue J, et al. Hepatic epithelioid haemangioendothelioma: is transplantation the only treatment option? *HPB (Oxford)*. 2010;**12**(8):546–553.
37. Desie N, Van Raemdonck DE, Ceulemans LJ, et al. Combined or serial liver and lung transplantation for epithelioid hemangioendothelioma: a case series. *Am J Transplant*. 2015;**15**(12):3247–3254.
38. Pallotti MC, Nannini M, Agostinelli C, et al. Long-term durable response to lenalidomide in a patient with hepatic epithelioid hemangioendothelioma. *World J Gastroenterol*. 2014;**20**(22):7049–7054.
39. Mascarenhas RC, Sanghvi AN, Friedlander L, et al. Thalidomide inhibits the growth and progression of hepatic epithelioid hemangioendothelioma. *Oncology*. 2004;**67**(5–6):471–475.
40. Soape MP, Verma R, Payne JD, et al. Treatment of hepatic epithelioid hemangioendothelioma: finding uses for thalidomide in a new era of medicine. *Case Rep Gastrointest Med*. 2015;**2015**:326795.
41. Semenisty V, Naroditsky I, Keidar Z, et al. Pazopanib for metastatic pulmonary epithelioid hemangioendothelioma—a suitable treatment option: case report and review of anti-angiogenic treatment options. *BMC Cancer*. 2015;**15**:402.
42. Kelly H, O'Neil BH. Response of epithelioid haemangioendothelioma to liposomal doxorubicin. *Lancet Oncol*. 2005;**6**(10):813–815.
43. Lakkis Z, Kim S, Delabrousse E, et al. Metronomic cyclophosphamide: an alternative treatment for hepatic epithelioid hemangioendothelioma. *J Hepatol*. 2013;**58**(6):1254–1257.
44. Kayler LK, Merion RM, Arenas JD, et al. Epithelioid hemangioendothelioma of the liver disseminated to the peritoneum treated with liver transplantation and interferon alpha-2B. *Transplantation*. 2002;**74**(1):128–130.
45. Stiles JM, Amaya C, Rains S, et al. Targeting of beta adrenergic receptors results in therapeutic efficacy against models of hemangioendothelioma and angiosarcoma. *PLoS One*. 2013;**8**(3):e60021.
46. Chevreau C, Le Cesne A, Ray-Coquard I, et al. Sorafenib in patients with progressive epithelioid hemangioendothelioma: a phase 2 study by the French Sarcoma Group (GSF/GETO). *Cancer*. 2013;**119**(14):2639–2644.
47. Agulnik M, Yarber JL, Okuno SH, et al. An open-label, multicenter, phase II study of bevacizumab for the treatment of angiosarcoma and epithelioid hemangioendotheliomas. *Ann Oncol*. 2013;**24**(1):257–263.
48. Theurillat JP, Vavricka SR, Went P, et al. Morphologic changes and altered gene expression in an epithelioid hemangioendothelioma during a ten-year course of disease. *Pathol Res Pract*. 2003;**199**(3):165–170.
49. Miller MA, Sandler AD. Elevated plasma vascular endothelial growth factor levels in 2 patients with hemangioendothelioma. *J Pediatr Surg*. 2005;**40**(5):e17–e19.
50. Errani C, Sung YS, Zhang L, et al. Monoclonality of multifocal epithelioid hemangioendothelioma of the liver by analysis of WWTR1-CAMTA1 breakpoints. *Cancer Genet*. 2012;**205**(1–2):12–17.
51. Calder CJ, Raafat F, Buckels JAC, et al. Orthotopic liver transplantation for type 2 hepatic infantile haemangioendothelioma. *Histopathology*. 1996;**28**(3):271–273.

52. Daller JA, Bueno J, Gutierrez J, et al. Hepatic hemangioendothelioma: clinical experience and management strategy. *J Pediatr Surg*. 1999;**34**(1):98–105.
53. Selby DM, Stocker JT, Waclawiw MA, et al. Infantile hemangioendothelioma of the liver. *Hepatology*. 1994;**20**(1, Pt 1):39–45.
54. Zhang Z, Chen HJ, Yang WJ, et al. Infantile hepatic hemangioendothelioma: a clinicopathologic study in a Chinese population. *World J Gastroenterol*. 2010;**16**(36):4549–4557.
55. Li DB, Si XY, Wan T, et al. A pooled analysis of treatment and prognosis of hepatic angiosarcoma in adults. *Hepatobiliary Pancreat Dis Int*. 2018;**17**(3):198–203.
56. Maluf D, Cotterell A, Clark B, et al. Hepatic angiosarcoma and liver transplantation: case report and literature review. *Transplant Proc*. 2005;**37**(5):2195–2199.
57. Grassia KL, Peterman CM. Clinical case series of pediatric hepatic angiosarcoma. *Pediatr Blood Cancer*. 2017;**64**(11):11.
58. Coulier B, Pierard F, Gielen I, et al. Hepatic angiosarcoma occurring 65 years after thorium dioxide (Thorotrast) exposure: imaging, surgical and histo-pathologic findings of a historical case. *JBR-BTR*. 2014;**97**(4):254–258.
59. Collins JJ, Jammer B, Sladeczek FM, et al. Surveillance for angiosarcoma of the liver among vinyl chloride workers. *J Occup Environ Med*. 2014;**56**(11):1207–1209.
60. Saleh HA, Tao LC. Hepatic angiosarcoma: aspiration biopsy cytology and immunocytochemical contribution. *Diagn Cytopathol*. 1998;**18**(3):208–211.
61. Kim B, Byun JH, Lee JH, et al. Imaging findings of primary hepatic angiosarcoma on gadoxetate disodium-enhanced liver MRI: comparison with hepatic haemangiomas of similar size. *Clin Radiol*. 2018;**73**(3):244–253.
62. Pickhardt PJ, Kitchin D, Lubner MG, et al. Primary hepatic angiosarcoma: multi-institutional comprehensive cancer centre review of multiphasic CT and MR imaging in 35 patients. *Eur Radiol*. 2015;**25**(2):315–322.
63. Groeschl RT, Miura JT, Oshima K, et al. Does histology predict outcome for malignant vascular tumours of the liver? *J Surg Oncol*. 2014;**109**(5):483–486.
64. Semelka RC, Nimojan N, Chandana S, et al. MRI features of primary rare malignancies of the liver: a report from four university centres. *Eur Radiol*. 2018;**28**(4):1529–1539.
65. Ringe B, Wittekind C, Bechstein WO, et al. The role of liver transplantation in hepatobiliary malignancy. A retrospective analysis of 95 patients with particular regard to tumour stage and recurrence. *Ann Surg*. 1989;**209**(1):88–98.
66. Penn I. Hepatic transplantation for primary and metastatic cancers of the liver. *Surgery*. 1991;**110**(4):726–734.
67. von Schönfeld J, Erhard J, Donhuijsen K, Breuer N. Hemangiosarcoma of the liver. The diagnostic difficulties and therapeutic possibilities. *Dtsch Med Wochenschr*. 1992;**117**(6):211–215.
68. Moreno-González E, Loinaz C, Gómez R, et al. Orthotopic liver transplantation in primary liver tumours. *J Surg Oncol Suppl*. 1993;**3**:74–77.
69. Rojter S, Villamil FG, Petrovic LM, et al. Malignant vascular tumours of the liver presenting as liver failure and portal hypertension. *Liver Transpl Surg*. 1995;**1**(3):156–161.
70. Awan S, Davenport M, Portmann B, Howard ER. Angiosarcoma of the liver in children. *J Pediatr Surg*. 1996;**31**(12):1729–1732.
71. Vennarecci G, Ismail T, Gunson B, McMaster P. Primary angiosarcoma of the liver. *Minerva Chir*. 1997;**52**(10):1141–1146.
72. Pichlmayr R, Weimann A, Tusch G, Schlitt HJ. Indications and role of liver transplantation for malignant tumours. *Oncologist*. 1997;**2**(3):164–170.
73. Pimentel Cauduro SK, Petrovic LM, Sodeman TC, et al. Unsuspected primary hepatic angiosarcoma associated with portal vein thrombosis complicating cirrhosis. *Liver Transpl*. 2002;**8**(11):1080–1081.
74. Dimashkieh HH, Mo JQ, Wyatt-Ashmead J, Collins MH. Pediatric hepatic angiosarcoma: case report and review of the literature. *Pediatr Dev Pathol*. 2004;**7**(5):527–532.
75. Walsh R, Harrington J, Beneck D, Ozkaynak MF. Congenital infantile hepatic hemangioendothelioma type II treated with orthotopic liver transplantation. *J Pediatr Hematol Oncol*. 2004;**26**(2):121–123.
76. Husted TL, Neff G, Thomas MJ, et al. Liver transplantation for primary or metastatic sarcoma to the liver. *Am J Transplant*. 2006;**6**(2):392–397.
77. Bismuth B, Castel H, Boleslawski E, et al. Primary sarcoma of the liver and transplantation: a case study and literature review. *Rare Tumours*. 2009;**1**(2):e31.
78. Matthaei H, Krieg A, Schmelzle M, et al. Long-term survival after surgery for primary hepatic sarcoma in adults. *Arch Surg*. 2009;**144**(4):339–344.
79. Geramizadeh B, Safari A, Bahador A, et al. Hepatic angiosarcoma of childhood: a case report and review of literature. *J Pediatr Surg* 2011;**46**(1):e9–e11.
80. Terzi A, Deniz EE, Haberal N, et al. Hepatic angiosarcoma and liver transplant: a report of 2 cases with diagnostic difficulties. *Exp Clin Transplant*. 2014;**12**(Suppl 1):126–128.
81. Xue M, Masand P, Thompson P, et al. Angiosarcoma successfully treated with liver transplantation and sirolimus. *Pediatr Transplant*. 2014;**18**(4):E114–E119.
82. Huerta-Orozco LD, Leonher-Ruezga KL, Ramírez-González LR, et al. Hepatic angiosarcoma and liver transplantation: case report and literature review. *Cir Cir*. 2015;**83**(6):510–515.
83. Pilbeam K, Eidenschink B, Sulciner M, et al. Success of chemotherapy and a liver transplant in a pediatric patient with hepatic angiosarcoma: a case report. *Pediatr Transplant*. 2019;**23**(4):e13410.
84. Konstantinidis IT, Nota C, Jutric Z, et al. Primary liver sarcomas in the modern era: resection or transplantation? *J Surg Oncol*. 2018;**117**(5):886–891.
85. Huang NC, Kuo YC, Chiang JC, et al. Hepatic angiosarcoma may have fair survival nowadays. *Medicine (Baltimore)*. 2015;**94**(19):e816.
86. Pierce DB, Johnson GE, Monroe E, et al. Safety and efficacy outcomes of embolization in hepatic sarcomas. *AJR Am J Roentgenol*. 2018;**210**(1):175–182.
87. Zhu YP, Chen YM, Matro E, et al. Primary hepatic angiosarcoma: a report of two cases and literature review. *World J Gastroenterol*. 2015;**21**(19):6088–6096.
88. Young RJ, Woll PJ. Anti-angiogenic therapies for the treatment of angiosarcoma: a clinical update. *Memo*. 2017;**10**(4):190–193.
89. Sindhu S, Gimber LH, Cranmer L, et al. Angiosarcoma treated successfully with anti-PD-1 therapy—a case report. *J Immunother Cancer*. 2017;**5**(1):58.
90. McMaster MJ, Soule EH, Ivins JC. Hemangiopericytoma. A clinicopathologic study and long-term followup of 60 patients. *Cancer*. 1975;**36**(6):2232–2244.
91. Enzinger FM, Smith BH. Hemangiopericytoma. An analysis of 106 cases. *Hum Pathol*. 1976;**7**(1):61–82.

92. Flores-Stadler EM, Chou P, Walterhouse D, et al. Hemangiopericytoma of the liver: immunohistochemical observations, expression of angiogenic factors, and review of the literature. *J Pediatr Hematol Oncol*. 1997;**19**(5):449–454.
93. Adams J, Lodge JP, Parker D. Liver transplantation for metastatic hemangiopericytoma associated with hypoglycemia. *Transplantation*. 1999;**67**(3):488–489.
94. Park MS, Patel SR, Ludwig JA, et al. Activity of temozolomide and bevacizumab in the treatment of locally advanced, recurrent, and metastatic hemangiopericytoma and malignant solitary fibrous tumor. *Cancer*. 2011;**117**(21):4939–4947.
95. Gill RM, Buelow B, Mather C, et al. Hepatic small vessel neoplasm, a rare infiltrative vascular neoplasm of uncertain malignant potential. *Hum Pathol*. 2016;**54**:143–151.
96. Joseph NM, Brunt EM, Marginean C, et al. Frequent GNAQ and GNA14 mutations in hepatic small vessel neoplasm. *Am J Surg Pathol*. 2018;**42**(9):1201–1207.
97. Walcott-Sapp S, Tang E, Kakar S, et al. Resection of the largest reported hepatic small vessel neoplasm. *Hum Pathol*. 2018;**78**:159–162.
98. Lazăr DC, Avram MF, Romoșan I, et al. Malignant hepatic vascular tumors in adults: characteristics, diagnostic difficulties and current management. *World J Clin Oncol*. 2019;**10**(3):110–135.
99. Ishak KG. Mesenchymal tumour of the liver. In: Okuda K, Peters RL, eds. *Hepatocellular carcinoma*. New York: John Wiley & Sons; 1976: 247–308.
100. Li DB, Si XY, Wan T, Zhou YM. A pooled analysis of treatment and prognosis of hepatic angiosarcoma in adults. *Hepatobiliary Pancreat Dis Int*. 2018;**17**(3):198–2036.
101. Hwang S, Lee SG, Lee YJ, et al. Prognostic impact of sarcomatous change of hepatocellular carcinoma in patients undergoing liver resection and liver transplantation. *J Gastrointest Surg*. 2008;**12**(4):718–724.
102. Nishi H, Taguchi K, Asayama Y, et al. Sarcomatous hepatocellular carcinoma: a special reference to ordinary hepatocellular carcinoma. *J Gastroenterol Hepatol*. 2003;**18**(4):415–423.
103. Kaneko J, Sugawara Y, Togashi J, et al. Sarcomatous change of hepatocellular carcinoma in a patient undergoing living donor liver transplantation. *Biosci Trends*. 2010;**4**(5):279–282.
104. Pichlmayr R, Weimann A, Tusch G, Schlitt HJ. Indications and role of liver transplantation for malignant tumours. *Oncologist*. 1997;**2**(3):164–170.
105. Sapisochin G, Fidelman N, Roberts JP, Yao FY. Mixed hepatocellular cholangiocarcinoma and intrahepatic cholangiocarcinoma in patients undergoing transplantation for hepatocellular carcinoma. *Liver Transpl*. 2011;**17**(8):934–942.
106. Park SE, Lee SH, Yang JD, et al. Clinicopathological characteristics and prognostic factors in combined hepatocellular carcinoma and cholangiocarcinoma. *Korean J Hepatobiliary Pancreat Surg*. 2013;**17**(4):152–156.
107. Bruix J, Sherman M. Management of hepatocellular carcinoma: an update. *Hepatology*. 2011;**53**(3):1020–1022.
108. Garcez-Silva MH, Gonzalez AM, Moura RA, Linhares MM, Lanzoni VP, Trivino T. Carcinosarcoma of the liver: a case report. *Transplant Proc*. 2006;**38**(6):1918–1919.
109. Kaneko J, Sugawara Y, Togashi J, et al. Sarcomatous change of hepatocellular carcinoma in a patient undergoing living donor liver transplantation. *Biosci Trends*. 2010;**4**(5):279–282.
110. Orlando G, Lai Q, Lerut J. Composite hepatocellular and hemangiosarcomatous tumour: the prognosis is determined by the sarcomatous component. *Hepatobiliary Pancreat Dis Int*. 2020;**19**(2):184–186.
111. Stocker JT, Ishak KG. Undifferentiated (embryonal) sarcoma of the liver: report of 31 cases. *Cancer*. 1978;**42**(1):336–348.
112. Weinberg AG, Finegold MJ. Primary hepatic tumours of childhood. *Hum Pathol*. 1983;**14**(6):512–537.
113. Webber EM, Morrison KB, Pritchard SL, Sorensen PH. Undifferentiated embryonal sarcoma of the liver: results of clinical management in one center. *J Pediatr Surg*. 1999;**34**(11):1641–1644.
114. Khan ZH, Ilyas K, Khan HH, et al. Unresectable undifferentiated embryonal sarcoma of the liver in an adult male treated with chemotherapy and orthotopic liver transplantation. *Cureus*. 2017;**9**(10):e1759.
115. Wei ZG, Tang LF, Chen ZM, Tang HF, Li MJ. Childhood undifferentiated embryonal liver sarcoma: clinical features and immunohistochemistry analysis. *J Pediatr Surg*. 2008;**43**(10):1912–1919.
116. Joshi SW, Merchant NH, Jambhekar NA. Primary multilocular cystic undifferentiated (embryonal) sarcoma of the liver in childhood resembling hydatid cyst of the liver. *Br J Radiol*. 1997;**70**:314–316.
117. Buetow PC, Buck JL, Pantongrag-Brown L, et al. Undifferentiated (embryonal) sarcoma of the liver: pathologic basis of imaging findings in 28 cases. *Radiology*. 1997;**203**(3):779–783.
118. Shehata BM, Gupta NA, Katzenstein HM, et al. Undifferentiated embryonal sarcoma of the liver is associated with mesenchymal hamartoma and multiple chromosomal abnormalities: a review of eleven cases. *Pediatr Dev Pathol*. 2011;**14**(2):111–116.
119. Weitz J, Klimstra DS, Cymes K, et al. Management of primary liver sarcomas. *Cancer* 2007;**109**(7):1391–1396.
120. Kim D-Y, Kim K-H, Jung S-E, Lee S-C, Park K-W, Kim W-K. Undifferentiated (embryonal) sarcoma of the liver: combination treatment by surgery and chemotherapy. *J Pediatr Surg*. 2002;**37**(10):1419–1423.
121. Lenze F, Birkfellner T, Lenz P, et al. Undifferentiated embryonal sarcoma of the liver in adults. *Cancer*. 2008;**112**(10):2274–2282.
122. Otte JB, Aronson D, Vraux H, et al. Preoperative chemotherapy, major liver resection, and transplantation for primary malignancies in children. *Transplant Proc*. 1996;**28**(4):2393–2394.
123. Chen LE, Shepherd RW, Nadler ML, Chapman WC, Kotru A, Lowell JA. Liver transplantation and chemotherapy in children with unresectable primary hepatic malignancies: development of a management algorithm. *J Pediatr Gastroenterol Nutr*. 2006;**43**(4):487–493.
124. Okajima H, Ohya Y, Lee KJ, et al. Management of undifferentiated sarcoma of the liver including living donor liver transplantation as a backup procedure. *J Pediatr Surg*. 2009;**44**(2):e33–e38.
125. Kelly MJ, Martin L, Alonso M, Altura RA. Liver transplant for relapsed undifferentiated embryonal sarcoma in a young child. *J Pediatr Surg*. 2009;**44**(12):e1–e3.
126. Dhanasekaran R, Hemming A, Salazar E, Cabrera R. Rare case of adult undifferentiated (embryonal) sarcoma of the liver treated with liver transplantation: excellent long-term survival. *Case Reports Hepatol*. 2012;**2012**:519741.
127. Plant AS, Busuttil RW, Rana A, Nelson SD, Auerbach M, Federman NC. A single-institution retrospective cases series of childhood undifferentiated embryonal liver sarcoma (UELS): success of combined therapy and the use of orthotopic liver transplant. *J Pediatr Hematol Oncol*. 2013;**35**(6):451–455.

128. Ismail H, Dembowska-Bagińska B, Broniszczak D, et al. Treatment of undifferentiated embryonal sarcoma of the liver in children—single center experience. *J Pediatr Surg*. 2013;**48**(11):2202–2206.
129. Walther A, Geller J, Coots A, et al. Multimodal therapy including liver transplantation for hepatic undifferentiated embryonal sarcoma. *Liver Transpl*. 2014;**20**(2):191–199.
130. Schluckebier D, McLin VA, Kanavaki I, Ansari M, Wildhaber BE. The role of liver transplantation in undifferentiated embryonal sarcoma of the liver in children. *J Pediatr Hematol Oncol*. 2016;**38**(6):495–496.
131. Techavichit P, Masand PM, Himes RW, et al. Undifferentiated embryonal sarcoma of the liver (UESL): a single-center experience and review of the literature. *J Pediatr Hematol Oncol*. 2016;**38**(4):261–268.
132. Shi Y, Rojas Y, Zhang W, et al. Characteristics and outcomes in children with undifferentiated embryonal sarcoma of the liver: a report from the National Cancer Database. *Pediatr Blood Cancer*. 2017;**64**(4):e26272.
133. Lerut J, Iesari S, Inostroza Núñez ME, et al. Adult-to-adult living-donor liver transplantation: the experience of the Université catholique de Louvain. *Hepatobiliary Pancreat Dis Int*. 2019;**18**(2):132–142.
134. Vinayak R, Cruz RJ Jr., Ranganathan S, et al. Pediatric liver transplantation for hepatocellular cancer and rare liver malignancies: US multicenter and single-center experience (1981–2015). *Liver Transpl*. 2017;**23**(12):1577–1588.
135. Calne RY, Williams R. Orthotopic liver transplantation: the first 60 patients. *Br Med J*. 1977;**1**(6059):471–476.
136. Saint-Paul MC, Gugenheim J, Hofman P, et al. [Leiomyosarcoma of the liver: a case treated by transplantation]. *Gastroenterol Clin Biol*. 1993;**17**(3):218–222.
137. Matthaei H, Krieg A, Schmelzle M, et al. Long-term survival after surgery for primary hepatic sarcoma in adults. *Arch Surg*. 2009;**144**(4):339–344.
138. Liang X, Xiao-Min S, Jiang-Ping X, et al. Liver transplantation for primary hepatic leiomyosarcoma: a case report and review of the literatures. *Med Oncol*. 2010;**27**(4):1269–1272.
139. Paganelli M, Beaunoyer M, Samson Y, et al. A child with unresectable biliary rhabdomyosarcoma: 48-month disease-free survival after liver transplantation. *Pediatr Transplant*. 2014;**18**(5):E146–E151.
140. Shen CH, Dong KR, Tao YF, et al. Liver transplantation for biliary rhabdomyosarcoma with liver metastasis: report of one case. *Transplant Proc*. 2017;**49**(1):185–187.
141. Guérin F, Minard-Colin TRV, Gaze MN, et al. Outcome of localized liver-bile duct rhabdomyosarcoma according to local therapy: a report from the European Paediatric Soft-Tissue Sarcoma Study Group (EpSSG)-RMS 2005 study. *Pediatr Blood Cancer*. 2019;**66**(7):e27725.
142. Perruccio K, Cecinati V, Scagnellato A, et al. Biliary tract rhabdomyosarcoma: a report from the Soft Tissue Sarcoma Committee of the Associazione Italiana Ematologia Oncologia Pediatrica. *Tumori*. 2018;**104**(3):232–237.
143. Urla C, Warmann SW, Sparber-Sauer M, et al. Treatment and outcome of the patients with rhabdomyosarcoma of the biliary tree: experience of the Cooperative Weichteilsarkom Studiengruppe (CWS). *BMC Cancer*. 2019;**19**(1):945.
144. Vaarwerk B, van der Lee JH, Breunis WB, et al. Prognostic relevance of early radiologic response to induction chemotherapy in pediatric rhabdomyosarcoma: a report from the International Society of Pediatric Oncology Malignant Mesenchymal Tumor 95 Study. *Cancer*. 2018;**124**(4):1016–1024.

20 Secondary neoplasms of the liver

Pål-Dag Line

Introduction

Secondary liver tumours are, as the name implies, tumours of non-hepatic origin due to metastatic spread from a primary tumour elsewhere. The liver is a frequent site of metastatic disease, and the extent of liver involvement and whether surgical removal is possible is usually decisive for the survival outcome of the patient. Some liver metastases are, however, due to the biological properties, stage, or aggressiveness of the primary tumour, not subjected to surgical therapy as the standard of care. Therefore, knowledge of the most important types of secondary liver tumours and therapeutic options are important. The following chapter provides an overview of the management of the most frequent secondary liver tumours with an emphasis on those that benefit from surgical therapy.

Aetiology and pathogenesis

Metastasis is a multistage process by which malignant cells detach from the primary tumour, invade vascular or lymphatic structures, and thereby migrate to a different tissue or organ. There are two main hypotheses explaining metastasis. The *seed and soil* hypothesis was introduced by Stephen Paget in 1889.[1] Klikk eller trykk her for å skrive inn tekst. He noted that in many cases the spread of malignant cells to certain organs could not be explained by anatomical topographical factors like blood supply alone and found an increased incidence of liver metastases in patients with advanced breast cancer. Against this background it was suggested the cancer cells behave analogously to seeds and the tissue of metastatic invasion acts as a fertile soil, implying that in order for metastasis to occur, crosstalk between cancer cells and the microenvironment of the organ is needed. The main features of this theory have been confirmed by recent studies, demonstrating that tissue-specific factors are essential for circulating tumour cells to successfully invade the organ and form metastatic lesions.

The mechanical hypothesis for metastasis relies on the fact that, for a range of tumour types, there is a clear relationship between the anatomical venous drainage territory and metastatic location.[2] The most typical phenomenon supporting this hypothesis is the high frequency of liver metastasis in cancers affecting the gastrointestinal system with venous drainage through the portal vein, thereby making the liver being the first microvascular bed that the circulating tumour cells encounter after entering the blood stream. In clinical reality, both mechanisms are at play, dependent on the primary tumour type. Finding circulating tumour cells is, however, not synonymous with established metastatic disease, as the majority of tumour cells entering the bloodstream are most likely to be eliminated. Essential for the formation of a metastatic lesion is the ability of the tumour cells to invade the host tissue through the vessel wall, establish a blood supply through angiogenesis, and evade the local immune response directed towards the malignant cells. Therefore, distinct molecular features of the particular cancer cell phenotype as well as host factors like adhesion molecules of the vascular endothelium and pro-tumorigenic phenotype of the immune cells in the microenvironment are important.

Epidemiology

Liver metastases are the most frequent types of malignant liver tumours, outnumbering primary liver cancers like hepatocellular carcinoma and cholangiocarcinoma by far. Assessment of the distribution of liver metastases with respect to the corresponding primary tumour type can be done on the basis of large-scale biopsy investigations. In a study published by de Ridder and co-workers from The Netherlands, histological data on 23,154 patients were analysed.[3] Carcinomas were found in 92% of the lesions, melanomas in 2.4%, and sarcomas in 1%. Adenocarcinoma was the most frequent carcinoma subtype followed by small cell carcinoma in 5.9%, neuroendocrine carcinoma in 4.6%, large cell carcinoma in 3.7%, and squamous cell carcinoma in 1.4%. Adenocarcinomas were typically originating from the gastrointestinal tract, most frequently from colorectal primaries. Small cell carcinoma was mostly associated with pulmonary primaries. Large cell carcinomas originated from the lung, gastrointestinal tract, and urological tract. Squamous histology was mainly from the lungs, oesophagus, and head and neck tumours.

Clinical features

The clinical picture is partly dependent on whether the patient has a primary tumour intact (synchronous liver metastasis) or whether the metastatic process occurs after the primary tumour has been removed. The term metachronous usually refers to liver metastases occurring 12 months or more after diagnosis of the primary. In synchronous disease, the clinical picture is often dominated by that of the primary tumour. Secondary liver tumours are by themselves often asymptomatic as long as the tumour load is moderate, consequently, delayed diagnosis is common. In tumours where the topographic location within the liver causes obstruction of the main biliary or vascular structures, corresponding clinical signs and symptoms like jaundice or vascular thrombosis may develop. When the hepatic tumour load is extensive, hepatomegaly and associated pain or discomfort can be a clinical sign and is often linked to advanced stages of disease where many of the patients might display general cancer-related symptoms like weight loss, general malaise, and loss of appetite.

Clinical investigations

A range of tumour markers are available for some of the secondary liver tumours in question. Since most patients have a known primary, the diagnosis itself is usually not the main clinical challenge. Radiological imaging is, however, imperative in the diagnostic evaluation of patients with secondary liver tumours and is also utilized to monitor treatment response. A distinct clinicopathological feature of malignant liver tumours is that the blood supply, unlike normal liver tissue, predominantly is derived from the hepatic artery, with very little portal vein perfusion. Hence, by timing contrast medium injection and image acquisition to record arterial as well as venous perfusion phases, the nature and dynamic changes of the vascular supply to liver lesions can be elucidated. Malignant liver tumours will, as a rule, display contrast enhancement through the arterial phase and a characteristic washout during the portovenous phase. Computed tomography (CT) scanning with intravenous contrast is usually the first choice of imaging in patients with secondary liver tumours. Image acquisition is done pre-infusion, during the arterial phase, and the portal venous phase and multiphase CT is a sensitive method for the detection of liver tumours as well as providing a useful anatomical mapping of where the lesions are located within the liver. The latter has clear consequences for possible surgical therapy. Furthermore, volumetric assessments of the liver with calculation of future liver remnant (FLR) volume can be performed relatively easily, which is essential for surgical planning. If the phasic contrast pattern of detected lesions for some reason appears atypical and a morphological diagnosis cannot be made, adding another different modality of imaging is recommended. Ultrasound scanning is largely used as a screening modality of the liver, but with added ultrasound-specific contrast medium it can be a useful diagnostic adjunct in this context. Intraoperative ultrasound has an important role in ensuring the detection of all metastatic lesions. As with all ultrasound investigations the results are, however, operator dependent. Magnetic resonance imaging (MRI) is particularly useful in fine tuning the diagnostic precision when needed. MRI is more sensitive than CT for detecting small metastatic lesions and may be particularly useful in distinguishing these from small benign lesions like cysts or haemangiomas.[4] Altered diffusion properties on MRI scanning provides unique features to distinguish tumours from benign lesions. In differential diagnosis against other tumour types, gadolinium-derived, liver-specific contrast medium offers a valuable diagnostic extension. In about 4%, the primary tumour type is not known, and an ultrasound-guided biopsy of the lesion is indicated. Various detailed immunohistochemical and/or genetic analyses might be required and, in a minority, the origin of the metastatic disease remains undetermined.

Positron emission tomography (PET) with the relevant tracer (^{18}F-fluorodeoxyglucose for most non-neuroendocrine cancers, octreotide, or ^{68}Ga-/^{64}Cu-DOTATATE-PET for neuroendocrine tumours (NETs)) are usually combined with CT and MRI. PET examination can be particularly useful in staging since it often can detect extrahepatic disease and also provide a functional measure related to metabolic activity in the malignant tissue.

Treatment: general principles

The treatment for secondary liver tumours relies on the exact tumour type and stage of the disease. The outcome will be dependent on whether or not resection of all sites of disease can be realistically performed. In general, the treatment principle for patients with secondary liver tumours is usually a combination of systemic therapy, surgery, ablation, or embolization, and these items may be combined to obtain maximal efficacy. Hence, all patients need to be evaluated by an experienced multidisciplinary team consisting of hepatobiliary surgeons, oncologists, pathologists, and radiologists. The specific choice of strategy is dependent on the type of primary tumour, disease stage, anatomical location of the metastases, and total hepatic tumour load. Some primary tumours, like pancreatic adenocarcinoma, are associated with a dire prognosis even without distant metastasis, and surgical resection of liver metastases from pancreatic adenocarcinoma is usually not recommended due to its doubtful benefit and short expected overall survival.

The criteria for resectability of liver metastases have undergone major development during the last few decades. Currently most liver surgeons consider a lesion resectable when the operation may result in total removal of all the metastatic lesions (R0 resection) and obtain an FLR with adequate functional volume, preserved vascular inflow and outflow, as well as biliary drainage. In many cases, the surgical options are restricted by a small FLR. The tolerable FLR volume may be as low as 25% in completely healthy liver parenchyma, but the safe threshold is considerably higher and approaches 40% in patients who have received extensive chemotherapy or have pre-existing liver disease.[5,6] Through the years, various methods to increase the FLR, and thereby resectability, have been introduced. Portal vein ligation or embolization will induce volume growth of the contralateral hemiliver over the course of 4–6 weeks. This technique may also be combined with two-stage hepatectomy during the first operation, thereby augmenting liver regeneration between the two procedures.[7] Two-stage hepatectomy with portal vein embolization/portal vein ligation is a safe procedure, but unfortunately, about 20% of the patients do not proceed to stage two, either due to insufficient FLR volume growth, or progressive disease in the interval.[8] Another, somewhat debated method in patients with small FLR is the so-called associating liver partition and portal vein ligation for staged hepatectomy (ALPPS).[9] This is also a two-staged procedure where the liver parenchyma is either partially or totally transected in the intended resection plane during the first stage without dividing any vascular or biliary structures, and the portal vein blood flow is redirected to the FLR through portal vein ligation or embolization. The liver is then left to regenerate, and volume growth checked by volumetry. When a sufficient FLR size is obtained, the second-stage hepatectomy is performed. Initially, the ALPPS procedure was associated with significant increments in procedure-related morbidity and mortality, but as the worldwide experience has increased and high-volume centres have gained experience, acceptable mortality and morbidity figures have been documented for the ALPPS procedure. The main advantages offered in ALPPS compared with portal vein embolization is more rapid and larger volume growth, and recent studies may indicate that this increases the resectability rate.[10] One problem in ALPPS is, however, that the rapid growth in volume is not necessarily accompanied by a corresponding equivalent increase in hepatic function. Thus, a too-short interstage interval in ALPPS increases the risk of postoperative liver failure following stage 2.[11,12] One way to assess hepatic function in this context is hepatobiliary scintigraphy with technetium-99m-labelled mebrofenin.[13]

Local ablation by radiofrequency or microwave can also be used to treat secondary liver lesions, and may play a role in a few small lesions, as an adjunct to surgery in patients with many metastases, or as an alternative in patients unfit for liver resection. The method is, however, restricted by a lesion diameter up to about 30 mm due to the fact that the delivered energy has a limited range. Larger blood vessels act as heat conduits and major biliary structures or neighbouring organs may further limit applicability.

Colorectal liver metastases

Colorectal cancer is the third most common cancer worldwide, and during the last three decades there has been a significant increase in its incidence, particularly in the younger age groups.[14,15] Metastases from colorectal cancer are the most common secondary liver tumours. About 50% of patients with colorectal cancer will develop liver metastases, either as synchronous or metachronous disease. Despite progress made in surgical technique, imaging technology, and systemic chemotherapy, only about 20–25% of the patients with Colorectal liver metastases (CRLMs) ultimately have resectable lesions. A range of factors are closely related to post-resection survival outcomes. Total tumour load in the liver, given as the number of lesions and diameter of the largest tumour, is significantly related to recurrence of disease and postoperative survival.[16] Elevated levels of carcinoembryonic antigen to greater than 200 ng/L are associated with more aggressive tumour biology. Right-sided primary tumours in general have a worse prognosis than left-sided and rectal tumours.[17] Mutation of the *BRAF* proto-oncogene, mucinous or signet ring cell differentiation, and undifferentiated histology are all negative prognostic factors associated with a worse outcome, and all these factors are more frequent in proximal colonic tumours. *KRAS* mutant status eliminates the use of epidermal growth factor inhibitor (cetuximab) therapy and is in itself associated with an increased risk of recurrence after liver resection. It is recommended to give all patients who can tolerate this chemotherapy prior to surgery, even though they seem resectable. A clear response to chemotherapy is a significant positive prognostic factor, and conversely, progression on chemotherapy is usually associated with a worse outcome. Recurrence after liver resection is common and occurs in around 50-70% of cases, and about half of them are located in the liver.[18] The results after repeat resections are reasonable in patients who do not have factors for aggressive tumour biology as outlined above.[19] In cases, with extensive disease burden in the liver that prohibits resection, patients may be downstaged through preoperative chemotherapy. Neoadjuvant chemotherapy may be beneficial in most patients. Effective regimens include 5-fluorouracil/leucovorin, capecitabine, oxaliplatin, and irinotecan. Antibody treatment with bevacizumab (antivascular endothelial growth factor antibody) and anti-epidermal growth factor antibodies (cetuximab, panitumumab) are also important additives, and may have a particular role in downstaging of patients. Locoregional therapies like ablation, chemoembolization, radioembolization, and arterial infusion therapy are widely used, but their place in standard potential curative care remains to be established.

Patients with non-resectable CRLM only have the option of palliative chemotherapy as standard of care. Despite recent advances in the development of chemotherapy and targeted agents, the expected 5-year overall survival for this palliative cohort is about 10%.[20] A range of scoring systems based on clinical factors exists for predicting recurrence and survival after liver resection for CRLM.[21,22] Given the alternative of only palliative chemotherapy, these scoring instruments are seldom used in clinical decision-making in individual patients, and every effort is made to make as many patients as possible resectable. There are a plethora of reports and studies on liver resection for CRLM. The 5-year survival rate in solitary metastases has been reported to be from 42% to 71%, but this represents a minority of the actual cohort.[23] The population outcome can be better assessed through registry studies like the LiverMetSurvey (https://livermetsurvey-arcad.org) which has data on more than 27,000 patients. The 5- and 10-year overall survival is 42% and 25%, respectively, with a 90-day operative mortality of 2.8%. Operated but not liver resected patients have a 5-year survival of 5%, whereas patients treated with ablation alone have a 5-year survival of 22%.

Liver transplantation for highly selected patients with non-resectable CRLM has been reported in the last 10 years.[24,25] Although the results have been promising, this is still a controversial and experimental therapy that should only be part of controlled prospective trials.

Neuroendocrine liver metastases

NETs are relatively rare, slow-growing cancers arising from neuroendocrine cell lineages, most often in the gastrointestinal tract or the respiratory system. The mode of presentation may be heterogeneous ranging from asymptomatic to the hormonal syndromes. The clinical course is usually indolent, due to the slow-growing nature of NETs. Liver metastasis is the most frequent metastatic manifestation with a rate of about 50% and the effective treatment of liver metastases dictates the outcome for these patients. The biological behaviour of these tumours is linked to histological grade with low grade (G1–G2) having far better prognosis than poorly differentiated (G3) and undifferentiated tumours (G4). Furthermore, the proliferation marker Ki67 (given as percentage of positive cells at histological examination) is closely linked to biological aggressiveness. Liver resection is the best treatment for NET liver metastases given that the lesions are resectable, and also leads to relief of

> **Box 20.1** Milan selection criteria for liver transplantation of patients with non-resectable liver metastases from neuroendocrine tumours
>
> - Low grade NET (G1–G2) confirmed on histology.
> - Primary tumour drained by portal system.
> - Primary tumour and all deposits radically removed in a separate operation before consideration for transplant.
> - Metastatic liver involvement <50% of liver volume.
> - Stable disease or response to treatment for at least 6 months prior to listing.
> - Age <60 years (relative criteria).
>
> Adapted with permission from Mazzaferro V, Sposito C, Coppa J, et al. The long-term benefit of liver transplantation for hepatic metastases from neuroendocrine tumors. Am J Transplant. 2016;16:2892–2902.

symptoms in patients with hormone active disease.[26] Unfortunately, only 10–20% of the patients can realistically obtain an R0 resection due to the fact that the diagnosis is often delayed, and many patients have multiple lesions with bi-lobar distribution. Recurrence is more common than in liver resection for CRLM, but due to the slow progression of disease in the majority of patients, reasonably long overall survival rates ranging from 50% to 75% at 5 years might be obtained. For highly selected patients with non-resectable NET liver metastases, liver transplantation can offer a potential cure. The available literature on liver transplantation for NET tumours displays great variability in overall survival and recurrence rates due to non-standardized transplant criteria and heterogeneous patient cohorts.[27] It is evident that stringent selection is necessary to avoid futile use of liver grafts that would negatively impact other patients on the waitlist. Liver transplantation should only be considered in patients with liver-only disease, indicating that radical resection of the primary and any other deposits is a requirement. An observation time after resection of the primary of at least 6 months is needed, and the tumours should demonstrate a response to systemic therapy. The latter is to exclude patients with aggressive tumour biology. Formally, only grade 1 and 2 tumours are considered, and some authors advocate a Ki67 rate below 10%. The Milan group published their experience in 2016 and did a propensity score matching against alternative therapy.[28] The 5- and 10-year overall survival rates were 97% and 89%, respectively, demonstrating a compelling survival benefit versus non-transplant treatment. The recurrence rate was only 13%, which is comparable to what is obtained in liver transplantation for HCC within established transplant criteria and new recurrences beyond 5 years of observation was not registered. The Milan criteria for liver transplantation in NET liver metastases are outlined in Box 20.1. In general, NET tumours do, however, often display an indolent, slow-growing nature. Therefore, it is advisable to follow up patients treated surgically over a long time with respect to recurrence of disease.

Non-colorectal, non-neuroendocrine liver metastases

Liver resection is the standard of care for patients with CRLM and patients with hepatic spread from NETs. For non-CRLM and non-NET liver tumours, the picture is less clear and the efficacy of surgical treatment somewhat undetermined, due to the large variety of different tumour types and associated biological features as well as the relative scarcity of larger systematic studies compared with NETs and CRLMs. Apart from gastrointestinal cancers, these tumours do not have portal venous drainage, and the dissemination is through the systemic route. Hence, more widespread and multifocal malignant disease could theoretically be anticipated in this heterogeneous cohort. When considering major surgical therapy in these patients, there is a need for optimal staging and selection criteria to avoid ineffective therapy in a seriously ill patient population.

Adam and colleagues published the largest study to date on liver resection in non-CRLM and non-NET liver tumours including 1452 patients from 41 European centres in 2006.[29] Based on multivariate prognostic factor analysis, a scoring system for risk stratification was developed where numeric points were set for six sets of variables (Table 20.1). Smaller cohort studies have, to a large extent, confirmed these findings, particularly with respect to main cancer types and the impact of the length of the disease-free interval. Analogously, whether the metastases are synchronous or metachronous has a prognostic impact. Patients with synchronous disease need to have a response to systemic therapy and remain stable over time to justify hepatic resection, further underlining the importance of assessing these patients in multidisciplinary teams. In the following, trends in survival outcomes for various tumour types are given in the order of which they appear in the literature.

Breast primary tumour

The liver is one of the predilection sites for metastatic disease in breast cancer and this was the largest group in the study by Adam et al.,[29] including 454 patients (31% of all). The 5- and 10-year overall survival was 41% and 22%, respectively, with a median survival of 45 months. Good response to chemotherapy and hormone-positive tumours are positive prognostic factors. Similar outcomes for breast cancer have been reported in other, smaller studies.[30,31]

Gastrointestinal primary tumour

This is a heterogeneous group covering the whole gastrointestinal tract, apart from colorectal cancer and NETs, and the criteria used in various studies are not standardized. It cannot be ruled out that there is a selection bias in the literature, meaning that the patients resected are not really representative of the ones regularly seen in the clinic. Hence the overall survival after resection is variable, and general recommendations are difficult to give and must be interpreted with some caution. The best outcome has been found in small bowel cancer with a 5-year overall survival of 49%. Pancreas cancer, other than ampullary primaries, tumours of the gastro-oesophageal junction, oesophagus, and head and neck cancers are associated with shorter median survival ranging from 14 to 18 months.

Urological and gynaecological primary tumours

Urological cancers do not metastasize to the liver very frequently. Good outcomes have been reported (in descending order) for adrenal, testicular, and renal cell carcinoma with 5-year survival of 66%, 51%, and 38%, respectively. Similar survival outcomes have been reported for ovarian and uterine primary tumours with 5-year survival of 50% and 35%, respectively. Testicular cancer is in a special position, since recent developments in chemotherapy yields very high curation rates for this tumour type.

Table 20.1 Prognostic score for survival after liver resection for non-colorectal, non-neuroendocrine liver metastasis according to Adam et al.

Prognostic variable	Scoring	Summary score	5-year survival (%)	Range (%)
		0	69	69–69
Extrahepatic metastases	1 point	1	54	46–62
Major hepatectomy	1 point	2	45	36–55
R2 resection	1 point	3	36	26–46
Patient age	<30 years = 0 30–60 years = 1 >60 years = 2	4	27	17–37
Disease-free interval from resection of primary to metastasis	>24 months = 0 12–24 months = 1 <12 months = 2	5	19	10–28
Breast cancer histology	0 points	6	12	5–19
Squamous histology	2 points	7	7	2–11
Melanoma histology	3 points	8	4	1–6
Any other histology	1 point	9	1	0–2
		10	0	0

Source: data from Adam R, Chiche L, Aloia T, et al. Hepatic resection for noncolorectal nonendocrine liver metastases: analysis of 1,452 patients and development of a prognostic model. *Ann Surg.* 2006;244:524–535.

Melanoma

Malignant melanoma can be subdivided in cutaneous, uveal, and choroidal. In general, these primary tumours can display an unpredictable clinical course. Patients with oligometastatic disease might be subject to surgical therapy, including liver resection or ablation, but concomitant distant metastasis is a contraindication, since there is no evident benefit of surgical therapy. The number of liver metastases might be difficult to assess on pretransplant imaging, as numerous small tumours, not readily visible on CT scans, are not uncommon. MRI is a logical adjunct in the preoperative workup. Peroperative ultrasound scanning might also be advisable to ascertain that no remnant tumour is left behind. The outcomes reported are highly variable ranging from 5-year survival rates of 20% to 81%, but the higher figures are based on small selective cohorts. The recurrence rates are also fairly high, and may appear late, explaining reduced survival expectations. Response to modern immunotherapy like ipilimumab and/or antibody towards programmed cell death receptor prior to surgery might possibly be used as a selection factor. In contrast, surgery first will reduce the tumour burden, possibly increasing the effect of systemic immunotherapy. These issues remain to be clarified.

Soft tissue and stromal tumours

This group consist of sarcomas and gastrointestinal stromal tumours (GISTs) and made up 14% of the histological subtypes in the study by Adam et al.[29] GIST tumours are characterized by immunoreactivity to the transmembrane tyrosine kinase receptor CD117. The introduction of the tyrosine kinase inhibitor imatinib has improved the outcomes in patients with GIST tumours. The most common soft tissue sarcoma type giving rise to liver metastasis is leiomyosarcoma. Both these primary tumours are associated with good survival after radical resection of liver metastases and the reported 5-year survival ranges from 55% to 70% for GIST, 48% for leiomyosarcoma, and 31% to 41% for other sarcomas.[32] The recurrence-free survival of 35.7% in GIST is by far superior to that of leiomyosarcoma (3.4%) and other sarcomas (21.4%).

Conclusion

Metastases constitute the most common malignant tumours of the liver. Surgical treatment is the only available potentially curative treatment option. Liver resection is the standard of care for CRLMs and liver metastases from NETs. Liver transplantation is an option for highly selected patients with non-resectable metastases from NETs. Secondary liver tumours arising from some other primaries can benefit from liver resection after proper staging and careful selection of patients with favourable tumour biology.

REFERENCES

1. Fidler IJ. The pathogenesis of cancer metastasis: the 'seed and soil' hypothesis revisited. *Nat Rev Cancer.* 2003;3(6):453–458.
2. Weiss L. Comments on hematogenous metastatic patterns in humans as revealed by autopsy. *Clin Exp Metastas.* 1992;10(3):191–199.
3. de Ridder J, de Wilt JHW, Simmer F, Overbeek L, Lemmens V, Nagtegaal I. Incidence and origin of histologically confirmed liver metastases: an explorative case-study of 23,154 patients. *Oncotarget.* 2015;7(34):55368–55376.
4. Granata V, Fusco R, de Lutio di Castelguidone E, et al. Diagnostic performance of gadoxetic acid-enhanced liver MRI versus multidetector CT in the assessment of colorectal liver metastases compared to hepatic resection. *BMC Gastroenterol.* 2019;19(1):129.
5. Guglielmi A, Ruzzenente A, Conci S, Valdegamberi A, Iacono C. How much remnant is enough in liver resection? *Digest Surg.* 2012;29(1):6–17.

6. Clavien P-A, Petrowsky H, DeOliveira ML, Graf R. Strategies for safer liver surgery and partial liver transplantation. *N Engl J Med*. 2007;**356**(15):1545–1559.
7. Kianmanesh R, Farges O, Abdalla EK, Sauvanet A, Ruszniewski P, Belghiti J. Right portal vein ligation: a new planned two-step all-surgical approach for complete resection of primary gastrointestinal tumors with multiple bilateral liver metastases. *J Am Coll Surg*. 2003;**197**(1):164–170.
8. Regimbeau JM, Cosse C, Kaiser G, Hubert C, Laurent C, Lapointe R, et al. Feasibility, safety and efficacy of two-stage hepatectomy for bilobar liver metastases of colorectal cancer: a LiverMetSurvey analysis. *HPB (Oxford)*. 2017;**19**(5):396–405.
9. Santibañes M de, Boccalatte L, Santibanes ED. A literature review of associating liver partition and portal vein ligation for staged hepatectomy (ALPPS): so far, so good. *Updates Surg*. 2017;**69**(1):9–19.
10. Sandstrom P, Røsok BI, Sparrelid E, Larsen PN, Larsson AL, Lindell G, et al. ALPPS improves resectability compared with conventional two-stage hepatectomy in patients with advanced colorectal liver metastasis: results from a Scandinavian Multicenter Randomized Controlled Trial (LIGRO Trial). *Ann Surg*. 2018;**267**(5):833–840.
11. Schadde E, Raptis DA, Schnitzbauer AA, et al. Prediction of mortality after ALPPS stage-1: an analysis of 320 patients from the international ALPPS Registry. *Ann Surg*. 2015;**262**(5):780–786.
12. Linecker M, Stavrou GA, Oldhafer KJ, et al. The ALPPS risk score. *Ann Surg*. 2016;**264**(5):1–9.
13. Olthof PB, Tomassini F, Huespe PE, et al. Hepatobiliary scintigraphy to evaluate liver function in associating liver partition and portal vein ligation for staged hepatectomy: liver volume overestimates liver function. *Surgery*. 2017;**162**(4):775–783.
14. Ferlay J, Soerjomataram I, Dikshit R, et al. Cancer incidence and mortality worldwide: sources, methods and major patterns in GLOBOCAN 2012. *Int J Cancer*. 2015;**136**(5):E359–E386.
15. Vuik FE, Nieuwenburg SA, Bardou M, et al. Increasing incidence of colorectal cancer in young adults in Europe over the last 25 years. *Gut*. 2019;**68**(10):1820–1826.
16. Allard MA, Adam R, Giuliante F, et al. Long-term outcomes of patients with 10 or more colorectal liver metastases. *Br J Cancer*. 2017;**117**(5):604–611.
17. Missiaglia E, Jacobs B, D'Ario G, et al. Distal and proximal colon cancers differ in terms of molecular, pathological, and clinical features. *Ann Oncol*. 2014;**25**(10):1995–2001.
18. D'Angelica M, Kornprat P, Gonen M, et al. Effect on outcome of recurrence patterns after hepatectomy for colorectal metastases. *Ann Surg Oncol*. 2010;**18**(4):1096–1103.
19. Shaw IM, Rees M, Welsh FKS, Bygrave S, John TG. Repeat hepatic resection for recurrent colorectal liver metastases is associated with favourable long-term survival. *Brit J Surg*. 2006;**93**(4):457–464.
20. Masi G, Vasile E, Loupakis F, et al. Randomized trial of two induction chemotherapy regimens in metastatic colorectal cancer: an updated analysis. *J Natl Cancer Inst*. 2011;**103**(1):21–30.
21. Fong Y, Fortner J, Sun RL, Brennan MF, Blumgart LH. Clinical score for predicting recurrence after hepatic resection for metastatic colorectal cancer: analysis of 1001 consecutive cases. *Ann Surg*. 1999;**230**(3):309–318.
22. Rees M, Tekkis PP, Welsh FKS, O'Rourke T, O'Rourke T, John TG. Evaluation of long-term survival after hepatic resection for metastatic colorectal cancer. *Ann Surg*. 2008;**247**(1):125–135.
23. Aloia TA, Vauthey J-N, Loyer EM, et al. Solitary colorectal liver metastasis: resection determines outcome. *Arch Surg*. 2006;**141**(5):460–466.
24. Hagness M, Foss A, Line P-D, et al. Liver transplantation for nonresectable liver metastases from colorectal cancer. *Ann Surg*. 2013;**257**(5):800–806.
25. Dueland S, Grut H, Syversveen T, Hagness M, Line P-D. Selection criteria related to long-term survival following liver transplantation for colorectal liver metastasis. *Am J Transpl*. 2019;**20**(2):530–537.
26. Reddy SK, Clary BM. Neuroendocrine liver metastases. *Surg Clin N Am*. 2010;**90**(4):853–861.
27. Moris D, Tsilimigras DI, Ntanasis-Stathopoulos I, et al. Liver transplantation in patients with liver metastases from neuroendocrine tumors: a systematic review. *Surgery*. 2017;**162**(3):525–536.
28. Mazzaferro V, Sposito C, Coppa J, et al. The long-term benefit of liver transplantation for hepatic metastases from neuroendocrine tumors. *Am J Transplant*. 2016;**16**(10):2892–2902.
29. Adam R, Chiche L, Aloia T, et al. Hepatic resection for noncolorectal nonendocrine liver metastases: analysis of 1,452 patients and development of a prognostic model. *Ann Surg*. 2006;**244**(4):524–535.
30. Lendoire J, Moro M, Andriani O, et al. Liver resection for non-colorectal, non-neuroendocrine metastases: analysis of a multicenter study from Argentina. *HPB (Oxford)*. 2007;**9**(6):435–439.
31. Schiergens TS, Lüning J, Renz BW, et al. Liver resection for non-colorectal non-neuroendocrine metastases: where do we stand today compared to colorectal cancer? *J Gastrointest Surg*. 2016;**20**(6):1163–1172.
32. Brudvik KW, Patel SH, Roland CL, Conrad C, Torres KE, Hunt KK, et al. Survival after resection of gastrointestinal stromal tumor and sarcoma liver metastases in 146 patients. *J Gastrointest Surg*. 2015;**19**(8):1476–1483.

21

Principles and techniques of liver resection

Philipp Kron and J. Peter A. Lodge

Introduction: basic principles of liver surgery

Indications for hepatic resection

The most common indication for liver resection in the West is colorectal liver metastases (CRLMs) but in the East it is hepatocellular carcinoma (HCC), due to its association with hepatitis B. The proportion of resections for HCC is increasing in the West due to immigration, despite rigorous policies for vaccination and treatment, and because of the association of HCC with chronic liver injury related to hepatitis C and alcohol. Cholangiocarcinoma, both perihilar and intrahepatic, are increasingly dealt with in major centres, but these tumours demand a more complex surgical approach due to significant vascular and biliary involvement. Other indications include neuroendocrine tumours and selected cases of renal, breast, gastric, sarcoma, and melanoma liver metastases (most usually those with localized disease confined to the liver after a long disease-free interval).

Benign liver tumours may also indicate a need for liver resection: hepatic adenomas more than 5 cm in diameter (due to the risk of haemorrhage or malignant change), focal nodular hyperplasia (due to pain or compression of adjacent structures), haemangiomas (due to pain or necrosis), or due to a diagnostic uncertainty. Benign biliary disease, including strictures, may also be an indication due to stone formation and recurrent ascending cholangitis. Traumatic liver laceration is increasingly rarely an indication due to the success of conservative management, including embolization for acute haemorrhage and biliary stents for bile leakage.

Contraindications for hepatic resection

Contraindications for liver resection are less specific and relate to failure of the anticipated risk:benefit ratio: risks of postoperative liver failure, comorbidities, or futility due to extrahepatic malignant disease.

Preoperative assessment

Assessment of resectability

The definition of resectability in hepatic surgery underlies a continuous flow. The boundaries have been constantly pushed and patients deemed to be unresectable previously are surgical candidates these days.[1] Essential in the preoperative surgical decision-making process are the requirements that the tumour can be removed *in toto* with clear resection margins (R0 resection) and that the liver remnant left behind (future liver remnant (FLR)) provides sufficient synthetic function. Therefore, a meticulous understanding and visualization of the tumour localization in relation to major vascular and biliary structures is crucial to preserve adequate vascular inflow, outflow, and biliary drainage following hepatic resection[2] (**Figure 21.1**). Thus, the aim of the preoperative assessment is to delineate the tumour burden and localization, define resectability, identify potential extrahepatic disease, and to elaborate a surgical plan.

Imaging

Computed tomography

Computed tomography (CT) is an economical and broadly available investigation to facilitate tumour assessment. CT scans have continuously been evolved, allowing a fast and exact anatomical acquisition with or without contrast. The application of contrast agents can help to further characterize lesions according to their enhancement patterns. Furthermore, CT imaging allows three-dimensional and vascular reconstructions as well as volumetric assessments for more complex resections. Therefore, CT-based reconstructions can facilitate preoperative planning such as the size and localization of the lesion, assessment of the potential resection margins, and the relationship of the lesion to surrounding vascular and biliary structures. This preoperative workup is of utmost importance for the safety of the patient and the understanding of the anatomy.

Magnetic resonance imaging

In contrast to CT, magnetic resonance imaging (MRI) uses the particular characteristics of water and fat to generate a high-resolution image based on the acquired differences in tissue. MRI can be very helpful in specific tumour-related characteristics, such as for further characterization of the liver lesions, especially when CT contrast is contraindicated or previous CT investigations are unclear. By adding diffusion-weighted imaging, MRI scans are able to further improve the detection rate of tumours and metastases. Additionally,

CHAPTER 21 Principles and techniques of liver resection

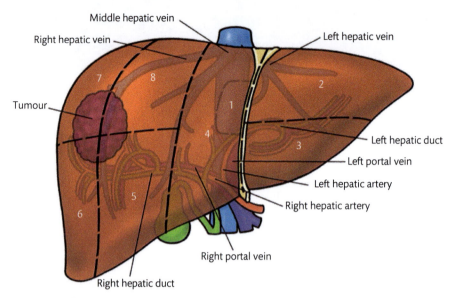

Figure 21.1 Preoperative assessment of respectability and planning of the extent of hepatic resection. Schematic illustration of the tumour location and its relationship to major vasculature and biliary structures.

by adding contrast, MRI scans can reduce false-positive findings.[3] MRI investigations themselves have the highest sensitivity and specificity currently, when compared to CT or positron emission tomography (PET)–CT scans.[4]

Positron emission tomography–computed tomography

PET-CT takes advantage of the increased glucose metabolism of vital tumour cells. The radioactive tracer used for PET scans is detected in high metabolic areas. Therefore, PET scans in liver surgery are used for preoperative staging, predominantly in detecting or excluding extrahepatic disease. However, an accurate anatomical delineation in PET-CT scans is difficult and this therefore cannot replace high-resolution CT imaging and MRI in the setting of preoperative anatomical planning.

The role of all of these imaging modalities is not only limited to preoperative staging; they are also used as surveillance scans post liver resection or as a tool to assess the tumour response to preoperative (neoadjuvant) chemotherapy.[5] For PET-CT, in the preoperative evaluation of the tumour response it is crucial that the chemotherapy-free interval is long enough to prevent an underestimation of the tumour burden.

Assessment of liver function and fitness for liver resection

Before any liver resection, it is essential to assess liver function, particularly in relation to the FLR. This is particularly important for patients with underlying parenchymal liver disease. It has long been recognized that patients with cirrhosis are at a high risk for both general anaesthesia and surgery because of the risk of acute deterioration in liver function (known as decompensation) postoperatively. Although originally it was thought that the risk of decompensation was only significant for major abdominal surgery, it is now recognized that even minor abdominal surgery or major surgery to other parts of the body is also associated with a significant risk of decompensation, resulting in an increased risk of perioperative death,

usually recorded in terms of 30- and 90-day mortality. Although sometimes difficult to quantify, when considering abdominal surgery on a patient with cirrhosis, this risk must be taken into account and the patient should be advised about it in a standard consent procedure. This is especially true if liver resection is going to be performed.

Several different scoring systems are used to assess liver disease, particularly in relation to assessment for the need for liver transplantation. The most commonly used is the Child–Pugh (also often called Child–Turcotte–Pugh) classification, which creates a score (A—low risk, B—moderate risk, C—high risk) based on five clinical features, originally developed in 1973. The five factors consist of three relating to synthetic function of the liver (bilirubin level, serum albumin, and international normalized ratio) and two relating to clinical assessment (degree of ascites and degree of hepatic encephalopathy). Critics of the Child–Pugh score have noted its reliance on clinical assessment, which may result in inconsistency in scoring. Others have suggested that its broad classifications of disease are impractical when determining priority for liver transplantation; nevertheless, it remains widely used. The Model for End-Stage Liver Disease (MELD) is a newer scoring system that has been developed to address some of the concerns with the Child–Pugh score, and the two systems are often used in conjunction to determine liver transplant policy and consideration of risk for surgical and radiological interventions. MELD is calculated from serum creatinine, bilirubin, and international normalized ratio along with the need for haemodialysis, and ranges from 6 (less ill) to 40 (gravely ill), with general agreement that the risk:benefit ratio for a liver transplant is appropriate for patients when the MELD is 15 or more (unless too sick). For liver transplantation in the UK, serum sodium is incorporated into the MELD score to create UKELD, which is thought to be more accurate. A UKELD score of 49 is needed to be eligible for a liver transplant.

The American Society of Anesthesiologists (ASA) classification is also used to stratify risk for surgery, developed in 1941 and subsequently modified. It is recognized that, although useful, the ASA classification cannot serve as a direct indicator of operative risk because it does not take into account the severity of the surgical procedure. ASA 1 is a normal healthy patient, ASA 2 is a patient with mild systemic disease, ASA 3 is a patient with a severe systemic disease that is not life-threatening but causes some functional limitation, ASA 4 is a patient with a severe systemic disease that is a constant threat to life, ASA 5 is a moribund patient who is not expected to survive the operation, and ASA 6 relates to brain death. A patient with cirrhosis should be considered ASA 3 as a minimum.

The presence of portal hypertension should also be taken into account. Nicoll[6] has presented guidelines for the management of the cirrhotic patient having surgery and included preoperative assessment (Child–Pugh and MELD score and assessment for portal hypertension) and discussion of risk of mortality and morbidity with patient and family: Child–Pugh A = about 10%, Child-Pugh A plus portal hypertension = about 30%, Child–Pugh B = about 30%, Child–Pugh C = about 75% risk.

As a general rule, for patients with parenchymal liver disease, to be fit enough to undergo liver resection they should be Child–Pugh A or B and without evidence of significant portal hypertension.

Volumetric and functional assessment

In order to further assess operative risk for patients undergoing liver resection, many expert centres routinely use liver volumetry studies and attempt functional assessment for both the whole liver and the FLR, which should range between 20% and 40% of healthy liver tissue. This measurement is usually based on CT scanning. Since liver volume is not equal to function, additional tools such as indocyanine green (ICG), LIMAX and hepatobiliary iminodiacetic acid (HIDA) can also be helpful to assess the estimated function, but these tools are not used universally. ICG is a special dye that binds to albumin and is homogeneously distributed in the blood. It is metabolized solely by the liver and excreted via the bile. Therefore, this test provides a good estimation to assess hepatic function preoperatively.[7] The LIMAX test assesses the function of cytochrome P450, which is only expressed in the liver parenchyma. This enzyme system is reduced in patients with liver disease and can indirectly be measured after metabolization of ^{13}C-methacetin in a non-invasive breath test.[8] The metabolism of technetium-99m-labelled HIDA is very similar to ICG and the predominantly hepatic uptake makes it suitable for functional assessment.

The FLR is also affected by neoadjuvant chemotherapy as this may impair immediate function and regenerative ability. Thus, timing for surgery becomes important and a delay of about 6 weeks after cessation of chemotherapy may be necessary to reduce the risk of postoperative liver failure. If the FLR is predicted to be inadequate, the resection should not proceed, but there are no current exact measurements that can be employed for this prediction.

Preoperative preparation (inadequate future liver remnant)

Portal vein embolization

Liver resection patients are at risk of postoperative liver insufficiency if the FLR is small or otherwise inadequate, as noted above. One way to combat this is consideration of preoperative portal vein embolization (PVE), which increases both FLR volume and function. However, tumours in the non-embolized segments of liver may progress more rapidly after PVE, so careful consideration also needs to be given to this aspect.

PVE was initially established for patients undergoing right hemi-hepatectomy, using radiological access via the left portal vein. Complications including left portal vein thrombosis encouraged a change to direct access to the right portal vein, with increased success and less complications. The alternative approach that has been used is direct surgical ligation of the right portal vein. Although perhaps more invasive, this is now commonly used in two stage liver surgery and recent studies have shown equal efficacy to PVE.[9]

For patients with disease in segment 4, removal of this segment with the right lobe (extended right hemihepatectomy/right hepatic trisectionectomy) may be required, typically leaving only segments 2 and 3 ±, 1 *in situ* and these segments frequently account for less than 20% of the total liver volume. For these patients, embolizing all of the liver to be resected (segments 4–8) and maximizing the hypertrophic stimulus to segments 2 and 3 is more appropriate but embolization of the segment 4 portal vein(s) is technically challenging, risks non-target embolization to the FLR and may be associated with increased complications. However, recent work has demonstrated that the addition of segment 4 PVE to right PVE is associated with useful increased hypertrophy of segments 2 and 3 compared with right PVE alone.[10] The mechanism may explain to some extent the extraordinary degree of FLR hypertrophy seen with rapid two-stage hepatectomy: associating liver partition and portal vein ligation for staged hepatectomy (ALPPS).

Hepatic vein embolization

Less work has been done with hepatic vein embolization; it is applicable when PVE fails to induce sufficient regeneration of the FLR. Several authors have now reported that the sequential application of HVE following PVE safely and effectively induces further FLR regeneration, at least in non-cirrhotic livers.

Surgical techniques for hepatic resection: principles

The role of liver-directed anaesthesia

Liver-directed anaesthesia has developed greatly in recent years, primarily with a concentration on low central venous pressure to reduce bleeding during liver parenchymal dissection. Whereas in the past a central venous line and arterial line were considered essential, along with epidural anaesthesia, the advent of better surgical techniques, and postoperative analgesia, including the routine use of wound catheters for local anaesthesia infusion, these are viewed as less essential today, except in the most major resections. However, in most cases, a urinary catheter is routinely placed for careful monitoring. A warm air flow device covers the patient as well as the use of a standard warming blanket underneath. Air–oxygen–desflurane-based anaesthesia is used in many centres as it has been shown to minimize the derangement of postoperative liver function, with infusions of *N*-acetyl cysteine and antioxidants to confer hepatic protection if prolonged major liver ischaemia is anticipated. Above all, an anaesthetist experienced with liver-directed anaesthesia is essential for major resectional surgery.

Intraoperative assessment of resectability

Planning

No battery of preoperative imaging replaces the definition of liver anatomy and tumour location by direct visualization and palpation at surgery. In addition, this is the best opportunity to finally consider the FLR. There is no doubt that experience enables the careful judgements needed in this demanding surgery: there is no place for liver resection outside expert centres.

Intraoperative ultrasound

Intraoperative ultrasound (IOUS) is a prerequisite in modern liver resection. After exploration of the abdominal cavity and mobilization of the liver, IOUS is routinely performed. The results gained during this intraoperative investigation may have a substantial impact on the surgical approach. The IOUS clearly defines the anatomy of the liver and the localization of the tumour, especially relationships to major vascular and biliary structures (Figure 21.2). Besides the pre-resection planning, the IOUS is a dynamic investigation and can be used during resection for further guidance and adaption of the resection plane to achieve a R0 resection in a parenchymal-sparing manner.[11,12]

Resection principles

Access

In most cases, access is gained through a 'reverse L' laparotomy incision under the right costal margin, and the use of mechanical retractors, although many resections can be done through a standard midline incision. Laparoscopic and robotic approaches are evolving.

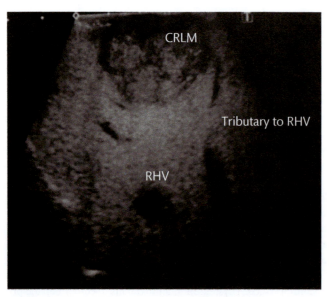

Figure 21.2 IOUS, CRLM, and its relation to vasculature.

Vascular isolation and ischaemia techniques

One main risk factor associated with poor outcome following hepatic resection is blood loss.[13] Therefore, inflow occlusion (portal triad clamping, known as the Pringle manoeuvre) has been used for more than 100 years to minimize blood loss during hepatic surgery and reduce morbidity and mortality eventually. However portal triad inflow occlusion itself causes an ischaemic injury in the potential FLR. Therefore, intermittent Pringle is used today with better results compared to the continuous Pringle manoeuvre.[14] A common routine is 15 minutes on followed by 5 minutes off. A liver with normal parenchyma should tolerate a total clamping time of 90 minutes and more whereas in diseased livers, this time is reduced. Another form of vascular isolation is hepatic vascular exclusion: besides portal triad, the inferior vena cava or hepatic veins are clamped. The hanging manoeuvre also has a place in this list of different techniques. The hanging manoeuvre causes a reduced blood flow on the one hand but facilitates resection in the right plane on the other. The principle of the hanging manoeuvre is simple. A tape is inserted in the groove on the right side of the middle hepatic vein and passed along the avascular plane in front of the retrohepatic cava to the caudal edge of the liver. By lifting the tape, the ideal transection plane can be identified and vessels and biliary structures can be easily recognized. Furthermore, the slight traction causes a certain outflow obstruction, paired with the applied Pringle leading to the principle of hepatic vascular exclusion.

Parenchymal transection

The use of ultrasonic dissection (CUSA, Valleylab, Inc., Boulder, CO, USA) or alternative appropriate parenchymal-dissection techniques reduce blood loss and postoperative bile leakage by allowing identification of significant structures during liver resection surgery. During the parenchymal transection, these vessels and ducts are divided and clipped or ligated. There are many new technologies available including Harmonic and Enseal (Ethicon, Johnson & Johnson), Ligasure (Medtronic), Lotus (Bowa Medical), and Erbejet (ERBE).

Anatomical versus non-anatomical resection

This remains an area for debate but in recent years there has been an increasing trend towards parenchymal-sparing techniques for CRLM and HCC surgery in particular to ensure survival through leaving an adequate FLR. Long-term outcomes do not appear to be compromised by this approach.

Resection margin

Much work has been done in recent years in order to define the question of adequate resection margins in liver resection. It is accepted that improved outcomes are associated with R0 resection, but the argument for 1 cm clearance is less firm as for CRLM 1 mm may be enough. There is also evidence that in hepatic resection for HCC vascular R1 status is not associated with inferior outcomes.[15] Once again, it is the preservation of an adequate FLR that is paramount.

Standard anatomical liver resections

Anatomical left-sided hepatic resections can be described as left lateral sectionectomy (resection of segments 2 and 3), left hemihepatectomy (resection of segments 2, 3, and 4 ± 1), and left

Resection principles 227

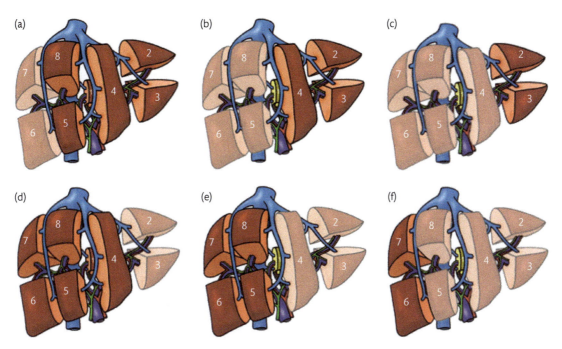

Figure 21.3 Standard anatomical liver resection. (a) Right posterior sectionectomy. (b) Right hemihepatectomy ± segment 1. (c) Right trisectionectomy ± segment 1. (d) Left lateral sectionectomy. (e) Left hemihepatectomy ± segment 1. (f) Left trisectionectomy ± segment 1.

hepatic trisectionectomy (resection of segments 2, 3, 4, 5, and 8 ± 1). Anatomical right-sided hepatic resections can be described as right posterior sectionectomy (resection of segments 6 and 7), right hemihepatectomy (resection of segments 5, 6, 7, and 8 ± 1) and right hepatic trisectionectomy (resection of segments 4, 5, 6, 7, and 8 ± 1). En bloc resection of the caudate lobe (segment 1) may be performed alone or in conjunction with anatomical hepatectomy for various diagnoses (Figure 21.3).

Anatomical liver resections

Left lateral sectionectomy

(See also Figure 21.3.) Left lateral sectionectomy is considered for tumours obliterating much of hepatic segments 2 and 3 or compromising the portal triad structures for these segments. A strictly anatomical approach is unnecessary and a lesser resection should usually be planned for more peripheral tumours as parenchymal-sparing techniques offer the patient a potential lifeline for re-resection if a further liver tumour occurs in the future. A resection of segment 2 or 3 individually or wedge excisions for smaller peripheral tumours can be performed. This can also be combined with a right liver resection. The use of modern parenchymal-dissection techniques negates the need for vascular control in most cases. If vascular control is needed, a simple Pringle manoeuvre should suffice. The segment 2 and 3 portal triad structures can be divided within the liver parenchyma using clamps and suture ligation or surgical staplers. The left hepatic vein is similarly divided, taking care not to compromise the middle hepatic vein at its common insertion into the inferior vena cava. This procedure, therefore, usually lends itself well to laparoscopic approaches.

Left hemihepatectomy

Portal triad dissection is commenced with cholecystectomy. After mobilization of the left liver (by division of the falciform and left triangular ligaments), the left portal vein and the left hepatic artery are divided separately at the base of the umbilical fissure, and a demarcation between the left and right hemilivers is observed. In cases planned for caudate lobe (segment 1) resection, the left portal vein and the left hepatic artery are divided at their origins to interrupt the blood supply to the caudate lobe. The most usual approach is intra-Glissonian (inside the Glissonian capsule that surrounds the portal triad structures) and no attempt is made to ligate or divide the left hepatic duct at this stage as variant anatomy is common and it is safer to divide the biliary tree later during liver parenchymal transection. The lesser omentum is divided (ligating any accessory left hepatic arterial branches). In cases of perihilar cholangiocarcinoma, these aspects are preceded by regional or extended (regional and para-aortic) lymphadenectomy along with division of the common bile duct within the superior aspect of the head of the pancreas to allow biliary excision, lymphadenectomy, and neurectomy of the portal triad region. If the caudate lobe is to be excised, it needs to be mobilized from the inferior vena cava, with ligation or suture of its short hepatic veins. No attempt is made to identify or isolate the left hepatic vein at this stage, as this introduces danger to the middle hepatic vein, which almost always has a common insertion into the inferior vena cava with the left hepatic vein.

During liver parenchymal transection, lifting the left lateral section ventrally will minimize the venous bleeding by reducing the 'central venous pressure' within the liver remnant. An intermittent Pringle manoeuvre may be used when necessary, and rarely hepatic vascular exclusion is needed with clamping of both the portal triad inflow and the major hepatic veins or inferior vena cava.

In most cases, it is usual to retain the hepatic duct confluence to avoid biliary injury. In cases with bile duct involvement, such as perihilar cholangiocarcinoma, resection and reconstruction between the right hepatic duct or the sectoral hepatic ducts and the jejunum is performed by Roux-en-Y hepaticojejunostomy.

Left hepatic trisectionectomy

After mobilization of both the right and the left liver, the left portal vein and the left hepatic artery are divided separately at the base of the umbilical fissure. In cases planned for caudate lobe (segment 1) resection, the left portal vein and the left hepatic artery are divided at their origins to interrupt the blood supply to the caudate lobe. The right anterior sectoral portal and arterial branches are divided separately by opening the right Glissonian sheath, if possible, or the entire right anterior sectoral portal pedicle can be isolated and divided at this stage, staying outside the Glissonian sheath. When the vessels are difficult to identify extrahepatically, they are divided during liver parenchymal transection. The lesser omentum is also divided. If the caudate lobe is to be excised, it needs to be mobilized from the inferior vena cava, with ligation or suture of its short hepatic veins. In this case, it is important to preserve any major inferior or middle right hepatic veins which may be draining segment 6. The hepatocaval confluence is then approached so that the middle and left hepatic veins can be isolated and slung together for subsequent division. If the right anterior sectoral portal vein and hepatic artery have been divided, then the middle and left hepatic veins should be divided immediately between vascular clamps or staplers. This division creates two distinct advantages: a clear line of demarcation appears at the junction of segments 6 and 7 with 5 and 8, and the extended left liver to be removed becomes considerably more mobile. If the right anterior sectoral portal vein and hepatic artery have not been divided, then division of the left and middle hepatic veins must wait until that point in the parenchymal transection, or the extended left liver will become congested, resulting in more difficult access and increased blood loss. All other aspects are as for left hemihepatectomy.

Right posterior sectionectomy

This operation is rarely performed, so a detailed description is not justified. Surgery begins with right liver mobilization and then ligation and division of the right posterior sectoral hepatic artery and portal vein using an intra-Glissonian approach or alternatively an extra-Glissonian approach for right posterior pedicle ligation and division. Parenchymal transection completes removal of hepatic segments 6 and 7, most usually with preservation of the right hepatic vein.

Right hemihepatectomy

Portal triad dissection is commenced with cholecystectomy and then ligation and division of the right hepatic artery and right portal vein. Mobilization of the right liver involves division of the ligamentum teres, falciform, coronary, and right triangular ligaments, exposing the bare area. The next step is ligation of the retrohepatic veins draining the right liver segments into the inferior vena cava and the hepatocaval ligament. Approximately 30% of patients will require division of a significant (>10 mm) inferior right hepatic vein and in 10% a significant middle right hepatic vein will also require division before finally dividing the right hepatic vein between clamps or staplers. If the caudate lobe is to be excised, it needs to be devascularized by ligation of small branches from the left portal vein and then mobilized from the inferior vena cava, with ligation or suture of its short hepatic veins. Parenchymal transection can then proceed to complete removal of hepatic segments 5–8 ± 1, with use of the Pringle manoeuvre as necessary.

Right hepatic trisectionectomy

Portal triad dissection is commenced with ligation and division of the cystic duct and artery, allowing access for ligation and division of the right hepatic artery and right portal vein. There should be no attempt to ligate and divide the hepatic artery or portal vein branches to hepatic segment 4 as this is arduous and risks damage to the left hepatic duct. If caudate lobectomy is planned, the left portal vein branches to segment 1 are identified at the base of the umbilical fissure and ligated and divided. Mobilization of the right liver and division of hepatic veins is as for right hemihepatectomy. Further retrohepatic veins are then divided to a point where it is possible to feel bimanually the planned hepatic transection plane (postero-anteriorly), determined by tumour extent. This simple manoeuvre adds considerable safety as it allows vascular control by bimanual pressure if there is difficulty during the subsequent hepatic parenchymal transection.

In cases of caudate lobectomy, the dissection is continued with ligation and division of the short veins draining segment 1 into the inferior vena cava, such that the caudate lobe is completely mobilized. Unless there is considerable tumour involvement of segment 1, it can be 'flipped' in front of the inferior vena cava, to the right, to allow bimanual palpation of the transection plane, again for vascular control.

No attempt is made to identify or isolate the middle hepatic vein at this stage as this introduces danger to the left hepatic vein. All points of further vascular or biliary division are carried out during parenchymal transection to prevent vascular or biliary injury to the residual liver segments (2, 3, ± 1) of the FLR.

During parenchymal transection, there may be a need for an intermittent Pringle manoeuvre or rarely hepatic vascular exclusion. Residual vascular and biliary division is done at appropriate stages of the hepatic transection; the middle hepatic vein is also ligated and divided. Parenchymal transection is completed by division of the right hepatic duct (or sectoral divisions) and then the caudate process. In cases with bile duct resection (e.g. perihilar cholangiocarcinoma), reconstruction between the left lateral sectional bile duct or the individual segment (or subsegmental) 2 and 3 bile ducts and the jejunum is performed by Roux-en-Y hepaticojejunostomy.

The liver remnant is fixed in position, by suturing the falciform ligament and ligamentum teres to the anterior abdominal wall to prevent kinking of the left hepatic vein, which may cause venous outflow obstruction.

Caudate lobectomy

Resection of segment 1 is rarely performed in isolation, so a detailed description is not justified. The major steps are as described above. It should be noted, however, that caudate lobe tumours present particular challenges due to proximity of both the portal triad and the major hepatic veins.

Vascular and biliary resection and reconstruction

Liver resection for tumours involving the porta hepatis or the hepatocaval confluence may require extra surgical techniques. Portal triad involvement is a particular challenge for perihilar cholangiocarcinoma and the operator needs to be prepared to resect and reconstruct the portal vein. Hepatic artery resection and reconstruction is described less commonly and is seen as a contraindication to resection by many. It can sometimes be too difficult to carry out a segmental hepatic artery reconstruction and portal vein arterialization has been described as a 'rescue procedure'.[16] Hepatic vein or inferior vena cava reconstruction may be needed for intrahepatic cholangiocarcinoma and HCC in particular. Biliary reconstruction is most often necessary for perihilar cholangiocarcinoma and is more straightforward with anastomosis of the residual hepatic ducts to the jejunum by Roux-en-Y hepaticojejunostomy.

Laparoscopic liver resection

The main advantages of laparoscopic surgery are a shorter hospital stay and reduced pain compared to equivalent open procedures. The first laparoscopic liver resections were reported in the 1990s.[17] Since then further endeavours have been made to facilitate laparoscopic liver resection and define clinical standards in hepatic resection.[18] Laparoscopic left lateral sectionectomy is already accepted as the standard for care. Further evidence will be needed comparing open and laparoscopic liver resections to define the clear role of each procedure.[19,20]

Robotic liver resection

Robotic surgery is further developing hepatic resection surgery. So far the evidence on robotic hepatic surgery is limited to relatively small numbers of cases worldwide and it is definitely too early to define its role in hepatic resection.[21] But robotic surgery is a fast and strongly expanding field that will have a major impact on this surgery in the future.

Innovative approaches

Synchronous versus staged resection for colorectal cancer

Concurrent resection of the liver for CRLM at the time of primary colorectal surgery has significant merit. Several studies have demonstrated no increase in postoperative morbidity and equivalent long-term survivals compared to staged surgery. In carefully selected patients there has been a demonstrable reduction in cumulative postoperative hospital stay, and thus a reduction in costs, but caution is urged for older patients and for larger liver or colorectal resections.

Liver-first approach for metastatic rectal cancer

First suggested by Mentha in 2008, the liver-first approach has gained popularity in recent years. It is particularly applicable in patients where the primary rectal cancer is controlled by neoadjuvant chemoradiotherapy and the CRLMs are of borderline resectability.[22] The advantage of the liver-first approach is that if there is a failure to proceed with the liver surgery then the patient is not subjected to colorectal resection unless symptoms occur.

Multistage stage liver resection

In patients with extensive bi-lobar liver disease and a marginal or too small FLR, multistage resection strategies offer potential cure. These concepts use the unique feature of the liver to regenerate.[23,24] Existing approaches for multistage liver resections are the classical two-stage hepatectomy approach or ALPPS. As well as clearing the FLR of metastases, the classical two-stage approach contains portal vein ligation or PVE of the diseased side in the first step followed by resection in the second step. The second step normally takes place 4–8 weeks after the initial treatment, provided that the FLR has increased appropriately.[24] By contrast, part of the first step in ALPPS besides portal vein ligation or PVE is hepatic parenchymal transection.[25] This additional element triggers an acceleration of liver growth permitting the second step within 7–14 days.[26–28]

Management of complications

Haemorrhage

Bleeding after hepatic surgery is a devastating but rare complication, affecting less than 1% of patients in experienced centres, and resolved by surgical re-exploration. Blood transfusion is avoided when possible as there is now considerable data to suggest that long-term outcomes may be compromised.

Abdominal collections

Postoperative fluid collections following hepatic surgery are much more common, affecting up to 30% of patients in major series. Typical symptoms are abdominal pain, tenderness, discomfort, fever, or increasing inflammatory markers. The treatment of choice is ultrasound or CT-guided percutaneous drainage so it is only rarely that surgical intervention will be needed.

Bile leak

Recent evidence estimates the rate of bile leaks following hepatic resection remains around 7–8%.[30,31] The evidence on risk factors associated with the incidence of bile leaks is scarce. There are a variety of methods to test the biliary system in the theatre, for example, injection of saline into the cystic duct or the 'white test', which uses diluted fat emulsion.[32] But the evidence is limited to small studies and high-volume randomized controlled trials are needed to clearly answer the question if any of these methods can significantly decrease the incidence of bile leaks post liver surgery.[33] Routine placement of intra-abdominal drains remains a point of argument for uncomplicated hepatic surgery as it may not prevent complications, but if present there may be no specific intervention needed.[34] A high percentage of bile leaks are treated by percutaneous drainage (Figure 21.4). Major high-output bile leaks can be treated with ERCP with or without stenting and sphincterotomy eventually, but this is rarely required. Bile leaks should be dealt with quickly as intra-abdominal bile collections are painful and can precipitate peritonitis.

Outcomes

Outcomes for hepatic surgery are almost entirely tumour specific: biological factors have more impact than surgical technique. Having said that, surgeon and centre effect data is accumulating: liver resection should only be done in expert centres in order to optimize immediate outcomes and to reduce complication rates and blood transfusion, both of which affect cancer-specific survival.

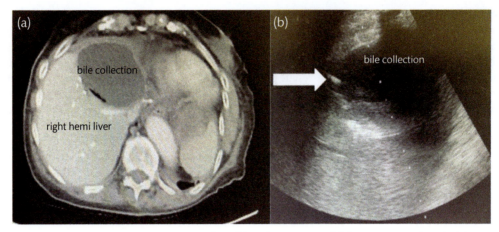

Figure 21.4 (a) CT scan showing a postoperative bile collection after left hemihepatectomy. (b) Percutaneous US-guided drainage of the collection with drain in place (white arrow).

REFERENCES

1. Mattar RE, Al-Alem F, Simoneau E, Hassanain M. Preoperative selection of patients with colorectal cancer liver metastasis for hepatic resection. *World J Gastroenterol*. 2016;**22**(2):567–581.
2. van Dam RM, Lodewick TM, van den Broek MA, et al. Outcomes of extended versus limited indications for patients undergoing a liver resection for colorectal cancer liver metastases. *HPB (Oxford)*. 2014;**16**(6):550–559.
3. Ong KO, Leen E. Radiological staging of colorectal liver metastases. *Surg Oncol*. 2007;**16**(1):7–14.
4. Niekel MC, Bipat S, Stoker J. Diagnostic imaging of colorectal liver metastases with CT, MR imaging, FDG PET, and/or FDG PET/CT: a meta-analysis of prospective studies including patients who have not previously undergone treatment. *Radiology*. 2010;**257**(3):674–684.
5. Mainenti PP, Romano F, Pizzuti L, et al. Non-invasive diagnostic imaging of colorectal liver metastases. *World J Radiol*. 2015;**7**(7):157–169.
6. Nicoll A. Surgical risk in patients with cirrhosis. *J Gastroenterol Hepatol*. 2012;**27**(10):1569–1575.
7. Okochi O, Kaneko T, Sugimoto H, Inoue S, Takeda S, Nakao A. ICG pulse spectrophotometry for perioperative liver function in hepatectomy. *J Surg Res*. 2002;**103**(1):109–113.
8. Guengerich FP, Krauser JA, Johnson WW. Rate-limiting steps in oxidations catalyzed by rabbit cytochrome P450 1A2. *Biochemistry*. 2004;**43**(33):10775–10788.
9. Pandanaboyana S, Bell R, Hidalgo E, et al. A systematic review and meta-analysis of portal vein ligation versus portal vein embolization for elective liver resection. *Surgery*. 2015;**157**(4):690–698.
10. Hammond CJ, Ali S, Haq H, et al. Segment 2/3 hypertrophy is greater when right portal vein embolisation is extended to segment 4 in patients with colorectal liver metastases: a retrospective cohort study. *Cardiovasc Intervent Radiol*. 2019;**42**(4):552–559.
11. Torzilli G, Montorsi M, Del Fabbro D, Palmisano A, Donadon M, Makuuchi M. Ultrasonographically guided surgical approach to liver tumours involving the hepatic veins close to the caval confluence. *Br J Surg*. 2006;**93**(10):1238–1246.
12. Torzilli G, Palmisano A, Del Fabbro D, et al. Contrast-enhanced intraoperative ultrasonography during surgery for hepatocellular carcinoma in liver cirrhosis: is it useful or useless? A prospective cohort study of our experience. *Ann Surg Oncol*. 2007;**14**(4):1347–1355.
13. Jarnagin WR, Gonen M, Fong Y, et al. Improvement in perioperative outcome after hepatic resection: analysis of 1,803 consecutive cases over the past decade. *Ann Surg*. 2002;**236**(4):397–406.
14. Kang KJ, Jang JH, Lim TJ, et al. Optimal cycle of intermittent portal triad clamping during liver resection in the murine liver. *Liver Transpl*. 2004;**10**(6):794–801.
15. Donadon M, Terrone A, Procopio F, et al. Is R1 vascular hepatectomy for hepatocellular carcinoma oncologically adequate? Analysis of 327 consecutive patients. *Surgery*. 2019;**165**(5):897–904.
16. Young AL, Prasad KR, Adair R, Abu Hilal M, Guthrie JA, Lodge JP. Portal vein arterialization as a salvage procedure during left hepatic trisectionectomy for hilar cholangiocarcinoma. *J Am Coll Surg*. 2008;**207**(5):e1–e6.
17. Mirnezami R, Mirnezami AH, Chandrakumaran K, et al. Short- and long-term outcomes after laparoscopic and open hepatic resection: systematic review and meta-analysis. *HPB (Oxford)*. 2011;**13**(5):295–308.
18. Buell JF, Cherqui D, Geller DA, et al. The international position on laparoscopic liver surgery: the Louisville Statement, 2008. *Ann Surg*. 2009;**250**(5):825–830.
19. Fretland AA, Kazaryan AM, Bjornbeth BA, et al. Open versus laparoscopic liver resection for colorectal liver metastases (the Oslo-CoMet Study): study protocol for a randomized controlled trial. *Trials*. 2015;**16**:73.
20. van Dam RM, Wong-Lun-Hing EM, van Breukelen GJ, et al. Open versus laparoscopic left lateral hepatic sectionectomy within an enhanced recovery ERAS(R) programme (ORANGE II-trial): study protocol for a randomised controlled trial. *Trials*. 2012;**13**:54.
21. Salloum C, Lim C, Malek A, Compagnon P, Azoulay D. Robot-assisted laparoscopic liver resection: a review. *J Visc Surg*. 2016;**153**(6):447–456.
22. Mentha G, Roth AD, Terraz S, et al. 'Liver first' approach in the treatment of colorectal cancer with synchronous liver metastases. *Dig Surg*. 2008;**25**(6):430–435.
23. Schnitzbauer AA, Lang SA, Goessmann H, et al. Right portal vein ligation combined with in situ splitting induces rapid left lateral liver lobe hypertrophy enabling 2-staged extended

right hepatic resection in small-for-size settings. *Ann Surg.* 2012;**255**(3):405–414.
24. Adam R, Miller R, Pitombo M, et al. Two-stage hepatectomy approach for initially unresectable colorectal hepatic metastases. *Surg Oncol Clin N Am.* 2007;**16**(3):525–536, viii.
25. Linecker M, Kambakamba P, Reiner CS, et al. How much liver needs to be transected in ALPPS? A translational study investigating the concept of less invasiveness. *Surgery.* 2017;**161**(2):453–464.
26. de Santibanes E, Clavien PA. Playing Play-Doh to prevent postoperative liver failure: the 'ALPPS' approach. *Ann Surg.* 2012;**255**(3):415–417.
27. Langiewicz M, Schlegel A, Saponara E, et al. Hedgehog pathway mediates early acceleration of liver regeneration induced by a novel two-staged hepatectomy in mice. *J Hepatol.* 2017;**66**(3):560–570.
28. Sandstrom P, Rosok BI, Sparrelid E, et al. ALPPS improves resectability compared with conventional two-stage hepatectomy in patients with advanced colorectal liver metastasis: results from a Scandinavian multicenter randomized controlled trial (LIGRO Trial). *Ann Surg.* 2018;**267**(5):833–840.
29. Fong Y, Blumgart LH. Hepatic colorectal metastasis: current status of surgical therapy. *Oncology (Williston).* 1998;**12**(10):1489–1498.
30. Brauer DG, Nywening TM, Jaques DP, et al. Operative site drainage after hepatectomy: a propensity score matched analysis using the American College of Surgeons NSQIP Targeted Hepatectomy Database. *J Am Coll Surg.* 2016;**223**(6):774–783.
31. Lam CM, Lo CM, Liu CL, Fan ST. Biliary complications during liver resection. *World J Surg.* 2001;**25**(10):1273–1276.
32. Li J, Malago M, Sotiropoulos GC, et al. Intraoperative application of 'white test' to reduce postoperative bile leak after major liver resection: results of a prospective cohort study in 137 patients. *Langenbecks Arch Surg.* 2009;**394**(6):1019–1024.
33. Linke R, Ulrich F, Bechstein WO, Schnitzbauer AA. The White-test helps to reduce biliary leakage in liver resection: a systematic review and meta-analysis. *Ann Hepatol.* 2015;**14**(2):161–167.
34. Gavriilidis P, Hidalgo E, de'Angelis N, Lodge P, Azoulay D. Re-appraisal of prophylactic drainage in uncomplicated liver resections: a systematic review and meta-analysis. *HPB (Oxford).* 2017;**19**(1):16–20.

22

Liver transplantation
General principles

Greg J. McKenna

Introduction

Liver transplantation is the widely accepted therapy for liver failure and complications associated with liver disease. What began in 1963 at the University of Colorado in the US as a controversial therapy for desperate patients with terminal liver failure has evolved over the decades into a successful procedure performed in almost 1200 transplant centres in more than 90 countries worldwide. Its increased application along with technical and pharmaceutical progress has helped survival at 1 year post transplant grow from 35% of recipients in 1978 to almost 95% of recipients 40 years later. The field continues to grow and in 2019, more than 35,000 liver transplants were performed worldwide.[1]

Pathophysiology of liver failure

The liver is complex, with a multitude of functions that include synthetic, metabolic, excretory, and immunoregulatory roles. Understanding the function of the liver and pathophysiology of liver injury allows for better managing liver failure and recognizing the role for liver transplantation in this disease (**Figure 22.1**).

Synthetic

The liver synthesizes many components including coagulation factors, albumin, and glucose (via gluconeogenesis). With the failure of synthetic function, liver failure can present as a coagulopathy as seen by an elevated international normalized ratio (INR), it can present as ascites, oedema, or anasarca due to decreased serum albumin, and can also present with severe hypoglycaemia in a setting of acute failure.

Metabolic

The liver metabolizes lactate converting it to pyruvate via the Cori cycle, and it deaminates amino acids via the ornithine cycle, converting the amine component into urea for excretion. The absence of these metabolic functions is why liver failure presents as metabolic acidosis from

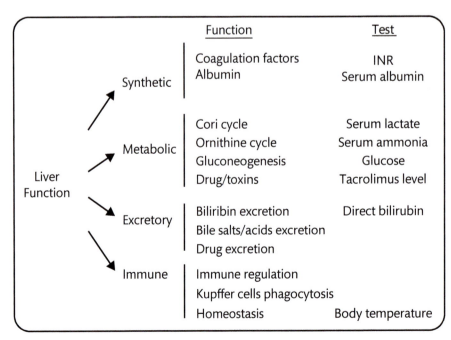

Figure 22.1 The liver has many functions, including synthetic, metabolic, excretory, and immunoregulatory roles. Various laboratory tests can be used to identify and track liver dysfunction.

an elevated serum lactate level, and also presents as encephalopathy from the hyperammonaemia and other unprocessed toxins.

Excretory

The liver clears bilirubin, and bile acids and it also removes detoxified drug products. In liver failure, excretory dysfunction can present clinically with jaundice due to the elevated serum bilirubin concentration that ultimately gets deposited in the skin.

Immunoregulatory

Immunoregulation is a key function of the liver. Hepatic macrophages called Kupffer cells (as well as dendritic cells and natural killer T cells) reside within the liver sinusoids, which are themselves lined by a fenestrated and very immunologically active layer of specialized endothelial cells, the liver sinusoidal endothelial cells (LSECs). The LSECs endocytose bacteria and foreign proteins coming from the portal system while Kupffer cells phagocytose bacteria and cellular components.[2] All of the non-parenchymal cells release cytokines and regulate an inflammatory response within the liver and immunomodulate throughout the body. When the liver fails, it alters the immune regulation function of the hepatic reticuloendothelial system, which leads to an increased risk of sepsis.[3]

During acute liver injury, the liver parenchymal cells replace necrotic and apoptotic cells through regeneration. However, when this injury is chronic, the regeneration process gradually fails and the wound healing mechanisms eventually replace healthy hepatocytes with nodular, fibrotic tissue resulting in cirrhosis. During this chronic injury, the LSECs lose their fenestration and become dysfunctional in a process called capillarization.[2] The LSECs lose the ability to regulate hepatic stellate cells and these cells become activated, differentiate into myofibroblasts, and produce an extracellular matrix in response to inflammatory cytokines.[2] The hepatic stellate cells along with the now activated Kupffer cells produce extracellular matrix and collagen resulting in hepatic fibrosis. The hepatic stellate cells also become contractile, which along with the fibrosis causes vasoconstriction which increases the intrahepatic vascular resistance. This leads to portal hypertension resulting in the ascites and variceal bleeding seen in advanced liver cirrhosis.[4] When fibrosis and intrahepatic resistance are significant enough to interfere with liver function, and when they cause these clinical manifestations of portal hypertension, a liver transplantation becomes necessary.

Candidate evaluation and selection

Following referral of a patient with liver disease to a transplant centre, a multidisciplinary evaluation is undertaken which typically has six steps and the whole process usually takes less than 1 week.

Indications

The first step is to identify those patients needing a liver transplant to survive, or having chronic cirrhosis with symptoms and complications of decompensation such as ascites, encephalopathy, variceal bleeding or the hepatorenal syndrome, which need a transplant.

Contraindications

The next step is to rule out any candidate with liver disease where the transplant will not improve long-term survival. Additionally, one needs to rule out patients having comorbid conditions that limit expected survival to an unacceptable level. This step includes a cardiac evaluation and stress test if cardiac risk factors are present, as well as a radiological screening to rule out any extrahepatic malignancies.

Screening

The goal of screening is to identify future risks related to immunosuppression. Because transplant patients require immunosuppression which can impact cancer and increase the risk of infection, candidates are screened for cancer risk using cross-sectional imaging as well as a colonoscopy, and in women specifically, a cervical smear (Pap test) and a mammogram.

Anatomical evaluation

Cross-sectional imaging is used to assess anatomy that might impact the transplant surgery, particularly vascular anatomy including portal vein thrombosis, collateral shunts, and calcifications and stenoses that might impact the inflow of the hepatic artery.

Psychiatric/social work assessment

Successful long-term allograft survival depends on recipient compliance with immunosuppression, as well as strong family social support. Psychiatric assessment evaluates compliance and the existence of substance abuse, and social work assessment helps determine available social supports as well as the impact of the future transplant on the recipient's social system.

Prioritization

Priority determines the need for a transplant. In the past, the waiting time was important in determining priority, but in the US since 2002, the Model for End-Stage Liver Disease (MELD) score has used an algorithm to determine 3-month mortality from three laboratory values (serum creatinine, total bilirubin, and INR), and this was further improved with the addition of serum sodium (Na) to yield the MELD-Na score. The algorithm produces a score from 6 to 40 that enables patients to be ranked based on mortality risk in an objective fashion, relatively free of bias, allowing the focus to be on patients most in need, regardless of waiting time. The goal is to transplant the patient most at risk of dying while on the waiting list.

Indications and contraindications

The current indications for liver transplant include irreversible hepatic failure from acute, subacute, and chronic causes, and this broad consideration is regardless of the specific aetiology of the liver disease.[5] In general, a potential recipient should have either (1) acute liver failure; (2) chronic decompensated cirrhosis with symptoms such as hepatic encephalopathy, variceal bleeding, ascites, or hepatorenal syndrome; (3) chronic liver disease with an increased mortality risk such as primary sclerosing cholangitis or inoperable liver tumours; or (4) a liver-based metabolic defect. To qualify for a liver transplant, the expected 1-year survival of a candidate should be less than 90% without a liver transplant being performed.[6]

The specific indications for liver transplant have changed significantly over the years. For decades, the most common indication for liver transplant was cirrhosis from hepatitis C virus (HCV), as well as alcoholic liver disease and chronic hepatitis B virus (HBV); however

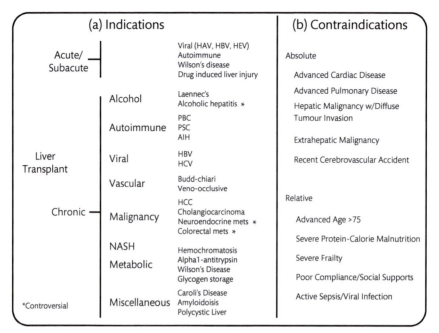

Figure 22.2 Liver failure is the main indication for a liver transplant and it can be classified as acute, subacute, and chronic. Many varied disease aetiologies can cause liver failure. The contraindications for liver transplant have changed markedly over the last five decades with few absolute contraindications remaining.

pharmacological innovations and socioeconomic demographic changes have dramatically shifted these indications.[7] Direct-acting antiviral HCV drugs have nearly eliminated HCV as an indication for transplantation in the US and Europe, decreasing from 34% of liver transplants in 2009 to 7.2% in 2019 in the US.[8] This decrease also coincided with a sharp rise in obesity with its associated non-alcoholic fatty liver disease, making non-alcoholic steatohepatitis (NASH) the sharpest increasing indication for transplant,[8] doubling from 14.6% of transplants in 2009 to 28.1% in 2019. At the same time, alcoholic liver disease has seen a similar marked increased indication for liver transplant from 18.1% in 2009 to 37.7% in 2019. The current indications for a liver transplant are outlined in Figure 22.2a.

The contraindications for liver transplant have similarly changed markedly over the last three decades, and many prior absolute contraindications in the past, like infections such as HIV and HBV as well as metastatic liver malignancies, are no longer contraindications today. As past absolute contraindications have evolved or else become more relative, the current absolute contraindications for liver transplant are (1) advanced cardiovascular disease, (2) hepatic malignancy with diffuse tumour invasion, (3) extrahepatic malignancy, and (4) recent cerebrovascular accident. The current contraindications for liver transplant are outlined in Figure 22.2b.

Liver malignancies have vacillated between being both indications and contraindications to liver transplant. Early experience with hepatocellular carcinoma (HCC) in the 1980s yielded high recurrence rates and poor 5-year survival, less than 35%, resulting in HCC being a contraindication to transplant.[9] Following the landmark 1996 study proposing the Milan criteria, HCC transplantation became indicated in patients with tumours having favourable features outlined in the Milan criteria and over the years these criteria have been expanded further to include larger HCCs with a worse prognosis.[10] Cholangiocarcinoma is the second most common liver tumour and it too was originally a contraindication to transplant due to poor survival. However in 2004, a protocol from the Mayo Clinic for liver transplant in a select population of patients with hilar cholangiocarcinoma, using neoadjuvant chemoradiotherapy prior to transplant, reported an improvement of the 5-year survival from 21% to 82%, and after further validation by other centres, selected hilar cholangiocarcinoma patients became accepted candidates for transplantation.[11,12] Similarly, transplant for intrahepatic cholangiocarcinoma (which represents 20% of all cholangiocarcinoma) was contraindicated given the historically poor long-term survival that ranged from 20% to 30%.[13] More recent research protocols for intrahepatic cholangiocarcinoma, using strict selection criteria of candidates based on tumour response to neoadjuvant chemoradiotherapy yielded excellent 5-year survival of up to 83% following liver transplant.[13,14] Finally, some metastatic liver tumours—long considered absolute contraindications—are now undergoing reconsideration as possible indications to liver transplant. Unresectable colorectal metastases have been transplanted in specific cases with a 5-year survival of 60%[13,15] and metastatic neuroendocrine tumours can have a 5-year survival of 90%[16] and both are being pushed as further expansions for indications for liver transplant.

Donor liver options

There are several different donor options for a liver allograft, and each has different benefits and risks. Donor liver allografts can come from both living donors and deceased donors.

Living donor liver transplantation

In living donation, a portion of a liver is resected and transplanted into the recipient, and either a right lobe or left lobe can be used, depending on the size of the lobe and size of the recipient.

Generally, the ratio of the donor graft weight to the recipient weight should be greater than 0.8% when selecting living donors and recipients.[17] Living donors make up 21% of liver transplants worldwide[1] and predominate in regions such as Asia where deceased donation options are limited. It affords the best statistical outcomes, and it allows for control over the timing of the transplant, to maximize recipient health status (see Chapter 24). These transplants are more technically difficult as the segment of the artery and bile duct are necessarily small and microvascular anastomotic techniques are used.

Deceased donor liver transplant

Deceased donor transplants use organs from donors that either meet 'brain death' criteria or from suitable donors who donate after cardiac death (DCD), with utilization of each type dependent on a country's local laws. For donation after brain death, the standard criteria donor is a healthy non-obese donor less than 60 years old, but donors meeting these criteria have become less common. Thus, increasing demand necessitates expansion of the acceptable criteria of donors after brain death to include elderly donors, HCV+ donors, and donors with increased liver steatosis, a group termed extended criteria donors. The use of extended criteria donor livers requires careful consideration of recipient factors, along with adjusting the surgical technique to minimize the implantation time, which enables a successful outcome. In some cases, a larger, good-quality standard criteria donor liver allograft can be divided into two separate lobes if two smaller recipients are available, and each lobe can be implanted into a separate recipient. With DCD liver donors, it is possible to significantly expand the donor pool given that the number of this donor type has the potential to be the most common; however these DCD allografts have an increased risk of graft failure from intrahepatic biliary strictures, termed ischaemic cholangiopathy, and are thus not suitable in every recipient.[18] Ischaemic cholangiopathy seen in DCD donors can be limited by reducing the ischaemia time of the donor allograft.

Organ allocation and priority

The increasing demand for liver transplants necessitates a priority and allocation strategy for donor allograft distribution, and because chronic liver disease is a life-threatening condition, allocation can be contentious; thus prioritization must be fair and equitable. In the US in 2002, the allocation protocols adopted the MELD score, a laboratory-based objective scoring system that uses three laboratory values (total bilirubin, serum creatinine, INR) to predict waiting list mortality in end-stage liver disease patients and subsequently prioritize patients based on that mortality risk (Figure 22.3). The MELD score was further refined in 2016 to incorporate a fourth lab value (sodium) resulting in the improved MELD-Na score, and work continues to improve the MELD score even further. In Europe there are no uniform allocation systems. Some countries use a centre-based allocation system based on clinical waiting time (e.g. Denmark, Finland, and Iceland), while other countries use a patient-directed allocation using the MELD score in conjunction with national allocation policies (e.g. Germany, Belgium, the Netherlands). Further European allocation systems include the Transplant Benefit Score (UK) made up of 28 donor and recipient variables, and the hybrid French Allocation Score (France) made up of donor and recipient variables as well as waiting time.[19] In Asia, there are very few deceased donor liver transplants performed; however, deceased donor allocation systems do exist including the patient-based Chinese Organ and Allocation Sharing System created in 2013,[20] as well as the MELD score used in Korea since 2016, and also a centre-directed allocation system used in India. When evaluating allocation systems as a whole, the goal of patient-directed allocation systems is to minimize the death of candidates while waiting for a liver transplant, focusing allocation on the greatest need. In contrast, centre-directed allocation systems opt to allocate transplants based on equal access for all candidates, and also strive to improve the overall efficiency of transplant outcomes.

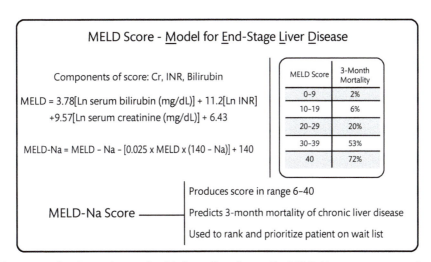

Figure 22.3 The MELD-Na score predicts 3-month mortality risk due to liver disease. The MELD-Na score uses a complex algorithm of four laboratory values to generate a score from 6 to 40 that is used to rank patients sequentially based on mortality risk. The goal is to identify those candidates most likely to die waiting for a liver transplant and prioritize those patients most in need.

Source: data from Wiesner R, et al. 'United Network for Organ Sharing Liver Disease Severity Score Committee. Model for end-stage liver disease (MELD) and allocation of donor livers', *Gastroenterology*. 2003 Jan;124(1):91–6; and OPTN/UNOS position paper, available from https://optn.transplant.hrsa.gov/media/1575/policynotice_20151101.pdf

Donor management

Selection

Donor quality has the greatest impact on allograft function, thus donor selection is important. The ideal deceased liver donor is one who was young, healthy, with no comorbid conditions, and no steatosis within the liver before death. However, improvements in trauma and critical care, and an ageing population, along with increased obesity with its concomitant metabolic syndrome and fatty liver disease, means the 'ideal donor' is rare, and more frequently the potential donors are older with more liver steatosis.[20] Both advanced donor age over 60 years and liver macrosteatosis greater than 30% decrease the tolerance of the donor liver to any ischaemia-reperfusion injury, and increases the risk of graft failure. The increased demand for donor organs necessitates consideration of these donor livers to increase supply making it paramount to have an effective donor allograft selection strategy. Several metrics have been devised to help describe and predict donor quality, including the Donor Risk Index (DRI) and the Eurotransplant Donor Risk Index (ET-DRI).[22] These metrics assess donor characteristics and recipient factors to predict donor organ quality and the impact on post-transplant outcomes.[23] The allografts classified as 'high risk' by these indexes are associated with an increased relative risk of allograft failure.[22]

Procurement

During a donor procurement a full laparotomy and sternotomy is performed through the midline. The potential donor allograft is assessed for quality including parenchymal fat content, fibrosis, and ischaemia, as well as assessment of the arterial vasculature. The intra-abdominal (and thoracic if necessary) structures are dissected and the retroperitoneum exposed using a Cattell–Braasch manoeuvre to visualize the vena cava and allow cannulation of the aorta. In a coordinated process between the donor operative teams, rapid cooling and delivery of an ice-cold high-potassium preservation fluid combined with rapid venous exsanguination is performed, allowing both arterial and portal venous flushing of the liver, all while the abdomen is filled with sterile ice. After complete flushing and cooling of the liver allograft the donor liver is expeditiously procured by dividing the ligament supports of the liver (falciform, left triangular, right triangular, and gastrohepatic ligaments). The common hepatic artery is identified and dissected completely to the coeliac artery and divided at the aorta, taking care to identify and avoid injury to any anatomical hepatic artery variants. The bile duct is isolated above the pancreas and divided, and the bile duct then flushed with iced saline. The portal vein is dissected up to behind the level of the pancreas and divided at the superior mesenteric vein and splenic vein confluence, and the infrahepatic and suprahepatic inferior vena cava are divided. The liver is extracted and placed on ice.

Preservation

Upon removal, the donor liver allograft must be quickly preserved and stored for transport from the site of the donor procurement to the recipient transplant centre. A 4°C ice-cold storage environment is used to slow the metabolic processes and cell breakdown within the liver allograft. The liver is stored in a high osmolality electrolyte solution which mimics the intracellular environment, limits cellular swelling, and prevents cold-induced cellular injury. High-potassium preservation solutions such as the University of Wisconsin solution and histidine–tryptophan–ketoglutarate solution are used for prolonged cold storage of allograft and have enabled a longer preservation time that allow procurements from longer distances.[24] More recently, machine perfusion systems have been developed using either hypothermic or normothermic perfusion fluids which allow prolonged storage and *ex situ* manipulation of the allograft prior to implantation of the allograft into the recipient.[25]

Liver transplant surgical procedure

Opening

Back table allograft preparation

Prior to the procedure, the donor allograft liver is removed from its cold storage, placed on sterile ice, and inspected on a back table in the recipient operating room. The fat and other residual tissue surrounding the liver allograft is cleared, and the donor liver vessels are dissected free from surrounding tissue to facilitate a quick implantation. The liver allograft is stored in University of Wisconsin solution in an ice slush for later implantation.

Incision

The recipient liver transplant incision is a right-sided subcostal incision with midline vertical extension ('L-shaped' or 'hockey-stick' incision). An alternative option is a bilateral subcostal incision, with a midline extension ('Mercedes-type' incision).

Retractor

The are many retractor options, but the Thompson retractor is preferable because the upper bars provide excellent diaphragmatic and suprahepatic exposure while the lower bars provide strong intestinal retraction to expose the hilum and infrahepatic inferior vena cava.

Hepatectomy

Initial exposure

The four hepatic ligaments are divided: (1) falciform ligament, which mobilizes the liver from the midline; (2) left triangular ligament, to mobilize the left lobe of the liver; (3) right triangular ligament, to mobilize the right lobe of the liver; and (4) gastrohepatic ligament, to separate the stomach from the liver.

Hilar dissection

With the liver retracted cephalad, the left and right branches of the hepatic artery are dissected and divided. The cystic duct is divided, which allows subsequent division of the common hepatic duct high in the hilum. The portal vein is isolated, dissected, and skeletonized circumferentially from the top of the pancreas up to the portal vein bifurcation (it is not divided at this point).

Hepatectomy/implantation

Following the hilar dissection there are two options for the hepatectomy and implantation, the caval replacement technique[26] and the piggyback technique[27,28] (**Figure 22.4**).

Liver transplant surgical procedure

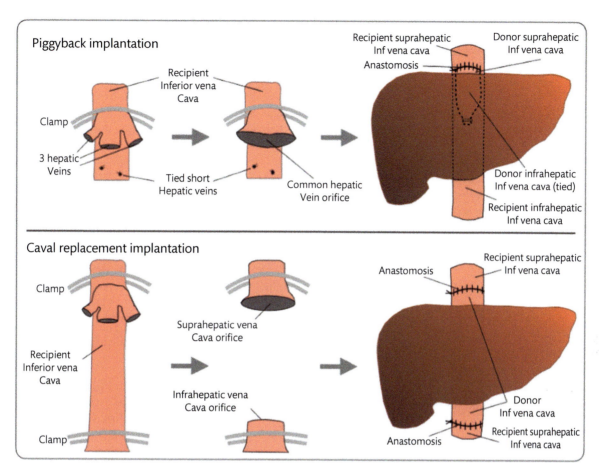

Figure 22.4 There are two options for implantation of a liver during a liver transplant—piggyback implantation and caval replacement implantation. The decision for each type is usually based on clinical parameters such as intraoperative haemodynamic stability, presence of portosystemic collaterals, size of donor allograft, and size/body habitus of recipient.

Option 1—caval replacement

The lateral margins of the infrahepatic inferior vena cava are dissected from the peritoneum bilaterally, dividing the right adrenal vein. This dissection is continued bilaterally from the immediately suprarenal inferior vena cava up to the suprahepatic inferior vena cava as it enters the diaphragm, and the retrocaval tissue is divided along its length to facilitate later vena cava clamp placement. The portal vein is clamped proximally and divided distally and the inferior vena cava clamped both below and above the liver. The inferior vena cava is then divided to allow removal of the liver along with its corresponding vena cava segment. The donor liver is removed from cold storage and brought onto the surgical field, and the donor liver suprahepatic vena cava is anastomosed end-to-end with the recipient suprahepatic vena cava using a running 4-0 Prolene suture. The donor liver infrahepatic vena cava is anastomosed end-to-end to the recipient infrahepatic vena cava with a running 4-0 Prolene suture. The portal veins of both the donor liver and recipient are shortened to avoid kinking and anastomosed end-to-end with a running 6-0 Prolene suture. The clamps are removed sequentially, first the suprahepatic clamp, next the infrahepatic clamp, and finally the portal vein clamp to reperfuse the liver. The reperfusion is done slowly to avoid a sudden rush to the heart of cold, acidotic blood from the new liver.

Option 2—piggyback technique

The liver is dissected off the inferior vena cava ligating the short hepatic veins that are between the liver and inferior vena cava, leaving the adrenal gland untouched. This dissection is taken up to the level of the hepatic veins. The portal vein is clamped and divided distally, the three hepatic veins are clamped distally on the inferior vena cava (leaving the inferior vena cava itself intact and patent and maintaining blood return to the heart), and the liver is removed. The bridges of the hepatic veins are divided to create one common orifice, and this hepatic vein orifice is anastomosed to the donor liver suprahepatic vena cava end-to-end with a running Prolene. The infrahepatic vena cava is ligated. The portal veins of both the donor liver and recipient are shortened and anastomosed end-to-end with a running 6-0 Prolene suture. The clamps are removed sequentially, first the suprahepatic clamp, next the infrahepatic clamp, and finally the portal vein clamp to reperfuse the liver. The reperfusion is done slowly to avoid a sudden rush to the heart of cold, acidotic blood from the new liver.

Hepatic artery and bile duct

Hepatic artery

The recipient proper hepatic artery is anastomosed end-to-end to the donor liver proper hepatic artery with a running 7-0 Prolene suture under magnification. (Note: if the donor liver has a replaced left hepatic artery variant anatomy, the donor anastomosis is at the coeliac axis.) The clamps are removed and the arterial flow in the liver is reperfused.

Bile duct

The donor bile duct is probed to define bifurcations, and the duct is divided above the cystic duct to shorten it, removing the cystic duct. There are two options for the biliary anastomosis. The most common, involving more than 80% of cases is the duct-to-duct anastomosis where the donor hepatic duct is anastomosed to the recipient hepatic duct end-to-end with 6-0 polydioxanone (PDS) sutures. The second option is a Roux-en-Y-hepaticojejunostomy, where a Roux limb is created from the jejunum and passed retrocolic and retrogastric to the donor hilum and a small jejunostomy is anastomosed to the donor duct with 6-0 PDS sutures.

Closure

Meticulous haemostasis is performed to ensure there is no bleeding from the retroperitoneum bare areas, nor from each of the anastomoses. The retractors are removed, and with the liver in its natural space, the hepatic artery and portal vein are inspected to ensure no kinking is present. The incision is closed in two layers laterally and one layer in the midline with 1-0 Prolene sutures, and the skin reapproximated with clips. The patient is brought to the intensive care unit postoperatively.

Complications

Liver transplantation is a complex surgery and complications are expected, in part because most organ allocation systems prioritize the sickest (and typically most debilitated) patients, because the transplanted allograft is of variable size and anatomy in relation to the recipient, and because the recipient must receive immunosuppression which limits wound healing and increases the infection risks in the recipient. The key to improving outcomes and reducing mortality following liver transplant involves effectively managing these complications.

Early detection of any complication is essential, and the clinical presentation for most are often non-specific, thus regular laboratory tests are the key for directing diagnostics and management (Figure 22.5). The liver enzymes aspartate transaminase and alanine transaminase identify hepatocyte breakdown as found in rejection, ischaemia, and viral infection, and alkaline phosphatase identifies biliary epithelium inflammation due to rejection or bile duct obstruction. Liver function tests such as INR, bilirubin, and lactate identify a component of liver function that is failing. Any elevated liver enzymes or liver function tests direct further diagnostic studies, such as a duplex ultrasound scan, or a liver biopsy. The results of these studies direct further diagnostics to identify the complication and subsequent management.

Allograft/parenchymal complications

Primary non-function (PNF)

PNF is a severe graft dysfunction related to ischaemia-reperfusion injury, and while the incidence has declined over the years, PNF is still the most feared post-transplant complication. Risk factors include a marginal donor allograft with high macrosteatosis,[29] advanced donor age, unstable donor, and prolonged allograft ischaemia, all of which render the liver more susceptible to ischaemia-reperfusion injury resulting in cell death and apoptosis.[30,31] Despite increased demand that necessitates the use of marginal organs, transplant centres have reduced the incidence of

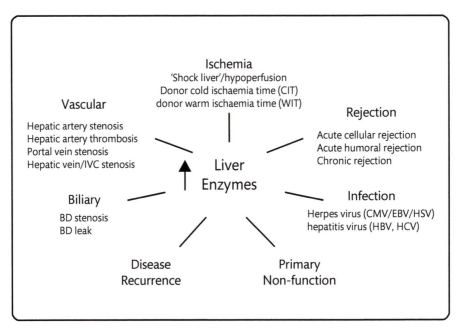

Figure 22.5 Most complications following a liver transplant result in elevations of the liver enzymes because anything that causes hepatocyte breakdown or loss, or biliary epithelial injury causes increases in the liver enzymes released into the bloodstream. Elevated liver enzymes are an excellent screening tool to initiate and guide further diagnostic tests and subsequent therapies. BD, bile duct; CMV, cytomegalovirus; HSV, herpes simplex virus.

PNF by adjusting practices to shorten ischaemia times, and optimizing recipient matching to mitigate the risk. PNF presents as a 'toxic liver syndrome' from a necrolysing liver, with hypoglycaemia, metabolic acidosis, coagulopathy, encephalopathy, hypothermia, and renal failure. PNF necessitates urgent retransplantation and management requires intensive care unit support with pressors, mechanical ventilation, and haemodialysis until the patient can be retransplanted. Even with retransplantation the 90-day mortality for PNF ranges from 54% to 73%.[31,32]

Vascular complication

Hepatic artery

Hepatic artery complications occur in 15% of recipients and are a major cause of mortality and graft loss. They are typically diagnosed by duplex ultrasound or angiography. Although 70% of the blood supply to the liver is from the portal vein, the sole blood supply to the biliary tree is via the hepatic artery, thus any complications of the hepatic artery have a profound impact on the bile ducts leading to strictures, necrosis, liver abscesses, and allograft dysfunction. Hepatic artery thrombosis (HAT) occurs in 1–9% of recipients[33–35] and risk factors for HAT include anastomotic technique errors, kinking, prolonged allograft ischaemia, and cytomegalovirus infection. The overall prognosis and management strategy is based on the timing of the HAT in relation to the transplant. HAT within the first month post transplant is defined as early, it makes up 30% of cases and carries a 30% mortality risk.

While early HAT typically requires retransplant, up to 15% can be treated through early revascularization by thrombectomy and thrombolysis. The remaining 70% of cases are defined as late and occur months to years post transplant. Because late HAT can occur in a setting of arterial collateralization, the presentation is often asymptomatic; however, biliary manifestations are still common. Management of late HAT involves treating any biliary strictures or hepatic abscesses that may result. HAT is a major cause graft loss with graft survival reported at 52% at 1 year and 27% at 5 years following the thrombosis.[35]

Other hepatic artery complications include stenosis which occurs in 2–13% of patients[36] and presents as elevated liver enzymes, and biliary complication such as biliary strictures and hepatic abscesses. Hepatic artery pseudoaneurysms occur in 1–2% of patients.[37] They typically arise near the anastomosis and are often due to mycotic infections, and while many are asymptomatic, they can present as abdominal pain. Outcomes for pseudoaneurysms are serious, with a mortality rate of 53% in those that rupture.[38] Both stenosis and pseudoaneurysms are resolved by either surgical revision using a donor iliac artery conduit, or venous interposition graft, or through endovascular stenting (Figure 22.6).[36]

Portal vein

Portal vein complications are much less frequent than arterial complications, occurring in 1–3% of recipients, but they are associated with high morbidity and risk of graft loss.[39] They are typically

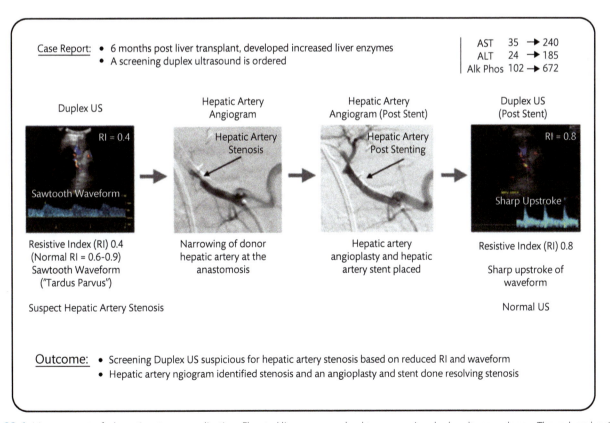

Figure 22.6 Management of a hepatic artery complication. Elevated liver enzymes lead to a screening duplex ultrasound scan. The reduced resistive index (RI) of 0.4 and the flattened sawtooth pattern of the duplex waveform ('tardus parvus waveform') are suspicious for a hepatic artery stenosis. The diagnosis is confirmed with a hepatic artery angiogram and it is treated with angioplasty and stenting of the hepatic artery. The success of the procedure is verified by a post-procedure duplex ultrasound scan which shows a normal waveform with a normal RI in the range of 0.6–0.9. If the endovascular stenting was unsuccessful, this stenosis would be managed with a surgical revision of the artery.

diagnosed by duplex ultrasound or computed tomography angiography. Portal vein thrombosis (PVT) occurs in 0.5–2% of patients and the clinical presentation depends on the timing. Early thrombosis is more frequent and results in gastrointestinal and variceal bleeding, ascites, severe allograft dysfunction, and graft failure. The presentation for late thrombosis depends on the extent of collateral circulation and presents as ascites, varices, and only rarely as graft failure. Risk factor for PVT includes anastomotic technique complications, kinking, stenosis, a small diameter portal vein, significant portosystemic collaterals, and portal vein reconstructions. For PVT in the first 72 hours, emergent surgical revision of the anastomosis is necessary to correct any kink, redundancy, or twist, and to thrombectomize and thombolyse any clot. If this is unsuccessful in re-establishing flow, retransplantation is necessary. Other PVTs occurring later in the first 30 days can also be managed using endovascular thrombectomy, thrombolysis, and stent placement. Late PVTs after the first 30 days that are symptomatic can be treated with systemic anticoagulation, stenting, or a transjugular intrahepatic portosystemic shunt.

Portal vein stenosis occurs most commonly at the anastomosis, affects less than 3% of recipients, and presents with findings consistent with portal hypertension including ascites, splenomegaly, and varices.[40] If found early, the stenosis can be treated with surgical revision of the anastomosis, otherwise interventional radiology including balloon dilation and portal vein stent placement are reported with success rates of 78%.[41–43]

Hepatic vein/vena cava

Liver allograft outflow obstruction through the hepatic veins can happen from kinking, stenosis, or thrombosis of the hepatic veins or the distal inferior vena cava, occurring in approximately 3% of patients.[44] It typically presents as ascites, lower limb oedema, hepatomegaly, and rarely the Budd–Chiari syndrome, and can sometimes progress to graft failure. Outflow obstruction results from anastomotic technique errors which lead to kinking or twisting and eventually to thrombosis. Hepatic vein outflow obstruction is more common in living donor transplants since the venous outflow orifice is smaller, and the partial segment size lends to twisting. Diagnosis is made with duplex ultrasound and is confirmed with a venogram combined with anastomotic pressure gradient measurements. Surgical revision of both hepatic vein and caval complications is rarely possible and endovascular approaches are the mainstay. Balloon dilation of the stenosis is nearly 100% successful, but the stenosis typically recurs necessitating serial dilations. Endovascular stent placement success is reported at 73–100%,[45] but this option is sometimes limited because of the stent potentially blocking nearby hepatic vein orifices. Retransplantation in this setting has a high mortality risk and therefore is a last resort. Caval stenosis can be avoided by using a piggyback implantation technique; however, implantation using as an orifice the confluence of the recipient hepatic vein can sometimes lead to hepatic vein obstruction and as such a side-to-side cavocavostomy has the lowest risk of outflow obstruction.[46]

Biliary complications

Bile duct complications are the most common post-transplant complication occurring in 5–30% of recipients, and they are a major source of morbidity in liver transplant recipients. The most common biliary complications are strictures and leaks, and an important element in the pathophysiology, as well as what guides the potential diagnostic studies, is the type of biliary reconstruction, either duct-to-duct anastomosis, or a Roux-en-Y hepaticojejunostomy.

Biliary strictures

Biliary strictures occur in up to 15% of liver recipients from weeks to years post transplant and presents as elevated liver enzymes (particularly alkaline phosphatase and bilirubin) and fever. Biliary strictures are classified as either anastomotic or non-anastomotic. Anastomotic strictures occur where the donor bile duct attaches to the recipient, and are usually caused by anastomotic technique factors, ischaemia, and rejection. The treatment is balloon dilation and stent placement, performed either endoscopically through endoscopic retrograde cholangiopancreatography or transheptically via percutaneous transhepatic cholangiography, progressively dilating with larger stents every 2 months on average for up to a year. This approach has a 75% success rate and those refractory to dilation are treated with surgical revision to a Roux-en-Y hepaticojejunostomy.[47] Non-anastomotic strictures are typically multiple, diffuse, and intrahepatic, and are caused by ischaemia such as from hepatic artery complications or prolonged warm and cold ischaemia of the donor allograft, or autoimmune causes such as primary sclerosing cholangitis.[48] Management is like anastomotic strictures, with biliary dilation and stent placement; however, it is more difficult due to the diffuse multiple nature and the location of the strictures within the liver, which precludes a surgical option and necessitates retransplantation.

Biliary leak

Biliary leaks occur in 2–20% of liver recipients and typically present in the days and weeks from transplant, with abdominal pain, fever, peritonitis, and elevated serum bilirubin level. Biliary leaks are related to anastomotic technique factors, tension on the anastomosis, distal obstruction, and ischaemic injury. Treatment is diversion of the bile via stents placed endoscopically by endoscopic retrograde cholangiopancreatography or transhepatic internal–external biliary diversion by percutaneous transhepatic cholangiography, in conjunction with percutaneous drainage of the leaked bile. This non-operative approach is successful in up to 85% of cases[49] and those not amenable to drainage are subsequently managed with surgical revision with a Roux-en-Y hepaticojejunostomy.

Immunological complications

Post-transplant lymphoproliferative disorder (PTLD)

PTLD is a B-cell proliferation that is initially promoted by an Epstein–Barr virus (EBV) infection, and results in an uncontrolled proliferation because immunosuppression inhibits the normal T-cell regulation of B-cell proliferation. Over time, these overproliferating B cells can develop mutations that make them malignant leading to a lymphoma.[50] PTLD is the second most common post-transplant malignancy. Initially PTLD is treated by ceasing immunosuppression and returning T-cell regulation. Rituximab, a monoclonal antibody that binds to CD-20 ligands found on B cells, depletes the proliferating B cells.[51] For more advanced malignancies, chemotherapy is needed and these have a worse prognosis.

Graft-versus-host disease

Graft-versus-host disease is a rare complication of liver transplant, affecting 0.1–2% of recipients, but is important because of its significant mortality exceeding 75%.[52,53] Graft-versus-host disease occurs when donor lymphocytes, which are transiting within the liver allograft, recognize recipient antigen as foreign and subsequently react. The disease presents as rash, diarrhoea, fever, and severe pancytopenia. This is problematic since these symptoms are non-specific and easily dismissed as drug side effects or other similarly benign explanations, which can delay diagnosis. Risk factors for graft-versus-host disease include close human leucocyte antigen matching between the recipient and donor, as well as a wide age discrepancy between a younger donor and older recipient. Diagnosis is made by the presence of donor lymphocyte chimerism of greater than 1% and given that survival is rare, there must be a high index of suspicion with these symptoms and therapy should be initiated upon suspicion since the confirmation chimerism studies can take time.[54] There is no consensus as to the best therapy, with some advocating withdrawing the immunosuppression to induce rejection while others advocate providing overimmunosuppression with steroids, interleukin (IL)-2 antagonists, and tumour necrosis factor-alpha inhibitors.[54,55]

Rejection

Acute rejection

Acute cellular rejection occurs in 15–25% of patients[56,57] with the majority occurring in the first 3 months post transplant. It occurs when recipient T cells recognize donor alloantigens[58] and induce a cytopathic immune response within donor tissue, with infiltration of the tissue by T cells and allograft dysfunction. This leads to cell breakdown and release of liver enzymes in the bloodstream, which heralds the rejection in the routine surveillance bloodwork. The gold standard for diagnosis is a percutaneous liver biopsy,[59] but newer technology includes biomarkers like circulating microRNAs. Treatment is with high-dose corticosteroids and increased maintenance immunosuppression. In approximately 10% of cases, the rejection is resistant to steroids and requires treatment with the T-cell-depleting polyclonal antibody antithymocyte globulin.

Chronic rejection

Chronic rejection is a progressive cholestatic disease that can lead to graft loss and typically develops months to years post transplant. It was more common in the past with ciclosporin-based maintenance immunosuppression but has decreased with tacrolimus-based immunosuppression[60] and has an incidence of 2–3%.[61,62] Chronic rejection is characterized on liver biopsy by bile duct loss ('vanishing duct syndrome') and intimal thickening and occlusion of the arteries ('obliterative arteriopathy').[63] While chronic rejection is more common in patients having multiple and severe acute cellular rejection episodes,[63] current evidence indicates a role for donor human leucocyte antigen-specific antibodies in chronic rejection.[64] Treatment is with increased immunosuppression and it can sometimes be reversible; however, retransplantation is needed in those who do not respond to therapy.

Infection

Infections are the most common post-transplant complication involving two-thirds of recipients in the first year post transplant, and this is because transplant candidates have significant underlying comorbidities and are also immunosuppressed. Bacterial infections occur most commonly in the first 2 months post transplant and stem from the complex nature of the transplant surgery, combined with the deconditioned state seen in many recipients. Most of these bacterial infections occur within the abdomen or in the biliary tree, but also include pneumonias and wound infections. There is increased incidence of viral and fungal infections because of the impact of immunosuppression and many occur because the patient is relatively over-immunosuppressed and/or malnourished. The incidence of post-transplant fungal infections is reported as 7–42% with *Candida* and *Aspergillus* species being the most common. Prophylaxis is routinely given in liver transplant recipients with antiviral agents such as valganciclovir given to prevent common viral infections such as cytomegalovirus and EBV, while prophylaxis for fungal infection typically uses nystatin for preventing *Candida* infection.[65]

Disease recurrence

In the past, disease recurrence was the primary cause of long-term allograft failure, notably from recurrent HCV and HBV; however, the development of antiviral therapies particularly for HCV has dramatically reduced this complication of disease recurrence. Recurrence of autoimmune liver diseases following liver transplant is common, occurring in 15–50% of liver recipients, with reports of recurrence ranging from 8% to 25% for autoimmune hepatitis (AIH), 10% to 34% for primary biliary cirrhosis, and 10% to 38% for primary sclerosing cholangitis.[66] Treatment of autoimmune disease recurrence involves increasing immunosuppression, adding or increasing corticosteroids, and, in the case of primary biliary cirrhosis, the addition of ursodeoxycholic acid. In addition, for recurrent primary sclerosing cholangitis, treatment of recurrence may involve dilation and stenting of isolated biliary strictures. While recurrent HCV is now practically eliminated, the rising incidence of NASH as an indication for transplant has also seen a marked rise in recurrence of fatty liver disease and NASH post transplant. Recurrent non-alcoholic fatty liver disease occurs in 70% of recipients transplanted for NASH, with 25–40% as recurrent NASH and 18–25% of patients with advanced fibrosis.[67,68] Risk factors for recurrence of NASH include lifestyle habits, metabolic syndrome, weight gain, genetics, and immunosuppression, and treatment involves managing the various risk factors.[69] In addition, much research has been directed towards future NASH pharmacological therapies, and the pipeline has many medications including anti-inflammatory and antifibrotic agents as well as lipogenesis inhibitors and intestinal microbiome manipulation options[70] that may work to limit disease recurrence from NASH.

Immunosuppression

The purpose of immunosuppression in liver transplantation is to inhibit the host alloimmune response to donor allograft antigens, and prevent rejection of the newly transplanted liver. The normal alloimmune response is a multistep cascade of cellular pathways leading to the activation and proliferation of T cells that have specificity to a particular foreign antigen (in the case of liver transplant, to the donor allograft antigens). The alloimmune response is defined in the 'three-signal model' which is a general outline to

CHAPTER 22 Principles and techniques of liver resection

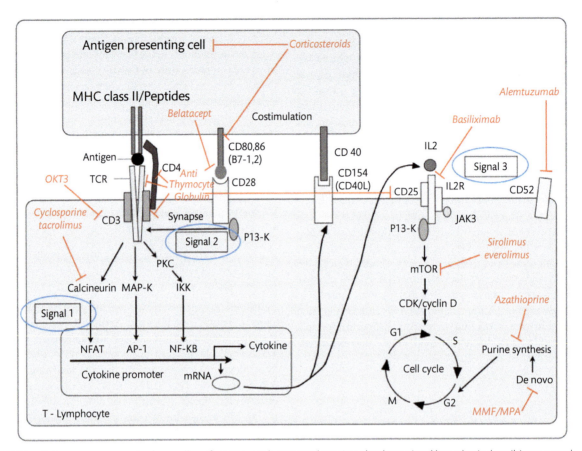

Figure 22.7 The alloimmune response to donor allograft antigens in liver transplantation, the three-signal hypothesis describing a complex multistep cascade that outlines the host response that leads to acute rejection. The various immunosuppression drugs act at various steps of the cascades to prevent T-cell proliferation. CDK, cyclin-dependent kinase; IL-2, interleukin 2; IL-2R, IL-2 receptor; JAK3, tyrosine kinase in signal transduction pathways; MHC, major histocompatibility complex; mRNA, messenger RNA; NFAT, AP-1, NF-kB, transcription factors; OKT3, the first monoclonal antibody created, used historically for rejection prophylaxis but has been discontinued; PI3-K, phosphoinositide 3-kinase, signal transducer enzyme; PKC, MAP-K, IkK, protein kinases in signal transduction pathways.
Reproduced with permission from McKenna G.J. et al. (2015) Chapter 91 'Induction and Maintenance of Immunosuppression', pp.1264–88, Fig. 91.1. In Busuttil R.W. & Klintmalm G.B. (2015) *Transplantation of the Liver*, 3rd Edition, Elsevier. Originally adapted from Hunt S.A. & Haddad F., 'The Changing Face of Heart Transplantation', *Journal of the American College of Cardiology*, Volume 52, Issue 8, 2008, pp.587–98, Fig 2.

simplify and describe what we realize now is a complex and overlapping interplay of signals (**Figure 22.7**). In this three-signal model, the antigen-presenting cell (APC) phagocytoses and subsumes foreign antigen, then displays and presents the antigen to the T cell where it binds the T-cell receptor (TCR). TCR binding triggers a cellular pathway cascade that leads to calcineurin activation which in turn triggers transcription factors in the nucleus to express genes for various cytokines including IL-2. This T-cell activation is termed 'signal 1', and for it to happen it also needs a concomitant 'signal 2' to occur, in which costimulatory molecules on T cells (i.e. CD28) bind their associated ligands on APCs (i.e. CD80) to activate kinases that in turn enhance the signal 1 cascade.[71] The cytokines released following activation in signal 1, particularly IL-2, binds the IL-2 receptor which is 'signal 3', and this binding activates the JAK–STAT signal transduction and also the mammalian target of rapamycin (mTOR) signal transduction pathway that controls the cell cycle through factors called cyclins.[72] These cyclins regulate the cell cycle to initiate mitosis and cell division which leads to proliferation of the T cells that have specific activity against the initial foreign antigen presented.

There are several classes of immunosuppression drugs, each of which acts on a different signal in the alloimmune response three-signal model:

Calcineurin inhibitors

Calcineurin inhibitors (CNIs) such as tacrolimus and ciclosporin are the mainstay of liver transplant immunosuppression and effect via signal 1. CNIs block TCR-mediated T-cell activation by inhibiting calcineurin, which ultimately inhibits the downstream transcription of cytokines like IL-2. CNIs have significant side effects and toxicities which are the downside of their long-term use, the most significant being their nephrotoxicity and neurotoxicity.[73]

Antimetabolites

This class of immunosuppressants include azathioprine and mycophenolate and block signal 3. They interfere with the synthesis of purines, a substrate that is needed for DNA synthesis and the cell cycle, and this ultimately blocks the lymphocyte proliferation that is necessary for an alloimmune response.[74] Unlike CNIs, the antimetabolites do not have any nephrotoxicity and the main side effects are cytopenias and gastrointestinal symptoms, particularly in the case of mycophenolate.

mTOR inhibitors

Sirolimus and everolimus are inhibitors of the mTOR complex and block the mTOR signal pathway which is part of signal 3. Normally the mTOR pathway controls homeostasis, adjusting cellular growth and cellular proliferation in response to local cellular conditions and nutrients.[75] The side effect profile reflects the numerous downstream effects of the complex mTOR pathway, and it includes impacts on wound healing, fibrosis, and cytopenias.[76,77]

Costimulatory molecules

The fusion protein belatacept is designed to mimic the CD28 ligand found on T cells, and this mimic binds the costimulatory molecule CD80 on APCs. This blockade prevents costimulatory molecule binding, blocking signal 2 and subsequently limits signal 1 pathway transduction. When a TCR is activated without co-stimulation due to this blockade, it also induces anergy or apoptosis of the T cell, further suppressing the alloimmune response.[78] Belatacept does not have the nephrotoxicity or cytopenias of other immunosuppressants but has viral-associated complications including PTLD in EBV− patients who later develop EBV, and an increased risk of JC virus infection that can cause a serious demyelinating disease called progressive multifocal leucoencephalopathy.[79]

Corticosteroids

As an original immunosuppressant, and still widely in use, corticosteroids have a role in both induction and maintenance immunosuppression for prophylaxis of rejection, as well as bolus therapy for treating an established rejection. Corticosteroids have a myriad of effects on all cells of the immune system and blocks signals 1, 2, and 3 of the alloimmune response.[80] They bind the glucocorticoid receptor within lymphocytes then pass into the nucleus and alter transcription of many inflammatory cytokines including IL-1 and IL-2, blocking cell division and lymphocyte proliferation.[81] Corticosteroids decrease B-cell levels and circulating T cells while also impacting T-cell differentiation. They also interfere with costimulatory molecule binding at CD80 on the APC and attenuate the costimulatory pathway.[82] The broad side effect profile of steroids limits their use in liver transplantation, including weight gain, diabetes, osteoporosis, hypertension, hyperlipidaemia, cataracts, acne, and altered wound healing. These side effects are why modern immunosuppression protocols are moving to steroid-free regimens, despite the effectiveness of steroids.

Biological anti-T-cell therapy

Several biological therapies exist that inhibit T-cell proliferation. Antithymocyte globulin is a polyclonal antibody that binds various ligands on T cells and B cells and blocks signals 1, 2, and 3 of the alloimmune response, with its main action to deplete T cells.[83] Alemtuzumab is a monoclonal antibody that binds CD-52 and depletes T cells, blocking signals 1 and 3.[84] Basiliximab is a chimeric antibody that binds the IL-2 receptor and blocks signal 3 of the alloimmune response and is a non-depleting antibody leaving the T-cell population intact.[85]

In the last five decades, few aspects of transplantation have evolved as much as immunosuppression, which has been the key to the field's success. There were few pharmacological immunosuppression options in the 1960s and 1970s and azathioprine and steroids were the choices—even radiation treatments and prophylactic splenectomy were tried in the hopes of augmenting these drugs. Acute rejection was a major cause of liver allograft failure, and 1-year survival peaked at 35% in 1978. However in 1979, a new drug called cyclosporine (now with the international non-proprietary name ciclosporin)—the first CNI—was introduced by Dr Roy Calne and by 1980, the 1-year survival jumped remarkably from 35% to almost 90%.[86,87] For the decades to follow, absolute avoidance of rejection using CNI became the focus; however, this myopic approach resulted in excellent short-term graft survival, but with long-term renal dysfunction from CNI nephrotoxicity affecting 40% of recipients at 5 years.[88] A large study from the Scientific Registry of Transplant Recipients (SRTR) of 36,849 liver recipients described 26% having stage 4 or worse chronic kidney disease with a glomerular filtration rate less than 30 mL/min at 10 years post transplant.[89] This chronic kidney disease has a major impact on long-term survival, and post-transplant renal dysfunction became the leading predictor of long-term mortality following liver transplant.[90]

Today, the goal of immunosuppression has evolved further to where it is no longer focused on absolute avoidance of rejection, but rather merely an intent to minimize rejection, and instead the primary focus is on avoiding nephrotoxicity and infections over the long term from overimmunosuppression. Immunosuppression strategies can be broadly divided into two phases, induction immunosuppression, and maintenance immunosuppression. Induction uses either corticosteroids, or an anti-T-cell antibody such as antithymocyte globulin or basiliximab to front-load immunosuppression, which allows avoiding higher doses of nephrotoxic CNIs. The maintenance phase of immunosuppression uses a CNI, in combination with a second agent like an antiproliferative such as mycophenolate or an mTOR inhibitor such as sirolimus, to minimize the CNI dosing. Over time, the long-term goal is a steady minimization of the CNI to the point where it can be discontinued, which is possible because the risk of rejection becomes much lower over time. Future immunosuppression strategies are likely to incorporate costimulatory blockade with using fusion protein biological therapies such as belatacept, to avoid CNIs from early on, suppressing the alloimmune response with minimal nephrotoxicity.

Outcomes

Improvements in surgical techniques, operative anaesthesia, post-transplant intensive care unit support, and the prevention and management of transplant complications, as well as pharmacological developments and an improved understanding of proper immunosuppression have enabled a steady improvement of both short-term and long-term successful outcomes. In the US, the most recent outcome data reported from the SRTR describe graft survival in deceased donor liver transplants at 1 year, 3 years, 5 years, and 10 years of 91.1%, 84.8%, 78.4%, and 57.4%, respectively, and the graft survival of living donor liver transplants were even better at 92.9%, 86.2%, 76.3%, and 67.9%, respectively.[57] Patient survival is similarly very good for both short- and long-term outcomes with patient survival at 1 year, 3 years, 5 years, and 10 years of 92.6%, 86.9%, 81.3%, and 60.5%, respectively[57] (Figure 22.8).

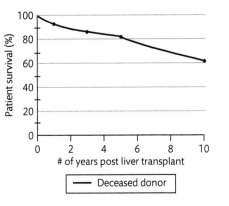
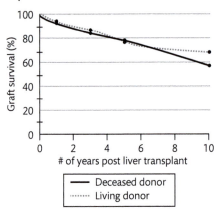

Figure 22.8 Liver transplant patient and graft survival outcomes in the US in 2019.
Source: data from Kwong AJ et al. OPTN/SRTR 2019 annual data report: liver. *Am J Transpl.* 2021;21(S2):208–315.

Future directions

Liver transplantation has evolved to become a standard procedure performed hundreds of times daily worldwide, with excellent surgical outcomes achieved. Despite the success so far, the field has two future goals. First, the successful management of recipients involves identifying and minimizing the post-transplant complications that impact long-term survival. Continued research and development of personalized biological-based immunosuppression options offers the hope of tailoring it to avoid the unwanted side effects and toxicities that impact survival. Second, the relentless increased demand for donor organs means a continued effort to expand a constrained supply. In the near term, that will mean further increasing living donation, and utilizing more extended criteria and DCD donors. However rapidly progressing stem cell, gene-editing, and three-dimensional printing technology means artificial donor livers may solve this supply issue in the future. Liver transplantation will continue to impact surgery and medicine going forward.

REFERENCES

1. Global Observatory on Donation and Transplantation. Homepage. n.d. http://www.transplant-observatory.org
2. Khanam A, Saleeb PG, Kottill S. Pathophysiology and treatment options for hepatic fibrosis: can it be completely cured? *Cells.* 2021;**10**(5):1097.
3. Poisson J, Lemoinne S, Boulanger C, et al. Liver sinusoidal endothelial cells: physiology and role in liver disease. *J Hepatol.* 2017;**66**(1):212–227.
4. Iwakiri Y. Pathophysiology of portal hypertension. *Clin Liver Dis.* 2014;**18**(2):281–291.
5. O'Leary JG, Lepe R, Davis GL. Indications for liver transplantation. *Gastroenterology.* 2008;**134**(6):1764–1776.
6. Cucceti A, Vukotic R, Andreone P, et al. Indications for liver transplantation. In: Pinna A, Ercolani G, eds. *Abdominal Solid Organ Transplantation.* Cham: Springer; 2015: 97–125.
7. Younossi ZM, Stepanova M, Younossi Y, et al. Epidemiology of chronic liver diseases in the USA in the past three decades. *Gut.* 2020;**69**(3):564–568.
8. Younossi ZM, Stepanova M, Ong J et al. Nonalcoholic steatohepatitis is the most rapidly increasing indication for liver transplantation in the United States. *Clin Gastroenterol Hepatol.* 2021;**19**(3):580–589.
9. Kulik L. Criteria for liver transplantation in hepatocellular carcinoma. *Clin Liv Dis.* 2015;**6**(4):100–102.
10. Mazzaferro V, Regalia E, Doci R, et al. Liver transplantation for the treatment of small hepatocellular carcinomas in patients with cirrhosis. *N Eng J Med.* 1996;**334**(11):693–700.
11. Gores GJ, Gish RG, Sudan D, Rosen CB, MELD Exception Study Group. Model for end-stage liver disease (MELD) exception for cholangiocarcinoma or biliary dysplasia. *Liver Transpl.* 2006;**12**(Suppl 3):S95–S97.
12. Heimbach JK, Gores GJ, Haddock MG, et al. Liver transplantation for unresectable perihilar cholangiocarcinoma. *Semin Liver Dis.* 2004;**24**(2):201–207.
13. Panayotova G, Lunsford KE, Latt NL, Paterno F, Guarrera JV, Pyrsopoulos N. Expanding indications for liver transplantation in the era of liver transplant oncology. *World J Gastrointest Surg.* 2021;**13**(5):392–405.
14. Lunsford KE, Javie M, Heyne K. Liver transplantation for locally advanced intrahepatic cholangiocarcinoma treated with neoadjuvant therapy: a prospective cases-series. *Lancet Gastroenterol Hepatol.* 2018;**3**(5):337–348.
15. Hughes CB, Humar A. Liver transplantation: current and future. *Abdom Radiol (N Y).* 2021;**46**(1):2–8.
16. Mazzaferro V, Pulvirenti A, Coppa J. Neuroendocrine tumours metastatic to the liver: how to select patients for liver transplantation? *J Hepatol.* 2007;**47**(4):460–466.
17. Hill MJ, Hughes M, Jie T, et al. Graft weight/recipient weight ratio: how well does it predict outcome after partial liver transplant? *Liver Transpl.* 2009;**15**(9):1056–1062.
18. Blok JJ, Detry O, Putter H, et al. Long-term results of liver transplantation from donation after circulatory death. *Liver Transpl.* 2016;**22**(8):1107–1114.
19. Muller P, Kabacam G, Vibert E, Germani G, Petrowsky H. Current status of liver transplantation in Europe. *Int J Surg.* 2020;**82S**:22–29.
20. Wu Y, Elliot R, Li, L, Tang T, Bai Y, Ma W. Cadaveric organ donation in China: a crossroads for ethics and sociocultural factors. *Medicine.* 2018;**97**(10):e9951.
21. deLemos AS, Vagefi PA. Expanding the donor pool in liver transplantation: extended criteria donors. *Clin Liver Dis (Hoboken).* 2013;**2**(4):156–159.

22. Feng S, Goodrich P, Bragg-Gresham JL, et al. Characteristics associated with liver graft failure: the concept of a donor risk index. *Am J Transplant*. 2006;**6**(4):783–790.
23. Flores A, Asrani SK. The donor risk index: a decade of experience. *Liver Transpl*. 2017;**23**(9):1216–1225.
24. Feng L, Zhao N, Yao X, et al. Histidine-tryptophan-ketoglutarate solution vs. University of Wisconsin solution for liver transplantation: a systematic review. *Liver Transpl*. 2007;**12**(8):1125–1136.
25. Xu J, Buchwald JR, Martins PN. Review of current machine perfusion therapeutics for organ preservation. *Transplantation*. 2020;**104**(9):1792–1803.
26. Starzl TE, Groth CG, Brettchneider L, et al. Orthotopic homotransplantation of the human liver. *Ann Surg*. 1968;**168**(3):398–415.
27. Tzakis A, Todo S, Starzl TE. Orthotopic liver transplantation with preservation of the inferior vena cava. *Ann Surg*. 1989;**210**(5):649–652.
28. Belghiti J, Panis Y, Sauvanet A, et al. A new technique of side-to-side caval anastomosis during orthotopic hepatic transplantation without inferior vena caval occlusion. *Surg Gynecol Obstet*. 1992;**175**(3):270–272.
29. Zhang QY, Zhang QF, Zhang DZ. The impact of steatosis on the outcome of liver transplantation: a meta-analysis. *Bio Res Int*. 2019;**2019**:3962785.
30. Hartog H, Hann A, Thamara M, Perera PR. Primary non-function of the liver allograft. *Transplantation*. 2022;**106**(1):117–128.
31. Uemura T, Randall HB, Sanchez EQ, et al. Liver retransplantation for primary nonfunction: analysis of a 20-year single-center experience. *Liver Transpl*. 2007;**13**(2):227–233.
32. Kulik U, Lehner F, Klempnauer J, Borlak J. Primary non-function is frequently associated with fatty liver allografts and high mortality after retransplantation. *Liver Int*. 2017;**37**(8):1219–1228.
33. Jain A, Costa G, Marsh W, et al. Thrombotic and non-thrombotic hepatic artery complications in adults and children following primary liver transplantation with long-term follow-up in 1000 consecutive patients. *Transpl Int*. 2006;**19**(1):27–37.
34. Bekker J, Ploem S, de Jong KP. Early hepatic artery thrombosis after liver transplantation: a systematic review of the incidence, outcome, and risk factors. *Am J Transplant*. 2009;**9**(4):746–757.
35. Mourad MM, Liossis C, Gunson BK, et al. Etiology and management of hepatic artery thrombosis after adult liver transplantation. *Liver Transpl*. 2014;**20**(6):713–723.
36. Piardi T, Lhuaire M, Bruno O, et al. Vascular complications following liver transplantation: a literature review of advances in 2015. *World J Hepatol*. 2016;**8**(1):36–57.
37. Fistouris J, Herlenius L, Backman L, et al. Pseudoaneurysm of hepatic artery following liver transplantation. *Transplant Proc*. 2006;**38**(8):2679–2682.
38. Volpin E, Pessaux P, Sauvanet A, et al. Preservation of the arterial vascularization after hepatic artery pseudoaneurysm following orthotopic liver transplantation: long term results. *Ann Transplant*. 2014;**19**:346–352.
39. Perez-Saborido B, Pacheco-Sanchez D, Barrera-Rebollo A, et al. Incidence, management, and results pf vascular complications after liver transplantation. *Transplant Proc*. 2011;**43**(3):749–750.
40. Schneider N, Scanga Ak Stokes L, Perri R. Portal vein stenosis: a rare yet clinically important cause of delayed-onset ascites after adult deceased donor liver transplantation: two case reports. *Transplant Proc*. 2011;**43**(10):3829–3834.
41. Wei BJ, Zhai RY, Wang JF, Dai DK, Yu P. Percutaneously portal venoplasty and stenting for anastomotic stenosis after transplantation. *World J Gastroenterol*. 2009;**15**(15):1880–1885.
42. Shibato T, Itoh K, Kibo T, et al. Percutaneous transhepatic balloon dilation of portal venous stenosis in patients with living donor liver transplantation. *Radiology*. 2005;**235**(3):1078–1083.
43. Zajko AB, Sheng R, Bron K, Reyes J, Nour B, Tzakis A. Percutaneous transluminal angioplasty of venous anastomotic stenoses complication liver transplantation: intermediate-term results. *J Vasc Interv Radiol*. 1994;**5**(1):121–126.
44. Schmitz V, Schoening W, Jelkmann I, et al. Different cava reconstruction techniques in liver transplantation: piggyback versus cava resection. *Hepatobiliary Pancreat Dis Int*. 2014;**13**(3):242–249.
45. Darcy MD. Management of venous outflow complications after liver transplantation. *Tech Vasc Interv Radiol*. 2007;**10**(3):240–245.
46. Bismuth H, Castaing D, Sherlock DJ. Liver transplantation by 'face-à-face' venacavaplasty. *Surgery*. 1992;**111**(2):151–155.
47. Kochhar G, Parungao JM, Hanouneh IA, Parsii MA. Biliary complications following liver transplantation. *World J Gastroenterol*. 2013;**19**(19):2841–2846.
48. Nishida S, Nakamura N, Kadono J, et al. Intrahepatic biliary strictures after liver transplantation. *J Hepatobiliary Pancreat Surg*. 2006;**13**(6):511–516.
49. Boeva I, Karagyozov PI, Tishkov I. Post-liver transplant biliary complications: current knowledge and therapeutic advances. *World J Hepatol*. 2021;**13**(1):66–79.
50. Green M, Michaels MG. Epstein-Barr virus infection and posttransplant lymphoproliferative disorder. *Am J Transplant*. 2013;**13**(Suppl 3):41–54.
51. Lauro A, Arpinati M, Pinna AD. Managing the challenge of PTLD in liver and bowel transplant recipients. *Br J Haematol*. 2015;**169**(2):157–172.
52. Akbulut S, Yilmaz M, Yilmaz S. Graft-versus-host disease after liver transplantation: a comprehensive literature review. *World J Gastroenterol*. 2012;**18**(37):5240–5248.
53. Cattrall MS, Langnas AN, Wisecarver JL, et al. Survival of graft-versus-host disease in a liver transplant recipient. *Transplantation*. 1994;**57**(8):1271–1274.
54. Murali AR, Chandra S, Stewart Z, et al. Graft versus host disease after liver transplantation in adults: a case series, review of literature and approach to management. *Transplantation*. 2016;**100**(12):2661–2670.
55. Lehner F, Becker T, Sybrecht L, et al. Successful outcome of acute graft-versus-host disease in a liver allograft recipient by withdrawal of immunosuppression. *Transplantation*. 2002;**73**(2):307–310.
56. Choudary NS, Saigal S, Bansal RK, Saraf N, Gautam D, Soin AS. Acute and chronic rejection after liver transplantation: what a clinician needs to know. *J Clin Exp Hepatol*. 2017;**7**(4):358–366.
57. Kwong AJ, Kim WR, Lake JR, et al. OPTN/SRTR 2019 annual data report: liver. *Am J Transplant*. 2021;**21**(Suppl 2):208–315.
58. Afzali B, Lombardi G, Lechler RI. Pathways of major histocompatibility complex allorecognition. *Curr Opin Organ Transpl*. 2008;**13**(4):438–444.
59. Rodriguez-Peralvarez M, Rico-Juri JM, Tsochatzis E, Burra P, De la Mata M, Lerut J. Biopsy-proven acute cellular rejection as an efficacy endpoint of randomized trials in liver transplantation: a systematic review and critical appraisal. *Transpl Int*. 2016;**29**(9):961–973.

60. Demetris AJ, Murase N, Lee RG. Chronic rejection: a general overview of histopathology and pathophysiology with emphasis on liver, heart, and intestinal allografts. *Ann Transpl.* 1997;**2**(2):27–44.
61. Blakomer K, Seaberg EC, Batts K. Analysis of the reversibility of chronic liver allograft rejection implications for a staging schema. *Am J Surg Pathol.* 1999;**23**(11):1328–1339.
62. Jain A, Demetris AJ, Kashyap R. Does tacrolimus offer virtual freedom from chronic rejection after primary liver transplantation? Risk and prognostic factors in 1048 liver transplantations with a mean follow-up of 6 years. *Liver Transpl.* 2001;**7**(7):623–630.
63. Neil DAH, Hubscher SG. Current views on rejection pathology in liver transplantation. *Transpl Int.* 2010;**23**(10):971–983.
64. O'Leary JG, Kaneku H, Susskind BM, et al. High mean fluorescence intensity donor-specific anti-HLA antibodies associated with chronic rejection post-liver transplant. *Am J Transplant.* 2011;**11**(9):1868–1876.
65. Cruciani M, Megoli C, Malena M, et al. Antifungal prophylaxis in liver transplant patients: a systematic review and meta-analysis. *Liver Transpl.* 2006;**12**(5):850–858.
66. Montano-Loza AJ, Bhanji RA, Wasilenko S, AL Mason AL. Systemic review: recurrent autoimmune liver diseases after liver transplantation. *Aliment Pharmacol Ther.* 2017;**45**(4):485–500.
67. Malik SM, Devera ME, Fontes P, Shaikh O, Sasatomi E, Ahmad J. Recurrent disease following liver transplantation for nonalcoholic steatohepatitis cirrhosis. *Liver Transpl.* 2009;**15**(12):1843–1851.
68. Bhati C, Idowu MO, Sanyal AJ, et al. Long-term outcomes in patients undergoing liver transplantation for nonalcoholic steatohepatitis-related cirrhosis. *Transplantation.* 2017;**101**(8):1867–1874.
69. Taneja S, Roy A. Nonalcoholic steatohepatitis recurrence after liver transplant. *Transpl Gastroenterol Hepatol.* 2020;**5**:24–30.
70. Sumida Y, Yoneda M. Current and future pharmacological therapies for NAFLD/NASH. *J Gatroenterol.* 2018;**53**(3):362–376.
71. Wakamatsu E, Mathis D, Benoist C. Convergent and divergent effects of costimulatory molecules in conventional and regulatory CD4+ T cells. *Proc Natl Acad Sci USA.* 2013;**110**(3):1023–1028.
72. Ross SH, Cantell DA. Signaling and function of interleukin-2 in T lymphocytes. *Ann Rev Immunol.* 2018;**36**(1):411–433.
73. Naesens M, Kuypers DRJ, Sarwal M. Calcineurin inhibitor nephrotoxicity. *Clin J Am Soc Nephrol.* 2009;**4**(2):481–508.
74. Allison AC, Eugui EM. Mechanisms of action of mycophenolate mofetil in preventing acute and chronic allograft rejection. *Transplantation.* 2005;**15**(2 Suppl):S181–S190.
75. McKenna GJ. Is it time to use de novo mTOR inhibitors posttransplant? *Curr Transpl Rep.* 2016;**3**(3):244–253.
76. McKenna GJ, Trotter JF, Klintmalm E, et al. Limiting hepatitis C virus progression in liver transplant recipients using sirolimus based immunosuppression. *Am J Transplant.* 2011;**11**(11):2379–2387.
77. McKenna GJ, Trotter JF, Klintmalm E, et al. Sirolimus and cardiovascular risk in liver transplantation. *Transplantation.* 2013;**95**(1):215–221.
78. Yeung MY, Grimmig T, Sayegh MH. Costimulation blockade in transplantation. *Adv Exp Med Biol.* 2019;**1189**:267–312.
79. Wekerle T, Grinyo JM. Belatacept: from rational design to clinical application. *Transpl Int.* 2012;**25**(2):139–150.
80. McEwen BS, Biron CA, Brunson KW, et al. The role of adrenocorticoids as modulators of immune function in health and disease: neural, endocrine and immune interactions. *Brain Res Rev.* 1997;**23**(1–2):79–133.
81. Coutinho AE, Chapman KE. The anti-inflammatory and immunosuppressive effects of glucocorticoids, recent developments and mechanistic insights. *Mol Cell Endocrinol.* 2011;**335**(1):2–13.
82. Giles AJ, Hutchinson MKND, Sonnemann HM, et al. Dexamethasone-induced immunosuppression: mechanisms and implications for immunotherapy. *J Immunotherapy Cancer.* 2018;**6**(1):51.
83. Mohty M. Mechanisms of action of anti-thymocyte globulin: T-cell depletion and beyond. *Leukemia.* 2007;**21**(7):1387–1394.
84. Morris PJ, Russell NK. Alemtuzumab (Campath-1H): a systematic review in organ transplantation. *Transplantation.* 2006;**81**(10):1361–1367.
85. Neuhaus P, Clavien PA, Kittur D, et al. Improved treatment response with basiliximab immunoprophylaxis after liver transplantation: results from a double-blind randomized placebo-controlled trial. *Liver Transpl.* 2002;**8**(2):132–142.
86. Starzl TE, Klintmalm GBG, Porter KA, Iwatsuki S, Schroter GPJ. Liver transplantation with use of cyclosporin A and prednisone. *N Eng J Med.* 1981;**305**(5):266–269.
87. Starzl TE, Klintmalm GBG, Iwatsuki S, Fernandez-Bueno C. Past and future prospects of orthotopic liver transplantation. *Arch Surg.* 1981;**116**(10):1342–1343.
88. Giusto M, Berenguer M, Merkel C, et al. Chronic kidney disease after liver transplantation. Pretransplantation risk factors and predictors during follow-up. *Transplantation.* 2013;**95**(9):1148–1153.
89. Ojo AO, Held PJ, Prok FK, et al. Chronic renal failure after transplantation of non-renal organ. *N Eng J Med.* 2003;**349**(10):931–940.
90. Watt KDS, Pederson RA, Kremers WK, Heimbach JK, Charlton MR. Evolution of causes and risk factors for mortality post-liver transplant: results of the NIDDK long-term follow-up study. *Am J Transplant.* 2010;**10**(6):1420–1427.

23
Paediatric liver transplantation

Mureo Kasahara

History

Paediatric liver transplantation (LT), a medical treatment with a relatively short history, was initiated in 1963 by T. E. Starzl et al. in the US.[1] Although the results were initially unsatisfactory, they have been remarkably improved because of advances in patient selection, surgical techniques, organ preservation methods, immunosuppressive therapy, and perioperative management, among others. In the US, approximately 600 paediatric deceased donor liver transplantations (DDLTs) are conducted annually; therefore, this can be considered an established medical treatment for patients with paediatric end-stage liver diseases. Paediatric LTs in Europe and the US are centred on DDLT by harvesting organs from brain-dead or cardiac arrest donors.

The shortage of size-matched cadaveric liver donors for paediatric recipients stimulated the development of technical innovations, based on the segmental anatomy of the liver, which facilitated transplanting parts of an adult cadaveric donor liver into smaller children. The technique of reduced size and split LT was developed and validated in the early 1990s.[2,3]

In Asian countries, the Organ Transplantation Law took effect in the 1990s, at which time DDLT became legally feasible. However, the demand of patients waiting for organ transplantations has not been sufficiently satisfied in Asian countries due to the shortage of deceased organ donors. With the background that there has been no progression in DDLT, LTs in Asia have been centred on living donor liver transplantations (LDLTs) using a partial liver from healthy relative donors. The concept of safety of LDLT has been validated by the *in situ* split procedure in heart beating cadaveric donors.[4] The first paediatric LDLT was performed on a boy with end-stage liver cirrhosis caused by biliary atresia by Raia et al. at San Paolo University, Brazil in 1989.[5] Unlike DDLT, LDLT has two major advantages. First, as organs are donated from healthy adults, it is possible to transplant organs with better viability compared to deceased donor organs that have been preserved in cold storage for a long time. It is possible to sufficiently evaluate potential donors prior to planned transplant surgery, and because of the short cold ischaemic time, it is possible to provide a liver with excellent quality and stable conditions for recipients in many cases. Second, depending upon the recipient's condition, it is possible to conduct elective surgery at the optimal time, even for patients who need very urgent transplantation such as acute liver failure (ALF). In contrast, the disadvantage of LDLT is that a liver resection for organ donation is required in healthy living donors despite there being no medical benefits. As donor deaths due to LDLT have been reported previously, it is difficult to guarantee the complete safety of living donors because they undergo medically unnecessary liver resection, which is a significantly invasive surgery.[6] LDLT should be done in an experienced centre specializing in hepatobiliary surgery and LT with special attention to the donor's safety.

Indications

Cholestatic liver disease

There are various indications for paediatric LT as seen in Table 23.1. According to the Japanese Liver Transplantation annual report, cholestatic liver diseases represented by biliary atresia accounted for 50% of cases.[7] Biliary atresia is an unexplained cholestatic liver disease occurring at a frequency of 1:5000 to 1:19,000 births and is a serious disease leading to cirrhosis from cholestasis. The Kasai procedure (portoenterostomy) was developed by Morio Kasai from Tohoku University, Japan, in the 1950s, and resulted in a dramatic improvement in the short-term survival rate.[8] However, the 20-year survival rate of autologous livers (without LT) following Kasai surgery is reportedly 49%, suggesting that LT is required to be performed in childhood for approximately half the patients as of now.[9]

Alagille syndrome (AGS), syndromic paucity of the intrahepatic bile ducts, is an autosomal dominant disorder, which is clinically defined by the presence of at least three of the following five major features: chronic cholestasis, congenital heart disease, peculiar facies, butterfly-like vertebrae, and a posterior embryotoxon. AGS is caused by a mutation in the Jagged1 gene (*JAG1*), which encodes a protein belonging to a family of ligands to the Notch receptor. The Jagged1 protein is important in determining cell differentiation and regulation of development of the biliary epithelium. The mutant *JAG1* gene varies in phenotypic expression, and there is no apparent relationship between the genotype and the clinical manifestation. AGS occurs in approximately 1:100,000 live births; however, the actual incidence is underestimated (Figure 23.1).

Table 23.1 Indications for paediatric liver transplantation

1. Chronic progressive liver disease	
a. Cholestatic liver disease	Biliary atresia, Alagille syndrome, primary sclerosing cholangitis, autoimmune hepatitis, chronic hepatic graft versus host disease, etc.
b. Vascular disease	Budd–Chiari syndrome, veno-occlusive disease, congenital absence of portal vein, etc.
c. Polycystic disease	Polycystic liver disease, Caroli disease, congenital hepatic fibrosis, etc.
2. Metabolic liver disease	
a. Disease that can cause cirrhosis	Alpha-1 antitrypsin deficiency, Wilson disease, haemochromatosis, tyrosinaemia, cystic fibrosis, primary familial intrahepatic cholestasis type II, neonatal intrahepatic cholestasis caused by citric deficiency, neonatal iron storage disease, glycogen storage disease, etc.
b. Disease that can cause extrahepatic manifestation	Hypercholesterolaemia, hyperlipoproteinemia, Crigler–Najjar syndrome, haemophilia, protein C deficiency, erythropoietic portoporphyria, citrullinemia, hyperoxaluria type 1, urea cycle defects (ornithine transcarbamylase deficiency, carbamoyl phosphate synthetase 1 deficiency, arginosuccinate synthetase deficiency), organic acidaemia) methylmalonic acidaemia, propionic acidaemia), mucopolysaccharidoses, etc.
3. Acute liver failure	Viral hepatitis, drug-induced hepatitis, mitochondrial hepatopathy, heat stroke, etc.
4. Hepatic neoplasm	Hepatoblastoma, haemangioendothelioma, hepatocellular carcinoma, etc.

As for living related donor selection in AGS, the problem of bile duct paucity in a genetically related donor has been reported.[10] Cardiac anomalies and the characteristic facies may or may not be present in family members with the disease, making diagnosis without pathological evidence or visualization of the biliary system difficult. Routine evaluation of magnetic resonance cholangiopancreatography during potential living donor evaluation for AGS transplantation should be necessary and percutaneous needle liver biopsy performed when other investigations are inconclusive. The prominent histological finding is paucity of the intralobular bile ducts (at least half of the portal triad has no bile ducts); however, magnetic resonance cholangiopancreatography can detect reduction in the diameter of biliary ducts. Parental mosaicism of Jagged1 mutations in families with AGS has been reported and may produce bile duct paucity in these donor candidates.[11]

Metabolic liver disease

Metabolic liver disease accounts for 10% of the total indication of LT. Metabolic liver disease can be divided into two groups: diseases that can cause cirrhosis (such as alpha-1 antitrypsin deficiency, Wilson disease, etc.) and those that cause extrahepatic manifestations (hypercholesterolaemia, urea cycle deficiency, etc.).[12] Metabolic liver disease is diagnosed by clinical symptoms, such as low activity after birth and vomiting, as well as blood sampling results, such as hyperammonaemia and acidosis. If medical treatment for metabolic failure is not successful, LT is occasionally indicated. The indications for LDLT were retrospectively evaluated according to a grading score system based on the guidelines recommended by the Japanese Ministry of Health, Labour and Welfare (Table 23.2).[13] The metabolic disorders were divided into groups based on the following: whether the disorder predominantly involved the liver (liver-oriented disease; Wilson's disease, urea cycle disorder, citrullinaemia, tyrosinaemia type 1, bile acid synthetic defects and Crigler–Najjar syndrome type 1) (Figure 23.2) or partly involved the liver, the effectiveness of conventional medical treatment, the quality of life, and the mental/physical status (Figure 23.3). Each parameter was classified into three scores. A score of over 10 points was defined as an absolute indication for LT, a score of 5–10 was defined as a relative indication, a score of 3–4 was defined as a prudent indication, and a score of less than 3 points was defined as a contraindication.

Acute liver failure

ALF is a life-threatening disease process characterized by the rapid onset of liver dysfunction, coagulopathy, and encephalopathy in patients without preceding chronic liver disease. The outcome of ALF in children is generally poor, especially in those younger than 12 months of age.[14] Several modalities of artificial liver support have been applied to ALF patients; however, the efficacy of them has not been well established.[15] Therefore, the modalities cannot be recommended until properly conducted randomized controlled trials show the effectiveness, and LT is the only effective treatment that has improved the outcome of ALF.[16] LT is considered when the recovery of liver function is not appropriate despite the aggressive supportive therapy for ALF. The common aetiologies for ALF in children differed from adults, were indeterminate in half of the patients, and related to acetaminophen overdose in 14%, metabolic 10%, viral and autoimmune 6%, ischaemic and non-acetaminophen drug induced in 5%, and some were combined with underlying liver disease[17] (Figure 23.4).

The early determination scoring system of the indications for LT proposed by the Intractable Hepato-Biliary Diseases Study Group of Japan (JIHBDSG) has been widely used in Japan to predict the outcomes for adults.[18] However, while the predictive accuracy, sensitivity, and specificity are acceptable at 78%, 80%, and 76%, respectively, applying this scoring system to children is still controversial, due to the lack of data. Therefore, a JIHBDSG scoring system applicable in children as well as highly sensitive and specific predictive indicators for outcome are needed in order to reduce the risk of unnecessary LT. Because of the rapid progression of liver deterioration in paediatric patients, the laboratory variables and clinical findings change over time. A previous study showed that the increase in the serum alpha-fetoprotein levels over 3 days after diagnosis with ALF reflected the hepatic regeneration in response to liver injury. Another study suggested a prognostic model, the ALF early dynamic model, superior to the King's College Hospital criteria, using 3-day changes in the independent prognostic factors associated with outcome.[19]

Hepatic malignancy

Hepatoblastoma is the most common malignant liver tumour in children, and is seen mostly in patients aged 2 years and under. Congenital anomalies are present in 5.5% of patients with hepatoblastoma. While a variety of histological patterns are noted, prognosis is primarily dependent on the surgical resectability of the tumour, with an overall survival rate of approximately 60%. Prognosis is better with the fetal-predominant type than with other types. Through combined improvements in imaging, surgical resection, and systemic chemotherapy, higher survival rates have been achieved. While disease-free patient survival rates have been

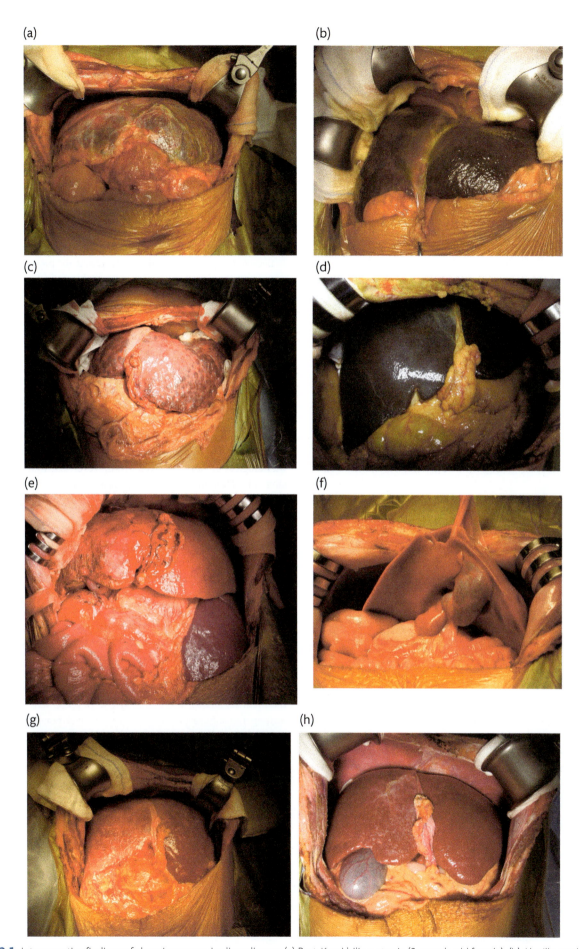

Figure 23.1 Intraoperative findings of chronic progressive liver disease. (a) Post-Kasai biliary atresia (8-month-old female). (b) Alagille syndrome (8-month-old female). (c) Primary sclerosing cholangitis (10-year-old female). (d) Chronic hepatic graft-versus-host disease, post bone marrow transplantation (18-year-old male). (e) Budd–Chiari syndrome (10-year-old male). (f) Congenital absence of portal vein, left-sided gall bladder (12-month-old female). (g) Caroli disease (7-year-old female). (h) Congenital hepatic fibrosis (14-year-old male).

Table 23.2 Scoring system for indication for liver transplantation for metabolic disorders (transplantation score)

	Score 5	Score 3	Score 1
Original disease			
Liver-oriented disease	O		
Previous case report		O	
Effectiveness of medical treatment			
Metabolic decompensation which necessitated hospitalization ≥6 times/year	O		
3–5 times/year		O	
Metabolic decompensation which necessitated admission ≥6 times/year			O
Metabolic decompensation which necessitated ICU care with apheresis ≥2 times/year	O		
Extremely poor response/adherence for medical treatment		O	
Poor response/adherence for medical treatment			O
Quality of life			
Nasogastric tube feeding/frequent meal		O	
Progressive neurological impairment		O	
Present status			
Good social interaction, full ambulation, partially impaired gross and fine motor skills, use of language, mildly delayed development, only modest learning deficits			O
Growth retardation (height <2.5 SD)			O
Continuous abnormal laboratory test (NH$_3$, lactate, base excess, liver function, cholesterol, glucose)			O
Score			**Liver transplantation**
≥10			Absolute indication
≥bsolute			Relative indication
>3 to <4			Prudent indication
<3			Contraindication

ICU, intensive care unit; SD, standard deviation.

dramatically improved by cisplatin chemotherapy regimens, LT remains an alternative curative treatment for patients whose liver tumour is unresectable following systemic chemotherapy or radical hepatectomy. Based on radiological findings, the PREtreatment EXTent of disease (PRETEXT) grouping grade III and IV could be an indication for LT[20] (**Figure 23.5**).

Immunosuppression

After successful transplantation, the recipients need lifelong immunosuppression therapy. Immunosuppression is administered with a calcineurin inhibitor (tacrolimus, ciclosporin) and low-dose steroids (**Figure 23.6**). Tacrolimus administration is started on the day before transplantation. The target whole blood trough level of tacrolimus is 10–12 ng/mL for the first 2 weeks, approximately 10 ng/mL for the following 2 weeks, and 8–10 ng/mL thereafter. Treatment with steroids is initiated at the time of graft reperfusion at a dose of 10 mg/kg, and tapered from 1 mg/kg/day to 0.3 mg/kg/day during the first month and withdrawn within the first 3 months. The patient, who receives an ABO-incompatible transplant, undergoes preoperative rituximab induction therapy 3–4 weeks prior to planned LT with plasma exchange in order to reduce anti-ABH antibody titre to less than ×64. The recipients less than 1.5 years of age, with an ABO-incompatible transplant have no preoperative treatment for ABO incompatibility.[21]

Graft size matching

Experience and technical improvements in relation to the left-side lobe donation have led to the use of further reducing left lateral segment (LLS) grafts and single segmental or hyper-reduced LLS grafts, in neonatal and infantile LDLT, to overcome the problems associated with large-for-size grafts.[22] The main problems in LT for young infants are the small size of the recipient's abdominal cavity and the insufficient blood supply to the graft, especially in patients without liver cirrhosis, portal hypertension, massive ascites, or hepatomegaly. Segmental grafts (segment 2/3) or reduced LLS (reducing thickness) grafts allow for the potential recipient pool to be expanded to include a greater number of infants, including smaller infants.

Although the indications for LT in young infants (including dominant fulminant hepatic failure, haemochromatosis, metabolic disease, etc.) are limited and differ from those in older infants, the rates of morbidity and mortality are considered to be high in comparison to older children because of the technical difficulty and their immunological immaturity. Recently, however, due to the advances in surgical techniques, immunosuppression, and perioperative management, young infants are increasingly listed for LT.

From the perspective of the graft shape, if the LLS of the donor was bulky, and its maximum thickness was larger than the anteroposterior diameter of the recipient's abdominal cavity, which was identified as the length from the inside abdominal wall to the front of the vertebra on axial computed tomography images, reducing the thickness of the LLS graft was considered. After isolating the donor left hepatic artery, hepatic duct, and portal branch, the hepatic parenchyma of the medial segment was transected at 5 mm to the right side of the falciform ligament without blood inflow occlusion or graft manipulation. The thickness of the LLSs of the donor grafts was reduced as necessary *in situ*. The determination of the transection plane for reduced LLS (in which the thickness of the LLS is reduced)—in which the main segment 2 and 3 branches were preserved—was made by intraoperative ultrasonography. In segment 2 monosegmentectomy, we confirmed that the entire length of the main left hepatic vein was preserved after the dissection of the Glissonian sheath in the umbilical portion of segment 3 on an intraoperative echography. Thereafter, the ventral thickness of the LLS was resected and discarded following the ligation of the arteries, portal structures, and bile ducts of the upward segment without vascular occlusion and with the preservation of the main segment 3 branch.

Hepatic artery reconstruction was performed using microvascular techniques in all cases. Portal reconstruction was performed with interrupted sutures in the anterior wall, without the use of an interpositional vein graft. Biliary reconstruction was achieved using Roux-en-Y hepaticojejunostomy. Primary abdominal closure was achieved without compression injury of the graft or respiratory failure[23] (**Figure 23.7**). The reduction of LLS technique could be applied for split DDLT as a bench surgery.[24] The discarded hepatic

Postoperative surgical complications

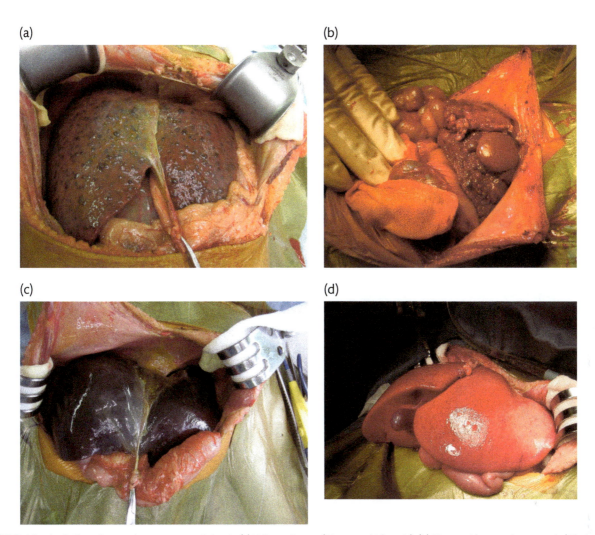

Figure 23.2 Metabolic liver disease that can cause cirrhosis. (a) Wilson disease (11-year-old female). (b) Neonatal haemochromatosis (19-day-old male). (c) Primary familial intrahepatic cholestasis type II (9-month-old male). (d) Glycogen storage disease type Ib (1-year-old male).

parenchyma was prepared for the 'hepatocyte transplantation programme' if informed consent was provided.[25]

Regarding the graft selection in paediatric LT, some recommendations could be possible (Figure 23.8). Although there are no clear border lines between the graft selection, one can find that the margins between the graft types would be 5 kg in reduced LLS, 25 kg in left lobe, and 50 kg in right lobe according to the our retrospective analysis (n = 500, paediatric LDLT series). The red spheres are patient mortalities for various reasons.

On the assumption that the graft has full function without any vascular complications, we realized that 50 g in a 25 kg recipient and 100 g in a 50 kg recipient will be crucial issue for graft selection, and subsequent graft survival. Therefore, the ideal graft selection could be as follows: reduced LLS: recipient BW less than 5.0 kg, left lobe: BW >25 kg and right lobe: BW>50 kg.

Postoperative surgical complications

Hepatic artery thrombosis

Sufficient hepatic arterial flow is indispensable for successful LT. Safe methods of hepatic arterial reconstruction have already been established in paediatric LDLT using microsurgical techniques.[26] Hepatic artery thrombosis (HAT) represents an uncommon complication of LT with the potential to cause graft loss and/or long-term patient morbidity.[27] Paediatric liver transplant recipients have historically had a higher incidence of HAT than adult recipients. The incidence of HAT is related to both technical and graft- related factors, such as prolonged cold ischaemic time, ABO incompatibility, rejection, anatomical site of arterial reconstruction, size of the donor artery, and the number of anastomoses.[28] Postoperatively, HAT frequently causes graft failure and death in up to 50% of cases. In the longer term, HAT correlates with the development of biliary complications such as strictures, bile leaks, severe biliary sepsis, and hepatic necrosis (Figure 23.9). It has been reported that early successful surgical revascularization was associated with significantly higher graft survival than failed or unattempted revascularization, and allowed the long-term salvage of grafts experiencing thrombosis before day 15 after paediatric transplantation.[29] Either revision surgical re-anastomosis or interventional radiological techniques have been applied for revascularization of the hepatic artery.

Regarding anticoagulation therapy following LT, heparin therapy is initiated in most centres usually by the third or fourth

CHAPTER 23 Paediatric liver transplantation

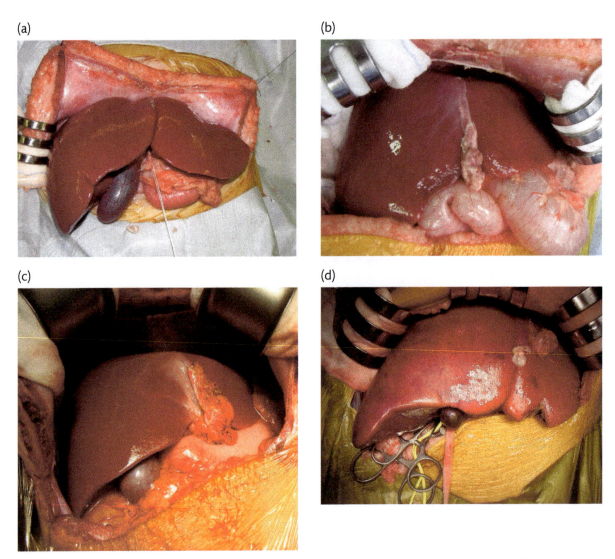

Figure 23.3 Metabolic liver disease that can cause extrahepatic manifestation. (a) Ornithine transcarbamylase deficiency (7-month-old male). (b) Carbamoyl phosphate synthetase I deficiency (5-month-old female). (c) Hyperoxaluria type I (20-month-old female). (d) Methylmalonic acidaemia (7-year-old female).

postoperative day (when the international normalized ratio returns to <1.5) as a standard 5 U/kg/h continuous infusion for 4 or 5 days or until oral aspirin (40 mg daily) is tolerated. Coagulation parameters from the new liver graft are allowed to normalize passively. Aspirin is commenced postoperatively when the child is able to take oral feeds and continued for 6 months.[28]

Portal vein thrombosis

Portal vein (PV) complications are the most frequent vascular complications in paediatric LTs. A retrospective study of PV complications among 521 paediatric LDLTs showed that the incidence of late-onset PV obstruction, defined as the complication after the first 3 months of LDLT, was 2.9% with graft survival of 60%.[30] The presentation of PV stenosis varies in symptoms; the most common is variceal bleeding, followed by recurrent ascites, rising liver function tests (increasing lactate dehydrogenase), pancytopenia, and splenomegaly.

In biliary atresia the native PV becomes sclerotic or hypoplastic and the PV flow may decrease at the time of LT, while the collateral vessels develop and provoke a further decrease in the PV flow. This negative spiral in PV circulation can complicate PV reconstruction at the time of LT. There have been several technical refinements reported in previous studies, including vein graft interposition, and longitudinal venoplasty; however, aside from the techniques of PV reconstruction, collateral interruption and sufficient PVF are crucial issues that can affect the initial graft function.[31]

The use of percutaneous transhepatic venoplasty of the PV stenosis after LT in paediatric patients was first described by Raby et al. in 1991.[32] After introduction of percutaneous PV venoplasty, the utility of this technique has been confirmed by other reports including long-term patency as well as efficacy of metallic stents in the cases with elastic stenosis. Although the utility of the transileocolic approach as well as the trans-splenic approach are reported, the majority of PV venoplasties are done in a percutaneous transhepatic retrograde fashion with an excellent success rate (**Figure 23.10**).

Postoperative surgical complications

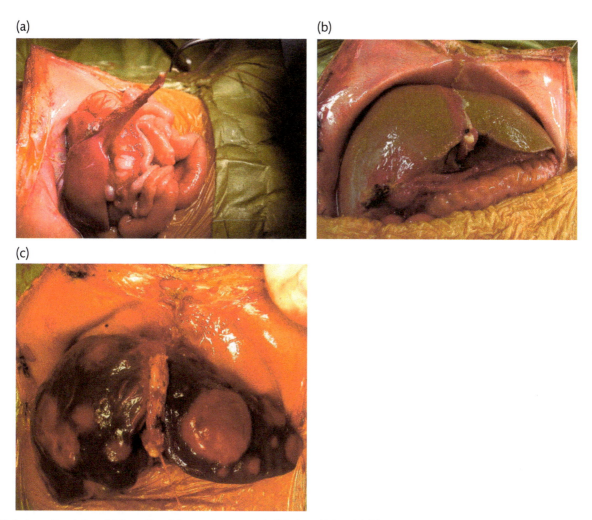

Figure 23.4 Acute liver failure. (a) Acute liver failure, unknown origin (22-day-old female). (b) Acute liver failure, mitochondrial hepatopathy (4-month-old female). (c) Acute liver failure, haemangioma (2-month-old male).

Hepatic vein stenosis

Hepatic vein stenosis can be a critical and sometimes life-threatening complication in paediatric LDLT. Outflow complication is rare in most series, but is clinically very serious and a difficult-to-manage problem when present. In adult DDLT using the whole liver, stenosis of the hepatic vein to the inferior vena cava anastomosis is uncommon, as a suprahepatic cavocaval anastomosis is typically employed. With the use of the piggyback technique, however, the incidence of a hepatic vein anastomotic complication has slightly increased.[33] In paediatric DDLT using split or reduced-size grafts,

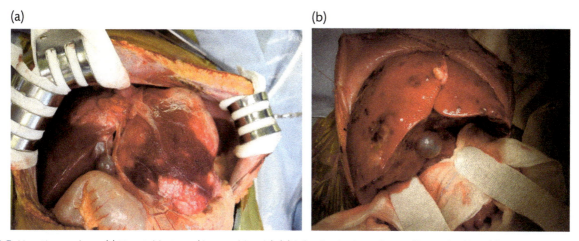

Figure 23.5 Hepatic neoplasm. (a) Hepatoblastoma (4-year-old male). (b) Infantile choriocarcinoma (2-month-old male).

CHAPTER 23 Paediatric liver transplantation

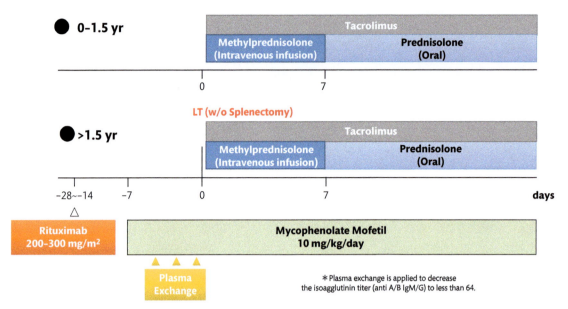

Figure 23.6 Current immunosuppression protocol for ABO-incompatible liver transplantation in Japan.

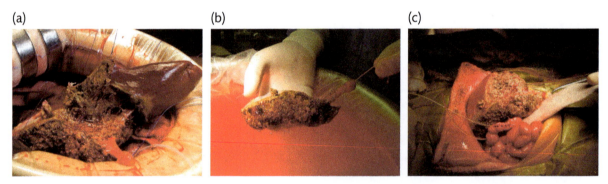

Figure 23.7 Primary abdominal closure in neonatal liver transplantation using reduced LLS graft. (a) Donor surgery. (b) Bench perfusion. (c) Recipient surgery.

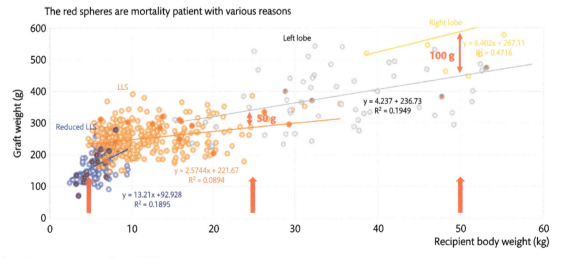

Figure 23.8 Graft selection in paediatric LDLT.

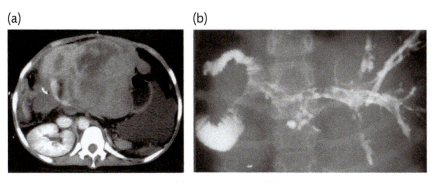

Figure 23.9 Imaging study following hepatic artery thrombosis. (a) Hepatic necrosis. (b) Ischaemic cholangiopathy.

the incidence of hepatic vein anastomotic complications is greater than than 8%, and in paediatric LDLT, the incidence of hepatic vein outflow complications ranges from 4.5% to 15.1%.[34,35]

A number of factors affect this incidence, including the vessel size, graft positioning, organ regeneration, and the length of the graft cuff. Several techniques for anastomosing the inferior vena cava to the hepatic veins have been reported, with the aim of minimizing the outflow obstruction. One such technique, initially described in 1991, involves the creation of a triangular anastomosis along the anterior surface of the inferior vena cava.[36]

The presentation of hepatic vein stenosis varies in symptoms; the most common are massive ascites, pleural effusion, and coagulopathy, followed by deterioration of the graft function. Hepatic vein stenosis immediately after LT is a surgical emergency and reoperation is necessary for correction. By contrast, late onset of hepatic vein stenosis can cause insidious deterioration of liver function and surgical correction is usually difficult because fibrotic changes develop around the anastomotic site. Thus, balloon angioplasty is considered as the first management steps for hepatic vein stenosis. However, some patients have had recurrences that required multiple interventions and should have been considered for the implantation of an inside metallic stent, which sometimes works in the long term (Figure 23.11). Surgical revision using the patch graft on the side wall of hepatic vein anastomosis may be another effective treatment option.[37]

Biliary stricture

The blood supply for the biliary anastomosis is a major concern in LDLT. The arterial blood supply of the biliary system has been described by several investigators. A previous study using fine casts showed that 60% of the arterial supply for the bile duct comes from caudal side through periduodenal arteries, 38% from the cranial side, and only 2% from the proper hepatic artery. The '3 o'clock', '9 o'clock', and retroportal arteries give rise to multiple arteriolar branches,[38] which form a free anastomosis within the wall of the bile duct. In the absence of any attachments in recipients of the transplanted liver, the blood supply to the graft bile duct is derived solely from the hepatic artery. The presence of bleeding from the graft and recipient bile duct at the time of anastomosis is critical. Histological examination of the disrupted duct-to-duct (DD) often shows the loss of the '3 o'clock' and '9 o'clock' intramural arteries on the recipient side. Preservation of the periductal microcirculation on the recipient duct and excellent hepatic artery reconstruction might be a key factor for a successful DD anastomosis, although most paediatric liver transplant recipients receive a Roux-en Y hepaticojejunostomy.

Biliary complications remain one of the most serious morbidities in LT. The incidence of biliary stricture in LDLT was reported to be 25–32%.[39,40] Biliary stricture in LDLT was higher than that of DDLT, which was reported to be 5–15%.[41] Biliary stricture is rarely the sole cause of graft loss, but it often leads to serious morbidity. Therefore, reliable and non-invasive tests for the early detection and

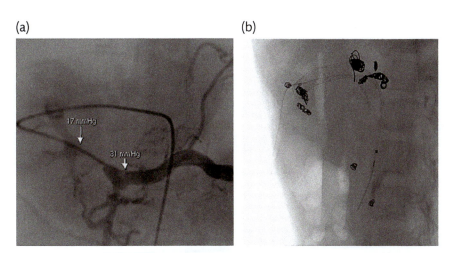

Figure 23.10 Percutaneous transhepatic venoplasty of the portal vein stenosis. (a) Transhepatic portography revealed long segmental obstruction of the PV trunk with prominent collaterals through the Roux-en-Y limb into the graft. (b) After balloon dilatation and stent placement.

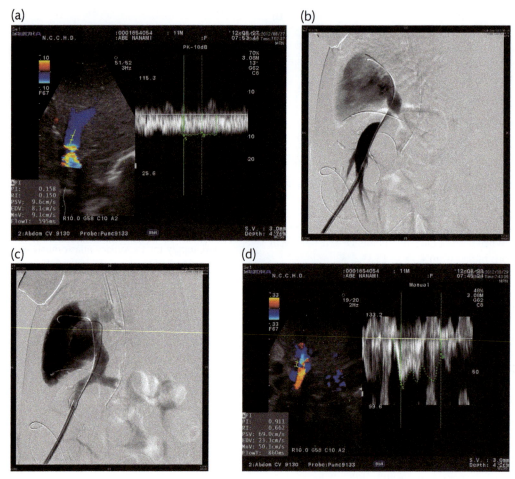

Figure 23.11 Treatment of hepatic vein stenosis with percutaneous transhepatic balloon dilatation. (a) Hepatic vein stenosis. (b) Percutaneous transhepatic hepatic venography. (c) Balloon dilatation. (d) Triphasic hepatic vein flow after hepatic vein dilatation.

differentiation of other complications from biliary stricture after paediatric LDLT are urgently needed. Hepatobiliary scintigraphy using technetium-99m-labelled N-pyridoxylmethyltryptophan (99mTc-PMT) provides comprehensive morphological and functional information about the hepatobiliary system (Figure 23.12).[42]

Patients with biliary stricture may be successfully treated with percutaneous transhepatic balloon dilatation and stenting catheter placement under general anaesthesia.

Outcome of paediatric liver transplantation

The survival rates observed in the recent paediatric LT series were excellent, nearly 80% at 20 years post LT.[43,44] Recently, adolescent age at the time of solid organ transplantation, not only for liver, but also kidney, heart, and lung, has been recognized as a risk factor for poor graft survival.[45,46] The graft survival was worse in adolescents (12 to <18 years) than in adults (≥18 years of age) even in LDLT, and the

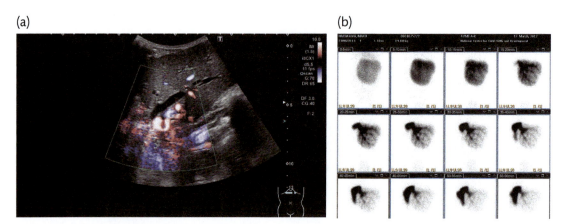

Figure 23.12 Biliary stricture. (a) Intrahepatic bile duct dilatation. (b) The dynamic image after 99mTc-PMT injection showed biliary stricture and a dilated intrahepatic bile duct. The biliary stricture case had 52.5% excretion until 60 min (cut-off >60%). Balloon dilatation and stenting were performed. There was a narrowing seen at the anastomosis.

corresponding crossing of the graft survival lines was demonstrated at 12 years post LDLT. With less ischaemia, improved donor selection, and controlled procedures, LDLT might lead to fewer adverse outcomes than DDLT.[47] It has been speculated that the increased risk of graft loss during adolescence among recipients of solid organ transplantation is due to a lack of adherence to immunosuppression, the transition from paediatric to adult care, and changes in health insurance coverage.[48,49] Japan has a universal healthcare system and most of the medical expenses before and after LT are covered by Japanese insurance benefits. As such, the influence of changes in health insurance coverage during adolescence may be less marked in Japan than in other countries without similar healthcare systems. The increased risk of graft loss during adolescence is most likely multifactorial, and prospective investigations of the transition process may be necessary to clarify these points.

The optimal timing for LT is crucial for achieving a successful outcome. Several studies have attempted to assess the influence of pre-LT variables on the outcome after LT. Gross et al. reported that the United Network for Organ Sharing status, liver allograft type, and pretransplant serum bilirubin level were significant predictors of patient survival, whereas the patient's age, weight, and a history of Kasai operations were not predictors.[50] Others found that growth failure, age less than 1 year, and immunosuppression regimen were predictors of mortality after LT; LT era and paediatric end-stage liver disease (PELD) score were not predictors.[51] The PELD score is calculated based on the age, growth failure, albumin, international normalized ratio, and total bilirubin level and is an excellent predictor for the outcome of paediatric LT patients. However, it has been reported that the PELD score does not accurately represent the true mortality risk associated with complications of portal hypertension, variceal bleeding, refractory ascites, and hepatopulmonary syndrome in the paediatric patient with end-stage liver disease. Early referral to a transplant centre should be considered when at least one complication of cirrhosis occurs during its natural history, regardless of the PELD/MELD score, as it allows the transplant centre to provide the most input possible regarding the management strategy for the recipient as well as potential donor candidates.

The paediatric population will possibly remain dependent on the additional LDLT programme to further reduce the waiting list mortality. Importantly, since the mortality of children on the waiting list has not entirely disappeared, LDLT should still be considered an additional option for paediatric candidates, even in DDLT-dominant countries. While we should continue to promote deceased donor organ transplantation, it may also be time to re-explore the outcomes after LDLT in context of the recent technical and medical improvements in this field with ensured living donor safety.

REFERENCES

1. Starzl TE, Marchioro TL, Vonkaulla KN, et al. Homotransplantation of the liver in humans. *Surg Gynecol Obstet*. 1963;**117**:659–676.
2. Otte JB, De Ville DeGoyet J, Sokel E, et al. Size reduction of the donor liver is a safe way to alleviate the shortage of size-matched organs in pediatric liver transplantation. *Ann Surg*. 1990;**211**(2):146–157.
3. Pichlmayer R, Ringe B, Gubernatis G, et al. [Transplantation of a donor liver to 2 recipients (splitting transplantation)--a new method in the further development of segmental liver transplantation]. *Langenbecks Arch Chir*. 1988;**76**:127–130.
4. Rogers X, Malago M, Gawad K, et al. In situ splitting of cadaveric livers. The ultimate expansion of a limited donor pool. *Ann Surg*. 1996;**224**(3):331–339.
5. Raia S, Nery JR, Mies S. Liver transplantation from live donors. *Lancet*. 1989;**2**(8661):497.
6. Cheah YL, Simpson MA, Pomposelli JJ, et al. Incidence of death and potentially life-threatening near-miss events in living donor hepatic lobectomy: a world-wide survey. *Liver Transpl*. 2013;**19**(5):499–506.
7. Umeshita K, Eguchi S, Egawa H, et al. Liver transplantation in Japan: registry by the Japanese liver transplantation society. *Hepatol Res*. 2019;**49**(9):964–980.
8. Kasai M, Kimura S, Asakura Y, et al. Surgical treatment of biliary atresia. *J Pediatr Surg*. 1968;**3**(6):655–675.
9. Nio M. Japanese biliary atresia registry. *Pediatr Surg Int*. 2017;**33**(12):1319–1325.
10. Kasahara M, Kuuchi T, Inomata Y, et al. Living-related liver transplantation for Alagille syndrome. *Transplantation*. 2003;**75**(12):2147–2150.
11. CeCile C, Tania AB, Ferechte ER, et al. Jagged1 gene expression during human embryogenesis elucidated the wide phenotypic spectrum of Alagille syndrome. *Hepatology*. 2000;**32**(3):574–581.
12. Kasahara M, Sakamoto S, Horikawa R, et al. Living donor liver transplantation for pediatric patients with metabolic disorders: the Japanese multicenter registry. *Pediatr Transplant*. 2014;**18**(1):6–15.
13. Baliga P, Alvarez S, Lindblad A, Zeng L. Posttransplant survival in pediatric fulminant hepatic failure: the SPLIT experience. *Liver Transpl*. 2004;**10**(11):1364–1371.
14. Dhawan A. Acute liver failure in children and adolescents. *Clin Res Hepatol Gastroenterol*. 2012;**36**(3):278–283.
15. Sakamoto S, Haga H, Egawa H, Kasahara M, Ogawa K, Takada Y, Uemoto S. Living donor liver transplantation for acute liver failure in infants: the impact of unknown etiology. *Pediatr Transplant*. 2008;**12**(2):167–173.
16. Squires RH Jr, Shneider BL, Bucuvalas J, et al. Acute liver failure in children: the first 348 patients in the pediatric acute liver failure study group. *J Pediatr*. 2006;**148**(5):652–658.
17. Naiki T, Nakayama N, Mochida S, et al. Novel scoring system as a useful model to predict the outcome of patients with acute liver failure: application to indication criteria for liver transplantation. *Hepatol Res*. 2012;**42**(1):68–75.
18. Schiodt FV, Ostapowicz G, Murray N, et al. Alpha-fetoprotein and prognosis in acute liver failure. *Liver Transpl*. 2006;**12**(12):1776–1778.
19. Kumar R, Shalimar, Sharma H, et al. Prospective derivation and validation of early dynamic model for predicting outcome in patients with acute liver failure. *Gut*. 2012;**61**(7):1068–1075.
20. Sakamoto S, Kasahara M, Mizuta K, et al. Nationwide survey of the outcomes of living donor liver transplantation for hepatoblastoma in Japan. *Liver Transpl*. 2014;**20**(3):333–346.
21. Kasahara M, de Ville de Goyet J. Reducing left liver lobe grafts, more or less? Don't throw out the baby with the bath water. … *Pediatr Transplant*. 2015;**19**(8):815–817.
22. Kasahara M, Sakamoto S, Shigeta T, et al. Reducing the thickness of left lateral segment grafts in neonatal living donor liver transplantation. *Liver Transpl*. 2013;**19**(2):226–228.

23. Kasahara M, Sakamoto S, Sasaki K, et al. Living donor liver transplantation during the first 3 month of life. *Liver Transpl.* 2017;**23**(8):1051–1057.
24. Sakamoto S, Sasaki K, Uchida H, et al. Ex vivo reduction of thickness in the left lateral section to tailor the graft size in infantile split deceased donor liver transplantation. *Liver Transplant.* 2018;**24**(3):428–431.
25. Enosawa S, Horikawa R, Yamamoto A, et al. Hepatocyte transplantation using a living donor reduced graft in a baby with ornithine transcarbamylase deficiency: a novel source of hepatocytes. *Liver Transpl.* 2014;**20**(3):391–393.
26. Inomoto T, Nishizawa F, Sasaki H, et al. Experiences of 120 microsurgical reconstruction of hepatic artery in living related liver transplantation. *Surgery.* 1996;**119**(1):20–26.
27. Heaton ND. Hepatic artery thrombosis: conservative management or retransplantation? *Liver Transpl.* 2013;**19**(Suppl 2):S14–S16.
28. Ziaziaris W, Darani A, Holland AJA, et al. Reducing the incidence of hepatic artery thrombosis in pediatric liver transplantation: effect of microvascular techniques and a customized anticoagulation protocol. *Pediatr Transplant.* 2017;**21**(4):e12917.
29. Ackermann O, Branchereau S, Franchi-Abella S. The long-term outcome of hepatic artery thrombosis after liver transplantation in children: role of urgent revascularization. *Am J Transplant.* 2012;**12**(6):1496–1503.
30. Ueda M, Oike F, Kasahara M, et al. Portal vein complication in pediatric living donor liver transplantation using left-side grafts. *Am J Transplant.* 2008;**8**(10):2097–2105.
31. Sakamoto S, Sasaki K, Kitajima T, et al. A novel technique for collateral interruption to maximize portal venous flow in pediatric liver transplantation. *Liver Transpl.* 2018;**24**(7):969–973.
32. Raby N, Karani J, Thomas S, O'Grady J, Williamus R. Stenosis of vascular anastomosis after hepatic transplantation: treatment with balloon angioplasty. *AJR Am J Roentgenol.* 1991;**157**(1):167–171.
33. Khorsandi SE, Athale A, Vilca-Melendez H, et al. Presentation, diagnosis, and management of early hepatic venous outflow complications in whole cadaveric liver transplant. *Liver Transpl.* 2015;**21**(7):914–921.
34. Tannuri U, Tannuri AC, Santos MM, Miyatani HT. Technique advance to avoid hepatic venous outflow obstruction in pediatric living-donor liver transplantation. *Pediatr Transplant.* 2015;**19**(3):261–266.
35. Sakamoto S, Ogura Y, Shibata T, et al. Successful stent placement for hepatic venous outflow obstruction in pediatric living donor liver transplantation, including a case series review. *Pediatr Transplant.* 2009;**13**(4):507–511.
36. Broelsch CE, Whitington PF, Emond JC, et al. Liver transplantation in children from living related donors. Surgical techniques and results. *Ann Surg.* 1991;**214**(4):428–437.
37. Akamatsu N, Sugawara Y, Kaneko J, et al. Surgical repair for late-onset hepatic venous outflow block after living-donor liver transplantation. *Transplantation.* 2004;**77**(11):1768–1770.
38. Northover JM, Terblanche J. A new look at the arterial supply of the bile duct in man and its surgical implications. *Br J Surg.* 1979;**66**(6):379–384.
39. Sharma S, Gurakar A, Jabbour N. Biliary strictures following liver transplantation: past, present and preventive strategies. *Liver Transpl.* 2008;**14**(6):759–769.
40. Kasahara M, Egawa H, Takada Y, et al. Biliary reconstruction in right lobe living-donor liver transplantation: comparison of different techniques in 321 recipients. *Ann Surg.* 2006;**243**(4):559–566.
41. Thethy S, Thomson B, Pleass H, et al. Management of biliary tract complications after orthotopic liver transplantation. *Clin Transplant.* 2004;**18**(6):647–653.
42. Fukuda A, Sakamoto S, Uchida H, et al. Hepatobiliary scintigraphy for the assessment of biliary stricture after pediatric living donor liver transplantation for hepaticojejunostomy reconstruction: the value of the excretion rate at 60 min. *Pediatr Transpl.* 2011;**15**(6):594–600.
43. Kasahara M, Umeshita K, Inomata Y, et al. Long-term outcomes of pediatric living donor liver transplantation in Japan: an analysis of more than 2200 cases listed in the registry of the Japanese Liver Transplantation Society. *Am J Transplant.* 2013;**13**(7):1830–1839.
44. McDiarmid SV, Anand R, Martz K, et al. A multivariate analysis of pre-, peri-, and post-transplant factors affecting outcome after pediatric liver transplantation. *Ann Surg.* 2011;**254**(1):145–154.
45. Bethany JF, Mourad D, Xun Z, Vikas RD, Conway J, Vicky NG. High risk of liver allograft failure during late adolescence and young adulthood. *Transplantation.* 2016;**100**(3):577–584.
46. Dharniharka VR, Lamb KE, Zheng J, et al. Across all solid organs, adolescent age recipients have worse transplant organ survival than younger age children: a US national registry analysis. *Pediatr Transplant.* 2015;**19**(5):471–476.
47. Kasahara M, Uneshita K, Inomata Y, et al. Long-term outcomes of pediatric living donor liver transplantation in Japan: an analysis of more than 2200 cases listed in the registry of the Japanese Liver Transplantation Society. *Am J Transplant.* 2013;**13**(7):1830–1839.
48. Abt PL, Rapaport-Kelz R, Desai NM, et al. Survival among pediatric liver transplant recipients: impact of segmental grafts. *Liver Transpl.* 2004;**10**(10):1287–1293.
49. Van Arendonk KJ, King EA, Orandi BJ, et al. Loss of pediatric kidney grafts during the 'high-risk age window': insights from pediatric liver and simultaneous liver-kidney recipients. *Am J Transplant.* 2015;**15**(2):445–452.
50. Goss JA, Shackleton CR, Swenson K, et al. Orthotopic liver transplantation for congenital biliary atresia-an 11-year single center experience. *Ann Surg.* 1996;;**224**(3):276–287.
51. Utterson EC, Shepherd RW, Sokol RJ, et al. Biliary atresia: clinical profiles, risk factors, and outcomes of 755 patients listed for liver transplantation. *J Pediatr.* 2005;**147**(2):180–185.

24

Live donor liver transplantation

Michele Finotti and Giuliano Testa

Introduction

For the past three decades, liver transplantation has been the treatment of choice for end-stage liver diseases and hepatocellular carcinoma (HCC). Recently other indications for liver transplantation have been proposed in the treatment of primary and secondary liver tumours, especially for colorectal liver metastases, in the so-called transplant oncology field.

Although the cure of hepatitis C has dramatically changed the landscape, liver transplantation still faces the problem of a large number of candidates and a shortage of deceased liver donors. To increase the donor pool and meet the need for liver grafts, alternative techniques such as the use of extended criteria donors and donation after cardiac death have been further implemented, with continued expansion of the clinical limits.

In this context, living donor liver transplantation (LDLT) has been a crucial additional source of grafts to deceased donor liver transplantation (DDLT), and, in selected cases, could be considered the first choice. The advantages of LDLT go beyond being an immediate source of a transplantable organ. There are clear advantages in terms of timing to intervention and long-term outcomes that significantly benefit the recipient of a LDLT. These advantages need to be critically weighed against the technically demanding surgeries of both donor and recipient and the ethical and safety issues involved in the living donation process.

Historical background

The concept and technical background of LDLT derives from the experience with reduced and split deceased donor liver transplant, especially in the paediatric population.

In the 1980s, liver transplantation in children accounted for only 10–15% of all liver replacements. However, the lack of adequate whole liver deceased donors matching the graft size for this population led to a pre-transplantation mortality of 25–50% in children.[1–3]

The deep knowledge of the liver anatomy, in particular of the vascular inflow/outflow and biliary tree structure, and the efforts of a few pioneers allowed the development of important alternative procedures to the use of the whole liver graft. The concept guiding the development of the idea that a liver graft can serve more than one recipient is based on the independence of the segmental liver units, since each segment is provided with its own vascular pedicle, bile duct, and venous drainage, and could in theory be used as a liver graft.

The reduced liver transplantation, first reported by Bismuth and Houssin in 1984,[1] starts with a standard liver procurement. On the bench, the liver is reduced into the left lateral segment (segments 2 and 3) or left lobe (segments 2–4), the most common segments used in paediatric recipients. In its original implementation the remaining right lobe was discarded.[3–6]

In 1988, Pichlmayr et al. reported the first split liver transplantation. The splitting consists of the division of the liver into two grafts: segments 2 and 3 for the paediatric recipient and segments 4–8 for adults. The liver splitting can be performed *ex vivo*, as firstly described, or *in situ*. Although no strong evidence exists in favour of either option, the *in situ* procedure (performed before the cold perfusion) is usually preferred. A better haemostasis and biliostasis in the resected liver surface and a short cold ischaemia time are the main advantages of *in situ* splitting; by contrast, the donor surgery is prolonged and a skilled surgical team is required.[1,7–10]

LDLT can be considered the sum of these techniques, associated with the progressive experience accumulated in reduced liver transplantation, split liver transplantation, liver resection, and medical management.[11,12]

In 1988, Raia et al.—pushed by the shortage of donors and by the high waiting list mortality (50% for adults and 73% for children)—performed the first two cases of LDLT. Left lateral segments (2 and 3) were provided by living donors and transplanted in paediatric recipients. The recipient's outcome was poor, but the donation process showed no complications.[13]

In 1990, Strong et al. reported the first successful LDLT in an 11-month-old child with biliary atresia. A left lobe was procured; segment 4 was discarded on the bench and segments 2 and 3 were transplanted into the recipient.[14]

Broelsch et al. in 1989 were the first to standardize the procedure of a left lateral hepatectomy and subsequent transplantation in children.[13] From there the history of paediatric LDLT was significantly written by the Asian countries led by Kyoto University in Japan.[12,13] LDLT had a rapid expansion in Asia, mainly driven by the reluctance of accepting the concept of brain death and the consequent lack of deceased donors.

The next milestone in the history of LDLT is represented by expansion to the adult population. The clinical need was still fuelled by the insufficient number of deceased donors and the growing number of patients on the liver transplant list. The first successful adult-to-adult LDLT was performed in 1993 using a left liver graft.[15] The first LDLT that used the right liver was performed in Kyoto and the first adult right liver LDLT was performed in Hong Kong in 1996.[16]

The LDLT application saw an initial progressive increase, paralleled by improvements in the surgical technique, donor safety, and competitive outcomes towards DDLT. Mirroring paediatric LDLT, adult LDLT has been the main form of liver transplantation in Asia and in most countries with a non-existing or undeveloped deceased donor system. Today, more than 90% of liver transplantations performed in Asia are from living donors, while, apart from a few exceptions, the procedure has not been embraced in most of Europe and North America.[17,18] As an example, in 2018, 401 LDLTs were performed in all of the US compared to the 1313 performed in India alone. The availability of deceased donors, the expansion of the deceased donor pool with donation after cardiac death, and extended criteria donors and clinical and ethical challenges associated with living donation are among the reasons for significantly different approaches between the Western world and Asia.

Ethical aspects of living donation

In the LDLT process, the balance of risks and benefits has to be weighed both in relation to the donors and the recipients. The initial question of clinical equipoise, is LDLT as good a therapy for end-stage liver disease as DDLT, has already been answered. Clearly LDLT offers outcomes that are as good if not superior to the ones seen in DDLT.[19] Moreover, the elimination of waitlist mortality in paediatric recipients and the additional alternative to deceased donors in the adult population represent the main benefit of LDLT for the recipient.[20–24]

But in LDLT, as pointed out by Cronin et al., the balance of risks and benefits has to be weighted both in relation to the donors and the recipients.[25] Once one has accepted the fact that living donation cannot be routinely performed with an absolute zero risk, the question remains how much risk is acceptable and how the risk of complications should be 'shared' between donor and recipient.[26] This concept is highlighted in the debate about using a left liver, where the risk for the donor is diminished but the risk of small for size in the recipient is increased, versus a right liver where the scenario is the opposite.[27–38]

While safety and freedom from coercion remain essential issues in the ethical debate surrounding living donation, much has been done in terms of improving the donor experience and the transplant community represented by the transplant professional societies continues to support living donation with shared initiatives with governmental agencies like the donor financial support offered through the National Living Donor Assistance programme in the US.[39]

Indications

General indications

The indications for LDLT are similar to those for DDLT. Figure 24.1 shows the main indications for LDLT in the US and in Japan.[40] The registry by the Japanese Liver Transplantation Society reported, from 1964 to 2017, 8795 LDLTs, mainly performed for cholestatic liver diseases (especially biliary atresia). Of note, the paediatric population were the most common recipients of LDLT, followed by patients between 50 and 59 years old (Figure 24.2). The Organ Procurement and Transplantation Network reported, from 1989 to date (April 2021), 7932 LDLTs, mainly for hepatocellular diseases.

In the Asian region, no international organ transplantation registry exists. However, an Asian Transplant Registry under the Asian Society of Transplantation is under development.[41]

Living donor liver transplantation and hepatocellular carcinoma

Since its inception, LDLT has been considered a viable option for patients affected by HCC. The simple fact that LDLT can significantly shorten the time from listing to transplantation has been seen as a very effective way to reduce the risk of patient dropout due to tumour progression. However, several studies suggest that LDLT is associated with a higher HCC recurrence rate, compared

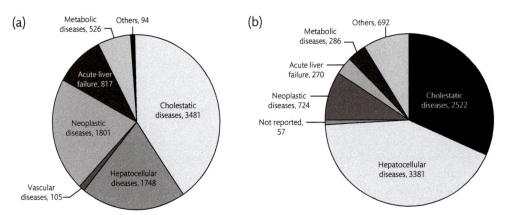

Figure 24.1 (a) Indications in Japan from 1964 to 2017 among 8795 LDLTs. (b) Indications in the US from 1989 to April 2021 among 7932 LDLTs.
(a) Source: data from Umeshita K et al. Liver transplantation in Japan: registry by the Japanese Liver Transplantation Society. *Hepatol Res.* 2019;49(9):964–980. (b) Source: data from Organ Procurement and Transplantation Network, https://optn.transplant.hrsa.gov/data/view-data-reports/national-data/

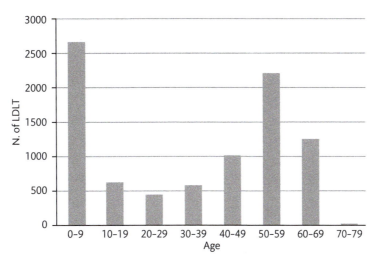

Figure 24.2 Age of LDLT recipients in Japan.
Source: data 1964–2017, from Umeshita K et al. Liver transplantation in Japan: Registry by the Japanese Liver Transplantation Society. *Hepatol Res.* 2019;49(9):964–980.

to DDLT, translating into a shorter disease-free and overall survival. The theoretical explanation of the increased incidence of tumour recurrence has pointed at the effect that liver regeneration after LDLT has on tumour growth. Especially in the case of small-for-size grafts, liver growth causes a rapid increase in growth factors and cytokines and a possible stimulation of HCC recurrence.[42–46] Insufficient tumour removal and HCC residue and dissemination in the recipient of a LDLT where the preservation of the native inferior vena cava and a longer hepatic artery and bile duct may be necessary, compared to DDLT, has also been called into question.[47,48] Furthermore, for LDLTs, the waiting time list is drastically reduced compared to DDLTs. The waiting time is useful, especially in HCC beyond the Milan criteria, to evaluate the HCC progression and to assess response to locoregional treatments, such as transarterial chemoembolization or ablative techniques (microwave ablation or radiofrequency ablation). In LDLTs this 'test of time' is significantly reduced, and the higher HCC recurrence might be the consequence of the inclusion of patient with aggressive HCC or HCC beyond Milan criteria.[42–46,48–57]

However, collected data are inconsistent, often due to the heterogeneity of the transplanted population, selection criteria, pre-transplantation treatment, time to transplantation, donor preservation, surgical technique, and post-liver transplantation management. Furthermore, the outcome evaluation starting not at the time of the liver transplantation but at the waitlist (intention-to-treat analyses) should be considered as another factor leading to different results among the published studies. It seems that patient selection more than technical issues is the most important factor in explaining the different HCC recurrence rate and overall survival in LDLT compared to DDLT.[58–61] Individual centre practices and experiences are then at the basis of the decision to adopt extended HCC criteria for patients who have access to LDLT compared to stricter ones for patients undergoing DDLT.[62,63]

In the past few years there has also been a renewed interest in addressing unresectable colorectal liver metastatic disease with liver transplantation. The Toronto group proposed a protocol to select patients affected by non-resectable colorectal liver metastases suitable for LDLT (NCT02864485). A modification of the RAPID technique has been proposed in patients with unresectable colorectal metastases who first undergo left hepatectomy and left lateral transplantation with a living donor graft and then to completion hepatectomy, once the small-for-size graft has grown to an appropriate mass and function.[64–66] Ongoing clinical trials are based on this technique (NCT02215889 and NCT04865471).

Inspired by the same concept, Konigsrainer et al. proposed a LDLT with two-stage hepatectomy in the recipient (LIVER-T(W)O-HEAL).[67] The previous techniques mixed the latest advances in hepatobiliary and liver transplantation surgery, using an association of LDLT, auxiliary partial orthotopic liver transplantation, and associating liver partition and portal vein ligation for staged hepatectomy (ALPPS) procedures.[68–70] These strategies do not affect the deceased donor pool and use the left liver lobe, reducing the risks for the donors.[71]

Donor evaluation

A proper donor selection is essential both for donor and recipient outcome. A prerequisite for a good outcome is that the donor can undergo hepatectomy with a lower risk and the recipient receives an appropriate graft.

Donor evaluation is typically made step by step, allowing the exclusion of unsuitable donors in the early phase to reduce as much as possible invasive and avoidable testing with a cost-effective approach.[23,72,73]

Many centres have adopted an electronic, internet-based screening tool that collects basic information such as age, height, weight, blood type, relationship with the donor, and basic medical, surgical, and social history.[74] Past major abdominal operations, medical comorbidities (diabetes, significant cardiac history), or obesity (body mass index >32 kg/m^2) may be sufficient initial elements to exclude the donation. Almost one-half to one-third of potential donors are ruled out at preclinical assessment. Most programmes have adopted a two-step consent process constituted first by informed consent to conduct the evaluation and second, after the evaluation has been completed and the candidate found

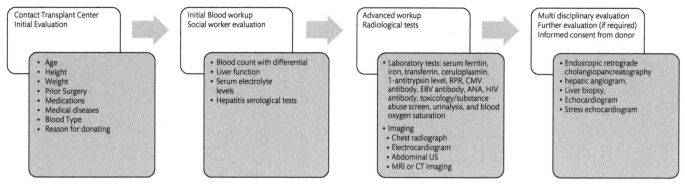

Figure 24.3 Donor evaluation for LDLT. ANA, antinuclear antibody; CMV, cytomegalovirus; EBV, Epstein–Barr virus; HIV: human immunodeficiency virus; RPR, rapid plasmin regain; US, ultrasound.

to be an appropriate donor, a final informed consent to proceed with the surgery. A multidisciplinary team (hepatologist, transplant surgeon, social workers, donor advocate) evaluates the candidate, reiterating pros and cons, characteristics of the surgery and hospital stay, time to recovery, and the incidence of complications (Figure 24.3).

Once the initial screening has been passed, the complete medical/social evaluation is conducted starting with complete blood work and continuing with thorough medical and social visits. If no contraindications arise, appropriate imaging studies to evaluate the liver anatomy and future liver remnant follow.

Imaging evaluation of the donor's liver through magnetic resonance imaging (MRI) and/or computed tomography (CT) abdominal scan is essential to estimate the liver volume with volumetry for both donor and recipient and to assess liver anatomy. The standard limits criteria for the right lobe donation are a donor remnant liver of at least 35% with at least 0.8% graft-to-recipient body weight ratio.[75] The limit of 0.8% is not considered absolute and a lower ratio down to 0.6% has been proposed when the donor is young (<40 years old) and the recipient clinical conditions permissible.[23,76,77] Standard liver volume formulas are also widely used in support or as an alternative to the graft-to recipient body weight ratio.[78–85]

CT angiography or MRI are routinely used to map the liver vascular inflow and outflow and the presence of anatomical variations. Magnetic resonance cholangiopancreatography is the imaging test of choice for the evaluation of the hepatic ducts. Most of the anatomical variants do not exclude living donation and can be managed by an experienced surgical team.[86,87] Liver biopsy is not routinely performed and it is usually indicated to confirm a suspected liver macrosteatosis (CT/MRI indicative for steatosis and/or body mass index >28 kg/m^2).[88–90] To obtain appropriately informed consent, the donor must be given the correct explanation of possible complications after donation. The reported overall donor complication incidence ranges between 15% and 40%, with major complications ranging between 1.6% and 3.2%.[91–98] Biliary complications, especially biliary strictures and bile leakages, are the most common issue after donation for LDLT.[91,99] Right lobe donor hepatectomy and left lateral liver procurement are not without risk, with a mortality rate of 0.4–0.6%, and 0.05–0.1% respectively.[100–103]

However, an actual estimation of mortality risk and causes of death is challenging due to a lack of an international registry for living liver donation.[104] In 2006 and 2008, a worldwide literature review revealed 14 and 33 living liver donor deaths, respectively.[105,106]

Donor deaths rates vary among the world: 0.3 deaths per 1000 donors in Japan and 2.3 deaths per 1000 donors in Europe.[107,108]

In 2012, a study based on 4111 live liver donors (66.9% right lobe donation) in the US followed up after donation for a mean of 7.6 years estimated the risk of death of 1.7 per 1000 donors. In particular, seven live liver donors died within the first 90 days after donation. To note, the risk of perioperative death and the long-term survival after liver donation was similar compared to matched live kidney donors and healthy individuals, respectively.[109] Most of the donor deaths seem to be related to the surgical procedure, but an accurate database would add detailed knowledge and could be key to reduce the donor risk.[35,101,108–115]

Surgical techniques

Donor and recipient hepatectomy are scheduled in simultaneous operating rooms, performed by two different surgical teams. In general, the donor hepatectomy starts prior to the recipient hepatectomy, allowing time to assess the donor anatomy and check any findings that contradict with the imaging studies.

Constant communication between the two surgical teams is essential at every surgical step, to coordinate and optimize the timing for both recipient and donor.

Donor hepatectomy

Donor hepatectomy can be performed through a laparotomy or minimally invasive approach (laparoscopic or robotic) according to the donor clinical and anatomical features and the centre expertise. Based on the presurgical evaluation, a left or right liver lobe donation can be harvested. Many centres are versatile in both right and left donor hepatectomies. The decision about the type of graft is usually driven by volume issues and at times by the anatomy of the donor liver. The left donor hepatectomy is considered less morbid but in general provides a smaller graft volume, shifting the risk of complications towards the recipient.

Both in the right and left hepatectomy, the procedure starts with an exploration of the abdomen. Depending on the centre's preference, intraoperative ultrasound and intraoperative cholangiography may be performed, to better determine the line of parenchymal transection and biliary anatomy. The surgical phases of the hepatectomy are universal, although the timing of each phase may vary according to the surgeon's preference. These phases include mobilization of the liver through dissection of the falciform and triangular ligaments, cholecystectomy, dissection of the hepatic artery and portal vein branches, control of the posterior hepatic veins, parenchymal transection, removal of the graft, and, finally, closure of the vascular and biliary stumps. Regarding the parenchymal transection, the most utilized instruments are the Cavitron and the Waterjet.

Left lateral segmentectomy

In the open left lateral segmentectomy, after dissection of the falciform and triangular ligaments, control of the left hepatic vein, and dissection of the left hepatic artery and portal vein, associated with control of the segment 4 hepatic portal branches, the liver parenchyma is transected within few millimetres from the falciform ligament.

When most of the parenchymal transection has been performed, the left hepatic duct is sharply cut.

A hanging manoeuvre may facilitate the last portion of the parenchymal transection. Lastly, the inflow vessels are clamped and cut, followed by the left hepatic vein.

Pitfalls of the open procedure are the proper dissection of the left hepatic vein that can be encircled with an umbilical tape which can be used for the hanging manoeuvre. The dissection of the left portal vein extends to include the tissue from its medial wall to the Arantius ligament and the control of the portal branches towards segment 4 by dissection of the round ligament and exposure of the recessus Rex. This last manoeuvre allows for a quick and almost bloodless hepatic parenchyma transection.

The left lateral segmentectomy can be performed through minimally invasive surgery (MIS), facilitated by the anterior position of the lobe and the limited number of anatomical variations.[116-118] Pitfalls in the MIS are the correct trocar placements, the precise cut of the left bile duct and the closure of the remnant bile duct, an adequate parenchymal dissection with the current laparoscopic device, and the Pfannenstiel incision.

The trocar placement is essential for optimal surgical vision. As described by Soubrane et al., a periumbilical trocar is used for the optics. With the correct triangulation, the other two trocars are placed. A fourth and a fifth trocar are positioned below the sternum and in the right flank, respectively, to allow proper exposure during the hepatectomy.[119]

The parenchymal dissection is performed as in open surgery, with ultrasound devices, avoiding blind stapling of liver parenchyma. The Hem-o-lok and vascular stapler can be used to control major intrahepatic vessels. The Pfannenstiel incision, used for the graft extraction, has to be performed carefully, to avoid bladder injury and postoperative haematomas, and provides excellent cosmetic results and good postoperative pain control. As in open surgery, hepatic duct division and closure of the remnant hepatic duct stump need to be performed with great care to avoid donor complications, such as biliary leakage or stricture.

Metal clips or Hem-o-lok, associated with real-time indocyanine green near-infrared fluorescence cholangiography, can help to identify the appropriate resection point and consequent closure of the remnant bile duct.[106,120] The robotic approach, thanks to the three-dimensional view, the stability, and the precision of the movements, may facilitate the previous steps compared to the laparoscopic technique.[121]

Right hepatectomy

The right hepatectomy (segments 5–8) starts either by immediately performing the cholecystectomy and the dissection of the right hepatic artery and right portal vein, or by first mobilizing the right liver by dissecting the right triangular ligament and exposing the lateral aspect of the infrahepatic vena cava. Most surgeons will perform an intraoperative cholangiogram, either through the cystic duct stump or through a longitudinal choledocotomy.[122] The mobilization of the liver from the vena cava and the control of the right hepatic vein are standard phases of any right hepatectomy. The difference is the preservation of any posterior hepatic vein with a diameter equal or greater than 5 mm. These hepatic veins can be clipped with Hem-o-lok clips and cut or left intact and then clamped at the time of graft extraction. As in the left hepatectomy, the line of parenchymal transection can be ascertained with a unilateral Pringle manoeuvre or by identifying and following the middle hepatic vein (MHV) with Doppler ultrasonography. Different instruments are used to transect the liver parenchyma, with most surgeons using either the WaterJet or the Cavitron. Large tributaries from segments 5 and 8 draining into the MHV should be preserved. In these cases, the Hem-o-lok clips are particularly useful. Most centres would refrain from including the entire MHV in the graft, as has been proposed by the Hong Kong Group, mainly because of concerns of leaving the donor with venous outflow based only on the left hepatic vein.[123-126] The hanging manoeuvre (a nylon tape is passed between the roots of the right hepatic vein and MHV, posterior to the caudate lobe) is often adopted to facilitate the parenchymal transection. The right hepatic duct is most often cut when most of the parenchymal transection has already been completed but severing of the hepatic duct prior to liver parenchymal transection has also been described.[122] When the liver transection is completed, the right hepatic artery, portal vein, and right hepatic vein are clamped and severed. As an alternative, a vascular stapler can be utilized especially for the venous structures.

Particular attention must be paid to the closure of the donor hepatic duct stump, to avoid postoperative leaks or strictures. In fact, in terms of the incidence of complications, biliary complications are still the most common after liver donation.[35,92,112,127-131]

Laparoscopic right hepatectomy in living donation has been proposed, firstly in a laparoscopic-assisted fashion and then in a pure laparoscopic technique.[132] The main limitation to the diffusion of the laparoscopic right hepatectomy compared to left hepatectomy is that is a challenging procedure, associated in some series with higher donor morbidity compared to open surgery.[133-136]

Pitfalls in the laparoscopic right hepatectomy are the correct mobilization of the right lobe; the identification of the frequent anatomical variations of the biliary and portal system, in particular early bifurcation of the right anterior and posterior bile ducts; and the correct plane of parenchymal and biliary transection.

Back table

The back table preparation of a living donor graft, especially the right liver, may require complex reconstructions mainly for the venous outflow, but also for the portal vein, the hepatic artery, and the hepatic duct. Reinforcing of the hepatic vein outflow with a segment of cryopreserved or stored vessel in the so-called fence technique has been promoted by the Asian group.[137-139] Joining of the right hepatic vein and MHV orifices has been described by the Hong Kong group when the right graft is procured with the entire MHV.[140] Different vein patches to obtain a single sewing surface when multiple posterior hepatic veins are present have been described by the Kyoto and Essen Groups.[141,142] Different types of material have been used to construct conduits to allow proper venous outflow from segment 5 and 8 tributaries: stored deceased vessels, appropriately fashioned recipient femoral veins, and Gore-Tex grafts.[138,143-151] A recent randomized trial showed a comparable patency rate between grafts with native and reconstructed MHV.[126]

Variant portal vein, hepatic artery, and biliary tract are not uncommon. Standard portal vein anatomy occurs in 70–85% of the patients. The most common variations, according to the Cheng classification, are types II–III and IV.[152-155] In the event of a double portal vein, different reconstruction techniques have been described: from the joining of the adjacent wall when the two lumens are close to each other, to a Y graft that can be constructed with an iliac vein graft from a deceased donor, to the portal vein of the recipient liver.[156] Double right hepatic artery can be encountered in 0.8–1% of the grafts.[157] In this case the reconstruction in a single inflow orifice can be performing by utilizing a cloacal technique, or utilizing a Y graft from stored deceased vessels. The problem with stored arterial vessels is the size mismatch with the graft hepatic arteries. One alternative option is to use the recipient right and left hepatic arteries Y graft to reconstruct the inflow.[158-161]

Two or even more hepatic ducts are not uncommon in a right graft (25–35% of grafts).[157,162] The reconstruction in a single orifice can be performed when the two ducts are close to each other. A good technique calls for the V-shaped incision of the mid portion of each medial wall and reconstruction in a cloaca fashion method. This technique helps the avoidance of the distortion of the orifice that is often the result of the simpler suturing of the medial walls.[131]

The left lateral and left liver grafts require much less attention on the back table, most often directed at the construction of a large single venous outflow orifice. In such cases a venous patch, usually with a stored deceased donor vessel, is the simplest method of reconstruction.[163]

Mono lateral and right posterior liver segments are not commonly used and require specific technical expertise for both the procurement and then the back table preparation.[164-171]

Recipient operation

The recipient hepatectomy is performed with caval preservation. In general, the hilar dissection demands greater preparation than in deceased donor transplantation. It is customary to extend the dissection to include longer segments of the right and left hepatic arteries and of the right and left portal vein. Unless a Roux-en-Y hepaticojejunostomy is planned, the hepatic duct should be dissected to include part of the hilar plate and the right and left confluence. Performing it in a sharp fashion when the inflow to the liver has already been taken can facilitate the dissection of the hilar plate. In this way an abundant amount of periductal tissue is left intact and a tedious dissection can be avoided.

The implantation of the right graft starts with the construction of the venous outflow. The anastomosis between the right hepatic vein of the graft and the recipient cava can be performed in a linear fashion, extending the recipient hepatic vein along the longitudinal axis of the cava or in a triangular fashion, extending the orifice of the recipient right hepatic vein towards the anterior surface of the vena cava. In the latter case three running sutures are used.[76] A posterior hepatic vein can be directly anastomosed through a separate cavotomy. When a venous conduit draining segment 5 and/or 8 is present, this can be anastomosed, preferably after graft reperfusion, to an appropriate size and length, to the common orifice of the recipient middle and left hepatic veins.[76,172] Portal inflow can be constructed using the main or the right branch of the portal vein. After reperfusion, the arterial anastomosis can be performed either with the microscope or with magnification loops. Smaller calibre arteries (<3 mm) might benefit from an interrupted instead of running suturing technique.[161,173,174] For the implantation of the left lateral or left liver grafts, most surgeons would prefer a triangulation of the venous outflow anastomosis, joining the orifices of the middle and left hepatic veins and then extending the opening towards the caudal–anterior portion of the vena cava wall.

Especially for a left lateral graft, particular attention must be paid to the proper orientation of the portal vein, to avoid its kinking.[76,172]

Different techniques have been proposed for the construction of the biliary anastomosis, probably a reflection of the still fairly high complication rate. Aside from specific centre preferences, both a duct-to-duct or a hepaticojejunostomy can be used. Since no single method has been proven to have a lower risk of complications than others, it remains the centre's preference whether to perform a running or interrupted suturing technique, to use re-absorbable or non-re-absorbable suture material, and finally whether to place a stent or not.[162,175]

Small-for-size syndrome and hepatic venous outflow management

The small-for-size syndrome (SFSS) is a clinical and laboratory condition precipitated by an insufficient liver graft volume, unable to meet the metabolic demands of the recipient.

Large volume ascites (>1 L), hyperbilirubinaemia, coagulopathy, encephalopathy (grade 3 or 4), and renal dysfunction are the clinical features of SFSS. However, a specific criterion to define SFSS is lacking and differences exist in the published literature.[176-182] Although left liver grafts in adult recipients are more prone to trigger a SFSS, this condition is present also after a right liver graft.

Graft- and recipient-related factors have been proposed on the pathogenesis of SFSS. Liver size is one of the main factors, and a graft less than or equal to 40–50% of standard liver volume (a graft-to-recipient weight ratio of <0.8%) is more often associated with SFSS development.[177]

Donor age and steatosis (>30%) are other donor factors that have been associated with SFFS. Critical recipient clinical conditions often reflected in a high Model for End-Stage Liver Disease (MELD) score have also been associated with SFFS syndrome.[181,183-186]

There are significant technical steps involving the construction and reconstruction of the venous outflow and the modulation of the portal inflow that have been proposed to mitigate the clinical impact of SFFS on the short- and long-term outcome of the recipients of such grafts.

The recognition of the importance of the MHV in the venous drainage of the right lobe was the first step to bring about all technical innovation aimed at avoiding graft congestion and consequent loss of functioning liver mass.[123,187] Today most programmes are very attentive at reconstructing large V5 and V8 tributaries and any large posterior hepatic veins.[76,172]

There are no MHV tributaries or posterior hepatic veins in a left graft but attention must be paid to the construction of a large venous outflow and a proper fashioning of a single orifice with the MHV and the left hepatic vein.[138,188-190] Moreover the inclusion of the caudate lobe and the preservation of its venous outflow has been described and proposed to increase the size of a left lobe graft.[191,192]

Modulation of the portal vein inflow is the other strategy utilized to mitigate the negative clinical impact of SFFS. While an adequate portal inflow is necessary to allow liver regeneration, portal hyperperfusion has been identified as a detrimental factor and a culprit of SFFS.[193-196] Different technical solutions have been proposed to decrease portal flow from creating temporary portocaval shunts, to ligation of the splenic artery and splenectomy.[196-214]

None of these technical modifications seems to routinely be successful in avoiding SFFS and it seems that a technically successful LDLT stands on the principles outlined by S. G. Lee in his comprehensive review: an adequate graft volume; a secure bile duct anastomosis to prevent leak, strictures, and sepsis; a sufficient inflow, avoiding portal flow steal, stenosis, or kinking; and a good outflow, with a wide ostium preventing liver congestion.[76]

Minimally invasive approach to live donation and future perspectives

In hepatobiliary surgery, MIS is considered the preferred approach in selected patients.[215] Compared to open surgery, MIS is associated with a shorter hospital stay, lower blood loss, lower need of transfusion, and better pain control.[216-218]

If MIS in minor hepatectomies (fewer than three segments) is considered the standard of care, laparoscopic major hepatic resections are still pilot procedures, due to the complex liver anatomy and the need for accurate bleeding control.[219] However, thanks to the good outcome and low morbidity of MIS in general and liver surgery, its application has started to be adopted in the field of living donation.[220]

In 1995, the first laparoscopic kidney graft procurement was performed with excellent outcomes.[221] Laparoscopic living donor left lateral sectionectomy, first reported by Cherqui et al. in 2002, is considered by many centres to be safe and feasible, with no additional donor mortality risk.[117,220,222,223] In contrast, laparoscopic right donor hepatectomy has been proposed only by a few centres in highly selected donors, often in a hybrid or hand-assisted fashion and with no clear benefits for donor recovery and decrease in complications.[132,220,224-234]

The robotic approach is considered the natural evolution of MIS.[235-238] In the robotic left lateral donor sectionectomy, first reported by Liao et al. in 2017, the outcomes are comparable in terms of morbidity and mortality, with lower blood loss rate and a shorter hospital stay.[239,240] Similar results are reported for robotic right lobe donor hepatectomy.[240-244] Although these results have been obtained in appropriately selected patients and by centres with robotic expertise, a much wider embracement of the robot in the living donor hepatectomy is foreseeable.

Most important improvements compared to laparoscopic technique are the more rapid learning curve and the three-dimensional imaging with a stable and high-definition view.[245] In particular, the robotic approach may help reduce the donor's biliary complication, thanks to the indocyanine green's fluorescent image—Firefly technology—that allows a clearer definition of the optimal hepatic duct division point[232,236,244,246] and an easier closure of the donor hepatic duct stump.[232,240,247]

The application of MIS in living donation seems to be safe and feasible.[248] Some of the doubts directed to a possible negative impact on recipient outcomes related to a longer warm ischaemia due to a more cumbersome extraction of the liver graft or the shorter length of the vessels, have not been supported by the reported data.[240-242,244]

REFERENCES

1. Busuttil RW, Goss JA. Split liver transplantation. *Ann Surg.* 1999;**229**(3):313–321.
2. Emond JC, Whitington PF, Thistlethwaite JR, et al. Transplantation of two patients with one liver. Analysis of a preliminary experience with 'split-liver' grafting. *Ann Surg.* 1990;**212**(1):14–22.
3. Jurim O, Csete M, Gelabert HA, et al. Reduced-size grafts—the solution for hepatic artery thrombosis after pediatric liver transplantation? *J Pediatr Surg.* 1995;**30**(1):53–55.
4. Emond JC, Whitington PF, Thistlethwaite JR, Alonso EM, Broelsch CE. Reduced-size orthotopic liver transplantation: use in the management of children with chronic liver disease. *Hepatology.* 1989;**10**(5):867–872.
5. Broelsch CE, Emond JC, Thistlethwaite JR, Rouch DA, Whitington PF, Lichtor JL. Liver transplantation with reduced-size donor organs. *Transplantation.* 1988;**45**(3):519–524.
6. Bismuth H, Houssin D. Reduced-sized orthotopic liver graft in hepatic transplantation in children. *Surgery.* 1984;**95**(3):367–370.
7. Hackl C, Schmidt KM, Susal C, Dohler B, Zidek M, Schlitt HJ. Split liver transplantation: current developments. *World J Gastroenterol.* 2018;**24**(47):5312–5321.
8. Cardillo M, De Fazio N, Pedotti P, et al. Split and whole liver transplantation outcomes: a comparative cohort study. *Liver Transpl.* 2006;**12**(3):402–410.
9. Zambelli M, Andorno E, De Carlis L, et al. Full-right-full-left split liver transplantation: the retrospective analysis of an early multicenter experience including graft sharing. *Am J Transplant.* 2012;**12**(8):2198–2210.
10. Angelico R, Trapani S, Spada M, et al. A national mandatory-split liver policy: a report from the Italian experience. *Am J Transplant.* 2019;**19**(7):2029–2043.
11. Otte JB, de Ville de Goyet J, Reding R, et al. Pediatric liver transplantation: from the full-size liver graft to reduced, split, and living related liver transplantation. *Pediatr Surg Int.* 1998;**13**(5–6):308–318.
12. Slooff MJ. Reduced size liver transplantation, split liver transplantation, and living related liver transplantation in relation to the donor organ shortage. *Transpl Int.* 1995;**8**(1):65–68.
13. Raia S, Nery JR, Mies S. Liver transplantation from live donors. *Lancet.* 1989;**2**(8661):497.
14. Strong RW, Lynch SV, Ong TH, Matsunami H, Koido Y, Balderson GA. Successful liver transplantation from a living donor to her son. *N Engl J Med.* 1990;**322**(21):1505–1507.

15. Hashikura Y, Makuuchi M, Kawasaki S, et al. Successful living-related partial liver transplantation to an adult patient. *Lancet.* 1994;**343**(8907):1233–1234.
16. Lo CM, Fan ST, Liu CL, et al. Extending the limit on the size of adult recipient in living donor liver transplantation using extended right lobe graft. *Transplantation.* 1997;**63**(10):1524–1528.
17. Nadalin S, Capobianco I, Panaro F, et al. Living donor liver transplantation in Europe. *Hepatobiliary Surg Nutr.* 2016;**5**(2):159–175.
18. Hibi T, Wei Chieh AK, Chi-Yan Chan A, Bhangui P. Current status of liver transplantation in Asia. *Int J Surg.* 2020;**82S**:4–8.
19. Singer PA, Siegler M, Whitington PF, et al. Ethics of liver transplantation with living donors. *N Engl J Med.* 1989;**321**(9):620–622.
20. Berg CL, Merion RM, Shearon TH, et al. Liver transplant recipient survival benefit with living donation in the model for endstage liver disease allocation era. *Hepatology.* 2011;**54**(4):1313–1321.
21. Olthoff KM, Smith AR, Abecassis M, et al. Defining long-term outcomes with living donor liver transplantation in North America. *Ann Surg.* 2015;**262**(3):465–475.
22. Laurence JM, Sapisochin G, DeAngelis M, et al. Biliary complications in pediatric liver transplantation: incidence and management over a decade. *Liver Transpl.* 2015;**21**(8):1082–1090.
23. Fisher RA. Living donor liver transplantation: eliminating the wait for death in end-stage liver disease? *Nat Rev Gastroenterol Hepatol.* 2017;**14**(6):373–382.
24. Mogul DB, Luo X, Bowring MG, et al. Fifteen-year trends in pediatric liver transplants: split, whole deceased, and living donor grafts. *J Pediatr.* 2018;**196**:148–153.
25. Cronin DC, 2nd, Millis JM, Siegler M. Transplantation of liver grafts from living donors into adults—too much, too soon. *N Engl J Med.* 2001;**344**(21):1633–1637.
26. Miller CM, Smith ML, Diago Uso T. Living donor liver transplantation: ethical considerations. *Mt Sinai J Med.* 2012;**79**(2):214–222.
27. de Villa VH, Lo CM, Chen CL. Ethics and rationale of living-donor liver transplantation in Asia. *Transplantation.* 2003;**75**(3 Suppl):S2–S5.
28. Malago M, Testa G, Marcos A, et al. Ethical considerations and rationale of adult-to-adult living donor liver transplantation. *Liver Transpl.* 2001;**7**(10):921–927.
29. Whitington PF. Living donor liver transplantation: ethical considerations. *J Hepatol.* 1996;**24**(5):625–627.
30. Mayer AD. The argument against live-donor liver transplantation. *J Hepatol.* 1996;**24**(5):628–630.
31. Broering DC, Sterneck M, Rogiers X. Living donor liver transplantation. *J Hepatol.* 2003;**38** Suppl 1:S119–S135.
32. Levitsky J, Gordon EJ. Living donor liver transplantation when deceased donor is not possible or timely: case examples and ethical perspectives. *Liver Transpl.* 2020;**26**(3):431–436.
33. Siegler M, Simmerling MC, Siegler JH, Cronin DC, 2nd. Recipient deaths during donor surgery: a new ethical problem in living donor liver transplantation (LDLT). *Liver Transpl.* 2006;**12**(3):358–360.
34. Shapiro RS, Adams M. Ethical issues surrounding adult-to-adult living donor liver transplantation. *Liver Transpl.* 2000;**6**(6 Suppl 2):S77–S80.
35. Ghobrial RM, Freise CE, Trotter JF, et al. Donor morbidity after living donation for liver transplantation. *Gastroenterology.* 2008;**135**(2):468–476.
36. Sotiropoulos GC, Radtke A, Molmenti EP, et al. Long-term follow-up after right hepatectomy for adult living donation and attitudes toward the procedure. *Ann Surg.* 2011;**254**(5):694–700.
37. Belghiti J, Liddo G, Raut V, et al. 'Inherent limitations' in donors: control matched study of consequences following a right hepatectomy for living donation and benign liver lesions. *Ann Surg.* 2012;**255**(3):528–533.
38. Gruttadauria S, Pagano D, Cintorino D, et al. Right hepatic lobe living donation: a 12 years single Italian center experience. *World J Gastroenterol.* 2013;**19**(38):6353–6359.
39. National Living Donor Assistance Center. Homepage. n.d. https://www.livingdonorassistance.org/
40. Umeshita K, Eguchi S, Egawa H, Haga H, Kasahara M, Kokudo N, et al. Liver transplantation in Japan: registry by the Japanese Liver Transplantation Society. *Hepatol Res.* 2019;**49**(9):964–980.
41. Jeong JC, Yuzawa K, Shroff S, et al. Development of the Asian Transplant Registry under the Asian Society of Transplantation. *Transplant Proc.* 2020;**52**(6):1634–1638.
42. Shi JH, Huitfeldt HS, Suo ZH, Line PD. Growth of hepatocellular carcinoma in the regenerating liver. *Liver Transpl.* 2011;**17**(7):866–874.
43. Yang ZF, Poon RT, Luo Y, et al. Up-regulation of vascular endothelial growth factor (VEGF) in small-for-size liver grafts enhances macrophage activities through VEGF receptor 2-dependent pathway. *J Immunol.* 2004;**173**(4):2507–2515.
44. Ninomiya M, Harada N, Shiotani S, et al. Hepatocyte growth factor and transforming growth factor beta1 contribute to regeneration of small-for-size liver graft immediately after transplantation. *Transpl Int.* 2003;**16**(11):814–819.
45. Man K, Fan ST, Lo CM, et al. Graft injury in relation to graft size in right lobe live donor liver transplantation: a study of hepatic sinusoidal injury in correlation with portal hemodynamics and intragraft gene expression. *Ann Surg.* 2003;**237**(2):256–264.
46. Efimova EA, Glanemann M, Liu L, et al. Effects of human hepatocyte growth factor on the proliferation of human hepatocytes and hepatocellular carcinoma cell lines. *Eur Surg Res.* 2004;**36**(5):300–307.
47. Zhang HM, Shi YX, Sun LY, Zhu ZJ. Hepatocellular carcinoma recurrence in living and deceased donor liver transplantation: a systematic review and meta-analysis. *Chin Med J (Engl).* 2019;**132**(13):1599–1609.
48. Liang W, Wu L, Ling X, et al. Living donor liver transplantation versus deceased donor liver transplantation for hepatocellular carcinoma: a meta-analysis. *Liver Transpl.* 2012;**18**(10):1226–1236.
49. Pinheiro RS, Waisberg DR, Nacif LS, et al. Living donor liver transplantation for hepatocellular cancer: an (almost) exclusive Eastern procedure? *Transl Gastroenterol Hepatol.* 2017;**2**:68.
50. Hu Z, Zhong X, Zhou J, et al. Smaller grafts do not imply early recurrence in recipients transplanted for hepatocellular carcinoma: a Chinese experience. *Sci Rep.* 2016;**6**:26487.
51. Bhangui P, Vibert E, Majno P, et al. Intention-to-treat analysis of liver transplantation for hepatocellular carcinoma: living versus deceased donor transplantation. *Hepatology.* 2011;**53**(5):1570–1579.
52. Ninomiya M, Shirabe K, Facciuto ME, et al. Comparative study of living and deceased donor liver transplantation as a treatment for hepatocellular carcinoma. *J Am Coll Surg.* 2015;**220**(3):297–304.
53. Samoylova ML, Dodge JL, Yao FY, Roberts JP. Time to transplantation as a predictor of hepatocellular carcinoma

54. Halazun KJ, Patzer RE, Rana AA, et al. Standing the test of time: outcomes of a decade of prioritizing patients with hepatocellular carcinoma, results of the UNOS natural geographic experiment. *Hepatology*. 2014;**60**(6):1957–1962.
55. Lai Q, Avolio AW, Lerut J, et al. Recurrence of hepatocellular cancer after liver transplantation: the role of primary resection and salvage transplantation in East and West. *J Hepatol*. 2012;**57**(5):974–979.
56. Allard MA, Sebagh M, Ruiz A, et al. Does pathological response after transarterial chemoembolization for hepatocellular carcinoma in cirrhotic patients with cirrhosis predict outcome after liver resection or transplantation? *J Hepatol*. 2015;**63**(1):83–92.
57. Kulik LM, Fisher RA, Rodrigo DR, et al. Outcomes of living and deceased donor liver transplant recipients with hepatocellular carcinoma: results of the A2ALL cohort. *Am J Transplant*. 2012;**12**(11):2997–3007.
58. Goldaracena N, Gorgen A, Doyle A, et al. Live donor liver transplantation for patients with hepatocellular carcinoma offers increased survival vs. deceased donation. *J Hepatol*. 2019;**70**(4):666–673.
59. Wong TCL, Ng KKC, Fung JYY, et al. Long-term survival outcome between living donor and deceased donor liver transplant for hepatocellular carcinoma: intention-to-treat and propensity score matching analyses. *Ann Surg Oncol*. 2019;**26**(5):1454–1462.
60. Fisher RA, Kulik LM, Freise CE, et al. Hepatocellular carcinoma recurrence and death following living and deceased donor liver transplantation. *Am J Transplant*. 2007;**7**(6):1601–1608.
61. Akamatsu N, Sugawara Y, Kokudo N. Living-donor vs deceased-donor liver transplantation for patients with hepatocellular carcinoma. *World J Hepatol*. 2014;**6**(9):626–631.
62. Lieber SR, Schiano TD, Rhodes R. Should living donor liver transplantation be an option when deceased donation is not? *J Hepatol*. 2018;**68**(5):1076–1082.
63. Bhangui P, Saigal S, Gautam D, et al. Incorporating tumor biology to predict hepatocellular carcinoma recurrence in patients undergoing living donor liver transplantation using expanded selection criteria. *Liver Transpl*. 2021;**27**(2):209–221.
64. Line PD, Hagness M, Berstad AE, Foss A, Dueland S. A novel concept for partial liver transplantation in nonresectable colorectal liver metastases: the RAPID concept. *Ann Surg*. 2015;**262**(1):e5–e9.
65. Dueland S, Line PD. Liver segment 2+3 living donation in liver transplantation for colorectal liver metastases. *Hepatobiliary Surg Nutr*. 2020;**9**(3):382–384.
66. Terpstra OT, Schalm SW, Weimar W, et al. Auxiliary partial liver transplantation for end-stage chronic liver disease. *N Engl J Med*. 1988;**319**(23):1507–1511.
67. Rauchfuss F, Nadalin S, Konigsrainer A, Settmacher U. Living donor liver transplantation with two-stage hepatectomy for patients with isolated, irresectable colorectal liver-the LIVER-T(W)O-HEAL study. *World J Surg Oncol*. 2019;**17**(1):11.
68. Nadalin S, Konigsrainer A, Capobianco I, Settmacher U, Rauchfuss F. Auxiliary living donor liver transplantation combined with two-stage hepatectomy for unresectable colorectal liver metastases. *Curr Opin Organ Transplant*. 2019;**24**(5):651–658.
69. Schnitzbauer AA, Lang SA, Goessmann H, et al. Right portal vein ligation combined with in situ splitting induces rapid left lateral liver lobe hypertrophy enabling 2-staged extended right hepatic resection in small-for-size settings. *Ann Surg*. 2012;**255**(3):405–414.
70. Schadde E, Ardiles V, Slankamenac K, et al. ALPPS offers a better chance of complete resection in patients with primarily unresectable liver tumors compared with conventional-staged hepatectomies: results of a multicenter analysis. *World J Surg*. 2014;**38**(6):1510–1519.
71. Konigsrainer A, Templin S, Capobianco I, et al. Paradigm shift in the management of irresectable colorectal liver metastases: living donor auxiliary partial orthotopic liver transplantation in combination with two-stage hepatectomy (LD-RAPID). *Ann Surg*. 2019;**270**(2):327–332.
72. Sharma A, Ashworth A, Behnke M, Cotterell A, Posner M, Fisher RA. Donor selection for adult-to-adult living donor liver transplantation: well begun is half done. *Transplantation*. 2013;**95**(3):501–506.
73. Nugroho A, Kim OK, Lee KW, et al. Evaluation of donor workups and exclusions in a single-center experience of living donor liver transplantation. *Liver Transpl*. 2017;**23**(5):614–624.
74. Roberts J, Webber A, Christensen H, et al. A web-based living kidney donor medical evaluation tool. *Am J Transplant*. 2013;**13**(Suppl 2):66.
75. Marcos A, Ham JM, Fisher RA, Olzinski AT, Posner MP. Single-center analysis of the first 40 adult-to-adult living donor liver transplants using the right lobe. *Liver Transpl*. 2000;**6**(3):296–301.
76. Lee SG. A complete treatment of adult living donor liver transplantation: a review of surgical technique and current challenges to expand indication of patients. *Am J Transplant*. 2015;**15**(1):17–38.
77. Marubashi S, Nagano H, Eguchi H, et al. Minimum graft size calculated from preoperative recipient status in living donor liver transplantation. *Liver Transpl*. 2016;**22**(5):599–606.
78. Urata K, Kawasaki S, Matsunami H, et al. Calculation of child and adult standard liver volume for liver transplantation. *Hepatology*. 1995;**21**(5):1317–1321.
79. Heinemann A, Wischhusen F, Puschel K, Rogiers X. Standard liver volume in the Caucasian population. *Liver Transpl Surg*. 1999;**5**(5):366–368.
80. Chouker A, Martignoni A, Dugas M, et al. Estimation of liver size for liver transplantation: the impact of age and gender. *Liver Transpl*. 2004;**10**(5):678–5*685.
81. Yu HC, You H, Lee H, Jin ZW, Moon JI, Cho BH. Estimation of standard liver volume for liver transplantation in the Korean population. *Liver Transpl*. 2004;**10**(6):779–783.
82. Chan SC, Liu CL, Lo CM, al. Estimating liver weight of adults by body weight and gender. *World J Gastroenterol*. 2006;**12**(14):2217–2222.
83. Hashimoto T, Sugawara Y, Tamura S, et al. Estimation of standard liver volume in Japanese living liver donors. *J Gastroenterol Hepatol*. 2006;**21**(11):1710–1713.
84. Kokudo T, Hasegawa K, Uldry E, et al. A new formula for calculating standard liver volume for living donor liver transplantation without using body weight. *J Hepatol*. 2015;**63**(4):848–854.
85. Tongyoo A, Pomfret EA, Pomposelli JJ. Accurate estimation of living donor right hemi-liver volume from portal vein diameter measurement and standard liver volume calculation. *Am J Transplant*. 2012;**12**(5):1229–1239.
86. Erbay N, Raptopoulos V, Pomfret EA, Kamel IR, Kruskal JB. Living donor liver transplantation in adults: vascular variants important in surgical planning for donors and recipients. *AJR Am J Roentgenol*. 2003;**181**(1):109–114.

87. Fulcher AS, Szucs RA, Bassignani MJ, Marcos A. Right lobe living donor liver transplantation: preoperative evaluation of the donor with MR imaging. *AJR Am J Roentgenol.* 2001;**176**(6):1483–1491.
88. Ryan CK, Johnson LA, Germin BI, Marcos A. One hundred consecutive hepatic biopsies in the workup of living donors for right lobe liver transplantation. *Liver Transpl.* 2002;**8**(12):1114–1122.
89. Fukumori T, Ohkohchi N, Tsukamoto S, Satomi S. The mechanism of injury in a steatotic liver graft during cold preservation. *Transplantation.* 1999;**67**(2):195–200.
90. Imber CJ, St Peter SD, Handa A, Friend PJ. Hepatic steatosis and its relationship to transplantation. *Liver Transpl.* 2002;**8**(5):415–423.
91. Lee JG, Lee KW, Kwon CHD, et al. Donor safety in living donor liver transplantation: the Korean organ transplantation registry study. *Liver Transpl.* 2017;**23**(8):999–1006.
92. Middleton PF, Duffield M, Lynch SV, et al. Living donor liver transplantation—adult donor outcomes: a systematic review. *Liver Transpl.* 2006;**12**(1):24–30.
93. Adcock L, Macleod C, Dubay D, et al. Adult living liver donors have excellent long-term medical outcomes: the University of Toronto liver transplant experience. *Am J Transplant.* 2010;**10**(2):364–371.
94. Lauterio A, Di Sandro S, Gruttadauria S, et al. Donor safety in living donor liver donation: an Italian multicenter survey. *Liver Transpl.* 2017;**23**(2):184–193.
95. Lo CM. Complications and long-term outcome of living liver donors: a survey of 1,508 cases in five Asian centers. *Transplantation.* 2003;**75**(3 Suppl):S12–S15.
96. Suh KS, Suh SW, Lee JM, Choi Y, Yi NJ, Lee KW. Recent advancements in and views on the donor operation in living donor liver transplantation: a single-center study of 886 patients over 13 years. *Liver Transpl.* 2015;**21**(3):329–338.
97. Shin M, Song S, Kim JM, et al. Donor morbidity including biliary complications in living-donor liver transplantation: single-center analysis of 827 cases. *Transplantation.* 2012;**93**(9):942–948.
98. Hwang S, Lee SG, Lee YJ, et al. Lessons learned from 1,000 living donor liver transplantations in a single center: how to make living donations safe. *Liver Transpl.* 2006;**12**(6):920–927.
99. Zimmerman MA, Baker T, Goodrich NP, et al. Development, management, and resolution of biliary complications after living and deceased donor liver transplantation: a report from the adult-to-adult living donor liver transplantation cohort study consortium. *Liver Transpl.* 2013;**19**(3):259–267.
100. Barr ML, Belghiti J, Villamil FG, et al. A report of the Vancouver Forum on the care of the live organ donor: lung, liver, pancreas, and intestine data and medical guidelines. *Transplantation.* 2006;**81**(10):1373–1385.
101. Cheah YL, Simpson MA, Pomposelli JJ, Pomfret EA. Incidence of death and potentially life-threatening near-miss events in living donor hepatic lobectomy: a world-wide survey. *Liver Transpl.* 2013;**19**(5):499–506.
102. Ratner LE, Sandoval PR. When disaster strikes: death of a living organ donor. *Am J Transplant.* 2010;**10**(12):2577–2581.
103. Rossler F, Sapisochin G, Song G, et al. Defining benchmarks for major liver surgery: a multicenter analysis of 5202 living liver donors. *Ann Surg.* 2016;**264**(3):492–500.
104. Mulligan DC. A worldwide database for living donor liver transplantation is long overdue. *Liver Transpl.* 2006;**12**(10):1443–1444.
105. Bramstedt KA. Living liver donor mortality: where do we stand? *Am J Gastroenterol.* 2006;**101**(4):755–759.
106. Ringe B, Strong RW. The dilemma of living liver donor death: to report or not to report? *Transplantation.* 2008;**85**(6):790–793.
107. Hashikura Y, Ichida T, Umeshita K, et al. Donor complications associated with living donor liver transplantation in Japan. *Transplantation.* 2009;**88**(1):110–114.
108. Trotter JF, Adam R, Lo CM, Kenison J. Documented deaths of hepatic lobe donors for living donor liver transplantation. *Liver Transpl.* 2006;**12**(10):1485–1488.
109. Muzaale AD, Dagher NN, Montgomery RA, Taranto SE, McBride MA, Segev DL. Estimates of early death, acute liver failure, and long-term mortality among live liver donors. *Gastroenterology.* 2012;**142**(2):273–280.
110. Abecassis MM, Fisher RA, Olthoff KM, et al. Complications of living donor hepatic lobectomy—a comprehensive report. *Am J Transplant.* 2012;**12**(5):1208–1217.
111. Saidi RF, Jabbour N, Li Y, Shah SA, Bozorgzadeh A. Is left lobe adult-to-adult living donor liver transplantation ready for widespread use? The US experience (1998–2010). *HPB (Oxford).* 2012;**14**(7):455–460.
112. Umeshita K, Fujiwara K, Kiyosawa K, et al. Operative morbidity of living liver donors in Japan. *Lancet.* 2003;**362**(9385):687–690.
113. Uchiyama H, Shirabe K, Nakagawara H, et al. Revisiting the safety of living liver donors by reassessing 441 donor hepatectomies: is a larger hepatectomy complication-prone? *Am J Transplant.* 2014;**14**(2):367–374.
114. Botha JF, Langnas AN, Campos BD, et al. Left lobe adult-to-adult living donor liver transplantation: small grafts and hemiportocaval shunts in the prevention of small-for-size syndrome. *Liver Transpl.* 2010;**16**(5):649–657.
115. Roll GR, Parekh JR, Parker WF, et al. Left hepatectomy versus right hepatectomy for living donor liver transplantation: shifting the risk from the donor to the recipient. *Liver Transpl.* 2013;**19**(5):472–481.
116. Cherqui D. Laparoscopic liver resection. *Br J Surg.* 2003;**90**(6):644–646.
117. Cherqui D, Soubrane O, Husson E, et al. Laparoscopic living donor hepatectomy for liver transplantation in children. *Lancet.* 2002;**359**(9304):392–396.
118. Scatton O, Katsanos G, Boillot O, et al. Pure laparoscopic left lateral sectionectomy in living donors: from innovation to development in France. *Ann Surg.* 2015;**261**(3):506–512.
119. Soubrane O, de Rougemont O, Kim KH, et al. Laparoscopic living donor left lateral sectionectomy: a new standard practice for donor hepatectomy. *Ann Surg.* 2015;**262**(5):757–761.
120. Ishizawa T, Bandai Y, Ijichi M, Kaneko J, Hasegawa K, Kokudo N. Fluorescent cholangiography illuminating the biliary tree during laparoscopic cholecystectomy. *Br J Surg.* 2010;**97**(9):1369–1377.
121. Troisi RI, Elsheikh Y, Alnemary Y, et al. Safety and feasibility report of robotic-assisted left lateral sectionectomy for pediatric living donor liver transplantation: a comparative analysis of learning curves and mastery achieved with the laparoscopic approach. *Transplantation.* 2021;**105**(5):1044–1051.
122. Testa G, Malago M, Porubsky M, et al. Hilar early division of the hepatic duct in living donor right hepatectomy: the probe-and-clamp technique. *Liver Transpl.* 2006;**12**(9):1337–1341.
123. Lo CM, Fan ST, Liu CL, et al. Adult-to-adult living donor liver transplantation using extended right lobe grafts. *Ann Surg.* 1997;**226**(3):261–269.

124. Gyu Lee S, Min Park K, Hwang S, et al. Modified right liver graft from a living donor to prevent congestion. *Transplantation*. 2002;**74**(1):54–59.
125. de Villa VH, Chen CL, Chen YS, et al. Right lobe living donor liver transplantation-addressing the middle hepatic vein controversy. *Ann Surg*. 2003;**238**(2):275–282.
126. Varghese CT, Bharathan VK, Gopalakrishnan U, et al. Randomized trial on extended versus modified right lobe grafts in living donor liver transplantation. *Liver Transpl*. 2018;**24**(7):888–896.
127. Broering DC, Wilms C, Bok P, et al. Evolution of donor morbidity in living related liver transplantation: a single-center analysis of 165 cases. *Ann Surg*. 2004;**240**(6):1013–1024.
128. Renz JF, Roberts JP. Long-term complications of living donor liver transplantation. *Liver Transpl*. 2000;**6**(6 Suppl 2):S73–S76.
129. Shah SA, Grant DR, McGilvray ID, et al. Biliary strictures in 130 consecutive right lobe living donor liver transplant recipients: results of a Western center. *Am J Transplant*. 2007;**7**(1):161–167.
130. Testa G, Malago M, Valentin-Gamazo C, Lindell G, Broelsch CE. Biliary anastomosis in living related liver transplantation using the right liver lobe: techniques and complications. *Liver Transpl*. 2000;**6**(6):710–714.
131. Gondolesi GE, Varotti G, Florman SS, et al. Biliary complications in 96 consecutive right lobe living donor transplant recipients. *Transplantation*. 2004;**77**(12):1842–1848.
132. Koffron AJ, Kung R, Baker T, Fryer J, Clark L, Abecassis M. Laparoscopic-assisted right lobe donor hepatectomy. *Am J Transplant*. 2006;**6**(10):2522–2525.
133. Kwon CHD, Choi GS, Kim JM, et al. Laparoscopic donor hepatectomy for adult living donor liver transplantation recipients. *Liver Transpl*. 2018;**24**(11):1545–1553.
134. Jeong JS, Wi W, Chung YJ, et al. Comparison of perioperative outcomes between pure laparoscopic surgery and open right hepatectomy in living donor hepatectomy: propensity score matching analysis. *Sci Rep*. 2020;**10**(1):5314.
135. Cho HD, Kim KH, Yoon YI, et al. Comparing purely laparoscopic versus open living donor right hepatectomy: propensity score-matched analysis. *Br J Surg*. 2021;**108**(7):e233–e234.
136. Hong SK, Tan MY, Worakitti L, et al. Pure laparoscopic versus open right hepatectomy in live liver donors: a propensity score-matched analysis. *Ann Surg*. 2022;**275**(1):e206–e212.
137. Sugawara Y, Makuuchi M, Imamura H, Kaneko J, Ohkubo T, Kokudo N. Outflow reconstruction in recipients of right liver graft from living donors. *Liver Transpl*. 2002;**8**(2):167–168.
138. Lee SG. Techniques of reconstruction of hepatic veins in living-donor liver transplantation, especially for right hepatic vein and major short hepatic veins of right-lobe graft. *J Hepatobiliary Pancreat Surg*. 2006;**13**(2):131–138.
139. Hwang S, Lee SG, Ahn CS, et al. Outflow vein reconstruction of extended right lobe graft using quilt venoplasty technique. *Liver Transpl*. 2006;**12**(1):156–158.
140. Lo CM, Fan ST, Liu CL, Wong J. Hepatic venoplasty in living-donor liver transplantation using right lobe graft with middle hepatic vein. *Transplantation*. 2003;**75**(3):358–360.
141. Mori A, Kaido T, Ogura Y, et al. Standard hepatic vein reconstruction with patch plasty using the native portal vein in adult living donor liver transplantation. *Liver Transpl*. 2012;**18**(5):602–607.
142. Malago M, Molmenti EP, Paul A, et al. Hepatic venous outflow reconstruction in right live donor liver transplantation. *Liver Transpl*. 2005;**11**(3):364–365.
143. Hwang S, Lee SG, Park KM, et al. Quilt venoplasty using recipient saphenous vein graft for reconstruction of multiple short hepatic veins in right liver grafts. *Liver Transpl*. 2005;**11**(1):104–107.
144. Ara C, Akbulut S, Ince V, et al. Circumferential fence with the use of polyethylene terephthalate (Dacron) vascular graft for all-in-one hepatic venous reconstruction in right-lobe living-donor liver transplantation. *Transplant Proc*. 2015;**47**(5):1458–1461.
145. Singhal A, Makki K, Chorasiya V, et al. Venous outflow reconstruction using a polytetrafluoroethylene (PTFE) graft in right lobe living donor liver transplantation: a single center study. *Surgery*. 2021;**169**(6):1500–1509.
146. Hong SK, Yi NJ, Cho JH, et al. Parietal peritoneum as a novel substitute for middle hepatic vein reconstruction during living donor liver transplantation. *Transplantation*. 2020;**105**(6):1291–1296.
147. Dayangac M, Taner CB, Balci D, et al. Use of middle hepatic vein in right lobe living donor liver transplantation. *Transpl Int*. 2010;**23**(3):285–291.
148. Kamel R, Hatata Y, Hosny K, Amer K, Taha M. Synthetic graft for reconstruction of middle hepatic vein tributaries in living-donor liver transplant. *Exp Clin Transplant*. 2015;**13**(Suppl 1):318–322.
149. Yi NJ, Suh KS, Lee HW, et al. An artificial vascular graft is a useful interpositional material for drainage of the right anterior section in living donor liver transplantation. *Liver Transpl*. 2007;**13**(8):1159–1167.
150. Hwang S, Jung DH, Ha TY, et al. Usability of ringed polytetrafluoroethylene grafts for middle hepatic vein reconstruction during living donor liver transplantation. *Liver Transpl*. 2012;**18**(8):955–965.
151. Lee KW, Lee DS, Lee HH, et al. Interpostion vein graft in living donor liver transplantation. *Transplant Proc*. 2004;**36**(8):2261–2262.
152. Yaprak O, Demirbas T, Duran C, et al. Living donor liver hilar variations: surgical approaches and implications. *Hepatobiliary Pancreat Dis Int*. 2011;**10**(5):474–479.
153. Covey AM, Brody LA, Getrajdman GI, Sofocleous CT, Brown KT. Incidence, patterns, and clinical relevance of variant portal vein anatomy. *AJR Am J Roentgenol*. 2004;**183**(4):1055–1064.
154. Cheng YF, Huang TL, Lee TY, Chen TY, Chen CL. Variation of the intrahepatic portal vein; angiographic demonstration and application in living-related hepatic transplantation. *Transplant Proc*. 1996;**28**(3):1667–1668.
155. Schmidt S, Demartines N, Soler L, Schnyder P, Denys A. Portal vein normal anatomy and variants: implication for liver surgery and portal vein embolization. *Semin Intervent Radiol*. 2008;**25**(2):86–91.
156. Lee SG, Hwang S, Kim KH, et al. Approach to anatomic variations of the graft portal vein in right lobe living-donor liver transplantation. *Transplantation*. 2003;**75**(3 Suppl):S28–S32.
157. Nakamura T, Tanaka K, Kiuchi T, et al. Anatomical variations and surgical strategies in right lobe living donor liver transplantation: lessons from 120 cases. *Transplantation*. 2002;**73**(12):1896–1903.
158. Marcos A, Ham JM, Fisher RA, Olzinski AT, Posner MP. Surgical management of anatomical variations of the

right lobe in living donor liver transplantation. *Ann Surg.* 2000;**231**(6):824–831.
159. Marcos A, Orloff M, Mieles L, Olzinski A, Sitzmann J. Reconstruction of double hepatic arterial and portal venous branches for right-lobe living donor liver transplantation. *Liver Transpl.* 2001;**7**(8):673–679.
160. Ahn CS, Lee SG, Hwang S, et al. Anatomic variation of the right hepatic artery and its reconstruction for living donor liver transplantation using right lobe graft. *Transplant Proc.* 2005;**37**(2):1067–1069.
161. Takatsuki M, Chiang YC, Lin TS, et al. Anatomical and technical aspects of hepatic artery reconstruction in living donor liver transplantation. *Surgery.* 2006;**140**(5):824–828.
162. Kasahara M, Egawa H, Takada Y, et al. Biliary reconstruction in right lobe living-donor liver transplantation: comparison of different techniques in 321 recipients. *Ann Surg.* 2006;**243**(4):559–566.
163. Concejero A, Chen CL, Wang CC, et al. Donor graft outflow venoplasty in living donor liver transplantation. *Liver Transpl.* 2006;**12**(2):264–268.
164. Strong R, Lynch S, Yamanaka J, Kawamoto S, Pillay P, Ong TH. Monosegmental liver transplantation. *Surgery.* 1995;**118**(5):904–906.
165. Srinivasan P, Vilca-Melendez H, Muiesan P, Prachalias A, Heaton ND, Rela M. Liver transplantation with monosegments. *Surgery.* 1999;**126**(1):10–12.
166. Shehata MR, Yagi S, Okamura Y, et al. Pediatric liver transplantation using reduced and hyper-reduced left lateral segment grafts: a 10-year single-center experience. *Am J Transplant.* 2012;**12**(12):3406–3413.
167. Rodriguez-Davalos MI, Arvelakis A, Umman V, et al. Segmental grafts in adult and pediatric liver transplantation: improving outcomes by minimizing vascular complications. *JAMA Surg.* 2014;**149**(1):63–70.
168. Hwang S, Lee SG, Lee YJ, et al. Donor selection for procurement of right posterior segment graft in living donor liver transplantation. *Liver Transpl.* 2004;**10**(9):1150–1155.
169. Yoshizumi T, Ikegami T, Kimura K, et al. Selection of a right posterior sector graft for living donor liver transplantation. *Liver Transpl.* 2014;**20**(9):1089–1096.
170. Sugawara Y, Makuuchi M. Right lateral sector graft as a feasible option for partial liver transplantation. *Liver Transpl.* 2004;**10**(9):1156–1157.
171. Sakuma Y, Sasanuma H, Miki A, et al. Living-donor liver transplantation using segment 2 monosegment graft: a single-center experience. *Transplant Proc.* 2016;**48**(4):1110–1114.
172. Sugawara Y, Makuuchi M, Akamatsu N, et al. Refinement of venous reconstruction using cryopreserved veins in right liver grafts. *Liver Transpl.* 2004;**10**(4):541–547.
173. Mori K, Nagata I, Yamagata S, et al. The introduction of microvascular surgery to hepatic artery reconstruction in living-donor liver transplantation—its surgical advantages compared with conventional procedures. *Transplantation.* 1992;**54**(2):263–268.
174. Uchiyama H, Hashimoto K, Hiroshige S, et al. Hepatic artery reconstruction in living-donor liver transplantation: a review of its techniques and complications. *Surgery.* 2002;**131**(1 Suppl):S200–S204.
175. Ishiko T, Egawa H, Kasahara M, et al. Duct-to-duct biliary reconstruction in living donor liver transplantation utilizing right lobe graft. *Ann Surg.* 2002;**236**(2):235–240.
176. Soejima Y, Shimada M, Suehiro T, et al. Outcome analysis in adult-to-adult living donor liver transplantation using the left lobe. *Liver Transpl.* 2003;**9**(6):581–586.
177. Dahm F, Georgiev P, Clavien PA. Small-for-size syndrome after partial liver transplantation: definition, mechanisms of disease and clinical implications. *Am J Transplant.* 2005;**5**(11):2605–2610.
178. Soejima Y, Taketomi A, Yoshizumi T, Uchiyama H, Harada N, Ijichi H, et al. Feasibility of left lobe living donor liver transplantation between adults: an 8-year, single-center experience of 107 cases. *Am J Transplant.* 2006;**6**(5 Pt 1):1004–1011.
179. Hill MJ, Hughes M, Jie T, Cohen M, Lake J, Payne WD, et al. Graft weight/recipient weight ratio: how well does it predict outcome after partial liver transplants? *Liver Transpl.* 2009;**15**(9):1056–1062.
180. Ikegami T, Yoshizumi T, Sakata K, et al. Left lobe living donor liver transplantation in adults: what is the safety limit? *Liver Transpl.* 2016;**22**(12):1666–1675.
181. Hernandez-Alejandro R, Sharma H. Small-for-size syndrome in liver transplantation: new horizons to cover with a good launchpad. *Liver Transpl.* 2016;**22**(S1):33–36.
182. Iesari S, Inostroza Nunez ME, Rico Juri JM, et al. Adult-to-adult living-donor liver transplantation: the experience of the Universite catholique de Louvain. *Hepatobiliary Pancreat Dis Int.* 2019;**18**(2):132–142.
183. Akamatsu N, Sugawara Y, Tamura S, Kaneko J, Matsui Y, Togashi J, et al. Impact of live donor age (>or=50) on liver transplantation. *Transplant Proc.* 2007;**39**(10):3189–3193.
184. Lo CM, Fan ST, Chan JK, Wei W, Lo RJ, Lai CL. Minimum graft volume for successful adult-to-adult living donor liver transplantation for fulminant hepatic failure. *Transplantation.* 1996;**62**(5):696–698.
185. Kiuchi T, Tanaka K, Ito T, et al. Small-for-size graft in living donor liver transplantation: how far should we go? *Liver Transpl.* 2003;**9**(9):S29–S35.
186. Masuda Y, Yoshizawa K, Ohno Y, Mita A, Shimizu A, Soejima Y. Small-for-size syndrome in liver transplantation: definition, pathophysiology and management. *Hepatobiliary Pancreat Dis Int.* 2020;**19**(4):334–341.
187. Lee S, Park K, Hwang S, et al. Congestion of right liver graft in living donor liver transplantation. *Transplantation.* 2001;**71**(6):812–814.
188. Kitajima T, Kaido T, Iida T, et al. Left lobe graft poses a potential risk of hepatic venous outflow obstruction in adult living donor liver transplantation. *Liver Transpl.* 2016;**22**(6):785–795.
189. Takemura N, Sugawara Y, Hashimoto T, et al. New hepatic vein reconstruction in left liver graft. *Liver Transpl.* 2005;**11**(3):356–360.
190. Suehiro T, Shimada M, Kishikawa K, et al. Impact of graft hepatic vein inferior vena cava reconstruction with graft venoplasty and inferior vena cava cavoplasty in living donor adult liver transplantation using a left lobe graft. *Transplantation.* 2005;**80**(7):964–968.
191. Hashimoto T, Sugawara Y, Tamura S, et al. One orifice vein reconstruction in left liver plus caudate lobe grafts. *Transplantation.* 2007;**83**(2):225–227.
192. Yamazaki S, Takayama T, Makuuchi M. The technical advance and impact of caudate lobe venous reconstruction in left liver: additional safety for living-related donor liver transplantation. *Transpl Int.* 2010;**23**(4):345–349.
193. Spitzer AL, Dick AA, Bakthavatsalam R, et al. Intraoperative portal vein blood flow predicts allograft and patient

survival following liver transplantation. *HPB (Oxford)*. 2010;**12**(3):166–173.
194. Fujimoto M, Moriyasu F, Nada T, et al. Influence of spontaneous portosystemic collateral pathways on portal hemodynamics in living-related liver transplantation in children. Doppler ultrasonographic study. *Transplantation*. 1995;**60**(1):41–45.
195. Ito T, Kiuchi T, Yamamoto H, et al. Changes in portal venous pressure in the early phase after living donor liver transplantation: pathogenesis and clinical implications. *Transplantation*. 2003;**75**(8):1313–1317.
196. Sanchez-Cabus S, Fondevila C, Calatayud D, et al. Importance of the temporary portocaval shunt during adult living donor liver transplantation. *Liver Transpl*. 2013;**19**(2):174–183.
197. Gruttadauria S, Mandala L, Miraglia R, et al. Successful treatment of small-for-size syndrome in adult-to-adult living-related liver transplantation: single center series. *Clin Transplant*. 2007;**21**(6):761–766.
198. Shimada M, Ijichi H, Yonemura Y, et al. The impact of splenectomy or splenic artery ligation on the outcome of a living donor adult liver transplantation using a left lobe graft. *Hepatogastroenterology*. 2004;**51**(57):625–629.
199. Sato Y, Kobayashi T, Nakatsuka H, et al. Splenic arterial ligation prevents liver injury after a major hepatectomy by a reduction of surplus portal hypertension in hepatocellular carcinoma patients with cirrhosis. *Hepatogastroenterology*. 2001;**48**(39):831–835.
200. Mitsumoto Y, Dhar DK, Yu L, et al. FK506 with portal decompression exerts beneficial effects following extended hepatectomy in dogs. *Eur Surg Res*. 1999;**31**(1):48–56.
201. Luca A, Miraglia R, Caruso S, Milazzo M, Gidelli B, Bosch J. Effects of splenic artery occlusion on portal pressure in patients with cirrhosis and portal hypertension. *Liver Transpl*. 2006;**12**(8):1237–1243.
202. Yoshizumi T, Mori M. Portal flow modulation in living donor liver transplantation: review with a focus on splenectomy. *Surg Today*. 2020;**50**(1):21–29.
203. Etesami K, Genyk Y. The increasingly limited basis for portal venous pressure modulation in living donor liver transplantation. *Liver Transpl*. 2018;**24**(11):1506–1507.
204. Emond JC, Goodrich NP, Pomposelli JJ, et al. Hepatic hemodynamics and portal flow modulation: the A2ALL experience. *Transplantation*. 2017;**101**(10):2375–2384.
205. Chan SC, Lo CM, Chok KS, et al. Modulation of graft vascular inflow guided by flowmetry and manometry in liver transplantation. *Hepatobiliary Pancreat Dis Int*. 2011;**10**(6):649–656.
206. Yoshizumi T, Taketomi A, Soejima Y, et al. The beneficial role of simultaneous splenectomy in living donor liver transplantation in patients with small-for-size graft. *Transpl Int*. 2008;**21**(9):833–842.
207. Yao S, Kaido T, Uozumi R, et al. Is portal venous pressure modulation still indicated for all recipients in living donor liver transplantation? *Liver Transpl*. 2018;**24**(11):1578–1588.
208. Ito K, Akamatsu N, Ichida A, et al. Splenectomy is not indicated in living donor liver transplantation. *Liver Transpl*. 2016;**22**(11):1526–1535.
209. Troisi R, Cammu G, Militerno G, et al. Modulation of portal graft inflow: a necessity in adult living-donor liver transplantation? *Ann Surg*. 2003;**237**(3):429–436.
210. Umeda Y, Yagi T, Sadamori H, et al. Preoperative proximal splenic artery embolization: a safe and efficacious portal decompression technique that improves the outcome of live donor liver transplantation. *Transpl Int*. 2007;**20**(11):947–955.
211. Moon DB, Lee SG, Hwang S, et al. Splenic devascularization can replace splenectomy during adult living donor liver transplantation - a historical cohort study. *Transpl Int*. 2019;**32**(5):535–545.
212. Ikegami T, Shirabe K, Nakagawara H, et al. Obstructing spontaneous major shunt vessels is mandatory to keep adequate portal inflow in living-donor liver transplantation. *Transplantation*. 2013;**95**(10):1270–1277.
213. Takada Y, Ueda M, Ishikawa Y, et al. End-to-side portocaval shunting for a small-for-size graft in living donor liver transplantation. *Liver Transpl*. 2004;**10**(6):807–810.
214. Troisi R, Ricciardi S, Smeets P, et al. Effects of hemi-portocaval shunts for inflow modulation on the outcome of small-for-size grafts in living donor liver transplantation. *Am J Transplant*. 2005;**5**(6):1397–1404.
215. Ciria R, Cherqui D, Geller DA, Briceno J, Wakabayashi G. Comparative short-term benefits of laparoscopic liver resection: 9000 cases and climbing. *Ann Surg*. 2016;**263**(4):761–777.
216. Guerron AD, Aliyev S, Agcaoglu O, et al. Laparoscopic versus open resection of colorectal liver metastasis. *Surg Endosc*. 2013;**27**(4):1138–1143.
217. Vanounou T, Steel JL, Nguyen KT, et al. Comparing the clinical and economic impact of laparoscopic versus open liver resection. *Ann Surg Oncol*. 2010;**17**(4):998–1009.
218. Nguyen KT, Geller DA. Outcomes of laparoscopic hepatic resection for colorectal cancer metastases. *J Surg Oncol*. 2010;**102**(8):975–977.
219. Abu Hilal M, Aldrighetti L, Dagher I, et al. The Southampton consensus guidelines for laparoscopic liver surgery: from indication to implementation. *Ann Surg*. 2018;**268**(1):11–18.
220. Cherqui D, Ciria R, Kwon CHD, et al. Expert consensus guidelines on minimally invasive donor hepatectomy for living donor liver transplantation from innovation to implementation: a joint initiative from the International Laparoscopic Liver Society (ILLS) and the Asian-Pacific Hepato-Pancreato-Biliary Association (A-PHPBA). *Ann Surg*. 2021;**273**(1):96–108.
221. Ratner LE, Ciseck LJ, Moore RG, Cigarroa FG, Kaufman HS, Kavoussi LR. Laparoscopic live donor nephrectomy. *Transplantation*. 1995;**60**(9):1047–1049.
222. Kim KH, Jung DH, Park KM, et al. Comparison of open and laparoscopic live donor left lateral sectionectomy. *Br J Surg*. 2011;**98**(9):1302–1308.
223. Soubrane O, Cherqui D, Scatton O, et al. Laparoscopic left lateral sectionectomy in living donors: safety and reproducibility of the technique in a single center. *Ann Surg*. 2006;**244**(5):815–820.
224. Rotellar F, Pardo F, Benito A, et al. Totally laparoscopic right-lobe hepatectomy for adult living donor liver transplantation: useful strategies to enhance safety. *Am J Transplant*. 2013;**13**(12):3269–3273.
225. Soubrane O, Perdigao Cotta F, Scatton O. Pure laparoscopic right hepatectomy in a living donor. *Am J Transplant*. 2013;**13**(9):2467–2471.
226. Han HS, Cho JY, Yoon YS, et al. Total laparoscopic living donor right hepatectomy. *Surg Endosc*. 2015;**29**(1):184.
227. Chen KH, Huang CC, Siow TF, et al. Totally laparoscopic living donor right hepatectomy in a donor with trifurcation of bile duct. *Asian J Surg*. 2016;**39**(1):51–55.
228. Takahara T, Wakabayashi G, Hasegawa Y, Nitta H. Minimally invasive donor hepatectomy: evolution from hybrid to pure laparoscopic techniques. *Ann Surg*. 2015;**261**(1):e3–e4.

229. Park JI, Kim KH, Lee SG. Laparoscopic living donor hepatectomy: a review of current status. *J Hepatobiliary Pancreat Sci*. 2015;**22**(11):779–788.
230. Samstein B, Griesemer A, Cherqui D, et al. Fully laparoscopic left-sided donor hepatectomy is safe and associated with shorter hospital stay and earlier return to work: a comparative study. *Liver Transpl*. 2015;**21**(6):768–773.
231. Rotellar F, Pardo F, Benito A, et al. Totally laparoscopic right hepatectomy for living donor liver transplantation: analysis of a preliminary experience on 5 consecutive cases. *Transplantation*. 2017;**101**(3):548–554.
232. Suh KS, Hong SK, Lee KW, et al. Pure laparoscopic living donor hepatectomy: focus on 55 donors undergoing right hepatectomy. *Am J Transplant*. 2018;**18**(2):434–443.
233. Samstein B, Griesemer A, Halazun K, et al. Pure laparoscopic donor hepatectomies: ready for widespread adoption? *Ann Surg*. 2018;**268**(4):602–609.
234. Broering DC, Elsheikh Y, Shagrani M, Abaalkhail F, Troisi RI. Pure laparoscopic living donor left lateral sectionectomy in pediatric transplantation: a propensity score analysis on 220 consecutive patients. *Liver Transpl*. 2018;**24**(8):1019–1030.
235. Tsung A, Geller DA, Sukato DC, et al. Robotic versus laparoscopic hepatectomy: a matched comparison. *Ann Surg*. 2014;**259**(3):549–555.
236. Choi GH, Chong JU, Han DH, Choi JS, Lee WJ. Robotic hepatectomy: the Korean experience and perspective. *Hepatobiliary Surg Nutr*. 2017;**6**(4):230–238.
237. Marino MV, Shabat G, Guarrasi D, Gulotta G, Komorowski AL. Comparative study of the initial experience in performing robotic and laparoscopic right hepatectomy with technical description of the robotic technique. *Dig Surg*. 2019;**36**(3):241–250.
238. Wu YM, Hu RH, Lai HS, Lee PH. Robotic-assisted minimally invasive liver resection. *Asian J Surg*. 2014;**37**(2):53–57.
239. Liao MH, Yang JY, Wu H, Zeng Y. Robot-assisted living-donor left lateral sectionectomy. *Chin Med J (Engl)*. 2017;**130**(7):874–876.
240. Troisi RI, Elsheikh Y, Alnemary Y, et al. Safety and feasibility report of robotic-assisted left lateral sectionectomy for pediatric living donor liver transplantation: a comparative analysis of learning curves and mastery achieved with the laparoscopic approach. *Transplantation*. 2021;**105**(5):1044–1051.
241. Chen PD, Wu CY, Hu RH, et al. Robotic liver donor right hepatectomy: a pure, minimally invasive approach. *Liver Transpl*. 2016;**22**(11):1509–1518.
242. Broering DC, Elsheikh Y, Alnemary Y, et al. Robotic versus open right lobe donor hepatectomy for adult living donor liver transplantation: a propensity score-matched analysis. *Liver Transpl*. 2020;**26**(11):1455–1464.
243. Broering DC, Zidan, A. Advancements in robotic living donor hepatectomy, review of literature and single-center experience. *Curr Transpl Rep*. 2020;**7**(5):324–331.
244. Rho SY, Lee JG, Joo DJ, et al. Outcomes of robotic living donor right hepatectomy from 52 consecutive cases: comparison with open and laparoscopy-assisted donor hepatectomy. *Ann Surg*. 2022;**275**(2):e433–e442.
245. Nota CL, Rinkes IHB, Molenaar IQ, van Santvoort HC, Fong Y, Hagendoorn J. Robot-assisted laparoscopic liver resection: a systematic review and pooled analysis of minor and major hepatectomies. *HPB (Oxford)*. 2016;**18**(2):113–120.
246. Chiow AKH, Rho SY, Wee IJY, Lee LS, Choi GH. Robotic ICG guided anatomical liver resection in a multi-centre cohort: an evolution from 'positive staining' into 'negative staining' method. *HPB (Oxford)*. 2021;**23**(3):475–482.
247. Chen PD, Wu CY, Wu YM. Use of robotics in liver donor right hepatectomy. *Hepatobiliary Surg Nutr*. 2017;**6**(5):292–296.
248. Iuppa G, Aucejo F, Miller C. Living donor robotic right hepatectomy is the future: or is it? *Liver Transpl*. 2016;**22**(11):1461–1462.

25 Non-operative management of liver lesions

T. Deepa Shree and Sandeep Botcha

Introduction

Liver malignancies stand sixth among the most common cancers and are the second leading cause of cancer-related mortality worldwide. Liver tumours can be primary or secondary, with the former starting in the liver and the secondaries arising in other organs (colon, breast, pancreas, ovary and lung) with subsequent spread to the liver.[1]

Hepatocellular carcinoma (HCC), cholangiocarcinoma, and sarcoma account for 6% of the total cancer burden worldwide with HCC being the commonest (accounting for 75–85%) primary liver cancer and its incidence is on the rise every year.[1,3,4]

Multiple forms of treatments are available for liver cancer. Transplantation and surgical resection of the liver remain the gold standard curative treatment options; however, only a limited number (15–20%) of patients are suitable candidates for these procedures due to advanced liver disease and/or associated comorbidities.[3,4]

Various minimally invasive interventional radiological procedures such as percutaneous ablative and catheter-based techniques have been developed and intensively investigated in patients with inoperable primary and secondary liver lesions. They are useful to downstage and bridge patients for surgical and transplant interventions, definitive curative intent in smaller lesions, and as primary palliative management improving survival outcomes and quality of life.[4,5] Their importance is also increasing in treating postsurgical (post hepatectomy/liver transplantation) tumour recurrence.

Several classification systems are available for non-operative management of each malignancy, with debate on the best available treatment options. Multidisciplinary assessment of the initial presentation, physical status of the patient, tumour characterization, and hepatic reserve are useful in optimizing candidate selection and achieving the maximum therapeutic response.[2,7]

The Barcelona Clinic Liver Cancer (BCLC) classification incorporates the essential multidisciplinary assessment (performance status, Child–Pugh score, tumour size/number/distribution, vascular invasion, extrahepatic spread of disease) and provides a recommended strategy and definitive management pathway based on tumour staging.[7] It is recommended by the American Association for the Study of Liver Diseases guidelines and endorsed by the European Association for the Study of the Liver panel of experts due to its prognostic ability.[2,7,8]

The recently proposed Hong Kong Liver Cancer staging classification provides treatment options for a wider population in early and advanced disease who still may be eligible for more aggressive treatments in comparison to the BCLC staging system.[2,8] Surgical resections play a larger role in the Hong Kong Liver Cancer staging treatment plan; however, due to high rates of liver cirrhosis and portal hypertension in the Western world, locoregional treatments play a primary role and should be optimized based on the tumour burden and distribution.[2,8]

A variety of image-guided locoregional interventional oncology therapies are available for treatment of liver lesions based on the disease staging and recommended treatment plan.

Non-operative interventional therapies

Interventional therapies are broadly classified into:

1. Percutaneous local ablation therapies:
   - Thermal ablation:
     Hyperthermic—radiofrequency ablation (RFA), microwave ablation (MWA), high-intensity focused ultrasound (HIFU), and laser-induced thermotherapy.
     Hypothermic—cryoablation.
   - Non-thermal ablation:
     Chemical ablation:
     - Percutaneous ethanol injection (PEI).
     - Percutaneous acetic acid injection.
     Irreversible electroporation.
2. Transarterial catheter-based therapies:
   - Bland embolization with particles/transarterial embolization (TAE).
   - Transarterial chemoembolization (TACE).
   - Radioembolization or selective internal radiation therapy.
3. Combination therapy.
4. Transvenous therapy:
   - Portal vein embolization (PVE).

Percutaneous local ablation therapies

These are minimally invasive procedures either performed percutaneously (mostly), laparoscopically, or through an open surgical approach (with intraoperative ultrasound guidance). Ablation involves direct administration of chemical or thermal energy to achieve necrosis within the tumour, minimizing damage to the adjacent structures and healthy hepatic parenchyma. It is used either as a curative or palliative treatment and is considered to be the best locoregional option in patients with focal early unresectable liver tumours.[6,13] It also has an important/effective role in treating liver secondaries.

Ablation therapies are of two types:

Thermal ablation:

- Hyperthermic—RFA, MWA, HIFU, and laser-induced thermotherapy.
- Hypothermic—cryoablation.

Non-thermal ablation:

- Chemical ablation—this involves percutaneous injection of chemical into the lesion:
  - PEI.
  - Percutaneous acetic acid injection.
- Irreversible electroporation.

Thermal ablation

Hyperthermic ablation

This involves percutaneous administration of thermal energy into the lesion. The thermal techniques used generate heat over 50–60° C within the targeted tissues causing irreversible intracellular protein damage resulting in coagulative necrosis.[6,13]

The temperature equilibrium depends on the type, quantity, and duration of energy delivered to a tissue. Thermal energy accumulation over the targeted area is proportional to the heat production, its conduction across adjacent tissues, and heat convection. The heat convection via the traversing large blood vessels (>3 mm) is called the 'heat sink effect'; due to this heat dissipation, complete necrosis of the nearby cells may not be possible leading to positive tumour margins which can lead to ineffective treatment.[12]

Radiofrequency ablation

RFA is a well-established percutaneous thermal therapy; it is included in management guidelines of multiple societies for treatment of liver lesions (primary and secondary) and is considered the gold standard among thermal ablative therapies which has a potential to alter patient outcomes.

RFA works on the principle of heat generation by inducing alternating high-frequency currents (radiofrequency (RF) waves) in the range of 200–1200 kHz onto the tissue causing ionic frictional agitation. The energy delivered relates to tissue impedance and is based on Ohm's law.[4,12,13]

The RF waves are produced by a RF generator, the thermal energy is deposited by a needle-shaped electrode (probe), and the circuit is closed by placing grounding pads on the patient (usually on the thighs) which cause heat production resulting in coagulative necrosis and scarring of the targeted tumour tissue. In background liver cirrhosis, the increased thickness of tissue surrounding the lesion acts as a thermal insulator and can prevent heat dispersion and is called the 'oven effect'.[6]

RFA is generally performed under ultrasound, computed tomography (CT) guidance, or a combination of both using monopolar, bipolar, or multipolar probes. Monopolar probes are used to treat lesions up to 3 cm. In larger lesions, a bipolar or a multipolar approach is effective, wherein two or more probes are placed around the tumour periphery, depositing a high-density field of concentric thermal energy, creating a central zone of ablation. In the multipolar application mode, up to six bipolar probes can be activated simultaneously by a single RF generator to generate temperatures over a larger area (up to 5 cm).[12,13] A faster and higher (>105° C) increase in temperature causes vaporization and carbonization of tissues which limits heat conduction and may result in a variable size, shape, and homogeneity of the ablation zone. Hence a slow and gradual rise in power is desired; alternatively, an internally cooled electrode design with cool-tip or RF energy pulsing can be used to prevent carbonization and efficient heat deposition.[4,5,6,13] Ideally, the ablative margin of 0.5–1.0 cm should be included for 360° surrounding the tumour for control and prevention of adjacent microscopic disease.[11,13]

Independent risk factors for tumour recurrence

- Tumour size: a size greater than 3 cm will require overlap ablations, which may leave some target areas untreated.
- Tumour location:
  - Near the intrahepatic vasculature: due to the heat sink effect and an overcautiousness of injury to the nearby vessel walls can cause reduced efficacy and metastasis of the disease.
  - Subcapsular location: due to a fear of injury to the adjacent organs as the probe is usually placed 5–10 mm beyond the tumour margin.
- Prolonged prothrombin time: prothrombin time greater than 3 seconds with dependent background liver cirrhosis or fibrosis.

In clinical practice, RFA outcomes can be improved by taking the above risk factors into consideration.

Advantages of RFA

- High local efficacy.
- Preserved healthy hepatic parenchyma outside the ablated zone.
- Safe repeating and reproducible potentiality.

Major disadvantages of RFA

- Heat sink effect—heat dissipation via adjacent major blood vessels, reducing its effectiveness/efficacy.
- Its ineffectiveness in targeting large tumours (>5 cm).

Complications

Early:

- Vascular: intraperitoneal bleeding, pseudoaneurysm formation, portal vein thrombosis, hepatic vein thrombosis, and hepatic infarction—less than 1%.
- Hepatic abscess (most common)—0.3–2%.
- Injury to adjacent structures: bile duct, gastrointestinal tract, gall bladder, and diaphragm (pneumothorax)—less than 1%.
- Skin burn.

Delayed (3–12 months after RFA):
- Biliary system: stricture, biloma, and haemobilia.
- Tumour seeding: along the needle tract, pleura, or peritoneum—0.2–1.4% (this can be minimized by tract ablation during needle withdrawal).

Nevertheless, the overall major complication rate of RFA ranges from 2.4% to 13.1% in comparison to the range of 9–22% for surgical resection.

Microwave ablation

MWA has been established as an optional thermal ablative treatment alternative to RFA. It works through the process of dielectric hysteresis,[14,17] that is, it generates thermal energy by using electromagnetic energy ranging between 915 MHz and 2.45 GHz., which excites electrical dipoles of water molecules to alternate along the induced electric field.[6,13] These oscillating water molecules cause frictional heating resulting in heat generation with subsequent coagulative necrosis of the targeted tissue.[12–14] Depending on the type of generator and needle used, an oval or elliptical zone of ablation is achievable. The water molecule excitation occurs over a larger radius with rapid, continuous, and uniform heat distribution and is directly proportional to the active electromagnetic energy applied.[5,13] The tissue penetration of MW energy is frequency dependent, with 915 kHz producing larger ablation zones and can reach temperatures of 160–180° C at the electrode tip.[12,13]

Microwaves are independent of current conduction which is seen in RFA. This property makes them less susceptible to charring, vaporization, and the 'heat sink effect', potentially achieving larger ablation volumes over a shorter time duration.[13,17] With evolution from the first to second generation of MWA systems larger (>5 cm), hotter, and faster rates of ablation are achievable.[11] As in RFA, the microwave generator can be used in mono-, bi-, or multipolar modes producing larger and quicker ablation zones.

Advantages of MWA
- No ground pads (required in RFA).
- Improved convection profile—no vaporization or charring.
- Higher intratumoural temperature with larger ablation volumes.
- Fewer needle placements with shorter/faster ablation times.
- Due to lesser potential for heat sink effect, its effect on perivascular tumours is better.

Due to its obvious advantages over RFA, its usability is increasing among interventionalists.[13]

Complications

Reported complication rate: 2.6–7.5%.[6]

- Skin burns.
- Liver capsular bleeds.
- Liver abscess.
- Ascites.
- Perforation of adjacent organs.
- Severe pain.

High-intensity focused ultrasound

This is a relatively new non-invasive technique of thermal ablation performed using magnetic resonance imaging (MRI) guidance. High-intensity focused acoustic energy (ultrasound waves) is targeted at a three-dimensional focal point creating local sound pressure, which is absorbed and converted to heat. This causes coagulative necrosis from combined hyperthermia and acoustic cavitation of targeted tissues with irreversible cellular death in the form of nuclear pyknosis, debris, and subsequent dissolution while sparing the surrounding structures.[11,13] Depending on the source's parameters, the focal point can be adjusted in a range of 1–5 mm in diameter and 10–50 mm in length.[13]

Drawbacks/disadvantages
- Complex set-up.
- High expense.
- Need for general anaesthesia—renders patients immobile and controls their respiration, while the patient is positioned prone in a water bath to remove the air between the transducer and target area.
- Time-consuming.

Complications

Observed in 13% of patients—skin or subcutaneous tissue injuries.

Studies

In one published study, 39 patients with cirrhosis Child A or B and unresectable HCC adjacent to the major hepatic veins were treated with HIFU. These patient/tumour characteristics would be ineligible for other ablation treatments such as RFA or PEI. Following one session of HIFU treatment, more than 50% of the patients developed complete tumour necrosis, indicating that HIFU can achieve complete tumour necrosis even when the lesion is located adjacent to major hepatic blood vessels. No major complications were observed and the overall survival rates at 1, 3, and 5 years were 75.8%, 49.8%, and 31.8%, respectively.[11]

In a similar study, Orsi et al. showed that in six HCC patients whose tumours were located in difficult locations (i.e. adjacent to a main hepatic blood vessel, heart, bowel, stomach, gall bladder, or bile ducts), treatment with HIFU achieved complete response in all patients without any complications.[11]

In combination with TACE, HIFU gives a 1-year survival rate of 42.9% for IVa stage patients (p <0.05 compared to patients receiving TACE only) and median reduction rates of 28.6%, 35.0%, 50.0%, and 50.0% of tumour sizes at 1, 3, 6, and 12 months, respectively.[5]

Zhang et al. treated 39 patients with HCC tumours within 1 cm of the main hepatic blood vessels with no major blood vessel injury observed in any subject. Morbidity from the procedure is also well tolerated in patients with cirrhosis.[13]

Laser-induced thermotherapy

This is a far less investigated hyperthermic ablative technique which uses optical fibre to transmit high-energy laser (Nd-YAG) radiation at near-infrared wavelength (600–1000 nm). This light is absorbed by targeted tissues and converted to heat with temperatures reaching up to 150° C, leading to substantial coagulative necrosis. Under magnetic resonance guidance, the optical fibre is inserted into the lesion through a percutaneously placed needle (removed after localization) and the thermocoagulation is monitored in real time using MRI for estimation of the extent of actual thermal damage.[5]

A multi-needle approach is essential to treat large lesions successfully (>5 cm) and is time-consuming in comparison to RFA and MWA.[5]

An advantage of using optical fibres is that it is well visualized on MRI, and the absence of metal also produces less streak artefacts on CT.[13]

A disadvantage is the limited energy penetration with inability to penetrate charred tissues.[13]

Due to its heavy reliance on thermal conduction, the heat sink phenomenon poses a larger problem requiring larger procedural times.[14] It is not currently used in clinical practice.

Study

Because with other ablative techniques, long-term success rates are related to tumour size, and an 82% complete response rate has been reported for lesions measuring 3.2 cm in diameter. In a series of 74 patients with small HCCs, survival rates at 1, 3, and 5 years were 99%, 48%, and 15%, respectively.[5]

Hypothermic ablation

This involves percutaneous administration of thermal energy into the lesion. Temperatures of −40° C are cytotoxic and seen to cause cell death. The thermal technique used generates extremely low temperatures within the targeted tissues that cause destruction of cellular structures and rupture of cellular membranes, thus resulting in tissue death.[11,14]

Cryoablation

This is a minimally invasive percutaneous ablative technique that uses rapid expansion of nitrogen or argon gas to cause rapid cooling. It uses freeze/thaw cycles, wherein during the freeze cycle the temperatures drop as low as −140° C followed by a slower thaw cycle with quick rise of temperature to 20–45° C. This causes intracellular ice crystal formation which results in rupture of the cell membranes and subsequent cell death of the targeted tissue.[6,11,13] The cellular integrity of the vessel wall is maintained during cryoablation; the vascular injury is due to blood stagnation with further microcirculation failure.[4,11]

Cellular death in cryoablation is influenced by various factors such as freezing rate and temperature, absolute depth of hypothermia, frequency of freeze/thaw cycles, and thaw rate.[5,13] The rapid cooling at the distal tip of the probe is independent of probe design and gas used.[13] Repeated freezing can improve its efficacy.[5] The real time ice-ball formation during the procedure allows precise evaluation of ablative zones and gives room for readjustment of needle positioning.[6]

The freeze/thaw cycle activates the antitumour immune response and can lead to a severe systemic reaction characterized by massive cytokine release and multiorgan failure and is called 'cryo-shock'.[11,13] The larger diameter of the current cryoprobes and the size (>5 cm) and location of tumours (inferior vena cava or major hepatic branch vessels) within the liver still pose a technical difficulty. The procedure is well tolerated under conscious sedation and can be a valuable option in patients who are poor candidates for anaesthesia.[6]

Potential adverse effects/complications

- Intraperitoneal haemorrhage—cracking of the liver surface during thawing of the ice-ball.

- Coagulopathy—thrombocytopenia and disseminated intravascular coagulation (more pronounced in background liver disease).
- Cryo-shock.

Studies

Based on a long-term follow-up study, cryosurgery could achieve a survival rate comparable to that of liver resection, in addition to reducing overall mortality and improving quality of life.[11]

Guo et al. reported 26 patients with HCCs of 10–14 cm in diameter receiving argon-helium cryotherapy after TACE. After this therapy, the average neoplasm necrosis rate was 28.7%, significantly higher than that of TACE only.[5]

One study reported a local recurrence rate for primary and metastatic liver tumours treated with cryotherapy versus RFA of 13.6 and 2.2%, respectively (p <0.01), and a much higher complication rate after cryotherapy (40.7 vs 3.3%; p <0.01). This and other similar studies have led to cryoablation being largely superseded by other ablative techniques.[14]

Non-thermal ablation

These ablation techniques do not rely on thermal effects and are most useful in treating centrally located tumours adjacent to bile ducts or vascular structures.

They are of two types:

- Chemical ablation:
  - PEI
  - Percutaneous acetic acid injection.
- Irreversible electroporation.

Chemical ablation

Involves percutaneous injection of a chemical into the lesion with resultant destruction of tumour cells.

Percutaneous ethanol injection

This is one of the first techniques devised to treat liver tumours and is usually performed under ultrasound guidance using a fine needle with injection of 95% ethanol. This causes cellular dehydration and protein denaturation resulting in coagulative necrosis of the tumour.[11,13] The volume of chemical agent to be administered depends on the radius of lesion (Box 25.1). The zone of ablation produced in PEI is not accurately predictable or reproducible and may

---

Box 25.1 Volume of chemical agent: calculation formula

$$V = 4/3\pi(r + 0.5)^3$$

V = volume of ethanol (in millilitres), r = radius of lesion (in centimetres).

As a safety margin, 0.5 is added to the radius—surrounding liver parenchyma all around the tumour as well as the tumour itself must be ablated.

Chemical injection to be stopped when high echogenic mass covering the tumour surpasses the edge by greater than 0.5 cm.

Source: data from Shiina S, et al. Percutaneous ethanol injection for hepatocellular carcinoma: 20-year outcome and prognostic factors. *Liver Int.* 2012;32(9):1434-1442; and Sun X, et al. Treatment of liver cancer of middle and advanced stages using ultrasound-guided percutaneous ethanol injection combined with radiofrequency ablation: a clinical analysis. *Oncol Lett.* 2016;11(3):2096-2100.

require multiple treatment sessions. The consistency of tissue, presence of septa/pseudo-capsule, and the degree of vascularity determines ethanol diffusion into the targeted tissue.[5,14] Due to the harder tissue consistency of liver metastases, diffusion of ethanol is not uniform and is considerably less effective in comparison to treatment of HCC lesions.[14] PEI is an effective treatment for a small HCC (<3 cm), but its overall therapeutic efficacy depends on the Child–Pugh score, BCLC staging, and serum alpha-fetoprotein levels devoid of tumour size. It is strongly recommended in HCC patients with small tumours (<1.5 cm) located near the major bile ducts, gall bladder, and diaphragm since they are not limited by a heat sink and have a safer profile.[11,13]

This technique is simple, safe, convenient, less costly, and reasonably effective; however, it is inferior to thermal ablation for most cases and is therefore not widely practiced.[13] In current practice, its applicability is limited to treatment of tumours near sensitive organs and tissues.[5]

Drawbacks

- High recurrence rate—usually around the tumour margin.
- Multiple injections.
- Large amounts of alcohol to achieve a better therapeutic effect—may cause cumulative damage and even cirrhosis in the hepatic parenchyma.
- High local progression rate of 17–38%.[5]

Complications (<5%)

- Intraperitoneal haemorrhage.
- Hepatic insufficiency or infarction.
- Biliary—gall bladder injury, bile duct necrosis, or biliary fistula.
- Portal vein thrombosis.
- Bowel or adjacent organ necrosis.[6,14]

Studies

It has been reported that in HCC patients whose tumour mass was less than 3 cm, a complete response rate of 70–80% and a 5-year survival of 40–60% have been achieved.[11]

Several randomized controlled trials have compared PEI vs. RFA in the treatment of small HCC. These trials have demonstrated an approximately 20% advantage for RFA vs. PEI in overall survival at 3–4 years, mainly as a result of a much lower incidence of local tumour recurrence in the RFA group. In addition, approximately threefold fewer treatment sessions were required for RFA compared to PEI. Two recent meta-analyses comparing RFA versus PEI echoed these sentiments, declaring RFA superior to PEI in the treatment of small HCC.[5]

However, Livraghi et al. reported that PEI could be applied in ≥5 cm liver tumours. They showed that for the 1,066 patients participating in their study, the 3-, 5- and 7-year survival rates were 72.3, 43.2 and 27.0%, respectively.[22]

Tumour recurrence and survival rates for RFA, PEI, and PAI [percutaneous acetic acid injection] in the treatment of HCC 3 cm in size or less, Child–Pugh A and B, were compared in a randomized trial involving 187 patients. Radiofrequency ablation was found to be superior, with local recurrence rates at 1 and 3 years of 10% and 14%, compared with 16% and 34% in the PEI group and 14% and 31% in the PAI group. Survival rates at 1 and 3 years were 93% and 74%, 88% and 51%, and 90% and 53% in the RFA, PEI, and PAI groups respectively. Cancer-free survival rates at 1 and 3 years were 74% and 43% in the RFA group, 70% and 21% in the PEI group, and 71% and 23% in the PAI group. Large tumour size (>2 cm) and high tumour grade were independent factors that correlated with local recurrence.[6]

Percutaneous acetic acid injection

Acetic acid is a chemical reagent that has better tissue diffusion capability than ethanol and was first reported by Ohnishi et al. The technique of percutaneous acetic acid injection is similar to PEI and is proposed as alternative to ethanol to achieve the same degree of tissue ablation with fewer number of treatment sessions (1–2 mL of acetic acid per tumour per session per week). It is a relatively simple and safe technique; however, it carries the risk of transient haemoglobinuria which can be contained by precautionary alkalinization of urine (administering intravenous fluids containing bicarbonates). Other adverse effects include fever, right upper abdominal pain (larger doses), segmental infarction, and metabolic acidosis.

Irreversible electroporation

IRE is a relatively new emerging non-thermal ablative technique which uses electrical pulses (short, repetitive, high voltage) targeted from multiple needle points that cause damage to cell membranes and apoptosis of targeted tumour tissue, while largely preserving the extracellular matrix.[13,17]

Its ablative zones are predictable in comparison to RFA and allow for preservation of tissue architecture and it can be used to treat tumours adjacent to central bile ducts or other vital structures (blood vessels and nerves). Kingham et al. showed no increase in recurrence when treating perivascular tumours.

Limited data is available in the use of IRE in hepatic tumours and is currently used to treat locally advanced pancreatic cancer. IRE followed by TACE has been studied in experimental porcine models with promising results showing enhanced intranuclear accumulation of doxorubicin in the reversible electroporation zone.[17]

IRE is seen to affect cardiac rhythm causing arrhythmias and also muscle contractions. These side effects can be mostly mitigated by using cardiac gating and paralytic agents.[13]

Additionally, it is technically cumbersome requiring the parallel placement of multiple probes, with slight deviations in alignment possibly resulting in failed treatment.

Currently, it is best used in small, unresectable, hepatic tumours that are also unsuitable for thermal ablation because of neighbouring vital structures.[13]

Transarterial catheter-based therapies

Rationale

The liver has a dual blood supply with almost 75% through the portal vein and 25% from the hepatic artery.[4] Hepatic malignancies derive their large blood supply from the hepatic artery, this allows selective intra-arterial administration of various drugs (chemotherapeutic agents, bland particles, or radioactive spheres) sparing the normal liver parenchyma. The terminal embolization results in ischaemia and necrosis of a tumour.[4,6,9]

Bland embolization with particles/transarterial embolization

Embolization refers to completely cutting off the vascular supply to a tumour. In TAE, the feeding hepatic arteries are occluded by injecting various intravascular emboli devoid of a chemotherapeutic agent which induces ischaemia and subsequent necrosis of the tumour. A variety of embolic agents like Gelfoam, polyvinyl alcohol (PVA) particles, and recently drug-eluting beads have been used.

Gelfoam consists of gelatin sponge particles which provide temporary (2–3 weeks) feeding vessel occlusion. Due to its large (1 mm) size, the particulate capacity to reach the tumour bed is sparse and may result in suboptimal embolization.[10] PVA particles range in size and can reach more distal arteriolar capillaries, providing more permanent occlusion.[10] Small-sized particles of 40–150 μm are the key for adequate penetration of the tumour microvasculature and distal tumoural bed occlusion.

Studies

Advocates of this catheter-based therapy claim that bland embolization may be equally effective as TACE for palliative treatment of primary liver cancer. Despite a trend toward improved survival with TACE, no study to date has demonstrated a difference in survival between the two techniques. A randomized trial comparing embolization (without chemotherapy) vs. symptomatic treatment in patients with hepatitis C virus-related liver disease and Child–Pugh class A liver function failed to demonstrate a 2-year survival advantage.[5]

Nicolini et al. reported that TAE using microspheres can achieve a complete response (CR), with evidence of devascularization of the tumour in 89% of cases. The definition of CR is an absence of peripheral enhancement in the arterial-phase CT images. However, the authors reported a local recurrence rate of 62% and development of additional tumours in 56% of patients. The time lag between assessment of CR and local recurrence of the tumour ranged from 3 months to 6 months. Nicolini et al. suggested the possibility of CT overestimation of tumour response and the small study sample as potential explanations for the high recurrence rate. Still, the study showed that TAE is a well-tolerated procedure for patients with early or intermediate HCC, causing no clinically significant deterioration in liver function.[6]

Transarterial chemoembolization

TACE combines intra-arterial cytotoxic drug administration to the tumour bed followed by embolization of the tumour vascularity using various embolic agents.[4,5,6,10,14,18]

The two most common methods of TACE are:

- Conventional TACE (C-TACE): TACE performed with lipiodol (iodinated poppy seed oil) as a carrying agent with embolic effect.
- Drug-eluting bead TACE (DEB-TACE): TACE performed with beads as carrying agents with an embolic effect.

Rationale

Administration of a chemotherapeutic drug mixed with a carrying agent (vector) results in increased contact time between the cytotoxic agent and the tumour with a higher drug concentration and retention within the tumour. This followed by an embolic agent results in destruction of the capillary beds (hypoxia) with subsequent extensive necrosis of the tumour.[5,10]

Indications

- HCC patients with good liver function reserve and no thrombosis in the portal vein trunk, who are incapable of having their tumours radically resected.
- Debulking the size of huge liver cancers for later resection.
- Palliative control of pain, bleeding, and arteriovenous fistula caused by the tumour.
- Preventive therapy after tumour resection.

Contraindications

Absolute contraindication: Bilirubin level greater than 3 mg/dL unless segmental injections can be performed.

Relatively contraindicated

- Main portal vein thrombosis (treated zone might develop extensive necrosis because of blocking of the entire blood supply to that specific area).
- Patients with liver function classified as Child–Pugh class C.
- Total liver involvement exceeding 50%.
- Bi-lobar tumours.
- Distant metastases.
- Glomerular filtration rate less than 40 mL/min/1.73 m^2.
- Arterioportal fistulae.

Complications (<1% of patients)

- Liver abscess.
- Liver failure.

C-TACE

In C-TACE ethiodized oil and a chemotherapeutic agent are mixed to create an oily emulsion. The ethiodized oil used is lipiodol. Due to its radiopaque nature, viscosity, and water insolubility it forms an excellent vector for intra-arterial microembolic agents as a whole.[6,13] The lipiodol is retained in the tumour due to the absence of Kupffer cells within in the tumour in comparison to normal liver parenchyma and may remain for weeks to months.[4,5] After administration of the oily emulsion, additional blocking material is injected for a complete embolic effect. Various embolic agents ranging from Gelfoam to microspheres are used with Gelfoam being the most commonly used material for end embolization.[13]

Multiple chemotherapeutic agents like cisplatin, doxorubicin, carboplatin, epirubicin, mitoxantrone, and mitomycin C are used alone or sometimes in combination[4,6] with mitomycin C, cisplatin, and doxorubicin being most commonly used.[12,19]

The TACE procedure is performed either segmentally or subsegmentally (super- selectively) as safely as feasible preserving the normal liver tissue.[13] As the administration of the oily emulsion passes through the peribiliary spaces, it enables a dual arterial and portal approach to the tumour with appearance of peribiliary-portal vein capillary stains as approximated end points of embolization.[18] As recanalization of the tumour occurs in the long term, further sessions of TACE can be repeated when residual disease is identified and planned focusing on the active tumour burden.[9,13]

Most patients experience postembolization syndrome comprising abdominal pain, nausea, fever, leucocytosis, and elevation of liver enzymes which lasts for about a week or two and is generally managed by conservative treatment.[4]

DEB-TACE

In DEB-TACE the chemotherapeutic agent is loaded on to beads containing and combining the carrying and embolic effect. This type of drug delivery system was introduced in 2006[20] and has the benefit of sustained drug release adsorbed to the bead surface over long periods of time maximizing their effectiveness with significant reduction in systemic toxicity.[4,5,6,10,19]

Drug-eluting microspheres are composed of biocompatible polymers such as PVA hydrogel and are hydrophilic and non-resorbable.[4–6] They are sulphonated to enable the binding of chemotherapeutic drugs using an ion exchange mechanism (positively charged parts of anthracyclines with anionic groups in their chemical structures) which enables controlled and sustained tumoural drug retention.[4,5,13,19]

Due to the important technical and scheduling drawbacks of C-TACE that have not yet been standardized with expected higher post-procedural pain score, the majority of interventionist are moving towards DEB-TACE when feasible.[20] However, the major drawback of C-TACE/DEB-TACE and its cause remains the same (Box 25.2).

As the beads' drug delivery is slow and sustained (half-life—150 hours (100–300 μm particles) and 1730 hours (700–900 μm particles)), a higher volume of drug (up to 150 mg of doxorubicin) can be administered devoid of decreased systemic side effects and rates of liver failure compared to C-TACE (lipiodol solution (half-life of 1 hour))[4,13,19] and this approach has both a cytotoxic and ischaemic effect leading to tumour/tumoural necrosis.[20] Super-selective drug administration of small-sized beads is usually preferred due to their deeper penetration and has a more effective embolic effect in comparison to larger beads without compromising patient safety.[13,21]

Balloon-occluded TACE (B-TACE)

B-TACE is a modification of C-TACE which was proposed by Irie et al. In B-TACE a micro-balloon is used to occlude the feeding vessel prior to drug administration. This shows a significant increase in lipiodol uptake and retention.[19]

Irie et al. attained higher tumour control rates and complete response rates in B-TACE (89.9%) in comparison to C-TACE (65.3%) in his study of 77 patients.[19]

Arai et al. and Ogawa et al. reported B-TACE superiority over C-TACE in response rates when miriplatin was used as the chemotherapeutic agent.[19]

Maruyama et al, showed high rates of adverse events and side effects when B-TACE was carried out using epirubicin with Irie et al. showing similar rates of adverse events using a doxorubicin plus mitomycin C combination.[19]

Currently, to avoid biliary and vascular injury caused by B-TACE, miriplatin is usually chosen as the anticancer drug because of its less hazardous damage against peripheral small vessels.[19]

Kawamura et al. described that visualization of the peripheral portal veins was significantly associated with high necrosis rates of tumours after B-TACE, which was also a well-known phenomenon in C-TACE.[19]

Transarterial radioembolization

Transarterial radioembolization (TARE) is a type of brachytherapy/interstitial radiotherapy/selective internal radiation therapy which involves the injection of microspheres labelled with a radioisotope into the hepatic artery.[6,9,12,13,18] TARE uses beta-emitting radioactive elements such as yttrium (Y), rhenium, or iodine-131 (^{131}I). ^{131}I-labelled iodinated poppy seed oil and ^{90}Y-loaded microspheres are the most frequently used compounds of which ^{90}Y treatment in particular is associated with low toxicity and is used primarily in clinical practice.[4,6,13] The pure beta-emitter radioisotope ^{90}Y is produced by means of neutron bombardment of ^{89}Y. It has an average energy of 0.9367 MeV and half-life of 64.2 hours with an average and maximal tissue penetration of 2.5 and 10 mm which decays to stable zirconium-90.[12,13,18]

Two types of US Food and Drug Administration-approved radioactive microspheres are currently available for intra-arterial drug delivery which differ in their particle make, size, and specific activity per particle. They are resin microspheres ^{90}Y (SIR-sphere, Sirtex Medical; average diameter/average specific activity 20–60 μm/50 Bq/sphere) which are approved for the treatment of colorectal metastases and glass microspheres; and ^{90}Y embedded within (Therasphere, BTG Corporation; average diameter/average specific activity 20–30 μm/2500 Bq/sphere) which are approved for treating HCC.[4,12,13] Due to its particle differences, a minimal embolic effect is noted with glass microspheres (approximately 1.2 million spheres to reach 3 GBq) versus a moderate embolic effect using resin microspheres (more homogeneous distribution; approximately 25 million spheres to reach 3 GBq).[4,9,12,18]

TARE combines a minimal embolic effect on tumour vascularity with cytotoxicity of radiation. The preferential deposition of microspheres and small range of ^{90}Y microspheres penetration of 1–2 mm within the tumour allows selective irradiation of the target tissue (reaching highly effective intratumoural radiation doses of 100–150 Gy for tumour destruction) rather than the normal hepatic parenchyma, thereby reducing the risk of radiation-induced liver disease.[4]

TARE involves two separate angiography procedures: mapping angiography and treatment angiography

Preparatory mapping angiography is performed as a separate procedure prior to TARE for evaluation of the arterial supply (collateral

---

Box 25.2 Drawbacks

Incomplete necrosis of tumour tissues is the major drawback of TACE. Why?
- Pathological examination of surgical specimens after TACE showed live cancer cells around most tumours.
- This is mainly due to drug resistance of tumour cells, incomplete tumour embolization, and re-established collateral blood supply.

Source: data from Chen X et al. Advances in non-surgical management of primary liver cancer. World J Gastroenterol. 2014;20(44):16630–16638.

flow to enteric and other non-target organs/direct hepatic arteriovenous shunts), planning treatment volumes necessary for radiation dosimetry, and calculation of the lung shunt fraction.[9,13,18]

This helps in proper planning and avoidance of severe and detrimental adverse effects of non-target extrahepatic radioembolization.[9]

In mapping angiography 2–5 mCi technetium-99m macro-aggregated albumin (99mTc-MAA) microspheres are injected into the planned treatment site (proper, right or left hepatic artery) followed by planar or single-photon emission computed tomography (SPECT) which maps the isotope deposition ensuring the targeted deposition, any sites of extrahepatic gastrointestinal hyperactivity, and calculating of the cumulative pulmonary dose. Pulmonary doses greater than 30 Gy per treatment or greater than 50 Gy cumulatively have been associated with the development of radiation pneumonitis.[9,18]

Coil embolization is indicated if arterial origins arise close to the drug injection site or super-selective catheterization cannot be achieved, which could lead to particles being taken up by extrahepatic organs, primarily the gastrointestinal tract. In addition, occlusion of some of the extrahepatic arteries to 'monopediculize' the tumour allows a single artery to be embolized.[9,18]

The radiation standard doses vary for resin and glass spheres and are calculated using the body surface area and the percentage of tumour invasion for the former and Medical Internal Radiation Dose methodology for the later.

The desired vial of ^{90}Y spheres is then ordered and delivered within a week's time and is calibrated accounting for its exponential decay.[4]

The aim of TARE is to treat the tumour and minimize exposure to healthy liver tissue. In treatment angiography, based on the tumour load, a single injection from the common hepatic artery or a single or sequential injection of ^{90}Y is performed accordingly in a slow and paced manner. Post administration of the calculated standard dose of radiation microspheres, a ^{90}Y Bremsstrahlung SPECT-CT imaging or a ^{90}Y positron emission tomography-CT imaging (internal pair production of ^{90}Y) is performed to ensure optimal sphere distribution.[18]

Standard treatments are usually delivered in a segmental, lobar, or bi-lobar fashion. Radiation segmentectomy is gaining popularity and uses a similar technique wherein usually two segments or fewer are targeted at higher doses (threshold dose of at least 190 Gy) of radiation in a more selective fashion.[13] This is being investigated as an alternative to PVE in the setting of extensive unipolar disease before hepatectomy.

TARE is usually a better tolerated procedure than TACE with reduced features of post-embolization syndrome (nausea, vomiting, abdominal pain, and fever),[19] providing a better quality of life.[4]

It has an added advantage of treating bi-lobar disease or extensive multifocal HCC even with portal vein invasion in a single session.[4]

A recent retrospective analysis demonstrated no difference in tumour response or survival between chemoembolization and radioembolization.[4]

Indications

- Similar to TACE.
- Bi-lobar disease.

Portal vein thrombosis is not a contraindication to radioembolization which has the potential to recanalize portal vein thrombosis resulting from tumour invasion.

Complications
Mild

- Skin irritation (via the falciform artery).
- Fatigue, lymphopenia, and rise in serum bilirubin.

Severe

(Non-targeted radiation can lead to 'bystander organ injury'—ischaemia/ulceration/necrosis of the stomach, gall bladder, and small bowel (via the gastric, cystic and duodenal arteries)).

- Pneumonitis.
- Hepatic abscess especially in diabetics and after a bilioenteric bypass.
- Radiation-induced cholecystitis, and biloma.
- Radiation hepatitis.
- Organ failure: liver and kidney.
- Deaths (2–3%) have been reported.

Studies
^{90}Y versus ^{131}I

A randomized controlled trial comparing ^{131}I-labelled iodinated poppy seed oil tare with best medical support in HCC patients having portal vein thrombosis showed a 6-month survival of 48% with treatment; in the best medical support arm, there were no survivors at 6 months. Chaudhury et al. reported a case of CR for a 4.7-cm HCC tumour with vascular involvement treated using sorafenib and ^{90}Y radioembolization. Comparing TACE with TARE, Salem et al. observed no significant difference in survival time (p = 0.42); however, the difference in time to progression was found to be clinically significant in favour of radioembolization (13.3 months for TARE vs 8.4 for TAE, p = 0.046). When comparing ^{131}I-labelled iodinated poppy seed oil tare with conventional TACE for unresectable HCC survival was similar for both treatments (6-month survival: 69.2% vs 65.6%), but with fewer side effects in the TARE group.[6]

TARE versus TACE

A comparative effectiveness study on outcomes following transarterial radioembolization and transarterial chemoembolization in a 245-patient adult HCC cohort showed that adverse events, clinical toxicities, response rate and time-to-tumour progression were improved with transarterial radioembolization. However there was no difference in overall survival between the two therapies.[9]

Transarterial radioembolization with ^{90}Y can deliver radiation doses as high as 150 Gy directly to the tumour. Doses this high cannot be safely accomplished by external beam radiation because of the effects on normal tissues. A comparative effectiveness study on outcomes following transarterial radioembolization and transarterial chemoembolization in a 245-patient adult HCC cohort showed that adverse events, clinical toxicities, response rate and time-to-tumour progression were improved with transarterial radioembolization. However, there was no difference in overall survival between the two therapies. While there is a growing body of literature for transarterial radioembolization in adults, very few data exist for transarterial radioembolization in paediatric patients.[9]

Combination therapy

Combination therapies are gaining popularity in the treatment of primary and secondary liver tumours with continued increases in evidence of safety and efficacy of percutaneous ablative and transarterial therapies.[14] The combination methods offer a synergistic strategy to widen the therapeutic benefit in large tumours.[14,11] Standard combination protocols are not available yet.

The commonly used treatment protocol is a combination of an ablative therapy with intra-arterial therapy. The most commonly used combinations are TACE prior to PEI (to render the tumour necrotic, and thus allow enhanced diffusion of the ethanol) and TACE prior to RFA (to cut off regional blood flow, reduces heat loss and improves the detrimental effect on the efficacy RFA).[5,10,14] With newer technologies devoid of the heat sink effect like MWA becoming popular, newer combinations are being performed. Recently TACE and immunotherapy anti-angiogenesis have been tried and could be applied for future clinical applications.[5]

Another ablative therapy combination is the use of RFA in combination with PEI. Few studies have demonstrated improved local tumour control and long-term survival with combination of RFA with PEI than performing RFA alone.[14]

Studies

In this study, patients with tumours larger than 3 cm were randomized to TACE, RFA, and TACE-RFA. The combination modality was superior in median survival (TACE-RFA at 37 months, TACE at 24 months vs. RFA at 22 months) and rate of objective tumour response (TACE-RFA at 54%, TACE at 35% vs. RFA at 36%).[5]

In another RCT that included 189 patients with tumours <7 cm, combined RFA and TACE resulted in better overall and tumour free survival than RFA alone. There are only cohort studies that compare TACE and RFA vs TACE alone and these have shown promising results that warrant adequately powered RCTs.[10] The positive findings in this study represent initial evidence in support for the use of combining local regional modalities to improve outcomes in patients with unresectable tumours.

Transvenous therapy

Portal vein embolization

PVE is a technique primarily used in patients who undergo extended liver resection. The portal blood flowing into the planned resected segments or lobe is cut off to increase the flow to the remaining liver, called the future liver remnant (FLR), resulting in hypertrophy of the remaining non-tumour-containing parenchyma and allowing safe extended liver resections. This technique is performed when the FLR is less than 20–30% of the initial total normal liver volume or less than 50% in fibrotic and cirrhotic livers.

Transhepatic puncture is predominantly performed over the trans-splenic approach for PVE.

In the transhepatic approach, the portal vein is punctured either through an ipsilateral or contralateral approach followed by embolization of the targeted segments. Various embolic particles (PVA), liquid (glue or alcohol) agents, and coils (large vessel occlusions) are deployed.

PVE acts as an adjuvant tool not only in primary liver tumours but also has the upmost importance in resection of metastatic liver disease which is often considered the best chance for cure.[12]

Side effects/complications

- Non-target embolization.
- Transient increase in white blood cell count.
- Fever.
- Abdominal discomfort.

Studies

Siriwardana et al. prospectively studied the effect of PVE on HCC recurrence in 34 patients who underwent curative liver resection after PVE and in 102 who underwent resection without PVE. The use of PVE increased the FLR from 23% to 34%. The study concluded that PVE can increase the resectability rate of HCC tumours considered initially unresectable because of insufficient FLR and that PVE has no deleterious oncological effect after major resection of HCC.[6]

Simoneau et al. studied the effect of PVE on the growth of liver metastases from colorectal tumours. They prospectively followed tumour growth in 109 patients who underwent right PVE, and 11 who did not. Tumour growth was significantly different between the groups, with the tumour volume increasing by 33.4% in the right lobe and 49.9% in the left lobe of the liver of the embolized group and decreasing by 34.8% in the right lobe of the liver and by 33.2% in the left lobe of the non-embolized group (p <0.001 in the right lobe, p = 0.022 in the left lobe). Despite these results, resectability was not affected. Similar data in HCC patients are lacking.[6]

Staging and management

Hepatocellular carcinoma

Interventional radiology is involved practically at each stage in the treatment of HCC as recommended in the European Association for the Study of the Liver–European Organisation for Research and Treatment of Cancer guidelines. It is even becoming more important as technological advances progress with the long-term assessment of its efficacy.[18]

Very early-stage HCC (BCLC classification stage 0)

Surgical resection remains the gold standard in treating non-cirrhotic patients with preserved liver function, normal bilirubin level, and devoid of significant portal hypertension. These patients have a 5-year survival rate of better than 75% and technique-related mortality rates of 1–3%.[7,8]

This procedure is suitable for candidates with suitable location for resection (central wide excision vs subcapsular wedge resection tumours) for preservation of maximal liver parenchyma and its function.[7,18]

Patients with small lesions (<2 cm) with an unsuitable surgical plane of resection which are not subcapsular or perivascular are offered RFA as a standard technique in most institutions.[7,18] A complete response rates of about 97% with 5-year survival rates of 68% were achieved in various studies.[7]

In recent times, RFA has challenged the role of surgical resection and Cho et al. concluded both techniques to be equally effective in treatment of very early HCC.[7] When there is limitation regarding both the above techniques, PEI can still be considered.

Early-stage HCC (BCLC classification stage A)

This includes patients with preserved liver function (Child–Pugh class A and B) having three or more lesions smaller than 3 cm. These patients when treated effectively have a 5-year survival rate estimate ranging from 50% to 75% with the possibility of long-term cure.[7,18]

Various management strategies such as resection, liver transplantation, and percutaneous ablation are in use. At present, percutaneous ablative techniques are preferred over others for tumour destruction. RFA is currently considered the best treatment option; however, MWA is emerging as a newer modality of choice due to its lower susceptibility to the heat sink effect.[7,18]

Recent reports of RFA on Child–Pugh class A disease with early-stage HCC showed that 5-year survival rates are as high as 51–64% and may reach 76% in patients who meet the BCLC criteria for surgical resection. The assessment of RFA over PEI on survival outcomes has been more controversial in the past; however, three independent meta-analyses that included all RCTs have confirmed survival benefit particularly for tumours larger than 2 cm. In lesions exceeding 3 cm but not over 5 cm, the effect of RFA to achieve tumour-free margins is decreased.

The BCLC classification has not proposed any line of treatment in those patients with a solitary large (5 cm) tumour. These patients deserve a special mention as they cannot undergo surgical resection nor qualify for transplantation. Currently available ablative modalities have been devoted towards achieving larger tumour burn areas; however, a combination of ablative and intra-arterial therapies provide the best results. In contrast, surgical resection is offered in a self-selected group with a low tendency for multifocal disease. Locoregional treatment plays an important role in patients waiting (>6 months to stall tumour progression) for liver transplantation.[7]

Intermediate-stage HCC (BCLC classification stage B–C)

This large heterogeneous population of patients consists of multinodular HCC with good clinical status and relatively well-preserved liver function without vascular invasion or extrahepatic spread. TACE is the recommended standard of care in these patients due to its demonstration of improved survival outcomes in comparison to the best supportive care or other suboptimal therapies in a meta-analysis of six randomized control trials.[7,18]

In patients who show no response in the treated tumour, after at least two sessions of TACE, other therapies such as ablation, systemic therapy, combination treatment, and radioembolization can be considered. Conversely, in patients with poor clinical status, radioembolization may represent an alternative.[18] Several phase I and II clinical trials investigating the efficacy of radioembolization in the treatment of HCC have shown a longer time to disease progression and lower toxicity.

Many authors equally emphasized the wide variety of BCLC stage B and attempted to form a subclassification:

1. The intermediate stage was subclassified into B1–B4, by Bolondi et al. based on tumour burden ('up-to-seven' criteria), liver function (Child–Pugh score 5–9), and performance status (Eastern Cooperative Oncology Group Performance Status (ECOG PS) 0 or 1).

TACE is the recommended treatment in the B1 class with ablation as an alternative option whereas supportive care, research trials, and liver transplantation was recommended for the B3 or B4 classes.[20]

2. Yamakado et al. proposed a novel subclassification based on tumour burden and Child–Pugh score in patients with BCLC stage B.

3. Kudo et al. published a subclassification based on tumour status (beyond Milan and within 'up-to-seven' criteria) and liver function (Child–Pugh score 5–7 or 8–9).

The Kinki criteria classified BCLC B stage into B1 (up to 7 cm; Child–Pugh score 5–7 and within 'up-to-seven'), B2 (beyond 'up-to-seven'; Child–Pugh score 5–7), and B3 (any tumour status; Child–Pugh score 8, 9, and beyond).[20]

4. Hiraoka et al. devised another subclassification using the ALBI score instead of the Child–Pugh classification for liver function estimation.

Though many classifications exist, TACE remains the mainstay of treatment in this population; however, its standardization on protocols has not yet been proposed.

Advanced stage (BCLC classification stage D)

This includes patients with cancer symptoms and/or vascular invasion or extrahepatic spread who have a short life expectancy (50% survival at 1 year).[7]

Multikinase inhibitors (like sorafenib) which show antiangiogenic and antiproliferative properties are considered the therapy of choice in these patients and have been seen to prolong median overall survival and median time to radiological disease progression. In a debatable selected group of patients in an advanced stage with limited disease (performance status = 1, without/minimal extravascular or extrahepatic disease, with portal vein invasion), intra-arterial treatments such as TACE and radioembolization are being tried and tested.

Patients with terminal-stage illness are only offered palliative care due to their generalized poor condition in all aspects from performance status to liver functions and have an overall life expectancy of less than 3 months. They are at a higher risk of decompensation after any of the procedures discussed.

A multidisciplinary approach is of upmost importance in the management of these patients of various stages. A team (including hepatologists, diagnostic radiologists, pathologists, transplant surgeons, surgical oncologists, interventional radiologists, medical oncologists, radiation oncologists, nurses, and palliative care professionals) has to work in an integrated manner to provide the best care to these patients through a multidisciplinary clinic with dedicated tumour board reviews.[8]

The best possible treatments should be offered to patients based on their disease status as a single or a succession of procedures throughout the course of the disease.[18]

Metastases

Colorectal cancer

Metastatic liver disease is a common cause of death in cancer patients with two-thirds of the mortality pertaining to colorectal cancer liver metastases.[12] Only 25% of patients are amenable to surgery (gold standard management) and have 5-year overall survival rates of about 50% with the most recent chemotherapeutic regimens providing better median survival times (up to 22 months) for colorectal cancer.

Locoregional therapies such as PVE, hepatic arterial infusion therapy (HAIC), percutaneous ablative techniques, and TAE (TACE and TARE) have not only provided curative treatment options in these patients who are not candidates for surgery, but also improved survival in the palliative setting.[12]

Non-resectable colorectal liver metastases are managed with systemic chemotherapy (HAIC) with or without biological agents in the current guidelines from the National Comprehensive Cancer Network.[7] The aim of HAIC is to increase drug concentrations in the tumour tissue, thereby eventually increasing response rates; however, the treatments are not well tolerated by the patients. First-line therapy using either FOLFOX (5-fluorouracil and oxaliplatin) or FOLFIRI (irinotecan with or without bevacizumab) with second-line therapy consisting of the other combination (i.e. oxaliplatin changed to irinotecan) are commonly used.[7]

Percutaneous thermal ablation is a viable option with similar overall survival rates as surgery and decreased complication rates for a defined number of lesions that are technically amenable to ablation. It can be applied wherever technically feasible to treat all visible disease at any given time point.

Arterial embolization is performed with irinotecan drug-eluting bead chemoembolization, and is associated with significant short-term toxicity, specifically intense abdominal pain during and immediately after administration. Due to the poor short-term tolerability of chemoembolization, ^{90}Y radioembolization has largely been favoured and in the salvage setting for colorectal cancer metastases has been shown to prolong survival.

Although patients in the radioembolization arm showed improved rates of objective tumour response and liver-specific progression, it did not result in an improvement on overall survival.

Neuroendocrine tumour metastasis (NET)

NETs are functional endocrine tumours which primarily metastasize to the liver. Surgical resection remains the mainstay curative treatment in NETs. Percutaneous ablation is used as a viable alternative when surgery is contraindicated as with multifocal disease or as an adjunct to treat satellite lesions that are outside the criteria of a simple resection.

HAIC combined with a somatostatin analogue or peptide receptor radionuclide therapy can be effective in settings of high-grade tumours or diffuse disease. Where NETs are not symptomatically controlled by HAIC in patients with low to medium-grade tumours, transarterial therapy is a feasible option.

Bland embolization, chemoembolization, and ^{90}Y radioembolization have all shown excellent efficacy in controlling symptoms and achieving reasonable tumour response rates without significant differences in overall survival. Although no proven survival benefits have been shown with radioembolization in comparison to bland embolization, it is associated with lower rates of systemic toxicity (postembolization syndrome and carcinoid crisis) and is preferred in settings of portal vein thrombosis.

Regardless of therapy, the survival rate is very promising, with average survival in many cohorts exceeding 5 years. Perseverance of hepatic reserve and arterial vasculature is important while treating patient with NETs for repetition of treatments.

Chemoembolization is also applied in cases of metastases from NET, breast cancer, and uveal melanoma.[12]

Other lesions

Haemangioma

Haemangiomas are one of the most common primary liver tumours with a reported prevalence ranging from 3% to up to 20%. Most lesions are detected incidentally, but lesions larger than 4 cm (giant haemangiomas) might be symptomatic and may require treatment due to their high risk of bleeding. Surgery is the mainstay treatment in lesions with optimal resection margins, although the complication rate is relatively high. Interventional techniques such as TAE or TACE using bleomycin have shown promising results. These techniques should be preferred as a standalone treatment or as a bridge prior to surgery for reduction of risk.[23]

Hepatic cysts

Hydatid cyst

This is an endemic parasitic disease caused by the tapeworm (*Echinococcus granulosus*). The cysts are most commonly localized in the liver (50–80%), followed by the lungs (5–30%). Hydatidosis can occur less frequently in the spleen, kidney, heart, bones, and central nervous system.[24,25] The disease can be fatal and can cause serious complications (rupture, infection, and anaphylaxis). Medical, surgical, and percutaneous drainage techniques are active treatment options for patients with hydatid liver disease.[24] Though surgery is a primary mode of management, due to its increased risk of morbidity and mortality, percutaneous management has been used in recent years.[25]

Percutaneous techniques such as PAIR or PAIDS (puncture and aspiration of cyst contents, injection of scolicidal agents, with re-aspiration or with catheter drainage and injection of sclerosing agents) as well as MoCaT (modified catheter technique), have been used for treatment of hydatid liver disease, with minimal morbidity.[24]

Procedure

Laboratory investigations such as blood counts, coagulation, and liver function are performed. Patients are monitored continuously for possible anaphylaxis throughout the procedure which is performed under intravenous sedation along with preprocedural antiallergic prophylaxis (diphenhydramine (10–50 mg/kg) and hydrocortisone sodium succinate (100 mg intravenously)).

Ultrasound guidance is used for puncture and may be combined with fluoroscopy when needed.

A puncture is made through the liver parenchyma carefully to prevent any possible leak of content, following which the cyst contents are aspirated and the cyst cavity is rinsed with normal saline (through the needle in PAIR or pigtail catheter in PAIDS).

A cystogram is performed to confirm that there is no communication between the biliary ducts and the cyst cavity. Scolicidal agents (20–30% hypertonic saline, albendazole solution, and 95% absolute alcohol) are administered at an estimated 25–35% (one-third) of cyst volume. After 15 minutes, the administered fluid is re-aspirated and the catheter is withdrawn. In case of modified catheter technique(MoCaT), the catheter is retained until the fluid drainage is less than 10 mL/day. A good practice is to monitor the patient for a period of 24 hours.

Follow-up

Routine sonographic examinations at the first week, 1 month, 3 months, and every 6 months thereafter.

The recurrence rate of percutaneous hydatid cysts treatment is in the range of 0–4%.

Simple hepatic cysts

These are formed as biliary malformations which do not communicate with the intrahepatic biliary tree and continue to secrete intraluminal fluid. They show a female predominance increasing in incidence over 50 years. Most cysts are less than 3 cm in diameter and are usually asymptomatic with patients having normal liver functions. Occasionally, these cysts are detected on ultrasound or CT and can be observed and may not require treatment. Cysts that are larger in size and causing a mass effect or clinical symptoms require attention for treatment.

Surgical fenestration can be performed, but it has limitations (cysts involving segments VII or VIII have higher recurrence rates) and rare possible complications (haemorrhage and biliary injury).

Percutaneous techniques of sclerotherapy have emerged as viable options to disrupt intracystic fluid secretion by destruction of the epithelial lining of the inner surface of the cyst wall. Under local anaesthesia and ultrasound guidance, using the Seldinger technique a drainage catheter is placed into the cyst cavity. A cystogram is performed to rule out any biliary, vascular, and peritoneal communication. The cyst is made to collapse by aspiration of the internal fluid, following which a sclerosing agent (ethanol, ethanolamine oleate, or minocycline hydrochloride) is injected and made to contact the inner cyst wall. After an indwelling time ranging from 120 to 240 minutes, the sclerosant is aspirated and the catheter is either removed or capped to see the response on subsequent acute follow-up. Due to its high recurrence rates, this form of management is best reserved for those patients who are not good candidates for surgery.[26]

Polycystic liver disease

This is an autosomal dominant genetic disease with development of multiple hepatic cysts. It presents in two forms, with or without polycystic kidney disease (autosomal dominant polycystic kidney disease (ADPKD)). As in simple cystic disease, patients with polycystic liver disease are usually asymptomatic and when symptoms do arise, they are mainly related to the volume of the enlarged liver and may present with pain, abdominal distention, dyspnoea, or early satiety. They show similar findings to a simple cyst as anechoic areas on ultrasound, as fluid density areas on CT, and as hyperintense areas on T2-weighted images devoid of other specific abnormal findings on MRI.

These cysts can uncommonly get infected, bleed, or rupture and can cause a mass effect on adjacent structures leading to cholestasis or portal hypertension. The need for treatment arises in symptomatic patients and those with immunocompromised status (ADPKD on dialysis/post renal transplantation). Surgical treatments such as partial liver resection and fenestration has been historically proposed, but are associated with high morbidity and mortality rates and liver transplantation is the only curative option.[26]

Minimally invasive options such as percutaneous sclerotherapy and drainage are aimed at emptying of cysts causing decompression and reduction of the liver size with disappointing results. Transcatheter therapies such as TAE are being tried as the cyst is mostly supplied from the hepatic arteries.[27]

Conclusion

With advances in imaging techniques and modalities, interventional radiology is now playing an important role in non-operative management of both primary and secondary liver malignancies through the various interventional therapies described.[2,4]

These therapies have minimal toxicity profiles, effective tumour response while preserving normal hepatic parenchyma, and help to significantly reduce disease progression in liver transplant candidates and prolong survival in non-transplant candidates.[4,13]

Although a definitive treatment is not available and the ideal choice of therapy continues to evolve with refined outcomes on studies and clinical trials (prospective and retrospective) performed, a reasonable selection of available treatment options based on tumour staging, patient age, and comorbidities play a key role in improving therapeutic outcome and overall survival.[11] In selective patient population, these minimally invasive therapies already offer survival rates that are comparable to that of surgery with the added benefits of improved quality of life, shortened recovery time, reduced costs, and lower morbidity.[5]

Knowledge of potential benefits and pitfalls of each therapeutic approach may allow the operator to tailor the therapy on a patient-to-patient basis producing maximum optimal outcomes.[4]

REFERENCES

1. Mohammadian M, Mahdavifar N, Mohammadian-Hafshejani A, Salehiniya H. Liver cancer in the world: epidemiology, incidence, mortality and risk factors. *WCRJ*. 2018;**5**(2):e1082.
2. Edwards M, MD, Padia SA. Locoregional management pathways for liver cancer: a practical approach to treating tumors in the liver caused by primary liver cancer, colorectal cancer, and neuroendocrine tumors. *Endovascular Today*. 2017;**16**(10):93–96.

3. Rawla P, Sunkara T, Muralidharan P, Raj JP. Update in global trends and aetiology of hepatocellular carcinoma. *Contemp Oncol (Pozn)*. 2018;**22**(3):141–150.
4. Shrimal A, Prasanth M, Kulkarni AV. Interventional radiological treatment of hepatocellular carcinoma: an update. *Indian J Surg*. 2012;**74**(1):91–99.
5. Loffroy R, Estivalet L, Favelier S, et al. Interventional radiology therapies for liver cancer. *Hepatoma Res*. 2016;**2**:1–9.
6. Molla N, AlMenieir N, Simoneau E, et al. The role of interventional radiology in the management of hepatocellular carcinoma. *Curr Oncol*. 2014;**21**(3):e480–e492.
7. Lencioni R, Crocetti L. Local-regional treatment of hepatocellular carcinoma. *Radiology*. 2012;**262**(1):43–58.
8. Marrero JA, Kulik LM, Sirlin CB, et al. Diagnosis, staging, and management of hepatocellular carcinoma: 2018 practice guidance by the American Association for the Study of Liver Diseases. *Hepatology*. 2018;**68**(2):723–750.
9. Lungren MP, Towbin AJ, Roebuck DJ, et al. Role of interventional radiology in managing pediatric liver tumors. Part 1: endovascular interventions. *Pediatr Radiol*. 2018;**48**(4):555–564.
10. Tsochatzis EA, Fatourou E, O'Beirne J, Meyer T, Burroughs AK. Transarterial chemoembolization and bland embolization for hepatocellular carcinoma. *World J Gastroenterol*. 2014;**20**(12):3069–3077.
11. Chen X, Liu H-P, Li M, Qiao L. Advances in non-surgical management of primary liver cancer. *World J Gastroenterol*. 2014;**20**(44):16630–16638.
12. Mahnken AH, Pereira PL, de Baère T. Interventional oncologic approaches to liver metastases. *Radiology*. 2013;**266**(2):407–430.
13. Holzwanger DJ, Madoff DC. Role of interventional radiology in the management of hepatocellular carcinoma: current status. *Chin Clin Oncol*. 2018;**7**(5):49.
14. Farrelly C, Ryan M. Advances in interventional radiology in the treatment of primary and metastatic liver cancer. *Eur Oncolog Dis*. 2007;**1**(2):68–72.
15. Yang B, Zou Jinghuai, Xia J, et al. Risk factors for recurrence of small hepatocellular carcinoma after long-term follow-up of percutaneous radiofrequency ablation. *Eur J Radiol*. 2011;**79**(2):196–200.
16. Crocetti L, de Baere T, Lencioni R. Quality improvement guidelines for radiofrequency ablation of liver tumours. *Cardiovasc Interv Radiol*. 2010;**33**(1):11–17.
17. Mu L, Chapiro J, Stringam J, Geschwind J-F. Interventional oncology in hepatocellular carcinoma: progress through innovation. *Cancer J*. 2016;**22**(6):365–372.
18. Aubé C, Bouvier A, Lebigot J, Vervueren L, Cartier V, Oberti F. Radiological treatment of HCC: interventional radiology at the heart of management. *Diagn Interv Imaging*. 2015;**96**(6):625–636.
19. Ikeda K. Recent advances in medical management of hepatocellular carcinoma. *Hepatol Res*. 2019;**49**(1):14–32.
20. Nouri YM, Kim JH, Yoon HK, Ko HK, Shin JH, Gwon DI. Update on transarterial chemoembolization with drug-eluting microspheres for hepatocellular carcinoma. *Korean J Radiol*. 2019;**20**(1):34–49.
21. Shiina S, Tateishi R, Imamura M, et al. Percutaneous ethanol injection for hepatocellular carcinoma: 20-year outcome and prognostic factors. *Liver Int*. 2012;**32**(9):1434–1442.
22. Sun X, Li RU, Zhang B, Yang Y, Cui Z. Treatment of liver cancer of middle and advanced stages using ultrasound-guided percutaneous ethanol injection combined with radiofrequency ablation: a clinical analysis. *Oncol Lett*. 2016;**11**(3):2096–2100.
23. Sindel HT. Hepatic giant hemagiomas; surgery or endovascular treatment? *Clin Surg*. 2017;**2**:1831.
24. Kahriman G, Ozcan N, Dogan S, Karaborklu O. Percutaneous treatment of liver hydatid cysts in 190 patients: a retrospective study. *Acta Radiol*. 2017;**58**(6):676–684.
25. Paksoy Y, Ödev K, Şahin M, Arslan A, Koç O. Percutaneous treatment of liver hydatid cysts: comparison of direct injection of albendazole and hypertonic saline solution. *AJR*. 2005;**185**(3):727–734.
26. Macedo FI. Current management of noninfectious hepatic cystic lesions: a review of the literature. *World J Hepatol*. 2013;**5**(9):462–469.
27. Wang MQ, Duan F, Liu FY, Wang ZJ, Song P. Treatment of symptomatic polycystic liver disease: transcatheter super-selective hepatic arterial embolization using a mixture of NBCA and iodized oil. *Abdom Imaging*. 2013;**38**(3):465–473.

26

Long-term outcomes following liver surgery

Yasuhito Iwao and Nigel D. Heaton

Introduction

The first anatomical liver resection was reported by Carl Langenbuch in 1888 who performed a limited resection of the left lateral segment.[1] The right and left hemi-lobes of the liver were identified by Hugo Rex in 1888[2] and James Cantlie in 1898.[3] The first anatomical right hepatectomy was performed by Ichiro Honjo in 1949[4] and subsequently Jean-Louis Lortat-Jacob in 1951.[5] Initially surgeons struggled with understanding of the liver anatomy, bleeding from the liver parenchyma, and complications such as biliary leak and liver dysfunction or post-resection liver failure. Inflow occlusion of the liver was described by James Pringle in 1908,[6] and used to manage hepatic trauma. The segmental nature of liver anatomy was initially described by Carl-Herman Hjortsjo in 1951[7] and by John E. Healey Jr and Paul C. Schroy in 1953,[8] and subsequently by Claude Couinaud in 1954[9] whose classification has been widely adopted. The first successful liver transplantation was reported by Thomas Starzl in 1967 and further stimulated understanding of haemostasis and specialist perioperative care.[10] The concept of anatomical resection for more limited segment or subsegment resection using intraoperative ultrasound[11] and the use of preoperative portal vein embolization to prevent small-for-size syndrome (SFSS)[12] were introduced by Masatoshi Makuuchi in the 1980s. The understanding of liver anatomy, advances in the use of haemostatic devices or agents, and cumulative experience of vascular reconstruction have led to increasingly advanced and complex liver resections. Laparoscopic major hepatectomy started in 2000[13] and robotic surgery is becoming established. Liver surgery has developed progressively over the last 60 years (summarized in Figure 26.1); however, it is only in the last 30 years that major hepatectomy has become commonplace. Reviewing long-term outcomes after liver surgery, data is available for 5- and 10-year follow-up, but little for 20 years and beyond. It was considered that patients who survived 5 years post hepatectomy free from cancer were 'cured'; however, late recurrence occurs and may be more frequent with the advent of more effective systemic therapies.

Long-term outcomes

The most significant contribution to long-term survival has been the continuous improvement in 30- and 90-day mortality. A number of factors contribute to this including improved pre-and perioperative imaging (early detection and intraoperative ultrasound detection), better patient selection, and improved perioperative management and surgical technique. Other factors associated with outcome include patient age and fitness, health of the liver, extent of liver resection, and the underlying primary cancer stage. Postoperative complications vary according to cancer type, presence of underlying liver disease, and extent of liver resection, and impact 3-month survival and will be discussed briefly. Longer-term survival depends on the tumour biology, progression of underlying liver disease, and late technical complications (nomenclature used for liver resections is the Brisbane 2000 terminology).[14]

Factors influencing early mortality

Patient factors which influence early mortality include age, cardiopulmonary disease, diabetes, obesity, renal insufficiency, malnutrition, viral hepatitis and steatohepatitis, raised serum bilirubin, thrombocytopenia, and cirrhosis. Surgical risk factors for liver surgery include blood loss and transfusion requirement, operative time, vascular resection, extent of resection, and the residual liver volume. Meticulous surgical technique is the key for major or complex resections where residual liver volume may be compromised. Preoperative drainage of obstructed bile ducts, liver volume manipulation, and nutritional support also impact early mortality and morbidity.

Early non-hepatic complications after liver surgery have also improved progressively over time. Enhanced recovery after surgery (ERAS) reduces the incidence of postoperative complications and length of hospital stay, but has no impact on mortality.[15] Liver surgery for elderly patients is not associated with a higher rate of general morbidity below and over 70 years, but is below and over

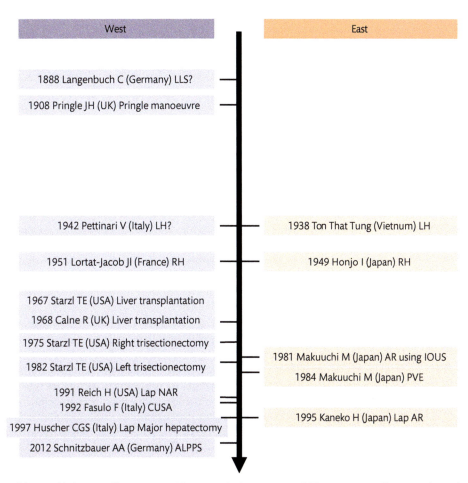

Figure 26.1 The history of the establishment of liver surgery. AR, anatomical resection; ALPPS, association of ligation of portal vein and parenchyma splitting; CUSA, cavitron ultrasonic surgical aspirator; IOUS, intraoperative ultrasonography; Lap, laparoscopic; LH, left hemi-hepatectomy; LLS, left lateral sectionectomy; NAR, non-anatomical resection; PVE, portal vein embolization; RH, right hemi-hepatectomy.

75 years, according to a systematic review and meta-analysis by Van Tuil et al.[16] However, none of the studies have shown any difference in long-term cancer survival between elderly and younger patients in the long term.

Little has been written about the long-term outcomes aside from patient survival. Cancer recurrence is probably the biggest determinant of medium-term survival up to 5 years. Beyond this the presence of underlying liver disease becomes an increasingly important factor impacting medium- to long-term survival. Progressive liver disease may be due to viral hepatitis, alcohol and non-alcoholic hepatitis, autoimmune liver diseases, and other causes of liver cirrhosis. The advent of effective antiviral therapies against hepatitis B or C has had a significant impact on long-term survival. Managing lifestyle health is essential in the management of the majority of causes of liver disease, particularly through diet, obesity, and diabetes and will protect the liver and improve survival outcomes for patients.

Surgical technique

Liver surgery is technically demanding to control bleeding and secure haemostasis, minimize parenchymal devascularization, and avoid vascular injury. Spolverato et al.[17] reported that over the era of 2000–2010 liver surgery in the US in high-volume institutions was associated with a lower risk of mortality due to lower complication rates and also better ability to rescue patients with major complications. The aim is to achieve bloodless surgery. The use of low central venous pressure with fluid restriction and head-up position requires experienced anaesthesiologists. Inflow occlusion with the Pringle manoeuvre is widely used,[6] although concern has been expressed of the potential for ischaemic injury. However, intermittent occlusion for 10 or 15 minutes followed by 5 or 10 minutes of reperfusion seems to avoid significant injury[18] and may be repeated for several cycles without problems. Makuuchi introduced the use of inflow occlusion liver resection in cirrhosis[19] and living donor hepatectomy.[20] Clamping can be extended to 30 minutes without complications as demonstrated by three randomized control trials using healthy candidates.[21–23] Total cumulative warm ischaemia time up to a maximum of 325 minutes has been reported without significant complications.[24] Multiple short duration of ischaemia–reperfusion cycles appear to precondition the liver.[25] There has been no evidence for the development of late cholangiopathy as a complication of inflow occlusion.

In contrast, total hepatic vascular exclusion, which controls both inflow and outflow, has not proved superior to the Pringle manoeuvre in terms of operative time, blood loss, or postoperative hospital stay.[26] The technique should be restricted to cases with a tumour thrombus within the inferior vena cava. Not all patients tolerate total hepatic vascular exclusion, and either infrarenal aortic clamping for up to 30 minutes[27] or venovenous bypass can be utilized in complex cases for restricted periods of time. In terms of long-term outcomes, warm ischaemia of the liver for up to 30 minutes is not regarded as critical because ischaemia–reperfusion injury to hepatocytes is reversible and recovery is rapid. There has been no evidence for the development of late cholangiopathy as a complication of inflow occlusion.

Complications

For good long-term outcomes after liver surgery optimal perioperative management is key to avoiding both liver-specific and general complications.

Small-for-size syndrome

SFSS and early liver failure are the most critical complications of liver surgery and are associated with a mortality of 50%.[28] SFSS is described as a critical shortfall in functioning liver volume and may arise due to multiple factors including preoperative overestimation of the future liver remnant (FLR) due to a background liver injury or disease and vascular complications of venous inflow or outflow.[29,30] Hepatic artery complications are less likely to produce SFSS, but are associated with liver abscess or biliary complications particularly if the common bile duct is divided. The incidence of SFSS and bile leakage in each type of liver resection are summarized in Table 26.1. Biliary non-anastomotic strictures or ischaemic cholangiopathy can occur as a consequence of vascular injury with refractory cholangitis especially when the extrahepatic biliary tree is excised.

Bile leak

Bile leakage is a common and significant morbidity. In the short term, endoscopic or percutaneous stenting may allow the bile leak to settle in the majority of cases. However, bile leak from a divided duct in a functioning liver remnant may persist for several months. An example is division of an unrecognized posterior right hepatic duct draining into the left hepatic duct during left hepatectomy. Various techniques have been used to plug refractory biliary leaks including ethanol ablation and glue.[31] The incidence of major bile leakage was reported as 30.5% in 609 liver resections which were combined with caudate resection and bilioenteric anastomoses. Lo et al. reported an 8.1% bile leak rate after 229 major and 118 minor hepatectomies in a single institution between 1989 and 1995.[32] Bile leak carried a higher risk of liver failure (35.7% vs 6.9%, p <0.001) and operative mortality (39.3% vs 6.0%, p <0.001). Risk factors for bile leak included prolonged operation time and left hepatectomies especially for trisegmentectomy. However, biliary fistulae are seldom a long-term problem except after division of the right posterior sectoral duct draining into the left hepatic duct as described previously which needs surgical reconstruction.

Biliary stricture

Biliary strictures may occur late and present with obstructive jaundice, liver dysfunction with cholestatic liver function tests, or cholangitis. Occasionally biliary obstruction may be due to recurrent tumour. Stones may form as a consequence of stasis related to a stricture or a sump. If a stricture is unrecognized, a later presentation with cholangitis or cholangitic liver abscesses may occur. Late complications are not systematically reported due in part to deaths of patients from cancer recurrence. As the number of long-term survivors increases, it is likely that there will be a small but significant incidence of biliary strictures, casts, and stone formation.

Biliary anastomotic stricture and reflux cholangitis usually occur late in the postoperative period. The frequency of cholangitis after biliary tract reconstruction has been reported at about 10% in the recent era[33] and 3.4% (4/117) by Bismuth et al. in 123 consecutive cases of Roux-en-Y hepaticojejunostomy for benign indications

Table 26.1 Summary of complications in each extent of liver surgery

	Mortality (%)	Small-for-size syndrome (%)	Bile leakage (%)	Others (%)
Left trisectionectomy[117]	9.7	15.0	12.4	–
Right trisectionectomy[119]	0.0	9.0	0.0	–
HPD[121]	9.7	20.7	22.0	POPF: 14.0
RH/Lap RH[123]	3.7/2.6	8.0/5.4	9.7/3.7	–
RH/Lap LH for donation[124]	0.2/0.4	–	1.7/3.3	–
LLS/Lap LLS[127]	–	–	0.0/1.4	DGE: 5.5[39]
LLS/LAP LLS for donation[128]	–	–	0.0/1.4	–
Anatomical resection[79]	1.8	–	1.0	–
Non-anatomical resection[79]	2.3	–	9.0	–
Repeated[63]	1.1	4.4	8.1	–
Two-staged hepatectomy[65]	11.3	2.4	4.3	–
ALPPS[68]	14.5	22	24	–

To simplify numbers, only the maximum incidence rates reported using reasonable population cohort were shown.
ALPPS, association of ligation of portal vein and parenchyma splitting; DGE, delayed gastric empty; HPD, hemi-hepatectomy with pancreaticoduodenectomy; Lap, laparoscopic; LH, left hemi-hepatectomy; LLS, left lateral sectionectomy; POPF, postoperative pancreatic fistula; RH, right hemi-hepatectomy; RT, right trisectionectomy.

between 1968 and 1974.[34] They reported that the prevalence of anastomotic strictures with hepaticojejunostomy was 0.85%.

Biliary strictures are treated using percutaneous transhepatic biliary drainage or double balloon endoscopic approaches. For recurrent strictures surgical reconstruction will be required.

Reflux cholangitis without anastomotic stricture is uncommon and reported as sump syndrome.[35] Marangoni et al. described six cases[36] which were managed by lengthening of the jejunal loop or by the creation of an antireflux valve. Alternatives include the use of probiotics or long-term prophylactic antibiotics.

Biliary non-anastomotic stricture or ischaemic cholangiopathy may occur as a consequence of arterial vascular injury, particularly if the extrahepatic bile duct is divided. If associated with recurrent cholangitis this may be difficult to manage and the patient will become malnourished and frail and die if not controlled.

Broncho-biliary fistula

This is a rare complication of hepatic resection that occurs days to years after surgery as a consequence of bile leak or stricture. Non-surgical interventions with endoscopic retrograde cholangiopancreatography or percutaneous transhepatic cholangiography can be successful if there is a distal stricture. Reoperation tends to be complicated with significant morbidity and mortality.[37]

Delayed gastric emptying

Delayed gastric emptying (DGE) or gastric stasis is most common following left-sided hepatectomy, possibly because the stomach is located next to the cut surface of the liver parenchyma and becomes adherent to it. Symptoms include nausea, vomiting, bloating, and epigastric discomfort and will usually settle without intervention. Patients can acquire DGE after left hepatectomy (25–28%), or left lateral segmentectomy (5.5%) and the likelihood of occurrence depends on the size of the cut surface ($p = 0.04$).[38,39] An incidence of 2% was reported after living donor hepatectomy from a Japanese cohort of 1841 donors.[40] Kim et al. found DGE in 1.2% of 500 living donor hepatectomies including following right liver resections.[41] Other causes of DGE include injury to the anterior branches of the vagus nerve, particularly the nerve of Latarjet which innervates the antrum and pylorus compromising antral contraction and relaxation of the pylorus. The presence of an accessory or replaced left hepatic artery is associated with nerve injury and this complication is presumably due to the greater extent of the dissection. The symptoms usually resolve after 6–8 weeks but occasional cases may persist long term. Endoscopic injection of botulism toxin at the pylorus may help with gastric emptying if symptoms persist. Reports of surgical re-exploration and lysis of adhesions with resolution of symptoms has been reported for stomach adherent to the liver cut surface. Others have described the use of omental flaps to cover the cut surface of the liver to prevent DGE.[38,39]

Diaphragmatic hernia

Acquired diaphragmatic hernias (DHs) are usually due to trauma. The incidence after liver surgery ranges from 0.6% to 6.2%. The incidence after living donor hepatectomy is 0.6–2.3% and 1.1–6.2% after resection for liver tumours.[42] They appear to be more common after right hepatectomy than left hepatectomy. Patients presenting with a combination of chest and abdominal symptoms should be suspected of having a DH and investigated urgently with chest X-ray and computed tomography scan. Esposito et al. found DHs in 2.3% of patients undergoing major hepatectomy for liver tumours presenting at a median of 14 months (4–31 months) post surgery.[43] The colon was the most commonly herniated bowel in 43% of cases. DHs were repaired as an emergency in 43% and bowel resection was performed in 28% of cases. DHs should be repaired as a semi-emergency even in asymptomatic cases to avoid bowel loss. The majority of cases occur on the right associated with the bare area herniating posteriorly into the chest and can be sutured directly. Approximately 20% require mesh to achieve secure closure and recurrence has been reported in 4%. Esposito et al. reviewed 28 patients described in the literature with 17 following liver resection for tumour and 11 after living donation at a mean of 19 months after surgery. One death occurred following perforation of the small bowel 3 months after surgery.[43] Potential risk factors for DH include resection for large tumours which stretch and weaken the diaphragm, direct injury during mobilization, and right phrenic injury isolating the right hepatic vein and suprahepatic inferior vena cava. It was most common after right hepatectomy presumably because of the space post resection with an incidence of 2.7%. It has also been reported in children after liver surgery and left lateral segment liver transplantation with an incidence of 2.8%.[44] Risk factors in children included left lateral segment graft, large-for-size grafts, ascites or postoperative ileus, delayed healing related to immunosuppression, and poor muscle mass related to malnutrition.[44] DH represents a significant late complication after right hepatectomy (for cancer and living donation) and when identified should be treated urgently to avoid major bowel loss.

Adhesions and small bowel obstruction

As the liver is located in the upper abdomen, small bowel obstruction is uncommon after liver surgery. The reported incidence is less than 1%. Pedersen et al. compared the incidence of small bowel obstruction after 79 laparoscopic and 208 open hepatectomies.[45] There were no cases of small bowel obstruction after laparoscopic compared to 3.3% after open surgery with 1.9% undergoing surgical intervention.

A rare form of bowel obstruction first reported by Chilaiditi in 1910[46] of hepato-diaphragmatic interposition of bowel has been described after right hepatectomy. The incidence of this syndrome has been estimated at 0.025–0.28% of the general population.

The addition of a Roux loop for biliary drainage may be associated long term with the risk of intussusception which usually occurs at the site of the jejunojejunostomy. It may be associated with underlying motility disorders. The incidence was 0.4% in a series of 2395 laparoscopic Roux en Y gastric bypasses performed in a single institution.[47] Patients present with abdominal colic and features of cholangitis or low-grade liver dysfunction and the abnormality is usually seen on computed tomography scanning. Surgical revision will resolve the problem unless there is a significant underlying motility disorder. Internal hernias may occur through the mesenteric defect if not closed at surgery or if sutures do not hold. Patients present with recurrent colicky pain and vomiting with low-grade liver dysfunction and surgical correction is always required.

Incisional hernia

Incisional ventral hernias are a common complication of abdominal surgery often requiring operative repair and are a cause of significant morbidity and financial cost. The incidence is lower after laparoscopic

(4.3%) compared to open liver surgery (10.1%).[48] In a study of 327 patients undergoing right hepatectomy, two groups of 118 patients undergoing open and 113 laparoscopic right hepatectomies were reviewed for incisional hernia.[49] The median time to hernia development was 40 months with open surgery having an incidence of incisional hernia of 11.5% versus 2.7% for laparoscopic surgery. The cost of repair differed significantly depending on incision type with Chevron the most expensive ($41,463 ± $5234) followed by midline ($15,729 ± $13,204) and subcostal ($7677 ± $1861). Risk factors for incisional hernias included male sex, body mass index (BMI) of at least 30 kg/m^2, and previous abdominal surgery. Hernia repair after open surgery was associated with a longer hospital stay, more complications, higher recurrence rates, and greater cost (threefold). Wabitsch et al. reported incisional hernia in 12% of 49 patients at a median of 26 months after laparoscopic liver resection.[50] Risk factors identified included umbilical site, poor performance status, and obesity with BMI greater than 25 kg/m^2. Kayashima et al. found incisional hernias in 31% of 192 patients after open hepatectomy for hepatocellular carcinoma (HCC) rising from 19.8% at 1 year to 38.8% at 5 years.[51] Multivariate analysis showed postoperative ascites, single layer mass closure with a running suture, and BMI greater than 25 kg/m^2. Nilsson et al. reviewed 256 patients undergoing liver resection for colorectal carcinoma liver metastases using computed tomography to identify incisional hernias.[52] The incidence was 30.5% although the majority were smaller than 1 cm and were most common in the midline part of the scar (85%) after a follow-up period of 13 months. Risk factors identified included preoperative chemotherapy of more than six cycles or bevacizumab, a monoclonal anti-vascular endothelial growth factor antibody with potential to impair wound healing and prior incisional hernia.

Evaluating quality of life after laparoscopic or open liver surgery in a randomized controlled trial, some aspects of quality of life were reduced 1 month after surgery in both arms. However, all aspects of quality of life had returned to preoperative levels 4 months after laparoscopic resections, in contrast to open surgery where recovery took much longer.[53]

Colorectal liver secondaries

This is the most common indication for liver resection in the West. Wagner et al. described the natural history in 252 patients with biopsy-proven colorectal liver secondaries (CRLS) and primary tumour resected between 1943 and 1976.[54] Thirty-nine had solitary and 31 patients had multiple lesions which could potentially have been resected. Median survival of those with solitary and multiple resectable lesions were 21 and 15 months, respectively. This was compared to the 5-year overall survival (OS) after hepatectomy for CRLS of 25% for 141 patients between 1948 and 1982. Stangl et al. analysed the OS of 484 patients who had palliative treatment for unresectable CRLS between 1980 and 1990.[55] Median OS was 7.5 months and 1-, 3-, and 5-year OSs were 31.3%, 2.6%, and 0.9%, respectively. The advent of systemic chemotherapy for unresectable metastatic colorectal carcinoma in the early 2000s achieved a median OS of 12 to 20 months.[56] Choti et al. reported a single institution experience from 1984–1999 of 226 patients who underwent 'curative' liver resection for CRLS.[57] The 5-year OS rose from era 1 (1984–1992) to era 2 (1993–1999) from 26% to 40%, in association with the use of systemic chemotherapy. Disease-free survival (DFS) improved concomitantly. Independent predictors of survival included the number of tumours less than three, clear resection margin, and a carcinoembryonic antigen (CEA) level less than 100 ng/mL. Over this time, postoperative length of stay (13 days vs 7 days), blood transfusion requirements (2.2 units per patient vs 1.0 unit per patient), morbidity (13% vs 23%), and mortality (2.2% vs 0%) have improved with changes to resection type (anatomical/non-anatomical, 62%/38% vs 80%/20%, respectively), use of intraoperative ultrasound (38% vs 79%), neoadjuvant chemotherapy (38% vs 62%), and improved preoperative imaging. The advent of neoadjuvant chemotherapy for the majority of patients led to parenchymal-sparing hepatectomy being considered more routinely. Hosokawa et al. compared outcomes between parenchyma-preserving hepatectomy and right hepatectomy for solitary small (<30 mm) CRLS using a multicentre cohort of 1720 patients between 2000 and 2015.[58] Parenchymal-sparing strategies were associated with lower rates of major complications (3% vs 10%) and 90-day mortality (1% vs 3%), with similar recurrence rates (36% vs 35%), and 5-year OS (63 vs 62%) and DFS (43 vs 41%). For patients with liver-only recurrence after resection, prior parenchymal-sparing hepatectomy allowed more patients to undergo repeat hepatectomy (67 vs 31%) and achieve higher 5-year OS (55 vs 23%). Fong et al. reported 10-year OS of 22% in a single-centre cohort of 1001 consecutive patients between 1985 and 1998.[59] Mortality within 30 days of hepatectomy was 2.8%. Risk factors for recurrent disease included lymph node positivity in the primary site, disease-free interval less than 12 months, multiple hepatic lesions, lesion more than 50 mm in size, and CEA greater than 200 ng/mL. Creasy et al. reported actual 10-year OS after liver resection of 24.4% in a cohort of 1211 patients with CRLS between 1992 and 2004 after excluding 90-day mortality (n = 35, 2.9%).[60] Of these, approximately one-quarter had undergone a further procedure for either intra- or extrahepatic recurrence. Factors associated with disease recurrence changed over time to include the presence of extrahepatic disease, positive resection margins, more than ten liver secondaries, and CEA level of greater than 200 ng/mL. To maximize benefits from surgery for CRLS, van Dam et al. proposed an expansion of the indications including number of tumours greater than four, bi-lobar disease, resectable extrahepatic lesions, and lesser surgical margin resections and reported 5-year OS of 33.2% in 129 patients with extended indications (1991–2010).[61] Subsequently, Allard et al. reported 5-year OS of 39% for 529 out of 12,406 patients (2005–2013) with expanded resection criteria with no limitation on size or number, unless a positive surgical margin was expected.[62]

Repeat hepatectomy is being increasingly performed in long-term survivors. Often patients have received multimodal therapies, in addition to surgery, which can make identification of anatomical landmarks difficult due to distortion difficulty of this procedure which is a result of the regeneration and hypertrophy of the residual liver. A systematic review and meta-analysis of repeat hepatectomy for CRLS showed that OS and mortality were not significantly different from first hepatectomy (hazard ratio (HR) 1.00 and p = 0.99, and odds ratio (OR) 1.13 and p = 0.79, respectively).[63] However, SFSS and bile leakage with fistula were more common, but without reaching statistical significance (OR 1.46 and p = 0.32, and OR 1.22 and p = 0.35, respectively). Wicherts et al. compared short-term outcomes between first, second, third, and fourth hepatectomy using a single-centre cohort of 1036 patients who underwent 1454 hepatectomy from 1990 to 2010.[64] They did not show increased mortality or morbidity up to the third hepatectomy. Long-term complications were not reported.

Two-stage hepatectomy (TSH) is utilized for patients with multiple tumours to try to achieve R0 resection while maintaining an adequate FLR. Regimbeau et al. reported outcomes after TSH in 869 patients out of 6655 patients with CRLS resected between 2000 and 2014.[65] Five-year OS and DFS on an intention-to-treat basis were found to be comparable to those after single hepatectomy (21.4% vs 32.4% and $p = 0.002$, and 21.6% vs 29.8% and $p = 0.39$, respectively). In a comparison between intended TSH and single hepatectomy, major complications were not significantly different (26.2% vs 24.1%, respectively, $p = 0.12$). More recent laparoscopic experience reported by Okumura et al. showed a favourable outcome of laparoscopic TSH in a study of 38 versus 48 (open surgery) patients between 2007 and 2017.[66] According to their propensity score matching study, there was no significant difference with regard to long-term survival or postoperative morbidity between laparoscopic and open approach although the groups were small.

Cumulative experience of TSH inspired the association of ligation of portal vein and parenchyma splitting (ALPPS) approach to try to perform curative surgery while maintaining patient safety.[67] While liver resections associated with portal vein embolization are reported to be safe outcome as regard with lesser complications, ALPPS appears to have relatively higher morbidity and mortality (73% vs 59% and $p = 0.16$, and 14% vs 7% and $p = 0.19$, respectively), despite greater hypertrophy of FLR in a meta-analysis of ALPPS.[68]

CRLS is potentially curable by liver surgery even with stage IV disease. The 5-year OS is a median 38% (16–71%), in a meta-analysis of patients treated in the late 1990s. Even with initially unresectable CRLS, 5-year OS of 33–50% can be achieved,[69] with modern systemic therapy. The roles of neoadjuvant or adjuvant therapy, the timing of surgery after systemic therapy, the role of surgery in the presence of extrahepatic diseases, and the potential place of liver transplantation for CRLS are evolving. Selected reports of long-term outcome after liver resection for CRLS are summarized in Table 26.2.

Hepatocellular carcinoma

In the East, liver resection for HCC has historically been more common than in the West, because of the prevalence of viral hepatitis and the relative lack of access to liver transplantation. Outcomes have continued to improve over time particularly with the advent of effective antiviral therapy. A large retrospective multicentre European study (all centres performed >50 resections) of 1467 patients from 1974 to 1999 reported a 30-day mortality of 10.6%[70] related to the aetiology and severity of liver disease, extent of resection, and study period. As with other cancers the authors concluded that early detection due to improvements in screening at-risk populations, preoperative imaging, patient selection, perioperative management, and surgical technique improved 5-year OS from 20% to 51% and DFS from 20% to 33%. A systematic review found actual 10-year OS of 7.2% following HCC resection from publications between 1987 and 2009.[71] Zheng et al. reported improved 90-day mortality of 6.1% after liver resection for HCC from a single institution of 212 consecutive patients between 1992 and 2006 in the US[72] with a 10-year survival of 23.6%.

There is a discrepancy in the outcomes of liver resection for HCC between the East and West.[73] Yang et al. considered surveillance and early-stage identification of HCC as a key factor. A Japanese nationwide study showed superior outcomes of liver resection for HCC with a 30-day surgical mortality of 1.6% between 2002 and 2003[74] and 0.9% between 2008 and 2009.[75] Other factors contributing to these results included patient selection, aetiology of underlying liver disease (particularly hepatitis B), and institutional guidelines, such as the Makuuchi criteria,[76] using indocyanine green testing.[77]

Improved long-term outcomes after liver resection for HCC in Japan can be observed for each stage of HCC. Results are shown in Table 26.3 of a Japanese cohort treated by liver resection between 1996 and 2007[75] and compared to a database representing

Table 26.2 Summary of survivals after liver surgery for liver secondaries

		3-year OS (%)	5-year OS (%)	10-year OS (%)	Median OS (months)	Median DFS (months)
CRLS	Resectable[69]	64.5	46	27.2	44	7.9
	Unresectable[69]	43.0	32	19.6	32	–
NELS	Resectable[105]		74	51	119	54
	Unresectable[105]		46	6	57	–
NCNNLS[106]		57	42	28[110]	49	21
Breast[106]		56	37	22[108]	36	22
Pancreatic[110]		40	31	18	26	
Gastric[110]		44	32	25	30	
Sarcoma[112]		68.2	58.1	35.2	725	31
GIST[110]		86	72	40	100	

To simplify numbers, only the maximum survivals reported using reasonable population cohort were shown. Some survival rates in *italic* were estimated from Kaplan–Meier curves provided in the articles by the author.
CRLS, colorectal liver secondaries; DFS, disease-free survival; GIST, gastrointestinal stromal tumours; NELS, neuroendocrine liver secondaries; NCNNLS, non-colorectal and non-neuroendocrine liver secondaries; OS, overall survival.

Table 26.3 Comparison of survival rates after liver surgery for each stage of hepatocellular carcinoma between Japan and the US

	UICC 8th	1-year OS	3-year OS	5-year OS	10-year OS	LCSGJ 6th
HCC		97.2%	90.0%	79.3%	51.0%	Stage I[88]
	Stage IA[91]	92.6%	82.4%	75.0%	–	
	Stage IB[91]	89.7%	75.0%	64.7%	–	
		94.9%	82.5%	70.5%	47.4%	Stage II[88]
	Stage II[91]	86.8%	70.6%	61.8%	–	
		87.2%	d67.3%	53.1%	30.9%	Stage III[88]
	Stage IIIA[91]	75.0%	48.5%	36.8%	–	
	Stage IIIB[91]					
		76.0%	48.6%	33.9%	–	Ruptured[96]
		63.2%	33.1%	–	–	IVCTT[98]
		56.8%	33.1%	24.9%	19.9%	PVTT[88]
		68.7%	42.2%	31.4%	18.9%	Stage IVA[88]
	Stage IVA[91]	64.7%	39.7%	30.9%	–	
	Stage IVB[91]					
		57.1%	31.7%	25.8%	19.3%	Stage IVB[88]

The survival rates from Japan were calculated based on the nationwide report published by the LCSGJ, whereas the survivals from the US included patients undergoing either resection or liver transplantation.[64] These survival rates in *italic* were estimated from Kaplan-Meier curves provided in the articles by the author.
IVCTT, inferior vena cava tumour thrombus; LCSGJ, the Liver Cancer Study Group of Japan; OS, overall survival; PVTT, portal vein tumour thrombus; UICC, Union for International Cancer Control.
Sources: data from Wicherts DA, de Haas RJ, Salloum C, et al. Repeat hepatectomy for recurrent colorectal metastases. *Br J Surg.* 2013;100:808–819; and Schnitzbauer AA, Lang SA, Goessmann H, et al. Right portal vein ligation combined with in situ splitting induces rapid left lateral liver lobe hypertrophy enabling 2-staged extended right hepatic resection in small-for-size settings. *Ann Surg.* 2012;255:405–414.

around 30% of the US population treated by either surgery (63%) or liver transplantation (37%) for HCC from 1998 to 2013. The Japanese cohort demonstrated better long-term outcome for early stage of HCC in comparison with the cohort from the US.[78] The difference in long-term outcome may be due to the preference for small anatomical rather than non-anatomical resections. Survival benefit with anatomical resection is probably due to the transportal spread of HCC[79,80] with 5-year OS and DFS compared to non-anatomical resection of 69% versus 56% and p = 0.018, and 38% vs 23% and p <0.001, respectively, from a meta-analysis (2001–2010).[79] All publications were retrospective and selection bias may have been present. In addition, patients undergoing non-anatomical resection usually have more severe background liver disease than those undergoing anatomical resection.[79,80] Of note, survival benefits from repeated liver resections for HCC were significantly inferior to those of salvage liver transplantation in a systematic review and meta-analysis.[81]

Other challenges include surgery for bleeding from ruptured HCC with a reported in-hospital mortality ranging from 25% to 100%.[82] These patients are more likely to present with liver dysfunction (12–42%) with an OS of 41.4%, 21.1%, and 13.3% at 1 year, 3 years, and 5 years, respectively.[83] Ruptured HCC treated by liver resection has a 1-year and 5-year OS of 76.0% and 33.9%, respectively. Macroscopic tumour thrombus in the hepatic or portal vein has been associated with poor prognosis. OS after hepatectomy for HCC with tumour thrombus in the main branch of portal vein was reported at 59.8% and 25% at 1 year and 5 years respectively.[75] Even if tumour thrombus reaches the inferior vena cava, 1-year and 3-year OS after liver resection are reported to be 63.2% and 33.1%, respectively.[84]

Prediction of prognosis of HCC has to combine both tumour stage and liver function. TNM staging remains of limited value,[85] other clinical scoring systems, such as the Okuda system in 1985,[86] the Cancer of the Liver Italian Program (CLIP) score in 1998,[87,88] Barcelona Clinic Liver Cancer (BCLC) systems in 1999,[89] and the albumin-bilirubin (ALBI) grade in 2015,[90] have been developed to try to guide treatment. Many validation studies for these prognostic scoring systems, and long-term survivals on each stage of each system are reported in the literature. In general, 5-year OS after liver resections for HCC without portal hypertension or hyperbilirubinaemia can be as high as 70%, while those after liver transplantation within Milan criteria are more than 70%.[91] HCC is invariably associated with chronic liver disease including hepatitis B and C, alcohol-related, steatohepatitis, autoimmune, and vascular aetiologies. The risk of further tumour in the residual liver is a long-term risk and provides a rationale for primary and salvage liver transplantation.

Intrahepatic cholangiocellular carcinoma

Intrahepatic cholangiocellular carcinoma (ICC) accounts for 5% of primary liver malignancy and comparable outcomes after liver surgery have not been reported. Five-year OS of 30.6% from the US was reported in a cohort of 1008 patients with HCC between 1998 and 2013[92] and 28.9% from a Japanese national cohort of 4436 patients from 1998 to 2009.[75] No difference was noted for each stage

Table 26.4 Comparison of survival rates of each stage of intrahepatic cholangiocellular carcinoma after liversurgery between Japan and the US

	UICC 8th	1-year OS	3-year OS	5-year OS	10-year OS	LCSGJ 6th
ICC		91.4 %	73.0 %	63.4 %	50.9 %	< 2cm[88]
	Stage IA[110]	87.3 %	69.1 %	60.0 %	-	
	Stage IB[110]	89.1 %	61.8 %	43.6 %	-	
		84.3 %	60.3 %	45.9 %	33.2 %	2 <, < 5 cm[88]
	Stage II[110]	81.8 %	50.9 %	32.7 %	-	
		67.2 %	40.5 %	31.0 %	19.9 %	> 5 cm[88]
		64.6 %	29.1 %	19.5 %	12.5 %	Multiple[88]
	Stage IIIA[110]	69.1 %	30.9 %	-	-	
	Stage IIIB[110]	65.5 %	23.6 %	12.7 %	-	
		61.2 %	30.6 %	19.4 %	0.0 %	N1[88]
		-	-	-	-	M1[88]
	Stage IV[110]	41.8 %	14.5 %	-	-	

These survival rates in *italic* were estimated from Kaplan–Meier curves provided in the articles by the author.
LCSGJ, the Liver Cancer Study Group of Japan; OS, overall survival; UICC, Union for International Cancer Control.
Sources: data from Wicherts DA, de Haas RJ, Salloum C, et al. Repeat hepatectomy for recurrent colorectal metastases. *Br J Surg.* 2013;100:808–819; and Kostakis ID, Machairas N, Prodromidou A, et al. Comparison between salvage liver transplantation and repeat liver resection for recurrent hepatocellular carcinoma: a systematic review and meta-analysis. *Transplant Proc.* 2019;51:433–436.

of disease between US and Japanese outcomes as shown[75,92] in Table 26.4. The morphological appearance of ICC was a survival factor in the Japanese cohort[93] which identified three variants including mass forming, periductal-infiltrating, and intraductal growth types. The 5-year survival based on histology was reported as 39% for the mass forming type, 69% for the intraductal growth type, and the poor prognosis of the periductal-infiltrating type.[94] Cholangiocellular carcinoma is also a newly defined biliary neoplasm with a gene expression profile suggesting it is a distinct biliary-derived entity,[95] with a 5-year survival rate of 75% in 29 patients after curative surgery.[96] ICC recurrence after surgery is reported as survival factor[97] and may be due to a multicentric carcinogenesis. Bagante et al. reported 10-year OS of 20.3% in an international study of 679 patients with ICC resected between 1990 and 2015.[98] Sahara et al. suggested a role for lymphadenectomy during liver resection for ICC, but this has not been accepted as definitely improving long-term outcome.[99]

Other liver secondaries

The management and prognosis of neuroendocrine tumour with liver secondaries (NETLS)[100] depends on the primary site of the neuroendocrine tumour,[101] its proliferation index, and hormonal profile. Surgery is indicated to debulk tumour volume and to control 'hormonal' symptoms.[102] Fairweather et al. reported 5-year and 10-year OS after liver resection for NETLS of 90% and 70%, respectively, in a single institutional cohort of 649 patients between 2003 and 2010.[103] Ruzzenente et al. reported better 10-year OS for G1–G2 compared to G3 of 58.8% versus 21.1%, respectively (p <0.001) in a Italian multicentre study of 238 patients (1990–2014).[104] Multiple other therapies have been utilized to manage NETLS. Surgery to resect the neuroendocrine tumour primary in patients with unresectable NETLS appears to improve OS based on a systematic review and meta-analysis.[105]

Whether non-colorectal and non-neuroendocrine tumour liver secondaries benefit from liver resection remains controversial.

The heterogeneity of the primary and the limited number of cases means that assessment of tumour biological behaviour has to be individualized. OS for this mixed population following liver resection at 3 and 5 years of 34–57% and 19–42%, respectively have been reported.[106]

Long-term outcomes in 73 patients after surgical resection for gastric cancer liver metastases (32 synchronous) were reported by Takemura et al.[107] The 1-, 3-, and 5-year survival was 84%, 50%, and 37%. Multivariate analysis identified serosal invasion by the primary and liver metastasis greater than 5 cm were associated with poor prognosis.

Breast cancer liver secondaries (BCLS) have become a more common indication for surgery with a reported OS of 49–68% at 3 years and 27–53% at 5 years.[106] Adam et al. found 5-year and 10-year OS of 41% and 22%, respectively, in a French multicentre review of 460 patients from 1983 and 2004.[108] Ruiz et al. compared outcomes between combinations of surgery and systemic therapies in 139 patients with BCLS from a single centre by propensity score matching test.[109] The conclusion was that liver resection for BCLS improved OS in selected cases. Sano et al. reported that OS and DFS were 41% and 21% at 5 years, and 28% and 15% at 10 years, respectively, in a multi-institutional Japanese cohort from 2001 to 2010.[110]

The indications for surgery of BCLS are poorly defined but patients with significant bony disease and those lacking disease control with systemic therapies are unlikely to benefit in the long term from surgery.[111] The long-term outcomes of liver resection for the most common liver metastases are summarized in Table 26.2, with another publication for non-colorectal and non-neuroendocrine tumour liver secondaries cited additionally.[112]

Benign or low-grade malignancies

Hepatocellular adenomatosis is characterized by the presence of more than ten hepatocellular adenomas. The median age at diagnosis is 39 years, and 94% have a history of oral contraceptive pill use. A germline *HNF1A* mutation should be excluded. Malignant transformation has been reported in 3% and tumour bleeding in 15% (usually the presenting problem). Five-year complication-free survival was reported at 87.5% by Barbier et al. reporting a single institutional cohort of 40 patients between 1991 and 2015.[113]

Hepatic angiomyolipoma is rarely characterized by malignancy with only 2.2% (2/92 cases) presenting with tumour recurrence after liver resection reported from a single centre from 2009 to 2016.[114] No tumour-related deaths have been reported. Symptomatic giant hepatic haemangiomas rarely cause problems such as haemorrhage or rupture, and are associated with the Kasabach–Merritt syndrome. Major complications and mortality were reported in 17.4% and 0.0%, respectively, by Qiu et al. in 730 patients with hepatic haemangioma removed surgically in one institution.[115] Liver cyst fenestration can be performed for symptomatic liver cystic lesions, and a laparoscopic approach has become the commonest form of surgery. Efficacy of this procedure has been reported at 90.2% (confidence interval (CI) 84.3–94.0%), with symptomatic recurrence of 9.6% (CI 6.9–12.8%) after a mean of 16.1 months, in a systematic review and meta-analysis.[116] Complications after fenestration were reported to be 10.8% (CI 8.1–13.9%), with 3.3% (CI 2.1–4.7%) being major, with a 1.0% (CI 0.5–1.6%) mortality.

Complications associated with types of liver resections

(The incidences of mortality and morbidities for each liver resection are summarized in Table 26.1.)

Extended liver resections

Left trisectionectomy is recognized as one of the more difficult liver resections and is associated with a high incidence of postoperative morbidity. Variations in outcomes in terms of morbidity and mortality have been reported, with 46.0% of morbidity and 9.7% of mortality in a single institution from the West,[117] and to 59.3% of morbidity and 1.2% mortality from Japan.[118] This resection leaves a small FLR, and preoperative optimization of the functional FLR and preoperative biliary drainage are key to low perioperative mortality. The use of portal vein embolization and hepatic vein occlusion has been shown to be associated with a significant increase in the FLR. Late portal vein stenosis or occlusion is a reported complication presenting with signs of portal hypertension and splenomegaly. The platelet count will be low but liver function tests will be relatively unaffected. Radiological intervention is with dilatation of the stenosis and, if required, stenting. Complete occlusion can be managed surgically with transposition of the proximal portal vein into the left portal vein within the Rex recess.

Right trisectionectomy is the most extreme liver resection and the indications remain limited.[119, 120] No significant difference has reported in mortality or major morbidity rate in these two procedures.[118] Extended hemi-hepatectomy combined with pancreaticoduodenectomy has been performed in patients with bile duct cancer with potentially curative resections. The morbidity and mortality have been reported to be 87.5% and 18.2% from the West[121] and 77.6% and 2.4% from Japan,[122] respectively.

Hemi-hepatectomies

Right hepatectomy is regarded as a technical gateway of major liver resection for the open approach in Japan, while laparoscopic right hepatectomy has not as yet been accepted as a routine procedure for hepatopancreatobiliary surgeons worldwide. Laparoscopic right hepatectomy done by laparoscopic experts was associated with significantly fewer complications than open surgery (Comprehensive Complications Index (CCI) 0.63 vs 4.42, respectively; p = 0.03).[123] In contrast, laparoscopic right hepatectomy for living donors did not demonstrate a statistically significant difference in the incidence of major complications (9.4% vs 15.1%, respectively; p = 0.36).[124] The incidence of major complications and CCI following laparoscopic and open left hepatectomy were 8.7% versus 12.2% and 10.6% versus 17.2% (p = 0.044 and 0.002, respectively).[125] For living donor resection, laparoscopic and open left hepatectomy had similar complication rates (1.7 vs 3.3%, respectively, p = 0.15).[126]

Left lateral sectionectomy is the simplest anatomical liver resection due to the thin and flat cut surface resulting from this hepatectomy. Surgery is invariably performed laparoscopically with a low incidence of complications except for DGE. No significant difference in outcome has been reported between laparoscopic and open left lateral sectionectomy with regard to major complications at 9.1% versus 7.6%, respectively,[127] or with regard to living donor hepatectomy at 1.4% versus 0.0%, respectively.[128]

Ex vivo liver resection and autotransplantation

This resection is performed in very few patients with unresectable tumours fit for surgery. R0 resection are reported in 60–90% of cases but outcomes are less satisfactory due to the high complications rate of about 25% and low survival at 3 years and beyond.[129]

REFERENCES

1. Langenbusch C. Ein fall von resection eines linksseitigen schnurlappens der leber. *Berl Kiln Wschr (Germany)*. 1888;**25**:37.
2. Rex H. Beitrage zur morphologie der saugerleber. *Morphol Jahrb*. 1888;**14**:517–616.
3. Cantlie J. On a new arrangement of the right and left lobes of the liver. *J Anat Physiol*. 1898;**32**:4–10.
4. Honjo I. [Subtotal resection of the right lobe of the liver] (in Japanese). *Syujutsu*. 1950;**4**:345–349.
5. Lortat-Jacob JL, Robert HG. Hepatectomie droite reglee. *Presse Med (French)*. 1952;**60**:549–551.
6. Pringle JH. Notes on the arrest of hepatic haemorrhage due to trauma. *Ann Surg*. 1908;**48**(4):541–549.
7. Hjortsjo CH. The topography of the intrahepatic duct systems. *Act Anat (Basel)*. 1951;**11**(4):599–615.
8. Healey JE Jr, Schroy PC. Anatomy of the biliary ducts within the human liver: analysis of the prevailing pattern of branches and the major variations of the biliary ducts. *Arch Surg*. 1953;**66**(5):599–616.
9. Couinaud C. Anatomic principles of left and right regulated hepatectomy: technics (in French). *Chir*. 1954;**70**(12):933–966.
10. Starzl TE, Groth CG, Brettschneider L, et al. Orthotopic homotransplantations of the human liver. *Ann Surg*. 1968;**168**(3):392–415.
11. Makuuchi M, Hasegawa H, Yamazaki S. Intraoperative ultrasonic examination for hepatectomy. *Jpn J Clin Oncol*. 1981;**11**:367–390.

12. Makuuchi M, Takayasu K, Takuma T, et al. Preoperative transcatheter embolization of the portal vein branch for patients receiving extended lobectomy due to the bile duct carcinoma (in Japanese). *Nihon Rinsyogeka Igakukaishi*. 1984;**45**:1558–1564.
13. Huscher CG, Lirici MM. Current position of advanced laparoscopic surgery of the liver. *J R Coll Surg Edinb*. 1997;**42**(4):219–225.
14. Terminology Committee of the International Hepato-Pancreato-Biliary Association. The Brisbane 2000 terminology of liver anatomy and resections. *HPB (Oxford)*. 2000;**2**(3):333–339.
15. Brustia R, Slim K, Scatton O. Enhanced recovery after liver surgery. *J Visceral Surg*. 2019;**156**:127–137.
16. van Tuil T, Dhaif AA, te Riele WW, van Ramshorst B, van Santvoort HC. Systemic review and meta-analysis of liver resection for colorectal metastases in elderly patients. *Dig Surg*. 2019;**36**(2):111–123.
17. Spolverato G, Ejaz A, Hyder O, Kim Y, Pawlik TM. Failure to rescue as a source of variation in hospital mortality after hepatic surgery. *Br J Surg*. 2014;**101**(7):836–846.
18. Gurusmy KS, Kumar Y, Pamecha V, Sharma D, Davidson BR. Ischaemic preconditioning for elective liver resections performed under vascular occlusion. *Cochrane DB Syst Rev*. 2009;21:CD007629.
19. Makuuchi M, Mori T, Gunven P, Yamazaki S, Hasegawa H. Safety of hemihepatic vascular occlusion during resection of the liver. *Surg Gynecol Obstet*. 1987;**164**(2):155–158.
20. Imamura H, Takayama T, Sugawara Y, et al. Pringle's manoeuvre in living donors. *Lancet*. 2002;**360**(9350):2049–2050.
21. Esaki M, Sano T, Shimada K, et al. Randomized clinical trial of hepatectomy using intermittent pedicle occlusion with ischaemic intervals of 15 versus 30 minutes. *Br J Surg*. 2006;**93**(8):944–951.
22. Kim YI, Fujita S, Hwang YJ, Chun JM, Song KE, Chun BY. Successful intermittent application of the Pringle maneuver for 30 minutes during human hepatectomy: a clinical randomized study with use of a protease inhibitor. *Hepatogastroenterology*. 2007;**54**(79):2055–2060.
23. van den Broek MAJ, Bloemen JG, Dello SAWG, van de Poll MCG, Olde Damink SWM, Dejong CHC. Randomized controlled trial analyzing the effect of 15 or 30 min intermittent Pringle maneuver on hepatocellular damage during liver surgery. *J Hepatol*. 2011;**55**(2):337–345.
24. Ishizaki Y, Yoshimoto J, Miwa K, Sugo H, Kawasaki S. Safety of prolonged intermittent Pringle maneuver during hepatic resection. *Arch Surg*. 2006;**141**(7):649–653.
25. Lloris-Carsi JM, Cejalvo D, Toledo-Pereyra LH, Calvo MA, Suzuki S. Preconditioning: effect upon lesion modulation in warm liver ischemia. *Transplant Proc*. 1993;**25**(6):3303–3304.
26. Belghiti J, Noun R, Zante E, Ballet T, Sauvanet A. Portal triad clamping or hepatic vascular exclusion for major liver resection—a controlled study. *Ann Surg*. 1996;**224**(2):155–161.
27. Svensson LG, Crawford ES, Hess KR, Coselli JS, Safi HJ. Experience with 1509 patients undergoing thoracoabdominal aortic operations. *J Vasc Surg*. 1993;**17**(2):357–370.
28. Tucker ON, Heaton N. The 'small for size' liver syndrome. *Curr Opin Crit Care*. 2005;**11**(2):150–155.
29. Balzan S, Belghiti J, Farges O, et al. The '50-50 criteria' on postoperative day 5—an accurate predictor of liver failure and death after hepatectomy. *Ann Surg*. 2005;**242**(2):824–829.
30. Rahbari NN, Garden OJ, Padbury R, et al. Posthepatectomy liver failure: a definition and grading by the International Study Group of Liver Surgery (ISGLS). *Surgery*. 2011;**149**(5):713–724.
31. Ito A, Ebata T, Yokoyama Y, et al. Ethanol ablation for refractory bile leakage after complex hepatectomy. *Br J Surg*. 2018;**105**(8):1036–1043.
32. Lo CM, Fan ST, Lim CN, et al. Biliary complications after hepatic resection: risk factors, management and outcome. *Arch Surg*. 1998;**133**(2):156.
33. Higuchi R, Takada T, Strasberg SM, et al. TG13 miscellaneous etiology of cholangitis and cholecystitis. *J Hepatobiliary Pancreat Sci*. 2013;**20**(1):97–105.
34. Bismuth H, Franco D, Corlette MB, Hepp J, et al. Longterm results of Roux-en-Y hepaticojejunostomy. *Surgery Gynaecology Obstetrics*. 1978;**146**:161–167.
35. Jones SA. The prevention and treatment of recurrent bile duct stones by transduodenal sphincteroplasty. *World J Surg*. 1978;2:473–485.
36. Marangoni G, Ali A, Faraj W, Heaton N, et al. Clinical features and treatment of sump syndrome following hepaticojejunostomy reflux of gastrointestinal content into the biliary tree above the anastomoses. *HBP Pancreat Dis Int*. 2011;**10**:261–264.
37. Liao GQ, Wang H, Hu QH, Tai S. A successful treatment of traumatic broncho-biliary fistula by endoscopic retrograde biliary drainage. *Chin J Traumatol*. 2012;**15**(1):59–61.
38. Igami T, Nishio H, Ebata T, Yokoyama Y, Sugawara G, Nagino M. Using the greater omental flap to cover the cut surface of the liver for prevention of delayed gastric emptying after left-sided hepatobiliary resection: a prospective randomized controlled trial. *J Hepatobiliary Pancreat Sci*. 2011;**18**(2):176–183.
39. Okano K, Asano E, Oshima M, et al. Omental flap wrapping with fixation to the cut surface of the liver for reducing delayed gastric emptying after left-sided hepatectomy. *Surg Today*. 2013;**43**(12):1425–1 432.
40. Umeshita K, Fujiwara K, Kiyosawa K, et al. Operative morbidity of living liver donors in Japan. *Lancet*. 2003;**362**(9385):687–690.
41. Kim SJ, Na GJ, Choi HJ, Yoo YK, et al. Surgical outcome of right living donors in living donor liver transplantation: single centre experience with 500 cases. *J Gastrointestinal Surg*. 2012;**16**(6):1160–1170.
42. Oh JW, Oh SN, Jung SE, Byun JY. Diaphragmatic hernia after living-donor right hepatectomy: an important late donor complication. *J Comput Assist Tomogr*. 2017;**41**(5):726–730.
43. Esposito F, Lim C, Salloum C, Osseis M, et al. Diaphragmatic hernia following liver resection: case series and review of the literature. *Ann Hepatobiliary Pancreat Surg*. 2017;**21**(3):114–121.
44. Cortes M, Tapura N, Khorsandi SE, Ibars EP, et al. Diaphragmatic hernia after liver transplantation in children: case series and review of the literature. *Liver Transpl*. 2014;**20**(12):1429–1435.
45. Pedersen R, Sung M, DiFronzo AL. Long-term nononcologic outcomes for laparoscopic liver resection: improvement over open hepatectomy? *Am Surg*. 2016;**82**(10):953–956.
46. Moaven O, Hodin RA. Chilaiditi syndrome: a rare entity with important differential diagnoses. *Gastroenterol Hepatol (N Y)*. 2012;**8**(4):276–278.
47. Elms L, Moon RC, Varnadore S, Teixeira AF, Jawad MA. Causes of small bowel obstruction after Roux-en-Y gastric bypass: a review of 2,395 cases at a single institution. *Surg Endosc*. 2014;**28**(5):1624–1628.
48. Kossler-Ebs JB, Grummich K, Jensen K, et al. Incisional hernia after laparoscopic or open abdominal surgery—a systematic review and meta-analysis. *World J Surg*. 2016;**40**(10):2319–2330.
49. Maxwell DW, Jajja MR, Hashmi SS, et al. The hidden costs of open hepatectomy: a 10-year, single institution series of right-sided hepatectomies. *Am J Surg*. 2020;**219**(1):110–116.

50. Wabitsch S, Schulz P, Fröschle F, et al. Incidence of incisional hernia after laparoscopic liver resection. *Surg Endosc.* 2021;**35**(3):1108–1115.
51. Kayashima H, Maeda T, Hanada N, Masuda T, et al. Risk factors for incisional hernia after hepatic resection for hepatocellular carcinoma in patients with cirrhosis. *Surgery* 2015;**158**:1667–1675.
52. Nilsson JH, Holka PS, Sturesson C. Retrospective incisional hernia after open resections for colorectal liver metastases—incidence and risk factors. *HPB (Oxford).* 2016;**18**:436–44.
53. Fretland AA, Dagenborg VJ, Waaler Bjornelv GM, et al. Quality of life from a randomized trial of laparoscopic or open liver resection for colorectal liver metastases. *Br J Surg.* 2019;**106**(10):1372–1380.
54. Wagner JS, Adson MA, van Heerden JA, Adson MH, Ilstrup DM. The natural history of hepatic metastases from colorectal cancer. *Ann Surg* 1984;**199**(5):502–508.
55. Stangl R, Altendorf-Hofmann A, Charnley RM, Scheele J. Factors influencing the natural history of colorectal metastases. *Lancet* 1994;**343**(8910):1405–1410.
56. Lee RM, Cardona K, Russell MC. Historical perspective: two decades of progress in treating metastatic colorectal cancer. *J Surg Oncol* 2019;**119**(5):549–563.
57. Choti MA, Sitamann JV, Tiburi MF, et al. Trends in long-term survival following liver resection for hepatic colorectal metastases. *Ann Surg* 2002;**235**(6):759–766.
58. Hosokawa I, Allard MA, Mirza DF, et al. Outcomes of parenchyma-preserving hepatectomy and right hepatectomy for solitary small colorectal liver metastasis: a LiverMetSurvey study. *Surgery* 2017;**162**(2):223–232.
59. Fong Y, Fortner J, Sun RL, Brennan MF, Blumgart MD. Clinical score for predicting recurrence after hepatic resection for metastatic colorectal cancer. *Ann Surg* 1999;**230**(3):309–321.
60. Creasy JM, Sadot E, Koerkamp BG, et al. Actual 10-year survival after hepatic resection of colorectal liver metastases: what factors preclude cure? *Surgery* 2018;**163**(6):1238–1244.
61. van Dam RM, Lodewick TM, van den Broek MAJ, et al. Outcomes of extended versus limited indications for patients undergoing a liver resection for colorectal cancer liver metastases. *HPB (Oxford).* 2014;**16**(6):550–559.
62. Allard MA, Adam R, Giuliante F, et al. Long-term outcomes of patients with 10 or more colorectal liver metastases. *Br J Cancer.* 2017;**117**(5):604–611.
63. Wurster EF, Tenckhoff S, Probst P, et al. A systemic review and meta-analysis of the utility of repeated versus single hepatic resection for colorectal cancer liver metastases. *HPB (Oxford).* 2017;**19**(6):491–497.
64. Wicherts DA, de Haas RJ, Salloum C, et al. Repeat hepatectomy for recurrent colorectal metastases. *Br J Surg* 2013;**100**(6):808–819.
65. Regimbeau JM, Cosse Cyril, Kaiser G, et al. Feasibility, safety and efficacy of two-stage hepatectomy for bilobar liver metastases of colorectal cancer: a LiverMetSurvey analysis. *HPB (Oxford).* 2017;**19**(5):396–405.
66. Okumura S, Goumard C, Gayet B, Fuks D, Scatton O. Laparoscopic versus open two-stage hepatectomy for bilobar colorectal liver metastases: a bi-institutional propensity score matched study. *Surgery.* 2019;**166**(6):959–966.
67. Schnitzbauer AA, Lang SA, Goessmann H, et al. Right portal vein ligation combined with in situ splitting induces rapid left lateral liver lobe hypertrophy enabling 2-staged extended right hepatic resection in small-for-size settings. *Ann Surg.* 2012;**255**(3):405–414.
68. Eshmuminov D, Raptis DA, Linecker M, Wirsching A, Lesurtel M, Clavien PA. Meta-analysis of associating liver partition with portal vein ligation and portal vein occlusion for two-stage hepatectomy. *Br J Surg.* 2016;**103**(13):1768–1782.
69. Adam R, Kitano K. Multidisciplinary approach of liver metastases from colorectal cancer. *Ann Gastroenterol Surg.* 2019;**3**(1):50–56.
70. Jaeck D, Bachellier P, Oussoultzoglou E, Weber JC, Wolf P. Surgical resection of hepatocellular carcinoma. Post-operative outcome and long-term results in Europe: an overview. *Liver Transplant.* 2004;**10**(2, Suppl 1):S58–S63.
71. Gluer AM, Cocco N, Laurence JM, et al. Systematic review of actual 10-year survival following resection for hepatocellular carcinoma. *HPB (Oxford).* 2012;**14**(5):285–290.
72. Zheng J, Kuk D, Gonen M, et al. Actual 10-year survivors after resection of hepatocellular carcinoma. *Ann Surg Oncol.* 2017;**24**(5):1358–1366.
73. Yang JD, Hainaut P, Gores GJ, Amadou A, Plymoth A, Roberts LR. A global view of hepatocellular carcinoma: trends, risk, prevention and management. *Nat Rev Gastroenterol Hepatol.* 2019;**16**(10):589–604.
74. Ikai I, Arii S, Okazaki M, et al. Report of the 17th nationwide follow-up survey of primary liver cancer in Japan. *Hepatol Res.* 2007;**37**(9):676–691.
75. Kudo M, Izumi N, Kubo S, et al. Report of the 20th nationwide follow-up survey of primary liver cancer in Japan. *Hepatol Res.* 2020;**50**(1):15–46.
76. Makuuchi M, Kosuge T, Takayama T, et al. Surgery for small liver cancers. *Sem Surg Oncol* 1993;**9**(4):298–304.
77. Takasaki T, Kobayashi S, Suzuki S, et al. Predetermining postoperative hepatic function for hepatectomies. *Int Surg.* 1980;**65**(4):309–313.
78. Kamarajah SK, Frankel TL, Sonnenda C, Cho CS, Nathan H. Critical evaluation of the American Joint Commission on Cancer (AJCC) 8th edition staging system for patients with hepatocellular carcinoma (HCC): a surveillance, epidemiology, end results (SEER) analysis. *J Surg Oncol.* 2018;**117**(4):644–650.
79. Huang X, Lu S. A meta-analysis comparing the effect of anatomical resection vs. non-anatomical resection on the long-term outcomes for patients undergoing hepatic resection for hepatocellular carcinoma. *HPB (Oxford).* 2017;**19**(10):843–849.
80. Shindoh J, Makuuchi M, Matsuyama Y, et al. Complete removal of the tumor-bearing portal territory decreases local tumor recurrence and improves disease-specific survival of patients with hepatocellular carcinoma. *J Hepatol.* 2016;**64**(3):594–600.
81. Kostakis ID, Machairas N, Prodromidou A, et al. Comparison between salvage liver transplantation and repeat liver resection for recurrent hepatocellular carcinoma: a systematic review and meta-analysis. *Transplant Proc.* 2019;**51**(2):433–436.
82. Yoshida H, Mamada Y, Taniai N, Uchida E. Spontaneous ruptured hepatocellular carcinoma. *Hepatol Res.* 2016;**46**(1):13–21.
83. Aoki T, Kokudo N, Matsuyama Y, et al. Prognostic impact of spontaneous tumor rupture in patients with hepatocellular carcinoma. *Ann Surg.* 2014;**259**(3):532–542.
84. Kokudo T, Hasegawa K, Matsuyama Y, et al. Liver resection for hepatocellular carcinoma associated with hepatic vein invasion: a Japanese nationwide survey. *Hepatology.* 2017;**66**(2):510–517.
85. Abou-Alfa GK, Pawlik TM, Vauthey JN, et al. Liver. In: Amin MB, Edge SB, Greene FL, eds. *AJCC Cancer Staging Manual.* 8th ed. New York: Springer; 2017: 287–293.

86. Okuda K, Ohtsuki T, Obata H, et al. Natural history of hepatocellular carcinoma and prognosis in relation to treatment—study of 850 patients. *Cancer*. 1985;**56**(4):918–928.
87. The Cancer of the Liver Italian Program investigators. A new prognostic system for hepatocellular carcinoma: a retrospective study of 435 patients. *Hepatology*. 1998;**28**(3):751–755.
88. Chevret S, Trinchet JC, Mathieu D, et al. A new prognostic classification for predicting survival in patients with hepatocellular carcinoma. *J Hepatol*. 1999;**31**(1):133–141.
89. Llovet JM, Bru C, Bruix J. Prognosis of hepatocellular carcinoma: the BCLC staging classification. *Semin Liver Dis*. 1999;**19**(3):329–338.
90. Johnson PJ, Berhane S, Kagebayashi C, et al. Assessment of liver function in patients with hepatocellular carcinoma: a new evidence-based approach—the ALBI grade. *J Clin Oncol*. 2015;**33**(6):550–558.
91. Forner A, Reig M, Bruix J. Hepatocellular carcinoma. *Lancet*. 2018;**391**(10127):1301–1314.
92. Kim Y, Moris DP, Zhang XF, et al. Evaluation of the 8th edition American Joint Commission on Cancer (AJCC) staging system for patients with intrahepatic cholangiocarcinoma: a surveillance, epidemiology, and end results (SEER) analysis. *J Surg Oncol*. 2017;**116**(6):643–650.
93. Yamamoto J, Kosuge T, Shimada K, et al. Intrahepatic cholangiocarcinoma: proposal of new macroscopic classification [in Japanese]. *Nihon Geka Gakkai Zasshi*. 1993;**94**(11):1194–1200.
94. Bosman FT, Carneiro F, Hruban RH, Theise ND. *World Health Organization Classification of Tumours of the Digestive System*. 4th ed. Lyon: International Agency for Research on Cancer; 2010.
95. Moeini A, Sia D, Zhang Z, et al. Mixed hepatocellular cholangiocarcinoma tumors: Cholangiolocellular carcinoma is a distinct molecular entity. *J Hepatol*. 2017;**66**(5):952–961.
96. Ariizumi S, Kotera Y, Katagiri S, et al. Long-term survival of patients with cholangiolocellular carcinoma after curative hepatectomy. *Ann Surg Oncol*. 2014;**21**(Suppl 3):S451–S458.
97. Zhang XF, Beal EW, Bagante F, et al. Early versus late recurrence of intrahepatic cholangiocarcinoma after resection with curative intent. *Br J Surg*. 2018;**105**(7):848–856.
98. Bagante F, Spolverato G, Weiss M, et al. Defining long-term survivors following resection of intrahepatic cholangiocarcinoma. *J Gastrointest Surg*. 2017;**21**(11):1888–1897.
99. Sahara K, Tsilimigras DI, Merath K, et al. Therapeutic index associated with lymphadenectomy among patients with intrahepatic cholangiocarcinoma: which patients benefit the most from nodal evaluation? *Ann Surg Oncol*. 2019;**26**(9):2959–2968.
100. Riihimaki M, Hemminki A, Sundquist K, Sundquist J, Hemminki K. The epidemiology of metastases in neuroendocrine tumors. *Int J Cancer*. 2016;**139**(12):2679–2686.
101. Dasari A, Shen C, Halperin D, et al. Trends in the incidence, prevalence, and survival outcomes in patients with neuroendocrine tumors in the United States. *JAMA Oncol*. 2017;**3**(10):1335–1342.
102. Kasai Y, Hirose K, Corvera CU, et al. Residual tumor volume discriminates prognosis after surgery for neuroendocrine liver metastasis. *J Surg Oncol*. 2020;**121**(2):330–336.
103. Fairweather M, Swanson R, Wang J, et al. Management of neuroendocrine tumor liver metastases: Long-term outcomes and prognostic factors from a large prospective database. *Ann Surg Oncol*. 2017;**24**(8):2319–2325.
104. Ruzzenente A, Bagante F, Bertuzzo F, et al. A novel nomogram to predict the prognosis of patients undergoing liver resection for neuroendocrine liver metastasis: an analysis of the Italian neuroendocrine liver metastasis database. *J Gastrointest Surg*. 2017;**21**(1):41–48.
105. Tsilimigras DI, Ntanasis-Stathopoulos I, Kostakis ID, et al. Is resection of primary midgut neuroendocrine tumors in patients with unresectable metastatic liver disease justified? A systematic review and meta-analysis. *J Gastrointest Surg*. 2019;**23**(5):1044–1054.
106. Takemura N, Saiura A. Role of surgical resection for non-colorctal non-neuroendocrine liver metastases. *World J Hepatol*. 2017;**9**(5):242–251.
107. Takemura N, Saiura A, Koga R, Arita J, et al. Long-term outcomes after surgical resection for gastric cancer liver metastasis: an analysis of 64 macroscopically complete resections. *Langenbecks Arch Surg* 2012;**397**(6):951–957.
108. Adam R, Chiche L, Aloia T, et al. Hepatic resection for noncolorectal nonendocrine liver metastases—analysis of 1452 patients and development of a prognostic model. *Ann Surg*. 2006;**244**(4):524–535.
109. Ruiz A, van Hillegersberg R, Siesling S, et al. Surgical resection versus systemic therapy for breast cancer liver metastases: results of a European case matched comparison. *Eur J Cancer*. 2018;**95**:1–10.
110. Sano K, Yamamoto M, Mimura T, et al. Outcomes of 1639 hepatectomies for non-colorectal non-neuroendocrine liver metastases: a multicentre analysis. *J Hepatobiliary Pancreat Sci*. 2018;**25**(11):465–475.
111. Yoo TG, Cranshaw I, Broom R, Pandanaboyana S, Bartlett A. Systematic review of early and long-term outcome of liver resection for metastatic breast cancer: is there a survival benefit? *Breast*. 2017;**32**:162–172.
112. Groeschl RT, Nachmany I, Steel JL, et al. Hepatectomy for noncolorectal non-neuroendocrine metastatic cancer: a multi-institutional analysis. *J Am Coll Surg*. 2012;**214**(5):769–777.
113. Barbier L, Nault JC, Dujardin F, et al. Natural history of liver adenomatosis: a long-term observational study. *J Hepatol*. 2019;**71**(6):1184–1192.
114. Yang X, Lei C, Qiu Y, et al. Selecting a suitable surgical treatment for hepatic angiomyolipoma: a retrospective analysis of 92 cases. *ANZ J Surg*. 2018;**88**(9):E664–E669.
115. Qiu J, Chen S, Wu H. Quality of life can be improved by surgical management of giant hepatic haemangioma with enucleation as the preferred option. *HPB (Oxford)*. 2015;**17**(6):490–494.
116. Bernts LHP, Echternach SG, Kievit W, Rosman C, Drenth JPH. Clinical response after laparoscopic fenestration of symptomatic hepatic cysts: a systematic review and meta-analysis. *Surg Endosc* 2019;**33**(9):691–704.
117. Farid SG, White A, Khan N, Toogood GJ, Prasad TKR, Lodge JPA. Clinical outcomes of left hepatic trisectionectomy for hepatobiliary malignancy. *Br J Surg*. 2016;**103**(3):249–256.
118. Natsume S, Ebata T, Yokoyama Y, et al. Clinical significance of left trisectionectomy for perihilar cholangiocarcinoma. *Ann Surg*. 2012;**255**(4):754–762.
119. Matsumoto N, Ebata T, Yokoyama Y, et al. Role of anatomical right hepatic trisectionectomy for perihilar cholangiocacinoma. *Br J Surg*. 2014;**101**(3):261–268.
120. Nagino M, Kamiya J, Arai T, Nishio H, Ebata T, Nimura Y. 'Anatomic' right hepatic trisectionectomy (extended right hepatectomy) with caudate lobectomy for hilar cholangiocarcinoma. *Ann Surg*. 2006;**243**(1):28–32.

121. Tran TB, Dua MM, Spain DA, et al. Hepato-pancreatectomy: how morbid? Results from the national surgical quality improvement project. *HPB (Oxford)*. 2015;**17**(9):763–769.
122. Ebata T, Yokoyama Y, Igami T, et al. Hepatopancreatoduodenectomy for cholangiocarcinoma: a single-center review of 85 consecutive patients. *Ann Surg*. 2012;**256**(2):297–305.
123. Yoon YI, Kim KH, Kang SH, et al. Pure laparoscopic versus open right hepatectomy for hepatocellular carcinoma in patients with cirrhosis—a propensity score matched analysis. *Ann Surg*. 2017;**265**(5):856–863.
124. Park J, Kwon CHD, Choi GS, et al. One-year recipient morbidity of liver transplantation using pure laparoscopic versus open living donor right hepatectomy: propensity score analysis. *Liver Transplant*. 2019;**25**(11):1642–1650.
125. Cipriani F, Alzoubi M, Fuks D, et al. Pure laparoscopic versus open hemihepatectomy: a critical assessment and realistic expectations—a propensity score-based analysis of right and left hemihepatectomies from nine European tertiary referral centers. *J Hepatobiliary Pancreat Sci*. 2020;**27**(1):3–15.
126. Coelho FF, Bernardo WM, Kruger JAP, et al. Laparoscopy-associated versus open and pure laparoscopic approach for liver resection and living donor hepatectomy: a systematic review and meta-analysis. *HPB (Oxford)*. 2018;**20**(8):687–694.
127. Wong-Lun-Hing EM, van Dam RM, van Breukelen GJP, et al. Randomized clinical trial of open versus laparoscopic left lateral hepatic sectionectomy within an enhanced recovery after surgery programme (ORANGE II study). *Br J Surg*. 2017;**104**(5):525–535.
128. Broering DC, Elsheikh Y, Shagrani M, Abaalkhail F, Troisi RI. Pure laparoscopic living donor left lateral sectionectomy in pediatric transplantation: a propensity score analysis on 220 consecutive patients. *Liver Transplant*. 2018;**24**(8):1019–1030.
129. Coco D, Leanza S. Ex vivo liver resection for liver tumors: last resort when conventional technique is not applicable. *World J Adv Res Rev*. 2021;**10**(2):6–9.

SECTION 2
The gall bladder and bile ducts

Diagnostic and therapeutic approaches for the biliary tree and gall bladder

27. Non-invasive imaging of the biliary tract 301
    Daniela Husarik and Cäcilia S. Reiner

28. Endoscopic diagnostic and treatment modalities of the biliary system 311
    Christoph Gubler and Frans Oliver The

29. Percutaneous biliary imaging and interventions 323
    Mathilde Vermersch, Alban Denys, and Naik Vietti Violi

30. Laparoscopic liver surgery 336
    Christian Hobeika, François Cauchy, and Olivier Soubrane

31. Pathogenesis and natural history of gallstones 348
    Veena Bheeman, Royce P. Vincent, and Ameet G. Patel

Specific conditions of the gall bladder

32. Acute and chronic cholecystitis 361
    Claire Goumard and Olivier Scatton

33. Post-cholecystectomy biliary injury 366
    Kayvan Mohkam, Jean-Yves Mabrut, Agnès Rode, and Mickaël Lesurtel

34. Biliary fistula, gallstone ileus, and Mirizzi syndrome 376
    Martin Palavecino and Juan Pekolj

35. Benign and malignant lesions of the gall bladder 391
    Anil K. Agarwal and Raja Kalayarasan

36. Medical and innovative therapies for biliary malignancies 415
    Sudha Kodali, Joy V. Nolte Fong, and R. Mark Ghobrial

The intrahepatic and extrahepatic bile ducts

37. Biliary atresia 423
    Priya Ramachandran

38. Neonatal cholestasis syndrome 433
    Priya Ramachandran

39. Acute cholangitis, recurrent cholangitis, and management of common bile duct calculi 437
    Haitham Triki and Karim Boudjema

40. Cystic diseases of the biliary system 446
    Stefan Heinrich

41. Primary sclerosing cholangitis 453
    James Neuberger

42. Malignant lesions of the extrahepatic biliary system 458
    Philippe Compagnon, Andrea Peloso, and Christian Toso

Non-invasive imaging of the biliary tract

Daniela Husarik and Cäcilia S. Reiner

Introduction

Non-invasive imaging of the biliary tract has been replacing invasive diagnostic imaging over the last decade with advancements in imaging techniques which have a higher quality and spatial resolution. This chapter discusses the various imaging techniques that can be used to evaluate the bile ducts and gall bladder, including ultrasound (US), computed tomography (CT), magnetic resonance imaging (MRI), and positron emission tomography (PET). In addition, technical considerations as well as advantages and disadvantages of the modalities will be emphasized. Typical imaging findings of biliary tract pathologies and potential pitfalls will be discussed and illustrated.

Spectrum of imaging modalities

Ultrasound

US is a non-invasive diagnostic modality that uses acoustic waves with a frequency above the human hearing capacity—1–30 megahertz (MHz)—to produce images. For imaging of the gall bladder and bile ducts at least 2.5–5 MHz are needed. The US waves are produced by piezoelectric elements in a handheld transducer and are partially reflected from layers where the acoustic impedance changes between different tissues. The reflected waves are then again received by the transducer where they are processed and transformed into images. B-mode images are two-dimensional cross-sectional images composed of dots of various shades of grey representing the US echoes created by tissues and organ boundaries. The brightness of each dot is determined by the amplitude of the returned echo signal. In normal bile as in other liquids, the US waves are not reflected, therefore the content of the gall bladder and bile ducts appear anechoic (dark).

For elective US of the gall bladder it is of advantage if the patients are fasting. Due to the superficial location of the gall bladder, visualization may only be limited due to large amounts of subcutaneous fat. The normal gall bladder can be up to 4 cm in diameter with a wall thickness of up to 2–3 mm.

The intrahepatic bile ducts run parallel to the adjacent, larger portal vein branches. In the liver hilum they can be more difficult to assess when there are large amounts of gas in the stomach or duodenum.

Contrast-enhanced ultrasound (CEUS) has been available for several years. The purely intravascular contrast medium (CM) for US is composed of microbubbles that can pass the capillaries and are formed by a stable phospholipid shell filled with an inert gas. A small amount (2 mL) of CM is injected intravenously and imaging can be performed for several minutes with low mechanical index techniques to avoid bursting of the microbubbles.

The wide availability and portability of the US machines are reasons why US is often the first imaging modality in diseases of the gall bladder and biliary tree.

The strengths of US include it being a live modality, the ability to dynamically and rapidly assess diseases at a relatively low cost, not having any known long-term harmful side effects, excellent spatial and temporal resolution, wide availability of the equipment, and the possibility of bedside imaging. Weaknesses are operator dependency, the inability to penetrate bone and gas, as well as limitations due to patient physique.

Computed tomography

CT is the most commonly used cross-sectional imaging tool and utilizes X-rays, depicting organs without superpositions. With modern multidetector spiral CT scanners, there is continuous rotation of the tube and detector around the patient while the table which the patient lies on moves through the gantry, capturing a gapless volume during a single breath hold.

Images from one acquisition can be reconstructed in the axial plane, but also in a coronal, sagittal, or curved plane. Minimum intensity projections are useful to depict low-attenuating structures such as the biliary system within higher-attenuating surrounding tissue such as the liver and pancreas.

In addition to an unenhanced scan, where calcified stones or haemorrhage can be detected as hyperdense structures, the use of iodinated intravenous contrast increases soft tissue contrast and is a crucial component of hepatobiliary CT imaging. Administering a total amount of 0.63 gI/kg of lean body weight using CM with iodine concentrations ranging from 270–400 mgI/mL results in diagnostic abdominal CT images.[1] The CM is commonly injected intravenously using an automatic power injector with a rate of 2.5–3.5 mL/s.

Thanks to fast scanning, multiple phases can be acquired including the late arterial phase (30–40 seconds post injection), the portal venous phase (50–90 seconds post injection), and the delayed phase (3–10 minutes post injection).[2]

For imaging of the biliary system, no oral contrast is given to optimize visualization of the common bile duct (CBD) without artefacts from contrast in the duodenum.

Many scanners have the ability to perform dual energy imaging, some with two tubes and detectors, others with tube voltage switching or dual layer detectors, all allowing for characterization of various tissues and stone composition.

The use of CT results in radiation exposure, which is a downside of the modality. Modern iterative reconstruction algorithms improve image quality allowing for imaging at lower radiation dose while maintaining diagnostic image quality. This has led to a significant decrease in radiation dose for CT over recent years.[3]

Strengths of CT are the wide availability and the fast image acquisition. Weaknesses include the involved radiation, relatively low soft tissue contrast, and limitations for the use of intravenous contrast in patients with reduced renal function or prior allergic reaction to the contrast agent.

Fluorodeoxyglucose-labelled positron emission tomography–computed tomography

PET is a modern non-invasive hybrid imaging technique. It requires the intravenous injection of a radiolabelled, positron-emitting radiopharmaceutical—in tumour imaging often F-18-fluorodeoxyglucose (FDG). After an uptake time of 45–60 minutes, hybrid imaging is performed by acquiring functional (PET) and anatomical images (CT) followed by co-registration of the images. The CT information is also used for attenuation correction of the PET images. As PET images have a limited spatial resolution and anatomical information, the co-registration with CT allows for exact anatomical correlation of increased uptake that certain tumours demonstrate due to high metabolic rates. Motion artefacts can result in a mismatch between PET and CT. FDG-PET/CT is used for staging and restaging of various tumours, including gall bladder carcinoma (GBC) and cholangiocarcinoma.

Magnetic resonance imaging

MRI including magnetic resonance cholangiopancreatography (MRCP) depicts conditions of the biliary system with a high diagnostic accuracy. In general, MRI provides high soft tissue contrast and the ability to excite or suppress specific tissue types such as water or fat. The visualization of the biliary tree relies on the selective excitation of water. Fat-suppressed heavily T2-weighted images are acquired showing the fluid-filled structures with bright signal and all background structures with very low-signal intensity. A stone, tumour, or stricture of the bile duct is depicted as a filling defect or narrowing of the fluid-filled bile duct on MRCP. The technique is a non-invasive method without the need of contrast injection. An advantage of MRCP is that it depicts the bile ducts proximal to the stenosis also in cases where retrogradely injected contrast agent at endoscopic retrograde cholangiopancreatography failed to pass the stenosis.

For MRCP two techniques can be used: the two-dimensional (2D) thick-slab MRCP and the three-dimensional (3D) multisection thin-slice MRCP. For 2D MRCP a single thick slab (50–150 mm) is acquired within a breath hold in an oblique coronal plane in different angles along the head–feet axis. This results in a 2D projection image of all fluid-filled structures within the slab. The disadvantage of this technique is that fluid-filled structures in the imaging plane such as the stomach, duodenum, and hepatic cysts, potentially obscure parts of the biliary tree. To minimize this effect a negative oral contrast agent can be used to darken the fluid in the stomach and duodenum (i.e. pineapple juice, iron-containing contrast agent). The 2D MRCP gives a quick overview of the biliary anatomy. However, in the 2D projection small intraductal stones or lesions may not be visible, because the adjacent fluid is projected over the intraductal lesion.

Therefore, the 3D MRCP covering the biliary tree with multiple thin slices is added to a complete biliary MRI protocol. The 3D MRCP is usually acquired during free breathing with respiratory triggering to overcome the breathing motion artefacts. With this method image information is acquired only at end expiration, which slows down the image acquisition, often lasting for around 5 minutes. The thin-slice 3D data set allows for image postprocessing including 3D reconstructions and volume rendering.

With the advent of hepatobiliary magnetic resonance (MR) contrast agents, which are excreted via the bile ducts, contrast-enhanced magnetic resonance cholangiography became possible. The available gadolinium-based contrast agents are gadobenate dimeglumine (Gd-BOPTA, MultiHance, Bracco) with a low biliary excretion rate of 4% and gadoterate dimeglumine (Gd-EOB-DTPA, Eovist or Primovist, Bayer HealthCare) with a higher biliary excretion rate of 50%. After entering the vascular and interstitial space, the contrast agent is transported into the hepatocytes followed by excretion into the bile resulting in intense enhancement of the liver parenchyma and the bile ducts during the hepatobiliary phase. This effect occurs 10–20 minutes after contrast injection of Gd-EOB-DTPA and 60–120 minutes after injection of Gd-BOPTA, which may provide more adequate biliary imaging in a shorter time using Gd-EOB-DTPA.[4] The uptake of Gd-EOB-DTPA is mediated through the same transporter as bilirubin uptake. In case of increased bilirubin levels greater than 5 mg/dL no hepatocyte phase may be achieved due to competing effects of the contrast agent and bilirubin, and the entire contrast agent may be excreted via the kidneys.

The biliary excretion of the contrast agent allows the visualization of the bile ducts on T1-weighted contrast-enhanced magnetic resonance cholangiography images, and morphological and functional assessment of the biliary tree. This method is helpful in the detection of bile duct injury and evaluation of biliary-enteric anastomoses including leakage, biloma, and strictures.[5]

Not only can the bile ducts be imaged with MRI, but also the surrounding structures and vessels. Dynamic imaging with acquisition of arterial, portal venous, delayed, and possibly hepatobiliary phase images is performed after intravenous injection of gadolinium-based contrast agents. For dynamic imaging either extracellular contrast agents or contrast agents combining the features of extracellular and hepatobiliary contrast agents can be used. Contrast-enhanced images allow for the evaluation of enhancement characteristics of biliary lesions and their relationship to adjacent vessels.

Diagnostic abilities of MRI are decreased in patients in poor clinical condition, as patients need to be more cooperative for MRI than for CT. Reduced breath-holding capacity, uncooperative patients, or massive ascites degrade image quality. Major advances have been made with shorter scan times and image acquisition under free breathing for these patients[6]; however, these techniques are not widely available yet. Furthermore, patients with cardiac pacemakers, neurostimulators, or metallic foreign bodies have limited access to MRI.

Spectrum of biliary diseases

Gall bladder

Cholecystitis

Acute cholecystitis is one of the most common causes for admission to a hospital for abdominal pain. Most cases of acute cholecystitis are due to biliary stones impacted in the gall bladder neck or cystic duct (90–95%) while only 5–10% of the cases are due to acalculous disease. The preferred modality for initial assessment of the gall bladder is US with the ability to triage whether further imaging is needed. The sonographic Murphy sign is a reliable indicator of acute cholecystitis with a high sensitivity.[7] Gall bladder wall thickening greater than 3 mm accompanied with gallstones has a high positive predictive value for the diagnosis of acute cholecystitis.[8] Additional findings on US are distention of the gall bladder greater than 40 mm as well as pericholecystic and perihepatic fluid.

CT is inferior to US for detecting biliary stones. In acute cholecystitis, findings on CT include wall thickening with pericholecystic inflammatory fat stranding and transient hyperenhancement of the hepatic gall bladder fossa. CT is the best technique for imaging possible complications of acute cholecystitis: in emphysematous cholecystitis, intramural or intraluminal gas can be seen, which can be mistaken for calcification on US or MRI. In gangrenous cholecystitis there can be irregular or discontinuous enhancement of the gall bladder wall on CT, accompanied by intraluminal membranes, and gas within the wall or lumen. Ischaemic necrosis can cause haemorrhage or micro-abscesses within the wall, resulting in intramural hyperintensity on fat-suppressed T2-weighted MR images. It is helpful to use intravenous contrast for CT and MRI to detect mural necrosis presenting as a lack of enhancement of the wall.[9] Gall bladder perforation can be difficult to diagnose, however the presence of extraluminal gallstones, gall bladder collapse with pericholecystic fluid, or abscess are useful indirect signs (Figure 27.1).

Gall bladder empyema can resemble sludge on all modalities and the findings need to be correlated with the history as well as clinical and laboratory findings.

In chronic cholecystitis there is thickening and fibrosis of the gall bladder wall, disrupting normal motility and resulting in a contracted appearance. Chronic cholecystitis can mimic GBC, especially in the form of xanthogranulomatous cholecystitis, where asymmetrical thickening of the gall bladder wall, a gall bladder mass, or an infiltrative mass can be present with heterogeneous contrast enhancement and hypoattenuating subserosal, intramural nodules pointing to the benign entity. A porcelain gall bladder is a rare manifestation of chronic cholecystitis best detected on CT as plaques of mural calcification, its association with GBC is between 11% and 33%.[7]

Other differential diagnoses for thickening of the gall bladder wall include systemic conditions such as hepatic, renal, or heart failure as well as with elevated portal or systemic venous pressure.

Gall bladder carcinoma

GBC is an uncommon disease in the West but common in India and other tropical countries and is the most common malignancy of the biliary tree. Early detection is essential for a favourable prognosis; however, indolent and non-specific clinical presentations with unspecific radiological features often preclude identification of GBC at an early stage. CT is important for the diagnosis and staging of GBC with a high accuracy for correct T-staging and predicting resectability by delineating hepatic and vascular invasion, lymphadenopathy, and distant metastases.[10,11] MRI with MRCP and multiphase contrast-enhanced imaging has up to 100% sensitivity for bile duct and vascular invasion.[12] PET/CT has the ability to detect unsuspected metastases.

On imaging, GBC can have three appearances[13,14]:

1. *A mass replacing or occupying the gall bladder lumen* (40–65%), often directly infiltrating the adjacent liver parenchyma with a heterogeneous, mostly hypoechoic signal on US. GBC is hypodense on unenhanced CT. On MRI, GBC is hypo- to

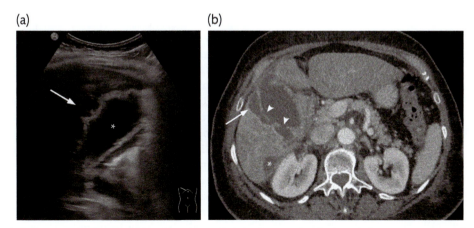

Figure 27.1 Perforated Cholecystitis. A 78-year-old female patient with 4-day history of acalculous cholecystitis, increasing C-reactive protein and leucocytes. (a) US showing an irregular configuration of the gall bladder (asterisk) with a thickened wall and adjacent hypoechoic areas in the liver (arrow), suggestive of abscess. (b) Axial CT in the portal venous phase confirming perforated cholecystitis with multiple disruptions of the gall bladder wall (arrowheads), and pericholecystic (arrow) and perihepatic (asterisk) abscess formation with rim enhancement.

isointense to the liver on T1-weighted images and moderately hyperintense on T2-weighted images. On CT and MRI, the tumours show irregular enhancement in the arterial phase with retention of contrast media due to fibrous stromal components during the portal venous and delayed phase. On PET/CT, GBC can be highly FDG avid, without being specific, as other malignant tumours can also show increased FDG uptake (Figure 27.2). Important differential diagnoses include liver lesions invading the gall bladder fossa (hepatocellular carcinoma, cholangiocellular carcinoma, and metastases).

2. If GBC presents as *focal or diffuse wall thickening* (20–30%), there is a broad differential diagnosis ranging from acute and chronic cholecystitis, to xanthogranulomatous cholecystitis, and to wall thickening due to systemic diseases. Diffuse symmetrical wall thickening is rather associated with non-neoplastic entities, while asymmetric, irregular, or extensive thickening with strong arterial enhancement is more common in GBC. FDG-PET cannot differentiate between benign inflammatory lesions and GBC.

3. GBC in an *intraluminal polyp* (15–5%) is usually larger than 1 cm and can have a thickened implantation base. On CEUS, GBC is sessile and enhances, differentiating it from biliary sludge or a clot with a high sensitivity and specificity.[15] Other differential diagnoses include adenomatous or hyperplastic cholesterol polyps, carcinoid, or metastases.

Bile ducts

Biliary stones

The role of imaging in biliary stones is to assess whether they are present, to evaluate their location, determine if they are a possible cause of the patient's symptoms, as well as evaluation of complications.

US is the best test for biliary stones with a high sensitivity and accuracy.[16] On US, gallstones are mobile, echogenic foci with posterior acoustic shadowing (Figure 27.3a). Non-shadowing structures are less likely to represent gallstones and include cholesterol polyps, sludge, adenomas, haematomas, and GBCs.

As not all stones are calcified and visible on CT, it is not commonly used as a first-line modality. On CT, gallstones may show hyper-, iso-, or hypoattenuation, depending on the composition of the stones. Advances in dual energy CT and postprocessing techniques to differentiate and quantify materials have increased the detectability of iso-attenuating stones.[17] For evaluation of complications such as perforation and bile stone ileus, CT is the modality of choice. If a gallstone impacted in the cystic duct or the infundibulum of the gall bladder compresses the CBD and causes biliary stasis, this phenomenon is called the Mirizzi syndrome.

In MR with MRCP, stones can be seen as filling defects in the gall bladder or biliary tree with a high sensitivity.

Choledocholithiasis is present in up to 20% of patients with cholelithiasis. US has a sensitivity of 73% and specificity of 91% for detecting CBD stones.[18] The distal CBD can be difficult to evaluate due to overlying bowel gas. A dilated extrahepatic bile duct larger than 6 mm can be reliably detected on US as an indirect sign for choledocholithiasis. A normal calibre CBD, however, does not exclude choledocholithiasis, with nearly half the patients with choledocholithiasis having a non-dilated CBD.[19] Furthermore, older patients may have a duct diameter greater than 6 mm as the diameter of the extrahepatic bile duct increases with age.

CT for the diagnosis of choledocholithiasis is usually not a definitive test (Figure 27.3b).

Non-invasive confirmatory diagnosis of choledocholithiasis can be made with MRI and MRCP (Figure. 27.3c). At the point of obstruction, an impacted biliary stone appears as a filling defect with a crescent of bile.[20] MRCP is also the preferred modality for assessing the intrahepatic stone burden. The use of a biliary contrast agent can provide added information about the degree of obstruction.

Cystic biliary lesions

Congenital biliary cysts are cystic dilatations of the biliary tree occurring in the extrahepatic bile ducts (= choledochal cysts), the intrahepatic bile ducts, or both, classified according to Todani.[21] In adult patients choledochal cysts may be incidentally detected on US or CT. Choledochal cysts bear a risk of biliary stones, recurrent cholangitis, biliary strictures, pancreatitis, secondary biliary cirrhosis, and an increased risk of cholangiocarcinoma and therefore should be surgically removed (Figure 27.4). If a focal dilatation or cystic lesion in the region of the extrahepatic bile duct is seen on US or CT, a choledochal cyst should be considered. The imaging method of choice to depict the full extension and anatomical details of congenital biliary cysts is MRI including MRCP. The cysts may contain calculi seen as signal voids on MRCP and are typically thin walled. Contrast-enhanced MR images should be added to detect focal or nodular contrast-enhanced thickening of the cyst wall, which could represent malignant transformation.[22] Differential diagnoses could be a pseudocyst in the head of the pancreas after pancreatitis, a duodenal diverticulum, other causes of bile duct dilatation (i.e. cholelithiasis, distal cholangiocarcinoma, inflammatory biliary stricture), and intraductal papillary neoplasms of the bile duct.

Intraductal papillary neoplasms of the bile duct (IPNBs) may appear as cystic lesions on imaging due to mucin hypersecretion analogous to intraductal papillary neoplasms of the pancreas.[23] Patients with IPNB have an increased risk of developing a cholangiocarcinoma. The mucin production may not only cause upstream dilatation, but also downstream to the lesion, which is described as a characteristic feature.[24] The imaging appearance of IPNB depends on the degree of papillary proliferation and mucin production. In case of predominant papillary proliferation, an IPNB appears as an intraductal mass. If mucin production is predominant, only lobar or segmental dilatation of the affected bile ducts is seen without a detectable mass. On US, CT, and MRI, segmental bile duct dilatation is seen, however mucin may not be detected, because it has the same appearance as bile. An intraductal mass can be identified in 41% of cases of IPNB with US.[25] Contrast enhancement of the lesion on CEUS, CT, or MRI may help to differentiate the mass from sludge or calculi; however, a differentiation from malignant tumours is not possible.[26] In general, MRI gives the most complete picture of IPNB owing to the advantages of MRCP. Diffusion-weighted MRI helps to distinguish the intraductal mass from calculi and improves tumour conspicuity.[27] Another differential diagnosis is a mucinous cystic neoplasm, which also produces mucin, but rarely shows communication with the biliary tree[28] (Figure 27.5).

Spectrum of biliary diseases

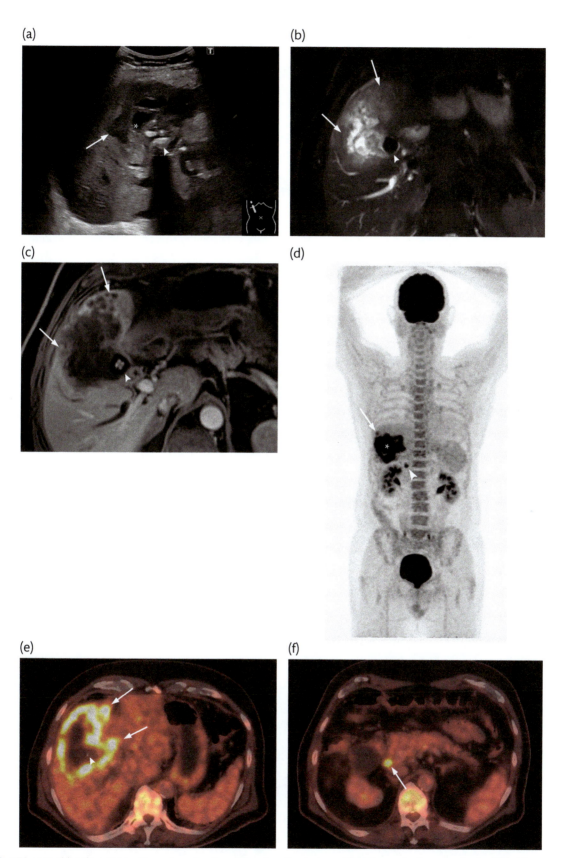

Figure 27.2 A 73-year-old male patient with unclear elevation of liver function tests and final diagnosis of metastasized gall bladder carcinoma. (a) US with heterogeneous mass in the gall bladder fossa with hyperechoic areas of calcification (arrowhead), anechoic cystic components (asterisk), and hypoechoic infiltration of the liver in the gall bladder fossa (arrow). (b) Irregular shaped mass with intermediate to high signal on axial T2-weighted, fat-suppressed axial MRI with infiltration of the liver (arrows) and hypointense stone in the gall bladder infundibulum (arrowhead). (c) The mass and the hepatic satellite noduli (arrows) demonstrate peripheral enhancement on axial T1-weighted, fat-suppressed MRI in the portal venous phase. (d) On a maximum intensity projection of the FDG-PET/CT, the high FDG uptake of the locally advanced gall bladder carcinoma (asterisk), a hepatic satellite nodule (arrow), and a lymph node metastasis (arrowhead) are apparent. Axial PET/CT shows intense FDG uptake in the gall bladder with hepatic extension of tumour (arrows in (e)) and of FDG-avid pancreaticoduodenal lymph node metastasis (arrow in (f)).

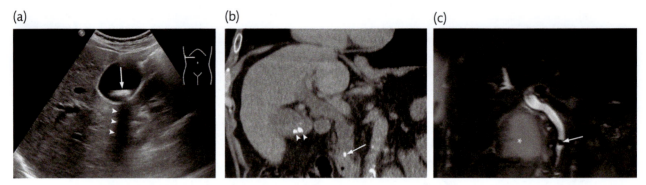

Figure 27.3 Biliary stones in three different patients. (a) On US in a 37-year-old female patient with intermittent right upper quadrant pain seen as a typical hyperechoic structure (arrow) in the gall bladder with posterior shadowing (arrowheads). (b) Cholecystolithiasis with calcified stones in the gall bladder (arrowheads) and choledocholithiasis with a calcified stone (arrow) in the distal common bile duct seen on coronal oblique reformatted unenhanced CT in an 81-year-old male patient with icterus. (c) Choledocholithiasis with a hypointense stone (arrow) in the common bile duct on coronal T2-weighed, fat-saturated MRI in a 78-year-old female patient with additional irregular thickened wall of the hydropic gall bladder (asterisk) due to carcinoma.

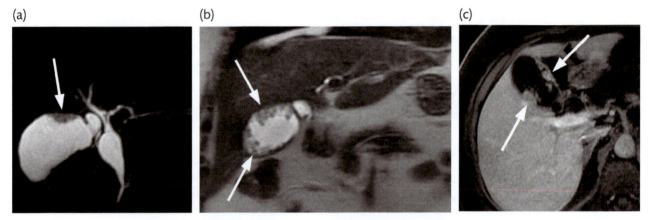

Figure 27.4 Choledochocele Todani type Ib and gall bladder cancer. A 58-year-old female patient with fusiforme dilatation of the extrahepatic bile duct on MRCP (a) diagnosed as choledochocele Todani type Ib. On T2-weighted coronal MRI the gall bladder cancer presents as a polypoid mass growing from the gall bladder wall into the lumen (b), showing strong contrast enhancement on T1-weighted fat-suppressed contrast-enhanced images (white arrows in (c)).

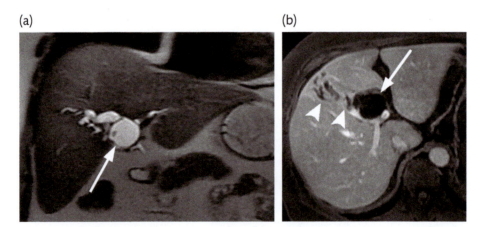

Figure 27.5 IPNB in a 59-year-old female patient. On the T2-weighted coronal image (a), a cystic lesion is seen in liver segment IVb (arrow in a). The lesion shows a T2-hypointense nodule and irregular wall enhancement on the T1-weighted contrast-enhanced image (white arrow in (b)). The segmental bile ducts distal to the lesion are widened (arrowheads in (b)) and probably communicate with the cystic lesion. The bright signal on T2-weighted images in the lesion and widened bile ducts corresponds to mucin produced by the IPNB.

Cholangitis

Inflammation of the bile ducts—cholangitis—includes various conditions, such as acute (ascending) cholangitis, pyogenic cholangitis, and primary and secondary sclerosing cholangitis, presenting with different imaging features.

In acute cholangitis, imaging by any modality may show dilated bile ducts with thickened bile duct walls with increased contrast enhancement on CT or MRI. Imaging is performed to identify the site and cause of obstruction and potential complications such as cholangitic abscesses. Abscesses are usually small and multiple and typically located at the site of biliary obstruction. They are hypoechoic on US, hypoattenuating on CT, and hyperintense on T2-weighted MRI.[29]

Primary and secondary sclerosing cholangitis are chronic inflammatory processes involving the wall of the intra- and extrahepatic bile ducts resulting in chronic obstructive jaundice. Primary sclerosing cholangitis (PSC) is an immune-mediated disease with intra- and extrahepatic bile duct inflammation leading to biliary fibrosis and liver cirrhosis. Imaging findings of PSC depend on the stage of disease. In early stages, focal biliary strictures alternate with bile ducts of normal calibre, but also dilated biliary segments may appear. In later stages the peripheral ducts become obliterated and the biliary tree may look like a 'pruned tree' on MRCP. Intrahepatic biliary stones may be present and depicted on US or CT. However, the narrowing and irregularity of the bile ducts are difficult to identify with these two techniques. In later stages liver parenchymal changes are seen with segmental or lobular atrophy with compensatory hypertrophy due to chronic biliary obstruction, caudate lobe hypertrophy, and wedge-shaped fibrotic areas.

With its high sensitivity and specificity,[30] MRCP is the imaging method of choice for primary evaluation of suspected PSC and follow-up imaging and should be favoured over endoscopic retrograde cholangiopancreatography, which is invasive and comes with an increased risk for complications in patients with PSC. MRI for PSC includes not only the MRCP, but also T2-, T1-weighted, diffusion-weighted, and contrast-enhanced images to diagnose potentially developing cholangiocarcinoma.

Cholangiocarcinoma

Cholangiocarcinoma (CC) is the second most common primary hepatobiliary malignancy. Imaging characteristics differ significantly, depending on the morphology and the location of the tumour. CC can be classified depending on the growth pattern (mass-forming—which will not be covered in this chapter—periductal infiltrating, and intraductal) and the location (intrahepatic peripheral and perihilar, 20%; extrahepatic, 80%). The diagnostic evaluation of CC can be challenging due to the heterogeneity of the tumours.[31] The role of cross-sectional imaging lies in primary diagnosis, local staging including evaluation of vascular infiltration, and search for metastases.

Periductal infiltrating

This type is usually seen as perihilar or extrahepatic CC.[32] On US, the tumours present with a narrowed or dilated bile duct without a well-defined mass. On CT, periductal infiltrating CC is characterized by a growth pattern along the bile duct without formation of an actual mass, and as in US, the ducts can be dilated or narrowed and demonstrate diffuse thickening with progressive enhancement. The strictures tend to be longer than benign strictures.

On MRI and MRCP, the wall thickening with progressive enhancement and narrowing of the affected segment can be seen with dilatation of the upstream intrahepatic bile ducts. Benign strictures tend to be shorter than malignant ones with regular margins, symmetrical narrowing, and no ductal enhancement. Tumour localization of extrahepatic CC is described by using the modified Bismuth–Corlette classification (Figure 27.6).

PET/CT for evaluation of CC is more useful for intrahepatic CC with higher sensitivity and specificity (83%) than for perihilar or extrahepatic CC.[33]

Intraductal growth

Tumours are characterized by alterations in duct calibre, usually duct ectasia with or without a visible mass on all imaging modalities. If a polypoid mass is seen, it is usually hyperechoic compared to the surrounding liver on US or hypoattenuating on pre-contrast CT with progressive enhancement over time on CT and MRI. Differential diagnoses include intraductal invasion by hepatocellular carcinoma (extraductal mass), hepatolithiasis (no enhancement, higher attenuation on CT), biliary cystadenoma or cystadenocarcinoma (intratumoural cysts that do not communicate with the biliary tree), or benign strictures.

Bile duct injuries

Postoperative bile duct injuries

Postoperative biliary strictures can be caused by misplaced clips, accidental ligation of an aberrant bile duct, fibrosis after recurrent inflammation, thermal injury, or stricture of the biliary–enteric anastomoses. The imaging feature in common is upstream biliary dilatation with a short narrowing and abrupt stricture. Metallic clips can be identified on gradient-echo sequences of MRI as a susceptibility artefact or on CT as a metallic structure at the site of the stricture. Complications of biliary–enteric anastomosis also include recurrent cholangitis, intrahepatic strictures, and stones. MRCP can be helpful when planning treatment of postoperative strictures and for depiction of intrahepatic strictures and stones. Biliary dilatation may be obstructive or nonobstructive in postoperative patients. Biliary-excreted contrast agent can provide information on the patency of a stricture or biliary–enteric anastomosis when contrast agent is seen in the duodenum or jejunum.[34]

Postoperative biliary leakage can occur due to transected bile ducts at cholecystectomy, leakage on the hemihepatectomy surface, biliary necrosis after liver tumour ablation, insufficiency of choledochocholedochostomy, or of biliary–enteric anastomosis. At imaging, fluid is seen at the site of the leak extending to the subhepatic space. Hepatobiliary contrast agents at MRI can help to localize the bile leak, distinguish bile collections from other fluid collections, and decide on the type of treatment[35] (Figure 27.7).

Traumatic bile duct injuries

Imaging findings of traumatic bile duct injuries are non-specific at CT, which is typically used as a first line imaging method in trauma patients. Non-specific findings include liver laceration, ascites, and

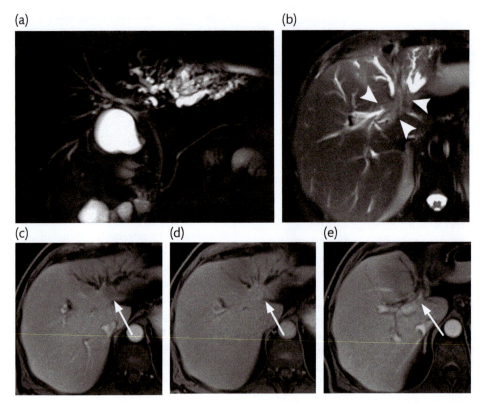

Figure 27.6 Hilar cholangiocarcinoma Bismuth type IIIb. A 64-year-old male patient with dilatation of the intrahepatic bile ducts, pronounced on the left side (a) with atrophy of the left liver lobe due to long-standing obstruction. On T2-weighted axial images the tumour is seen as a slightly hyperintense lesion growing along the bile ducts to the right and left side (arrowheads in (b)). On contrast-enhanced images (c, d) the tumour is visible as a mass (arrow) with irregular margin and progressive contrast-enhancement from portal venous (c) to late phase (d). In the portal venous phase narrowing of the left portal vein branch is seen (arrow in (e)) as a result of tumour infiltration.

intra- or perihepatic, hypoattenuating fluid collections increasing in size over time suggesting biloma. MR cholangiography with hepatobiliary contrast agent increases the diagnostic accuracy in detecting the site of bile leakage compared to non-contrast enhanced MRCP.[36]

Post-transplantation cholangiopathy

Post-transplantation cholangiopathy is typically caused by biliary ischaemia leading to necrosis, bile duct dilatation, and bilomas. Ultimately, ischaemic cholangiopathy presents with a pattern of alternating biliary dilatation and stricture. In addition, biliary casts

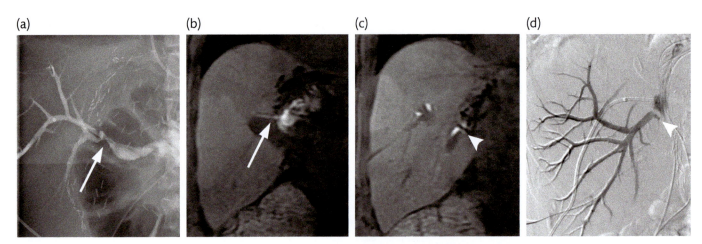

Figure 27.7 Biliary leak from the right posterior bile duct after left hemihepatectomy for a Klatskin tumour. Cholangiography via a percutaneous drain in the right anterior bile duct shows a narrow hepaticojejunostomy without a biliary leak. Nevertheless, a biliary leak was suspected clinically and an MRI with hepatobiliary phase images (b, c) was acquired. The arrow in (b) points to the right anterior bile duct not showing a leak. The arrowhead in (c) points to hepatobiliary contrast medium right next to the right posterior bile duct at the sight of anastomosis. The biliary leak was confirmed on percutaneous cholangiography via the right posterior bile duct (arrowhead in (d)), which was not visible during the first cholangiography (a). During this procedure a drain was placed over the anastomotic leak.

Spectrum of biliary diseases

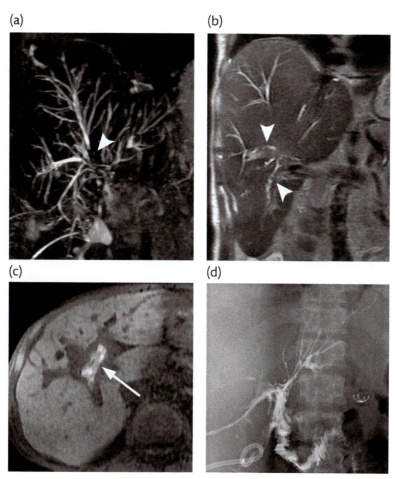

Figure 27.8 Post-liver transplantation ischaemic cholangiopathy. MRCP (a) shows dilated intrahepatic bile ducts of irregular calibre with signal loss in a central bile duct segment (arrowhead in (a)) and multiple stenoses in the left intrahepatic bile ducts. T2-weighted coronal image shows irregular calibre of bile ducts in segment VI (arrowheads in (b)). A similar picture is seen on percutaneous cholangiography (d). On T1-weighted fat-suppressed image (c), central intrahepatic bile ducts are filled with T1-bright biliary cast.

can develop, where debris of biliary mucosa and bile form into a mass-like hardened material in the intra- and/or extrahepatic bile ducts—the biliary cast syndrome. US is often the first imaging modality used, where early changes of chemical cholangiopathy are very subtle. In general, MRI is the non-invasive imaging method of choice depicting post-transplantation biliary complications with a high sensitivity and specificity.[37] A biliary cast is seen as a filling defect on MRCP with a sensitivity and specificity of 55–70% and 97–98%, respectively.[38] When adding T1-weighted fat-saturated MR images where a biliary cast appears as a bright structure, sensitivity increases to 90–95% for diagnosing biliary cast syndrome[38] (Figure 27.8).

REFERENCES

1. Zanardo M, Doniselli FM, Esseridou A, et al. Abdominal CT: a radiologist-driven adjustment of the dose of iodinated contrast agent approaches a calculation per lean body weight. *Eur Radiol Exp.* 2018;**2**(1):41. doi:10.1186/s41747-018-0074-1
2. Kartalis N, Brehmer K, Loizou L. Multi-detector CT: liver protocol and recent developments. *Eur J Radiol.* 2017;**97**:101–109. doi:10.1016/j.ejrad.2017.10.026
3. Higaki T, Nakamura Y, Fukumoto W, Honda Y, Tatsugami F, Awai K. Clinical application of radiation dose reduction at abdominal CT. *Eur J Radiol.* 2019;**111**:68–75. doi:10.1016/j.ejrad.2018.12.018
4. Dahlström N, Persson A, Albiin N, Smedby O, Brismar TB. Contrast-enhanced magnetic resonance cholangiography with Gd-BOPTA and Gd-EOB-DTPA in healthy subjects. *Acta Radiol.* 2007;**48**(4):362–368.
5. Lee NK, Kim S, Lee JW, et al. Biliary MR imaging with Gd-EOB-DTPA and its clinical applications. *Radiographics.* 2009;**29**(6):1707–1724.
6. Yoon J-H, Nickel MD, Peeters JM, Lee JM. Rapid imaging: recent advances in abdominal MRI for reducing acquisition time and its clinical applications. *Korean J Radiol.* 2019;**20**(12):1597–1615.
7. O'Connor OJ, Maher MM. Imaging of cholecystitis. *Am J Roentgenol.* 2011;**196**(4):W367–W374. doi:10.2214/AJR.10.4340
8. Ralls PW, Colletti PM, Lapin SA, et al. Real-time sonography in suspected acute cholecystitis. Prospective evaluation of primary and secondary signs. *Radiology.* 1985;**155**(3):767–771. doi:10.1148/radiology.155.3.3890007
9. Watanabe Y, Nagayama M, Okumura A, et al. MR imaging of acute biliary disorders. *RadioGraphics.* 2007;**27**(2):477–495. doi:10.1148/rg.272055148
10. Kim SJ, Lee JM, Lee JY, et al. Accuracy of preoperative T-staging of gallbladder carcinoma using MDCT. *Am J Roentgenol.* 2008;**190**(1):74–80. doi:10.2214/AJR.07.2348

11. Kalra N, Suri S, Gupta R, et al. MDCT in the staging of gallbladder carcinoma. *Am J Roentgenol.* 2006;**186**(3):758–762. doi:10.2214/AJR.04.1342
12. Kim JH, Kim TK, Eun HW, et al. Preoperative evaluation of gallbladder carcinoma: efficacy of combined use of MR imaging, MR cholangiography, and contrast-enhanced dual-phase three-dimensional MR angiography. *J Magn Reson Imaging.* 2002;**16**(6):676–684. doi:10.1002/jmri.10212
13. Kanthan R, Senger J-L, Ahmed S, Kanthan SC. Gallbladder cancer in the 21st century. *J Oncol.* 2015;**2015**:1–26. doi:10.1155/2015/967472
14. Furlan A, Ferris JV, Hosseinzadeh K, Borhani AA. Gallbladder carcinoma update: multimodality imaging evaluation, staging, and treatment options. *Am J Roentgenol.* 2008;**191**(5):1440–1447. doi:10.2214/AJR.07.3599
15. Serra C, Felicani C, Mazzotta E, et al. CEUS in the differential diagnosis between biliary sludge, benign lesions and malignant lesions. *J Ultrasound.* 2018;**21**(2):119–126. doi:10.1007/s40477-018-0286-5
16. Bortoff GA, Chen MYM, Ott DJ, Wolfman NT, Routh WD. Gallbladder stones: imaging and intervention. *RadioGraphics.* 2000;**20**(3):751–766. doi:10.1148/radiographics.20.3.g00ma16751
17. Soesbe TC, Lewis MA, Xi Y, et al. A technique to identify isoattenuating gallstones with dual-layer spectral CT: an ex vivo phantom study. *Radiology.* 2019;**292**(2):400–406. doi:10.1148/radiol.2019190083
18. Molvar C, Glaenzer B. Choledocholithiasis: evaluation, treatment, and outcomes. *Semin Intervent Radiol.* 2016;**33**(4):268–276. doi:10.1055/s-0036-1592329
19. Hunt DR. Common bile duct stones in non-dilated bile ducts? An ultrasound study. *Australas Radiol.* 1996;**40**(3):221–222. doi:10.1111/j.1440-1673.1996.tb00389.x
20. Baron RL, Tublin ME, Peterson MS. Imaging the spectrum of biliary tract disease. *Radiol Clin North Am.* 2002;**40**(6):1325–1354. doi:10.1016/S0033-8389(02)00045-3
21. Todani T, Watanabe Y, Narusue M, Tabuchi K, Okajima K. Congenital bile duct cysts: classification, operative procedures, and review of thirty-seven cases including cancer arising from choledochal cyst. *Am J Surg.* 1977;**134**(2):263–269.
22. Banks JS, Saigal G, D'Alonzo JM, Bastos MD, Nguyen NV. Choledochal malformations: surgical implications of radiologic findings. *Am J Roentgenol.* 2018;**210**(4):748–760.
23. Ainechi S, Lee H. Updates on precancerous lesions of the biliary tract: biliary precancerous lesion. *Arch Pathol Lab Med.* 2016;**140**(11):1285–1289.
24. Wu C-H, Yeh Y-C, Tsuei Y-C, et al. Comparative radiological pathological study of biliary intraductal tubulopapillary neoplasm and biliary intraductal papillary mucinous neoplasm. *Abdom Radiology (N Y).* 2017;**42**(10):2460–2469.
25. Lee SS, Kim M-H, Lee SK, et al. Clinicopathologic review of 58 patients with biliary papillomatosis. *Cancer.* 2004;**100**(4):783–793.
26. Liu LN, Xu HX, Zheng SG, et al. Ultrasound findings of intraductal papillary neoplasm in bile duct and the added value of contrast-enhanced ultrasound. *Ultraschall Med.* 2015;**36**(6):594–602.
27. Yoon HJ, Kim YK, Jang KT, et al. Intraductal papillary neoplasm of the bile ducts: description of MRI and added value of diffusion-weighted MRI. *Abdom Imaging.* 2013;**38**(5):1082–1090.
28. Kim HJ, Yu ES, Byun JH, et al. CT differentiation of mucin-producing cystic neoplasms of the liver from solitary bile duct cysts. *Am J Roentgenol.* 2014;**202**(1):83–91.
29. Feldman MK, Coppa CP. Noninvasive imaging of the biliary tree for the interventional radiologist. *Tech Vasc Interv Radiol.* 2015;**18**(4):184–196.
30. Dave M, Elmunzer BJ, Dwamena BA, Higgins PDR. Primary sclerosing cholangitis: meta-analysis of diagnostic performance of MR cholangiopancreatography. *Radiology.* 2010;**256**(2):387–396.
31. Olthof S-C, Othman A, Clasen S, Schraml C, Nikolaou K, Bongers M. Imaging of cholangiocarcinoma. *Visc Med.* 2016;**32**(6):402–410. doi:10.1159/000453009
32. Vanderveen KA. Magnetic resonance imaging of cholangiocarcinoma. *Cancer Imaging.* 2004;**4**(2):104–115. doi:10.1102/1470-7330.2004.0018
33. Chung YE, Kim M-J, Park YN, et al. Varying appearances of cholangiocarcinoma: radiologic-pathologic correlation. *RadioGraphics.* 2009;**29**(3):683–700. doi:10.1148/rg.293085729
34. Reiner CS, Merkle EM, Bashir MR, Walle NL, Nazeer HK, Gupta RT. MRI assessment of biliary ductal obstruction: is there added value of T1-weighted gadolinium-ethoxybenzyl-diethylenetriamine pentaacetic acid-enhanced MR cholangiography? *Am J Roentgenol.* 2013;**201**(1):W49–W56.
35. Melamud K, LeBedis CA, Anderson SW, Soto JA. Biliary imaging: multimodality approach to imaging of biliary injuries and their complications. *Radiographics.* 2014;**34**(3):613–623.
36. Kantarcı M, Pirimoglu B, Karabulut N, et al. Non-invasive detection of biliary leaks using Gd-EOB-DTPA-enhanced MR cholangiography: comparison with T2-weighted MR cholangiography. *Eur Radiology.* 2013;**23**(10):2713–2722.
37. Boraschi P, Donati F, Pacciardi F, et al. Gadoxetate disodium-enhanced MR cholangiography for evaluation of biliary-enteric anastomoses: added value beyond conventional T2-weighted images. *Am J Roentgenol.* 2019;**213**(3):W123–W133.
38. Kinner S, Umutlu L, Dechêne A, et al. Biliary complications after liver transplantation: addition of T1-weighted images to MR cholangiopancreatography facilitates detection of cast in biliary cast syndrome. *Radiology.* 2012;**263**(2):429–436.

28

Endoscopic diagnostic and treatment modalities of the biliary system

Christoph Gubler and Frans Oliver The

Introduction

Besides radiological imaging techniques such as transabdominal ultrasound, computed tomography, and magnetic resonance imaging, there are two endoscopic modalities with which one can examine the biliary system. The oldest technique is endoscopic retrograde cholangiopancreatography (ERCP) which was introduced in the 1960s.[1] About one decade later, the first experience with endosonography or endoscopic ultrasound (EUS) was reported.[2] With the introduction of magnetic resonance cholangiopancreatography (MRCP) in addition to EUS, the use of ERCP shifted more and more to a solely therapeutic technique. The reason for this is mainly because it is accompanied by a significant risk of complications. This does not only imply morbidity but also (although seldomly) mortality.

Endosonography

EUS combines flexible endoscopy with a high-resolution ultrasound transducer mounted on the tip of the instrument. High frequencies allow an impressive resolution with, however, only limited tissue penetration depth. Therefore, only distinct regions or lesions limited to the vicinity of the echo-endoscope can be characterized accurately.

Most of these devices come with a side viewing optic, and their angulation and resolution do not therefore meet the current standards of regular video endoscopes. These limitations hinder adequate routine examination of the luminal surface. With respect to their sonographic characteristics, two different types of echo-endoscopes are currently commercially available: (1) those equipped with a radial transducer (Figure 28.1a) which display a 360° angle view (Figure 28.1b). These enable accurate local tumour staging (infiltration depth and delineation)[3–5]; and (2) devices equipped with a linear probe (Figure 28.1c) which has a more restricted viewing angle (Figure 28.1d). As these devices are also fitted with a therapeutic-sized and elevator-equipped working channel (Figure 28.2a), these linear echo-endoscopes combine viewing beyond the mucosal surface with a range of interventions. The most commonly performed intervention is the fine needle aspiration or fine needle biopsy (Figure 28.2b) providing cytological or even histological conformation of a suspected diagnosis. More advanced and therapeutic EUS-guided interventions applicable to the biliary system will be discussed later in this chapter.

To further differentiate vital tissue from necrosis, sludge, and liquids or discriminate tumours and fibrotic lesions, contrast-enhanced EUS, which involves injecting an intravenous contrast agent or elastography, can be applied (Figure 28.3).

With respect to the biliary system, sensitivity and specificity of endosonography are highest in the distal two-thirds of the common bile duct (CBD). In addition, one can visualize the proximal one-third of the CBD, gall bladder, and left liver lobe (segments II, III and IV). This, however, may be done with a loss of sensitivity and specificity.

Finally, for staging biliary neoplasia as in other predominantly haemato-oncological disease manifestations in the upper abdomen and mediastinum, endosonography (with or without collection of cytological or histological proof) can be of great value.

Endoscopic retrograde cholangiopancreatography

To optimize inspection of the papilla of Vater (Figure 28.4b) and enable cannulation of its orifice, a flexible instrument with a side viewing optic is required (Figure 28.4a). This so-called duodenoscope has a large-bore therapeutic working channel equipped at the distal end with an elevator (Figure 28.4c). The latter enables working angle optimization of devices inserted through the working channel accessing the biliary system (Figure 28.4c,d). There is a wide range of devices available for interventions in the biliary tree as well as the pancreatic ducts (i.e., Wirsung and Santorini). Besides the basic papillotome, diagnostic catheters and guidewires, extraction balloons, dilatation balloons, cytology brushes, lithotripsy baskets, biopsy forceps, electrohydraulic or laser lithotripsy catheters, and stents are some examples of these accessories (Figure 28.5).

CHAPTER 28 Endoscopic diagnostic and treatment modalities of the biliary system

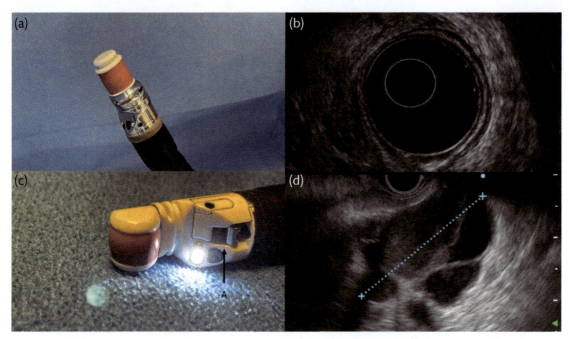

Figure 28.1 (a) Radial echo-endoscope with radial transducer. (b) Typical image generated with radial echo-endoscope with 360 degree scanning plane. (c) Linear echo-endoscope with elevator equipped therapeutic working channel (A). (d) Typical image generated with linear echo-endoscope.

Peroral cholangioscopy

In certain clinical settings, direct imaging of the biliary tree, enabling real-time visualization of its luminal surface and contents, can be of great diagnostic and therapeutic help (Figure 28.6).

Several solutions have been developed over the years, which turned out to be relatively fragile and challenging to use. In addition, imaging quality was somewhat poor. For this reason, cholangioscopy remained a not widely used procedure and was only performed in specialized centres. Recently, Boston Scientific has developed a plug and play system with a relatively robust videoscope and much better imaging quality, called SpyGlass (Figure 28.7). At present this mother–baby system is the only one commercially available and its use is no longer limited to a small number of expert centres. Although large-volume experience and subsequent data are still scarce, there are several recognized indications like difficult bile duct stone management and strictures of unknown aetiology.[6-9]

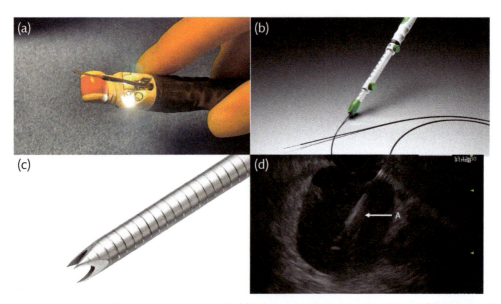

Figure 28.2 (a) Linear echo-endoscope with cytology puncture needle (b) inserted through the working channel. (c) Histological biopsy needle which has a three-headed tip and a specially designed surface. (d) Endosonographic image while puncturing a cystic lesion. The needle is well visualized, marked with the arrow (A).
Panels (c) and (d) provided courtesy of Boston Scientific. Copyright 2019 © Boston Scientific Corporation or its affiliates. All rights reserved.

Peroral cholangioscopy 313

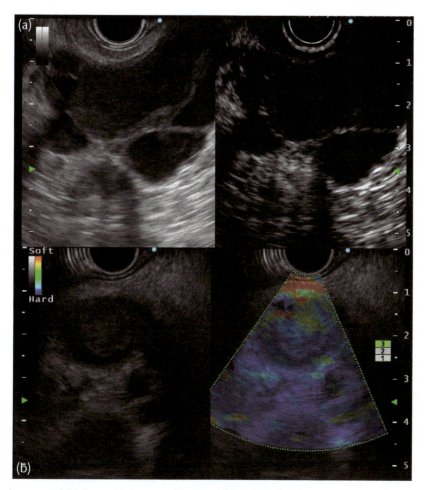

Figure 28.3 (a) Contrast endosonography, left panel is the normal image while on the right side contrast enhancement is visualized of the same area. (b) Shows elastography. With a colour spectrum as displayed in the left upper corner, the stiffness of the interrogated tissue is visualized.

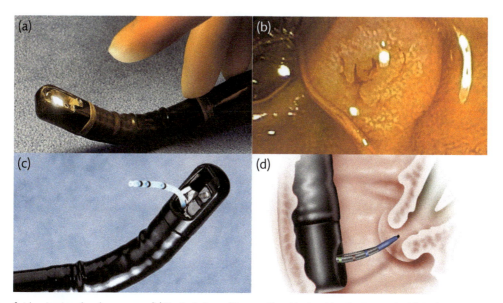

Figure 28.4 (a) Tip of side-viewing duodenoscope. (b) Typical view of the papilla with the side-viewing optic. (c) Catheters or other devices inserted through the working channel can be steered by using the elevator in addition to steering aides. (d) Position of the duodenoscope in the duodenum, while inserting the papillotome into the orifice of the papilla major.
Panel (d) provided courtesy of Boston Scientific. Copyright 2019 © Boston Scientific Corporation or its affiliates. All rights reserved.

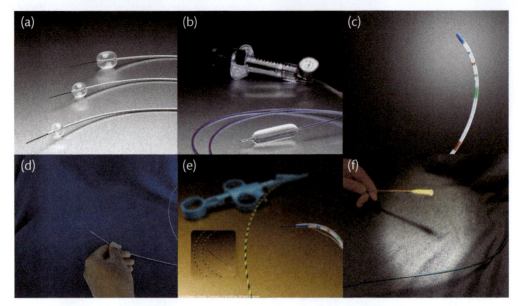

Figure 28.5 Some of the typical devices used during an ERCP procedure. From top left, clockwise to bottom left: extraction balloons in different sizes, dilatation balloon, pre-cut catheter fully covered SEMS, papillotome, and basket.
Panels (a), (b), (c), and (e) provided courtesy of Boston Scientific. Copyright 2019 © Boston Scientific Corporation or its affiliates. All rights reserved.

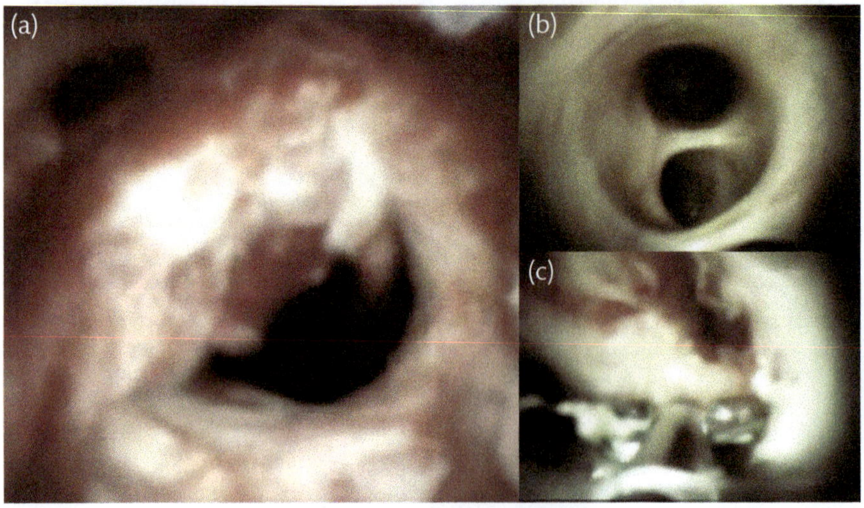

Figure 28.6 (a) Cholangioscopic image of a malignant biliary stenosis. (b) Cholangioscopic image of a normal intrahepatic biliary tree. (c) Image of a biopsy taken during a cholangioscopic procedure, evaluating intraductal pathological stricture.

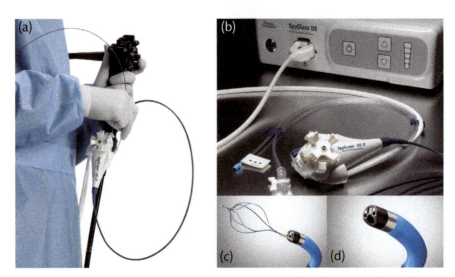

Figure 28.7 (a) Mother–baby cholangioscope system attached to the duodenoscope and inserted through the working channel of the duodenoscope. (b) The only currently commercially available cholangioscope system is called the SpyGlass DS II and contains a plug and play controller with light source and a disposable single-use cholangioscope.
Material provided courtesy of Boston Scientific. Copyright 2019 © Boston Scientific Corporation or its affiliates. All rights reserved.

Therapeutic endoscopic modalities in biliary disease

Historically, ERCP was the first and is still the predominant therapeutic endoscopic modality in biliary pathology. The first successful peroral attempts to visualize the biliary tree and pancreatic duct go back to 1965.[1] Endoscopic papillotomy and bile stone extraction were the first described therapeutic milestones in endoscopic biliary intervention and were described in 1973.[10] In the decades afterwards other through-the-scope devices were developed, expanding the potential of ERCP.

Bleeding, perforation, and post-ERCP pancreatitis (PEP) remain complications which can be potentially lethal.[11,12] PEP is the most frequently observed complication with a reported incidence of 5–7%.[11] Its course in most cases (93%) is mild to moderate[12]; 7% are classified as severe and result in prolonged hospitalization and, in some cases, additional invasive interventions.[12]

It is not that long ago that therapeutic endosonography got its place in biliary endoscopy. To date, ante- as well as retrograde biliary drainage and gall bladder decompression using EUS guidance are considered to be therapeutic options with a limited number of indications.[13–15]

Indications for endoscopic retrograde cholangiopancreatography

As mentioned earlier, in general, ERCP should only be performed with a therapeutic intent. The most common reasons to perform an ERCP are biliary stone disease and benign and malignant biliary intraductal strictures.

Less frequent indications comprise postoperative bile duct leakage, ampullectomy (endoscopic resection of papillary adenomas), radiofrequency ablation of intraductal tumours or uncovered self-expandable stent dysfunction, and photodynamic therapy of unresectable cholangiocarcinomas.

Biliary access

In the past, cannulating the major papilla, accessing the CBD, was performed with a catheter or sphincterotome using contrast medium to verify the (correct) position. As unintentional cannulation of the pancreatic duct is not a rare occurrence and injecting contrast into the pancreatic duct is a major risk factor for PEP, this technique has mostly been replaced by guidewire-guided cannulation.[16] After cannulation and visualizing the biliary tree with contrast (cholangiography), a papillotomy can be performed to enable easier future access or extraction of bile duct stones (Figure 28.8) In addition, in cases of recurrence, bile duct stones can migrate into the duodenum spontaneously.

A sphincterotome is a catheter with a slightly bent tip equipped with a metal wire which can be bent to generate a bowstring image. The letter enables the sphincter muscle to be cut using an electrocautery device. Alternatively, endoscopic balloon dilatation can be performed, decreasing the risk of post-procedural bleeding but significantly increasing the risk of a PEP.[17,18]

Biliary stone disease

Choledocholithiasis is the most common indication for performing an ERCP. The approach by which successful stone removal is achieved depends mainly on their size. Stones up to 10 mm in diameter can sometimes pass spontaneously into the duodenum.[19] It is, however, common practice to extract the stone(s), not waiting for their spontaneous passage. This is mostly done using an extraction balloon or basket after cutting the papilla (i.e. papillotomy). Larger stones often need a different strategy using other devices. In case of difficult stone management, multiple interventions might even be required. In these cases, one or multiple plastic endoprostheses are needed to ensure adequate biliary drainage in between interventions. In addition to this draining capacity, these endoprostheses expose the

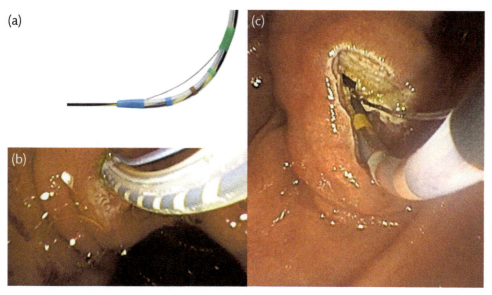

Figure 28.8 (a) Standard papillotome with guidewire inserted through its wire channel. (b) The papillotome is inserted into the bile duct through the orifice of the Papilla major. The angle of the tip can be changed by shortening the equipped snare, facilitating cannulation. (c) When correctly positioned, electric current is applied to cleave the sphincter of Oddi.
Panel (a) provided courtesy of Boston Scientific. Copyright 2019 © Boston Scientific Corporation or its affiliates. All rights reserved.

impacted stones to mechanical friction.[20,21] The latter approach, with or without the use of medical agents like ursodeoxycholic acid, can downsize stones making extraction in a later stage easier.[22,23]

When the size of the stone exceeds the diameter of the sphincterotomy and/or distal CBD, dilatation of the latter two or fragmentation of the first is required. Stone fragmentation can be performed using mechanical lithotripsy, electrohydraulic lithotripsy, laser lithotripsy, or extracorporeal shockwave lithotripsy.

When patients present with a sepsis or cholangitis, antibiotic therapy and fluid resuscitation should be the first-line therapy.[24,25] Depending on the clinical response and the potential presence of a coagulopathy, primary biliary decompression using a fully covered self-expandable metal stent (SEMS) or endoprosthesis without sphincterotomy should be considered as a bridge to sphincterotomy and stone extraction under more optimal circumstances.[25,26]

Stricturing bile duct disease

To ensure the right choice of draining method, the number, location, extent, and preferably aetiology of strictures should be known prior to the intervention.[26,27] It should be emphasized that in hilar or proximal segmental stenosis, contrasting and thereby contaminating the wrong segment is likely to influence prognosis. Therefore, adequate imaging should precede any draining procedure, defining a draining plan.

Biliary strictures, depending on their nature and extent, can be treated with dilatation, stenting, radiofrequency ablation, or a combination of these methods. When the diagnosis is not clear, it is recommended to obtain cytology or histology prior to treatment.[27] With respect to its choice, this is defined based on the above-mentioned characteristics. Going into detail of all the modalities is not within the scope of this chapter so an overview of the type of biliary stent and where to use them will be given. Biliary stents can be subdivided into plastic endoprostheses and SEMS. The latter are available with, without, and with a partial covering of the metal meshes. Uncovered SEMS should not be used in stenosis of unknown origin and benign or malignant diseases with a curative intent.

In extrahepatic malignant stenoses, SEMS are associated with a lower risk of stent dysfunction, fewer repetitive interventions, and longer patient survival (in palliative settings), when compared with plastic endoprostheses. When comparing covered and uncovered SEMS, placement of the first is related to more frequent stent migration.[26]

Plastic endoprostheses are the stents of choice when draining perihilar and intrahepatic stenoses of benign or malignant aetiology when a surgical resection is foreseen. In a palliative setting, uncovered SEMS show a higher success rate and fewer repetitive interventions therefore improving quality of life.[26]

In case of perihilar and intrahepatic peripheral stenoses, depending on the local experience, either percutaneous transhepatic cholangiography and percutaneous biliary drainage or an endoscopic retrograde strategy should be chosen. Ideally, these more complex dilemmas are treated in expert centres and after multidisciplinary case discussions.

Iatrogenic bile duct leakage

Bile duct injury is an occasional surgical complication in addition to another traumatic cause. Leakage of the cystic duct remnant is the most frequently described. Less common causes are biliary anastomotic insufficiency and perioperative liver/bile duct injury. Endoscopic treatment (e.g. ERCP with papillotomy and/or stent placement) in these settings is highly effective with reported success rates of over 90%.[28] Although evidence is mainly from retrospective data, it shows fairly consistently that papillotomy alone often suffices and might even result in fewer procedures and earlier hospital discharge when compared to biliary stent placement in addition to papillotomy. A two-step algorithm (i.e. starting with a papillotomy only, adding a stent when leakage persist over time) is therefore justifiable.

Biliary intervention in altered anatomy

When conventional ERCP fails or either surgical alteration of the anatomy or a duodenal stenosis hinders access to the papilla, percutaneous transhepatic cholangiography and subsequent intervention including percutaneous biliary drainage are currently the standard of care. However, EUS-guided biliary access as a patient-friendly alternative is receiving growing attention.[29,30]

In a world where obesity is a significant and growing health problem,[31,32] patients who have undergone bariatric surgery in the past are not uncommon. Gaining access to the papilla after a Roux-en-Y gastric bypass might be challenging. The classical approach (i.e. reaching the duodenum and papilla via the jejunojejunostomy) utilizes a single or double balloon or a spiral fitted overtube endoscope. The papilla identification rate using this technique is 90% whereas successful cannulation and therapeutic success are reported to be 77% and 73% respectively.[33] In comparison, a laparoscopic-assisted ERCP identifies the papilla in 97% of cases and cannulation and therapeutic success rates are 95% and 87%, respectively.[33] Although success is high, this procedure is associated with a significant additional complication risk. ERCP-related adverse events occur in approximately 6–8%, which is comparable to that in conventional ERCP. Non-ERCP-related adverse events in laparoscopic-assisted procedures, however, account for 19%. Besides this considerable adverse event rate, laparoscopic-assisted procedures can also be a logistical challenge. Organizing a surgical, anaesthesiology, endoscopy, and radiology team with their equipment all at the same time in one operating room has been proven to be cumbersome. In this perspective, gaining access to the disconnected stomach remnant using endosonographic guidance is an attractive alternative (**Figure 28.9**).

Depending on its urgency, the procedure can be executed in a one- or two-step fashion. The first step is generating a fistula between the stomach pouch and the stomach remnant. This is done by puncturing the stomach remnant from the pouch and deploying a 20 mm diameter lumen-apposing metal stent (LAMS) between the two orifices (**Figure 28.10**). The second step is the actual ERCP itself (**Figure 28.11**). In urgent cases, such as during cholangiosepsis, one can dilate the newly made access with a balloon and proceed with the actual ERCP in the same procedure. This single-procedure approach might coincide with an increased risk of complication including stent dislodgment. No larger prospective studies are currently available comparing these techniques.

Patients who have undergone a Billroth II distal gastrectomy or pancreaticoduodenectomy in the past and are in need of a biliary intervention also require a different endoscopic approach. In the case

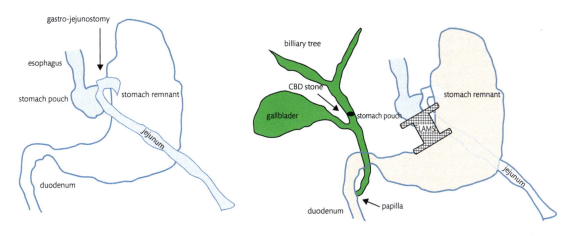

Figure 28.9 Accessing major papilla after gastric bypass surgery. (left image) Situation after Roux-en-Y bariatric surgery. (right image) Step 1, after placement of a 20 mm LAMS enabling endoscopic access to the stomach remnant.

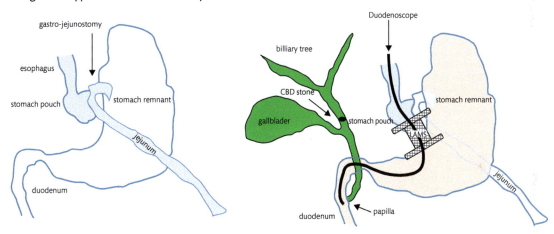

Figure 28.10 Step 2 after placement of a LAMS between pouch and stomach remnant performing ERCP (right image).

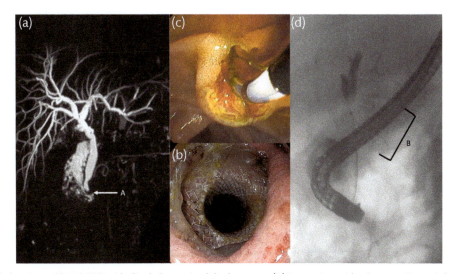

Figure 28.11 (a) MRCP showing a dilated CBD with distal obstructing bile duct stone (A) in a patient with a Roux-en-Y gastric bypass. MRCP as an endosonographic assessment of the CBD is not possible in this altered anatomy. (b) After EUS-guided placement of a LAMS between the stomach pouch and the stomach remnant (step 1), the gastric antrum and duodenum can be reached in step 2 with a normal duodenoscope and a regular papillotomy can be performed. (c, d) Cannulated bile duct and cholangiogram. The duodenum is reached via the LAMS (B) between stomach pouch and remnant.

CHAPTER 28 Endoscopic diagnostic and treatment modalities of the biliary system

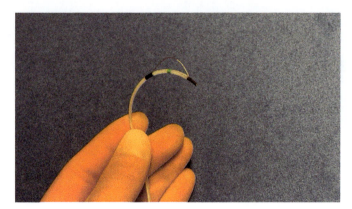

Figure 28.12 Billroth II papillotome with a snare that is pushed out of the insulated sheath instead of shortening it, hereby enabling cleavage of the sphincter.

of a Billroth II gastrectomy, a therapeutic gastroscope or a paediatric colonoscope is used instead of a side-viewing duodenoscope. After intubation of the blind-loop, identification and cannulation of the papilla is relatively easy. A specially designed papillotomy catheter (Figure 28.12) is used to cut the sphincter muscle. Other than that, the through-the-scope devices used are the same as in normal ERCP procedures. After pancreaticoduodenectomy and Roux-en-Y reconstructive surgery, a balloon/spiral enteroscope or paediatric colonoscope is used to reach the hepaticojejunostomy. The EUS-guided transgastric approach, as discussed below, can be considered in cases where metastatic disease causes biliary obstruction.

The transgastric gall bladder drainage, hepatico-gastrostomy and hepatico-duodenostomy are three other examples of minimal invasive internal biliary drainage, using EUS guidance (Figure 28.13). These are not standard procedures and should only be performed in carefully selected instances, predominantly in palliative oncological settings and expert centres. Depending on the number and level of stenosis one should choose the optimal approach. In general, distal locally advanced bile duct obstructions in which the papillary region is inaccessible are most suitable for transduodenal drainage generating an hepatico-duodenostomy. A hepatico-gastrostomy, however, is also suitable in such a situation. In tumours invading the proximal CBD and upwards, transduodenal biliary access is not possible. In such settings, a hepatico-gastrostomy can be the alternative strategy to percutaneous biliary drainage. In case of intrahepatic multiple segmental stenoses, EUS-guided biliary drainage generally has no place.

Endoscopic modalities in rare hepatobiliary diseases

General remarks

An in-depth discussion of hepatobiliary disease and its consequences on bile duct integrity lies beyond the scope of this chapter. Endoscopic therapeutic principles are basically discussed in the paragraph on stricturing bile duct disease. If and at what timepoint endoscopic intervention is needed should be evaluated on an individual basis. Furthermore, one should always be aware of the fact that infectious inflammatory bile duct disease and biliary neoplastic disease can mimic one another.

Autoimmune cholangiopathy

Autoimmune cholangitis is the perfect example of the above-mentioned diagnostic pitfall.[34,35] This predominantly immunoglobulin G4 (IgG4)-mediated disease can be the spitting image of a cholangiocellular carcinoma.[36] Both being rare diseases and difficult to confirm cyto- or histologically in the pre-treatment workup, they are challenging entities to diagnose (Figure 28.14). Autoimmune cholangiopathy may be part of a systemic disease but can also present itself as isolated sclerosing cholangitis.[37] The latter, in most cases, coincides with autoimmune pancreatitis.[38] When patients present themselves with painless jaundice, a more cholestatic than hepatocellular laboratory test result, and matching imaging with a dominant biliary stricture, a malignancy is generally suspected. In addition to tumour markers, it is advised to determine the IgG subtypes (in particular IgG4) and assess diagnostic criteria using validated scores such as the Mayo Clinic's HISORt-criteria.[39,40] Although IgG4 is elevated (>1.4 g/L)

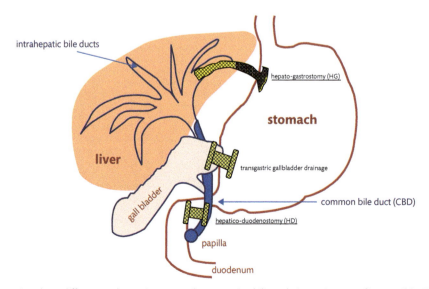

Figure 28.13 Cartoon illustrating three different endoscopic approaches restoring biliary drainage in case of impossible ERCP.

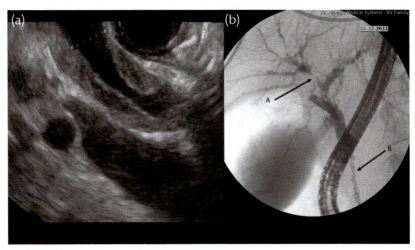

Figure 28.14 (a) EUS image of a typical biliary wall thickening seen in autoimmune sclerosing cholangiopathy, responsible for strictures (in this case localized in the CBD). (b) Cholangiogram with intrahepatic strictures without pre-stenotic dilatation and a dominant stricture of the CBD with pre-stenotic dilatation (type 2b).

in 70% of patients with IgG4-related disease, only 22% who had an elevated serum IgG4 met criteria for an autoimmune cholangitis-pancreatitis. Moreover, in a large cohort study 13% of patients with elevated IgG4 levels were diagnosed with a malignancy.[41,42] These numbers illustrate the diagnostic dilemma as well as the need for an accurate diagnostic workup and better diagnostic markers. Ultimately, obtaining cytology and/or histology of the dominant stricture is vital in order to establish the correct diagnosis. Cholangioscopy might improve histology acquisition, and in the process allow visual examination of the stricture(s) and biliary tree.[43,44]

Autoimmune cholangitis/cholangiopathy can be subclassified based on the distribution of strictures (Figure 28.15). There are four subtypes, type 1 having the highest incidence.[45] Type 1, 2, and 3 have distal CBD stricturing in common, which often reflects pancreatic involvement. Type 3 and especially type 4 can mimic cholangiocarcinoma and therefore the latter should be ruled out as described above. If, during initial diagnostic assessment, cytology and/or histology does not confirm malignancy (especially when the IgG4 is elevated), a short diagnostic steroid trial should be considered before moving to surgery.[46,47]

Parasitic infections of the biliary tract

Parasitic involvement of the biliary system is a rarity[48] and clinical situations where endoscopic intervention is needed even more so. The most relevant pathogens residing in the intra- and extrahepatic bile ducts are *Ascaris lumbricoides* (the adult worm can get up to

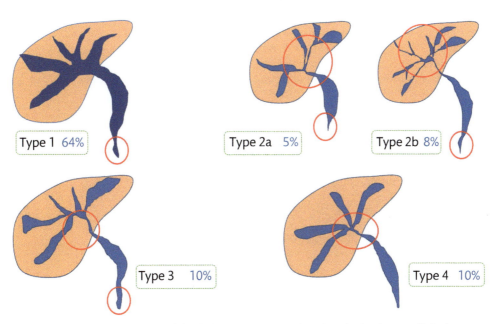

Figure 28.15 Classification according to interpretation of the cholangiogram/MRCP, based on the distribution of bile duct strictures. Type 1 with an extrahepatic stricture only (mimicking a distal cholangiocarcinoma or pancreatic head carcinoma); type 2a: intrahepatic biliary strictures with pre-stenotic dilatation and extrahepatic bile duct stenosis and type 2b comprising diffuse intrahepatic strictures without obvious pre-stenotic dilatation and extrahepatic stricture manifestation; type 3 cholangiopathy presents with hilar strictures and an extrahepatic biliary obstruction; finally type 4 has only hilar strictures which makes it a differential diagnostic challenge in which a perihilar cholangiocarcinoma has to be ruled out.

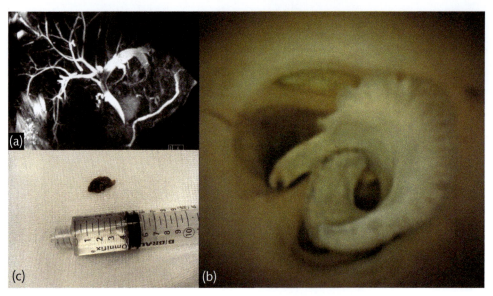

Figure 28.16 (a) MRCP with dilatation of the left intrahepatic biliary tree with a filling defect in the hilar region. (b) *F. hepatica* caught during cholangioscopy and (c) after retrieval with a basket.

35 cm long), *Fasciola hepatica* (30 mm), *Clonorchis sinensis* (20 mm), and *Opisthorchis viverrine* (7 mm). The first is a relatively common intestinal resident but can also access the CBD through the major papilla. This may lead to biliary obstruction and subsequent symptoms. *C. sinensis* and *O. viverrine* are small flukes which are common in Asia and eastern Europe. After ingestion of raw freshwater fish containing these parasites, they are able to penetrate the human body, migrating to the peripheral smaller intrahepatic bile ducts. Here they trigger a local inflammation, with bile duct wall thickening and dilatation. This infection is mostly asymptomatic and seldom needs endoscopic diagnostic aid or intervention. However, depending on the length and/or infection load, this may lead to colicky abdominal pain, cholangitis, or abscess formation. *F. hepatica* favours the larger hilar and distal bile ducts causing cholestasis and pain (**Figure 28.16**). In these cases, biliary decompression is required, warranting a papillotomy and extraction using a basket or balloon. Finally, one should bear in mind that unrecognized, chronic, or otherwise untreated infections with these pathogens increase the risk for developing a cholangiocellular carcinoma.[49,50]

Intraductal papillary neoplasm of the bile duct

Intraductal papillary mucinous neoplasms are cystic lesions of the main duct or its side branches of the pancreas. Both have the potential to transform into a malignancy, the latter being less oncogenic.

Within the bile ducts similar luminal lesions with malignant potential can be found. The incidence of such a so-called intraductal papillary neoplasm of the bile duct (IPNB) is significantly lower than its pancreatic counterpart.[51,52] It is associated with hepatolithiasis and liver fluke infestation, due to which it is seen predominantly in Far Eastern countries.

Patients with IPNB present with painless jaundice or cholangitis and cross-sectional imaging displays bile duct dilatation, irregular intraluminal masses with late arterial contrast enhancement, and porto-venous washout (**Figure 28.17**). Beside

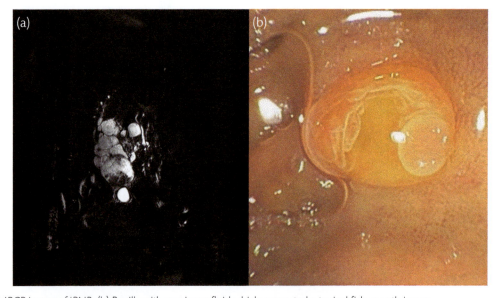

Figure 28.17 (a) MRCP image of IPNB. (b) Papilla with mucinous fluid which generated a typical fish-mouth image.

non-invasive imaging, ERCP preferably with cholangioscopy can provide histological conformation as well as video imaging. The latter can show a typical image and be of great help delineating the resection margins.

Because of its occlusive nature in addition to the significant malignant potential, IPNBs are considered an indication for surgical resection.[53] In patients not fit for surgery, local endoscopic therapy, meaning ERCP with radiofrequency ablation, can be discussed on a case-by-case basis in addition to symptomatic decompression using stents.[54]

Acknowledgements

Images Figure 28.2 panels (b) and (c); Figure 28.4 panel (d); Figure 28.5 panels (a), (b), (c), and (e); Figure 28.7 were kindly provided courtesy of Boston Scientific. Copyright 2019 © Boston Scientific Corporation or its affiliates. All rights reserved.

REFERENCES

1. Rabinov KR, Simon M. Peroral cannulation of the ampulla of Vater for direct cholangiography and pancreatography. Preliminary report of a new method. *Radiology*. 1965;**85**(4):693–697. DOI: 10.1148/85.4.693
2. Lutz H, Rosch W. Transgastroscopic ultrasonography. *Endoscopy*. 1976;**8**(4):203–205. DOI: 10.1055/s-0028-1098414
3. Krill T, Baliss M, Roark R, et al. Accuracy of endoscopic ultrasound in esophageal cancer staging. *J Thorac Dis*. 2019;**11**(Suppl 12):S1602–S1609. DOI: 10.21037/jtd.2019.06.50
4. Botet JF, Lightdale CJ, Zauber AG, et al. Preoperative staging of gastric cancer: comparison of endoscopic US and dynamic CT. *Radiology*. 1991;**181**(2):426–432. DOI: 10.1148/radiology.181.2.1924784
5. Tio TL, Cohen P, Coene PP, Udding J, den Hartog Jager FC, Tytgat GN. Endosonography and computed tomography of esophageal carcinoma. Preoperative classification compared to the new (1987) TNM system. *Gastroenterology*. 1989;**96**(6):1478–1486. DOI: 10.1016/0016-5085(89)90515-5
6. Bukhari M, Chen YI, Gutierrez OB, Khashab MA. Direct per-oral cholangioscopy with electrohydraulic lithotripsy for primary severe hepatolithiasis. *VideoGIE*. 2017;**2**(9):241–243. DOI: 10.1016/j.vgie.2017.02.009
7. Galetti F, Moura DTH, Ribeiro IB, et al. Cholangioscopy-guided lithotripsy vs. conventional therapy for complex bile duct stones: a systematic review and meta-analysis. *Arq Bras Cir Dig*. 2020;**33**(1):e1491. DOI: 10.1590/0102-672020190001e1491
8. Woo YS, Lee JK, Oh SH, et al. Role of SpyGlass peroral cholangioscopy in the evaluation of indeterminate biliary lesions. *Dig Dis Sci*. 2014;**59**(10):2565–2570. DOI: 10.1007/s10620-014-3171-x
9. Yan S, Tejaswi S. Clinical impact of digital cholangioscopy in management of indeterminate biliary strictures and complex biliary stones: a single-center study. *Ther Adv Gastroenterol Endosc*. 2019;**12**:2631774519853160. DOI: 10.1177/2631774519853160
10. von Ackeren H, Henning H, Soehendra N. [Experiences with papillotomy]. *Zentralbl Chir*. 1973;**98**(6):191–199.
11. Mergener K. Complications of endoscopic and radiologic investigation of biliary tract disorders. *Curr Gastroenterol Rep*. 2011;**13**(2):173–181. DOI: 10.1007/s11894-011-0179-7
12. Freeman ML, Nelson DB, Sherman S, et al. Complications of endoscopic biliary sphincterotomy. *N Engl J Med*. 1996;**335**(13):909–918. DOI: 10.1056/nejm199609263351301
13. Canakis A, Baron TH. Relief of biliary obstruction: choosing between endoscopic ultrasound and endoscopic retrograde cholangiopancreatography. *BMJ Open Gastroenterol*. 2020;**7**(1):e000428. DOI: 10.1136/bmjgast-2020-000428
14. Salerno R, Davies SEC, Mezzina N, Ardizzone S. Comprehensive review on EUS-guided biliary drainage. *World J Gastrointest Endosc*. 2019;**11**(5):354–364. DOI: 10.4253/wjge.v11.i5.354
15. Fabbri C, Luigiano C, Lisotti A, et al. Endoscopic ultrasound-guided treatments: are we getting evidence based—a systematic review. *World J Gastroenterol*. 2014;**20**(26):8424–8448. DOI: 10.3748/wjg.v20.i26.8424
16. Tse F, Yuan Y, Moayyedi P, Leontiadis GI. Guidewire-assisted cannulation of the common bile duct for the prevention of post-endoscopic retrograde cholangiopancreatography (ERCP) pancreatitis. *Cochrane Database Syst Rev*. 2012;**12**(12):CD009662. DOI: 10.1002/14651858.CD009662.pub2
17. Liu Y, Su P, Lin S, et al. Endoscopic papillary balloon dilatation versus endoscopic sphincterotomy in the treatment for choledocholithiasis: a meta-analysis. *J Gastroenterol Hepatol*. 2012;**27**(3):464–471. DOI: 10.1111/j.1440-1746.2011.06912.x
18. Baron TH, Harewood GC. Endoscopic balloon dilation of the biliary sphincter compared to endoscopic biliary sphincterotomy for removal of common bile duct stones during ERCP: a metaanalysis of randomized, controlled trials. *Am J Gastroenterol*. 2004;**99**(8):1455–1460. DOI: 10.1111/j.1572-0241.2004.30151.x
19. Gao J, Ding XM, Ke S, et al. Anisodamine accelerates spontaneous passage of single symptomatic bile duct stones ≤ 10 mm. *World J Gastroenterol*. 2013;**19**(39):6618–24. DOI: 10.3748/wjg.v19.i39.6618
20. Jang DK, Lee SH, Ahn DW, et al. Factors associated with complete clearance of difficult common bile duct stones after temporary biliary stenting followed by a second ERCP: a multicenter, retrospective, cohort study. *Endoscopy*. 2020;**52**(6):462–468. DOI: 10.1055/a-1117-3393
21. Lee TH, Han JH, Kim HJ, Park SM, Park SH, Kim SJ. Is the addition of choleretic agents in multiple double-pigtail biliary stents effective for difficult common bile duct stones in elderly patients? A prospective, multicenter study. *Gastrointest Endosc*. 2011;**74**(1):96–102. DOI: 10.1016/j.gie.2011.03.005
22. Han J, Moon JH, Koo HC, et al. Effect of biliary stenting combined with ursodeoxycholic acid and terpene treatment on retained common bile duct stones in elderly patients: a multicenter study. *Am J Gastroenterol*. 2009;**104**(10):2418–2421. DOI: 10.1038/ajg.2009.303
23. Nishizawa T, Suzuki H, Takahashi M, Kaneko H, Suzuki M, Hibi T. Effect of ursodeoxycholic acid and endoscopic sphincterotomy in long-term stenting for common bile duct stones. *J Gastroenterol Hepatol*. 2013;**28**(1):63–67. DOI: 10.1111/jgh.12012
24. Miura F, Okamoto K, Takada T, et al. Tokyo Guidelines 2018: initial management of acute biliary infection and flowchart for acute cholangitis. *J Hepatobiliary Pancreat Sci*. 2018;**25**(1):31–40. DOI: 10.1002/jhbp.509
25. Manes G, Paspatis G, Aabakken L, et al. Endoscopic management of common bile duct stones: European Society of Gastrointestinal Endoscopy (ESGE) guideline. *Endoscopy*. 2019;**51**(5):472–491. DOI: 10.1055/a-0862-0346
26. Dumonceau JM, Heresbach D, Deviere J, et al. Biliary stents: models and methods for endoscopic stenting. *Endoscopy*. 2011;**43**(7):617–626. DOI: 10.1055/s-0030-1256315

27. Mansour JC, Aloia TA, Crane CH, Heimbach JK, Nagino M, Vauthey JN. Hilar cholangiocarcinoma: expert consensus statement. *HPB (Oxford)*. 2015;**17**(8):691–699. DOI: 10.1111/hpb.12450
28. Chandra S, Murali AR, Masadeh M, Silverman WB, Johlin FC. Comparison of biliary stent versus biliary sphincterotomy alone in the treatment of bile leak. *Dig Dis*. 2020;**38**(1):32–37. DOI: 10.1159/000499872
29. Kahaleh M, Artifon EL, Perez-Miranda M, et al. Endoscopic ultrasonography guided drainage: summary of consortium meeting, May 21, 2012, San Diego, California. *World J Gastroenterol*. 2015;**21**(3):726–741. DOI: 10.3748/wjg.v21.i3.726
30. Jirapinyo P, Lee LS. Endoscopic ultrasound-guided pancreatobiliary endoscopy in surgically altered anatomy. *Clin Endosc*. 2016;**49**(6):515–529. DOI: 10.5946/ce.2016.144
31. Wang BC, Furnback W. Modelling the long-term outcomes of bariatric surgery: a review of cost-effectiveness studies. *Best Pract Res Clin Gastroenterol*. 2013;**27**(6):987–995. DOI: 10.1016/j.bpg.2013.08.022
32. Nguyen NT, Masoomi H, Magno CP, Nguyen XM, Laugenour K, Lane J. Trends in use of bariatric surgery, 2003-2008. *J Am Coll Surg*. 2011;**213**(2):261–266. DOI: 10.1016/j.jamcollsurg.2011.04.030
33. Tonnesen CJ, Young J, Glomsaker T, et al. Laparoscopy-assisted versus balloon enteroscopy-assisted ERCP after Roux-en-Y gastric bypass. *Endoscopy*. 2020;**52**(8):654–661. DOI: 10.1055/a-1139-9313
34. Geary K, Yazici C, Seibold A, Guzman G. IgG4-related cholangiopathy and its mimickers: a case report and review highlighting the importance of early diagnosis. *Int J Surg Pathol*. 2018;**26**(2):165–173. DOI: 10.1177/1066896917730902
35. Oh HC, Kim MH, Lee KT, et al. Clinical clues to suspicion of IgG4-associated sclerosing cholangitis disguised as primary sclerosing cholangitis or hilar cholangiocarcinoma. *J Gastroenterol Hepatol*. 2010;**25**(12):1831–1837. DOI: 10.1111/j.1440-1746.2010.06411.x
36. Swensson J, Tirkes T, Tann M, Cui E, Sandrasegaran K. Differentiating IgG4-related sclerosing cholangiopathy from cholangiocarcinoma using CT and MRI: experience from a tertiary referring center. *Abdom Radiol (NY)*. 2019;**44**(6):2111–2115. DOI: 10.1007/s00261-019-01944-1
37. Zen Y, Kawakami H, Kim JH. IgG4-related sclerosing cholangitis: all we need to know. *J Gastroenterol*. 2016;**51**(4):295–312. DOI: 10.1007/s00535-016-1163-7
38. Nishimori I, Otsuki M. Autoimmune pancreatitis and IgG4-associated sclerosing cholangitis. *Best Pract Res Clin Gastroenterol*. 2009;**23**(1):11–23. DOI: 10.1016/j.bpg.2008.11.017
39. Chari ST. Diagnosis of autoimmune pancreatitis using its five cardinal features: introducing the Mayo Clinic's HISORt criteria. *J Gastroenterol*. 2007;**42**(Suppl 18):39–41. DOI: 10.1007/s00535-007-2046-8
40. van Heerde MJ, Buijs J, Rauws EA, et al. A comparative study of diagnostic scoring systems for autoimmune pancreatitis. *Pancreas*. 2014;**43**(4):559–564. DOI: 10.1097/MPA.0000000000000045
41. Culver EL, Sadler R, Simpson D, et al. Elevated serum IgG4 levels in diagnosis, treatment response, organ involvement, and relapse in a prospective IgG4-related disease UK cohort. *Am J Gastroenterol*. 2016;**111**(5):733–743. DOI: 10.1038/ajg.2016.40
42. Masamune A, Kikuta K, Hamada S, et al. Nationwide epidemiological survey of autoimmune pancreatitis in Japan in 2016. *J Gastroenterol*. 2020;**55**(4):462–470. DOI: 10.1007/s00535-019-01658-7
43. Itoi T, Kamisawa T, Igarashi Y, et al. The role of peroral video cholangioscopy in patients with IgG4-related sclerosing cholangitis. *J Gastroenterol*. 2013;**48**(4):504–514. DOI: 10.1007/s00535-012-0652-6
44. Ishii Y, Serikawa M, Tsuboi T, et al. Usefulness of peroral cholangioscopy in the differential diagnosis of IgG4-related sclerosing cholangitis and extrahepatic cholangiocarcinoma: a single-center retrospective study. *BMC Gastroenterol*. 2020;**20**(1):287. DOI: 10.1186/s12876-020-01429-2
45. Kamisawa T, Nakazawa T, Tazuma S, et al. Clinical practice guidelines for IgG4-related sclerosing cholangitis. *J Hepatobiliary Pancreat Sci*. 2019;**26**(1):9–42. DOI: 10.1002/jhbp.596
46. Chari ST, Takahashi N, Levy MJ, et al. A diagnostic strategy to distinguish autoimmune pancreatitis from pancreatic cancer. *Clin Gastroenterol Hepatol*. 2009;**7**(10):1097–1103. DOI: 10.1016/j.cgh.2009.04.020
47. Moon SH, Kim MH, Park DH, et al. Is a 2-week steroid trial after initial negative investigation for malignancy useful in differentiating autoimmune pancreatitis from pancreatic cancer? A prospective outcome study. *Gut*. 2008;**57**(12):1704–1712. DOI: 10.1136/gut.2008.150979
48. Lim JH. Liver flukes: the malady neglected. *Korean J Radiol*. 2011;**12**(3):269–279. DOI: 10.3348/kjr.2011.12.3.269
49. Steele JA, Richter CH, Echaubard P, et al. Thinking beyond Opisthorchis viverrini for risk of cholangiocarcinoma in the lower Mekong region: a systematic review and meta-analysis. *Infect Dis Poverty*. 2018;**7**(1):44. DOI: 10.1186/s40249-018-0434-3
50. Xia J, Jiang SC, Peng HJ. Association between liver fluke infection and hepatobiliary pathological changes: a systematic review and meta-analysis. *PLoS One*. 2015;**10**(7):e0132673. DOI: 10.1371/journal.pone.0132673
51. Onoe S, Ebata T, Yokoyama Y, et al. A clinicopathological reappraisal of intraductal papillary neoplasm of the bile duct (IPNB): a continuous spectrum with papillary cholangiocarcinoma in 181 curatively resected cases. *HPB (Oxford)*. 2021;**23**(10):1525–1532. DOI: 10.1016/j.hpb.2021.03.004
52. Sakai Y, Ohtsuka M, Sugiyama H, et al. Current status of diagnosis and therapy for intraductal papillary neoplasm of the bile duct. *World J Gastroenterol*. 2021;**27**(15):1569–1577. DOI: 10.3748/wjg.v27.i15.1569
53. Krawczyk M, Ziarkiewicz-Wroblewska B, Podgorska J, et al. Intraductal papillary neoplasm of the bile duct—a comprehensive review. *Adv Med Sci*. 2021;**66**(1):138–147. DOI: 10.1016/j.advms.2021.01.005
54. Delaney S, Zhou Y, Pawa S, Pawa R. Intraductal papillary neoplasm of the left hepatic duct treated with endoscopic retrograde cholangiopancreatography guided radiofrequency ablation. *Clin J Gastroenterol*. 2021;**14**(1):346–350. DOI: 10.1007/s12328-020-01284-4

Percutaneous biliary imaging and interventions

Mathilde Vermersch, Alban Denys, and Naik Vietti Violi

Introduction

Percutaneous bile duct imaging and interventions can be performed for various conditions and these allow for multiple diagnostic and therapeutic procedures. They require preprocedural planning including a knowledge of the patient's history, laboratory test results, and a review of the ongoing medications as well as evaluation of the indications, contraindications, and potential complications of each procedure. The large panel of bile duct interventions will be oriented depending upon the malignant or benign nature of the obstruction. These interventions can be performed by interventional radiologists alone or in collaboration with gastroenterologists as in the rendez-vous technique before surgery for biliary drainage in the context of a tumoural stricture.

Before the procedure

Intervention planning

Each intervention has proper indications and contraindications that have to be reviewed before any procedure is planned (Table 29.1). Coagulation abnormalities have to be checked and corrected if needed: according to the Cardiovascular and Interventional Radiological Society of Europe recommendations, the limits for biliary intervention are an international normalized ratio less than 1.5, activated partial thromboplastin time less than 60 seconds, prothrombin ratio greater than 50%, and platelet count greater than 50,000/mm^3.[1] While aspirin doses less than 100 mg can generally be continued, oral antiplatelet therapy has to be withhold 5 days before the intervention, and anticoagulant therapy has to be switched for fractionated heparin, withholding two doses for 24 hours before the intervention. Platelet transfusions are given if needed. For the newer anticoagulants, in the absence of strong evidence, the consensus is to wait for a time lapse of five half-lives of a particular agent.[2]

The presence of an anaesthesia team during the intervention is generally needed to ensure patient sedation, analgesia, and immobility. Moreover, haemodynamic surveillance and general anaesthesia are required in case of complex interventions potentially at risk of bleeding or septicaemia.[3] In these cases, a preprocedural visit by the anaesthetist and fasting are required.

As for all interventional radiology interventions, biliary procedures should be performed in an area close to the operative room with high attention to sterility. The Society of Interventional Radiology guidelines recommend prophylactic antibiotics for all patients undergoing percutaneous biliary drainage.[4] Biliary infections are due to *Escherichia coli* and *Clostridium* species in 75%, while *Enterococcus*, *Klebsiella*, and *Streptococcus* and various yeasts can also be found. While no consensus exists regarding the first choice of antibiotic, a beta-lactam or a third-generation cephalosporin are commonly used. Ampicillin and sulbactam are alternatives against *Enterococcus*. The antibiotic prophylaxis should be started before the procedure in order to get a sufficient intrabiliary concentration.

Except in case of emergency, the interventional radiologist should explain and discuss the details with the patient and obtain informed consent before the procedure.

Non-invasive imaging of the biliary tree

Before any percutaneous procedure, a precise revision of any previous imaging is required. These include ultrasound (US), computed tomography (CT), and magnetic resonance cholangiopancreatography (MRCP) and will allow the identification of any biliary tree anatomical variations and the procedure planning according to disease involvement. Furthermore, cross-sectional imaging, particularly MRCP, identifies the nature of the obstruction in more than 90%[5] of the cases. On imaging, benign obstructions are more likely to be regular, symmetrical, and involve short bile duct segments while malignant obstructions tend to be irregular, asymmetrical, and involve long segments. When cross-sectional imaging fails to find the nature of the obstruction, bile duct biopsy is required.

Additional to the nature of the obstruction, cross-sectional imaging helps to define the level of the obstruction which can be high or low. By definition, a high bile obstruction is located above or at the common hepatic duct while a low bile obstruction involves the common bile duct (e.g. below the insertion of the cystic duct). High biliary obstructions can be classified according to their

Table 29.1 Percutaneous biliary interventions—indications and contraindications

Procedure	Indications	Contraindications
PC	Anatomic characterization Diagnosis and disease extension	Coagulopathy Allergy to iodinated contrast media Massive ascites
Percutaneous transcatheter brush biopsy	Diagnose cause of biliary stricture	Coagulopathy Sepsis, cholangitis
PBD	Cholangitis Symptoms related to jaundice (pruritus, anorexia, nausea) Decrease serum bilirubin before chemotherapy Bile leak	Same as PC Multiple segmental or sub-segmental isolations (drainage unlikely to provide palliation except for pruritus)
Percutaneous balloon dilatation	Definitive treatment of benign strictures	Same as PBD Sepsis, cholangitis
Percutaneous metallic stent placement	Definitive treatment of malignant strictures Exclude bile leak	Same as PBD Sepsis, cholangitis Surgical candidates

PBD, percutaneous bile duct drainage; PC, percutaneous cholangiography.
Adapted with permission from Rocio Perez-Johnston, Amy R. Deipolyi, Anne M. Covey, 'Percutaneous Biliary Interventions', *Gastroenterology Clinics of North America*, Volume 47, Issue 3, 2018, pp 621–641.

extension using the Bismuth–Corlette classification. This classification was initially developed for treatment decisions in hilar cholangiocarcinomas.[6] Obstruction can also be classified according to its degree.[7] A *complete obstruction* is the isolation of one segment, without contrast passing through the obstruction. *Effective isolation* is when the isolated duct is opacified during cholangiography but not adequately drained. *Impending isolation* is when the segment is currently both opacified and drained but an occlusion is expected in the near future. Because of potential contamination of these ducts during cholangiography, both impending and effective isolated ducts are at risk of infection.

Interventions

Access

Biliary intervention can be done percutaneously with interventional radiology or endoscopically with endoscopic retrograde cholangiopancreatography (ERCP).[8]

Low obstructions are usually managed using ERCP as a single-stent placement can drain the entire bile tree. Percutaneous interventions are the second choice, reserved for situations where ERCP is contraindicated (postoperative conditions) or has not been successful. Conversely, the percutaneous approach is the first choice in case of high biliary obstructions for the following reasons: (1) it allows targeted biliary segment drainage and (2) compared to ERCP, percutaneous drainage does not necessarily disrupt the ampulla, allowing it to retain its sphincter function and isolate the bile tree from the enteric bacterial flora with a corresponding decreased risk of cholangitis. Additionally, the percutaneous approach allows sterile sampling of the bile while digestive germs will contaminate ERCP sampling. Of note is that not all dilated bile duct segments require drainage. For example, in case of chronic biliary obstruction, the liver parenchyma in the affected segment will develop atrophy.[9] Drainage of these segments has to be reserved for refractory cholangitis as the benefit in terms of liver function is low.

In the presence of ascites, the liver can be displaced from the abdominal wall, increasing the technical difficulty of the procedure and risk of complications (especially bleeding).[10] Further, there is a risk of ascitic leak from the percutaneous access site. Preprocedural paracentesis is an efficient but transitory solution. A left-sided biliary tree approach (anterior epigastric) is an alternative to avoid or decrease the volume of cutaneous ascites leak and reduce the risk of bleeding complications.

Percutaneous access to the biliary system is achieved via the creation of a parenchymal tract across the liver to access a peripheral bile duct under US or fluoroscopic guidance.[11] A 21 G styled needle is used to access a peripheral duct allowing introduction of a 0.018-inch guidewire into the biliary tree. The needle is then exchanged to a coaxial set and access has to be secured. According to the location of the obstruction, a left- or right-sided approach can be made. A right-sided approach is classically chosen for common hepatic or common bile duct obstruction as the majority of the bile is drained via the right-sided system. In case of a left-sided approach, US guidance is preferred. The access should be central enough to get stable access into the bile duct and easy access to the occlusion but as peripheral as possible to reduce the risk of arterial damage with consequent haemorrhagic complications. Once the puncture is made, bile can be collected and sent for bacteriological analysis if infection is suspected. During any bile duct intervention, attention has to be given to avoid over-distension on the biliary tract by limiting the opacification and introducing a catheter above the stenosis to reduce tension on the pre-stenotic segment.[11]

Percutaneous bile duct biopsy/brush

Bile duct tumours are generally too small to present specific radiological characteristics or to be targeted by percutaneous biopsy. They present with indirect signs of biliary obstruction. The differential diagnosis between a benign or malignant stricture is sometimes difficult, particularly in patients with chronic bile duct diseases such as primary stenosing cholangitis that can lead to either benign or malignant strictures. Consequently, a percutaneous approach is a reliable tool as it allows, in the same procedure, tissue sampling and release of the obstruction.

Tissue sampling can be performed using either brush cytology and forceps biopsy (Figure 29.1). Both techniques have a limited sensitivity, with a high variation between reports (26–92%).[12] The use of flow cytometry and fluorescent *in situ* hybridization has been proposed to increase the diagnostic performance of conventional cytology.[13] The consensus is to combine brush cytology and forceps biopsy in the same procedure and to consider repeating the procedure in case of a high suspicion of malignancy with negative cytology and biopsy results.

Percutaneous drainage

The technical success of biliary drainage is 70% and 95% for non-dilated and dilated bile ducts, respectively.[4] The first step for drainage consists of passing across the stenosis. Hydrophilic guidewires are used and the anatomy of the stenosis will then determine the choice between a curved or straight distal guidewire as well as its degree

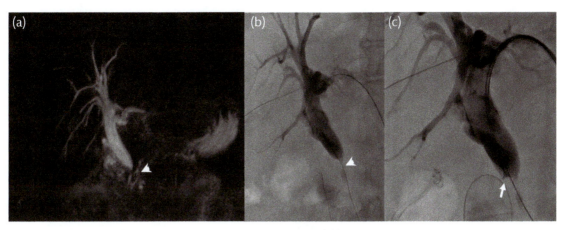

Figure 29.1 A 65-year-old woman with mass suspicion of the head of the pancreas. (a) MRI showed an important bile duct dilatation due to a stricture in the inferior third of the common bile duct (arrowhead). (b) Cholangiography performed after percutaneous puncture of bile duct confirmed the stenosis crossed by the guide (arrowhead). (c) A biopsy was performed using forceps biopsy confirming pancreatic adenocarcinoma (arrow).

of rigidity. Once passed, the guidewire is placed far away past the stenosis to ensure stability and dilatation of the stenosis can be performed with dilatators of increasing diameters or balloons to allow drainage. Opacification of the opposite side of the stenosis is useful to gain appropriate information for planning the following intervention. Evaluation of the entire biliary tree including the sphincter and the duodenum is useful to exclude a potential second stenosis along the biliary tree. The choice between drainage only or primary stent placement will depend on various elements including the cause and level of the stenosis, any evidence of infection in the bile duct, the presence of haemobilia, as well as the future therapeutic options (surgery or palliative management).[11]

Internal–external versus external drainage

Biliary drains are of two types, which differ in function and indications: external biliary drains (EBDs) or internal–external biliary drains (IEBDs).[7] The EBD is a catheter located in the biliary system which drains percutaneously into a bag. An IEBD has an external drain that extends into the biliary tree, distal to the occlusion until it reaches the bowel. The former preserves the competence of the ampulla and isolates the biliary tree from the bowel flora.

Compared to the IEBD, the EBD is more prone to dislocation and cannot be capped. With external drainage, the patient is at risk of excessive fluid loss leading to hypovolaemia and electrolyte disturbances. It is preferred in the following clinical conditions: (1) an obstruction cannot be passed at the time of drainage; (2) in cholangitis, an EBD can be preferred over an IEBD as it requires less manipulation; (3) where the obstruction has been relieved, an EBD can be left until effective drainage is confirmed (used as 'safety catheter').

The IEBD has the advantages of being more stable and allowing versatility of drain positioning. By capping the external drainage, physiological bile excretion is simulated. An IEBD is indicated in the following situations: (1) for initial biliary drainage when the diagnosis is not known; (2) preoperatively; (3) internal–external biliary drainage can be performed initially before internal drainage to decrease the bilirubin to a target level; (4) metallic stent occlusion; (5) in case of a bilioenteric anastomosis stenosis allowing progressive dilatation; and (6) access for local therapy (brachydynamic or photodynamic therapy).

Percutaneous bile duct dilatation

Once the stenosis has been crossed, bile duct dilatation can be performed using an angioplasty balloon. Of note is that balloon dilatation is contraindicated in case of active infection. In this situation, the dilatation should be performed once the infection is controlled. The balloon diameter should be at least the same as the bile duct before and after the stenosis. It is also possible to oversize it up to 25–30%. The balloon should be inflated in the middle of the stenosis. The criteria for the success of dilatation are spontaneous contrast passage and less than 20–30% residual stenosis.[14] An IEBD is then left for 2 weeks up to longer than 6 months according to each group.[15,16] The rate of restenosis is relatively high after dilatation, with at least 30% of patients requiring more than one treatment.[15] In case of repeated stenosis, a cutting balloon dilatation technique has been described which has shown improved results compared to a standard balloon dilatation.[17] These balloons have four longitudinal blades that can effectively incise scars or zones of fibrosis. Compared to standard balloons, no additional complications have been described. Balloon dilatation is not indicated in case of the stenosis of a recent (<1 month) postoperative bilioenteric anastomosis which is more likely due to oedema.

In case of a complex stricture, the collaboration of gastroenterologists may be needed to pass through the occlusion. The 'rendezvous technique' is a combination of percutaneous cholangiography and ERCP that is used in cases of complete bile duct obstruction (**Figure 29.2**). The concomitant antegrade and retrograde access facilities safe recanalization, with a decreased risk of bleeding and perforation.[18] In these procedures, a close collaboration between the interventional radiology and gastroenterology teams is mandatory.

Percutaneous stent placement

Percutaneous stents can be placed through a biliary obstruction in one procedure: a primary biliary stent (PS) or an IEBD can be initially placed with secondary conversion into a stent (SS), classically several weeks later (**Figure 29.3**). Initially, a safety stent is usually left in place and capped to ensure an adequate flow through the stent. In case there is suspicion of an inadequate flow (manifesting clinically with abdominal pain, fever or leakage), the safety catheter can be

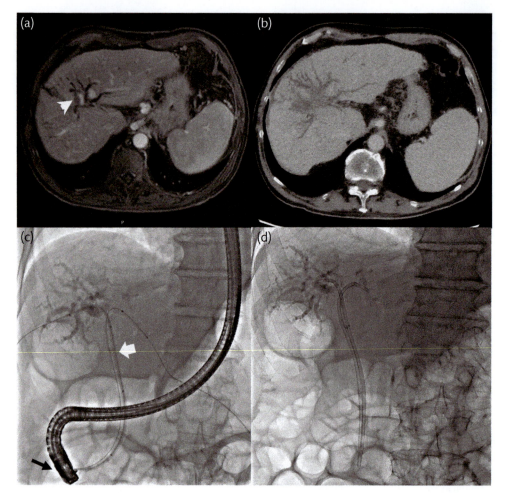

Figure 29.2 A 66-year-old man with biliary stenosis secondary to microwave thermal ablation close to biliary convergence. (a) MRI showed a left intrahepatic bile duct dilatation upstream to the thermoablation site (arrowhead). (b) Bile duct dilatation predominant on left upstream of the thermoablation site was also visible on CT scan with minimum intensity projection axial reconstruction. (c) Drainage using the rendezvous technique was decided for left and right drainage. An endoscope was placed in the second duodenum (black arrow), percutaneous puncture of the right and the left biliary ducts were performed and the wire guides introduced percutaneously were recovered by the endoscopist. Plastic stents were then inserted into the bile duct on the guides (white arrow). (d) Post procedural control was satisfactory.

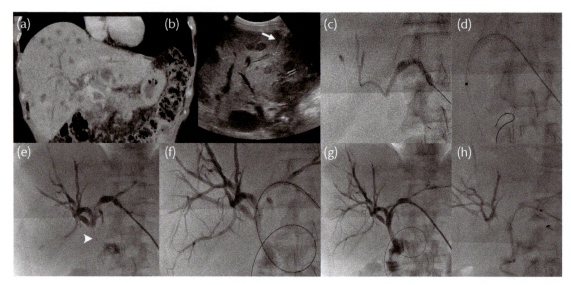

Figure 29.3 A 50-year-old man with adenocarcinoma in the head of the pancreas and multiple liver metastases responsible for a common bile duct stenosis. (a) Coronal reconstruction of a CT scan performed at portal venous phase showed intrahepatic bile duct dilatation. (b) Puncture of a distal left bile duct was performed under ultrasound using a 21 G needle (arrow). (c) Injection into the needle was made to confirm bile duct puncture. (d) A guidewire was pushed until the common bile duct and the sheath was introduced. (e) Cholangiography confirmed the stenosis (arrowhead). (f) A metallic stent was placed in the middle of the stenosis and (g) cholangiography confirmed its permeability. Finally, (h) an IEBD was placed into the stent to control the permeability 1 day later.

Postprocedural considerations

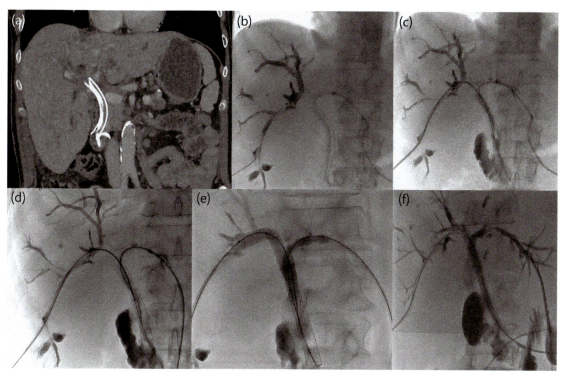

Figure 29.4 A 65-year-old man with adenocarcinoma in the head of the pancreas and liver metastases responsible for a bile duct dilatation. A stent was placed into the common bile duct and a left IEBD was left in place. Coronal reconstruction of a CT scan performed at portal venous phase showed right intrahepatic bile duct dilatation (a) and a decision was made to make a bilateral drainage. (b) Puncture of a distal right bile duct was performed and cholangiography confirmed central stenosis with isolation of both hepatic ducts. (c) A guide was passed through the stenosis and stent until the duodenum on both sides. (d) Y stenting was then performed: two stents were placed into both sides and (e) were dilated with balloon simultaneously. (f) Cholangiography confirmed the great permeability of the stents.

uncapped for external drainage. Additionally, the safety catheter can be used for contrast injection in order to perform diagnostic cholangiography allowing identification of cause for stent dysfunction that could include inadequate stent expansion, papillary dysfunction or inadequate bowel peristalsis. Safety stents can usually be removed 24 hours after placement.[19] Even if there is no consensus in favour of PS or SS regarding stent patency and patient survival,[20] compared to PS, SS has a higher rate of complications including haemobilia, cholangitis and sepsis.[21]

Metallic stents are indicated in patients with active malignancies and limited life expectancy or patients with no other acceptable alternative. Metallic stents can be bare or covered. Bare stents with narrow interstices are typically indicated in malignant conditions as they limit tumour in-growth, and decrease stent migration and the risk of cystic or pancreatic duct obstruction. However, bare stents are definitive: they cannot be changed. For this reason, when used in benign conditions, covered stents which can be changed and removed are preferred.[22] The changing and removal of a covered stent is done by ERCP and cannot be performed percutaneously. In case of stent occlusion, additional drainage is required. An additional stent or catheter can be placed. Sometimes, a new stent can be placed throughout the interstices of an occluded stent.

In case of central occlusion with the isolation of both hepatic ducts, bilateral drainage may be needed. Two different configurations can be performed: 'T' or 'Y' stenting. In a T-stenting configuration, two stents are placed from a single access: one is placed side to side (left to right) and the second one is placed down into the common bile duct or across the ampulla.[23] A Y-stenting configuration refers to stents side by side (right and left), parallel across the confluence. The Y configuration is the most preferred alternative in case of bilateral obstruction and allows easier reintervention in case of stent obstruction[24] (Figure 29.4).

Postprocedural considerations

Complications

Major complications of percutaneous biliary intervention include sepsis, haemorrhage, pleural transgression, and death. The rate of complications is between 3% and 10%.[10,25] Mortality rates range between 0.1% and 0.8%, mainly due to sepsis and haemorrhage.[26,27] The rate of complications has been shown to be higher in patients with non-dilated intrahepatic bile ducts.[10]

Haemorrhagic complications

Haemorrhagic complications can be divided according to their origin: arterial or venous. This will determine the degree of the emergency, as arterial bleeding requires immediate attention while venous or portal are usually self-limiting. Bleeding into the digestive system will not be evident immediately and manifest as melaena and a decrease in haemoglobin levels. Conversely, blood in the drainage bag can be seen easily and its colour (dark/bright red) can be helpful to differentiate the origin of the bleed.

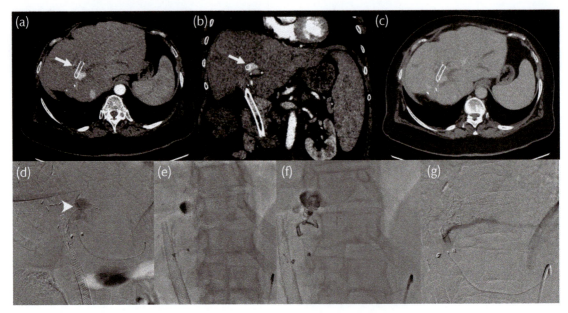

Figure 29.5 A 70-year-old woman with rectal adenocarcinoma with liver metastases. The patient benefited from right hepatectomy complicated with biliary stenosis which occurred due to tumoural invasion. A biliary stent was placed by endoscopy and the patient returned to the emergency department due to jaundice and a decrease in haemoglobin level. (a, b) A CT scan performed at arterial phase showed a pseudoaneurysm of the hepatic artery partially into the stent (arrow). (c) At portal venous phase, new dilatation of the intrahepatic bile duct secondary to stent occlusion by pseudoaneurysm was evident. (d) Arteriography confirmed the presence of a pseudoaneurysm (arrowhead). (e, f) The pseudoaneurysm and the upstream artery were progressively embolized using coils. (g) Arteriography confirmed the exclusion of the pseudoaneurysm.

Arterial bleeding

In case of arterial bleeding, a pseudoaneurysm or arterio-biliary fistula should be specifically searched for with cross-sectional imaging or arteriography as it is the main arterial complication. The management of a pseudoaneurysm or arterio-biliary fistula requires interventional radiology with intra-arterial access and coiling of the afferent artery (Figure 29.5).

Venous or portal bleeding

Due to the access through the liver, damage to the small portal or hepatic veins is almost inevitable. For this reason, a more peripheral access is always preferred in order to cross the smallest vessels possible. When a more central puncture is needed, the rate of complications is higher. Venous or portal haemorrhage occurs frequently when the drainage catheter moves backward and retracts along the liver track allowing a communication between the catheter and veins within the liver parenchyma. A secure sealed positioning of the catheter is important to prevent this complication and diagnostic cholangiography may help to identify the problem. Replacement of the catheter with adequate positioning and sealing is usually sufficient for peripheral venous bleeding while more central veins may require coil embolization. Upsizing the catheter to provide tamponade is also helpful.

Sepsis

Access to the biliary tree is a clean or contained procedure, depending on the patient's condition and careful asepsis should be maintained throughout. Cholangitis is largely an iatrogenic disease—the result of contamination of the biliary tree during the procedure. Sepsis is considered to be related to mechanical manipulation like biliary over-distension with contrast injection and bile duct to blood vessel connection due to the catheter tracking through the liver parenchyma. Aspiration through an IEBD should be avoided due to the risk of sepsis by contamination of the bile duct by the digestive contents. Biliary tree interventions have to be covered with preprocedural antibiotics with the goal of avoiding sepsis and shock. In case of signs of sepsis and shock (temperature >38° C, tachycardia (>90 bpm), hypotension (<90 mm Hg in systolic blood pressure or a drop of >40 mm Hg), increased respiratory rate), the control of the source of infection, broad-spectrum systemic antibiotic therapy, volume resuscitation, and cardiopulmonary support are appropriate measures. When sepsis persists despite antibiotic therapy, additional procedures should be considered to drain blocked or isolated ducts.[28]

Transpleural access to biliary system

Careful preprocedural planning should be done in order to avoid pleural transgression that can lead to bile in the thorax or a pneumothorax. Cutaneous puncture has to be located below the 10th to 11th intercostal space, at the mid-axillary line in order to avoid these complications. The puncture site should carefully controlled using US and/or fluoroscopic guidance. This position is also subject to limit the rate of tube retraction secondary to respiratory movements. In case of a bile leak into the thorax, the drain has to be left in place for 4–6 weeks in order to allow the formation of a fibrous track, avoiding the leak of bile into the chest. The patient will remain at risk of recurrence. Management of pneumothorax is conventional, by placing a chest tube in order to allow the lung to re-expand. See Figure 29.6.

Transcolonic access to biliary system

Careful preprocedural planning is helpful to avoid transcolonic access. If this occurs the patient will manifest with symptoms of colonic perforation and/or a pericolonic abscess. Cross-sectional imaging

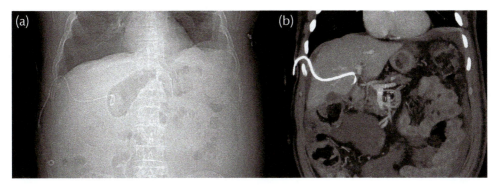

Figure 29.6 A 72-year-old man with adenocarcinoma of the head of the pancreas with bile duct occlusion and intrahepatic bile duct dilatation requiring drainage. After percutaneous drainage, the patient complained of thoracic pain. A chest X-ray was performed showing a suspicious transpleural biliary drain (a), and was confirmed with CT showing transpleural passage of the biliary drain responsible for a bilothorax (b). The drain was then removed and another percutaneous drainage using an inferior access was performed.

will help confirm the diagnosis. Management of transcolonic access is surgical with early or delayed segmental colonic resection. Immediate drain removal is contraindicated because of the risk of a fistula.

Tube displacement

Biliary catheter displacement or retraction will manifest most often with bleeding or bile leak from the cutaneous access site. A tube displacement before formation of a fibrous track is a risk for a biliary leak into the peritoneal cavity with subsequent biliary peritonitis. Early recognition of tube displacement can be corrected by introducing a guidewire and changing the drain. When it is not possible, a new biliary access procedure should be performed.

Catheter occlusion

Catheter occlusion usually manifests either with infection or with bile leak from the cutaneous access site. Flushing the catheter with saline can clear the obstruction. Using a guidewire or changing catheters are other options.

Postprocedural follow-up

The first aim of postprocedural management is to explain and teach biliary drain management to the patient and his or her caregivers. Particular attention should be paid to an early detection of complications. The biliary drain should be flushed using saline twice a day and the catheter may be changed routinely every 8–12 weeks.

Indications for bile duct interventions

Malignant biliary obstruction

When a tumour grows and obstructs bile duct flow, at any point from the liver to bowel, it is a malignant bile duct obstruction (Figure 29.7). This manifests as jaundice, pruritus, and alcoholic stools, leading to significant morbidity and mortality as well as a negative impact on the quality of life.[29] The most frequent causes of a malignant biliary obstruction are secondary to cholangiocarcinoma, gall bladder cancer, pancreatic cancer, or metastatic disease.

Cholangiocarcinoma can be divided in three types: distal, perihilar, and intrahepatic.[30] The distal type is the most frequent constituting 40–60% of the total, while the perihilar type represents 30–50% of cases and the intrahepatic type 10%.[31]

Bile duct biopsy

Cross-sectional imaging does not always allow differentiation between malignant and benign bile duct occlusion. In these cases, biopsy is required to make a diagnosis. This can be done using different techniques: bile cytology, bile duct brush biopsy, and forceps biopsy. The latter two are specially indicated in case of suspicion of a cholangiocarcinoma or an intraluminal metastasis. Both techniques have a sensitivity ranging from 40% to 70% meaning that a negative biopsy does not exclude a diagnosis and a repeat biopsy is often needed until the diagnosis is established.[40]

When occlusion is not associated with a mass lesion, percutaneous fine needle aspiration can be performed using a notched needle directed to the stricture. The sensitivity of fine needle aspiration has been reported to be higher than brush biopsy (77% vs 44%, respectively), making this technique an alternative when the first biopsy is inconclusive.[41] The main concern of this technique is the risk of complications related to the structures crossed while targeting the lesion; however, initial reports do not describe a high complication rate with fine needle biopsy.[41]

Preoperative drainage

Preoperative drainage in surgical candidates with malignant bile duct obstruction is controversial. It was initially thought that preoperative drainage allowed reduction of inflammation, improvement of liver function, reduction in postoperative complications, and improvement in outcome.[32] However, further evaluation including meta-analysis and prospective series evidenced either no difference or even worse outcomes in patients with preoperative drainage including a longer postoperative hospital stay[33] and higher rate of serious adverse events due to bile contamination.[34] When performed, percutaneous drainage has shown a lower morbidity compared to the endoscopic approach.[35] In addition to the risk of bleeding and infection, tumour spread by seeding along the catheter has been reported in up to 3.8% of patients after an R0 resection.[36] In all cases, if the tumour is surgically resectable, a metallic stent is contraindicated because it cannot be removed. If preoperative drainage is necessary, only percutaneous IEBD or an endoscopic plastic stent should be deployed.

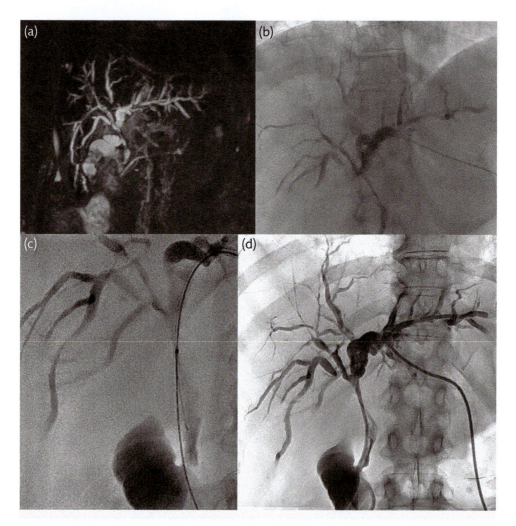

Figure 29.7 A 62-year-old woman with intrahepatic bile duct dilatation, suspicious for cholangiocarcinoma. (a) MRI showed common bile duct stenosis with intrahepatic bile duct dilatation predominant on left side. After percutaneous puncture of the left branch (b), a cytobrush was advanced to the stenosis to make a cytology (c). An IEBD was then placed. (d) Final cholangiography showed multifocal disease. Cytology was revealed to be positive for cholangiocarcinoma.

Inoperable tumour

In patients with unresectable tumours, the palliative options are surgical bypass, percutaneous drainage or stenting, and endoscopic stenting. The former is associated with a higher duration of patency compared to the two non-surgical options.[37] However, due to perioperative morbidity and mortality as well as an impact on the quality of life of patients with advanced cancer, a less invasive procedure with a shorter hospital stay is often the best option.

The Bismuth classification of obstructions is useful for the treatment option decision: unless there is a contraindication, Bismuth I and II are treated using ERCP given its less invasive nature. In Bismuth III and IV, a percutaneous approach is indicated as it has shown a higher success rate than ERCP, with a lower risk of cholangitis and no difference in terms of pancreatitis, overall complications, and 30-day mortality.[38,39]

Benign biliary obstruction

Benign bile duct stricture

The most common cause of a benign bile duct stricture is related to an operative procedure[42] (Figure 29.8). The treatment option in this benign condition is bile duct dilatation using a balloon and/or a stent. Low bile duct strictures without bilioenteric anastomoses are treated via ERCP while high bile duct strictures and patients with bilioenteric anastomoses are treated percutaneously.

In short segment strictures, involving the main bile duct, balloon dilatation has been shown to be the first option as short-term patency is around 90% while the long-term patency rate is up to 74%.[15,43,44] Peripheral, long segment strictures, post surgical anastomotic oedema are less likely to respond to balloon dilatation. Other strategies should then be considered.[42]

Biliary stones

ERCP is the first choice of treatment for the extraction of stones in the bile duct (Figure 29.9). The percutaneous approach should be reserved for patients with biliopancreatic anastomoses or other contraindications to ERCP, intrahepatic stones, large impacted stones, or after ERCP failure.[45] Two kinds of stones have to be differentiated as their management differs: intraductal stones are the result of stasis in the hepatic duct secondary to distal obstruction and are pigment or brown stones.[46] These stones are not calcified. They can be removed by balloon maceration, retrieval by basket and a choledoscope, or by sweeping after duct stricture dilatation. On the other hand, calcified biliary stones arise from gall bladder. Due to their calcified

Indications for bile duct interventions | 331

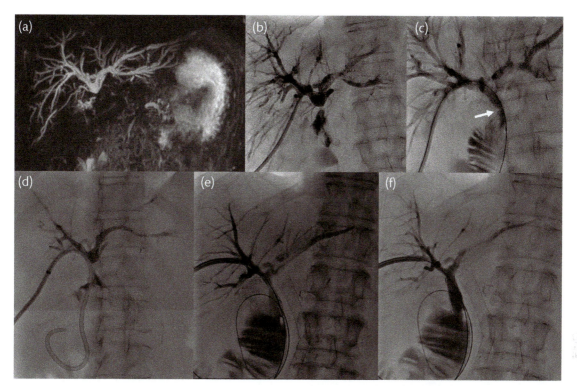

Figure 29.8 A 61-year-old woman with postoperative status after pancreaticoduodenectomy with biliary–enteric anastomosis. The patient was admitted for multiple episodes of cholangitis. (a) MRI showed bile duct stenosis at the level of the anastomosis. (b) Cholangiography performed after percutaneous puncture of bile duct confirmed the stenosis. Percutaneous bile duct dilatation was initially performed. (c) A balloon was inflated in the middle of the stenosis and the stricture was clearly visible during dilatation (arrow). (d) An IEBD was then placed for 6 months. Due to persistence of stenosis at 6 months, a stent was placed through biliary obstruction. (e) Persistence of stenosis was visible when the stent was placed. (f) Dilatation of the stent with balloon was then performed allowing an adequate flow through the stent. Note that the second stent visible on the images (d), (e), and (f) is a portal stent for portal recanalization.

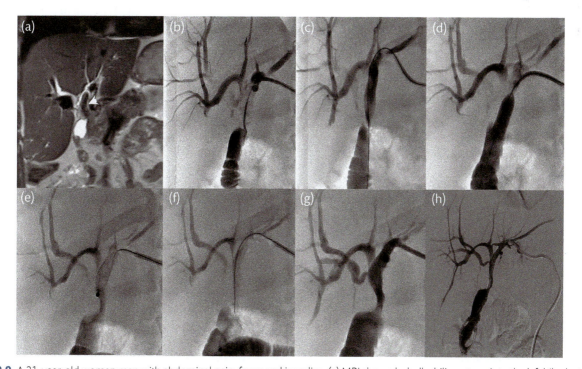

Figure 29.9 A 31-year-old woman man with abdominal pain, fever, and jaundice. (a) MRI showed a bulky biliary stone into the left bile duct (arrowhead). (b) Cholangiography performed after percutaneous puncture of the left bile duct confirmed biliary stones into the left and the common biliary ducts. (c, d) First, a balloon was used to push the stones from the bile duct to the duodenum thanks to a back-and-forth movement (Fogarty technique). Unfortunately, a balloon was not sufficient to remove the bulky biliary stone. (e, f) Then, a Dormia catheter was used to pick the stone and release it into the duodenum. (g) Immediate control after the procedure was satisfactory and the IEBD was left in place. (h) Cholangiography performed 2 days later confirmed the absence of a residual biliary stone and resolution of bile duct dilatation.

composition, they cannot be macerated. When measuring less than 5 mm they can be swept into the duodenum after dilating the distal obstruction. Stones 5–10 mm in size required papillotomy, which can be performed percutaneously using an 8 mm diameter angioplasty balloon.[47] Larger stones are removed after fragmentation performed by litotrispy.[45]

Percutaneous biliary stone removal has a success rate of 90% for common bile duct stones and 60% for intrahepatic stones. Large or multiple stones may require multiple removal sessions. The main causes of treatment failure are impacted stones, intrahepatic ductal strictures, and an inability to fragment the stones. The rate of complication is 6.8%, mainly sepsis and perihepatic bilioma.[48]

Chronic pancreatitis and choledocholithiasis

Pancreatitis is a frequent cause of bile duct stricture, which is found in up to 46% of patients with chronic pancreatitis. The most frequently affected location is the intrapancreatic portion of the common bile duct.[49] Signs of chronic pancreatitis such as pancreatic calcification, parenchymal atrophy, or ductal dilatation suggest the origin. In this context, the appearance of a new bile duct dilatation has to be considered with high suspicion of pancreatic cancer before concluding that it is due to chronic pancreatitis.

Obstruction related to choledocholithiasis can be secondary to the presence of the stone itself or to a stricture developed secondary to chronic obstruction leading to scarring or fibrosis.[50]

Whatever the cause, these obstructions are generally in the distal bile duct and the obstruction should be handled with ERCP being the first choice. Percutaneous intervention will be reserved in case of ERCP failure or a complex situation such as that following a bilioenteric anastomosis.

Primary sclerosing cholangitis

Primary sclerosing cholangitis is a chronic progressive disease that manifests as serial alternating strictures and dilatations along the intra- and extrahepatic biliary tree.[51] One-half of the patients will develop a dominant stricture during the course of the disease. When it happens, the diagnostic differential is critical as it can be due to cholangiocarcinoma or a sequela of cholangitis and stone disease.[52] The first imaging tool for diagnosis is MRCP. ERCP is the first choice for patients who require intervention, while the percutaneous approach is considered in case of ERCP failure.

IgG4-related sclerosing cholangitis

IgG4-related sclerosing cholangitis is part of the spectrum of IgG4-related diseases which include autoimmune pancreatitis, retroperitoneal fibrosis, and sialadenitis. A high value of IgG4-positive plasma cell infiltrate and the presence of retroperitoneal fibrosis are diagnostic. Imaging characteristics include one of the following patterns: (1) distal strictures, (2) diffuse intra- and extrahepatic strictures, (3) hilar and distal common bile duct strictures, and (4) isolated hilar strictures.[53] The need for percutaneous intervention will depend on each pattern and the degree of disease involvement. Intervention is only considered a second choice after medical treatment which is sufficient in the most cases.

Post-liver transplant biliary complications

Biliary complications, mainly leaks and strictures, occur in 22–33% of patients after liver transplantation.[54,55] Leaks are treated with drainage allowing healing of the breach. Bile strictures are seen in 15–18% of cases and are classified according to their location: anastomotic or non-anastomotic.[54,55] Anastomotic strictures are related to tension at the surgical anastomosis, ischaemia, or duct size mismatch between the donor and recipient. Non-anastomotic strictures are secondary to ischaemia inducing multifocal strictures along the biliary tree. The main causes are a compromised arterial flow (due to stenosis or thrombosis), prolonged cold ischaemia before liver transplantation, infection, rejection, or recurrent primary sclerosing cholangitis.[56]

MRCP is the imaging tool of choice for diagnosis of post-liver transplant biliary complications with a reported sensitivity of 96% and specificity of 94%.[57] Treatment options include balloon dilatation and stent placement. Because of the postoperative status with Roux-en-Y anastomosis, the percutaneous approach is usually indicated. This is effective in treating post-liver transplant biliary strictures with 1- and 3-year patency rates of 94% and 45% after balloon dilatation, respectively, with a better outcome for non-ischaemic compared to ischaemic strictures.[58] In this setting, a knowledge of the exact post-surgical status is important to decide the best management option and be aware of contraindications for the endoscopic approach.[59]

Infection

HIV cholangiopathy is seen in patients with CD4 counts less than 100 cells/mm^3 and considered to be a type of sclerosing cholangitis. Associated opportunistic infection (cytomegalovirus or *Cryptosporidium*) can also contribute to biliary inflammation. Manifestations can be similar to primary sclerosing cholangitis with multiple intra- and extrahepatic strictures, isolated long extrahepatic stenosis, or ampullary stenosis.[60]

Recurrent pyogenic cholangitis is seen in patients with chronic parasitic or Gram-negative infection. Additional environmental factors such as malnutrition seem to be contributory. It is prevalent almost exclusively in Southeast Asia. In patients with this condition, multiple intrahepatic strictures are associated with intraductal pigment stones. The strictures are usually located in the posterior segment of the right lobe or the lateral segment of the left lobe.[61] Complications include abscesses, fistulae, and bilomas.

Iatrogenic bile duct injuries

Iatrogenic bile duct injuries are infrequent but serious complications after hepatobiliary surgery or abdominal trauma[62] (Figure 29.10). Interdisciplinary management of these patients is required with interventional radiology playing a central role in their diagnosis, classification, and treatment for mainly biliary leaks.

The most common leak locations are from the cystic duct or ducts of Luschka (accessory subvesicular bile ducts) after cholecystectomy, the biliary anastomosis after liver transplantation, and surgical bed in partial hepatectomy with extended left hepatectomy and caudate lobe resection.[63]

The diagnosis is made using cross-sectional imaging that demonstrates a perihepatic fluid collection. In case of doubt or to help locate the leak, an MRI using liver-specific contrast (gadoxetic acid, Eovist/Primovist, Bayer) can be performed with acquisition of the hepatobiliary phase where contrast will opacify the biliary tree.[64]

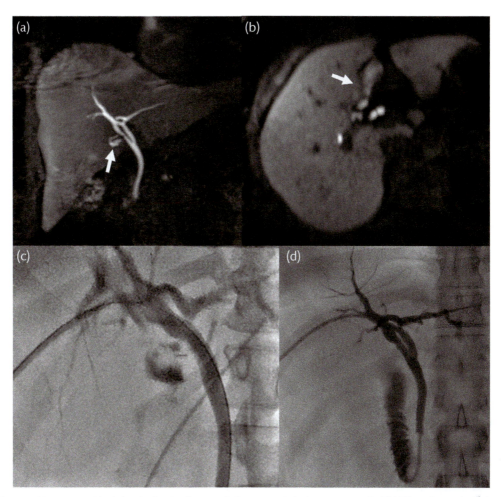

Figure 29.10 A 32-year-old woman with abdominal pain after gastric bypass and cholecystectomy. (a, b) MRI performed with intravenous injection of gadoxetic acid (Primovist/Eovist) at hepatobiliary phase showed leakage of contrast agent (arrow) due to a common bile duct injury. (c) Cholangiography performed after percutaneous puncture of the right bile duct confirmed contrast leakage. An IEBD was placed. (d) A control at 2 months with IEBD showed that the injury was resolved and no leakage was observed on cholangiography.

Minor leaks usually resolve with conservative management. Leaks of greater magnitude will require drainage of bilomas and biliary diversion, usually performed in a two-stage approach: first drainage and control of the biloma, then biliary diversion. In refractory leaks, the duct can be sclerosed with ethanol or cyanoacrylate.[65]

Drainage of the gall bladder

Gall bladder puncture is done under ultrasound control. After catheter placement, bile can be collected for bacteriological analysis and the drainage catheter is left in place for 3 weeks. A trans-hepatic access is recommended in order to prevent the risk of biliary leakage.[66] Complications are usually minor and have been described in 3–13%. The main ones are pain or catheter migration. Major complications as haemorrhage, bile peritonitis, or pneumothorax have also been described (<5%).[67] To limit haemorrhage, a 8 Fr diameter drain is recommended.

The main indications for percutaneous gall bladder drainage are acalculous cholecystitis in intensive care unit patients, gallstone cholecystitis in non-operable patients, and cholecystitis secondary to cystic duct occlusion (mostly secondary to tumour involvement).

In order to avoid bile leakage after drain retrieval, track maturation is essential so at least 3 weeks of drainage is needed.[66]

Future directions

Current research on malignant biliary obstruction focuses on suppressing local tumour growth thus reducing stent occlusion rate and improving survival. A few groups have presented results on intraductal radiofrequency ablation and shown that the technique is safe and seems to improve long-term patency of self-expanding metallic stents. This needs to be confirmed in a larger series.[68–71] Another approach is to place drug-coated self-expanding metallic stents with the aim of providing a local anti-tumoural effect to prevent obstruction from tumour growth.[72]

Conclusion

Percutaneous biliary access allows a large variety of interventions including diagnosis, drainage, dilatation, and stenting of bile duct tree and gall bladder. Careful pre-procedure planning is essential in order to improve technical success and to limit the risk of potential life-threatening complications. Percutaneous bile duct interventions are now part of patient management in a large range of benign and malignant conditions from cure to palliation.

REFERENCES

1. Patel IJ, Davidson JC, Nikolic B, et al. Consensus guidelines for periprocedural management of coagulation status and hemostasis risk in percutaneous image-guided interventions. *J Vasc Interv Radiol*. 2012;**23**(6):727–736.
2. Patel IJ, Davidson JC, Nikolic B, et al. Addendum of newer anticoagulants to the SIR consensus guideline. *J Vasc Interv Radiol*. 2013;**24**(5):641–645.
3. Wang L, Yu WF. Obstructive jaundice and perioperative management. *Acta Anaesthesiol Taiwan*. 2014;**52**(1):22–29.
4. Burke DR, Lewis CA, Cardella JF, et al. Quality improvement guidelines for percutaneous transhepatic cholangiography and biliary drainage. *J Vasc Interv Radiol*. 2003;**14**(9 Pt 2):S243–S2436.
5. Suthar M, Purohit S, Bhargav V, Goyal P. Role of MRCP in differentiation of benign and malignant causes of biliary obstruction. *J Clin Diagn Res*. 2015;**9**(11):TC08–TC12.
6. Bismuth H, Corlette MB. Intrahepatic cholangioenteric anastomosis in carcinoma of the hilus of the liver. *Surg Gynecol Obstet*. 1975;**140**(2):170–178.
7. Perez-Johnston R, Deipolyi AR, Covey AM. Percutaneous biliary interventions. *Gastroenterol Clin North Am*. 2018;**47**(3):621–641.
8. Duan F, Cui L, Bai Y, Li X, Yan J, Liu X. Comparison of efficacy and complications of endoscopic and percutaneous biliary drainage in malignant obstructive jaundice: a systematic review and meta-analysis. *Cancer Imaging*. 2017;**17**(1):27.
9. Hann LE, Getrajdman GI, Brown KT, et al. Hepatic lobar atrophy: association with ipsilateral portal vein obstruction. *AJR Am J Roentgenol* 1996;**167**(4):1017–1021.
10. Weber A, Gaa J, Rosca B, et al. Complications of percutaneous transhepatic biliary drainage in patients with dilated and nondilated intrahepatic bile ducts. *Eur J Radiol*. 2009;**72**(3):412–417.
11. Brown KT, Covey AM. Management of malignant biliary obstruction. *Tech Vasc Interv Radiol*. 2008;**11**(1):43–50.
12. Boos J, Yoo RJ, Steinkeler J, et al. Fluoroscopic percutaneous brush cytology, forceps biopsy and both in tandem for diagnosis of malignant biliary obstruction. *Eur Radiol*. 2018;**28**(2):522–529.
13. Singh A, Gelrud A, Agarwal B. Biliary strictures: diagnostic considerations and approach. *Gastroenterol Rep (Oxf)*. 2015;**3**(1):22–31.
14. Kapoor BS, Mauri G, Lorenz JM. Management of biliary strictures: state-of-the-art review. *Radiology*. 2018;**289**(3):590–603.
15. Cantwell CP, Pena CS, Gervais DA, Hahn PF, Dawson SL, Mueller PR. Thirty years' experience with balloon dilation of benign postoperative biliary strictures: long-term outcomes. *Radiology*. 2008;**249**(3):1050–1057.
16. Savader SJ, Cameron JL, Lillemoe KD, Lund GB, Mitchell SE, Venbrux AC. The biliary manometric perfusion test and clinical trial—long-term predictive value of success after treatment of bile duct strictures: ten-year experience. *J Vasc Interv Radiol*. 1998;**9**(6):976–985.
17. Saad WE, Davies MG, Saad NE, et al. Transhepatic dilation of anastomotic biliary strictures in liver transplant recipients with use of a combined cutting and conventional balloon protocol: technical safety and efficacy. *J Vasc Interv Radiol*. 2006;**17**(5):837–843.
18. Bukhari MA, Haito-Chavez Y, Ngamruengphong S, Brewer Gutierrez O, Chen YI, Khashab MA. Rendezvous biliary recanalization of complete biliary obstruction with direct peroral and percutaneous transhepatic cholangioscopy. *Gastroenterology*. 2018;**154**(1):23–25.
19. Thornton RH, Frank BS, Covey AM, et al. Catheter-free survival after primary percutaneous stenting of malignant bile duct obstruction. *AJR Am J Roentgenol*. 2011;**197**(3):W514–W518.
20. Inal M, Aksungur E, Akgul E, Oguz M, Seydaoglu G. Percutaneous placement of metallic stents in malignant biliary obstruction: one-stage or two-stage procedure? Pre-dilate or not? *Cardiovasc Intervent Radiol*. 2003;**26**(1):40–45.
21. Chatzis N, Pfiffner R, Glenck M, Stolzmann P, Pfammatter T, Sharma P. Comparing percutaneous primary and secondary biliary stenting for malignant biliary obstruction: a retrospective clinical analysis. *Indian J Radiol Imaging*. 2013;**23**(1):38–45.
22. Venbrux AC, Osterman FA, Jr. Percutaneous management of benign biliary strictures. *Tech Vasc Interv Radiol*. 2001;**4**(3):141–146.
23. Karnabatidis D, Spiliopoulos S, Katsakiori P, Romanos O, Katsanos K, Siablis D. Percutaneous trans-hepatic bilateral biliary stenting in Bismuth IV malignant obstruction. *World J Hepatol*. 2013;**5**(3):114–119.
24. Chandrashekhara SH, Gamanagatti S, Singh A, Bhatnagar S. Current status of percutaneous transhepatic biliary drainage in palliation of malignant obstructive jaundice: a review. *Indian J Palliat Care*. 2016;**22**(4):378–387.
25. Altekruse SF, Henley SJ, Cucinelli JE, McGlynn KA. Changing hepatocellular carcinoma incidence and liver cancer mortality rates in the United States. *Am J Gastroenterol*. 2014;**109**(4):542–553.
26. Smith TP, Ryan JM, Niklason LE. Sepsis in the interventional radiology patient. *J Vasc Interv Radiol*. 2004;**15**(4):317–325.
27. Halpenny DF, Torreggiani WC. The infectious complications of interventional radiology based procedures in gastroenterology and hepatology. *J Gastrointestin Liver Dis*. 2011;**20**(1):71–75.
28. Yarmohammadi H, Covey AM. Percutaneous biliary interventions and complications in malignant bile duct obstruction. *Chin Clin Oncol*. 2016;**5**(5):68.
29. Sauvanet A, Boher JM, Paye F, et al. Severe jaundice increases early severe morbidity and decreases long-term survival after pancreaticoduodenectomy for pancreatic adenocarcinoma. *J Am Coll Surg*. 2015;**221**(2):380–389.
30. Razumilava N, Gores GJ. Classification, diagnosis, and management of cholangiocarcinoma. *Clin Gastroenterol Hepatol*. 2013;**11**(1):13–21.
31. DeOliveira ML, Cunningham SC, Cameron JL, et al. Cholangiocarcinoma: thirty-one-year experience with 564 patients at a single institution. *Ann Surg*. 2007;**245**(5):755–762.
32. Denning DA, Ellison EC, Carey LC. Preoperative percutaneous transhepatic biliary decompression lowers operative morbidity in patients with obstructive jaundice. *Am J Surg*. 1981;**141**(1):61–65.
33. Pitt HA, Gomes AS, Lois JF, Mann LL, Deutsch LS, Longmire WP, Jr. Does preoperative percutaneous biliary drainage reduce operative risk or increase hospital cost? *Ann Surg*. 1985;**201**(5):545–553.
34. Fang Y, Gurusamy KS, Wang Q, et al. Pre-operative biliary drainage for obstructive jaundice. *Cochrane Database Syst Rev*. 2012;**9**:CD005444.
35. Al Mahjoub A, Menahem B, Fohlen A, et al. Preoperative biliary drainage in patients with resectable perihilar cholangiocarcinoma: is percutaneous transhepatic biliary drainage safer and more effective than endoscopic biliary drainage? a meta-analysis. *J Vasc Interv Radiol*. 2017;**28**(4):576–582.
36. Kim KM, Park JW, Lee JK, Lee KH, Lee KT, Shim SG. A comparison of preoperative biliary drainage methods for perihilar cholangiocarcinoma: endoscopic versus percutaneous transhepatic biliary drainage. *Gut Liver*. 2015;**9**(6):791–799.

37. Wongkonkitsin N, Phugkhem A, Jenwitheesuk K, Saeseow OT, Bhudhisawasdi V. Palliative surgical bypass versus percutaneous transhepatic biliary drainage on unresectable hilar cholangiocarcinoma. *J Med Assoc Thai*. 2006;**89**(11):1890–1895.
38. Choi J, Ryu JK, Lee SH, et al. Biliary drainage for obstructive jaundice caused by unresectable hepatocellular carcinoma: the endoscopic versus percutaneous approach. *Hepatobiliary Pancreat Dis Int*. 2012;**11**(6):636–642.
39. Moole H, Dharmapuri S, Duvvuri A, et al. Endoscopic versus percutaneous biliary drainage in palliation of advanced malignant hilar obstruction: a meta-analysis and systematic review. *Can J Gastroenterol Hepatol*. 2016;**2016**:4726078.
40. Tapping CR, Byass OR, Cast JE. Cytological sampling versus forceps biopsy during percutaneous transhepatic biliary drainage and analysis of factors predicting success. *Cardiovasc Intervent Radiol*. 2012;**35**(4):883–889.
41. Gonzalez-Aguirre A, Covey AM, Brown KT, et al. Comparison of biliary brush biopsy and fine needle biopsy in the diagnosis of biliary strictures. *Minim Invasive Ther Allied Technol*. 2018;**27**(5):278–283.
42. Fidelman N. Benign biliary strictures: diagnostic evaluation and approaches to percutaneous treatment. *Tech Vasc Interv Radiol*. 2015;**18**(4):210–217.
43. Kocher M, Cerna M, Havlik R, Kral V, Gryga A, Duda M. Percutaneous treatment of benign bile duct strictures. *Eur J Radiol*. 2007;**62**(2):170–174.
44. Janssen JJ, van Delden OM, van Lienden KP, et al. Percutaneous balloon dilatation and long-term drainage as treatment of anastomotic and nonanastomotic benign biliary strictures. *Cardiovasc Intervent Radiol*. 2014;**37**(6):1559–1567.
45. Copelan A, Kapoor BS. Choledocholithiasis: diagnosis and management. *Tech Vasc Interv Radiol*. 2015;**18**(4):244–255.
46. Carey MC. Pathogenesis of gallstones. *Recenti Prog Med* 1992;**83**(7–8):379–391.
47. Stokes KR, Clouse ME. Biliary duct stones: percutaneous transhepatic removal. *Cardiovasc Intervent Radiol* 1990;**13**(4):240–244.
48. Ozcan N, Kahriman G, Mavili E. Percutaneous transhepatic removal of bile duct stones: results of 261 patients. *Cardiovasc Intervent Radiol*. 2012;**35**(3):621–627.
49. Abdallah AA, Krige JE, Bornman PC. Biliary tract obstruction in chronic pancreatitis. *HPB (Oxford)*. 2007;**9**(6):421–428.
50. Shi EC, Ham JM. Benign biliary strictures associated with chronic pancreatitis and gallstones. *Aust N Z J Surg*. 1980;**50**(5):488–492.
51. Tischendorf JJ, Hecker H, Kruger M, Manns MP, Meier PN. Characterization, outcome, and prognosis in 273 patients with primary sclerosing cholangitis: a single center study. *Am J Gastroenterol*. 2007;**102**(1):107–114.
52. Chapman R, Fevery J, Kalloo A, et al. Diagnosis and management of primary sclerosing cholangitis. *Hepatology*. 2010;**51**(2):660–678.
53. Nakazawa T, Ohara H, Sano H, Ando T, Joh T. Schematic classification of sclerosing cholangitis with autoimmune pancreatitis by cholangiography. *Pancreas*. 2006;**32**(2):229.
54. Llado L, Fabregat J, Baliellas C, et al. Surgical treatment of biliary tract complications after liver transplantation. *Transplant Proc*. 2012;**44**(6):1557–1559.
55. Gunawansa N, McCall JL, Holden A, Plank L, Munn SR. Biliary complications following orthotopic liver transplantation: a 10-year audit. *HPB (Oxford)*. 2011;**13**(6):391–399.
56. Buis CI, Verdonk RC, Van der Jagt EJ, et al. Nonanastomotic biliary strictures after liver transplantation, part 1: radiological features and risk factors for early vs. late presentation. *Liver Transpl*. 2007;**13**(5):708–718.
57. Jorgensen JE, Waljee AK, Volk ML, et al. Is MRCP equivalent to ERCP for diagnosing biliary obstruction in orthotopic liver transplant recipients? A meta-analysis. *Gastrointest Endosc*. 2011;**73**(5):955–962.
58. Giampalma E, Renzulli M, Mosconi C, Ercolani G, Pinna AD, Golfieri R. Outcome of post-liver transplant ischemic and nonischemic biliary stenoses treated with percutaneous interventions: the Bologna experience. *Liver Transpl*. 2012;**18**(2):177–187.
59. Llado L, Figueras J. Techniques of orthotopic liver transplantation. *HPB (Oxford)*. 2004;**6**(2):69–75.
60. Bilgin M, Balci NC, Erdogan A, Momtahen AJ, Alkaade S, Rau WS. Hepatobiliary and pancreatic MRI and MRCP findings in patients with HIV infection. *AJR Am J Roentgenol*. 2008;**191**(1):228–232.
61. Jain M, Agarwal A. MRCP findings in recurrent pyogenic cholangitis. *Eur J Radiol*. 2008;**66**(1):79–83.
62. Flum DR, Cheadle A, Prela C, Dellinger EP, Chan L. Bile duct injury during cholecystectomy and survival in Medicare beneficiaries. *JAMA*. 2003;**290**(16):2168–2173.
63. Sakamoto K, Tamesa T, Yukio T, Tokuhisa Y, Maeda Y, Oka M. Risk factors and managements of bile leakage after hepatectomy. *World J Surg*. 2016;**40**(1):182–189.
64. Camacho JC, Coursey-Moreno C, Telleria JC, Aguirre DA, Torres WE, Mittal PK. Nonvascular post-liver transplantation complications: from US screening to cross-sectional and interventional imaging. *Radiographics*. 2015;**35**(1):87–104.
65. Carrafiello G, Ierardi AM, Piacentino F, Cardim LN. Percutaneous transhepatic embolization of biliary leakage with N-butyl cyanoacrylate. *Indian J Radiol Imaging*. 2012;**22**(1):19–22.
66. Hatzidakis A, Venetucci P, Krokidis M, Iaccarino V. Percutaneous biliary interventions through the gallbladder and the cystic duct: what radiologists need to know. *Clin Radiol*. 2014;**69**(12):1304–1311.
67. Ginat D, Saad WE. Cholecystostomy and transcholecystic biliary access. *Tech Vasc Interv Radiol*. 2008;**11**(1):2–13.
68. Laleman W, van der Merwe S, Verbeke L, et al. A new intraductal radiofrequency ablation device for inoperable biliopancreatic tumors complicated by obstructive jaundice: the IGNITE-1 study. *Endoscopy*. 2017;**49**(10):977–982.
69. Acu B, Kurtulus Ozturk E. Feasibility and safety of percutaneous transhepatic endobiliary radiofrequency ablation as an adjunct to biliary stenting in malignant biliary obstruction. *Diagn Interv Imaging*. 2018;**99**(4):237–245.
70. Alis H, Sengoz C, Gonenc M, Kalayci MU, Kocatas A. Endobiliary radiofrequency ablation for malignant biliary obstruction. *Hepatobiliary Pancreat Dis Int*. 2013;**12**(4):423–427.
71. Dolak W, Schreiber F, Schwaighofer H, et al. Endoscopic radiofrequency ablation for malignant biliary obstruction: a nationwide retrospective study of 84 consecutive applications. *Surg Endosc*. 2014;**28**(3):854–860.
72. Jang SI, Kim JH, You JW, et al. Efficacy of a metallic stent covered with a paclitaxel-incorporated membrane versus a covered metal stent for malignant biliary obstruction: a prospective comparative study. *Dig Dis Sci*. 2013;**58**(3):865–871.

30

Laparoscopic liver surgery

Christian Hobeika, François Cauchy, and Olivier Soubrane

Introduction

The first successful laparoscopic liver resection (LLR) was reported in 1993 but the diffusion of this approach has long been limited due to initial technical limitations, absence of specific laparoscopic devices for liver surgery, concerns about patients' safety (especially with the risk of gas embolism and uncontrollable haemorrhage), uncertainty regarding its oncological validity (risk of incomplete resection, especially in segments of difficult access), and a long learning curve explained by the need for an expertise in both liver and laparoscopic surgery. Hence, it is only in the 2000s that the first large series reporting on the safety and feasibility of LLRs was released.[1] To date, tens of thousands of LLRs have been performed worldwide and both the feasibility and safety of this approach have now been demonstrated.[2-4] In this setting, LLR is now considered standard practice for various procedures such as left lateral sectionectomy and limited wedge resections in the so-called easy segments. Despite its important diffusion, LLR accounts for less than 40% of liver resections. This minimally invasive approach remains a skill-demanding technique, which requires an expert environment and favourable clinical situations to be safely performed.

This chapter aims to provide an overview of the current status of LLR and describes the main technical insights to safely adopt this new technique.

Assessment and transmission of laparoscopic liver resection

Outcomes following LLR

The literature reporting the benefits of laparoscopy on short-term outcomes following liver resection has been prolific during the two past decades.[4] By definition, LLR provides a minimal access to a procedure, thus preserving the abdominal wall from large incisions. Still, advantages allocated to LLR go beyond the limitation of the risks of wound complications.[5] As a result of its minimally invasive nature, LLR has been reported to reduce intraoperative blood loss, postoperative complications, postoperative pain, and hospital stay.[6-7] Moreover, the theoretical benefits of LLR in patients with cirrhosis have been studied, explaining why hepatocellular carcinoma (HCC) still represents the most frequent indication for LLR.[8] Specifically, the reduced intraoperative blood loss, decreased incidence of liver-specific complications, and improved postoperative cardiorespiratory rehabilitation are all arguments in favour of a minimally invasive approach in patients with cirrhosis. In this setting, LLR seems to improve the tolerance of these patients, especially regarding the recovery of postoperative liver function.[9,10]

All these encouraging results have promoted the worldwide diffusion of this innovative technique and LLR has progressively become the standard practice for minor liver resection.[3] Despite a slow technical development, indications have been extended even for advanced procedures in complex clinical situations, provided there is substantial expertise in both liver and laparoscopic surgery.[4,11] However, at this stage of LLR development, the importance of its benefit is hard to affirm given the small number of randomized controlled trials available. In this setting, there is a need to promote adequate assessment of LLR results, especially regarding advanced procedures as well as in patients with underlying liver disease.[12]

Oncological endpoints and textbook outcomes in LLR

Liver resection mainly concerns patients with malignant disease. Logically, the prerequisite for the development of LLR was to ensure at least similar oncological results using the laparoscopic approach as compared to the open approach.[13,14] In fact, assessment of innovative techniques, such as LLR, has reinforced the use of various quality indicators in surgical oncology such as intraoperative blood loss, postoperative morbidity, margins, lymph node dissection, tumour spillage, and rehabilitation/time to return to chemotherapy.[15] With the exception of laparoscopic lymphadenectomy, which has not yet been appropriately evaluated, the laparoscopic approach seems to successfully achieve these endpoints as well as the open approach.[15]

As mentioned above, the laparoscopic approach has been repeatedly reported to reduce blood loss and improve postoperative outcomes.[4] Despite the technical difficulty of LLR and the lack of tactile feedback, equivalent margins and margin widths seem to be achieved with LLR.[15] By its mini-invasive nature, the laparoscopic approach is intrinsically a no-touch procedure. In association with the caudal approach, which abrogates the need of primary liver mobilization in major right-sided resections, LLR reduces the risk of tumour spillage.[16] Altogether, these endpoints are all individual criteria accounting for the quality of care, which are summarized in the recent concept of textbook outcome,[12] a composite measure of overall quality of surgical care.[17] Patients who achieve a textbook outcome following liver resection accumulate all favourable criteria and thus have an ideal hospitalization. By enhancing the overall surgical environment reflected by the rate of textbook outcome, the laparoscopic approach could be a vector of improvement in the field of oncological liver surgery.[18]

Learning curve, classification systems, and benchmarking in LLR

LLR is a skill-demanding technique, which has rapidly raised the questions of reproducibility and transmission to new adopters.[19,20] With the intention to promote the safe progression of the technique, various studies have described and defined learning curves and technical prerequisites to safely start a programme of LLR.[21-23] Above all, the paramount requirement is to perform LLR in a surgical environment with substantial expertise in both laparoscopic and liver surgery.[4] The techniques and devices employed in LLR are continuously evolving.[24] Moreover, indications for LLR have been widely extended through its development to malignant lesions, patients with comorbidities and underlying liver diseases,[12] and even in living donors.[11] Finally, it seems that new trainees get used more easily to LLR than the previous generation of pioneers and early adopters.[20] Obviously, the emergence of international programmes of proctorship and of fellow skills curricula will improve the standardization and the transmission of LLR.[25,26] Altogether, the previously described cut-offs of minor and major LLR defining expertise in LLR now all have a limited relevance in routine practice.

In parallel with the learning curve models, several classification or scoring systems have emerged to stratify the technical difficulty of LLR procedures.[27-30] It has been consensually acknowledged that safe diffusion of LLR requires a stepwise progression from so-called easy LLR (new adopters) to advanced level of LLR (expert surgeons).[4] While the calibration and validation of these classifications remain poor, some are practical to use and helpful in routine practice as well as in clinical research.[31] Interestingly, research specifically involving LLR has allowed us to overcome the traditional binary minor/major classification of liver resection previously used in open liver surgery, which has in turn led to a more refined classification of open liver resection procedures.[32,33] Likewise, there is no consensual and relevant definition of centre of expertise in LLR. In fact, such a worldwide definition (based on LLR volume) is hardly addressable because the LLR caseload widely varies according to healthcare policies and geographical repartition of HPB centres in each country. In contrast, the recent concept of benchmarking in surgery has been reported to be highly relevant and to provide indicators of best practice for a specific surgical procedure.[34] Applying this concept to LLR could help providing reference values, and define expert practice across centres.[12]

The three main indications for laparoscopic liver resection

Colorectal cancer liver metastasis

Colorectal cancer liver metastases (CRLM) are the most common indications for liver resection.[4] Anatomical resection is not recommended for CRLM and simple wedge resections with sufficient margin width provide satisfactory oncological results.[35] Thus, small tumours located in easily accessible anterolateral segments of the liver represent ideal indications for LLR. In fact, LLR represents an attractive technique for the CRLM patient by improving the feasibility of sequential liver–colorectal procedures as well as two step-hepatectomy strategies and/or repeated hepatectomy for CRLM recurrences.[36] Moreover, CRLM patients are likely to be younger and without advanced liver diseases as compared to those with primary liver cancers. In addition to the prolific literature of low level of evidence in favour of LLR in CRLM patients, two randomized controlled trials have shown the superiority of LLR in CRLM patients.[6,7] They have highlighted advantages of LLR regarding the rate of complications, length of hospital stay, and quality of life. LLR in CRLM patients is clearly becoming a standard of care in their management.

Nevertheless, several limitations against LLR have to be mentioned. First, the absence of tactile feedback and challenging completion of state-of-the-art ultrasonography examination may limit the use of LLR.[37] Second, bi-lobar and multiple tumours can represent challenging situations because of the need for extensive liver mobilization and suboptimal patient installation to achieve adequate exposure of both sides of the liver.[38] Finally, chemotherapy-associated liver injuries, especially sinusoidal obstruction syndrome, are associated with increased intraoperative bleeding, decreased efficiency of pedicle clamping, and patients' tolerance to major resection.[39] In this setting, LLR remains ideally indicated for pauci-nodular and unilobar CRLM accessible to wedge resections or qualifying for formal major resection in patients who have received less than six cycles of chemotherapy.[40] In turn, the increased technical difficulty to perform wedge resection in posterosuperior segments under laparoscopy should not favour major resections at the expense of parenchymal-sparing strategies, which remains of paramount importance in the management of these patients.[41]

Hepatocellular carcinoma

HCC is the most frequent primary liver tumour worldwide and occurs in the vast majority of the cases on a background of underlying liver disease.[42] Liver transplantation, liver resection, and tumour ablation are the most efficient curative treatments. In liver resection, preoperative evaluation of the liver function, degree of fibrosis, and severity of portal hypertension are the cornerstone of the pretherapeutic evaluation of these patients regardless of the surgical approach. The laparoscopic approach yields several theoretical benefits in the specific context of HCC patients, explaining why HCC is still the main indication for LLR.[9] However, at this stage of development, the level of evidence regarding these specific advantages remains low. Specifically, the role of the minimally invasive nature of the approach on the preservation of collateral circulation and thus the reduced risk of postoperative liver function decompensation remains debated. While no randomized trials focusing on the role of laparoscopy in the subset of HCC patients have been released to date, the laparoscopic approach seems to improve the overall surgical environment of HCC patients.[18] Indeed, as measured by the textbook outcome, HCC patients who undergo LLR cumulate more frequently multiple quality criteria (negative margins, no transfusion, no complications, no prolonged hospital stays, and no readmission), which altogether seem to improve their long-term prognosis.

In fact, HCC patients can benefit the most from the promising advantages of the laparoscopic approach especially regarding liver-related complications. In turn, these patients represent a technical challenge in LLR.[12] Indeed, indications for easy wedge resection in HCC patients are scarce, likely to be replaced by the upcoming techniques of radiological ablation.[43] In the vast majority of cases, liver resection for HCC aims to remove all the tumour-bearing portal territory.[44] Thus, when the underlying liver function allows, HCC patients require at least an anatomical segmentectomy or sectionectomy if not a major resection to be performed. In addition, the underlying liver disease distorts the liver anatomy. Liver mobilization and the exposure of both the hepatic pedicle and the transection plane can become very difficult. The fibrotic texture of the parenchyma decreases the efficiency of the Cavitron ultrasonic surgical aspirator (CUSA) and the portal hypertension increases bleeding. Altogether, the parenchymal transection can require prolonged and multiple pedicle intermittent clampings. In addition, the need for a volume optimization strategy using portal vein embolization is frequent, especially in case of major right-sided resection. Consequently, the induced atrophy of the right liver modifies the direction of the middle hepatic vein from the sagittal to the frontal plane, which may increase the difficulty for correct exposure.[45]

Altogether, HCC summarizes most of the difficulties met in LLR and emphasizes the need for expertise in both laparoscopic and HPB surgery when approaching these patients. Large series of LLR in HCC patients have emphasized the increased operative risk of these patients despite the laparoscopic approach.[10] While HCC patients probably benefit from this innovative approach, their perioperative evaluation and the anticipation of the intraoperative difficulties remain of primary importance.

Living donor

Liver resection in living donors logically represents the most debated indication for LLR. The increased technical difficulty associated with the reduced tactile feedback in LLR questions the benefit:risk equation for such an indication, especially in countries where living donor liver transplantation is not common.[46] In contrast, living donors are young, healthy patients with normal underlying liver parenchyma and may represent ideal surgical candidates for a successful laparoscopic approach, as demonstrated by the fact that these patients represent the reference population for the definition of benchmark values for major resections. These patients would benefit most from the minimally invasive nature of LLR. In fact, one large international and multicentre cohort study has demonstrated the feasibility of LLR in living donors without compromising the donors' safety. The reported short-term results were similar to the defined benchmark values in open right and left hepatectomy.[11]

Laparoscopic living donor hepatectomy remains one of the most common indications for hybrid/hand-assisted LLR. Indeed, only half of the patients currently undergo LLR using a full laparoscopic approach.[11] Indeed, there are specific difficulties in the LLR living donor, which could be intimidating and dissuasive in the attempt of full laparoscopic procedures.[47,48] First, the interruption of the portal and arterial flow in the retrieved hemiliver (future recipient's graft) should be delayed as late as possible during parenchymal transection to reduce the time of ischaemia. This can increase the difficulty to progress during parenchymal transection. Second, the intraoperative understanding of donor anatomy is of paramount importance. While accurate preoperative imaging evaluation is essential to identify abnormal vascular or biliary anatomy, intraoperative exploration and understanding can be challenging under LLR. Third, liver mobilization and specimen extraction remain very skill-demanding steps, especially in the setting of right hepatectomy, both occurring at the end of the procedure when the surgeon's fatigue and weariness are pushed to their limits. Yet, these steps require meticulous and maximum attention to avoid injury to the future graft.

Altogether, the living donor procedure is probably the most leading-edge LLR indication.[49] While it has become a standard practice for adult-to-child donation, it is likely that its results will improve with further experience for adult-to-adult donation.[11,50] Interestingly, the assessment of this indication will lead to the refinement of new end points in liver surgery such as quality of life, body image, and willingness to donate and could provide important arguments in favour of the laparoscopic approach.

Surgical approach in laparoscopic liver resection

Loss of praxis for a magnified view

In laparoscopic surgery, the surgeon's vision is digitalized by the camera connected to the optics of the laparoscope and displayed on a screen. The laparoscope is positioned below the liver and the vision is oriented upwards along a very horizontal oblique axis called the 'caudal view'. Through the camera, the view is magnified allowing a detailed visualization of the anatomical structures while restrained by the focal length and the laparoscope's angle (0°, 30°, or 45°). Overall, LLR does not allow a global vision of the operative field. The comprehensive understanding of the operative field lies on the assistant's (who may the first assistant surgeon, a physician assistant, or a scrub nurse) abilities to shoot, centre, stabilize, and anticipate the anatomical region of interest. In addition, the feasibility of LLR is strongly related to the technological refinement of the devices (e.g. camera's definition, 4K resolution, three-dimensional, flexible optic, and screen size of the monitor).[51,52] Moreover, LLR is characterized by the amount of intra-abdominal fluids, not only blood, but also wet fog and carbon particles that frequently spoil the lens of the optics, requiring frequent cleaning to maintain an optimal view.

In contrast to the optimal view of the operative field, all surgical skills are performed using long and rigid instruments through the differently placed trocars, while direct prehension of the anatomical structures is not possible. In this setting, every step of a liver procedure is more skill demanding as compared to the standard open approach, especially in some extreme positions with limited triangulation of the instruments and the laparoscope. As an example, the first steps of LLR development have gone through hybrid and/or hand-assisted techniques, which were characterized by a planned conversion to laparotomy during the procedure. In such a technique, the completion of the procedure can be performed under direct manual control.[53]

From the anterior to the caudal approach

The association of a restrained and caudal field of view with a limited praxis have led to some necessary refinements in the surgeon's approach in LLR. Even the steps of liver procedures considered easy by open approach such as the liver mobilization, cholecystectomy, and Pringle manoeuvre can be more challenging in LLR. The limited abilities to expose the liver with prehensive instruments, to reach highly located anatomical structures, such as the hepato-caval confluent, and to manage blood-impregnated operative fields have led to the conventional approaches being questioned. Indeed, both conventional and anterior approaches with transhepatic/intrahepatic control of the Glissonian pedicles[54] seem significantly challenging, especially in the context of underlying liver disease.[10,55] Moreover, the so-called posterosuperior segments (4a, 8, 7, 1/9) are considered as difficult locations despite their minor extent[4] as they require an extensive mobilization of the liver.[56] In contrast, the magnified caudal view of the liver in LLR seems particularly relevant to perform primary vascular control.

Altogether, these considerations have led to the conceptualization of the caudal approach in LLR defined according to four technical steps.[16,57] First, the caudal view with the optimal triangulation of instruments allows for a precise intrafascial pedicular dissection or extrafascial supra-hilar Glissonian pedicles to perform vascular inflow control of either the hemiliver or section before parenchymal transection thus ensuring oncological safety. Second, in the case of right hepatectomy, parenchymal transection is performed without mobilization of the liver, which is in favour of the 'no-touch' oncological criteria. Third, at the end of the parenchymal transection, the anterolateral aspect of the inferior vena cava is exposed, allowing for safe control and dissection of the right hepatic vein(s). The totally devascularized hemiliver can be safely mobilized from a medial to lateral direction. Finally, the specimen is placed in a plastic bag and externalized through a remote extraction site.

All these technical considerations related to LLR development have led to the refinement of the classification of liver procedures in terms of difficulty. In turn, the standard dichotomization between minor and major resection have become obsolete in the modern era of liver surgery.[33,58] As an example, some major resections such as a formal left hepatectomy appear to be technically more accessible compared to segment 7 or 8 unisegmentectomies.[31] Moreover, procedures with advanced difficulty have been reported to be associated with jeopardized outcomes in patients. In fact, the level of technical difficulty has to be analysed as a separate indicator in addition to the extent of the liver resection for the assessment of patients' quality of care in LLR.[59]

Patient position and pneumoperitoneum

Patient and surgeon position

To be optimal, laparoscopic liver parenchymal transection should be aligned with the optical trocar and surgeon vision, with one operative port on each side to achieve triangulation. Figure 30.1 shows an example of installation for laparoscopic right hepatectomy and the principle of triangulation.[16,60,61] In the French position, the patient is placed in a supine position with the surgeon standing between split legs. This position can be used for all procedures performed in supine patients, such as left lateral sectionectomy or major hepatectomies. The advantages of this position include the possibility to align the surgeon's eyes with the optic and monitor, thus respecting the principle of triangulation and avoiding any shift in angle of vision (Figure

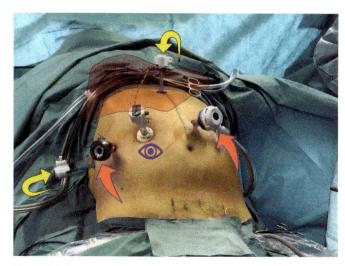

Figure 30.1 Port sites and location of remote incision for specimen externalization. The optical trocar (blue eye) is aligned with the transection plane (Cantlie line in this case of right hepatectomy); two 12 mm operative trocars (red arrows) in triangulation with the optics; two 5 mm trocars (yellow arrows) for suction and retraction by the assistant.

30.1). This position is also probably more relaxing for surgeons, which is an important issue in long-lasting procedures.

A head-up tilt (reverse Trendelenburg) of 10–15° is also required.[61] In this position, the blood flow return to the heart is mechanically reduced by gravity, which further helps maintaining a low (<5 mmHg) central venous pressure. The reverse Trendelenburg position also improves exposure by gravitationally shifting visceral structures downwards, away from the liver. By contrast, semi-/partial/full left lateral or even semi-prone positions, which also use gravity and optimize surgical ergonomics have been developed for LLR of posterosuperior lesions. The latter are considered 'difficult locations' for LLR. For example, Ikeda and colleagues developed a new LLR approach using a semi-prone position. The patient is set in the left lateral position and surgeons stand at the left side, rotating the operating table by 20–25° from the semi-prone position.

Pneumoperitoneum and trocar placement

As for other laparoscopic procedures, the primary concept of LLR is to insufflate a pneumoperitoneum (with carbonic gas) to create a sufficient intra-abdominal space of work. There are two opposed described techniques to create the pneumoperitoneum, called the entry techniques: direct trocar insertion without previous pneumoperitoneum (the 'Hasson' open entry) versus direct insufflation using a Veress needle (the Veress needle entry).[62] The open entry involves performing a minimally invasive laparotomy (1–2 cm) and introducing the first trocar into the abdominal cavity under direct vision. Through this first trocar, which usually serves as the optic trocar during the procedure, the carbonic gas is progressively insufflated to create an adequate pneumoperitoneum (from 10 to 14 mmHg). In contrast, the Veress needle technique involves direct percutaneous puncture of the abdominal cavity and insufflation of the pneumoperitoneum. Controversies continue to exist between the two techniques. While the open entry seems safer regarding the risk of visceral injuries using the Veress needle, the mini laparotomy can be challenging to perform in obese patients.[63]

CHAPTER 30 Laparoscopic liver surgery

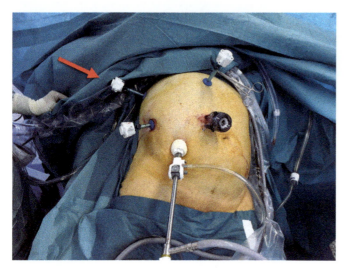

Figure 30.2 An additional transthoracic trocar (red arrow) may help for resection in the posterosuperior segments.

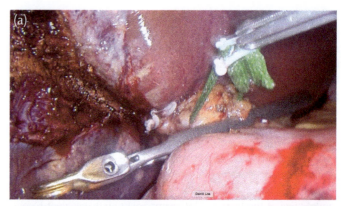
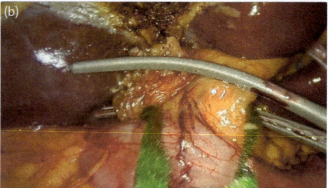
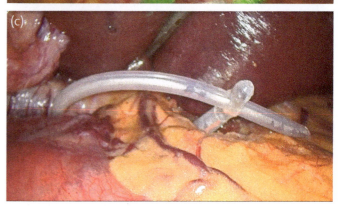

Figure 30.3 Intraoperative view of Pringle manoeuvre with different technique: (a) intracorporeal large bulldog clamp. (b) Extracorporeal aortic clamp passing through the abdominal wall. (c) Loop using a Foley catheter as reported by Huang et al.[68]

Trocar placements for the assistants are determined on the basis of surgeons' preference and intraoperative view after positioning the optical trocar. The number of trocars used generally ranges from four to five, while the use of an epigastric port is variable between teams. While single-port laparoscopy has been reported for various LLR procedures, its relevance remains debated. The optical trocar is more often positioned above the umbilicus and the distance from the umbilicus varies considerably. When approaching posterosuperior segments, a transthoracic access using intercostal ports with or without conventional abdominal access may be useful (Figure 30.2).

Vascular control

Vascular clamping in LLR

Vascular clamping techniques are efficient tools in liver surgery to reduce overall intraoperative blood loss and facilitate parenchymal transection in LLR as well as in standard open liver resection.[64] Indeed, vascular clamping provides a bloodless operative field and facilitates immediate control of vessel injuries. Different techniques of intermittent or continuous clamping techniques depending on the location and the approach of the inflow or outflow elements have been described.

These vascular controls and clamping are used to reduce the intraoperative blood loss but also to determine the limits of the part of the liver to be resected using the ischaemia demarcation of the segments of interest. Yet, parenchymal transection and management of bleeding are skill demanding especially in advanced procedures and may be intimidating for new adopters of the technique. Hence, mastering laparoscopic inflow clamping is a prerequisite to progress in LLR.

Pedicular control or Pringle manoeuvre

The Pringle manoeuvre (Figure 30.3) was first described in 1908 in the context of bleeding control in liver trauma. It is the most efficient and routinely used technique for inflow clamping in liver resection. Similar to the open approach, the laparoscopic Pringle manoeuvre is an 'en masse' clamping of the hepatoduodenal ligament. This could be performed using some atraumatic flexible clamp or more frequently using a tourniquet. With the exception of total vascular exclusion, this inflow clamping is usually intermittent with various reported timings (15–5, 10–5, or 10–10 minutes) to minimize induced ischaemic injury.[64] The specificity of the laparoscopic approach relies on the fact that the surgeon has not direct access to the clamp or the tourniquet. In this setting, the Pringle laparoscopic manoeuvre may use extracorporeal or totally intracorporeal techniques.[65–67]

To control the hepatic pedicle, the lesser sac is opened and a grasping forceps, a dissector, or an atraumatic clamp is introduced through the most lateral right trocar. Then, the grasper is passed through the foramen of Winslow, behind the hepatic pedicle to encircle the hepatoduodenal ligament with an umbilical tape (used for the tourniquet). In the extracorporeal technique, the umbilical tape is pulled to the halfway point and brought out extracorporeally via the closest port. The two ends of the tape are positioned through the tourniquet. The trocar is removed and reintroduced so that the tourniquet is adjacent to the trocar and does not interfere with instrument exchange. Another possibility is to bring the tape down to a remote site such as the distant supra-pubic incision. Otherwise, direct clamping of the hepatoduodenal ligament using a large vascular clamp (through a trocar or not) is an alternative extracorporeal technique.

In the totally intracorporeal technique, the tape is passed through a 10–12 cm tourniquet which is pushed into the abdominal cavity. Then, the ends of the tape are cut after having joined the two tips with a clip placed few centimetres above the tourniquet. In this setting, the clamping system is switched totally intracorporeally. The Pringle manoeuvre is done under direct vision using a Mayo clamp (in the extracorporeal technique) or a heavy-duty clip (in the intracorporeal technique) to cinch the tourniquet around the hepatoduodenal ligament stopping the inflow.

An effective, easy, and practical alternative intracorporeal Pringle manoeuvre has been reported by Huang et al. using one 14 Fr Foley catheter shortened to 15 cm with a side-hole at the tip. It is introduced into the abdomen.[68] Then, the tail is pulled out through the side-hole to make a loop to encircle the hepatoduodenal ligament. The Pringle manoeuvre is done by tightening the loop above the cross perpendicularly.

Supra-hilar controls

In case of major liver resections, prior vascular control and clamping of the resected hemiliver emphasizes the transection plane using the ischaemic demarcation line and decreases intraoperative blood loss during parenchymal transection. In LLR, the caudal approach helps the surgeon to perform such vascular control, while an intrahepatic (during the transection) control and section of the hemiliver inflow pedicle can be challenging.[54] There are two opposed techniques to perform such extrahepatic hemiliver inflow control: the intrafascial and the extrafascial approach.

The intrafascial approach is an extrahepatic dissection of the lateral aspect of the hepatic pedicle to reach and individualize the portal and arterial first division branches of the hemiliver of interest, below the hilar plate.[16,69] This approach allows for an exhaustive evaluation and understanding of the anatomy thus ensuring oncological safety regarding a suspicion of tumoural vascular invasion. It is the first choice in case of vascular and biliary involvement in the context of hilar tumours and/or in case of anatomical variations of portal, arterial, or biliary distribution (Figure 30.4). In contrast, the meticulous dissection can be challenging and thus there is a risk of vascular or biliary injury. In LLR, the magnified caudal view helps to achieve adequate control of the portal bifurcation and even, in most cases, the second division branches (helpful for posterior sectionectomy or central hepatectomy). Nevertheless, some clinical situations such as repeated hepatectomy with prior history of pedicular dissection can increase the difficulty of this intrafascial approach, which may become even more hazardous. In such situations, an extrafascial approach can be more appropriate to avoid the risk related to an extensive dissection of the hepatic pedicle.

Two techniques of the extrafascial approach which are applied to LLR have been described: the supra-hilar approach and the Glissonian approach. The supra-hilar one is an extension of the Hepp and Couinaud manoeuvre.[70,71] It involves the detachment and the

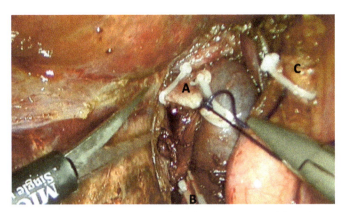

Figure 30.4 Intraoperative view of intrafascial dissection of the right hepatic pedicle during laparoscopic right hepatectomy in a case of type III portal vein bifurcation. A: right anterior branch of the portal vein to be divided (note the double control with ligature plus secured clip). B: stump of the distant right posterior portal vein. C: stump of the branch of the middle hepatic artery.

lowering of the hilar plate for en masse encircling of the left or right pedicles.[72] The Glissonian approach was first described by Takasaki et al. and Launois et al. and widely popularized by Machado et al. especially in the context of LLR.[73–76] This approach defined pairs of landmarks in the liver capsule according to the hilar plate and the liver sulcus. Each pair of landmarks theoretically encircle the Glissonian pedicle of interest. In this setting, small incisions and introduction of a vascular clamp through a pair of landmarks allow an effective and selective en masse clamping of the Glissonian pedicle without extensive dissection. Obviously, these Glissonian techniques should never be used in cases of suspected hilar involvement of the tumour and thus for perihilar cholangiocarcinoma. For major resection, the rate of technical success of this technique is about 70–75%.[77,78] In addition, this Glissonian approach has also been described for selective clamping of the third division of Glissonian branches.[75]

Outflow controls and the hanging manoeuvre

The hanging manoeuvre was first described by Belghiti et al. for formal right hepatectomy.[79] This is a practical and efficient procedure, which facilitates parenchymal transection through both the conventional and anterior approaches for major liver resections. Briefly, the hanging manoeuvre involves placing, a surgical tape or a nasogastric tube through Couinaud's avascular tunnel.[80,81] The hanging manoeuvre improves the understanding of the surgical plan, refines the exposure of the posterior part of the transection (especially during the anterior approach), and compresses the parenchyma, thus decreasing or controlling venous bleeding. Finally, it facilitates incision of the very last section of the posterior liver capsule and protects from surgical injuries both the vena cava and its spigelian collaterals. While initially described for formal right hepatectomy, the location of the tube can be further adjusted according to the liver procedure.[82] Thus, these modified hanging manoeuvres provide safe control of the outflow during laparoscopic liver procedures.[82] In fact, the laparoscopic caudal approach allows for better visual control and exposure of the posterior part of the parenchymal transection and anterolateral aspect of the vena cava during major resection.[57] The advantages allocated to the hanging manoeuvre are somehow offset by

CHAPTER 30 Laparoscopic liver surgery

the laparoscopic approach and the former is not performed on a systematic basis. Nevertheless, it allows for improvements in second-stage hepatectomies.[83,84]

While more challenging, the hanging manoeuvre can be performed by the laparoscopic approach. Both approaches are described according to the side of which the tube is initially placed: the conventional 'down-to-up' or craniocaudal approach and the 'up-to-down' approach (more similar to the open approach). In fact, both approaches are complementary.[85] While the 'down-to-up' way is more practical by the laparoscopic approach, the 'up-to-down' is safer in complex situations such as in obese patients or those with underlying liver disease. In routine practice, the avascular tunnel of Couinaud is created using repeated dissection on both sides (i.e. the areas of the hepatocaval confluence and the right side of the vena cava at the posterior aspect of segment 6). A 10 mm trocar is required to be placed in the epigastric area. After dissection of the falciform ligament and the hepatocaval confluent, the termination of the hepatic vein is dissected carefully. Then, the plane between the right and the middle hepatic vein is blindly opened using a laparoscopic dissector or even a long vascular clamp of open surgery (after removing the trocar) through the epigastric port. This dissection should be vertical, in line with the anterior aspect of the vena cava (the dissector directed towards the feet of the patient) to avoid injuries of the right or middle hepatic vein armpits. At the lower end, the anterior and right aspects of the infrahepatic vena cava is dissected by opening the parietal peritoneum. The first Spiegel collaterals from segments 1 and 6 serve as a landmark so that the dissection of the Couinaud's tunnel using the dissector is made medially to this vein. At the upper end, the dissection is performed vertically, along the anterior aspect of the vena cava and directed upward, to the xiphoid process, to avoid injury to the vena cava. Finally, the tube or tape can be introduced to complete the laparoscopic hanging manoeuvre. Of note, all these procedures do not require any liver mobilization.

Parenchymal transection techniques

Determination of the transection plane

The exposure in a V-shape of the parenchymal section, especially in advanced and major resection, can be very challenging. In this setting, trocar placement should be optimized according to the anticipated surgical plan (triangulation rule). Thus, very specific considerations should be provided in the preoperative imagines.[61] Thereafter, the transection plane should be assessed intraoperatively using ultrasonography. Indeed, ultrasonography is an efficient and practical tool providing several important decision-making parameters such as extent and number of lesions and its landmarks with anatomical structures.[86] In fact, identification of the hepatic veins and Glissonian pedicles is mandatory especially in anatomical resections. Intraoperative fluorescence imaging techniques using systemic indocyanine green injection is an alternative tool, which could refine the determination of the transection plane.[87]

Parenchymal transection

Parenchymal transection starts with the opening of both the capsule and superficial layer of the liver (up to 2 cm deep) along the previously drawn transection plane, as far as the exposure allows.[88] During this phase, there is usually no major vessel or bile duct. This step can be performed using ultrasonic shears only without pre-coagulation and CUSA dissection. Triggering the ultrasonic shears before completely closing the device improves haemostasis. Transection of the deeper parenchyma should be performed cautiously with meticulous dissection and exposure of both intra-parenchymal vascular and biliary structures. The concomitant use of an ultrasonic dissector (CUSA EXcel, IntegraTM Life Sciences Corporation, NJ, USA) and bipolar forceps is efficient and provides safe and bloodless progression (Table 30.1 indicates the main instruments available

Table 30.1 Instruments for laparoscopic liver parenchymal transection

Instruments	Way of use	Disadvantage	Example
Transection device			
CUSA	Separate parenchyma	–	Cusa Excel
Water-jet	Separate parenchyma	Easy to blur the lens	Helix Hydro-Jet
Energy device		–	
Precoagulators	Blind	Structure injury	Radiotherapy-assisted device
Ultrasonic shears	Blind or elective use	Not applicable for vessels larger than 5 mm	Harmonic Ultracision
Bipolar	Elective or crush Sealing or transection tool	–	Bipolar forceps
Sealing device	Elective coagulation or crush Section after coagulation (<7 mm)	Caution of large vessel structure	Ligasure Enseal Thunderbeat
Sealing simultaneous or sequential section	Elective or crush Efficient on small branches of the vena cava (<7 mm)	Caution of large vessel structure	Thunderbeat
Others			
Clips	Suturing large structures	–	Hem-o-lok
Stapler	Cutting and suturing large structures	–	Echelon Flex Endopath Staplers

The description about 'Energy diveice' is based on Scatton et al. (2015).[46]
Reproduced with permission from Yoh T, Cauchy F, Soubrane O. Techniques for laparoscopic liver parenchymal transection. *Hepatobiliary Surg Nutr.* 2019 Dec;8(6):572–581.

for parenchyma division). Moreover, the 'Tissue Select' mode of the CUSA is a useful pulsatile mode for major vessels dissection. It slows down parenchymal transection and avoids vein injuries.

Vessel transection

Small vessels (diameter ≤2 mm) are diathermically sealed using sealing devices (such as Thunderbeat or a Harmonic scalpel) and then divided. Larger vessels (3–7 mm in diameter) are divided with sealing devices or clips where appropriate after exposure. Significant hepatic veins or Glissonian pedicles are dissected then taped allowing for traction and good positioning of the clips or suture. This process allows for preventing clips or suture from untying, breaking, and slipping. Almost all cases are then double clipped using Hem-o-lok (Weck Closure Systems, NC, USA) and divided by straight scissors. A vascular stapler is used for the division of large structures already dissected (Figure 30.5). For major hepatectomy, transection of the large hepatic veins is performed with a laparoscopic vascular stapler. Proper identification and isolation of the hepatic veins may represent the most difficult aspect of these procedures (c.f. 'Tissue Select' mode). For example, in laparoscopic right hepatectomy, the right hepatic vein is gently encircled after transection of the liver parenchyma and then hung up using a dedicated tape as mentioned earlier.

Management of bleeding

Minimizing blood loss during parenchymal transection

Minimizing intraoperative blood loss and efficient management of acute bleeding related to large vessel injury has always been a crucial point in liver surgery.[89] The technical difficulty related to the laparoscopic approach increases the challenge of bleeding management. A bloody operative field impacts the surgeon's vision, notably because the red colour absorbs light. Thus, maintaining a dry operative field is mandatory to safely progress under laparoscopy throughout parenchymal transection. Some basic principles help minimizing intraoperative blood loss such as the association of pneumoperitoneum of 10–12 mmHg with low central venous pressure (<5 mmHg), which reduces the venous engorgement of the liver and therefore the risk of backflow bleeding during transection.[4] Several studies have reported that a low central venous pressure is well tolerated and that the theoretical risk of gas embolism remains low.[90]

Management of acute bleeding

In addition to intermittent inflow clamping (described above), which is the cornerstone technique favouring bleeding control, there are several techniques which may help to control an acute bleed related to large vessel injuries. First, compression for several minutes using small gauze pads allows for a step back, to clean the operative field, improve the camera view, and peacefully analyse the situation.[89] In some cases, this compression can be sufficient to stop the bleeding, especially in the case of a venous injury.[91] When encountering bleeding from small vessels, bipolar forceps coagulation or direct clipping of the exposed vessel are simple techniques. When encountering bleeding from a large vessel such as a hepatic vein, portal vein, or even the inferior vena cava, a direct suture can be attempted after achieving prior temporary control using a clip, a vascular clamp, or a grasper.[61] The 'grab and stitch' technique is the most efficient technique and may require an additional trocar if needed. Fibrin-based haemostatic agents and sealants (e.g. TachoSil, Nycomed Linz, Austria) seem to be less suitable in LLR. In fact, positioning patch agents that are not designed for the laparoscopic approach, may be technically difficult. Of note, the magnified view allows for detailed and meticulous haemostasis of the parenchymal transection. Therefore, the use of these agents could become meaningless in this setting.

Conversion to open resection

Definition of conversion

Conversion is defined as the requirement of a non-scheduled laparotomy during LLR. Thus, hybrid and/or hand-assisted LLR are not considered under this terminology. During the early steps of development, conversion represented the failure of the laparoscopic approach and therefore became an indicator of technical feasibility of LLR procedures. Hence, conversion raised the concepts of learning curve, surgeon, and centre expertise in LLR. Conversion still occurs routinely despite the advanced expertise in LLR, especially in technically demanding procedures and should be considered as a part of the technique. As an example, some of the classification systems of LLR difficulty were based on the conversion rate, as well as blood loss and operative time. Moreover, the benchmarked rate of conversion varied from 7.2% for left lateral sectionectomy to 29.8% for right hepatectomy.

Causes of conversion

Conversion should be considered as a consequence of an unexpected event that prevents the safe completion of the procedure by laparoscopy. The reported causes of conversion are multiple and can be arbitrary dichotomized into 'unfavourable life-threatening events' and 'unfavourable findings' that are not directly related to the patient's clinical tolerance.[92] This dichotomization has a direct influence on the outcome of the converted patient. Indeed, it has been reported that patients converted for 'unfavourable life-threatening event' (such as uncontrolled bleeding) had an increased morbidity while those converted for 'unfavourable findings' did not. Routinely, uncontrolled intraoperative bleeding is the most frequent cause

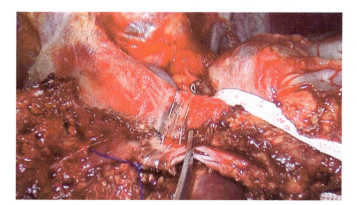

Figure 30.5 Section of the left hepatic vein after stapling using unilateral vascular stapler in a living liver donor.

of conversion and the laparoscopic management of intraoperative bleeding is an important concern of the hepatopancreatobiliary surgeon especially in an early experience of LLR. Nevertheless, teams with substantial experience have reported that even massive bleeding related to hepatic vein injuries can be safely managed by the laparoscopic approach using vascular controls and appropriate suturing skills.[89]

Risk factors of conversion

Various clinical situations (i.e. risk factors) have been reported to increase the risk of conversion during LLR such as age, American Society of Anesthesiologists classification, body mass index, tumour size, previous liver resection, biliary reconstruction, neoadjuvant chemotherapy, and underlying liver disease.[20,93] All these factors are acknowledged to increase intraoperative difficulty, especially regarding the risk of bleeding, and to jeopardize postoperative outcomes in both open and laparoscopic approaches. These risk factors of conversion were defined during the development of LLR and are likely to change and/or evolve with increase expertise in LLR and its worldwide diffusion.[12] Current predictors of conversion have not yet been appropriately identified. In this setting, whether a subset of patients will benefit from straight open surgery instead of LLR with high risk of conversion remains unknown.

Timing of conversion

The ideal timing for conversion is not clearly defined and relies on several factors and especially on the clinical intraoperative tolerance of the patients. In case of bleeding, it has been reported that intraoperative blood loss is not an accurate indicator for conversion, while the requirement of transfusion seems to be a more relevant indicator of an unfavourable intraoperative process.[89] Likewise, the oncological quality of the liver resection should not be impaired by the surgical approach and, therefore, conversion should be considered in case of doubt regarding oncological margins, location/involvement of the tumours, and presence of unanticipated metastasis.

While conversion to laparotomy can be regarded as an indicator of technical failure, it should be considered as a consequence of an unfavourable intraoperative event, when continuing the laparoscopic approach would not be feasible or safe.[92] In this setting, the morbidity associated with the conversion in LLR series is largely related to the cause of the conversion. Hence, delaying or avoiding conversion at all costs could worsen patients' outcomes.[94,95]

Technique for conversion

The first choice of surgical site incision for conversion is usually the same incision for a similarly scheduled open liver procedure. It is mainly a J-shape or subcostal incision. Conversion into laparotomy must improve and optimize both the understanding and exposure of the operative field thus allowing for a quick and efficient management of the cause of the conversion (e.g. stopping the bleeding). In this setting, the incision should be at least as large as for a scheduled open liver resection. In some cases, when the mobilization of the liver is achieved, the conversion may be performed through a median, sub-umbilical incision. The need for conversion is always a stressful situation in the operative theatre. All required material for conversion and open surgery should be anticipated for all LLR procedures and ready for use. As far as possible, bleeding should be controlled using compression or clamping before conversion. In the best scenario, the instrument used to control the bleeding should be maintained by a senior surgeon while another senior surgeon performs the incision.

Extraction sites

Short-term results related to the choice of extraction site

Three extraction sites have been described in LLR and include supra-pubic, midline, and subcostal incisions.[96] With the exception of converted patients, a subcostal incision for the extraction is not routinely recommended because its use may compromise all advantages related to the laparoscopic approach regarding postoperative pain, complications, and rehabilitation, especially respiratory recovery.[96] Therefore, the first choices for specimen extraction are mostly supra-pubic transverse or midline incisions despite the very low risk of postoperative incisional hernia of the subcostal incision.[16,96]

Long-term results and postoperative incisional hernia

The rate of postoperative hernia is one of the most important end points influencing the choice of the extraction site.[97] While it is an under-reported complication, especially in the context of patients followed for malignant diseases, incisional hernias can seriously affect functional and cosmetic outcomes and therefore the quality of life of the patients.[97,98] Moreover, the treatment of these hernias is likely to require extensive surgical parietal procedures and the use of a prosthetic mesh.[99] Current evidence in surgery suggests that one-layer incisions, such as a midline incision, increase the risk of incisional hernia, while after subcostal or transverse incisions it is rare. In this setting, a supra-pubic transverse incision appears to be the first choice of extraction site in LLR by cumulating a decreased impact on short-term outcomes (comparatively to subcostal incision) and a decreased risk of incisional hernia (compared to a midline incision).[96] Moreover, recent series suggested that using a previous incision site for extracting the specimen is associated with an increased risk of incisional hernia and should be avoided.

Supra-pubic transversal or Pfannenstiel incision and specimen extraction

The Pfannenstiel incision appears to be a cosmetic and versatile incision with a negligible incisional hernia rate, thereby representing the best alternative to the classical incisions for specimen extraction in LLR as well as in laparoscopic colorectal surgery.[100] The incision should be marked in the supra-pubic skin fold and measured between 6 and 12 cm according to the size of the specimen. At the end of the procedure, the anterior sheath of the rectus abdominus muscles is incised transversally (6–12 cm), centred on the middle line. Then, the anterior sheath of rectus muscles is peeled from the muscular plan on both sides of the incision allowing for more flexibility to spread the rectus muscle. In the majority of the cases, this dissection allows for stretching and separating the rectus muscles without cutting them to extract the specimen. Finally, a plastic bag is introduced using a trocar through the parietal peritoneum between the rectus muscles and under a maintained pneumoperitoneum.

Conclusion

The laparoscopic approach is an innovative minimally invasive technique, which has gained worldwide popularity and acceptance among HPB surgeons. The technical difficulty of this new technique requires a stepwise initiation, from easy to advanced LLRs. The safe learning of LLR requires a familiarity with intimidating situations such as bleeding, conversion, and clamping techniques. Despite a profuse literature reporting the results of LLR, this technique remains a surgical innovation requiring further validation, especially for complex procedures. In fact, indications for LLR are likely to keep on extending and will undoubtedly inspire new innovations such as augmented reality and robotic-assisted surgery.

REFERENCES

1. Buell JF, Cherqui D, Geller DA, et al. The international position on laparoscopic liver surgery: the Louisville Statement, 2008. *Ann Surg*. 2009;**250**(5):825–830.
2. Ban D, Tanabe M, Kumamaru H, et al. Safe dissemination of laparoscopic liver resection in 27,146 cases between 2011 and 2017 from the National Clinical Database of Japan. *Ann Surg*. 2021;**274**(6):1043–1050.
3. Wakabayashi G, Cherqui D, Geller DA, et al. Recommendations for laparoscopic liver resection: a report from the second international consensus conference held in Morioka. *Ann Surg*. 2015;**261**(4):619–629.
4. Abu Hilal M, Aldrighetti L, Dagher I, et al. The Southampton Consensus Guidelines for Laparoscopic Liver Surgery: from indication to implementation. *Ann Surg*. 2018;**268**(1):11–18.
5. Bhangu A, Ademuyiwa AO, Aguilera ML, et al. Surgical site infection after gastrointestinal surgery in high-income, middle-income, and low-income countries: a prospective, international, multicentre cohort study. *Lancet Infect Dis*. 2018;**18**(5):516–525.
6. Robles-Campos R, Lopez-Lopez V, Brusadin R, et al. Open versus minimally invasive liver surgery for colorectal liver metastases (LapOpHuva): a prospective randomized controlled trial. *Surg Endosc*. 2019;**33**(12):3926–3936.
7. Fretland ÅA, Dagenborg VJ, Bjørnelv GMW, et al. Laparoscopic versus open resection for colorectal liver metastases: the OSLO-COMET randomized controlled trial. *Ann Surg*. 2018;**267**(2):199–207.
8. Cipriani F, Fantini C, Ratti F, et al. Laparoscopic liver resections for hepatocellular carcinoma. Can we extend the surgical indication in cirrhotic patients? *Surg Endosc*. 2018;**32**(2):617–626.
9. Prodeau M, Drumez E, Duhamel A, et al. An ordinal model to predict the risk of symptomatic liver failure in patients with cirrhosis undergoing hepatectomy. *J Hepatol*. 2019;**71**(5):920–929.
10. Hobeika C, Fuks D, Cauchy F, et al. Impact of cirrhosis in patients undergoing laparoscopic liver resection in a nationwide multicentre survey. *Br J Surg*. 2020;**107**(3):268–277.
11. Soubrane O, Eguchi S, Uemoto S, et al. Minimally invasive donor hepatectomy for adult living donor liver transplantation: an international, multi-institutional evaluation of safety, efficacy and early outcomes. *Ann Surg*. 2022;**275**(1):166–174.
12. Hobeika C, Fuks D, Cauchy F, et al. Benchmark performance of laparoscopic left lateral sectionectomy and right hepatectomy in expert centers. *J Hepatol*. 2020;**73**(5):1100–1108.
13. Cheung TT, Poon RTP, Yuen WK, et al. Long-term survival analysis of pure laparoscopic versus open hepatectomy for hepatocellular carcinoma in patients with cirrhosis: a single-center experience. *Ann Surg*. 2013;**257**(3):506–511.
14. Fretland ÅA, Dagenborg VJ, Waaler Bjørnelv GM, et al. Quality of life from a randomized trial of laparoscopic or open liver resection for colorectal liver metastases. *Br J Surg*. 2019;**106**(10):1372–1380.
15. Yoh T, Cauchy F, Soubrane O. Oncological resection for liver malignancies: can the laparoscopic approach provide benefits? *Ann Surg*. 2022;**275**(1):182–188.
16. Soubrane O, Schwarz L, Cauchy F, et al. A conceptual technique for laparoscopic right hepatectomy based on facts and oncologic principles: the caudal approach. *Ann Surg*. 2015;**261**(6):1226–1231.
17. Merath K, Chen Q, Bagante F, et al. A multi-institutional international analysis of textbook outcomes among patients undergoing curative-intent resection of intrahepatic cholangiocarcinoma. *JAMA Surg*. 2019;**154**(6):e190571.
18. Hobeika C, Nault JC, Barbier L, et al. Quality of surgical care has a significant impact on the probability of cure for early stage HCC occurring on cirrhosis. *JHEP Rep*. 2020;**2**(6):100153.
19. Cherqui D, Soubrane O. Laparoscopic liver resection: an ongoing revolution. *Ann Surg*. 2017;**265**(5):864–865.
20. Halls MC, Alseidi A, Berardi G, et al. A comparison of the learning curves of laparoscopic liver surgeons in differing stages of the IDEAL paradigm of surgical innovation: standing on the shoulders of pioneers. *Ann Surg*. 2019;**269**(2):221–228.
21. Nomi T, Fuks D, Kawaguchi Y, Mal F, Nakajima Y, Gayet B. Learning curve for laparoscopic major hepatectomy. *Br J Surg*. 2015;**102**(7):796–804.
22. van der Poel MJ, Besselink MG, Cipriani F, et al. Outcome and learning curve in 159 consecutive patients undergoing total laparoscopic hemihepatectomy. *JAMA Surg*. 2016;**151**(10):923–928.
23. Vigano L, Laurent A, Tayar C, Tomatis M, Ponti A, Cherqui D. The learning curve in laparoscopic liver resection: improved feasibility and reproducibility. *Ann Surg*. 2009;**250**(5):772–782.
24. McCulloch P, Altman DG, Campbell WB, et al. No surgical innovation without evaluation: the IDEAL recommendations. *Lancet*. 2009;**374**(9695):1105–1112.
25. Krenzien F, Schöning W, Brunnbauer P, et al. The ILLS laparoscopic liver surgery fellow skills curriculum. *Ann Surg*. 2020;**272**(5):786–792.
26. Broering DC, Berardi G, El Sheikh Y, Spagnoli A, Troisi RI. Learning curve under proctorship of pure laparoscopic living donor left lateral sectionectomy for pediatric transplantation. *Ann Surg*. 2020;**271**(3):542–548.
27. Kawaguchi Y, Fuks D, Kokudo N, Gayet B. Difficulty of laparoscopic liver resection: proposal for a new classification. *Ann Surg*. 2018;**267**(1):13–17.
28. Halls MC, Berardi G, Cipriani F, et al. Development and validation of a difficulty score to predict intraoperative complications during laparoscopic liver resection. *Br J Surg*. 2018;**105**(9):1182–1191.
29. Ban D, Tanabe M, Ito H, et al. A novel difficulty scoring system for laparoscopic liver resection. *J Hepatobiliary Pancreat Sci*. 2014;**21**(10):745–753.
30. Tanaka S, Kawaguchi Y, Kubo S, et al. Validation of index-based IWATE criteria as an improved difficulty scoring system for laparoscopic liver resection. *Surgery*. 2019;**165**(4):731–740.

31. Kawaguchi Y, Tanaka S, Fuks D, et al. Validation and performance of three-level procedure-based classification for laparoscopic liver resection. *Surg Endosc.* 2020;**34**(5):2056–2066.
32. Kawaguchi Y, Hasegawa K, Tzeng C-WD, et al. Performance of a modified three-level classification in stratifying open liver resection procedures in terms of complexity and postoperative morbidity. *Br J Surg.* 2020;**107**(3):258–267.
33. Viganò L, Torzilli G, Troisi R, et al. Minor hepatectomies: focusing a blurred picture: analysis of the outcome of 4471 open resections in patients without cirrhosis. *Ann Surg.* 2019;**270**(5):842–851.
34. Gero D, Muller X, Staiger RD, et al. How to establish benchmarks for surgical outcomes?: a checklist based on an international expert Delphi consensus. *Ann Surg.* 2022;**275**(1):115–120.
35. de Haas RJ, Wicherts DA, Flores E, Azoulay D, Castaing D, Adam R. R1 resection by necessity for colorectal liver metastases: is it still a contraindication to surgery? *Ann Surg.* 2008;**248**(4):626–637.
36. Okumura S, Goumard C, Gayet B, Fuks D, Scatton O. Laparoscopic versus open two-stage hepatectomy for bilobar colorectal liver metastases: a bi-institutional, propensity score-matched study. *Surgery.* 2019;**166**(6):959–966.
37. Viganò L, Ferrero A, Amisano M, Russolillo N, Capussotti L. Comparison of laparoscopic and open intraoperative ultrasonography for staging liver tumours. *Br J Surg.* 2013;**100**(4):535–542.
38. Fuks D, Nomi T, Ogiso S, et al. Laparoscopic two-stage hepatectomy for bilobar colorectal liver metastases. *Br J Surg.* 2015;**102**(13):1684–1690.
39. Duwe G, Knitter S, Pesthy S, et al. Hepatotoxicity following systemic therapy for colorectal liver metastases and the impact of chemotherapy-associated liver injury on outcomes after curative liver resection. *Eur J Surg Oncol.* 2017;**43**(9):1668–1681.
40. De Gottardi A, Rautou P-E, Schouten J, et al. Porto-sinusoidal vascular disease: proposal and description of a novel entity. *Lancet Gastroenterol Hepatol.* 2019;**4**(5):399–411.
41. Okumura S, Tabchouri N, Leung U, M, et al. Laparoscopic parenchymal-sparing hepatectomy for multiple colorectal liver metastases improves outcomes and salvageability: a propensity score-matched analysis. *Ann Surg Oncol.* 2019;**26**(13):4576–4586.
42. European Association for the Study of the Liver. EASL Clinical Practice Guidelines: management of hepatocellular carcinoma. *J Hepatol.* 2018;**69**(1):182–236.
43. Doyle A, Gorgen A, Muaddi H, et al. Outcomes of radiofrequency ablation as first-line therapy for hepatocellular carcinoma less than 3 cm in potentially transplantable patients. *J Hepatol.* 2019;**70**(5):866–873.
44. Shindoh J, Makuuchi M, Matsuyama Y, et al. Complete removal of the tumor-bearing portal territory decreases local tumor recurrence and improves disease-specific survival of patients with hepatocellular carcinoma. *J Hepatol.* 2016;**64**(3):594–600.
45. Goumard C, Komatsu S, Brustia R, Fartoux L, Soubrane O, Scatton O. Technical feasibility and safety of laparoscopic right hepatectomy for hepatocellular carcinoma following sequential TACE-PVE: a comparative study. *Surg Endosc.* 2017;**31**(5):2340–2349.
46. Scatton O, Katsanos G, Boillot O, et al. Pure laparoscopic left lateral sectionectomy in living donors: from innovation to development in France. *Ann Surg.* 2015;**261**(3):506–512.
47. Soubrane O, Perdigao Cotta F, Scatton O. Pure laparoscopic right hepatectomy in a living donor. *Am J Transplant.* 2013;**13**(9):2467–2471.
48. Sánchez-Cabús S, Cherqui D, Rashidian N, et al. Left-liver adult-to-adult living donor liver transplantation: can it be improved? A retrospective multicenter European study. *Ann Surg.* 2018;**268**(5):876–884.
49. Cherqui D, Soubrane O, Husson E, M, et al. Laparoscopic living donor hepatectomy for liver transplantation in children. *Lancet Lond Engl.* 2002;**359**(9304):392–396.
50. Soubrane O, de Rougemont O, Kim K-H, et al. Laparoscopic living donor left lateral sectionectomy: a new standard practice for donor hepatectomy. *Ann Surg.* 2015;**262**(5):757–761.
51. Hong SK, Shin E, Lee K-W, et al. Pure laparoscopic donor right hepatectomy: perspectives in manipulating a flexible scope. *Surg Endosc.* 2019;**33**(5):1667–1673.
52. Kawai T, Goumard C, Jeune F, Komatsu S, Soubrane O, Scatton O. 3D vision and maintenance of stable pneumoperitoneum: a new step in the development of laparoscopic right hepatectomy. *Surg Endosc.* 2018;**32**(8):3706–3712.
53. Hasegawa Y, Koffron AJ, Buell JF, Wakabayashi G. Approaches to laparoscopic liver resection: a meta-analysis of the role of hand-assisted laparoscopic surgery and the hybrid technique. *J Hepato-Biliary-Pancreat Sci.* 2015;**22**(5):335–341.
54. Ton-That-Tung, Nguyen-Duong-Quang. [Segmentary hepatectomy by transparenchymatous vascular ligation]. *Presse Med.* 1965;**73**(52):3015–3017.
55. Liu CL, Fan ST, Cheung ST, Lo CM, Ng IO, Wong J. Anterior approach versus conventional approach right hepatic resection for large hepatocellular carcinoma: a prospective randomized controlled study. *Ann Surg.* 2006;**244**(2):194–203.
56. Scuderi V, Barkhatov L, Montalti R, et al. Outcome after laparoscopic and open resections of posterosuperior segments of the liver. *Br J Surg.* 2017;**104**(6):751–759.
57. Yoh T, Cauchy F, Kawai T, et al. Laparoscopic right hepatectomy using the caudal approach is superior to open right hepatectomy with anterior approach and liver hanging maneuver: a comparison of short-term outcomes. *Surg Endosc.* 2020;**34**(2):636–645.
58. Strasberg SM, Belghiti J, Clavien P-A, et al. The Brisbane 2000 terminology of liver anatomy and resections. *HPB.* 2000;**2**(3):333–339.
59. Tzeng C-WD, Vauthey J-N. Evaluation of new classifications for liver surgery: can anatomic granularity predict both complexity and outcomes of hepatic resection? *Ann Surg.* 2018;**267**(1):24–25.
60. Goumard C, Farges O, Laurent A, et al. An update on laparoscopic liver resection: the French Hepato-Bilio-Pancreatic Surgery Association statement. *J Visc Surg.* 2015;**152**(2):107–112.
61. Yoh T, Cauchy F, Soubrane O. Techniques for laparoscopic liver parenchymal transection. *Hepatobiliary Surg Nutr.* 2019;**8**(6):572–581.
62. Yerdel MA, Karayalcin K, Koyuncu A, et al. Direct trocar insertion versus Veress needle insertion in laparoscopic cholecystectomy. *Am J Surg.* 1999;**177**(3):24724–24729.
63. Powell-Brett S, Richardson M, Super P, Singhal R. Veress needle creation of pneumoperitoneum: a safe technique. *Obes Surg.* 2020;**30**(5):2026–2027.
64. Rahbari NN, Wente MN, Schemmer P, et al. Systematic review and meta-analysis of the effect of portal triad clamping on outcome after hepatic resection. *Br J Surg.* 2008;**95**(4):424–432.
65. Piardi T, Lhuaire M, Memeo R, Pessaux P, Kianmanesh R, Sommacale D. Laparoscopic Pringle maneuver: how we do it? *Hepatobiliary Surg Nutr.* 2016;**5**(4):345–349.
66. Dua MM, Worhunsky DJ, Hwa K, Poultsides GA, Norton JA, Visser BC. Extracorporeal Pringle for laparoscopic liver resection. *Surg Endosc.* 2015;**29**(6):1348–1355.

67. Laurenzi A, Cherqui D, Figueroa R, Adam R, Vibert E, Cunha AS. Totally intra-corporeal Pringle maneuver during laparoscopic liver resection. *HPB (Oxford)*. 2018;**20**(2):128–131.
68. Huang J-W, Su W-L, Wang S-N. Alternative laparoscopic intracorporeal Pringle maneuver by Huang's loop. *World J Surg*. 2018;**42**(10):3312–3315.
69. Couinaud C. [Leading principles for controlled hepatectomies] [author's transl]. *Chir Memoires Acad Chir*. 1980;**106**(2):136–142.
70. Hepp J, Couinaud C. [Approach to and use of the left hepatic duct in reparation of the common bile duct]. *Presse Med*. 1956;**64**(41):947–948.
71. Kim JH, Kim H. Laparoscopic right hemihepatectomy using the Glissonean approach: detachment of the hilar plate (with video). *Ann Surg Oncol*. 2021;**28**(1):459–464.
72. Lazorthes F, Chiotasso P, Chevreau P, Materre JP, Roques J. Hepatectomy with initial suprahilar control of intrahepatic portal pedicles. *Surgery*. 1993;**113**(1):103–108.
73. Takasaki K, Kobayashi S, Tanaka S, Saito A, Yamamoto M, Hanyu F. Highly anatomically systematized hepatic resection with Glissonean sheath code transection at the hepatic hilus. *Int Surg*. 1990;**75**(2):73–77.
74. Launois B, Sutherland FR, Harissis H. A new technique of Hepp-Couinaud hepaticojejunostomy using the posterior approach to the hepatic hilum. *J Am Coll Surg*. 1999;**188**(1):59–62.
75. Machado MAC, Surjan RC, Basseres T, Schadde E, Costa FP, Makdissi FF. The laparoscopic Glissonian approach is safe and efficient when compared with standard laparoscopic liver resection: results of an observational study over 7 years. *Surgery*. 2016;**160**(3):643–651.
76. Machado MA, Makdissi F, Surjan R. Laparoscopic glissonean approach: making complex something easy or making suitable the unsuitable? *Surg Oncol*. 2020;**33**:196–200.
77. Mouly C, Fuks D, Browet F, et al. Feasibility of the Glissonian approach during right hepatectomy. *HPB (Oxford)*. 2013;**15**(8):638–645.
78. Figueras J, Lopez-Ben S, Lladó L, et al. Hilar dissection versus the 'glissonean' approach and stapling of the pedicle for major hepatectomies: a prospective, randomized trial. *Ann Surg*. 2003;**238**(1):111–119.
79. Belghiti J, Guevara OA, Noun R, Saldinger PF, Kianmanesh R. Liver hanging maneuver: a safe approach to right hepatectomy without liver mobilization. *J Am Coll Surg*. 2001;**193**(1):109–111.
80. Couinaud C. [Surgical anatomy of the liver. Several new aspects]. *Chir Memoires Acad Chir*. 1986;**112**(5):337–342.
81. Ogata S, Belghiti J, Varma D, et al. Two hundred liver hanging maneuvers for major hepatectomy: a single-center experience. *Ann Surg*. 2007;**245**(1):31–35.
82. Kim JH, Kim H. Modified liver hanging maneuver in laparoscopic major hepatectomy: the learning curve and evolution of indications. *Surg Endosc*. 2020;**34**(6):2742–2748.
83. Brustia R, Scatton O, Perdigao F, El-Mouhadi S, Cauchy F, Soubrane O. Vessel identifications tags for open or laparoscopic associating liver partition and portal vein ligation for staged hepatectomy. *J Am Coll Surg*. 2013;**217**(6):e51–e55.
84. Scatton O, Katsanos G, Soubrane O. Two-stage hepatectomy: tape it and hang it, while you can. *World J Surg*. 2012;**36**(7):1647–1650.
85. Dokmak S, Aussilhou B, Rebai W, Cauchy F, Belghiti J, Soubrane O. Up-to-down open and laparoscopic liver hanging maneuver: an overview. *Langenbecks Arch Surg*. 2020;**406**(1):19–24.
86. Araki K, Conrad C, Ogiso S, Kuwano H, Gayet B. Intraoperative ultrasonography of laparoscopic hepatectomy: key technique for safe liver transection. *J Am Coll Surg*. 2014;**218**(2):e37–e41.
87. Ishizawa T, Saiura A, Kokudo N. Clinical application of indocyanine green-fluorescence imaging during hepatectomy. *Hepatobiliary Surg Nutr*. 2016;**5**(4):322–328.
88. Otsuka Y, Kaneko H, Cleary SP, Buell JF, Cai X, Wakabayashi G. What is the best technique in parenchymal transection in laparoscopic liver resection? Comprehensive review for the clinical question on the 2nd International Consensus Conference on Laparoscopic Liver Resection. *J Hepatobiliary Pancreat Sci*. 2015;**22**(5):363–370.
89. Nassar A, Hobeika C, Lamer C, et al. Relevance of blood loss as key indicator of the quality of surgical care in laparoscopic liver resection for colorectal liver metastases. *Surgery*. 2020;**168**(3):411–418.
90. Pan Y-X, Wang J-C, Lu X-Y, et al. Intention to control low central venous pressure reduced blood loss during laparoscopic hepatectomy: a double-blind randomized clinical trial. *Surgery*. 2020;**167**(6):933–941.
91. Abu Hilal M, Underwood T, Taylor MG, Hamdan K, Elberm H, Pearce NW. Bleeding and hemostasis in laparoscopic liver surgery. *Surg Endosc*. 2010;**24**(3):572–577.
92. Halls MC, Cipriani F, Berardi G, et al. Conversion for unfavorable intraoperative events results in significantly worse outcomes during laparoscopic liver resection: lessons learned from a multicenter review of 2861 cases. *Ann Surg*. 2018;**268**(6):1051–1057.
93. Cauchy F, Fuks D, Nomi T, et al. Risk factors and consequences of conversion in laparoscopic major liver resection. *Br J Surg*. 2015;**102**(7):785–795.
94. Costi R, Scatton O, Haddad L, et al. Lessons learned from the first 100 laparoscopic liver resections: not delaying conversion may allow reduced blood loss and operative time. *J Laparoendosc Adv Surg Tech A*. 2012;**22**(5):425–431.
95. Hobeika C, Fuks D. Reply regarding: Benchmark performance of laparoscopic left lateral sectionectomy and right hepatectomy in expert centers. *J Hepatol*. 2021;73(6):1576.96. Guilbaud T, Feretti C, Holowko W, et al. Laparoscopic major hepatectomy: do not underestimate the impact of specimen extraction site. *World J Surg*. 2020;**44**(4):1223–1230.
97. Lee L, Mata J, Droeser RA, et al. Incisional hernia after midline versus transverse specimen extraction incision: a randomized trial in patients undergoing laparoscopic colectomy. *Ann Surg*. 2018;**268**(1):41–47.
98. Forester B, Attaar M, Donovan K, et al. Short-term quality of life comparison of laparoscopic, open, and robotic incisional hernia repairs. *Surg Endosc*. 2020;**35**(6):2781–2788.
99. Al Chalabi H, Larkin J, Mehigan B, McCormick P. A systematic review of laparoscopic versus open abdominal incisional hernia repair, with meta-analysis of randomized controlled trials. *Int J Surg Lond Engl*. 2015;**20**:65–74.
100. Rausa E, Bonitta G, Bonavina L. Comment on 'Is Pfannenstiel incision the 'one-size-fits-all' solution for specimen retrieval in colorectal surgery?' *Ann Surg*. 2019;**270**(2):e37–e38.

31

Pathogenesis and natural history of gallstones

Veena Bheeman, Royce P. Vincent, and Ameet G. Patel

Introduction

Gallstone disease is a common gastrointestinal disorder. The prevalence ranges between 5% and 20%.[1] The incidence is 0.6–1.39% per year in the European population. The spectrum of presentation ranges from completely asymptomatic in the majority, to symptomatic gallstone disease along with its complications. Surgery forms the main basis of treatment in those that require intervention.[2,3] Gallstones and their complications are responsible for one-third of emergency surgical admissions in the UK.[4] The rates of urgent cholecystectomy range from 0.2% to 35% across England.[5] The National Institute for Health and Care Excellence (NICE) 2014 guidelines state that asymptomatic stones in a normal gall bladder with a normal biliary tree require no intervention. Patients with symptomatic stones should be offered a laparoscopic cholecystectomy, preferably in the day care setting.[6]

Epidemiology

The prevalence is highest in the West, and the incidence increases with age. This is likely to be explained partly by the longer life expectancy in this region.[1] Women develop gallstones two to three times more frequently than men.[2]

Gallstone prevalence is highest in people of Northern European descent, in Hispanics and Native Americans, lower in Asia, and least of all in Africa.[7] It is interesting to note that some epidemiological factors resulting in gallstone development favour gall bladder cancer as well, although the full extent of the association whether genetic or environmental remains to be understood.[8]

The more affluent regions of the world have a preponderance, up to 85% of cholesterol stones, whereas pigment and mixed stones are more prevalent in the less affluent countries.[9] However, these epidemiological demarcations have blurred in the last few decades with the East adopting the Western lifestyle. There has also been a rise in the incidence of gallstones in general, and cholesterol stones particularly in those groups known to have a low prevalence. A recent study from Germany showed that the prevalence of gall bladder stones was 3.8% in 2002 and went up to 10.8% in 2013.[10] The Japan Gall Stone Study Group also found a prevalence of 10%, which was traditionally believed to be under 5%, as well as an increased proportion of cholesterol stones.[11]

Pathogenesis

Several factors contribute to the formation of gallstones, and they are discussed more in detail below. Bile is 95% water and contains primarily cholesterol, phospholipids, bile salts, proteins, and bilirubin.[12] The different types of gallstones form by different mechanisms. Normally, bile acids and phospholipids keep cholesterol in its soluble form. The process of crystallization occurs when the factors favouring stone formation or pro-nucleating factors dominate those that prevent it. A genetic predisposition, compounded by increased cholesterol secretion, leading to supersaturated bile and poor motility of the gall bladder are the main pro-nucleating factors that favour cholesterol stone formation. Similarly, pigment stones occur due to excess bilirubin formation. Mixed stones contain both cholesterol and pigments occurring against a background of infections.[13]

Risk factors for development of gallstones

There are several risk factors, both modifiable and non-modifiable, that contribute to gall stone disease (Table 31.1).

Non-modifiable risk factors

Age

As age increases, the duration of exposure of the gall bladder to pro-nucleating factors increases. In the elderly, regardless of sex, there is decreased bile acid production and increased cholesterol secretion.[1] Such a decrease in bile acid production is due to a reduction in the action of the rate-limiting enzyme of bile acid synthesis.[14,15]

Table 31.1 Non-modifiable and modifiable risk factors

Non-modifiable risk factors	Modifiable risk factors
1. Increasing age 2. Female sex 3. Gene mutations and hereditary factors	1. Lifestyle associations: • A high-calorific intake • Low-calcium diet • Low vitamin C • Smoking • Lack of alcohol intake • Reduced physical activity • Rapid weight loss 2. Metabolic syndrome 3. Pharmacological associations: • Oral contraceptives • Parenteral nutrition • Lipid-lowering agents 4. Inflammatory bowel disease 5. Mechanical factors: • Gallbladder dysmotility • Slow intestinal transit • Spinal cord injuries

Sex

Women, in the reproductive age group, demonstrate a significant preponderance to gallstone disease, a difference that narrows as age increases. Parity seems to have a direct correlation. Higher parity at a younger age is associated with an increased risk of development of gallstones.[16] However, women tend to have a more uncomplicated course when compared to men.[17]

The hyper-oestrogenic state induced by pregnancy causes an upregulation of low-density lipoprotein receptors, causing larger amounts of cholesterol to enter the hepatic pool, an increase in cholesterol biosynthesis, and increased biliary secretion of cholesterol.[18,19] Gallstones and their complications are the second most common non-obstetric emergency, seen in up to 12% of pregnant women. It is estimated that 3% of women in the US require a cholecystectomy in their first year after delivery. The rate of development of complications is high. Maternal gall stone pancreatitis has an alarmingly high mortality rate of 37%.[20]

Genetic factors

Twin studies have shown that 25% of the various presentations of gallstone disease have a genetic background.[21] In a recent meta-analysis of two genome-wide association studies involving 27,174 cases and 736,838 controls, 21 novel gallstone-associated variants were identified at 20 loci. The most significant example of this is, perhaps, mutations in the hepatic ATP-binding cassette transporters, ABCG5 and ABCG8, which are necessary for hepatic cholesterol transport. Such variants could be responsible for 25% of gallstones. Specific variants contribute to different populations. Missense mutations in the apical sodium-dependent bile acid transporter (ASBT) are associated with a greater risk of gallstone disease and shed light on the role of the intestinal compartment of the enterohepatic circulation of bile acids in gallstone disease susceptibility.[22,23] In addition, epigenetic mechanisms affecting gene expression may be involved where environmental and gene–environment interactions are involved.[24]

Lifestyle associations

Cholesterol gallstones are most commonly caused by an intake of a high-calorific foods, low dietary fibre, and a sedentary lifestyle.[25,26] Other factors that compound this problem are a diet low in calcium and vitamin C. An increase in coffee consumption decreases the risk by increasing the enterohepatic circulation of bile salts.[27] While smoking has minimal effects on gall stone formation, alcohol consumption may have a protective effect.[28] Modaine et al. attributed this to both rapid postprandial gall bladder emptying and accelerated gall bladder filling, probably caused by an increase in sphincter of Oddi pressures.[29]

The metabolic syndrome

The components of the metabolic syndrome are atherogenic dyslipidaemia, hypertension, insulin resistance, a pro-inflammatory state, and a prothrombotic state. Gallstones are associated with the above conditions because of alterations in bile acid metabolism and gall bladder motility, inflammation, and decreased bowel movement.[30,31] Biliary lipids are derived from lipoproteins. The synthesis, uptake, and degradation of plasma lipoproteins occur in the liver. Interestingly, while bile is the only mechanism of elimination of cholesterol from the body and most gallstones are made of cholesterol, there is no definitive association between serum lipid levels and gallstones with the notable exception of hypertriglyceridemia. Nearly all patients with hypertriglyceridaemia have supersaturated gall bladder bile even if they have a normal body mass index.[32]

Insulin resistance leads to poor gall bladder motor function, and also increases cholesterol synthesis and its excretion in bile.[33] Diabetics are at a higher risk of the development of the more severe complications of gallstone disease and of surgical intervention.[34] Mahapure et al. recently showed that diabetes could be associated with intraoperative difficulties and prolonged surgical time.[35] Additionally, the rates of mortality and morbidity due to surgery are higher when acutely ill. Thus, surgery is indicated sooner rather than later once symptoms develop.[36]

Several studies have shown that the mere presence of gallstones can herald the onset of adverse cardiovascular events. Zhao et al. in a systematic review published in 2019 determined that the presence of gallstones was associated with a 1.24-fold increase in prevalence and a 1.23-fold increase in the incidence for cardiovascular disease, coronary artery disease, and stroke—which are all established end points of the metabolic syndrome.[37]

Pharmacological associations

Oral contraceptive pills

The long-term use of oral contraceptives and oestrogen therapies is thought to be associated with an increased risk of gallstone disease. Both oestrogen and progesterone are implicated, albeit through different mechanisms. Oestrogen increases the hepatic cholesterol pool and progesterone decreases gall bladder motility.[38] A recent systematic review and meta-analysis that included 19 studies 556,620 participants found that the pooled relative risk of oral contraceptive intake and cholelithiasis risk was 1.19 (95% confidence interval (CI) 0.97–1.45), while the relative risk for hormone replacement therapy was 1.79 (95% CI 1.61–2.00).[39] Etminan et al. in a large retrospective study looked at 2,721,014 women who were using an oral contraceptive containing ethinyl oestradiol combined with a progestin during 1997–2009. They found a small, statistically significant increase in the risk of gall bladder disease associated with desogestrel, drospirenone, and norethindrone compared with levonorgestrel.[40]

Parenteral nutrition

Several mechanisms underlie the increase in gall stone formation in patients on long-term parenteral nutrition. The lack of gastrointestinal stimuli for both biliary secretion and gall bladder motility, and changes in bile acid metabolism like the excessive intestinal production of secondary bile salts deoxycholate and lithocholate have been implicated. In addition, the varying proportions of individual components of parenteral nutrition formulations such as the increase in the percentage of lipids or amino acid imbalances can also prove lithogenic. Lastly, the underlying condition warranting parenteral nutrition may contribute to one or more factors resulting in gallstones, such as cholestasis. All of the above are most significantly seen in those patients that have nil oral intake, have had ileal resections, have short bowel syndrome, and those on long-term narcotics and anticholinergics.[41]

Lipid-lowering agents

The fibric acid derivatives are potent inhibitors of acyl coenzyme A (CoA) cholesterolacyl transferase (ACAT) and cause increase secretion of cholesterol in the bile thereby favouring gall stone formation.[42] On the other hand, the statins have a protective effect by reducing biliary cholesterol excretion by the inhibition of 3-hydroxy-3-methyl-glutaryl coenzyme-A reductase (HMG CoA reductase).[43]

Inflammatory bowel disease

The prevalence of gallstones in patients with Crohn's disease has been found to be 13–34% in literature.[44] The most important mechanism underlying gall stone formation in these patients is thought to be the reduced enterohepatic circulation of bile acids due to resection of the terminal ileum or due to functional loss due to the inflammatory process. The relative excess of cholesterol then results in super-saturation and cholesterol stone formation.[45,46] However, there is evidence to suggest that such changes to the enterohepatic circulations are transient and that increased bile acid absorption in the colon then occurs.[47,48] Another mechanism is the increased excretion of bilirubin resulting in pigment stones.[49] In addition, the need for parenteral nutrition can result in gallstones by the mechanisms outlined above.[50]

The relationship of gallstone disease with ulcerative colitis appears less certain. Some studies show a correlation in the more severe and extensive cases of ulcerative colitis, while most show none.[51]

Mechanical factors

Gall bladder dysmotility

Gall bladder motility is modulated by several neural and hormonal factors. In response to food intake, the gall bladder has a triphasic response. There are two phases of emptying separated by a refilling phase.

The liver secretes approximately 1000 mL of bile a day at a secretory pressure of 30 cmH$_2$O. In the fasting state, the pressure at the sphincter of Oddi is 12–15 cmH$_2$O and the pressure within the common bile duct is 12 cmH$_2$O. The pressure within the gall bladder is about 10 cmH$_2$O. This gradient ensures that bile fills in the gall bladder in the fasting state.[52,53]

Cholecystokinin (CCK) is the main hormonal modulator of gall bladder motility. It is secreted by the I cells in the duodenum. It functions as a hormone and a neurotransmitter. At least four different forms have been identified in circulation. CCK release is triggered by luminal acid, fats, and amino acids. It has an excitatory effect on gall bladder smooth muscles and an inhibitory effect on the neural fibres to the sphincter of Oddi, thereby facilitating gall bladder emptying.[54,55] See Figure 31.1. The effect of CCK is calcium dependent. It is enhanced by hypercalcaemia and is inhibited by the addition of calcium-channel blocking agents.[56]

Neural control of gall bladder motility comes from the hepatic branch of the anterior vagus, which is parasympathetic, and sympathetic supply is from the coeliac plexus through the right phrenic nerve and the hepatic plexus.[57] The autonomic plexuses are situated in the muscular and the submucosal layers. The vagus and its cholinergic neurons maintain the fasting tone of the gall bladder.[58] The sympathetic system causes gall bladder relaxation when pre-treated with CCK.[59]

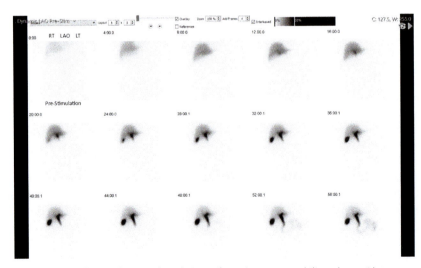

Figure 31.1 Hepatobiliary iminodiacetic acid scan: showing slow drainage from the common biliary duct, with tracer persisting up to 1 hour after its administration, suggestive of sphincter of Oddi dysfunction.

Pharmacological modifiers of gall bladder motility

Somatostatin and its long-acting analogue octreotide block the action of CCK on the gall bladder mucosa. Long-term use interferes with post-prandial emptying of the gall bladder, which subsequently results in its dilatation.[60]

Prostaglandins have a prokinetic effect on the gall bladder. Nonsteroidal anti-inflammatory drugs such as indomethacin abolish prostaglandin production. While this results in a decreased tone of the gall bladder, as expected, it also promotes gall bladder emptying, a phenomenon that is possibly explained by the inhibitory effect of the drug on the sphincter of Oddi.[61,62]

Erythromycin has a prokinetic effect mediated by both serotoninergic and adrenergic pathways. This effect is blocked by atropine and ondansetron, a serotonin 5-HT3 receptor antagonist. Amino acid infusions cause gall bladder emptying, probably mediated by CCK release. The same is true of intravenous lipids, but the mechanism remains to be determined. Cholestyramine is an anion exchange resin that probably causes gall bladder emptying by triggering CCK release via reduced negative feedback from bite salts in the gut on CCK release.[63]

Slow intestinal transit

Regardless of the cause, intestinal hypomotility results in gall stone formation by virtue of increased deoxycholate concentration in the bile which results in cholesterol supersaturation. Deoxycholate is formed in the colon from the bile salts that escape enterohepatic circulation. Thus, an increase in deoxycholate indicates an inefficient enterohepatic circulation.[64] In diabetes, the autonomic neuropathy affects both small intestinal transit and gall bladder motility.[65,66]

Spinal injuries

While the parasympathetic stimulus from the vagus is the predominant secretomotor neurological input, loss of sympathetic innervation in spinal injuries, especially above the tenth thoracic vertebra, is known to cause gall bladder dysmotility and subsequent development of gall stones. The exact action of the sympathetic nervous system on gall bladder motility is poorly understood. A certain degree of dysmotility in the form of slower emptying does occur. Decreased intestinal transit leading to an abnormal enterohepatic circulation, and metabolic changes causing abnormal biliary lipid secretion are also implicated.[67–70]

Gallstones and the biliary microbiome

Intestinal dysbiosis is believed to play a role in the development of gallstone disease. Several studies are being done to investigate the microbiome in order to recognize patterns that could be predictive of various gastrointestinal disorders.[71] The biliary microbiome is similar to that of the duodenum. Interestingly, the microbiome of the oral cavity has bearing on the development of gallstones. Certain oral bacteria can disrupt the synthesis of nitric oxide, the cofactor of endothelial nitric oxide synthase, thereby decreasing the expression of the antioxidant protein NRF2 increasing the amount of reactive oxygen species. Patients with gallstones have a high level of oxidative stress in the gall bladder mucosa, resulting in altered gall bladder absorption and secretion of bile components such as mucins and glycoproteins. This may contribute to bile supersaturation and formation (or progression) of gallstones. Wu et al. studied the microbiomes of the gut, bile, and gallstones and found an increase in proteobacteria and a decrease in *Faecalibacterium*, *Lacnospira*, and *Roseburia* species in those with gallstones.[72] Delayed colonic transit with an increase in Gram-positive anaerobic bacteria causing increased 7α-dehydroxylation activity can result in elevation of lithogenic secondary bile acid deoxyxholate.[73] The cholecystectomy has been found to alter the microbiota of different parts of the gastrointestinal tract, probably mediated by an abnormal intestinal flow pattern of bile acids, increasing the risk for cancers of the stomach, small intestine, and colon.[71,74]

The correlation between *Helicobacter* species infection and cholelithiasis and cholecystitis has been researched extensively. The three commonest species implicated are *Helicobacter pylori*, *H. bilis*, and *H. hepaticus*. The underlying mechanisms are thought to be related to increased calcium precipitation by the action of urease, increased release of inflammatory cytokines interleukin 1 and 6, and tumour necrosis factor alpha, and the similarity of the CagA protein on the surface of *Helicobacter* to glycoprotein aminopeptidases, which are pro-nucleating factors in the biliary tree.[75–77] The data on the association of *Helicobacter* species infection and gallstones is rather heterogeneous. Attaallah et al. studied ninety-four consecutive patients with symptomatic gallstone disease. Urease tests and gastroscopy were performed before cholecystectomy. After cholecystectomy, the gall bladder tissue was subjected to urease testing, Giemsa, and immunohistochemical staining. The latter tests confirmed *H. pylori* in the gall bladder mucosa in 35 patients (37%). The rapid urease test was positive in the gastric mucosa in 47 patients (59%), and it was positive in the gall bladder mucosa in 21 patients (22%). In 15 patients, both gastric and gall bladder tested positive with the urease test. There was significant correlation of the rapid urease test in both gall bladder and gastric mucosa (p = 0.0001).[78] Takahashi et al. analysed 15,551 Japanese adults without a past medical history of gastrectomy, cholecystectomy, *H. pylori* eradication, and utilization of proton pump inhibitors, antidiabetic drugs, or anticholesterol drugs. A further group of 1057 subjects with a history of *H. pylori* eradication were analysed separately. The gallstone prevalence among *H. pylori*-negative patients was 4%, 5% in those with *H. pylori* eradication, and 6% in those with active infection.[79] *H. pylori* may also play a role in the complications of gall stone disease.[71,80]

Bariatric surgery and gall stones

Obesity is one of the most consistently associated risk factors for gallstone disease. Bariatric surgeries have revolutionized the management of those with morbid obesity.[81] When rapid weight loss occurs following these procedures, increased cholesterol secretion into the bile favours the development of gall stones in up to 30% of these patients.[2,82] Uy et al. in a meta-analysis of five randomized controlled trials with a total of 521 subjects concluded that the rates of gallstone formation with ursodeoxycholic acid was 9% compared to 28% with placebo.[83] Talha et al. demonstrated a fall in gallstone formation from 22% to 6.5%.[84] Various studies have tried to arrive at the optimal dose of the drug required.[84] Ursodeoxycholic acid at a dose 500–600 mg for a period of 6 months following surgery is found to reduce the incidence of gallstones (odds ratio 0.25 (95% CI 0.17–0.38); p <0.00001).[85,86] The ongoing UPGRADE trial in the Netherlands is currently investigating the effect of 900 mg of ursodeoxycholic acid versus placebo on gallstone formation in patients undergoing bariatric surgery and should help clarify things further.[87]

Pathogenesis of gall stone formation

Gallstones occur when pro-nucleating factors overwhelm the ability of bile to keep the substances like cholesterol and bilirubin in a soluble form[12]. Gallstones have been classified into several types and subtypes. One systematic classification divided them into eight types and more than ten subtypes. They are cholesterol stones, pigment stones, calcium carbonate stones, phosphate stones, calcium stearate stones, protein stones, cystine stones, and mixed stones (Figure 31.2).

Spectroscopic techniques to analyse stone composition have been in use for several decades. Recent advances in these methods have yielded more precise elemental analyses and have added to our understanding of the composition of gallstones. This allows for more accurate identification of the types of stones.[89] The three most common types are cholesterol stones, pigment stones, and mixed stones.

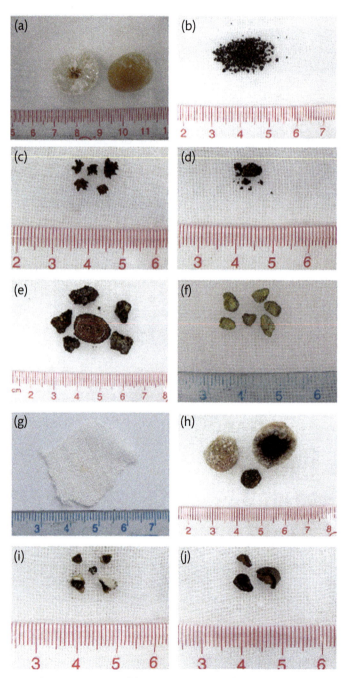

Figure 31.2 The appearance of each type of gall bladder stone. (a) Cholesterol stone. (b) Pigment stone. (c) Calcium carbonate stone. (d) Phosphate stone. (e) Calcium stearate stone. (f) Protein stone. (g) Cystine stone. (h) Cholesterol–bilirubinate mixed stone. (i) Bilirubinate–calcium carbonate mixed stone. (j) Bilirubinate–phosphate mixed stone.

Reproduced from Qiao T, Ma RH, Luo XB, Yang LQ, Luo ZL, Zheng PM. The systematic classification of gallbladder stones. *PLoS One.* 2013;8(10):e74887. Published 2013 4 Oct, under a Creative Commons Attribution 3.0 License (https://creativecommons.org/licenses/by/3.0/).

Cholesterol stones

These stones are essentially those that contain more than 90% cholesterol. They are soft, yellow to brown or grey stones with a predominantly smooth surface with a lamellar arrangement of tightly stacked cholesterol crystals.[90] The fundamental mechanism contributing to this type of stone is bile super-saturation with cholesterol, that is, an increase in the ratio of cholesterol to bile acids and phospholipids.

Three enzymes are involved in achieving this balance between cholesterol and the bile acids and phospholipids:

- HMG CoA reductase.
- Acyl Co A cholesterol acyl transferase.
- 7α hydroxylase (CYP7A1).

HMG CoA reductase catalyses the rate-limiting step in the biosynthesis of cholesterol and other isoprenoids (Figure 31.3). Hypercholesterolaemia, most commonly brought about by dietary excess, causes an increase in the activity of HMG CoA reductase, which translates into increased hepatic secretion of cholesterol into the bile.[91]

Acyl CoA cholesterol acyl transferase is involved in the esterification of excessive intracellular cholesterol. The cholesterol esters are then either stored in the cytosol or secreted into circulation in conjunction with lipoproteins. The gene responsible for this enzyme's activity in humans is the *ACAT2* gene coding for the enzyme ACAT2. The gene is expressed in liver and small intestine.[92,93] Its deficiency in the liver can increase cholesterol availability for biliary

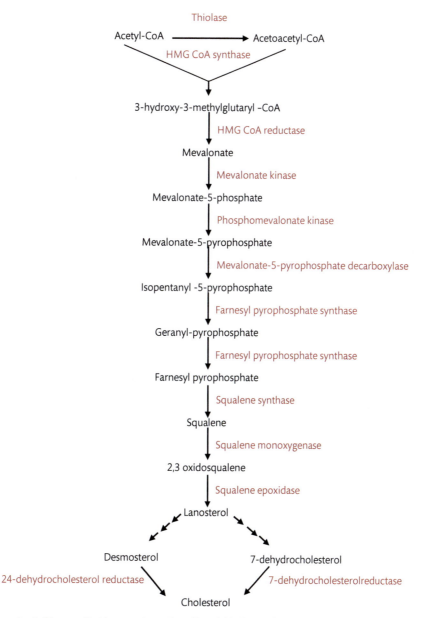

Figure 31.3 Cholesterol biosynthesis. The rate-limiting step is catalysed by HMG-CoA reductase. It takes 19 reactions for lanosterol to be converted into cholesterol.

Sources: data from Cerqueira NM, Oliveira EF, Gesto DS, et al. Cholesterol biosynthesis: a mechanistic overview. *Biochemistry*. 2016;55(39):5483–5506; Porter FD, Herman GE. Malformation syndromes caused by disorders of cholesterol synthesis. *J Lipid Res*. 2011;52(1):6–34; and Stromsten A, von Bahr S, Bringman S, et al. Studies on the mechanism of accumulation of cholesterol in the gallbladder mucosa. Evidence that sterol 27-hydroxylase is not a pathogenetic factor. *J Hepatol*. 2004;40:8–13.

secretion, thereby increasing the risk of gallstones and its deficiency in the intestine decreases the risk of gallstones by decreasing biliary cholesterol output in liver.[94]

The cholesterol thus secreted is carried in four ways in the bile:

- The vast majority as mixed micelles with a lecithin and cholesterol core with bile salts surrounding them.
- Vesicles with bilayers of cholesterol and phospholipids.
- Simple micelles containing cholesterol and bile acids.
- Cholesterol–lipoprotein complex.[98]

Bile salts monomers, when secreted from the liver cells, also stimulate the secretion of cholesterol and lecithin from the liver cell membrane in the form of small unilamellar vesicles. The bile salts then coalesce with the vesicles to form mixed micelles. However, within the hepatic bile ducts, this process remains incomplete due to the dilute nature of bile and about 90% of the cholesterol is carried in the form of vesicles. As the bile becomes more and more concentrated in the gall bladder, the cholesterol is rendered more soluble. Hence, most of the cholesterol in the gall bladder is carried as mixed micelles in normal individuals. In the hypercholesterolemic state, when more cholesterol is secreted into bile in comparison to bile acids and lecithin, more cholesterol remains in vesicles that combine to form large multilamellar cholesterol-rich vesicles. Crystallization of cholesterol can then occur in a matter of hours.[99] Such nucleation is the first essential step in stone formation.

It is important to distinguish the nucleation of cholesterol crystals, that is, the initial formation of a crystal, from crystal growth and stone formation. It is probable that different factors determine these two processes.[100] In the normal gall bladder, such crystals are washed out with the flow of bile. When gall bladder motility is affected, this clearing mechanism is not effective.[101] Reduced intestinal motility is also implicated in reduced gall bladder mucin clearance. This results in the mixing of cholesterol crystals and thickened gall bladder mucoprotein and bridges the gap between nucleation and stone formation.[102] When bile contains excessive calcium, bilirubin precipitates and calcification of gallstones occurs.[103]

Pigment stones

Pigment stones may be black or brown in colour. The black stones are amorphous and brittle and are made up of spherical or irregular bilirubinate particles of different sizes, loosely clumped together.[104] They occur when there is excessive haem turnover from red blood cell breakdown as can be seen in chronic haemolytic conditions like the thalassaemias, hereditary spherocytosis, sickle cell disease, and cirrhosis of the liver.[105] Patients with haemolytic syndromes are prone to developing gallstones at an early age. The rate of development of symptoms is also higher because the duration of harbouring the stones is longer. Finally, in sickle cell anaemia, the symptoms of a vaso-occlusive crisis mimic those of symptomatic gallstones.[106]

Mixed stones

The brown pigment stones, also referred to as mixed stones, are soft, greasy, and more commonly found primarily in the bile duct. They contain two or more of the eight primary components. Their shape and microstructure vary based on the composition. They are most commonly seen in association with infections of the biliary tract. This is best exemplified by Asiatic cholangiohepatitis, but not limited to it. Bacteria in the biliary tree release beta-glucuronidases that cleave glucuronic acid from bilirubin. In its unconjugated form, the latter precipitates into calcium bilirubinate, thereby leading to stone formation. Polymerization then occurs, with progressive enlargement of the stone. It is not known if polymerization occurs at the pigment level or if it is a function of the precipitated calcium bilirubinate.[107,108]

Gallstones and gall bladder carcinoma

The association of gallstones with gall bladder cancer has long been suggested by their similar epidemiological determinants.[109] The commonest prerequisite for this cancer is a chronically inflamed gall bladder. Gallstones usually predate cancer by about 20 years. A Swedish study recently reposted the overall incidence of gall bladder cancers in patients with gallstones to be 0.5%.[110] A large cohort study of 396,720 patients conducted in South Korea showed that gallstones were significantly associated with an increased risk of gall bladder cancer and subsequent mortality.[111]

However, our understanding at this point is far from complete, as evidenced by the rising incidence of these cancers in younger individuals who have not had long-standing gallstones. Many recent studies have tried to provide robust evidence of the strength of such an association. This insight would help determine which patients would benefit from a prophylactic cholecystectomy, since gall bladder cancers, although of a relatively low incidence, contribute to a disproportionately high number of cancer deaths due to late detection.[112,113]

A recent study from India used data from a gall bladder cancer case–control study done at Tata Memorial Hospital and used 26 genetic variants identified in a genome-wide association study of 27,174 gallstone cases and 736,838 controls of European ancestry in a complementary observational and Mendelian randomization analysis to assess the presence of such an association. The odds ratio for the development of gall bladder cancer in the presence of gall stone was found to be 1.3–1.6.[114]

The natural history of gallstones

Since the first account of gallstones by a Florentine pathologist in the fifteenth century, the symptoms and evolution of gallstone disease have been studied extensively.[115] Early studies into the subject mostly involved case series with retrospective data and reports based on autopsies. When ultrasonography came into popular use as a reliable means of diagnosing gall stones, it became simpler to identify asymptomatic stones. A few studies that identified gall stones by various means and followed them up to ascertain the natural history of gallstones (Table 31.2).

Asymptomatic gallstones

The vast majority of gallstones are asymptomatic.[124] There is an overwhelming body of evidence to support this.[119–123] An interesting study by Schwab et al. looked at fetal gallstones and their natural history. Fetal incidence of gallstones is around 0.45%. They identified 34 fetuses with gallstones from 300,000 obstetric sonograms. They followed a subset of 17 children for 3–20 years. None developed

Table 31.2 Studies of the natural history of gall stones

Authors, study year range	Sample size	Diagnostic modality	Follow-up (years)	Symptoms New onset	Symptoms Evolution of symptoms	Surgery
Comfort et al.,[116] 1925-1934	112 (A)	Incidental during Surgery	10-20	51 (46%)	50% (Rec)	24/51 (47%) (S)
Lund et al.,[117] 1936-1950	478 (A&S)	X-ray, OCG	5-20	–	136/478 (28%) (Rec)	120/478 (25%) 96/478 (20%) (A)
Thistle et al.,[118] 1972	193 (A)	USG	2	60/193 (31%)	41/60 (69%) (Rec)	7/60 (12%) (S)
Sama et al.,[119] 1982	132 108 (A) 24 (S)	USG	5	14/108 (13%)	15/24 (63%) (Rec)	20/108 (19%) (A) & 2/24 (8%) (S)
Gracie and Ransohoff,[120] 1982	123 (A)	USG	10	18/123 (15%)	–	–
Attili et al.,[121] 1981-1984	151 118 (A) 33 (S)	USG & OCG	10	30/118 (26%)	16/33 (49%) (Rec)	28/118 (24%) (A) & 15/33 (45%) (S)
Thwayeb et al.,[122] 2004	109 (A)	USG	18	31/109 (28%)	–	10/78 (13%) (A) & 29/31 (16%) (S)
Festi et al.,[123] 2010	806 580 (A) 94 (MS) 119 (SS)	USG	9	61 (11%) (MS) 66 (11%) (SS)	(MS) 55/94 (58%) resolved, ↑ 25%, stable 17% (SS) 62/119 (52%) resolved, ↓ 17% stable 31%	41% (A) 17% (MS) 41% (SS)

↓, decrease; ↑, increase; A, asymptomatic; HPE: histopathological examination increase; decrease; MS, mild symptoms; OCG, oral cholecystogram; Lap, laparotomy; Rec, recurrent symptoms; S, symptomatic; SS, severe symptoms; USG, ultrasonogram; X-ray, plain radiograph of the abdomen.

sequelae of cholelithiasis.[126] While this is a small study of a demographic traditionally not associated with gall stones, it adds to the body of evidence supporting the benign nature of gallstone disease.

Patients with asymptomatic stones require no follow-up imaging or intervention.[6] Yet, 10–40% of these patients are subjected to surgery.[117,119,121–123] Lifestyle modifications are often all that is required. Increased physical activity lowers the risk of progression to cholecystectomy.[127] The use of gallstone dissolution therapies may delay symptom onset or lead to dissolution of stones to a variable extent. Unfortunately, the adverse side effects in the form of diarrhoea and musculoskeletal pain and the long-term requirement of dissolution therapy diminish compliance.[128]

There are a few coexisting conditions where a prophylactic cholecystectomy is indicated. They include the so-called porcelain gall bladder, associated large polyps, diabetes, states of immunosuppression, and haemolytic anaemias.[128] In addition, it is indicated for those undergoing solid organ transplantation, which is increasingly done all over the world. This is in anticipation of a delay in diagnosis of complications due to the immunosuppressed state. These complications are expected to have much worse implications in these patients. In addition, drugs like ciclosporin and tacrolimus are lithogenic.[129]

Symptomatic gallstones

The current consensus is that incidentally discovered gallstones produce symptoms 20% of the time.[1,125] In Table 31.2, this number is higher in some of the earlier studies with rates of up to 45%. This is reflective of an era where the only conclusive method of identification of gallstones was either during surgery or at autopsy. Typical symptoms along with cholecystographic evidence of a nonfunctioning gall bladder and plain abdominal radiographs were used for diagnosis. The number of patients with symptoms attributed to gallstones may not be entirely accurate. Following the advent of the ultrasonogram, the diagnostic accuracy increased and the detection rate of gallstones was seen to be more reflective of the current scenario.

While the current NICE guidelines suggest that the laparoscopic cholecystectomy be offered for symptomatic gallstones, there is plenty of evidence to suggest that uncomplicated symptomatic gallstones can be managed conservatively. McSherry et al. expressed their conviction that if safe and effective cholelitholytic medicines were to come into clinical practice, more of these patients could be spared surgery.[130] Ursodeoxycholic acid was approved for use in the US approximately 3 years later in December 1987.[131] In the study by Festi et al. (Table 31.2), a group of 856 patients were studied for a mean period of 9 years; 580 (73%) of them were asymptomatic and 317 (37%) symptomatic. Of the asymptomatic group, 452 (78%) remained asymptomatic. In those who were symptomatic to begin with, interestingly, resolution of symptoms was seen in 165 (52%). However, Festi et al. found that of the 189 cholecystectomies performed, 41% were in asymptomatic subjects.[124] The pressing question then, is whether surgery is required at all in uncomplicated symptomatic gallstones. In order to address this at the present time, the C-Gall study is being conducted across 20 NHS hospitals with 430 participants comparing laparoscopic cholecystectomy with conservative management in adults with uncomplicated symptomatic gallstones.[132]

The threshold for early intervention may be lowered those with limited access to healthcare in order to avoid complications. Lastly, in those patients with vague dyspepsia with no discernible cause, a prophylactic cholecystectomy can improve the quality of life if the symptoms are distressing enough to begin with.[133]

The changing landscape of laparoscopic cholecystectomy

The now ubiquitous laparoscopic cholecystectomy, with its standardization and reproducibility, while giving us a simpler and less morbid form of treatment, has likely reduced the threshold for surgery. It is thus prudent to keep revisiting the natural history of gallstones in this context. However, as important as it is to recognize this, it is equally important to recognize those situations where readmissions for recurrent symptoms may mean higher morbidity and increased costs to the healthcare system.[134]

From 1995 to 2013, Allie et al. looked at 711,406 cholecystectomies performed in New York State; 637,308 (90%) were laparoscopic. The overall frequency of cholecystectomy did not increase during this time. The incidence of calculous cholecystitis declined by 20% (p <0.0001) between 1995 and 2013, while other diagnoses such as biliary colic, gallstone pancreatitis, and acalculous cholecystitis increased in incidence. Outpatient laparoscopic cholecystectomies saw a sharp increase from 0.2% in 1995 to 49% in 2013, going up over 320-fold. It is interesting to note the decrease in the rate of acute cholecystitis over this interval, as the rates of outpatient cholecystectomies increased exponentially. This may be reflective of an early intervention to cholecystectomy at a lower threshold. The overall cholecystectomy complication rate was 9%. The authors concluded that caution must be exercised in the management of benign biliary disease as the complication rate was high.[135] Other authors, such as Sakofaras et al. observed that while the procedure has simplified the treatment of gall stone disease, it has also broadened the indications for cholecystectomy. This filters down to the referral system where more general practitioners and gastroenterologists now have a lower threshold for referring for elective laparoscopic cholecystectomy. The latter may require re-evaluation in view of the predominantly benign nature of the natural history of uncomplicated gallstones.[136]

The timing of the cholecystectomy and its ramifications in terms of conversion rate, postoperative complications, and the attendant length of hospital stay has been studied in great detail.[137,138] For patients on a waitlist, the recurrence of symptoms while they wait for surgery ranges between 5% and 39%. These patients may be readmitted up to ten times. Factoring in the costs of readmissions and including associated morbidity, the early laparoscopic cholecystectomy emerges as the intervention of choice in the acute setting.[139–143]

Conclusion

The majority of gallstones remain asymptomatic.[1,144] One in five patients with asymptomatic gallstones develop symptoms. The incidence of symptoms are a risk factor in themselves for recurrent symptoms.[144] At this time, in the symptomatic patient, early laparoscopic cholecystectomy is the treatment of choice.[134–143] The association of gallstones with gall bladder carcinoma remains to be completely determined.[109–114] Formation of gallstones is multifactorial, with lifestyle and diet having major influence as reflected by the higher incidence of adverse cardiac events and overall mortality in the presence of gallstones.[145,146]

REFERENCES

1. Gurusamy KS, Davidson BR. Gallstones. *BMJ.* 2014;**348**:g2669.
2. Lammert F, Gurusamy K, Ko CW, et al. Gallstones. *Nat Rev Dis Primers.* 2016;**2**:16024.
3. Shabanzadeh D. Incidence of gallstone disease and complications. *Curr Opin Gastroenterol.* 2018;**34**(2):81–89.
4. NHS Digital. Hospital Episode Statistics Admitted Patient Care England (2013–2014). Health and Social Care Information Centre; 2015. https://www.hscic.gov.uk/catalogue/PUB16719
5. AUGIS/ASGBI J. Pathway on management of acute gallstone diseases. 2015. https://www.augis.org/wp-content/uploads/2014/05/Acute-Gallstones-Pathway-Final-Sept-2015.pdf
6. National Institute for Health and Care Excellence (NICE). Gallstone Disease: diagnosis and management. Clinical guideline [CG188]. 2014. https://www.nice.org.uk/guidance/cg188
7. Shaffer EA. Epidemiology and risk factors for gallstone disease: has the paradigm changed in the 21st century? *Curr Gastroenterol Rep.* 2005;**7**(2):132–140.
8. Schmidt M, Marcano-Bonilla L, Roberts, L. Gallbladder cancer: epidemiology and genetic risk associations. *Chin Clin Oncol.* 2019;**8**(4):4.
9. Everhart JE, Ruhl CE. Burden of digestive diseases in the United States. Part III: liver, biliary tract and pancreas. *Gastroenterology.* 2009;**136**(4):1134–1144.
10. Kratzer W, Klysik M, Binzberger A, Schmidberger J. Gallbladder stone incidence and prevalence in Germany: a population-based study. *Z Gastroenterol.* 2021;**59**(8):859–864.
11. Tazuma S. Epidemiology, pathogenesis and classification of biliary stones (common bile duct and intrahepatic). *Best Pract Res Clin Gastroenterol.* 2006;**20**(6):1075–1083.
12. Boyer JL. Bile formation and secretion. *Compr Physiol.* 2013;**3**(3):1035–1078.
13. Singh VK, Jaswal BS, Sharma J, Rai PK. Analysis of stones formed in the human gall bladder and kidney using advanced spectroscopic techniques. *Biophys Rev.* 2020;**12**(3):647–668.
14. Einarsson K, Nilsell K, Leijd B, et al. Influence of age on secretion of cholesterol and synthesis of bile acids in the liver. *N Engl J Med.* 1985;**313**(5):277–282.
15. Bertolotti M, Gabbi C, Anzivino C, et al. Age-related changes in bile acid synthesis and hepatic nuclear receptor expression. *Eur J Clin Invest.* 2007;**37**(6):501–508.
16. Novacek G. Gender and gallstone disease. *Wien Med Wochenschr.* 2006;**156**(19–20):527–533.
17. Bailey KS, Marsh W, Daughtery L, Hobbs G, Borgstrom D. Gender disparities in the presentation of gallbladder disease. *Am Surg.* 2019;**85**(8):830–833.
18. Valdivieso V, Covarrubias C, Siegel F, et al. Pregnancy and cholelithiasis: pathogenesis and natural course of gallstones diagnosed in early puerperium. *Hepatology.* 1993;**17**(1):1–4.
19. Vazquez MC, Rigotti A, Zanlungo S. Molecular mechanisms underlying the link between nuclear receptor function and cholesterol gallstone formation. *J Lipids.* 2012;**2012**:547643.
20. Hess E, Thumbadoo RP, Thorne E, McNamee K. Gallstones in pregnancy. *Br J Hosp Med (Lond).* 2021;**82**(2):1–8.
21. Katsika D, Grjibovski A, Einarsson C et al. Genetic and environmental influences on symptomatic GD: a Swedish study of 43,141 twin pairs. *Hepatology.* 2005;**42**:1138–1143.
22. Ferkingstad E, Oddsson A, Gretarsdottir S, et al. Genome-wide association meta-analysis yields 20 loci associated with gallstone disease. *Nat Commun.* 2018;**9**(1):5101.
23. Rebholz C, Krawczyk M, Lammert F. Genetics of gallstone disease. *Eur J Clin Invest.* 2018;**48**(7):e12935.
24. Di Ciaula A, Wang DQ, Bonfrate L, Portincasa P. Current views on genetics and epigenetics of cholesterol gallstone disease. *Cholesterol.* 2013;**2013**:298421.
25. Njeze GE. Gallstones. *Niger J Surg.* 2013;**19**(2):49–55.

26. Di Ciaula A, Wang DQ, Portincasa P. Cholesterol cholelithiasis: part of a systemic metabolic disease, prone to primary prevention. *Expert Rev Gastroenterol Hepatol*. 2019;**13**(2):157–171.
27. Martínez García RM, Jiménez Ortega AI, Salas-González MD, Bermejo López LM, Rodríguez-Rodríguez E. Intervención nutricional en el control de la colelitiasis y la litiasis renal [Nutritional intervention in the control of gallstones and renal lithiasis]. *Nutr Hosp*. 2019;**36**(3):70–74.
28. Shabanzadeh DM, Novovic S. Alcohol, smoking and benign hepato-biliary disease. *Best Pract Res Clin Gastroenterol*. 2017;**31**(5):519–527.
29. Modaine P, Davion T, Capron D, Capron JP. Etude échographique de la motricité vésiculaire du sujet sain. Reproductibilité de la méthode et effet de l'alcool [Ultrasound study of gallbladder motility in healthy subjects. Reproducibility of the method and effect of alcohol]. *Gastroenterol Clin Biol*. 1993;**17**(11):839–844.
30. Grundy SM, Brewer HB, Cleeman JI, Smith SC, Lenfant C. Definition of metabolic syndrome: report of the National Heart, Lung, and Blood Institute/American Heart Association conference on scientific issues related to definition. *Circulation*. 2004;**109**(3):433–438.
31. Latenstein CSS, Alferink LJM, Darwish Murad S, Drenth JPH, van Laarhoven CJHM, de Reuver PR. The association between cholecystectomy, metabolic syndrome, and nonalcoholic fatty liver disease: a population-based study. *Clin Transl Gastroenterol*. 2020;**11**(4):e00170.
32. Ahlberg J. Serum lipid levels and hyperlipoprotinaemia in gallstone patients. *Acta Chir Scand*. 1979;**145**(6):373–377.
33. Shabanzadeh DM, Sorensen LT, Jorgensen T. Determinants for gallstone formation—a new data cohort study and a systematic review with meta-analysis. *Scand J Gastroenterol*. 2016;**51**(10):1239–1248.
34. Ziaee SA, Fanaie SA, Khatib R, Khatibzadeh N. Outcome of cholecystectomy in diabetic patients. *Indian J Surg*. 2005;**67**:87–89.
35. Mahapure KS, Metgud SC. Effect of diabetes mellitus on operative outcome following laparoscopic cholecystectomy: a one year cross sectional study at tertiary care hospital. *Arch Int Surg*. 2019;**9**(3):78.
36. Łącka M, Spychalski P, Obłój P, et al. Costs of elective vs emergency cholecystectomy in diabetic patients. *Eur J Trans Clin Med*. 2020;**3**(2):37–43.
37. Zhao SF, Wang AM, Yu XJ, Wang LL, Xu XN, Shi GJ. Association between gallstone and cardio-cerebrovascular disease: systematic review and meta-analysis. *Exp Ther Med*. 2019;**17**(4):3092–3100.
38. George ED, Schluger LK. Special women's health issues in hepatobiliary diseases. *Clin Fam Pract*. 2000;**2**(1):155–169.
39. Wang S, Wang Y, Xu J, Chen Y. Is the oral contraceptive or hormone replacement therapy a risk factor for cholelithiasis. *Medicine*. 2017;**96**(14):e6556.
40. Etminan M, Delaney JA, Bressler B, Brophy JM. Oral contraceptives and the risk of gallbladder disease: a comparative safety study. *CMAJ*. 2011;**183**(8):899–904.
41. Angelico M, Della Guardia P. Review article: hepatobiliary complications associated with total parenteral nutrition. *Aliment Pharmacol Ther*. 2000;**14**(2):54–57.
42. Caroli-Bosc FX, Gall PL, Pugliese P, et al. Role of fibrates and HMG-CoA reductase inhibitors in gallstone formation. *Dig Dis Sci*. 2001;**46**(3):540–544.
43. Lioudaki E, Ganotakis ES, Mikhailidis DP. Lipid lowering drugs and gallstones: a therapeutic option? *Curr Pharm Des*. 2011;**17**(33):3622–3631.
44. Fraquelli M, Losco A, Visentin S, et al. Gallstone disease and related risk factors in patients with Crohn disease: analysis of 330 consecutive cases. *Arch Intern Med*. 2001;**161**(18):2201–2204.
45. Fagagnini S, Heinrich H, Rossel JB, et al. Risk factors for gallstones and kidney stones in a cohort of patients with inflammatory bowel diseases. *PLoS One*. 2017;**12**(10):e0185193.
46. Dowling RH, Bell GD, White J. Lithogenic bile in patients with ileal dysfunction. *Gut*. 1972;**13**(6):415–420.
47. Lapidus A, Einarsson K. Effects of ileal resection on biliary lipids and bile acid composition in patients with Crohn's disease. *Gut*. 1991;**32**(12):1488–1491.
48. Färkkilä MA. Biliary cholesterol and lithogeneity of bile in patients after ileal resection. *Surgery*. 1988;**104**(1):18–25.
49. Brink MA, Slors JF, Keulemans YC, et al. Enterohepatic cycling of bilirubin: a putative mechanism for pigment gallstone formation in ileal Crohn's disease. *Gastroenterology*. 1999;**116**(6):1420–1427.
50. Damião AO, Sipahi AM, Vezozzo DP, Gonçalves PL, Fukui P, Laudanna AA. Gallbladder hypokinesia in Crohn's disease. *Digestion*. 1997;**58**(5):458–463.
51. Zhang FM, Xu CF, Shan GD, Chen HT, Xu GQ. Is gallstone disease associated with inflammatory bowel diseases? A meta-analysis. *J Dig Dis*. 2015;**16**(11):634–641.
52. Hallenbeck GA. Biliary and pancreatic pressures. In: Code CF, ed. *The Handbook of Physiology VI: The Alimentary Canal, Vol 2 (Secretion)*. Washington, DC: American Physiological Society; 1968: 1007–1010.
53. Kjellgren K. Persistence of symptoms following biliary surgery. *Ann Surg*. 1960;**152**:1026–1036.
54. Everson GT. Gallbladder function in gallstone disease. *Gastroenterol Clin North Am*. 1980;**20**(1):85–110.
55. Patankar R. Gallbladder motility, gallstones, and the surgeon. *Dig Dis Sci*. 1995;**40**(11):2323–2335.
56. Malagelada JR, Holtermuller KH, Sizemore GW, Go VLW. The influence of hypercalcemia on basal and CCK stimulated pancreatic, gallbladder, and gastric functions in man. *Gastroenterology*. 1976;**71**(3):405–408.
57. Williams PL, Warwick R, Dyson M, Bannister LM. *Gray's Anatomy*. 37th ed. London: Churchill Livingstone; 1989.
58. Sutherland SD. Tile neurons of the gallbladder and gut. *J Anat*. 1967;**101**(4):701.
59. Strah KM, Melendez RL, Pappas TN, Debes HT. Interactions of vasoactive intestinal polypeptide and cholecystokinin octapeptide on the control of gallbladder contraction. *Surgery*. 1986;**99**(4):469–473.
60. Neri M, Cuccurullo, F, Marzio L. Effect of somatostatin on gallbladder volume and small intestinal motor activity in humans. *Gastroenterology*. 1990;**98**(2):316–321.
61. Kotwall CA, Clanachan AS, Bale HP. Effect of prostaglandins on motility of gallbladders removed from patients with gallstones. *Arch Surg*. 1984;**119**(6):709–712.
62. O'Donnell LID, Wilson P, Guest P, et al. Indomethacin and postprandial gallbladder emptying. *Lancet*. 1992;**339**(8788):269
63. Van Erpecum KJ, Venneman NG, Portincasa P, Vanberge-Henegouwen GP. Review article: agents affecting gall-bladder motility—role in treatment and prevention of gallstones. *Aliment Pharmacol Therapeut*. 2000;**14**(Suppl 2):66–70.
64. Marcus SN, Heaton KW. Deoxycholic acid and the pathogenesis of gall stones. *Gut*. 1988;**29**(4):522–533.
65. Nakeeb A, Comuzzie AG, Al-Azzawi H, et al. Insulin resistance causes human gallbladder dysmotility. *J Gastrointest Surg*. 2006;**10**(7):940–949.
66. Van Erpecum KJ, Van Berge-Henegouwen GP. Gallstones: an intestinal disease? *Gut*. 1999;**44**(3):435–438.

67. Apstein MD, Dalecki-Chipperfield K. Spinal cord injury is a risk factor for gallstone disease. *Gastroenterology.* 1987;**92**(4):966–968.
68. Moonka R, Stiens SA, Resnick WJ, et al. The prevalence and natural history of gallstones in spinal cord injury. *J Am Coll Surg.* 1999;**189**(3):274–281.
69. Tandon RK, Garg PK & Jain RK. Increased incidence of biliary sludge in high spinal cord injury. *Gastroenterology.* 1995;**108**:A438.
70. Rotter K, Larraín C. Gallstones in spinal cord injury (SCI): a late medical complication? *Spinal Cord.* 2003;**41**(2):105–108.
71. Grigor'eva IN, Romanova TI. Gallstone disease and microbiome. *Microorganisms.* 2020;**8**(6):835.
72. Wu T, Zhang Z, Liu B, Hou D, Liang Y, Zhang J, Shi P. Gut microbiota dysbiosis and bacterial community assembly associated with cholesterol gallstones in large-scale study. *BMC Genomics.* 2013;**14**:669.
73. Thomas LA, Veysey MJ, Murphy GM, et al. Octreotide induced prolongation of colonic transit increases faecal anaerobic bacteria, bile acid metabolising enzymes, and serum deoxycholic acid in patients with acromegaly. *Gut.* 2005;**54**(5):630–635.
74. Yoon WJ, Kim HN, Park E, et al. The impact of cholecystectomy on the gut microbiota: a case-control study. *J Clin Med.* 2019;**8**(1):79.
75. Belzer C, Kusters JG, Kuipers EJ, van Vliet AH. Urease induced calcium precipitation by Helicobacter species may initiate gallstone formation. *Gut.* 2006;**55**(11):1678–1679.
76. Kasprzak A, Szmyt M, Malkowski W, et al. Analysis of immunohistochemical expression of proinflammatory cytokines (IL-1α, IL-6, and TNF-α) in gallbladder mucosa: comparative study in acute and chronic calculous cholecystitis. *Folia Morphol (Warsz).* 2015;**74**(1):65–72.
77. Maurer KJ, Ihrig MM, Rogers AB, et al. Identification of cholelithogenic enterohepatic helicobacter species and their role in murine cholesterol gallstone formation. *Gastroenterology.* 2005;**128**(4):1023–1033.
78. Attaallah W, Yener N, Ugurlu MU, Manukyan M, Asmaz E, Aktan AO. Gallstones and concomitant gastric Helicobacter pylori infection. *Gastroenterol Res Pract.* 2013;**2013**:643109.
79. Takahashi Y, Yamamichi N, Shimamoto T, et al. Helicobacter pylori infection is positively associated with gallstones: a large-scale cross-sectional study in Japan. *J Gastroenterol.* 2014;**49**(5):882–889.
80. Wang L, Chen J, Jiang W, et al. The relationship between helicobacter pylori infection of the gallbladder and chronic cholecystitis and cholelithiasis: a systematic review and meta-analysis. *Can J Gastroenterol Hepatol.* 2021;**2021**:8886085.
81. Sjöström L. Review of the key results from the Swedish Obese Subjects (SOS) trial—a prospective controlled intervention study of bariatric surgery. *J Intern Med.* 2013;**273**(3):219–234.
82. Guzmán HM, Sepúlveda M, Rosso N, San Martin A, Guzmán F, Guzmán HC. Incidence and risk factors for cholelithiasis after bariatric surgery. *Obes Surg.* 2019;**29**(7):2110–2114.
83. Uy MC, Talingdan-Te MC, Espinosa WZ, Daez ML, Ong JP. Ursodeoxycholic acid in the prevention of gallstone formation after bariatric surgery: a meta-analysis. *Obes Surg.* 2008;**18**(12):1532–1538.
84. Talha A, Abdelbaki T, Farouk A, et al. Cholelithiasis after bariatric surgery, incidence, and prophylaxis: randomized controlled trial. *Surg Endosc.* 2020;**34**:5331–5337.
85. Magouliotis DE, Tasiopoulou VS, Svokos AA, et al. Ursodeoxycholic acid in the prevention of gallstone formation after bariatric surgery: an updated systematic review and meta-analysis. *Obes Surg.* 2017;**27**(11):3021–3030.
86. Machado FHF, Castro Filho HF, Babadopulos RFAL, Rocha HAL, Rocha JLC, Moraes Filho MO. Ursodeoxycholic acid in the prevention of gallstones in patients subjected to Roux-en-Y gastric bypass1. *Acta Cir Bras* 2019;**34**(1):e20190010000009.
87. Boerlage TCC, Haal S, Maurits de Brauw L, et al. Ursodeoxycholic acid for the prevention of symptomatic gallstone disease after bariatric surgery: study protocol for a randomized controlled trial (UPGRADE trial). *BMC Gastroenterol.* 2017;**17**(1):164.
88. Qiao T, Ma RH, Luo XB, Yang LQ, Luo ZL, Zheng PM. The systematic classification of gallbladder stones. *PLoS One.* 2013;**8**(10):e74887.
89. Singh VK, Jaswal BS, Sharma J, Rai PK. Analysis of stones formed in the human gall bladder and kidney using advanced spectroscopic techniques. *Biophys Rev.* 2020;**12**(3):647–668.
90. Friesen JA, Rodwell VW. The 3-hydroxy-3-methylglutaryl coenzyme-A (HMG-CoA) reductases. *Genome Biol.* 2004;**5**(11):248.
91. Chang TY, Chang CC, Lin S, Yu C, Li BL, Miyazaki A. Roles of acyl-coenzyme A: cholesterol acyltransferase-1 and -2. *Curr Opin Lipidol.* 2001;**12**(3):289–296.
92. Suggi S, Lin S, Ohgami N, Chang CCY, Chang TY. Roles of endogenously synthesized sterols in the endocytic pathway *J Biol Chem.* 2006;**281**(32):23191–23206.
93. Buhman KK, Accad M, Novak S, et al. Resistance to diet-induced hypercholesterolemia and gallstone formation in ACAT2-deficient mice. *Nat Med.* 2006;**6**(12):1341–1347.
94. Berg JM, Tymoczko JL, Stryer L. Section 26.2, Cholesterol is synthesized from acetyl coenzyme A in three stages. In: *Biochemistry.* 5th ed. New York: WH Freeman; 2002. https://www.ncbi.nlm.nih.gov/books/NBK22350/
95. Cerqueira NM, Oliveira EF, Gesto DS, et al. Cholesterol biosynthesis: a mechanistic overview. *Biochemistry.* 2016;**55**(39):5483–5506.
96. Porter FD, Herman GE. Malformation syndromes caused by disorders of cholesterol synthesis. *J Lipid Res.* 2011;**52**(1):6–34.
97. Stromsten A, von Bahr S, Bringman S, et al. Studies on the mechanism of accumulation of cholesterol in the gallbladder mucosa. Evidence that sterol 27-hydroxylase is not a pathogenetic factor *J Hepatol.* 2004;**40**(1):8–13.
98. Sahlin S, Thyberg P, Ahlberg J, Angelin B, Einarsson K. Distribution of cholesterol between vesicles and micelles in human gallbladder bile: influence of treatment with chenodeoxycholic acid and ursodeoxycholic acid. *Hepatology.* 1991;**13**(1):104–110.
99. Carey MC. Formation of cholesterol gallstones: the new paradigms. In: Paumgartner G, Stichl A, Gerok W, eds. *Trends in Bile Acid Research*. Dordrecht: Kluwer Academic Publishers; 1989: 259–281.
100. Bouchier IAD. Gallstone formation. *Keio J Med.* 1992;**41**(1):1–5.
101. Everson GT. Gallbladder function in gallstone disease. *Gastroenterol Clin North Am.* 1991;**20**(1):85–110.
102. Strasberg SM, Toth JL, Gallinger S, Harvey PR. High protein and total lipid concentration are associated with reduced metastability of bile in an early stage of cholesterol gallstone formation. *Gastroenterology.* 1990;**98**(3):739–746.

103. Moore EW. Biliary calcium and gallstone formation. *Hepatology.* 1990;**12**(3 Pt 2):206S–214S.
104. Soloway RD, Trotman BW, Ostrow JD. Pigment gallstones. *Gastroenterology.* 1977;**72**(1):167–182.
105. Maki T. Pathogenesis of calcium bilirubinate gallstones: role of E. coli, 0-glucuronidase, and coagulation by inorganic ions, polyelectrolytes, and agitation. *Ann Surg.* 1966;**165**:90–100.
106. Stephens CG, Scott RB. Cholelithiasis in sickle cell anemia: surgical or medical management. *Arch Intern Med.* 1980;**140**:648–651.
107. Stewart L, Oesterle AL, Erdan I, Griffiss JM, Way LW. Pathogenesis of pigment gallstones in Western societies: the central role of bacteria. *J Gastrointest Surg.* 2002;**6**(6):891–903.
108. Boonyapisit ST, Trotman BW, Ostrow JD. Unconjugated bilirubin, and the hydrolysis of conjugated bilirubin, in gallbladder bile of patients with cholelithiasis. *Gastroenterology.* 1978;**74**:70–74.
109. 5. Henley SJ, Weir HK, Jim MA, et al. Gallbladder cancer incidence and mortality, United States 1999–2011. *Cancer Epidemiol Biomarkers Prev.* 2015;**24**(9):1319–1326.
110. Bertran E, Heise K, Andia ME, et al. Gallbladder cancer: incidence and survival in a high-risk area of Chile. *Int J Cancer.* 2010;**127**(10):2446–2454.
111. Muszynska C, Lundgren L, Lindell G, Andersson R, Nilsson J, Sandström P, Andersson B. Predictors of incidental gallbladder cancer in patients undergoing cholecystectomy for benign gallbladder disease: results from a population-based gallstone surgery registry. *Surgery.* 2017;**162**(2):256–263.
112. Ryu S, Chang Y, Yun KE, Jung HS, Shin JH, Shin H. Gallstones and the risk of gallbladder cancer mortality: a cohort study. *Am J Gastroenterol.* 2016;**111**(10):1476–1487.
113. Rawla P, Sunkara T, Thandra KC, Barsouk A. Epidemiology of gallbladder cancer. *Clin Exp Hepatol.* 2019;**5**(2):93–102.
114. Mhatre S, Richmond RC, Chatterjee N, et al. The role of gallstones in gallbladder cancer in India: a Mendelian prophylactic cholecystectomy is indicated for randomization study. *Cancer Epidemiol Biomarkers Prev.* 2021;**30**(2):396–403.
115. De. Evolution of cholecystectomy: a tribute to Carl August Langenbuch. *Indian J Surg.* 2004;**66**(2):97–100.
116. Comfort MW, Gray HK, Wilson JM. The silent gallstone: a ten to twenty year follow-up study of 112 cases. *Ann Surg.* 1948;**128**(5):931–937.
117. Lund J. Surgical indications in cholelithiasis: prophylactic choleithiasis: prophylactic cholecystectomy elucidated on the basis of long-term follow up on 526 nonoperated cases. *Ann Surg.* 1960;**151**(2):153–162.
118. Thistle JL, Cleary PA, Lachin JM, Tyor MP, Hersh T. The natural history of cholelithiasis: the National Cooperative Gallstone Study. *Ann Intern Med.* 1984;**101**(2):171–175.
119. Barbara L, Sama C, Morselli Labate AM, et al. A population study on the prevalence of gallstone disease: the Sirmione Study. *Hepatology.* 1987;**7**(5):913–917.
120. Gracie WA, Ransohoff DF. The natural history of silent gallstones: the innocent gallstone is not a myth. *N Engl J Med.* 1982;**307**(13):798–800.
121. Attili AF, De Santis A, Capri R, Repice AM, Maselli S. The natural history of gallstones: The GREPCO experience. *Hepatology.* 1995;**21**(3):656–660.
122. McSherry CK, Ferstenberg H, Calhoun, WF, Lahman, EMA, Virshup M. The natural history of diagnosed gallstone disease in symptomatic and asymptomatic patients. *Ann Surg.* 1985;**202**(1):59–63.
123. Thwayeb, Y, Hernandez Siverio Gonzalez, N, Gutierrez Garcia, R. (2013). Natural history of asymptomatic gallstones. a prospective 18-year follow-up. *East J Med.* 2013;**9**(2):57–62.
124. Festi D, Reggiani ML, Attili AF, et al.. Natural history of gallstone disease: expectant management or active treatment? Results from a population-based cohort study. *J Gastroenterol Hepatol.* 2010;**25**(4):719–724.
125. Shabanzadeh DM. Incidence of gallstone disease and complications. *Curr Opin Gastroenterol.* 2018;**34**(2):81–89.
126. Schwab ME, Braun HJ, Feldstein VA, Nijagal A. The natural history of fetal gallstones: a case series and updated literature review. *J Matern Fetal Neonatal Med.* 2022;**35**(24):4755–4762.
127. Leitzmann MF, Rimm EB, Willett WC, et al. Recreational physical activity and the risk of cholecystectomy in women. *N Engl J Med.* 1999;**341**(11):777–784.
128. Obeid NR, Todd SR.Management of asymptomatic gallstones. In: Eachempati S, Reed R II, eds. *Acute Cholecystitis.* Cham: Springer; 2015. https://doi.org/10.1007/978-3-319-14824-3_6
129. Dobosz Ł, Kobiela J, Danielewicz R, Śledziński Z, Dębska-Ślizień A. Gallbladder pathologies in kidney transplant recipients: single-center experience and a review of the literature. *Ann Transplant.* 2018;**23**:572–576.
130. McSherry Charles K, Ferstenberg, HM, Calhoun, WF, Lahman EMA, Virshup M. *Ann Surg.* 1985;**202**(1):69–74.
131. Food and Drug Administration (FDA). Actigall: FDA-Approved Drugs. 2018. https://www.accessdata.fda.gov/drugsatfda_docs/label/2018/019594s21lbl.pdf
132. NHS Health Research Authority. C-gall. 2016. https://www.hra.nhs.uk/planning-and-improving-research/application-summaries/research-summaries/c-gall/
133. Mentes BB, Akin M, Irkorucu O, Tatlicioglou E, Ferahkose Z, Yildirim A, Maral I. Gastrointestinal quality of life in patients with symptomatic or asymptomatic cholelithiasis before and after laparoscopic cholecystectomy. *Surg Endosc.* 2001;**15**(11):1267–1272.
134. Di Ciaula A, Portincasa P. Recent advances in understanding and managing cholesterol gallstones [version 1; peer review: 2 approved]. *F1000Research.* 2018;**7**(F1000 Faculty Rev):1529. https://doi.org/10.12688/f1000research.15505.1
135. Alli VV, Yang J, Xu J, et al. Nineteen-year trends in incidence and indications for laparoscopic cholecystectomy: the NY State experience. *Surg Endosc.* 2017;**31**(4):1651–1658.
136. Sakorafas GH, Milingos D, Peros G. Asymptomatic cholelithiasis: is cholecystectomy really needed? a critical reappraisal 15 years after the introduction of laparoscopic cholecystectomy. *Dig Dis Sci.* 2007;**52**(5):1313–1325.
137. Gurusamy KS, Samraj K. Early versus delayed laparoscopic cholecystectomy for acute cholecystitis. *Cochrane Database Syst Rev.* 2006;**4**(4):CD005440.
138. Lau H, Lo CY, Patil NG, Yuen WK. Early versus delayed-interval laparoscopic cholecystectomy for acute cholecystitis: a metaanalysis. *Surg Endosc.* 2006;**20**(1):82–87.
139. Wiggins T, Markar SR, MacKenzie H, et al. Optimum timing of emergency cholecystectomy for acute cholecystitis in England: population-based cohort study. *Surg Endosc.* 2019;**33**(8):2495–2502.

140. Siddiqui T, MacDonald A, Chong PS, Jenkins JT. Early versus delayed laparoscopic cholecystectomy for acute cholecystitis: a meta-analysis of randomized clinical trials. *Am J Surg.* 2008;**195**(1):40–47.
141. Brazzelli M, Cruickshank M, Kilonzo M, et al. Clinical effectiveness and cost-effectiveness of cholecystectomy compared with observation/conservative management for preventing recurrent symptoms and complications in adults presenting with uncomplicated symptomatic gallstones or cholecystitis: a systematic review and economic evaluation. *Health Technol Assess.* 2014;**18**(55):1–101, v–vi.
142. Kerwat D, Zargaran A, Bharamgoudar R, Arif N, Bello G, Sharma B, Kerwat R. Early laparoscopic cholecystectomy is more cost-effective than delayed laparoscopic cholecystectomy in the treatment of acute cholecystitis. *Clinicoecon Outcomes Res.* 2018;**10**:119–125.
143. Saeb-Parsy K, Mills A, Rang C, Reed JB, Harris AM. Emergency laparoscopic cholecystectomy in an unselected cohort: a safe and viable option in a specialist centre. *Int J Surg.* 2010;**8**(6):489–493.
144. Shabanzadeh DM, Sørensen LT, Jørgensen T. A prediction rule for risk stratification of incidentally discovered gallstones: results from a large cohort study. *Gastroenterology.* 2016;**150**(1):156–167.
145. Fairfield CJ, Wigmore SJ, Harrison EM. Gallstone disease and the risk of cardiovascular disease. *Sci Rep.* 2019;**9**(1):5830.
146. Shabanzadeh DM, Sørensen LT, Jørgensen T. Gallstone disease and mortality: a cohort study. *Int J Public Health.* 2017;**62**(3):353–360.

32

Acute and chronic cholecystitis

Claire Goumard and Olivier Scatton

Introduction

Cholecystitis remains the main risk factor for bile duct injury (BDI) during cholecystectomy. While the paradigm of gall bladder surgery has evolved to a full mini-invasive approach, the incidence of BDI has remained steady over the last decades, ranging from 0.1% to 0.6%.[1] Now young surgeons and trainees are more used to mini-invasive than open cholecystectomy, and efforts have been put in place to develop safe alternatives to conversion in case of intraoperative difficulties. In this chapter, we will summarize the specifics of cholecystectomy in the context of cholecystitis and develop the recommended alternatives to standard retrograde cholecystectomy, keeping in mind that safety first is the key to prevent BDI and its dramatic consequences.

Preoperative management

When to operate for cholecystitis?

International recommendations on the diagnosis and treatment of cholecystitis have been published previously. The most commonly used among the surgical hepatopancreatobiliary community are the Tokyo Guidelines, which are regularly updated.[2-4]

The diagnosis of acute cholecystitis (AC) according to the Tokyo Guidelines relies on the association of a minimum of two out of three basic parameters: clinical local signs of inflammation (pain, Murphy's sign), systemic signs of inflammation (fever, elevated C-reactive protein, and/or white blood count), and imaging signs of AC. Associating those parameters carry a high sensitivity and specificity for the diagnosis of AC, while remaining basic and cost-effective.[5] The severity of AC is categorized into three levels: grade I—mild, grade II—moderate, and grade III—severe, which is associated with a worse prognosis. In brief, severe AC is associated with organ dysfunction, moderate AC is defined by marked signs of inflammation and/or duration of complaints for longer than 72 hours, and mild AC applies to all remaining cases.[5]

Based on this classification, the Tokyo Guidelines recommend in grade I (mild) patients a laparoscopic cholecystectomy (Lap-C) within 7 days (best within 72 hours) of onset of symptoms, and in grade II (intermediate) patients an emergent Lap-C if the performance status is good and the laparoscopic technique available. In case of poor patient performance status, either early biliary drainage or delayed/elective Lap-C are recommended. In grade III (severe) patients, emergent biliary drainage is recommended except in cases of a well-preserved patient condition who is a low surgical risk, where a Lap-C can be proposed in advanced centres.[2]

For chronic cholecystitis, there is no consensus on the timing for cholecystectomy; however, the key point is to rule out a gall bladder cancer, which may commonly present as chronic cholecystitis. Therefore, dedicated magnetic resonance imaging must be liberally performed in case of an atypical presentation of cholecystitis.

Which preoperative imaging is required?

The recommended imaging modality for the diagnosis of AC remains abdominal ultrasound, which combines a very good sensitivity and specificity to cost-effectiveness and simplicity.[5,6] A thickening of the gall bladder wall (≥4 mm), enlargement of the gall bladder (long axis ≥8 cm, short axis ≥4 cm), gallstones or retained debris, fluid accumulation, and infiltration of the fatty tissue around the gall bladder are the common signs observed. Computed tomography scanning and magnetic resonance imaging are only recommended in case of diagnostic uncertainty on ultrasound, and computed tomography scanning is particularly useful for the diagnosis of gangrenous or emphysematous cholecystitis.[5,6]

Operative technique and surgical options

Laparoscopic gold standard technique

Lap-C is the recommended technique for cholecystectomy in AC, even though the risks of conversion and BDI have been reported to be higher in this context of pedicular inflammation causing tissue retraction and an unclear vision of the gall bladder plate anatomy.[7,8] While not contraindicating the laparoscopic approach, these risks must be kept in mind and anticipated prior to surgery.

There is no consensus on the method of entry or the number of ports. However, in the presence of a cholecystitis, we recommend prioritizing exposure and ergonomics over aesthetics due to the potential difficulty and increased length of surgery.[4,9] Therefore, four ports including one 12 mm operating trocar allow proper triangulation

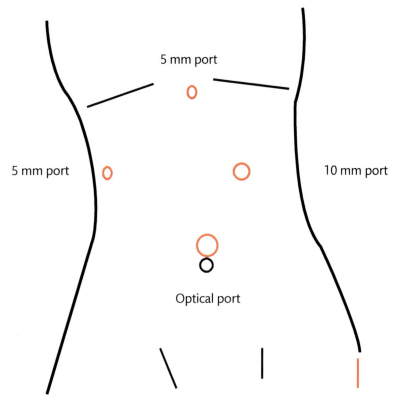

Figure 32.1 Trocar placement for a laparoscopic cholecystectomy in the presence of a cholecystitis.

and dissection in good conditions with the use of a 10 mm dissector which facilitates duct or vessel identification (Figure 32.1).

The open trocar insertion, with peritoneum cutting under direct vision, has been acknowledged as a safe entry method.[9] However, the method of entry should be tailored to the patient's characteristics, and blind pneumoperitoneum inflation using the Veress needle may be more appropriate in obese patients, or in some patients with predictable adhesions.

One important first step is exploration and careful exposure of the gall bladder itself. While an easy phase during most scheduled Lap-C procedures, the presence of cholecystitis increases the difficulty of this first step but also allows an evaluation of the severity of local inflammation. Severe cholecystitis is usually associated with an absence of direct visualization of the gall bladder itself, which is covered by the omentum, transverse colon, and/or duodenum (the 'curtain sign') (Figure 32.2). The denser and more inflamed these adhesions are, the more severe the cholecystitis will be.[4] If dividing these adhesions without significant bleeding is unlikely and the identification of the surrounding anatomical structures due to intense inflammation is not possible, a quick conversion to open surgery should be done in order to prevent a colonic or duodenal injury.

As soon as the gall bladder is identified and safely dissected from the surrounding organs, it may be decompressed externally using a Veress needle for aspiration (or a cholangiography needle).[4] This early drainage allows (1) an improvement in the Calot's triangle exposure by emptying the gall bladder's pouch, and (2) obtaining bile sampling for bacteriological examination. The needle insertion site may then be simply cauterized to avoid any leak. If the gall bladder is not distended (retracted) without causing interference with the field of view, this step may be avoided.

A gauze piece may be carefully inserted and placed below the gall bladder to absorb blood and/or bile or to collect any spilled stones.

The choice of an energy device depends mostly on the surgeon's habits, and there is a low level of evidence to recommend one source of energy compared with another with regard to safety.[9] However, monopolar cautery has been associated with thermal biliary tree injuries and more frequent gall bladder perforation.[10] In our team, we

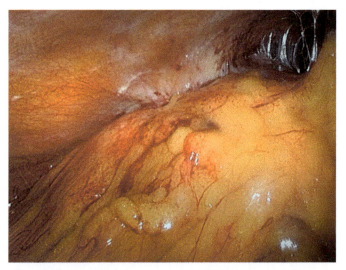

Figure 32.2 Laparoscopic vision when entering the abdominal cavity in the presence of a severe cholecystitis: the gallbladder is not visible and surrounded by severe adherences with adjacent organs.

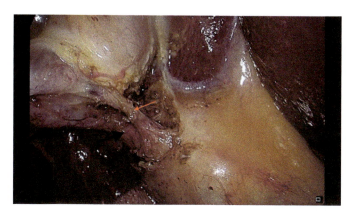

Figure 32.3 CVS in a case of cholecystitis. The cystic duct is identified with a black arrow, the cystic artery with a red arrow.

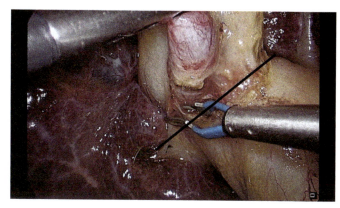

Figure 32.4 Imaginary line (in black) between Rouvière's sulcus and the base of segment 4 delineating the safe anatomical region above which the dissection should be performed.

prefer the bipolar cautery and scissors to monopolar electrocoagulation. The use of ultrasonic devices has also been reported to be safe and may be associated with a shorter operative time in classic cholecystectomy procedures. More generally, all energy devices carry an inherent risk for thermal injuries and the surgeon should be familiar with the specific complications associated with the type of energy used.

If the pedicular inflammation is moderate, a 'classic' retrograde cholecystectomy with prior identification of arterial and biliary structures within the cystic plate may be attempted. The safety of this dissection not only depends on the severity of tissue inflammation, but also on the surgeon's experience and assessment.

The gall bladder should be retracted superiorly by the fundus and laterally by the Hartmann's pouch to create an optimal angle between the cystic and the common bile duct, in order to properly dissect the hepatocystic triangle and obtain the critical view of safety (CVS)[4,11] (Figure 32.3).

The importance of obtaining the CVS during any cholecystectomy has been recently emphasized through the Research Institute Against Cancer of the Digestive System (IRCAD) recommendations on safe laparoscopic cholecystectomy.[9] The CVS has been previously described by Strasberg et al., and must comprise the three following elements: (1) hepatocystic triangle is cleared of fat and fibrous tissues, (2) the lower one-third of the gall bladder is separated from the liver to expose the cystic plate, and (3) two and only two structures should be seen entering in the gall bladder.[9,11] During this step, the use of a 10 mm hand dissector may be helpful.

In the context of cholecystitis, this step is a cornerstone of BDI prevention, and any failure to obtain a clear CVS should lead to surgical strategy modifications such as calling a colleague for help, performing an intraoperative cholangiogram, opting for a partial cholecystectomy, or conversion to laparotomy.

One additional key point is to identify Rouviere's sulcus to keep away from the elements of the right part of the hilum (right hepatic artery, right portal vein, right bile duct). Pedicular retraction may shorten significantly the distance between the vascular and biliary structures, and BDIs are often associated with right hepatic artery injuries. According to the Tokyo Guidelines, a safe procedure is to identify Rouvière's sulcus and the base of segment 4 and perform all surgical procedures above the imaginary line connecting these two landmarks[4] (Figure 32.4).

In case of persistent haemorrhage, it is recommended to achieve haemostasis primarily by compression and avoid an excessive use of the electrocautery or clips.[4]

After obtaining a proper CVS, the cystic artery and duct may be divided and closed. Prior to closing the cystic duct, the absence of a residual stone must be checked by mechanical pressure (using a grasper) and/or cholangiography when in doubt. As the tissue inflammation usually thickens the cystic duct wall, clips may not be sufficient to obtain a solid closure. Therefore, the operator must be prepared to add sutures, or even for replacing the incomplete clips. Replacing poorly positioned, multiple clips by sutures may avoid a postoperative cystic stump fistula. One must keep in mind that tissue inflammation and retraction may shorten the cystic duct and retract the common bile duct, and care must be taken to avoid any common bile duct stenosis due to large sutures or clips. Any doubt about the integrity of the common bile duct should indicate intraoperative cholangiography.

The detachment of the gall bladder bed may be difficult in severe cholecystitis, where tissue inflammation merges planes. Hence, the fragile liver bed offers less resistance than the thickened gall bladder wall and is easily detached by traction, causing significant bleeding. One way to overcome this problem is to expose the inner layer of the subserosal layer (ss I-layer) of the gall bladder, as described by Honda et al.[12] After opening the serosa (or the covering peritoneal sheath) the whole subserosal outer layer (the fat tissue) is stripped away en bloc from the subserosal inner layer. The exposed plane is then followed bluntly towards the fundus (Figure 32.5).

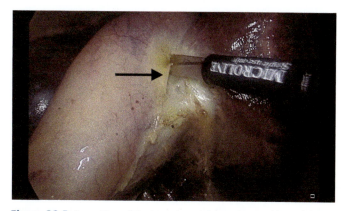

Figure 32.5 Exposition of the inner layer of the subserosal layer (black arrow) of the gall bladder.

Particular attention must be paid to abdominal irrigation and cleaning prior to closing the patient. A spilled stone may happen easily, and if not retrieved may be responsible for a postoperative collection. In case of severe pedicular inflammation, a drain may be placed behind the cystic stump to retrieve any postoperative leak.

Dome-down cholecystectomy

The dome-down (fundus-first/antegrade) technique is an alternative to the classic retrograde approach when the triangle of Calot is severely inflamed, whose dissection would involve a significant risk of BDI. As highlighted by the IRCAD guidelines, the requirements for a safe dome-down cholecystectomy are the following:

- A clear understanding of the anatomy of the cystic and hilar plates is mandatory.
- The dissection should be maintained along the subserosal inner layer to avoid vascular and/or biliary injury (Figure 32.5). In other words, the dissection should be as close to the gall bladder wall as possible. The fundus-first technique has been associated with 'extreme' BDI after plane misidentification when performed in patients with severe biliary inflammation. Therefore, if the subserosal inner layer cannot be exposed around the Calot's triangle, further dissection should be abandoned, and a subtotal cholecystectomy may be preferred to prevent vasculobiliary injury.[9]

Subtotal cholecystectomy

Although the CVS is recommended for achieving safety standards during cholecystectomy, pushing on with blind dissection within highly inflamed tissue may risk BDI and major vascular injuries. Therefore, surgeons must be aware that changing the surgical strategy promptly may result in lowering the risk of BDI. In this context, partial or subtotal cholecystectomy has been acknowledged to be a safe alternative technique in difficult cholecystectomy.[9,13,14]

During subtotal cholecystectomy, the gall bladder is opened along its axis up to the gall bladder neck, and emptied of stones so that the cystic duct is identified from the inside. It may be occluded due to stones or inflammation, and the help of a probe can be used with caution. The careful removal of all gall bladder stones is important for avoiding any postoperative collection.

Strasberg et al. described two types of subtotal cholecystectomy depending on the closure or not of the gall bladder remnant[14]:

1. Subtotal fenestrating cholecystectomy (no full-thickness gall bladder remnant existing): the remaining gall bladder neck is left open. The mucosa is usually ablated, and the cystic duct may be closed from the inside with a purse-string suture, while taking care not to suture the common bile duct. This approach may result in a postoperative biliary fistula, which resolves spontaneously in most cases.
2. Subtotal reconstituting cholecystectomy (existence of a gall bladder remnant): the remaining gall bladder is closed with sutures. This approach, due to the persistence of a gall bladder remnant, may result in new stone formation, and expose the patient to the risk of recurrent cholecystitis with a possibly challenging reoperative cholecystectomy, although this is a rare event (<5% in published series).

A drain should be left close to the gall bladder remnant in any case, to help the management of a postoperative biliary fistula.

Performing a subtotal cholecystectomy should be described in the operative report and the patient should be informed that a portion of the gall bladder is in place.[9]

Open approach

Although the development of surgical expertise and the use of bailout procedures allow us to perform even difficult cholecystectomies by laparoscopy, conversion to open surgery remains a safe option in case of unclear anatomy or complex situations. Young surgeons have less experience in the open than the laparoscopic approach, making the safety of an open conversion questionable compared to laparoscopic bailout procedures. However, any young surgeon has to be prepared to face a situation of open cholecystectomy.

An open cholecystectomy usually requires a subcostal right incision, which may be enlarged depending on the operative findings.

The gall bladder area may be pushed anteriorly by placing one or several compresses behind the right liver for better exposure. The assistant placed on the left of the patient retracts the surrounding organs and fat tissue (Figure 32.6).

The surgical steps are then similar to Lap-C. Proper exposure of the Calot's triangle by retracting the gall bladder's neck in order to obtain the CVS is critical.

When the CVS cannot be obtained in safe conditions, one must consider bailout procedures similar to laparoscopic surgery. The fundus-first approach must be associated with clear vision of the anatomy of the hilar plate and follow the subserosal inner layer of the gall bladder. If these conditions cannot be achieved safely, a subtotal cholecystectomy is a safest option. All the stones must be carefully removed in this case.

The place of intraoperative cholangiography

There is no consensus on the role of intraoperative cholangiography during Lap-C for cholecystitis. Despite an abundant literature, there

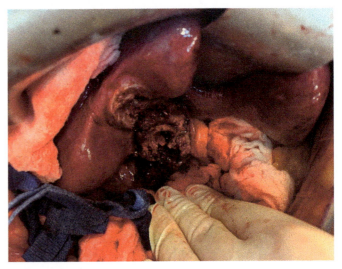

Figure 32.6 Example of an open cholecystectomy for severe cholecystitis. In this case, the chosen technique was a dome-down, partial fenestrating cholecystectomy.
Reproduced courtesy of Dr Laurent Genser, Department of Metabolic Surgery, Sorbonne University, Institute of Cardiometabolism and Nutrition (ICAN), Inserm, Paris, France, and Dr Chetana Lim, Department of Hepatobiliary Surgery and Liver Transplantation, Sorbonne Université, Hôpital Pitié-Salpêtrière, Assistance Publique-Hôpitaux de Paris, France.

is currently no evidence that systematic cholangiography could prevent BDI.[9,15] Therefore, intraoperative cholangiography may be used only in situations of unclear biliary anatomy. Near-infrared fluorescence cholangiography has been reported safe and may be an interesting alternative to classic intraoperative cholangiography in the near future.[9,16]

Postoperative care

In contrast to planned Lap-C, where 1-day surgery is usually achieved with an excellent outcome, the postoperative course after cholecystectomy for cholecystitis benefits from closer monitoring.

Secondary collections, or bile leaks, may happen after a complex cholecystectomy, especially in the case of a subtotal cholecystectomy where the cystic duct is left open. The majority of biliary fistulae resolve spontaneously through the drain. Otherwise, endoscopic management via endoscopic retrograde cholangiopancreatography and stent placement usually resolves the leak.[13]

Acknowledgements

We would like to thank Dr Laurent Genser and Dr Chetana Lim for kindly providing the picture used for Figure 32.6.

REFERENCES

1. Flum DR, Cheadle A, Prela C, Dellinger EP, Chan L. Bile duct injury during cholecystectomy and survival in medicare beneficiaries. JAMA. 2003;**290**(16):2168–2173.
2. Mayumi T, Okamoto K, Takada T, et al. Tokyo Guidelines 2018: management bundles for acute cholangitis and cholecystitis. J Hepatobiliary Pancreat Sci. 2018;**25**(1):96–100.
3. Joseph B, Jehan F, Dacey M, et al. Evaluating the relevance of the 2013 Tokyo Guidelines for the diagnosis and management of cholecystitis. J Am Coll Surg. 2018;**227**(1):38–43.
4. Wakabayashi G, Iwashita Y, Hibi T, et al. Tokyo Guidelines 2018: surgical management of acute cholecystitis: safe steps in laparoscopic cholecystectomy for acute cholecystitis (with videos). J Hepatobiliary Pancreat Sci. 2018;**25**(1):73–86.
5. Yokoe M, Hata J, Takada T, et al. Tokyo Guidelines 2018: diagnostic criteria and severity grading of acute cholecystitis (with videos). J Hepatobiliary Pancreat Sci. 2018;**25**(1):41–54.
6. Kiewiet JJS, Leeuwenburgh MMN, Bipat S, Bossuyt PMM, Stoker J, Boermeester MA. A systematic review and meta-analysis of diagnostic performance of imaging in acute cholecystitis. Radiology. 2012;**264**(3):708–720.
7. Archer SB, Brown DW, Smith CD, Branum GD, Hunter JG. Bile duct injury during laparoscopic cholecystectomy: results of a national survey. Ann Surg. 2001;**234**(4):549–558.
8. Strasberg SM. Error traps and vasculo-biliary injury in laparoscopic and open cholecystectomy. J Hepatobiliary Pancreat Surg. 2008;**15**(3):284–292.
9. Conrad C, Wakabayashi G, Asbun HJ, et al. IRCAD recommendation on safe laparoscopic cholecystectomy. J Hepatobiliary Pancreat Sci. 2017;**24**(11):603–615.
10. Janssen IMC, Swank DJ, Boonstra O, Knipscheer BC, Klinkenbijl JHG, van Goor H. Randomized clinical trial of ultrasonic versus electrocautery dissection of the gallbladder in laparoscopic cholecystectomy. Br J Surg. 2003;**90**(7):799–803.
11. Strasberg SM, Brunt LM. Rationale and use of the critical view of safety in laparoscopic cholecystectomy. J Am Coll Surg. 2010;**211**(1):132–138.
12. Honda G, Iwanaga T, Kurata M, Watanabe F, Satoh H, Iwasaki K. The critical view of safety in laparoscopic cholecystectomy is optimized by exposing the inner layer of the subserosal layer. J Hepatobiliary Pancreat Surg. 2009;**16**(4):445–449.
13. Elshaer M, Gravante G, Thomas K, Sorge R, Al-Hamali S, Ebdewi H. Subtotal cholecystectomy for 'difficult gallbladders': systematic review and meta-analysis. JAMA Surg. 2015;**150**(2):159–168.
14. Strasberg SM, Pucci MJ, Brunt LM, Deziel DJ. Subtotal cholecystectomy—'fenestrating' vs 'reconstituting' subtypes and the prevention of bile duct injury: definition of the optimal procedure in difficult operative conditions. J Am Coll Surg. 2016;**222**(1):89–96.
15. Flum DR, Dellinger EP, Cheadle A, Chan L, Koepsell T. Intraoperative cholangiography and risk of common bile duct injury during cholecystectomy. JAMA. 2003;**289**(13):1639–1644.
16. Ishizawa T, Bandai Y, Ijichi M, Kaneko J, Hasegawa K, Kokudo N. Fluorescent cholangiography illuminating the biliary tree during laparoscopic cholecystectomy. Br J Surg. 2010;**97**(9):1369–1377.

33 Post-cholecystectomy biliary injury

Kayvan Mohkam, Jean-Yves Mabrut, Agnès Rode, and Mickaël Lesurtel

Introduction

Biliary injury is the most common severe complication of cholecystectomy. Despite increasing experience with laparoscopic surgery, the incidence of iatrogenic biliary injury associated with laparoscopic cholecystectomy remains two to three times greater than that of open cholecystectomy (0.4–0.6% vs 0.2–0.3%).[1–3] When compared with open surgery, biliary injuries sustained during laparoscopic cholecystectomy are more likely to present earlier, are more proximal, more often associated with persistent bile leaks, and usually closer to the porta hepatis with concomitant vascular injury.[4] This results in significant patient morbidity and mortality, requiring complex and costly management and leads to an impaired quality of life.[5] In a retrospective chart review of more than 800,000 patients undergoing laparoscopic cholecystectomy in the US, more than 80% of patients with common bile duct (CBD) injury required operative intervention with an average 1-year cost of more than $60,000. Patients with CBD injury have an increased mortality of 7.2% and 14.5% at 1 year and 5 years, respectively, compared to the general population.[6] Single-incision laparoscopic cholecystectomy seems to be associated with an even higher rate of bile duct injury (0.72%).[7] Finally, robotic cholecystectomy does not seem to improve safety although is costlier in comparison with laparoscopic cholecystectomy.[8]

More modern data sets have, however, begun showing similar risks of CBD injury after laparoscopic and open surgery.[9]

Risk factors

The main risk factors identified in the literature are anatomical factors, nature of the pathology, and surgeon dependent factors.[10]

Anatomical variants include low insertion of the right posterior sectoral duct, cystic duct opening into the right hepatic duct, and right hepatic artery (RHA) looping into the Calot's triangle. Awareness of common variant anatomy and careful dissection with division of the cystic duct and artery close to the gall bladder should be kept in mind.

Acute cholecystitis, acute biliary pancreatitis, a severely scarred or shrunken gall bladder, impacted gallstone in the infundibulum, short cystic duct, and Mirizzi syndrome are the main pathologies which carry a risk of biliary injury.

Finally, the operator-dependent factors are associated with the learning curve, errors of perception, overlooking of safety protocols, and conditions. From an extensive experience in repair of biliary injuries, Strasberg identified four error traps in laparoscopic and open cholecystectomy.[11] The most common cause of misidentification results from the 'infundibular technique' error trap. This error is associated with severe inflammation hiding the cystic duct and which obliterates the Calot's triangle making the common hepatic duct appear to be part of the gall bladder wall (Figure 33.1). The 'fundus-down' cholecystectomy (anterograde dissection) has been associated with vasculobiliary injuries. It usually occurs at open cholecystectomy after conversion. The two other error traps are due to failure to perceive the presence of an aberrant right hepatic duct on cholangiography and injury to the CBD in the case of a 'parallel union' cystic duct. Interestingly, it has been shown that the cognitive misperception of anatomy is so compelling that injuries are seldom recognized at the time of surgery and the operation may be thought to be normal.[12]

Associated vascular injury

Biliary injuries are potentially accompanied by vascular injuries, which may worsen the bile duct injury and cause liver ischaemia. According to cadaveric studies, vascular injuries would occur in 7–10% of cholecystectomies without clinical consequence.[13] This incidence seems higher in patients with biliary injury, ranging from 12% to 47%.[14,15]

According to Strasberg,[16] 'a vasculobiliary injury is an injury to both a bile duct and a hepatic artery and/or portal vein; the bile duct injury may be caused by operative trauma, be ischaemic in origin or both, and may or may not be accompanied by various degrees of hepatic ischaemia'.

The most frequent of these injuries is an occlusion of the RHA or of a replaced RHA.[14] Reflow after occlusion of the RHA occurs from the left side through the hilar marginal artery and hilar plexus, which act as a collateral arterial route.[17] As opposed to an RHA injury alone, any RHA injury associated with a bile duct injury may preclude compensatory collateral flow through marginal arteries when the RHA is occluded. This may explain the 10% slow hepatic infarction seen after occlusion of the RHA.[16] Therefore, the use of the Hepp–Couinaud

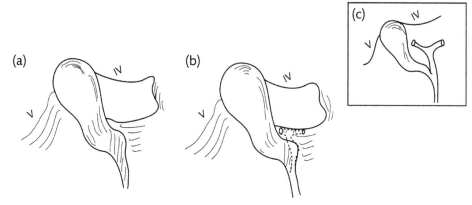

Figure 33.1 Misidentification of the cystic duct (CD)/common hepatic duct (CHD) in case of inflammation of the pedicle of the gallbladder where the common bile duct (CBD) is fused with the cystic duct (CD) and hidden behind him. (a) What is seen. (b) What is reality. (c) Normal anatomy.

technique to perform the biliary repair at, or above, the hilar level should allow success.[14] Additionally, in the face of an RHA occlusion, consideration should be given to delaying biliary repair because repair of the artery is rarely feasible and the overall benefit unclear. Indeed, opportunities for repair are limited, both because it must be performed within a short time after the injury, ideally within hours, and because the injury is frequently too severe to be repaired.

Finally, injuries involving the portal vein or the common or proper hepatic arteries are much less common, but have more serious effects including rapid infarction of the liver. The potential important consequences of vasculobiliary injuries justify that assessment of the hepatic arteries should be part of the investigation of all major biliary injuries. To do so, enhanced-computed tomography with arterial phase has replaced invasive angiography.[18]

Biliary injury classifications

The classification should provide an anatomical description of the biliary injury, help group the lesions according to severity of prognosis, provide information on the mechanisms involved, guide therapy, and allow a comparison of outcomes between series.

More than 15 classification systems of biliary injury encountered during cholecystectomy have been published which describe a spectrum ranging from minor cystic duct leaks to complete transection, or complex injuries of the CBD with or without a concomitant vascular injury.[19,20] None of them is ideal because most current versions fail to deal with all aspects of the injury which will influence short- and long-term prognosis.[10]

The two most popular and widely used classifications remain the Bismuth and the Strasberg classifications (which is an extension of the former), probably because they give a good anatomical picture of the lesion and are easy to remember.[11,21] The Bismuth classification was initially described for biliary strictures and then extended to injuries.[21] It is based on the lowest level at which healthy biliary mucosa is available for anastomosis. The classification is intended to help the surgeon to choose the appropriate repair technique. Strasberg's classification is stratified from classes A to E, class E injuries being further subdivided into E1 to E5 according to Bismuth's classification system[11] (Table 33.1 and Figure 33.2).

More recently, Fingerhut et al. under the auspices of the European Association for Endoscopic Surgery have proposed a composite all-inclusive classification, which divides the injuries into three easy-to-remember overall categories known by the mnemonic ATOM: anatomy (A), time of detection (TO), and mechanism (M).[22] While this classification combines all information on biliary injury, it remains complex and has not yet gained wide acceptance.

Table 33.1 Comparison of Bismuth and Strasberg classifications of biliary injury

Biliary anatomy	Bismuth	Strasberg
Cystic duct leak or leak from small ducts in liver bed	-	A
Occlusion of an aberrant RHD	-	B
Transection without ligation of an aberrant RHD	-	C
Lateral injury to CBD (<50% circumference)	-	D
CHD stricture, stump >2 cm	Type 1	E1
CHD stricture, stump <2 cm	Type 2	E2
Hilar stricture, no residual CHD, confluence is preserved	Type 3	E3
Hilar stricture, involvement of confluence, loss of communication between RHD and LHD	Type 4	E4
Stricture of low-lying right sectorial duct (alone or with concomitant CHD stricture)	Type 5	E5

CBD: common bile duct; CHD: common hepatic duct; LHD: left hepatic duct; RHD: right hepatic duct.

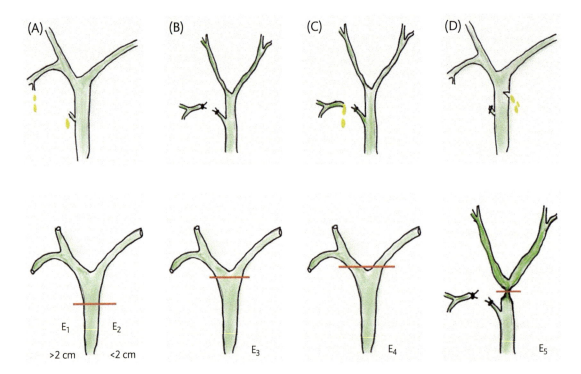

Figure 33.2 Comparison of Bismuth and Strasberg classifications of biliary injury.

Workup of a patient with biliary injury

Management should be guided by an optimal workup. It depends on the timing of recognition of injury, the extent of biliary injury, the patient's condition, and the availability of surgical expertise. When biliary injury is recognized or suspected during cholecystectomy, the best effort should be made to get a clear picture of the biliary anatomy by direct cholangiography either through the cystic duct or through the biliary injury itself. However, about 70% of injuries are diagnosed postoperatively.[10] Even more useful than reviewing the operating notes, it is paramount to talk to the primary surgeon if possible.

If emergency surgery in this setting has been done for peritoneal lavage and drainage in order to control sepsis associated with the biliary fistula, there is no role for diagnostic exploratory laparotomy/re-laparoscopy to only delineate biliary anatomy. The aims of radiological investigations are to correctly identify the damage, its extension, and severity, and to plan a therapeutic strategy. The enhanced-abdominal computed tomography scan is the main investigation that allows the identification of perihepatic fluid collections, free ascites, biliary obstruction with upstream dilatation, and any associated vascular injuries, such as to the RHA.

Magnetic resonance cholangiopancreatography (MRCP) is a non-invasive tool which allows the delineation of biliary anatomy. It can be completed with sequences injected with a hepatobiliary specific contrast agent (ideally gadolinium ethoxybenzyl diethylenetriamine pentaacetic acid (Gd-EOB-DTPA) if available) for comparison with MRCP to detect bile leaks and determination of biliary anatomy.[23,24] Finally, if the primary surgeon has left any biliary drain within the injury or at its contact, a simple cholangiogram through this drain may be attempted to see the biliary tree for comparison with MRCP. Close attention should be given to not miss a sectoral duct injury which should be specifically sought for (**Figure 33.3**).

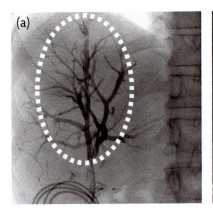
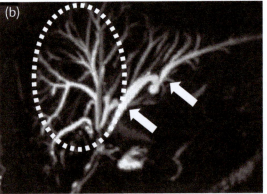

Figure 33.3 Magnetic resonance cholangiopancreatography (b) showing a left hepatic duct (arrows) which was not opacified on a cholangiography (a) performed through a biliary drain left by the surgeon in the right antero-medial duct (dotted circle).

Invasive endoscopic retrograde cholangiopancreatography (ERCP) has the disadvantage of allowing assessment of the biliary tree anatomy only distally to any injury but may have the benefit of performing a curative intervention at the time of diagnosis.[25]

Therapeutic management of post-cholecystectomy bile duct injury

The management of post-cholecystectomy biliary injury is complex, due to several factors:

- An inflammatory surgical field caused by a prolonged bile leak against a potential background of cholecystitis/pancreatitis.
- Small non-dilated bile ducts, resulting in difficult percutaneous access or surgical anastomosis.
- Possibly associated vascular injury and/or ischaemic injury of the biliary system.

Several therapeutic options exist, including surgical repair, endoscopic, and interventional radiological procedures, which could be used either separately or in combination with each other. The most important is probably to encourage a culture of safety in laparoscopic cholecystectomy to decrease the risk of biliary injury.

How to prevent bile duct injury during laparoscopic cholecystectomy

The risk of biliary injury has persisted over time despite the growing number of methods intended to reduce its occurrence including obtaining the critical view of safety (CVS) after Calot's triangle dissection,[26] performing intraoperative cholangiography (IOC), using landmarks, and developing efforts to facilitate surgical education, training, and mentorship.[27] Biliary injury during laparoscopic cholecystectomy most often occurs as a result of misidentification of the common bile or hepatic duct or the RHA instead of the cystic duct. Indeed, the CBD is usually thought to be the cystic duct then injured. An international Delphi consensus study, headed by the SAGES safe cholecystectomy task Force,[28] identified the most important safety factors in laparoscopic cholecystectomy as the following: establishing the CVS, understanding the anatomy, adequate exposure, ability to call a senior colleague for help, and recognizing when to convert or abandon. Strasberg[29] recently proposed a three-step conceptual roadmap for avoiding biliary injury in laparoscopic cholecystectomy which consists of (1) obtaining a safe anatomical identification of the cystic structures whenever operative findings permit, (2) not to proceed to a total cholecystectomy when conditions do not permit secure identification, and (3) to proceed towards a safe 'bail-out' procedure.

For our team, the standard of care for laparoscopic cholecystectomy consists of obtaining the CVS which has reached the status of being a worldwide accepted concept for a secure identification of the anatomical structures, and to perform routine IOC. CVS should not be considered as a method of dissection, but as a method of target identification before clipping or dividing any structures: the targets being the cystic duct and the cystic artery. Obtaining the CVS consists of clearing Calot's triangle of fat and fibrous tissue (without requiring a CBD exposure), and visualizing two (cystic artery and cystic duct) and only two anatomical structures entering the gall bladder after separating the lower (one-third) part of the gall bladder from the cystic plate (Figure 33.4). To achieve the CVS, effective retraction of the gall bladder is mandatory to develop a plane in the Calot's triangle area (decompression of any distended gall bladder with needle aspiration should be done if necessary) and dissection has to be started high on the gall bladder from the posterior leaf of the peritoneum covering it. The 2018 Tokyo Guidelines emphasized that dissection has to be strictly located above (on the ventral side of) the imaginary line connecting the base of the left medial section (segment IV) and the roof of Rouviere's sulcus[30] (Figure 33.4). Importantly, dissection should always be kept close to the gall bladder maintaining the plane of dissection within the subserosal layer throughout cholecystectomy. There is no standard way of performing dissection to achieve the CVS but any appropriate use of energy devices is important: a hook cautery on low settings is usually adopted but hydro-dissection and bipolar cautery have our favour in case of inflammation. In case of haemorrhage, avoiding excessive use of electrocautery or clipping is of major importance to limit the risk of bile duct and/or vascular injury. In this instance, temporary haemostasis by compression followed by selective and precise haemostasis represent the rules to limit the risk of biliary injury.

In a difficult laparoscopic cholecystectomy due to an impacted gallstone in the confluence of the cystic and hepatic ducts, severe inflammation, and/or fibrosis of the gall bladder neck and surrounding organs, the CVS strategy should be challenged. Further dissection may expose the patient to an increased risk of biliary injury which is significantly correlated with the severity grade of acute cholecystitis.[31]

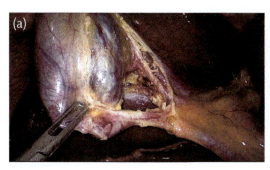 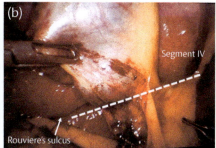

Figure 33.4 (a) Critical view of safety. (b) Dissection of the Calot's triangle which has to be strictly located above the imaginary line connecting the base of the left medial section (Segment IV) and the roof of Rouviere's sulcus.

When operative findings do not permit secure anatomical identification, CVS cannot be safely obtained, and surgeons have to adopt an alternative surgical strategy. Either performing an IOC or abandoning the operation and deciding on bail-out procedures are advocated in this situation. Depending on skills, experience, and training, the time to bail-out may differ among surgeons. Calling a senior surgical colleague for advice is recommended in this situation.

IOC may be useful to confirm the course of bile ducts, but also to peroperatively detect biliary injury, while there is no clear consensus on this. Indeed, no randomized study has ever demonstrated any efficacy of performing IOC in decreasing the risk of biliary injury. Such a randomized trial is, however, highly unlikely to take place because the incidence of biliary injury is so low that more than 5000 patients would be required in each arm. Interestingly, in a recent Swedish case–control study[5] the intention to perform an IOC halved the risk of biliary injury during cholecystectomy. We strongly consider that surgeons should be able to estimate the need for IOC but also to perform and to be able to interpret (e.g. anomalous bile duct) the results. In our team, the policy to perform routine use of IOC for learning and training in order to reduce the risk of biliary injury has been advocated for open cholecystectomy then maintained over time for the laparoscopic approach.

In a difficult cholecystectomy where achievement of the CVS itself appears dangerous because of severe inflammation, adhesions, or changes in orientation, surgeons should be prepared to switch to bail-out procedures and we consider that laparoscopic subtotal cholecystectomy is a useful and effective alternative. Subtotal fenestrating cholecystectomy, which precludes any second operation (contrary to surgical tube cholecystostomy), consists of performing an incision in the gall bladder to remove all impacted gallstones and to perform ablation of the residual mucosa of the remaining gall bladder. The cystic duct of the remnant gall bladder is left open close to an abdominal drain. Any postoperative biliary fistula usually stops spontaneously in a few days without a need for an endoscopic sphincterotomy. However, this fenestrating procedure avoids any risk of encountering residual or recurrent gallstones in a remnant gall bladder when and if a reconstituting cholecystectomy is performed.

The fundus-first technique (dome-down cholecystectomy) represents an alternative way of dissection of the gall bladder by laparotomy. It consists of separating the gall bladder from the cystic plate in an anterograde way before approaching the Calot's triangle. This technique has not been adequately studied regarding whether it is useful in avoiding or reducing the risk of biliary injury during the laparoscopic approach.

Our policy for open conversion has evolved over time. We do not currently consider conversion as a specific bail-out procedure. Indeed, no randomized controlled trial has ever investigated advantages and disadvantages of converting to open cholecystectomy. However, if subtotal laparoscopic cholecystectomy is not feasible in a safe way, then open conversion can be undertaken in order to perform a subtotal rather than a total cholecystectomy.[32] Although conversion to an open cholecystectomy was the only recommendation of the 2013 Tokyo Guidelines in case of difficult laparoscopic cholecystectomy for acute cholecystitis, the current revision identified subtotal cholecystectomy, conversion to open, and fundus-first technique as specific bail-out procedures.[30]

Therapeutic options

Surgical repair

Biliodigestive anastomosis

In the event of a complete division of the main bile duct, the standard repair procedure is represented by a hepaticojejunostomy using a 70 cm transmesocolic Roux-en-Y loop, which could be performed in various ways, depending on the level of the damage.

In most cases, a biliodigestive anastomosis at the level of the main convergence extended to the left duct according to the Hepp–Couinaud technique represents the preferred option, especially when the stump is short (<2 cm between the convergence and the cut edge).[21] The principle of this procedure relies on the fact that it uses the left bile duct, which is long and horizontal, and allows a larger anastomosis to be performed. The procedure requires a lowering of the hilar plate followed by dissection of the left bile duct and performance of a latero-lateral anastomosis using a Roux-en-Y loop. Extended dissection of the left bile duct is avoided, especially along its inferior aspect, in order to prevent associated vascular deprivation of biliary tissues. Therefore, the left duct is divided on its anterior aspect, starting from the common hepatic channel stump, and the anastomosis is performed using interrupted absorbable monofilament 4/0 or 5/0 sutures (Figure 33.5).

When the distance between the biliary convergence and the stump is of 2 cm or more, a standard hepaticojejunostomy

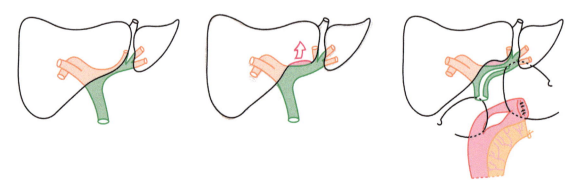

Figure 33.5 After lowering of the hilar plate, hepaticojejunostomy on the biliary convergence extended to the left bile duct according to Hepp–Couinaud procedure using a Roux-en-Y loop.

Therapeutic options 371

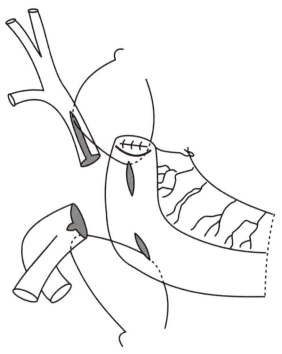

Figure 33.6 Separated biliodigestive anastomoses on the right and left hepatic ducts using a single Roux-en-Y loop.

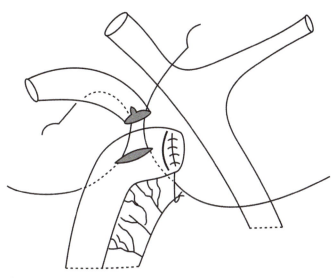

Figure 33.7 Isolated injury of the right postero-lateral duct (Strasberg's type B or C) repaired by a bilio-digestive anastomosis using a Roux-en-Y loop.

using a Roux-en-Y loop could be performed. The anterior aspect of the bile duct could be divided in order to create a patch and enlarge the anastomosis.[21] If the main bile duct stump diameter, however, remains narrow, the Hepp–Couinaud procedure offers the best results and should be preferred over a standard hepaticojejunostomy.[33]

When the roof of the biliary convergence is injured, the main difficulty is to gain access to the right hepatic duct, due to its short extrahepatic segment. Moreover, the two sectional right ducts often converge into the right hepatic duct less than 1 cm before the bile duct convergence, and therefore, it is often necessary to perform three separate anastomoses (i.e. the anteromedial, the posterolateral, and the left ducts). To do so, the cystic plate together with a small portion of segments IV and V should be divided.[34,35] Once the right duct has been isolated, several procedures could be done: performing two (or sometimes three) biliodigestive anastomoses on each hemiliver or section (using the left, anteromedial, and posterolateral ducts, separately)[36,37] (Figure 33.6); repair of the convergence roof followed by a hepaticojejunostomy using a Roux-en-Y loop; or a portoenterostomy.[34] In the event of an isolated injury of the posterolateral duct (Strasberg's type B or C), a biliodigestive anastomosis using a Roux-en-Y loop represents the standard procedure (Figures 33.7 and 33.8).

Alternative modalities of surgical biliary repair

Other modalities of surgical repair have been described, but these are seldom performed. For injuries of the distal CBD, hepaticoduodenostomy

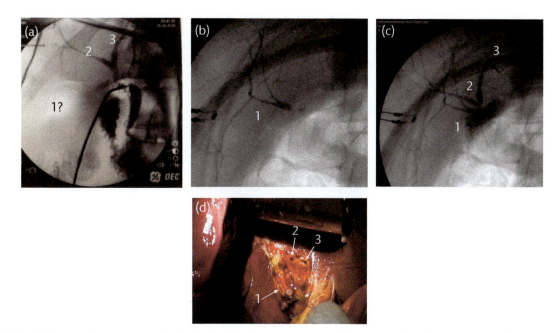

Figure 33.8 Early bile duct repair on postoperative day 2 after complete common hepatic duct section during laparoscopic cholecystectomy (Strasberg E4). (a) Peroperative cholangiography showing missing posterolateral duct (1), anteromedial duct (2), and left duct (3). (b) Opacification of the posterolateral duct only (1). (c) Opacification of all bile ducts. (d) Exposition of the three bile ducts before repair with a hepaticojejunostomy using a Roux-en-Y loop.

has been proposed, but this has a risk of biliary-gastric reflux, and therefore, such a repair should not be recommended as routine.[38] In the case of a lateral injury of the CBD, a suture secured by a drain (T-tube or transcystic) may be performed. When the injured CBD segment is short, with no substantial loss of tissue, a duct-to-duct repair can be performed, although such repairs result in higher rates of strictures in the long term.[39]

Hepatectomy

Elective liver resections do not represent the commonest procedures performed in the setting of bile duct injury, and primary biliary repair should remain the first-line treatment. However, in some cases, a liver resection aiming to remove a fibrotic section or lobe may be indicated. Such indications include hepatic atrophy, severe bile duct stricture causing intrahepatic cholelithiasis, and/or repeated episodes of cholangitis, with or without an associated vascular injury of the concerned hepatic segment.[40,41]

Use of surgical drains

Due to the inflammatory context usually encountered in the setting of post-cholecystectomy bile duct injury, biliary transanastomotic drains are widely used. Such drains could be externalized either using a transhepatic or transjejunal route. They offer access to the biliary tree and allow postoperative cholangiography to be performed.[36] However, there is currently no evidence regarding their efficacy to diminish the rate of anastomotic stricture after surgical repair.[42]

Surgical approach

Due to its complexity, surgical repairs of bile duct injuries are widely performed through a classical open approach, either through a right subcostal or J-shaped incision. The laparoscopic approach could be used for a peritoneal lavage when a two-step procedure (lavage combined with drainage of any injured bile duct, followed by late surgical repair), while it does not seem appropriate for surgical repair. The robotic approach, however, may represent a promising approach for surgical repair, but further studies are warranted to evaluate its safety.[43,44]

Timing and referral

When should the surgical repair be performed, and where should the patient be managed (i.e. in the same centre where the cholecystectomy was performed or in a tertiary referral centre) are the two main questions to be asked following any bile duct injury.

Several studies have suggested the high impact of the timing of repair on postoperative and long-term outcomes of surgical repair[45-48] but due to inconsistent findings, the best timing for surgical repair remains controversial. Typically, timing of repair could be divided into three categories: early (0–7 days post biliary injury), intermediate (1–6 weeks post biliary injury), and late (6 weeks to 6 months).[49] Early repairs are supposedly associated with better outcome when compared to intermediate repair,[48,50] provided they are performed by hepatopancreatobiliary (HPB) specialists. One important factor that must be considered in the event of early biliary injury repair is the surgeon's expertise. Post-cholecystectomy biliary injury mostly occurs among patients with non-dilated bile ducts, making any attempt of immediate surgical repair difficult, and early repairs must therefore be reserved for expert HPB surgeons. As such, it is recommended that general surgeons not expert in the field of HPB surgery and who identify a biliary injury intraoperatively do not attempt to repair the injury themselves, but rather insert a drain within and/or along the injured duct(s), and refer the patient to an expert centre without delay.

Unfortunately, the diagnosis of biliary injury is often delayed, and thus associated with difficult local conditions related to prolonged leakage and peritonitis, which represent independent predictors of poor surgical results.[50,51] In such situations, delaying surgery must be preferred in order to perform the anastomosis on non-inflamed tissues. To allow for it, an external biliary drain should be placed in each divided bile duct, in addition to perihepatic drainage to avoid biloma formation.

Liver transplantation

Ultimately, biliary damage may result in irreversible liver injury caused by secondary biliary cirrhosis and repeated episodes of cholangitis; in such cases, liver transplantation may represent the only viable option and should be discussed ideally before the occurrence of acute liver failure.[52,53]

Interventional radiology

Interventional radiological procedures represent a safe alternative to surgical procedures, allowing a minimally invasive modality for managing both leakage and strictures.[54] They may also precede and/or be used in combination with surgical or endoscopic procedures.[54]

Each procedure starts with a cholangiography, using a pre-existing or percutaneous transhepatic drain. The percutaneous transhepatic biliary drainage may be challenging because of the non-dilated biliary tree. Whenever possible, it should be internalized in the digestive segment (the duodenum or the jejunum in case of a Roux-en-Y reconstruction). Passing the drain through the fully sectioned duct is only possible during the first weeks after the biliary injury, and sometimes requires the use of the 'rendezvous technique' (Figure 33.9). Internalization consists of closing the drain allowing the bile to flow along the physiological path, while decreasing the risk of accidental drain removal. In addition to biliary drainage, any biloma should be drained simultaneously to treat sepsis and avoid prolonged local inflammation.

The management of strictures requires prolonged drainage, and drains should be changed at regular intervals in order to increase the drain size (to at least 15 Fr), until cholangiographic control shows disappearance of the stricture.

Endoscopy

Similar to radiological drainage, the endoscopic management of biliary injury aims to place a drain across the injured bile duct under ERCP. In addition to covering the biliary defect, sphincterotomy results in a decrease of pressure gradient between the biliary system and the duodenum, thus favouring bile flow through the papilla (Figure 33.10).

The treatment usually lasts 1 year, due to the necessity for changing drains every 3 months to avoid stent obstruction and cholangitis, and an average number of five procedures are required before healing.[55]

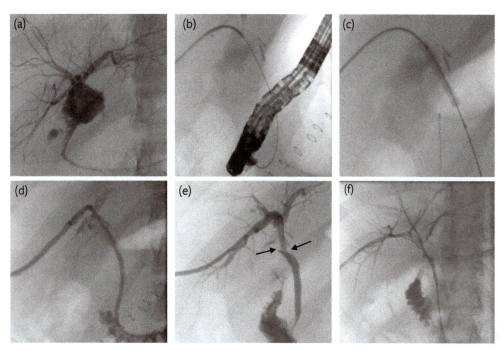

Figure 33.9 Interventional radiology stepwise approach to cure a post-cholecystectomy Strasberg E1 biliary injury. (a) Percutaneous external drainage of a biloma and cholangiography obtained by reflux after opacification of the biloma; the main duct is not depicted. (b) One-stage 'rendezvous' technique between percutaneous transhepatic cholangiography drainage (PTCD) and ERCP to bridge the bile duct defect and internalize the PTCD. (c) During the same procedure, balloon dilatation of the biliary stricture. (d) Final cholangiography through the PTCD. (e) One-month cholangiography control with up-sizing of the PTCD. The injured duct segment (arrows) is short and irregular but not stenotic. (f) Six-month cholangiography control with guidewire still in place. PTCD was removed after 6 months of calibration showing no residual stenosis of the injured common hepatic duct.

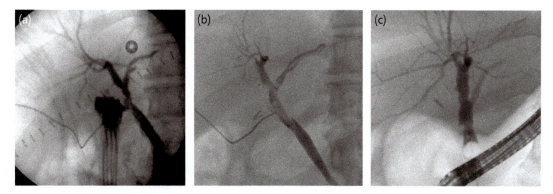

Figure 33.10 Post-cholecystectomy Strasberg D biliary injury (lateral injury to CBD). A T-tube was put in the injury during index surgery. (a) Bile leakage around the T-tube drained through a multi-tubular drain. (b) Cholangiography through the T-tube after inserting an endoscopic biliary plastic stent through ERCP. Bile leakage was solved, and T-tube was closed and removed 2 months later. (c) Six-month endoscopic cholangiography showing good results, plastic stent was removed.

Outcome after treatment

Postoperative morbidity

Overall, surgical management of biliary injury remains a morbid procedure with a rate of postoperative complications ranging from 26% to 42%, and a 1–4% rate of 90-day mortality.[1,47,56,57] The main specific 30-day complication observed after surgical repair is represented by cholangitis, which occurs in up to 10% of patients, followed by anastomotic biliary leakage (6%), intra-abdominal deep abscess related to the biloma (5%), and abdominal wall abscesses (3–8%). Up to 11% of patients require a surgical reintervention; however, most complications can be managed by the percutaneous or endoscopic approach, such as percutaneous transhepatic bile duct drainage, placement of an intra-abdominal pigtail drain, or biliary stenting.[56,57]

Long-term results

If performed in tertiary referral centres, approximately 90% of patients after surgical repair of a biliary injury will have satisfactory long-term results.[58,59] However, one third of them will develop late complications, including delayed anastomotic strictures (occurring after a median delay of 63 months), whereas 14% will present with repeat episodes of cholangitis, which may occur after an initial asymptomatic period of several years.[58,60] Long-term treatment failures may be managed by both minimally invasive (percutaneous dilatation or stent placement) or surgical procedures (repeat bilioenteric reconstruction).

Conclusion

In summary, the management of post-cholecystectomy biliary injury must preferentially comply with some key principles: management in a tertiary expert centre, early referral within hours/days after diagnosis of biliary injury, multidisciplinary approach involving hepatobiliary surgeons, interventional radiologists, and endoscopists experts in ERCP procedures, and handover to a new surgical team who was not involved in the initial management.

REFERENCES

1. Ismael HN, Cox S, Cooper A, Narula N, Aloia T. The morbidity and mortality of hepaticojejunostomies for complex bile duct injuries: a multi-institutional analysis of risk factors and outcomes using NSQIP. *HPB (Oxford)*. 2017;19(4):352–358.
2. Dixon JA, Morgan KA, Adams DB. Management of common bile duct injury during partial gastrectomy. *Am Surg*. 2009;75(8):719–721.
3. Fragulidis G, Marinis A, Polydorou A, et al. Managing injuries of hepatic duct confluence variants after major hepatobiliary surgery: an algorithmic approach. *World J Gastroenterol*. 2008;14(19):3049–3053.
4. Chaudhary A, Manisegran M, Chandra A, Agarwal AK, Sachdev AK. How do bile duct injuries sustained during laparoscopic cholecystectomy differ from those during open cholecystectomy? *J Laparoendosc Adv Surg Tech A*. 2001;11(4):187–191.
5. Boerma D, Rauws EA, Keulemans YC, et al. Impaired quality of life 5 years after bile duct injury during laparoscopic cholecystectomy: a prospective analysis. *Ann Surg*. 2001;234(6):750–757.
6. Fong ZV, Pitt HA, Strasberg SM, et al. Diminished survival in patients with bile leak and ductal injury: management strategy and outcomes. *J Am Coll Surg*. 2018;226(4):568–576.
7. Joseph M, Phillips MR, Farrell TM, Rupp CC. Single incision laparoscopic cholecystectomy is associated with a higher bile duct injury rate: a review and a word of caution. *Ann Surg*. 2012;256(1):1–6.
8. Strosberg DS, Nguyen MC, Muscarella P 2nd, Narula VK. A retrospective comparison of robotic cholecystectomy versus laparoscopic cholecystectomy: operative outcomes and cost analysis. *Surg Endosc*. 2017;31(3):1436–1441.
9. Halbert C, Pagkratis S, Yang J, et al. Beyond the learning curve: incidence of bile duct injuries following laparoscopic cholecystectomy normalize to open in the modern era. *Surg Endosc*. 2016;30(6):2239–2243.
10. Bharathy KG, Negi SS. Postcholecystectomy bile duct injury and its sequelae: pathogenesis, classification, and management. *Indian J Gastroenterol*. 2014;33(3):201–215.
11. Strasberg SM. Error traps and vasculo-biliary injury in laparoscopic and open cholecystectomy. *J Hepatobiliary Pancreat Surg*. 2008;15(3):284–292.
12. Way LW, Stewart L, Gantert W, et al. Causes and prevention of laparoscopic bile duct injuries: analysis of 252 cases from a human factors and cognitive psychology perspective. *Ann Surg*. 2003;237(4):460–469.
13. Halasz NA. Cholecystectomy and hepatic artery injuries. *Arch Surg*. 1991;126(2):137–138.
14. Alves A, Farges O, Nicolet J, Watrin T, Sauvanet A, Belghiti J. Incidence and consequence of an hepatic artery injury in patients with postcholecystectomy bile duct strictures. *Ann Surg*. 2003;238(1):93–96.
15. Wudel LJ Jr., Wright JK, Pinson CW, et al. Bile duct injury following laparoscopic cholecystectomy: a cause for continued concern. *Am Surg*. 2001;67(6):557–563.
16. Strasberg SM, Helton WS. An analytical review of vasculobiliary injury in laparoscopic and open cholecystectomy. *HPB (Oxford)*. 2011;13(1):1–14.
17. Mays ET, Wheeler CS. Demonstration of collateral arterial flow after interruption of hepatic arteries in man. *N Engl J Med*. 1974;290(18):993–996.
18. Gorsi U, Gupta P, Kalra N, et al. Multidetector computed tomography evaluation of post cholecystectomy complications: a tertiary care center experience. *Trop Gastroenterol*. 2015;36(4):236–243.
19. Lau WY, Lai EC. Classification of iatrogenic bile duct injury. *Hepatobiliary Pancreat Dis Int*. 2007;6(5):459–463.
20. Stewart L, Robinson TN, Lee CM, Liu K, Whang K, Way LW. Right hepatic artery injury associated with laparoscopic bile duct injury: incidence, mechanism, and consequences. *J Gastrointest Surg*. 2004;8(5):523–530.
21. Bismuth H, Majno PE. Biliary strictures: classification based on the principles of surgical treatment. *World J Surg*. 2001;25(10):1241–1244.
22. Fingerhut A, Dziri C, Garden OJ, et al. ATOM, the all-inclusive, nominal EAES classification of bile duct injuries during cholecystectomy. *Surg Endosc*. 2013;27(12):4608–4019.
23. Hamad MA, Nada AA, Abdel-Atty MY, Kawashti AS. Major biliary complications in 2,714 cases of laparoscopic cholecystectomy without intraoperative cholangiography: a multicenter retrospective study. *Surg Endosc*. 2011;25(12):3747–3751.
24. Cieszanowski A, Stadnik A, Lezak A, et al. Detection of active bile leak with Gd-EOB-DTPA enhanced MR cholangiography: comparison of 20-25 min delayed and 60–180 min delayed images. *Eur J Radiol*. 2013;82(12):2176–2182.
25. Copelan A, Bahoura L, Tardy F, Kirsch M, Sokhandon F, Kapoor B. Etiology, diagnosis, and management of bilomas: a current update. *Tech Vasc Interv Radiol*. 2015;18(4):236–243.
26. Strasberg SM, Brunt LM. The critical view of safety: why it is not the only method of ductal identification within the standard of care in laparoscopic cholecystectomy. *Ann Surg*. 2017;265(3):464–465.
27. Pucher PH, Brunt LM, Davies N, et al. Outcome trends and safety measures after 30 years of laparoscopic cholecystectomy: a systematic review and pooled data analysis. *Surg Endosc*. 2018;32(5):2175–2183.
28. Pucher PH, Brunt LM, Fanelli RD, Asbun HJ, Aggarwal R. SAGES expert Delphi consensus: critical factors for safe surgical practice in laparoscopic cholecystectomy. *Surg Endosc*. 2015;29(11):3074–3085.
29. Strasberg SM. A three-step conceptual roadmap for avoiding bile duct injury in laparoscopic cholecystectomy: an invited perspective review. *J Hepatobiliary Pancreat Sci*. 2019;26(4):123–127.
30. Wakabayashi G, Iwashita Y, Hibi T, et al. Tokyo Guidelines 2018: surgical management of acute cholecystitis: safe steps in laparoscopic cholecystectomy for acute cholecystitis (with videos). *J Hepatobiliary Pancreat Sci*. 2018;25(1):73–86.

31. Tornqvist B, Waage A, Zheng Z, Ye W, Nilsson M. Severity of acute cholecystitis and risk of iatrogenic bile duct injury during cholecystectomy, a population-based case-control study. *World J Surg.* 2016;**40**(5):1060–1067.
32. Iwashita Y, Hibi T, Ohyama T, et al. Delphi consensus on bile duct injuries during laparoscopic cholecystectomy: an evolutionary cul-de-sac or the birth pangs of a new technical framework? *J Hepatobiliary Pancreat Sci.* 2017;**24**(11):591–602.
33. Mercado MA, Chan C, Orozco H, Tielve M, Hinojosa CA. Acute bile duct injury. The need for a high repair. *Surg Endosc.* 2003;**17**(9):1351–1355.
34. Mercado MA, Vilatoba M, Contreras A, et al. Iatrogenic bile duct injury with loss of confluence. *World J Gastrointest Surg.* 2015;**7**(10):254–260.
35. Strasberg SM, Picus DD, Drebin JA. Results of a new strategy for reconstruction of biliary injuries having an isolated right-sided component. *J Gastrointest Surg.* 2001;**5**(3):266–274.
36. Johnson SR, Koehler A, Pennington LK, Hanto DW. Long-term results of surgical repair of bile duct injuries following laparoscopic cholecystectomy. *Surgery.* 2000;**128**(4):668–677.
37. Nordin A, Halme L, Makisalo H, Isoniemi H, Hockerstedt K. Management and outcome of major bile duct injuries after laparoscopic cholecystectomy: from therapeutic endoscopy to liver transplantation. *Liver Transpl.* 2002;**8**(11):1036–1043.
38. Moraca RJ, Lee FT, Ryan JA Jr, Traverso LW. Long-term biliary function after reconstruction of major bile duct injuries with hepaticoduodenostomy or hepaticojejunostomy. *Arch Surg.* 2002;**137**(8):889–893.
39. Lau WY, Lai EC, Lau SH. Management of bile duct injury after laparoscopic cholecystectomy: a review. *ANZ J Surg.* 2010;**80**(1–2):75–81.
40. Laurent A, Sauvanet A, Farges O, Watrin T, Rivkine E, Belghiti J. Major hepatectomy for the treatment of complex bile duct injury. *Ann Surg.* 2008;**248**(1):77–83.
41. Perini MV, Herman P, Montagnini AL, et al. Liver resection for the treatment of post-cholecystectomy biliary stricture with vascular injury. *World J Gastroenterol.* 2015;**21**(7):2102–2107.
42. Mercado MA, Chan C, Orozco H, et al. To stent or not to stent bilioenteric anastomosis after iatrogenic injury: a dilemma not answered? *Arch Surg.* 2002;**137**(1):60–63.
43. Dokmak S, Amharar N, Aussilhou B, et al. Laparoscopic repair of post-cholecystectomy bile duct injury: an advance in surgical management. *J Gastrointest Surg.* 2017;**21**(8):1368–1372.
44. Giulianotti PC, Quadri P, Durgam S, Bianco FM. Reconstruction/repair of iatrogenic biliary injuries: is the robot offering a new option? Short clinical report. *Ann Surg.* 2018;**267**(1):e7–e9.
45. Dageforde LA, Landman MP, Feurer ID, Poulose B, Pinson CW, Moore DE. A cost-effectiveness analysis of early vs late reconstruction of iatrogenic bile duct injuries. *J Am Coll Surg.* 2012;**214**(6):919–927.
46. de Reuver PR, Grossmann I, Busch OR, Obertop H, van Gulik TM, Gouma DJ. Referral pattern and timing of repair are risk factors for complications after reconstructive surgery for bile duct injury. *Ann Surg.* 2007;**245**(5):763–770.
47. Sahajpal AK, Chow SC, Dixon E, Greig PD, Gallinger S, Wei AC. Bile duct injuries associated with laparoscopic cholecystectomy: timing of repair and long-term outcomes. *Arch Surg.* 2010;**145**(8):757–763.
48. Thomson BN, Parks RW, Madhavan KK, Wigmore SJ, Garden OJ. Early specialist repair of biliary injury. *Br J Surg.* 2006;**93**(2):216–220.
49. A European-African HepatoPancreatoBiliary Association (E-AHPBA) Research Collaborative Study management group; other members of the European-African HepatoPancreatoBiliary Association Research Collaborative. Post cholecystectomy bile duct injury: early, intermediate or late repair with hepaticojejunostomy—an E-AHPBA multi-center study. *HPB (Oxford).* 2019;**21**(12):1641–1647.
50. Dominguez-Rosado I, Sanford DE, Liu J, Hawkins WG, Mercado MA. Timing of surgical repair after bile duct injury impacts postoperative complications but not anastomotic patency. *Ann Surg.* 2016;**264**(3):544–553.
51. Schmidt SC, Settmacher U, Langrehr JM, Neuhaus P. Management and outcome of patients with combined bile duct and hepatic arterial injuries after laparoscopic cholecystectomy. *Surgery.* 2004;**135**(6):613–618.
52. de Santibanes E, Pekolj J, McCormack L, et al. Liver transplantation for the sequelae of intra-operative bile duct injury. *HPB (Oxford).* 2002;**4**(3):111–115.
53. Parrilla P, Robles R, Varo E, et al. Liver transplantation for bile duct injury after open and laparoscopic cholecystectomy. *Br J Surg.* 2014;**101**(2):63–68.
54. Mastier C, Valette PJ, Adham M, et al. Complex biliary leaks: effectiveness of percutaneous radiological treatment compared to simple leaks in 101 patients. *Cardiovasc Intervent Radiol.* 2018;**41**(10):1566–1572.
55. Pitt HA, Sherman S, Johnson MS, et al. Improved outcomes of bile duct injuries in the 21st century. *Ann Surg.* 2013;**258**(3):490–499.
56. Sicklick JK, Camp MS, Lillemoe KD, et al. Surgical management of bile duct injuries sustained during laparoscopic cholecystectomy: perioperative results in 200 patients. *Ann Surg.* 2005;**241**(5):786–792.
57. Stilling NM, Fristrup C, Wettergren A, et al. Long-term outcome after early repair of iatrogenic bile duct injury. A national Danish multicentre study. *HPB (Oxford).* 2015;**17**(5):394–400.
58. AbdelRafee A, El-Shobari M, Askar W, Sultan AM, El Nakeeb A. Long-term follow-up of 120 patients after hepaticojejunostomy for treatment of post-cholecystectomy bile duct injuries: a retrospective cohort study. *Int J Surg.* 2015;**18**:205–210.
59. Lillemoe KD, Melton GB, Cameron JL, et al. Postoperative bile duct strictures: management and outcome in the 1990s. *Ann Surg.* 2000;**232**(3):430–441.
60. Stewart L, Way LW. Laparoscopic bile duct injuries: timing of surgical repair does not influence success rate. A multivariate analysis of factors influencing surgical outcomes. *HPB (Oxford).* 2009;**11**(6):516–522.

Biliary fistula, gallstone ileus, and Mirizzi syndrome

Martin Palavecino and Juan Pekolj

Biliary fistula

Biliary fistula is defined as an abnormal communication between the biliary tree and the body surface or a viscera. Anatomically, a fistula has three components: an orifice in the biliary tree, an orifice on the opposite side of the fistula, and a fistulous tract between both orifices.[1,2]

According to the location of the non-biliary end, fistulae are classified as external when the skin is the distal end of the tract (biliocutaneous fistula), and internal when the distal end is another organ (e.g. bilioenteric fistula).[2]

Primary or spontaneous fistulae are the result of the evolution of the disease without previous medical interventions. The main causes are stones, peptic ulcers, tumours, and parasites. Secondary fistulae occur after a surgical or a medical procedure. An example of this type of fistula is secondary to a bile duct injury during a laparoscopic cholecystectomy.[1,2]

In this chapter, internal biliary fistulae secondary to gallstones and gall bladder chronic inflammatory processes will be described. An accurate diagnosis prior to the treatment selection is paramount. Open surgery and mini-invasive techniques are options for transient or definitive treatment of biliary fistulae. Sepsis, the patient's performance status, level of the biliary injury, and the involvement of gastrointestinal structures define the complexity and type of the treatment and results.[1-4]

Biliary fistula secondary to gallstones

The incidence of biliary fistula secondary to gallstones (BFSG) is directly related to the time of evolution of the symptoms. The range is between 1% and 2% of patients with symptomatic gallstones and rises to 4.7% to 5.7% in Latin America.[2,4,5]

It still represents a diagnostic and therapeutic challenge with a high mortality rate. This is because it occurs predominantly in elderly, fragile, and morbid patients.

The most frequent BFSGs are cholecystoduodenal fistulae (80%), cholecystocolonic fistulae 15%, cholecystogastric fistulae (1%), and the remaining 4% are combined or rare fistulae (choledochoduodenal fistulae and Mirizzi syndrome (MS)).[2-6]

The incidence of BFSG in a series of laparoscopic cholecystectomy is variable from 0.2% to 0.9%. In the Hospital Italiano series, of 6107 laparoscopic cholecystectomies, the BFSG rate was 0.6%.[3]

BFSG are most common in women (3:1), 80% are older than 60 years of age, and more than 60% of them have a history of abdominal pain longer than 5 years.[2-5]

Pathophysiology

The spontaneous formation of a bilioenteric fistula (primary biliary fistula) results from a chronic pericholecystic inflammation due to cholecystitis. Recurrent inflammation secondary to a voluminous gallstone (>2.5 cm) determines the onset of a bilioenteric fistula. The development of adhesions between the gall bladder and the duodenum (60–86%), colon, or stomach is the result of this chronic process. Due to the anatomical proximity, the duodenum is the most frequent place involved. Necrosis produced by a voluminous gallstone on the biliary wall causes progressive erosion into the wall of any gastrointestinal structure and the formation of a fistula. This process requires a significant duration of time, frequently with mild symptoms, and may explain why this clinical scenario is usually found in elderly patients (Figure 34.1).

Cholecystoduodenal fistula is the most frequent, followed by a cholecystocolonic fistula; this situation is probably due to the anatomical relationship between the gall bladder and the other organ.[2-6]

Clinical manifestations

Abdominal pain is the most frequent symptom. The association of abdominal distension and vomiting may suggest gallstone ileus (GI). The presence of jaundice is observed in patients with MS. Signs and symptoms of cholangitis are developed by the bacterial overgrowth due to the presence of intestinal contents in the biliary tree.[2,4,5]

Cholecystocolonic fistulae alter the enterohepatic circulation, causing a malabsorption syndrome with chronic diarrhoea and weight loss. The triad of cholecystocolonic fistulae is pneumobilia, chronic diarrhoea, and vitamin K malabsorption. Severe cholangitis may be present if the biliary tree is obstructed with colonic reflux of stools with a high bacterial load. The obstruction of the sigmoid colon by a stone is a rare situation.[7,8]

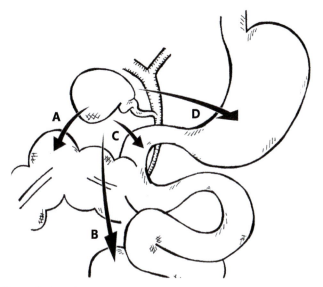

Figure 34.1 Different types of internal biliary fistulae due to gallstones. A: cholecystocolonic. B: cholecystojejunal. C: cholecystoduodenal. D: cholecystogastric.

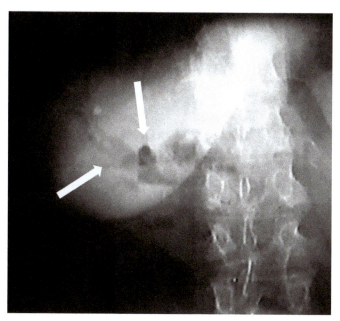

Figure 34.2 Abdominal X-ray with massive presence of air in the biliary tree (white arrows). A cholecystocolonic fistula was suspected.

The treatment should be defined and performed as soon as possible, to avoid the potential development of severe cholangitis and sepsis. Cholecystectomy and closure of the fistulous communication is the recommended procedure.

Diagnosis

Because of non-specific symptoms of BFSG, preoperative diagnosis is difficult and is performed in only 30% of patients.[2,4,5]

Preoperative diagnosis is essential to ensure an adequate management of the case. Its failure may expose the surgeon to intraoperative challenges, changes, and an increased complexity of the surgical technique in an aged and fragile patient.

To evaluate patients with an acute abdomen, abdominal radiography and abdominal ultrasound (US) are the images performed in the emergency setting. Unfortunately, both approaches have a low sensitivity to diagnose a BFSG. For this reason, a computed tomography (CT) scan is mandatory to identify the cause of the abdominal pain, defining the localization and size of the migrated stones.[2,4,9]

Abdominal X-ray has a low sensitivity. The main finding in non-complicated cases is air in the biliary tree (pneumobilia) (Figure 34.2). In the cases of massive pneumobilia, a cholecystocolonic fistula has to be suspected (Figure 34.3). The rest of the findings are related to the GI and will be described in other paragraphs.

Transabdominal US has a high sensitivity to diagnose gallstones (96%). A retracted gall bladder, with thickening of its walls and the presence of air within the gall bladder lumen, are findings that suggest the presence of a BFSG.[2,4,9]

A CT scan is the most accurate and useful radiological image. The interphase between the gall bladder and the compromised viscus is usually not clearly seen but the presence of stones and air in the biliary tree are well defined. Some typical signs of BFSG are gall bladder with thickened walls, retracted gall bladder, pneumobilia, unidentified interphase between the gall bladder and the gastrointestinal tube, fistulous communication, and presence of stones outside the biliary tree (Figure 34.4).[2,4,9]

Magnetic resonance cholangiopancreatography (MRCP) defines precisely and with high accuracy the anatomy, the presence of gallstones, and the compromise of the biliary tree. Common bile duct stones are present in up to 40% of the cases.

When US reveals contact between the gall bladder and structures of the gastrointestinal tract, with no clear interphase in an elderly female patient, a BFSG should be suspected. A CT scan should be done, and if the patient is jaundiced, a MRCP will be useful.[2,4,9]

Treatment

For many years, in the management of BFSG, open surgery was considered as the preferred approach. However, in the last decade the minimally invasive approach has been increasingly applied. Upper and lower gastrointestinal endoscopy is indicated as an alternative to resolve GI.[2–5,7,10–14]

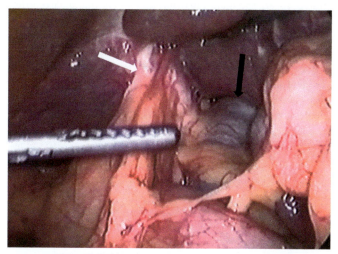

Figure 34.3 Intraoperative laparoscopic view. A fistula (white arrow) between the gall bladder fundus and the colonic hepatic flexure was found. A common bile duct stone (black arrow) was present the biliary tree.

CHAPTER 34 Biliary fistula, gallstone ileus, and Mirizzi syndrome

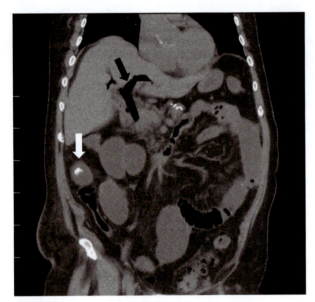

Figure 34.4 CT scan with air in the biliary tree (black arrow), and a calcified stone in the small bowel (white arrow) in a case of cholecystoduodenal fistula.

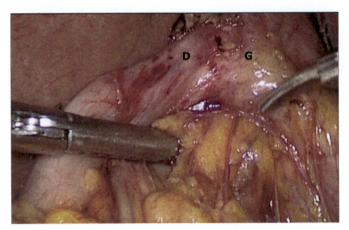

Figure 34.5 Laparoscopic intraoperative view of a cholecystoduodenal fistula. A fistula between the gall bladder fundus (G) and the duodenum (D) was found.

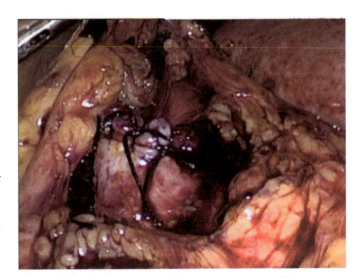

Figure 34.6 Laparoscopic view of the complete closure of the duodenal hole.

The number of small series of laparoscopic approaches is increasing and their results have been encouraging (Table 34.1). With these results, the laparoscopic approach should be strongly considered in selected cases, always performed by well-trained surgeons in complex biliary surgery. In a well fit patient, surgical treatment is mandatory.

Preoperative assessment of the biliary damage, the presence of stones in the biliary tree, and the involvement of the alimentary tract is necessary. Anatomical distortions associated with chronic inflammation and the difficult exposure of anatomical structures, increases the risk of a bile duct injury during cholecystectomy.

The main intraoperative findings are dense inflammatory adhesions around the gall bladder and a shrunken and fibrotic gall bladder, which is firmly stuck to the adjacent organs.

Dense and heavy local adhesions make the procedure difficult and time-consuming. In laparoscopic procedures, bleeding and bowel perforations are the main cause for conversion. Bile duct injuries and residual stones are the main complications. The rate of complications, conversions, and reoperations have a direct relationship with the accuracy of the preoperative assessment.[2-5,7,10-14]

After a meticulous and careful adhesiolysis, the fistulous tract has to be identified and transected with scissors or a stapler. The enteral defect is repaired by hand sewing (Figures 34.5 and 34.6).

In elective cases, the objective is the cholecystectomy and closure of the fistulous tract. In complicated cases, like GI, the objective is to resolve the bowel transit (and the gall bladder is left *in situ*). The cholecystectomy and closure of the fistulous communication may be performed during the same (one-stage) or in a different procedure (two-stage surgery).[2-5,7,10-16]

Laparoscopic management of BFSG is tedious and hazardous. However, in experienced hands, is safe, feasible, and associated with a rapid postoperative recovery.

The anatomy of Calot's triangle can not usually be clearly identified. In these cases, a cholangiography (by direct puncture of the gall

Table 34.1 Results of the authors' series of laparoscopic treatment of bilioenteric fistulas

Type of fistula	n	% of the cases	Efficacy (%)	Conversion rate. n/%	Morbidity
Cholecystoduodenal	21	56.7	90.5	2 (9.5)	3 (14.2)
MS type II	12	29.7	66.7	4 (33.3)	5 (41.6)
Cholecystocolonic	4	10.8	100	0	0
Combined	1	2.7	0	1 (100)	0

Gallstone ileus

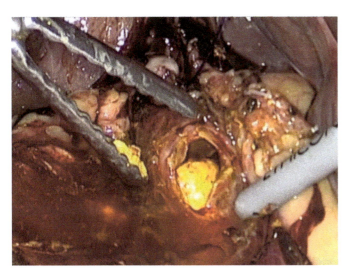

Figure 34.7 Stones in the common bile duct. The case was successfully treated with a laparoscopic choledochotomy.

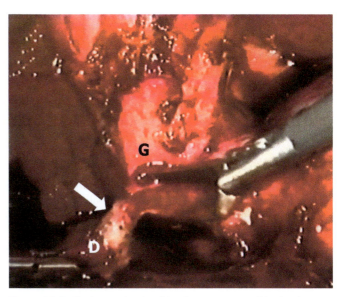

Figure 34.9 Cholecystoduodenal fistula. Transection of the fistulous tract (white arrow) with scissors. D, duodenum; G, gall bladder.

bladder), and partial or subtotal cholecystectomy are the principal tools to avoid an injury to the biliary tract.

In our experience, stones in the biliary tree are found in 40% of the cases of BFSG. These findings are related to the duration of the symptoms. The laparoscopic approach is effective with a high rate of clearance of the biliary tree (Figures 34.7 and 34.8).[3]

Conversion to open surgery in frail patients will increase the risk of postoperative morbidity and mortality.

The published series on laparoscopic surgery for BFSG report better outcomes, due to significant differences in the operative time, blood loss, length of stay, complications, and mortality.

Technical tips for a successful laparoscopic procedure

1. Experience in advanced laparoscopic surgery. Master laparoscopic suturing skills.
2. BFSG should be suspected preoperatively.
3. Meticulous dissection and adhesiolysis.
4. No energy devices in the dissection and sectioning of the fistulous tract (Figure 34.9).
5. Explore the sinus tract and the visceral hole.
6. Identify the anatomical structures in the porta hepatis.
7. Intraoperative cholangiography (via direct puncture of the gall bladder).
8. Confirm stone clearance of the biliary tree and rule out bile duct injury.[3]

Gallstone ileus

Introduction

GI is a rare surgical disease and is a mechanical bowel obstruction due to an impaction of a biliary stone. It is an uncommon and potentially severe complication of gallstones, but it represents only 1% of all cases of small bowel obstruction; however, it forms 25% of non-strangulated cases in elderly patients. It is a rare condition and difficult to diagnose. The management should be tailored for each patient, as there are many therapeutic options, with their own advantages and disadvantages.[17–20]

The ideal treatment remains controversial, being that the main surgical manoeuvre is enterolithotomy. Cholecystectomy and closure of the fistula can be performed during the same procedure or a couple of months afterwards (one-stage or two-stage surgery).[17–20]

Minimally invasive treatments, such as laparoscopy and endoscopy, are applied more frequently in these clinical situations. An attempt to decrease morbidity and mortality in this group of elderly patients is mandatory.[21–23]

Definition

GI is a mechanical bowel obstruction due to one or more gallstones migrating from the biliary tree and impacting within the gastrointestinal tract.

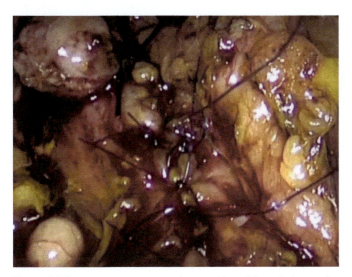

Figure 34.8 Laparoscopic primary closure without biliary drainage of a choledochotomy.

Epidemiology

GI is a relatively rare complication of cholelithiasis. Only 0.3–0.5% of patients with gallstones have this complication and it represents only 30–35 cases per million admissions.

Less than 1% of intestinal obstruction cases are due to GI.[2,4,20]

GI has a higher frequency in women (72–90%) and in an elderly population, with an age range between 60 and 84 years in American patients.[1,2,4,17,18]

Pathophysiology

GI occurs due to the impaction of a stone in the bowel, after the migration of the stones through a biliodigestive fistula.

The spontaneous formation of a biliary–enteric fistula (primary biliary fistula) is usually the result of a chronic pericholecystic inflammation due to repeated episodes of cholecystitis. Recurrent inflammation due to a large gallstone (>2.5 cm) determines the onset of a bilioenteric fistula. The development of adhesions between the gall bladder and the duodenum (60–86%), colon, or stomach is the result of this chronic process. Because of its anatomical proximity, the duodenum is the most frequent place involved. Necrosis produced by the compression of a gallstone on the biliary wall results in a progressive erosion of the gastrointestinal tube's wall and the formation of a fistula. This process requires a significant amount of time, frequently with the presence of mild symptoms. This may explain why this scenario is most frequently found in elderly patients.

The stone passes through the fistula and migrates through the gastrointestinal tract up to a stenotic or narrow area, where it impacts and occludes the visceral lumen.[17–20]

The location of the fistula, the size of the gallstone, and the diameter of the lumen of the bowel will determine whether or not an impaction will occur.

The most common place of impaction is the terminal ileum or the ileocaecal valve (50–75%) because of their relatively narrow lumen and potentially less active peristalsis. Other places where obstruction can occur are the proximal ileum and jejunum (20–40%), and the stomach and duodenum (10%). In the case of a fistula between the gall bladder and colon, the impaction occurs more frequently in the sigmoid but represents a rare event.[17–20,24]

The impaction in the stomach or duodenum causes a Bouveret's stomach outlet syndrome.[15–17,25] Some causes of bowel stenosis as Crohn's or diverticular disease, explain rare places of stone impaction.[17]

At the site of impaction, due to the pressure generated against the bowel wall, it may develop ischaemia and necrosis, even perforation followed by peritonitis.

The faceted morphology of the stones may be predictive of recurring GI. This is based on the concept that each facet implies a multiplicity of stones, which should alert the surgeon, during exploration, of the possibility of further stones in the remaining bowel.[2,4,17]

Clinical manifestations

The clinical presentation of GI depends on the site of impaction and time of evolution (may be an acute, intermittent, or chronic clinical presentation). As a bowel occlusion, the most common symptoms are nausea, vomiting, and epigastric pain. Abdominal distension is related to the place of the impaction. Lower levels of obstruction are associated with more prominent distension.[17–19]

A history of prior biliary symptoms is present in between 27% and 80% of patients. Usually, patients are elderly and have comorbidities. Some degree of dehydration and jaundice are often present. Fever is related to cholangitis or peritonitis. Physical examination may be non-specific. Abdominal distension, tenderness, and high-pitched bowel sounds are frequently found.[17–20]

The type of the vomiting is related to the place and time of evolution of the obstruction.

When the obstruction is located in the upper gastrointestinal tract, the vomit is mainly of gastric content, becoming feculent when the distal ileum is obstructed.

Diagnosis

The symptoms and signs of GI are mostly non-specific and explain why patients arrive at the emergency room several days after the onset of symptoms.[2,4,17,18] According to different series, a correct preoperative diagnosis has been made in only 30–75% of the cases.

The laboratory tests are non-specific. High white cell counts and abnormalities in liver function tests are related to retrograde cholangitis, associated with the reflux of digestive contents through the fistula to the biliary tree. The diagnosis is usually based on the findings of imaging studies.

X-ray

The typical findings on X-rays are signs of intestinal obstruction, pneumobilia (air in the biliary tree), and gallstones in non-typical locations. These findings were described by Rigler in 1941.[9,17] The presence of two of these three signs has been considered to be pathognomonic and are present in 20–50% of the cases (Figures 34.10–34.12).

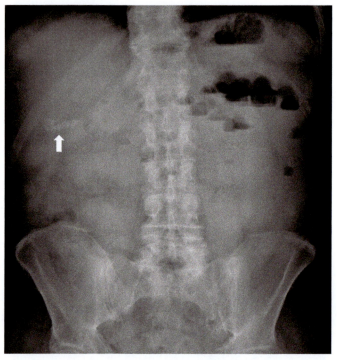

Figure 34.10 Abdominal X-ray in a GI. Dilated small bowel with air fluid levels. In the right upper quadrant, the white arrow shows calcified gallstones.

Gallstone ileus

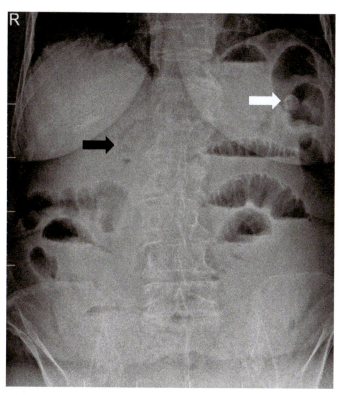

Figure 34.11 Abdominal X-ray in a GI. Dilated small bowel with air fluid levels. Air in the biliary tree (black arrow) and a calcified stone (white arrow) are seen. These findings are the Rigler's triad.

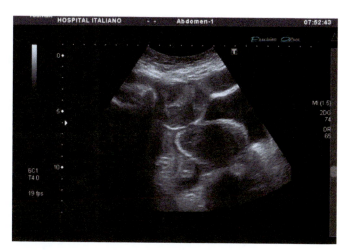

Figure 34.13 Abdominal US with dilated small bowel loops, transverse image. Unspecific finding in a GI.

X-ray shows dilated small bowel loops and high-density endoluminal images suggestive of a stone. Calcified stones are exceptional.

Abdominal ultrasound

A US study is able to show gallstones, presence of air in the biliary tree (pneumobilia), a contracted gall bladder, associated choledocholithiasis, distended small bowel, and an impacted gallstone.[17–20] Sometimes, US is inconclusive (Figures 34.13 and 34.14).

Computed tomography

CT is considered the best study for most of the cases of GI, with a 93% sensitivity, 100% specificity, and 93% accuracy.[17–20]

CT has the highest sensitivity to demonstrate the signs of Rigler's triad. The location of the obstruction, the size of the stone, the presence of the fistula, and abdominal complications secondary to the occlusion are more easily defined with a CT scan (Figure 34.15).

When preoperative diagnosis is possible, the management of the patient is easier. It is also important to define the potential mini-invasive approach by endoscopy or laparoscopy.

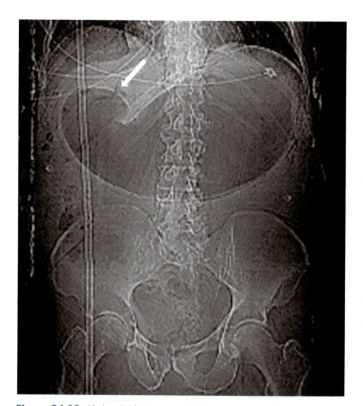

Figure 34.12 Abdominal X-ray in a GI. Massive gastric dilatation in a case of Bouveret's obstruction outlet stomach syndrome.

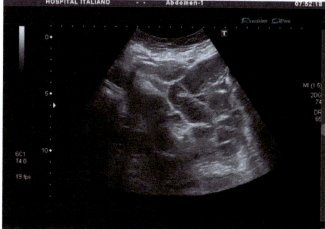

Figure 34.14 Abdominal US with dilated small bowel loops, longitudinal image. Unspecific finding in a GI.

CHAPTER 34 Biliary fistula, gallstone ileus, and Mirizzi syndrome

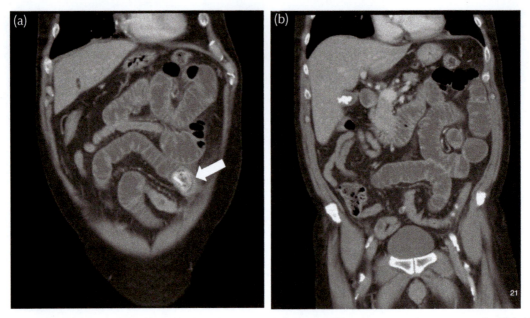

Figure 34.15 (a) CT scan showing dilated small bowel and an obstructive calcified stone. (b) In the same patient, a retracted gall bladder with calcified stones is seen.

In Bouveret syndrome, findings in the CT scan include the presence of a gastroduodenal mass, gas in the gall bladder, inflammatory changes in the area, oral dye in the gall bladder, evidence of the fistula, and a thickened gall bladder wall.[15,16,25] (Figures 34.16 and 34.17). Migrated stones are defined with precision using the CT scan (Figures 34.18 and 34.19).

Magnetic resonance cholangiopancreatography

MRCP may be useful in selected cases, when CT is not diagnostic. The anatomical characteristic of the biliary tree, gall bladder, and the presence of stones and a fistula are well defined using this study.[9,17]

Also, it is possible to define the location of the obstruction (Figures 34.20 and 34.21).

Endoscopy

Endoscopy is a useful study in upper and lower bowel obstructions caused by a gallstone. Also, this approach may even be therapeutic. In cases of Bouveret syndrome, it is a very accurate way to confirm the cause of the obstruction and potentially solve the problem[15,16,25] (Figure 34.22).

In the cases where the obstruction is located in the sigmoid colon, endoscopy is an excellent tool to confirm the cause of the obstruction, and the diagnosis of the type of stenosis (inflammatory or tumourous).[17,24]

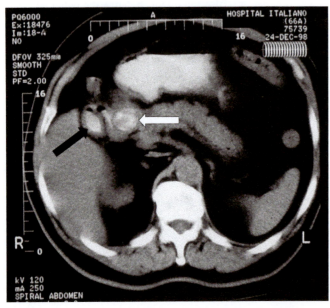

Figure 34.16 GI as Bouveret syndrome. White arrow: calcified stone in the duodenum. Black arrow: oral contrast and air in the gall bladder.

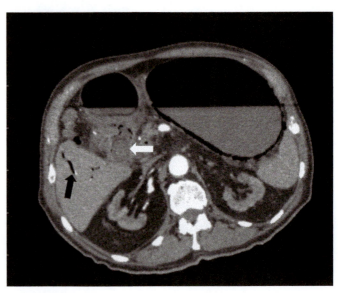

Figure 34.17 GI as Bouveret syndrome. White arrow: stone in duodenum. Black arrow: air in the biliary tree.

Gallstone ileus

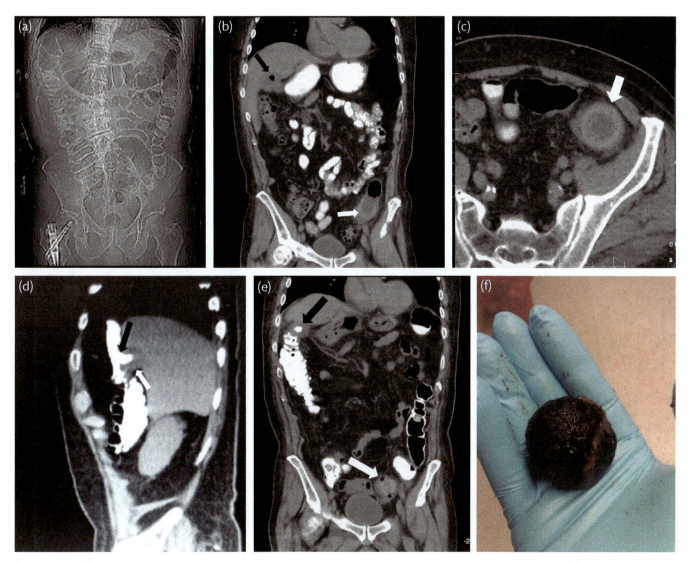

Figure 34.18 (a) Abdominal X-ray with evidence of obstruction in the sigmoid colon with dilatation of the rest of the colon. (b) Air in the gall bladder (black arrow) and a stone in the sigmoid colon. (c) More detail of the stone (white arrow). (d) Fistulous tract (black arrow) between the hepatic flexure of the colon and the gall bladder (white arrow). (e) Oral radiographic contrast inside the gall bladder. (f) The stone removed through a colotomy.

Treatment

Spontaneous resolution rate of GI is low, and the delay in the resolution may worsen the patient's general condition.

This is a surgical problem associated with high morbidity and mortality rates when compared to other causes of bowel obstruction. The mortality described in different series has been up to 27%, and the morbidity up to 50% of the cases. However, a most recent publication, on 3268 patients with GI, reported better results in terms of mortality rate (6.6%). This improvement was related to a better and earlier diagnosis, and improvement in the management of the patients.

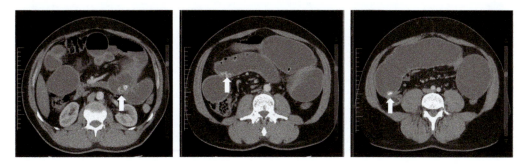

Figure 34.19 Small gallstones (white arrow) in different loops of the small bowel. A small stone was impacted in an inflammatory stenosis in the distal ileum causing a GI.

CHAPTER 34 Biliary fistula, gallstone ileus, and Mirizzi syndrome

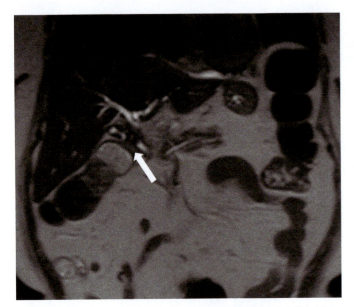

Figure 34.20 MRCP in a GI, with adhesions of a retracted gall bladder to the transverse colon.

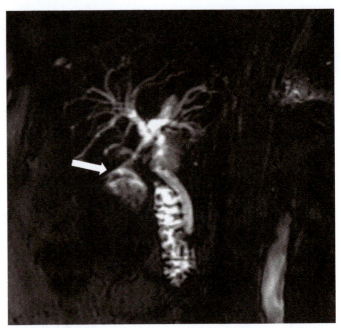

Figure 34.21 MRCP with hepatobiliary contrast. A leakage from the biliary tree into the transverse colon confirms a bilioenteric fistula.

This is a geriatric disease. Most of the patients are elderly and frail with comorbidities. Diagnosis is difficult and late, and this is, in part, the cause of the bad general status, grade of dehydration, and electrolyte abnormalities, factors that explain the high mortality rate in this population.[17–20,26]

Preoperative improvement of the hydration and electrolyte balance, and management of comorbid conditions are mandatory.

Surgery is the most frequent therapeutic approach. Nowadays, laparoscopy is an interesting minimally invasive option to decrease

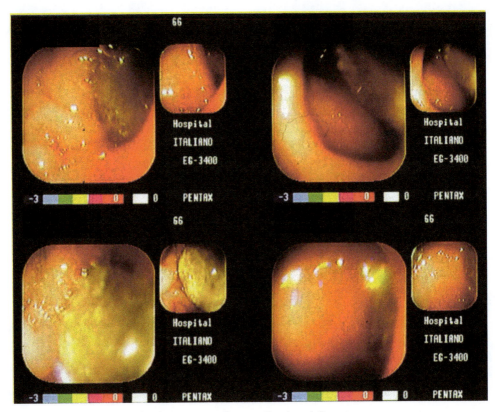

Figure 34.22 GI as Bouveret syndrome. A gastroduodenoscopy confirms a yellow large biliary stone.

morbidity and mortality. In some selected cases of upper or lower GI, the endoscopic approach is under development.[21-23]

Open surgery

Which procedure is the best option to treat GI is still a matter of debate? Possible options are (1) enterolithotomy alone, (2) two-stage surgery (enterolithotomy in an emergency setting and cholecystectomy performed a few months later), and (3) one-stage surgery (enterolithotomy, cholecystectomy, and fistula repair at the same time).[17,19,20,22]

Several factors should be considered before choosing the appropriate approach. The patient's general status and the duration of obstruction are the most important prognostic factors. The main goal is to solve the intestinal obstruction. The adequate selection of the approach should also be based on the site of the gallstone impaction. The patient's age and comorbidity are variables that may contraindicate a radical procedure as one-stage surgery. Because of its low incidence of complications, enterolithotomy is the best option in frail patients and remains the most common surgical treatment in most cases. In a published review, this procedure was performed in 62% of 3268 patients.[20] Through a surgical exploration (open or laparoscopic), the site of the obstruction is identified. The rest of the small bowel must be inspected to rule out another stone inside of the small bowel that could be a cause of recurrent GI. The impacted stone is mobilized and milked proximally to an area where the visceral wall is in a better condition, with less oedema. A longitudinal incision is made on the antimesenteric border and the stone is removed through gentle manoeuvres. The bowel is closed transversally. Bowel resection is sometimes necessary, particularly in the presence of ischaemia, perforation, or stenosis.

Two-stage surgery is recommended by surgeons who argue that fistula diversion is time-consuming and technically demanding. Spontaneous fistula closure can occur in more than 50% of the cases (when the gall bladder is free of stones and the cystic duct remains patent). The recurrence rate of GI is low, ranging between 5% and 8%. The mortality of enterolithotomy is less than 5%.[2,17,18,20] The two-stage surgery adds a second procedure to the enterolithotomy, to remove the fistulous tract and to perform the cholecystectomy.[27] Demonstration of persistent gallstones in postoperative studies, new onset of symptoms, cholangitis due to the persistence of a fistula, or recurrent GI are clear indications for this strategy. Evaluation of associated common bile duct stones is mandatory. In our own experience, 40% of the patients with spontaneous biliodigestive fistulae had stones in the main biliary ducts. The recommended time between both stages is not clearly defined and experienced surgeons propose a period ranging from 4 weeks to 6 months. The mortality of this approach was 2.9%.[20]

One-stage surgery is justified only in highly selected cases, for patients in good general condition who are able to safely undergo a prolonged operation. This approach is particularly useful also in cases with severe acute cholecystitis, gall bladder gangrene, or the presence of stones in the gall bladder. This strategy is associated with the highest mortality (8%). Enteric or biliary leakage after fistula closure are the specific complications of this approach. In the previously mentioned publication, the one-stage procedure was performed in only 19% of GI cases.[20,26,27]

The location of the impaction has a key role in the selection of the surgical approach. An impaction in the small bowel allows us to discuss the three options according to the above-described criteria. However, an impaction in the duodenum will drive us to perform a one-stage surgery due to a compromise of the local structures. In the case of impaction in the colon, this also pushes us to a one-stage procedure due to the cholangitis caused by the fistula between the colon and the gall bladder. However, surgeons should judge the feasibility of the one-stage surgery on the basis of patient's general condition. This intraoperative dilemma is difficult to solve, and the different described variables should be taken into account.[19,20] Table 34.2 describes surgical options and variables to select each of them.

Four factors were identified that increase mortality rate: (1) age, (2) comorbidities, (3) delayed diagnosis and treatment, and (4) postoperative recovery and general complications. The most common complication is acute kidney injury in 30% of the patients. Local complications occur in 20% of the patients (leaks, abscesses, wound infection).[20]

Laparoscopic approach

Open surgery, for the treatment of GI, is associated with significant morbidity (20–50%) and mortality (7–18%).

Open surgery is still the most used approach; however, laparoscopy is more frequently selected and used by experienced surgeons (Figure 34.23). The better results in laparoscopy than in open surgery encourage the use of a minimally invasive approach for GI. The use of laparoscopy in acute small bowel obstruction has been associated with better results: shorter postoperative course, shorter length of stay, and lower morbidity when compared to open surgery.[17,21,22]

Table 34.2 Three main surgical options for the treatment of gallstone ileus

	Indications	Advantages	Disadvantages	Place of obstruction
Enterolithotomy	Fragile patient Short life expectancy Multiple comorbidities	Short operative time Low morbidity and mortality	Recurrence of ileus and biliary symptoms Cholangitis Carcinogenesis?	Small bowel
Two-step surgery	Healthier patient Long life expectancy	Conservative in the emergency All is finally resolved	Two procedures	Small bowel
One-step surgery	Healthier patient Young patient Tissues in good conditions Trained surgeon	One surgery Prevents future gallstone events	Complex surgery High morbidity and mortality Long procedure Risky in elderly and fragile patients	Small bowel Duodenum/stomach Colon

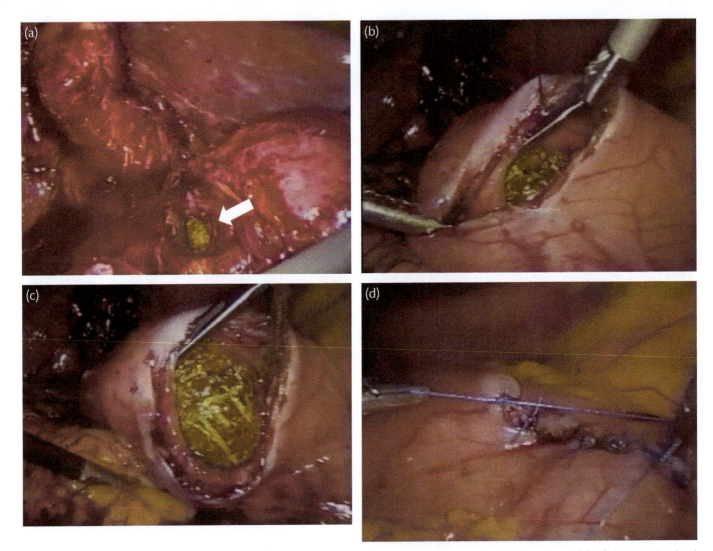

Figure 34.23 Laparoscopic treatment of Bouveret syndrome. (a) Duodenal hole in anterior face of duodenum (white arrow) (b, c) The giant duodenal stone was removed laparoscopically through the pylorus, by an incision on anterior wall of the stomach. A one-stage surgery was performed. (d) Closure of the anterior gastric wall.

All the minimally invasive approach advantages should be offered to patients with GI.

The experience in minimally invasive surgical treatment of GI is still poor; adequate management in low-risk patients is the first step towards improving the results.

For enterolithotomy, a laparoscopic-assisted procedure makes the surgery faster. Once the segment of the bowel where the stone is impacted is identified, it is taken out of the abdominal cavity through a small abdominal incision. The enterotomy is performed, the stone is removed and the incision in the bowel is sutured. This extracorporeal approach is faster and avoids potential contamination of the peritoneal cavity due to the spillage of intestinal contents[17,21,22] (Figure 34.24).

In the laparoscopic approach, an early recovery and low mortality are expected. Some series of the laparoscopic two-stage treatment indicate that this approach has better results.

The laparoscopic two-stage procedure was found to be an efficient and safe approach for the management of GI. The operative time for the first stage is shorter than that required for the one-stage procedure; all this results in another advantage for elderly patients.[22]

Endoscopic approach

Gallstones causing gastroduodenal or colonic obstruction may be amenable for an endoscopic treatment option. The success is related to the experience of the operator and to the size of the stone. The success rate of the endoscopic management was less than 10% at the beginning of the experience.[17,23,24] Many cases of successful endoscopic management of Bouveret syndrome have been described, by removing the obstructive stone, combining endoscopic manoeuvres and lithotripsy.[2,4,17] Biliary stenting reduces the pressure in the fistulous tract, increasing the spontaneous closure of the fistula.

Due to the large size of the stones, some kind of lithotripsy is necessary. This could be performed mechanically, by electrohydraulic waves or using a laser. The main advantage of the laser is the precise targeting of the impacted stone with reduced risk of organ perforation.[17,21,22]

These endoscopic methods should be considered in high-risk patients. In the endoscopic treatment of stones located in the stomach or duodenum, the fragmentation of the stone in small pieces is recommended, to avoid the possibility of distal impaction of gallstone fragments.

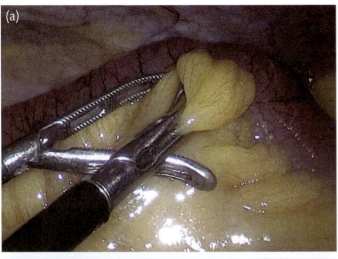
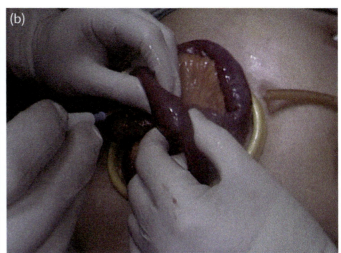
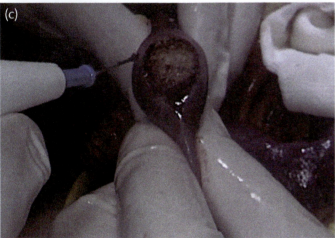

Figure 34.24 Laparoscopic-assisted enterolithotomy. (a) Identification of the loop with the impacted stone. (b) Exteriorization of the loop. (c) Longitudinal enterotomy to remove the stone.

Currently, endoscopy and lithotripsy are considered first-line strategies (Figure 34.25). In case of failure of the endoscopic approach, surgery must be performed without delay, to avoid impairment in the patient's status and potential abdominal complications.

Mirizzi syndrome

The MS is a rare condition in biliary surgery. It was first described in 1948 by an Argentinian surgeon, Pablo Mirizzi.[28] This syndrome is present when a large stone is impacted in Hartmann's pouch and the stone compresses the main bile duct. The described situation requires many years to develop and in its final stages, the MS is characterized by a complete communication (fistula) between the gall bladder and the main bile duct. In some countries, like Argentina, the incidence is rather high (around 2%)[3] and in countries like the US, the incidence below 0.2%.[29] The MS classification has been modified by Csendes. He described four types[30] (Figure 34.26):

- Type I: no fistula, compression of the main hepatic duct by the stone.
- Type II: fistula between the gall bladder and the main hepatic duct, the communication comprises less than 33% of its diameter.
- Type III: same as II but with a communication between 33% and 66% of its diameter.
- Type IV: same as III but with a communication larger than 66% of its diameter.

Almost 20 years later, Csendes[31] modified his own classification by adding type V. This last type includes any type of MS associated with any bilioenteric fistula (cholecystoduodenal, cholecystogastric, or cholecystocolonic; all of them described previously).

Since the development of complex laparoscopic biliary procedures, this approach has been increasingly used for the treatment of MS. A thorough examination of the biliary tree anatomy by preoperative radiological assessment and the possibility to perform intraoperative cholangiography by direct injection of dye into the gall bladder overcome the lack of Calot's triangle visibility and the inability to identify the critical view of safety as described by Dr Strasberg.[32] However, in order to be able to perform this procedure safely, skills in advanced biliary laparoscopy are mandatory. So, with an accurate preoperative evaluation and in centres with a high volume of biliary and laparoscopic surgery, the MS can be laparoscopically approached.[33]

CHAPTER 34 Biliary fistula, gallstone ileus, and Mirizzi syndrome

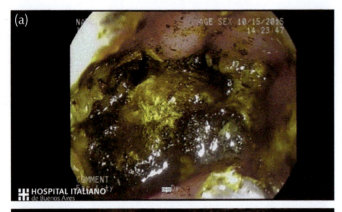

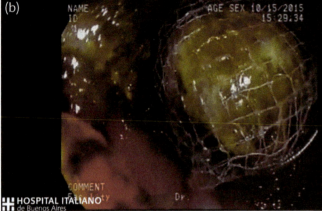

Figure 34.25 (a) An impacted biliary stone in the sigmoid colon after endoscopic lithotripsy. (b) Removal of fragments of the stone.

Diagnosis

MS should be considered when patients present with abdominal pain, jaundice, and symptomatic gall bladder stones. Laboratory tests and radiological studies should be performed. In the blood tests, a high bilirubin (predominantly direct bilirubin) and a high alkaline phosphatase level are expected; in cases presenting with cholangitis, a high white cells count might be present. Diagnostic imaging is the key to diagnose this syndrome, and different options are available:

- US: a stone impacted in Hartmann's pouch or into the main bile duct, dilatation of the intrahepatic bile ducts, and normal distal bile duct.
- CT scan: same findings, malignancy has to be ruled out.
- MRCP: provides the most accurate anatomy of the biliary tree, also useful to assess the presence of malignant disease (Figure 34.27).
- ERCP: necessary in patients with moderate to severe cholangitis.

If malignancy is still suspected or preoperative assessment is not clear, a diagnostic laparoscopy with laparoscopic US is mandatory.

In some cases, the diagnosis is not suspected preoperatively, and the patient is surgically approached. A MS has to be suspected when Calot's triangle is not easily found, and a critical view of safety is not achieved. In this situation, a cholangiogram by direct injection of the gall bladder is necessary. If cholangiography is not available, a laparoscopic cholecystostomy should be deferred and the patient needs to be sent to a centre with experience in the management of complex biliary cases. Subtotal cholecystectomy is not recommended since the anatomy is unclear.

Treatment

The adequate approach to treat these patients depends on the presence or not of cholangitis. In cases with mild cholangitis, antibiotic treatment is indicated. In cases with moderate or severe cholangitis, a minimally invasive procedure should be performed, either ERCP or a percutaneous transhepatic biliary drainage. A surgical procedure is performed depending on the type of MS. In those cases, with no cholangitis or once the cholangitis is solved, a surgical procedure in needed to solve the problem. The preferred approach is laparoscopy. The surgical procedure has to be selected according to the type (according to the Csendes classification):[34]

Type I

For type I, primary closure of the main bile duct is recommended. Once the cholangiography (by direct injection of the gall bladder) confirms the presence of this type, the gall bladder should be opened, and the stone removed. A second cholangiography can be performed through the cystic duct. Once the anatomy is clear, the gall bladder has to be resected. Choledochoscopy can also be performed to evaluate the presence of stones in the main bile duct. Once the case is completed, the cystic duct can be closed by an intracorporeal knot. Clips are not recommended due to the diameter of the duct and the tissue frailty. If a knot is not feasible because the cystic duct

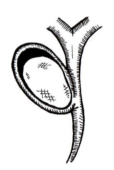 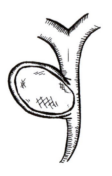 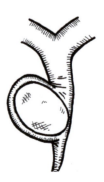 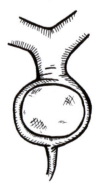

Figure 34.26 Csendes' classification of MS. Four types as described in the text.

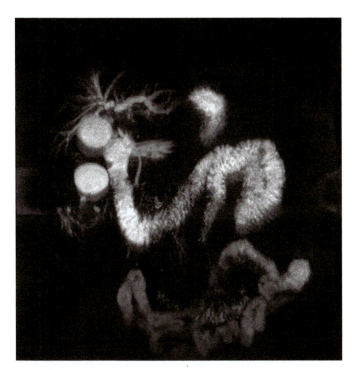

Figure 34.27 MRCP showing an obstruction below the biliary confluence, with mild dilatation of the intrahepatic bile duct and a normal distal main hepatic duct.

is too short, separate stitches of 5/0 or 6/0 polypropylene are needed to close the stump.

Type II

Once type II MS is confirmed by cholangiography, the distal portion of the Hartmann's pouch has to be left in place. In order to accomplish this, the gall bladder needs to be opened and the stone removed. The gall bladder has to be resected. The pouch is used to create a patch to safely close the main bile duct with no strictures; for this purpose, separate 4/0 or 5/0 stitches are needed. A T-tube or other biliary drainage should be placed to achieve a low pressure in the bile duct.

Type III and IV

For the types III and IV MS, a Roux-en-Y hepaticojejunostomy is necessary. Since the common bile duct lacks lateral wall, there is no chance of creating a patch using the gall bladder (like in type II).

As always, cholangiography is mandatory. It can be performed by a direct injection of the gall bladder. The gall bladder stump has to be opened and the stone removed; the common bile duct must be dissected. Once the bile duct is completely encircled (above the fistula with the gall bladder), it has to be cut with no-energy devices (use only Metzenbaum scissors). The gall bladder needs to be completely removed to improve the surgical field. A side-to-side Roux-en-Y can be performed using staples, 70 cm distal to the hepaticojejunostomy. The long limb of the Roux-en-Y loop is placed side to end to the bile duct. An enterotomy is carried out and a single-layer end-to-side anastomosis between the bile duct and the jejunum is performed, using a 4/0 polypropylene or a polydioxanone running suture. A drainage has to be left in place in all cases.

Conclusion

A BFSG is an internal spontaneous communication between the biliary tree and mainly with structures of the gastrointestinal tube. Preoperative diagnosis is crucial and still challenging. CT scan is most frequently used due to its diagnostic accuracy. In most cases, the laparoscopic approach performed by a well-trained surgeon is the treatment of choice. All the advantages of the minimally invasive approach are also seen in this particularly elderly population. Alternative endoscopic procedures are effective in upper and lower obstructions of the gastrointestinal tract by biliary stones.

GI is a mechanical bowel obstruction due to an impaction of a stone. It represents less than 1% of all obstructions. It affects mostly older female patients. This is a high morbidity and mortality scenario. Four main reasons have been found to be related to the high mortality rates: (1) age, (2) comorbidities, (3) delay in diagnosis and treatment, and (4) difficult postoperative recovery and general complications. The best diagnostic tool is an abdominal CT scan. The main therapeutic objective is to release the obstruction. Surgical enterolithotomy is the most frequently used procedure. Two-stage surgery and one-stage surgery have specific indications. The laparoscopic approach is increasingly used; its applicability in these complex cases is safe and effective when is performed by experienced surgeons. The endoscopic approach has selective indications in some gastroduodenal and colonic obstructions.

MS is a fistula between the gall bladder and the main bile duct. The degree of communication (size of the fistula) determines the specific treatment. For type I MS, since there is no communication, a laparoscopic cholecystectomy with primary closure of the cystic duct is feasible. In type II, due to the lack of cystic duct, a patch using the Hartmann's pouch needs to be performed to close the fistula, with or without any biliary drainage. In type III and IV, a Roux-en-Y hepaticojejunostomy is necessary to successfully repair this syndrome. In all cases the laparoscopic approach is preferred with experienced surgeons.

Acknowledgements

We thank Maria Eugenia Fratantoni, MD, for collaborating on some of the illustrations.

REFERENCES

1. Dorrance HR, Lingam MK, Hair A, Oien K, O'Dwyer PJ. Acquired abnormalities of the biliary tract from chronic gallstone disease. *J Am Coll Surg*. 1999;**189**(3):269–273. doi:10.1016/S1072-7515(99)00126-X
2. Crespi M, Montecamozzo G, Foschi D. Diagnosis and treatment of biliary fistulas in the laparoscopic era. *Gastroenterol Res Pract*. 2016;**2016**:6293538. doi:10.1155/2016/6293538
3. Pekolj J, Facs M, Quiñónez E, Mazza O, Arbués G, De Santibañes E. Tratamiento laparoscópico de las fístulas biliodigestivas y del síndrome de Mirizzi. *Revista Argent Cirug*. 2006;**90**(3/4):142–151.
4. Inukai K. Gallstone ileus: a review. *BMJ Open Gastroenterol*. 2019;**6**(1):e000344. doi:10.1136/bmjgast-2019-000344

5. Li XY, Zhao X, Zheng P, Kao XM, Xiang XS, Ji W. Laparoscopic management of cholecystoenteric fistula: a single-center experience. *J Int Med Res*. 2017;**45**(3):1090–1097. doi:10.1177/0300060517699038
6. Wu MB, Zhang WF, Zhang YL, Mu D, Gong JP. Choledochoduodenal fistula in mainland China: a review of epidemiology, etiology, diagnosis and management. *Ann Surg Treat Res*. 2015;**89**(5):240–246. doi:10.4174/astr.2015.89.5.240
7. Gibreel W, Greiten LL, Alsayed A, Schiller HJ. Management dilemma of cholecysto-colonic fistula: case report. *Int J Surg Case Rep*. 2018;**42**:233–236. doi:10.1016/j.ijscr.2017.12.017
8. Abbasi S, Khan DB, Khandwala K, Raza R, Wasim A. Cholecystocolonic fistula case presentation. *Cureus J Med Sci*. 2019;**11**(6):1–7. doi:10.7759/cureus.4874
9. Aldo C, Lorenzo M, Olgerta L, Alberto C, Licia U, Melchiore G. Rolling in the deep: imaging findings and diagnostic pearls in gallstone ileus. *Surg Reg Pract*. 2020;**2020**:1421753. doi:10.1155/2020/1421753
10. Angrisani L, Corcione F, Tartaglia A, et al. Cholecystoenteric fistula (CF) is not a contraindication for laparoscopic surgery. *Surg Endosc*. 2001;**15**(9):1038–1041. doi:10.1007/s004640000317
11. Ibrahim IM, Wolodiger F, Saber AA, Dennery B. Treatment of cholecystocolic fistula by laparoscopy. *Surg Endosc*. 1995;**9**(6):728–729. doi:10.1007/BF00187951
12. Nixon SJ, Mirghani MM. Laparoscopic management of cholecystenteric fistula. *Br J Surg*. 1995;**82**(5):675–676. doi:10.1002/bjs.1800820537
13. Targarona EM, Andrade E, Balagué C, Ardid J, Trías M. Mirizzi's syndrome. *Surg Endosc*. 1997;**11**(8):842–845. doi:10.1007/s004649900467
14. Moreno Ruiz FJ, del Rey Moreno A, Suescun García RM, et al. Treatment of cholecystoduodenal fistula in the era of laparoscopy. *Rev Esp Enfermedades Dig*. 2001;**93**(11):715–720.
15. Rodriguez Romano D, Moreno Gonzalez E, Jiménez Romero C, et al. Duodenal obstruction by gallstones (Bouveret's syndrome). Presentation of a new case and literature review. *Hepatogastroenterology*. 1997;**44**(17):1351–1355.
16. Malvaux P, Degolla R, Saint-Hubert M, Farchakh E, Hauters P. Laparoscopic treatment of a gastric outlet obstruction caused by a gallstone (Bouveret's syndrome). *Surg Endosc*. 2002;**16**(7):1108–1109. doi:10.1007/s004640042033
17. Nuño-Guzmán CM, Marín-Contreras ME, Figueroa-Sánchez M, Corona JL. Gallstone ileus, clinical presentation, diagnostic and treatment approach. *World J Gastrointest Surg*. 2016;**8**(1):65–76. doi:10.4240/wjgs.v8.i1.65
18. Jakubauskas M, Luksaite R, Sileikis A, Strupas K, Poskus T. Gallstone ileus: management and clinical outcomes. *Medicina (Kaunas)*. 2019;**55**(9):598. doi:10.3390/medicina55090598
19. Bakhshi G, Chincholkar R, Agarwal J, Gupta M, Gokhe P, Nadkarni A. Gallstone ileus: dilemma in the management. *Clin Pract*. 2017;**7**(3):977. doi:10.4081/cp.2017.977
20. Halabi WJ, Kang CY, Ketana N, et al. Surgery for gallstone ileus: a nationwide comparison of trends and outcomes. *Ann Surg*. 2014;**259**(2):329–335. doi:10.1097/SLA.0b013e31827eefed
21. Mirza Gari MK, Eldamati A, Foula MS, Al-Mulhim AM, Abdulmomen AA. Laparoscopic management for gallstone ileus, case report. *Int J Surg Case Rep*. 2018;**51**:268–271. doi:10.1016/j.ijscr.2018.09.004
22. Inukai K, Tsuji E, Takashima N, Yamamoto M. Laparoscopic two-stage procedure for gallstone ileus. *J Minim Access Surg*. 2019;**15**(2):164. doi:10.4103/jmas.JMAS_88_18
23. Shah-Khan S, Vallabh H, Cardinal J, Nasr J. Novel use of an endoscopic suturing device to repair a cholecystoduodenal fistula. *ACG Case Reports J*. 2017;**4**(1):e121. doi:10.14309/crj.2017.121
24. Farkas N, Kaur V, Shanmuganandan A, et al. A systematic review of gallstone sigmoid ileus management. *Ann Med Surg*. 2018;**27**:32–39. doi:10.1016/j.amsu.2018.01.004
25. Kalwaniya DS, Arya SV, Guha S, et al. A rare presentation of gastric outlet obstruction (GOO)—the Bouveret's syndrome. *Ann Med Surg*. 2015;**4**(1):67–71. doi:10.1016/j.amsu.2015.02.001
26. Conzo G, Mauriello C, Gambardella C, et al. Gallstone ileus: one-stage surgery in an elderly patient: one-stage surgery in gallstone ileus. *Int J Surg Case Rep*. 2013;**4**(3):316–318. doi:10.1016/j.ijscr.2012.12.016
27. Tartaglia D, Bakkar S, Piccini L, et al. Less is more: an outcome assessment of patients operated for gallstone ileus without fistula treatment. *Int J Surg Case Rep*. 2017;**38**:78–82. doi:10.1016/j.ijscr.2017.07.007
28. Mirizzi, PL. Sindrome del conduct hepatico. *J Int Chir*. 1948;**8**:731–777. http://ci.nii.ac.jp/naid/10013548373/en/
29. Erben Y, Benavente-Chenhalls LA, Donohue JM, et al. Diagnosis and treatment of Mirizzi syndrome: 23-year mayo clinic experience. *J Am Coll Surg*. 2011;**213**(1):114–119. doi:10.1016/j.jamcollsurg.2011.03.008
30. Csendes A, Diaz JC, Burdiles P, Maluenda F, Nava O. Mirizzi syndrome and cholecystobiliary fistula: a unifying classification. *Br J Surg*. 1989;**76**(11):1139–1143. doi:10.1002/bjs.1800761110
31. Beltran MA, Csendes A, Cruces KS. The relationship of Mirizzi syndrome and cholecystoenteric fistula: validation of a modified classification. *World J Surg*. 2008;**32**(10):2237–2243. doi:10.1007/s00268-008-9660-3
32. Strasberg SM, Hertl M, Soper NJ. An analysis of the problem of biliary injury during laparoscopic cholecystectomy. *J Am Coll Surg*. 1995;**180**(1):101–125.
33. Senra F, Navaratne L, Acosta A, Martínez-Isla A. Laparoscopic management of type II Mirizzi syndrome. *Surg Endosc*. 2020;**34**(5):2303–2312. doi:10.1007/s00464-019-07316-6
34. Palavecino M, Pekolj J. Laparoscopic treatment of Mirizzi's syndrome. In: Asbun H, Geller D, eds. *ACS Multimedia Atlas of Surgery: Liver Surgery Volume*. Woodbury, CT: Ciné-Med; 2014: chapter 7.

35

Benign and malignant lesions of the gall bladder

Anil K. Agarwal and Raja Kalayarasan

Introduction

Gall bladder cancer (GBC), the most common biliary tract cancer, shows significant regional variations in its incidence.[1,2] While incidental GBC is common in Western countries, primary GBC still accounts for a considerable proportion in endemic regions. Since its first description in 1877, GBC has been considered to be an aggressive tumour with a dismal outcome.[3] Alfred Blalock's writing that 'in malignancy of the gallbladder when a diagnosis can be made without exploration, no operation should be performed, as much as it only shortens the patient's life' highlights the widely prevalent nihilistic approach towards GBC.[4] However, recent studies have shown better survival rates after multidisciplinary management of GBC, with radical surgery being the mainstay.[5-8] Because of the relative rarity of the disease, there is still a controversy regarding the optimal management of GBC, including using a minimally invasive approach. As cholecystectomy is a commonly performed surgical procedure, the gall bladder (GB) is one of the most common specimens encountered in surgical pathology laboratories. While chronic cholecystitis will be the common pathological finding, incidental diagnosis of another pathology is not uncommon.[9] Hence a knowledge of the various benign and premalignant pathologies affecting the GB is essential to differentiate them from GBC. The current chapter will provide an updated overview of the various benign and malignant lesions affecting the GB, focusing on the surgical management of GBC and addressing various controversies regarding this.

Benign lesions of the gall bladder

Benign lesions of the GB are relatively common, and the majority are GB polyps.[10-12] These are elevated lesions of the GB wall that project into the lumen. They are common incidental findings detected during abdominal ultrasonography (USG), with an estimated prevalence of approximately 5% in the global population. Polyps are broadly classified into being benign and neoplastic based on their malignant potential (Table 35.1). Neoplastic polyps include benign adenomatous polyps that can potentially transform into GBC. Based on their pathological features, they are also classified as being true and pseudo polyps. A cholesterol polyp is the most common pseudopolyp, followed by focal adenomyomatosis and an inflammatory polyp. Most GB polyps are benign. While adenomas are the most common benign neoplastic polyp, GBC often presents initially as a polyp. Unlike in colonic polyps, the adenoma–carcinoma sequence is not the predominant malignant pathway. However, evidence suggests that a small proportion of GBC arises from pre-existing adenomas.[13] As GBC is an aggressive tumour, the aim of clinical evaluation of a patient with a GB polyp is focused on differentiating a true polyp from a pseudopolyp and not missing an early GBC. The challenge in clinical practice is to achieve the above-mentioned aim without increasing the rate of unnecessary cholecystectomies with their possible associated complications.

Investigations

Ultrasonography

Transabdominal USG is the commonly used investigation for the evaluation of a GB polyp. The absence of posterior acoustic shadowing and fixity of the lesion after USG done in two positions differentiates a polyp from a stone. Cholesterol polyps that form due to the deposition of triglycerides and cholesterol esters within macrophages in the lamina propria appear echogenic without a visible stalk giving rise to a 'ball on the wall' appearance.[14] The focal form of adenomyomatosis usually presents as a polyp involving the fundus. The intramural diverticula filled with inspissated bile appear as anechoic areas on USG that differentiate it from a GBC. Occasionally adenomyomatosis produces twinkling or comet-tail artefacts at USG when the intramural diverticula contain sludge or stones.[15] Inflammatory polyps do not have typical imaging features and a definitive preoperative diagnosis is challenging. Adenomas are less echogenic and typically demonstrate internal vascularity on Doppler USG. The USG features suggestive of malignancy in a patient with adenomatous polyp are a solitary polyp larger than 10 mm, a broad-based polyp, and a focal wall thickening of more

Table 35.1 Types of gall bladder polyps

Benign	Neoplastic
• Cholesterol polyps • Inflammatory polyps • Hyperplastic polyps • Haemangioma • Xanthogranuloma • Heterotopic gastric tissue • Heterotopic intestinal tissue	Benign: • Adenoma • Myoma • Papilloma • Fibroma • Lipoma • Granular cell tumour Malignant: • Carcinoma • Carcinoid tumours • Sarcoma • Mucinous cystadenoma

than 3 mm. High-resolution USG that operates at a greater frequency (5–7 MHz) compared to the conventional transabdominal USG (2–5 MHz) is more accurate in identifying hypoechoic spots in neoplastic polyps.[16]

Endoscopic USG which uses a much higher-frequency probe (5–12 MHz) is considered to be more accurate than transabdominal USG in differentiating neoplastic from non-neoplastic polyps.[17,18] However, its accuracy is lower in polyps smaller than 10 mm, where the decision-making is controversial.[19] Endoscopic USG is more sensitive in detecting hypoechoic foci that are observed in 91% of neoplastic polyps compared to only 11% of non-neoplastic polyps. However, as it is an invasive investigation, its use is limited to situations in which a transabdominal USG cannot rule out a neoplastic polyp or in patients in whom malignancy is suspected.

Computed tomography and magnetic resonance imaging

Computed tomography (CT) is indicated in large polyps (>1 cm), especially when the suspicion of GBC is high. It is primarily used for the staging of GBC.[20] CT is not an appropriate investigation for either the primary diagnosis or follow-up of GB polyps because of the radiation exposure. Magnetic resonance imaging (MRI) is usually not recommended for evaluating a GB polyp unless a CT is contraindicated, as in conditions like renal failure. Malignant GB polyps are often hyperintense, whereas benign lesions are moderately intense or hypointense.[21] A lower apparent diffusion coefficient value is reported in malignant lesions compared to benign polyps on diffusion-weighted MRI.

In summary, transabdominal USG, especially contrast-enhanced or high-resolution USG, is the primary investigation recommended for the diagnosis of polyps. Endoscopic USG and cross-sectional imaging (CT/MRI) are reserved for suspicious lesions.

Management

The management of GB polyps is controversial due to a lack of high-quality evidence and considerable heterogeneity in the published literature. The two main indications for surgery in a patient with a GB polyp are the presence of symptoms and the risk of malignancy.[22,23] Currently, a polyp size of greater than 10 mm on radiological imaging is considered to be a significant risk factor for malignancy. However, malignancy has been reported in polyps less than 10 mm in size. Hence all polyps measuring between 4 and 10 mm should be kept under regular surveillance using transabdominal USG.[22] The recommended interval is two initial 6-monthly scans followed by yearly scans up to 5 years. Polyps that reach 10 mm or increase in size by more than 2 mm during surveillance mandate cholecystectomy. Although malignancy has not been reported in polyps smaller than 4 mm, there is still such a risk in true polyps; hence surveillance but at a lower frequency (1, 3, and 5 years) is recommended. It is essential to understand that the surveillance and treatment plan should be tailored for individual patients based on other risk factors like solitary polyps, sessile morphology, age more than 50 years, associated gallstones, primary sclerosing cholangitis, and compliance to follow-up (Figure 35.1).

The laparoscopic approach is preferred for cholecystectomy in patients with a GB polyp like any other benign GB pathology. All cholecystectomy specimens should be cut open and examined.[24] If there is any suspicion of malignancy, a frozen section examination should be performed. In patients with a suspected malignant polyp, a laparoscopic approach has earlier been considered to be a contraindication due to reports of tumour recurrence at port sites following laparoscopic cholecystectomy for GBC. As discussed in the later part of the chapter, the concept of minimally invasive surgery for GBC has evolved over time and a suspicion of malignancy is no longer a contraindication for a laparoscopic approach.[25] In those patients with suspicion of GBC, the GB should be removed with the small wedge (2 cm) of the liver so that the cystic plate is not breached, and the specimen sent for frozen section examination.[26] If the frozen section turns out to be malignant, then a lymphadenectomy part of the radical cholecystectomy should be performed using the open or laparoscopic approach according to the available expertise and philosophy of the surgical team.

Gall bladder cancer

Epidemiology and risk factors

As stated earlier, GBC is the most common malignancy of the biliary tract.[1] It is the only cancer of the digestive tract that is more common in females. The global incidence of GBC shows a significant variation with geographical region and ethnicity.[27] Countries like Chile, Bolivia, India (the Northern states), Pakistan, Nepal, South Korea, Thailand, and Japan have a high incidence of GBC, with native South Americans and those of Indian ethnicity increasing the predisposition in the developed countries. Cholelithiasis is considered to be a significant risk factor for GBC. Although a direct causal relationship has not been established, chronic irritation due to gallstones combined with local production of carcinogens such as secondary bile acids results in metaplasia of the GBC mucosa followed by dysplasia and carcinoma.[28,29] A large size and long duration of gallstone presence might increase the risk of GBC. Association of chronic infection by *Salmonella* (*S. typhi* and *S. paratyphi*) or *Helicobacter* (*H. pylori* and *H. bilis*) and heavy metal ingestion (filtered in the bile) with GBC is also perhaps a cause of chronic inflammation as seen with gallstones.[30,31] The high risk of malignancy (10–50%) reported earlier with porcelain GB has been challenged by recent studies, but the real risk is less than 10%, with stippled calcification of the mucosa representing a higher risk compared to diffuse calcification. Despite the lower risk of malignancy, cholecystectomy is recommended in medically fit patients with a porcelain GB especially in high incidence areas.[32] Obesity and female sex increase

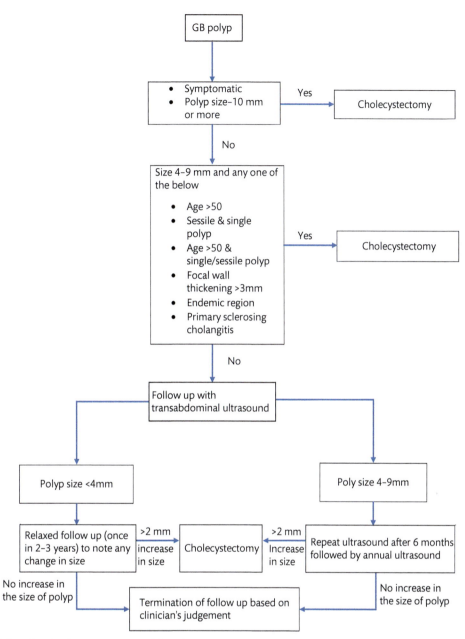

Figure 35.1 Proposed algorithm for the management of GB polyps.

the risk due to elevated oestrogen levels causing supersaturation of bile with cholesterol, thereby increasing the risk of gallstones.[33] True GB polyps, primary sclerosing cholangitis, and an anomalous pancreaticobiliary duct junction are other risk factors for GBC.[34]

Pathology

Adenocarcinoma is the most common histological type and others contribute to less than 10% of GBC (Box 35.1). While some reports suggest that patients with squamous variants of GBC and neuroendocrine carcinoma have a poorer prognosis compared to adenocarcinoma, it is often due to their advanced stage at presentation and their overall survival is comparable to patients with adenocarcinoma at a similar pathological stage.[35] Similarly, the papillary variant of GBC is associated with a relatively better prognosis as it tends to be less invasive. However, when it does become invasive, its prognosis resembles other histological types at similar pathological stages.[36]

Clinical features

The clinical presentation of GBC shows a distinct difference in different geographical areas. While primary GBC with the symptomatic presentation is more common in high-incidence areas like India and other Asian countries, an asymptomatic incidental diagnosis is common in the West.[37,38] In a 2016 study from Korea comparing the differences in clinical outcomes of GBC patients operated in two different time periods, the percentage of patients with asymptomatic presentation increased from 14% to 35%.[39] The authors attributed this shift in the presentation to the improvement in imaging technology and early detection of GBC. However, in countries like

CHAPTER 35 Benign and malignant lesions of the gall bladder

> **Box 35.1** Pathological types of gall bladder cancer
>
> **Epithelial tumours**
> - Adenocarcinoma
> - Biliary type.
> - Intestinal type.
> - Gastric foveolar type.
> - Adenosquamous carcinoma.
> - Squamous cell carcinoma.
> - High-grade neuroendocrine carcinoma.
> - Small cell neuroendocrine carcinoma.
> - Mixed adenoneuroendocrine carcinoma.
> - Mucinous adenocarcinoma.
> - Clear cell adenocarcinoma.
> - Signet ring cell carcinoma.
> - Undifferentiated carcinoma.
> - Intraductal papillary neoplasm with an associated invasive carcinoma.
> - Mucinous cystic neoplasm with an associated invasive carcinoma.
>
> **Mesenchymal tumours**
> - Embryonal rhabdomyosarcoma.
> - Leiomyosarcoma.
> - Malignant fibrous histiocytoma.
> - Angiosarcoma.
>
> **Other tumours**
> - Melanoma.
> - Carcinoid.

India, Pakistan, and Nepal, symptomatic presentation and locally advanced GBC remain common.

Investigations

USG examination of the abdomen is the initial investigation in patients with no evidence of metastatic disease on clinical evaluation. Cross-sectional imaging in the form of CT or MRI abdomen is performed in patients with no evidence of disseminated disease on the USG scan of the abdomen. MRI abdomen with MRCP is preferred in patients with biliary obstruction. Some studies have reported that a positron emission tomography (PET) scan is more sensitive in detecting metastatic disease compared to conventional imaging and can change management in up to 25% of patients deemed resectable on conventional imaging.[40] However, PET is not specific for identifying peritoneal carcinomatosis. Also, distant lymph node metastasis detected on PET should be confirmed with histopathological examination as coexistent tuberculosis is not uncommon, especially in tropical countries.[41] In this scenario, labelling nodes as metastatic without histopathological confirmation might deny the patient a chance for a cure. With the currently available evidence, PET cannot be routinely recommended in all GBC patients and is reserved for patients with locally advanced disease on cross-sectional imaging or those requiring extended resection beyond the standard radical cholecystectomy. Patients with evidence of distant (coeliac, superior mesenteric, and aortocaval) nodes on cross-sectional imaging should undergo image-guided fine-needle aspiration cytology and their involvement precludes curative resection.[42] Upper gastrointestinal endoscopy and colonoscopy are indicated in patients with suspected duodenal and colonic involvement. Preoperative bowel preparation might be required in patients with colonic involvement. Significantly elevated tumour marker levels (carbohydrate antigen (CA) 19-9 and carcinoembryonic antigen) in the absence of biliary obstruction might predict metastatic disease.

Current management of gall bladder cancer

GBC is an aggressive tumour and over the last two decades or so several centres (especially from the East—Japan/Korea) have reported promising stage-based results following an aggressive surgical approach.[5-8] The use of less radical treatment has been an important factor for poor long-term outcomes in addition to the aggressive nature of the tumour in some of the reported experiences. The widespread prevalence of the nihilistic approach towards the management of GBC in the West is highlighted by the analysis of the Surveillance, Epidemiology, and End Results (SEER) database of GBC. Of the 2835 patients, only 8.6% of GBC patients underwent an en bloc resection, and lymphadenectomy was performed only in 5.3% of patients. Appropriate surgical management is critical to achieving a good long-term outcome. It will be discussed under the following headings.

1. Changes in the current American Joint Committee on Cancer (AJCC)/ Union for International Cancer Control (UICC) staging and its limitations.
2. Role of staging laparoscopy (SL).
3. Preoperative and intraoperative evaluation of interaortocaval (IAC) lymph node metastasis.
4. Extent of lymphadenectomy.
5. The extent of liver resection.
6. Optimum management of T2 tumours in the light of a recent subclassification.
7. Appropriate management of GBC patients with extrahepatic adjacent organ involvement.

Staging

The commonly used staging system for GBC is the AJCC/UICC tumour, node, and metastasis (TNM) staging system. The current edition of TNM staging (eighth edition) differs from the seventh edition in the following important aspects (Table 35.2 shows the UICC version)[43-46]:

- T2 disease that includes tumour invasion of the perimuscular connective tissue is now subdivided into two groups: T2a includes tumours on the peritoneal side of the GB and those on the hepatic side of the GB are classified as T2b.
- The N classification has been changed from a location-based to a number-based definition. In the seventh edition, N1 includes nodes along the hepatoduodenal ligament and N2 includes coeliac, periduodenal, peripancreatic, IAC, and superior mesenteric artery nodes. In the current eighth edition, N1 is defined as an involvement of one to three nodes and N2 as four or more positive nodes. Harvesting of at least six lymph nodes is recommended for adequate nodal staging.

The subclassification of T2 tumours into T2a and T2b was based on recent reports highlighting tumour location to be an important prognostic factor.[47–50] The hepatic side of the GB lacks a serosa and is attached directly to the liver by loose connective tissue. Its venous

Table 35.2 Comparison of seventh and eighth editions of UICC staging for gall bladder cancer (changes in eighth edition are *italicized*)

7th UICC staging	8th UICC staging
T–primary tumour T1 Tumour invades lamina propria or muscular layer T1a Tumour invades lamina propria T1b Tumour invades muscular layer T2 Tumour invades perimuscular connective tissue; no extension beyond serosa or into liver T3 Tumour perforates the serosa (visceral peritoneum) and/or directly invades the liver and/or one other adjacent organ or structure, such as stomach, duodenum, colon, pancreas, omentum, extrahepatic bile ducts T4 Tumour invades main portal vein or hepatic artery or invades two or more extrahepatic organs or structures	**T–primary tumour** T1 Tumour invades lamina propria or muscular layer T1a Tumour invades lamina propria T1b Tumour invades muscular layer T2 Tumour invades perimuscular connective tissue; no extension beyond serosa or into liver *T2a Tumour invades perimuscular connective tissue on the peritoneal side, with no extension to the serosa* *T2b Tumour invades perimuscular connective tissue on the hepatic side, with no extension into the liver* T3 Tumour perforates the serosa (visceral peritoneum) and/or directly invades the liver and/or one other adjacent organ or structure, such as stomach, duodenum, colon, pancreas, omentum, extrahepatic bile ducts T4 Tumour invades main portal vein or hepatic artery or invades two or more extrahepatic organs or structures
N–regional lymph nodes NX Regional lymph nodes cannot be assessed N0 No regional lymph node metastasis N1 Regional lymph node metastasis (including nodes along the cystic duct, common bile duct, common hepatic artery, and portal vein)	**N–regional lymph nodes** NX Regional lymph nodes cannot be assessed N0 No regional lymph node metastasis *N1 Metastases to 1–3 regional nodes* *N2 Metastasis to 4 or more regional nodes*
M–distant metastasis M0 No distant metastasis M1 Distant metastasis	**M–distant metastasis** M0 No distant metastasis M1 Distant metastasis

Reproduced with permission from Sobin LH, Gospodarowicz MK, and Wittekind C, *TNM Classification of Malignant Tumours*, 7th edition, UICC/Wiley-Blackwell, 2009, pp.119–120; and Brierley, JD, Gospodarowicz MK, and Wittekind C, *TNM Classification of Malignant Tumours*, 8th edition, UICC/Wiley-Blackwell, 2017, pp. 85–86.

drainage is by short cystic veins that directly communicate with the intrahepatic portal veins. Also, the lymphatic drainage of the hepatic side is towards the intrahepatic portion. In contrast, the peritoneal side of the GB is usually drained by one or two cystic veins that generally terminate in the venous plexus at the hepatic hilum. Also, the lymphatic drainage of T2a tumours is towards the hepatoduodenal ligament. As the hepatic side tumours are associated with a poorer prognosis compared to those on the peritoneal side, the subclassification of T2 tumours was introduced in the current AJCC classification. The management implication of this subclassification is discussed in the later part of this chapter.

The fifth to the seventh editions of the AJCC classification used the nodal location as the basis for the staging of the lymph node metastases as recent studies have shown that the number of involved lymph nodes rather than their location more accurately determines prognosis. A number-based definition is used in the current classification. Retrieval of at least six lymph nodes is recommended as studies have shown that number as a critical lymph node count cut-off that can improve risk stratification and staging quality.[44] However, we have observed that the number of retrieved lymph nodes may be less than six despite adequate lymphadenectomy especially in patients with incidental GBC and varies based on several factors including T stage and extent of inflammation/infection (empyema) in the GB. Also, it is crucial to understand that N1 and N2 classification in the eighth edition is based on the number of positive regional lymph nodes equivalent to the N1 classification in the seventh edition. Metastasis to the distant lymph nodes (equivalent to N2 in the seventh edition) is grouped along with other distant metastases into M1. A limitation of the current AJCC classification is the retropancreatic nodes (station 13a), usually included as part of a standard lymphadenectomy in many Eastern centres, which have been excluded from the regional node classification.[51] Also, TanyN2M0 and TanyNanyM1 are both classified as stage IVB in the current classification. However, studies have shown that patients with early T-stage N2 disease (T1–2N2M0) included in stage IVB as per the current classification have a better survival than the advanced T-stage N2 disease (T3–4N2M0). Hence, the inclusion of both groups of patients in stage IVB needs to be re-evaluated.[52]

Staging laparoscopy

Despite advances in imaging technology, a significant number of patients with GBC have radiologically occult metastatic disease detected at the time of surgical exploration. With improvements in interventional radiology and endoscopic techniques, palliative surgery is rarely required in patients with GBC. Hence, SL, a minimally invasive tool, can preclude morbidity related to a non-therapeutic laparotomy. Among hepatobiliary malignancies, the yield of SL is high for GBC. In a large series of 409 patients with primary GBC, SL avoided non-therapeutic laparotomy in 23% of patients.[53] Although the yield of SL was high in locally advanced GBC, approximately 11% of patients with early GBC (T1 and T2) had radiologically occult metastatic disease. Hence, a routine SL is recommended in all patients with primary GBC. However, the indications for SL in patients with incidental gall bladder cancer (IGBC) are not as well defined. Patients with IGBC tend to have a higher failure rate with SL. In the series reported by Butte et al., SL detected metastatic disease in only two of the 46 IGBC patients included in the study with an overall yield of 4.3%.[54] The proposed reasons for the relatively low yield of SL in this group of patients are that most IGBC patients who present after simple cholecystectomy have a relatively early-stage disease with perhaps a lower incidence of distant metastases. Also, intra-abdominal adhesions from the previous surgery, especially after open cholecystectomy, can interfere with a proper assessment by SL. Often SL is done through a single umbilical port. Missing a few detectable metastases in our experience made us realize that the use of additional ports during SL would help to perform adhesiolysis and visualize potential blind spots like the undersurface of the liver. We usually perform two-port laparoscopy; the second port allows visualization of blind areas and helps in taking a biopsy for histopathological examination of the detected metastases. Additional port(s) are placed for IAC lymph node biopsy or if laparoscopic radical cholecystectomy (LRC) is planned. While the addition of laparoscopic USG might improve the yield and accuracy of SL by detecting parenchymal liver metastasis, improvement in preoperative imaging has limited its routine use. Targeting high-risk IGBC patients like those with advanced T-stage tumours, bile spillage during the index cholecystectomy, or late presentation after index cholecystectomy might improve the yield of SL in these patients. In our practice, despite its lower yield (than in primary GBC), a routine SL is preferred in IGBC patients also as it is associated with less morbidity and does not significantly contribute to prolonged operative time or cost.

Evaluation of an inter-aortocaval lymph node metastasis

IAC lymph node (station 16b1) involvement is generally considered to be a sign of advanced disease with a dismal prognosis, equivalent to metastatic disease.[54-57] However, some series do not consider 16b1 lymph node metastasis to be a contraindication for radical resection. The reason for variable survival outcomes reported in patients with positive 16b1 lymph node metastases could be due to the differences in the pathway of lymphatic spread. A very small group of patients with a skip metastasis to the 16b1 lymph nodes without significant lymphadenopathy in other stations might benefit from radical surgery especially if R0 resection can be achieved with a radical cholecystectomy. However, in the majority of GBC patients, it portends a poor prognosis. Except in patients with isolated 16b1 lymph node metastasis, its involvement is considered to be a contraindication for curative resection. Hence, preoperative evaluation and routine intraoperative sampling of IAC nodes is recommended.

The proposed criteria for diagnosing a metastatic lymph node on cross-sectional imaging are size greater than 10 mm, round shape, and a heterogeneous internal architecture. However, a significant proportion of positive IAC lymph nodes are missed on preoperative imaging. The reported sensitivity and positive predictive value of a preoperative CT scan with image-guided fine-needle aspiration cytology in identifying metastatic IAC lymph nodes is 14.7% and 33.3%, respectively. We started using endoscopic USG examination for a guided fine-needle aspiration cytology for preoperative detection of metastatic IAC nodes, especially in patients with no safe window to target these nodes using the percutaneous approach.[58] A routine biopsy of the IAC lymph node (16b1) is recommended before proceeding with radical resection as it prevented non-therapeutic radical resection with its associated morbidity in 18.6% of patients deemed resectable on preoperative imaging and SL. While IAC lymph node metastasis was commoner in locally advanced tumours (clinical T3 and T4), even patients with early-stage tumours (clinical T1 and T2) were also found to have lymph node metastasis, though with much lower incidence. Traditionally it is done by the open approach. After duodenal Kocherization, lymph nodes in the IAC region below the level of the left renal vein are excised and sent for frozen section examination. In our later part experience, we included laparoscopic IAC lymph node sampling as part of SL to improve its yield and thus avoid non-therapeutic laparotomy.[59] Subsequently, with the use of the laparoscopic approach for the treatment of GBC, it became an integral part of SL before proceeding for LRC. The proposed algorithmic approach for the evaluation of IAC lymph nodes (Figure 35.2) can be used in all GBC patients except in selected good-risk patients with skip metastasis to IAC nodes or limited locoregional disease who can be taken up for radical resection.

Radical surgery for gall bladder cancer

The two essential components of radical surgery for GBC are:

1. Adequate lymphadenectomy.
2. Adequate liver resection.

In patients with extrahepatic adjacent organ involvement, en-bloc resection of the involved viscera is recommended to achieve an R0 resection.

Lymphadenectomy for gall bladder cancer

GBC has a strong propensity for lymph node metastases. The incidence of lymph node metastasis can be as high as 40% for T2 tumours, and overall, 45–85% of patients with GBC have lymph node involvement.[60] Hence an adequate lymphadenectomy is an integral part of radical surgery for GBC patients with stage T1b or higher. The lymphatic plexuses in the wall of the GB course through its medial and lateral walls and terminate in the cystic node and pericholedochal nodes, respectively. From here, the lymphatics follow one of the three pathways.[61]

- The cholecysto-retropancreatic pathway: the primary lymphatic pathway which converges at the retroportal lymph node.
- The cholecysto-coeliac pathway: the lymphatics from the GB wall travel to the left via the hepatoduodenal ligament to reach the coeliac nodes.
- The cholecysto-mesenteric pathway: the lymphatics travel anterior to the portal vein and connect with the nodes at the root of the mesentery.

These three pathways converge at the IAC lymph nodes near the left renal vein. While this is the most common route of lymphatic spread from the GB, extensive connections exist between the various lymphatic vessels, including a direct spread to the IAC nodes from the pericholedochal nodes.

Lymph node involvement is an important prognostic factor in GBC, and thus a complete lymphadenectomy is an integral component of any radical surgery. As mentioned earlier, para-aortic lymphadenectomy is not routinely recommended for curative resection of GBC. The standard lymphadenectomy for GBC involves clearance of the nodes from the hepatoduodenal ligament, skeletonizing the vascular structures and the bile ducts to remove nodes anterior and posterior to the head of the pancreas and the hepatic artery until its origin from the coeliac axis. However, most Western centres do not include retropancreatic nodes as part of the standard lymphadenectomy for GBC. A recent Japanese study reported that the survival of GBC patients with positive retropancreatic nodes is like N1 disease (one to three total positive nodes), especially in patients with T1/T2 disease. Hence, in patients with early-stage tumours with a lower nodal disease burden, the retropancreatic nodes should be cleared even if pancreatoduodenectomy is required for

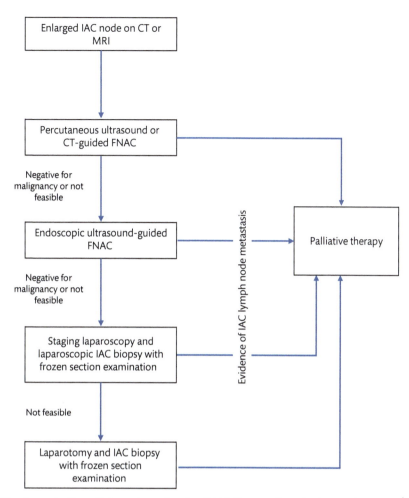

Figure 35.2 Proposed algorithm for evaluation of interaortocaval nodes. FNAC, fine-needle aspiration cytology.

nodal clearance as it behaves like a regional node. Even in patients with locally advanced disease, dissection of the retropancreatic node is recommended and it can often be performed without adding a pancreatoduodenectomy. In patients with advanced T-stage or greater nodal burden (N2 disease), requiring major hepatectomy and pancreatoduodenectomy to clear retropancreatic nodes, it is associated with inferior survival. However, in carefully selected patients extended radical surgery can be performed to clear these nodes. Recently lymph node ratio has been proposed as an independent prognostic factor.[62,63] Patients with a lymph node ratio of more than 0.5 have poor survival and a significantly higher probability of developing a distant recurrence.

Extent of liver resection

The liver is the commonly involved adjacent viscus in GBC and its involvement occurs by direct extension, haematogenous spread, or lymphatic permeation. Hepatic resection for GBC has two primary purposes.

1. To resect tumours that have directly invaded the liver from the GB bed.
2. To prevent micrometastases that may recur around the GB bed.

The extent of liver resection in GBC can range from 2 cm wedge, anatomical segment IVb/V (as per the Japanese nomenclature IVb is termed as IVa) resection or major hepatectomy. The extent of liver resection is determined by:

1. The location of the tumour (fundus or neck).
2. The morphological pattern of liver involvement.
3. Degree of vascular/bile duct involvement.

The technique of segment IVb/V resection

Anatomical segments IVb (anterior) and V resection involves two critical steps[64]:

1. Identification of the transection line between segment IVa and segment IVb.
2. Identification of the transection line between segments V and VI.

The transection line between segments IVa and IVb can be delineated by clamping the IVb pedicle in the umbilical fissure. When there is an extrahepatic origin of the IVb pedicle, it is a relatively straightforward procedure to loop and clamp the pedicle. However, when there is an intrahepatic origin, control of the pedicle is achieved after parenchymal transection to the right of the falciform ligament. One needs to ensure that the segment IVa pedicle is not inadvertently included (ensured by trial clamping of the pedicle before division). Also, as there may be more than one IVb pedicle, careful analysis of the preoperative cross-sectional imaging and reconstruction using image processing software will facilitate intraoperative identification. If the line of demarcation is not clear after clamping the IVb pedicle, temporary clamping of the middle hepatic artery might better delineate the ischaemic line of demarcation.

Identification of the ischaemic line between segments V and VI can be achieved by one of the following three methods.

1. Temporary clamping of the right posterior pedicle using a vascular clamp at the level of Rouvier's sulcus. Looping of the right posterior pedicle is not recommended to prevent iatrogenic damage.
2. When the parenchymal transection along the right side of the falciform ligament reaches towards the anterior Glissonian pedicle, the segment V pedicle can be isolated.
3. Use of intraoperative USG to identify the right hepatic vein and mark the line of transection between segments V/VIII and VI/VII.

In methods 1 and 3, the superior extent of the segment V transection can be delineated by joining the horizontal line of demarcation between segments IVa and IVb with the vertical line of demarcation between the anterior and posterior sectors. As with any other liver resection, central venous pressure should be kept low to minimize bleeding.

Segment IVb/V resection or a wedge?

The rationale of segment IVb/V resection in GBC is based on anatomical studies demonstrating venous drainage from the GB predominantly into segments IVb and V. It has been postulated that central inferior bi-subsegmentectomy (segment IVb and V) may prevent early micrometastasis via the cystic vein. Yoshikawa et al., in their analysis of 201 patients with GBC, demonstrated the superiority of segment IVb/V resection over wedge resection in achieving a curative procedure in patients with liver invasion less than 20 mm.[65] On the other hand, a few reports have shown that a bi-subsegmentectomy is not effective in preventing liver metastasis.[66,67] In the Japanese nationwide survey of T2 GBC patients, there was no significant difference in the overall survival between patients who underwent wedge resection and segment IVb/V liver resection.[68] There was no increased incidence of recurrence in segment IVB/V among patients who underwent wedge resection. Hence, both wedge resection of the GB bed and 'segment IVb and V resection' are oncologically acceptable procedures provided an R0 resection is achieved. However, in patients with limited liver infiltration, segment IVb/V resection facilitates R0 resection. In our centre we prefer to perform segment IVb/V resection both in the open and laparoscopic methods as it is a more standardized procedure to achieve negative margins in patients with T3 tumours. Also, in T2 patients it has a theoretical advantage of taking care of micrometastasis in segments IVB/V. Only in patients with an intraoperative low index of suspicion of GBC, the GB is removed with a wedge of the liver and sent for frozen section histopathology.

Extended hepatectomy

Patients with extensive liver infiltration or GB neck tumours with vascular or biliary involvement may require an extended resection in the form of an extended right hepatectomy to achieve a curative resection. However, morbidity and mortality rates are increased after extended hepatic resection. Kondo et al., in their series of 68 patients with stage III/IV, GBC reported a 50% morbidity and an operative mortality of 18% following extensive surgical resections.[55] The most important cause of mortality was postoperative hepatic failure. The use of preoperative biliary drainage combined with portal vein embolization has been shown to augment the size of the future liver remnant and prevent postoperative hepatic failure-related morbidity.[69,70] The chapter authors' preferred approach is to perform segment IVa preserving extended right hepatectomy in patients requiring extended right hepatectomy and have uninvolved segment IVa to maximize the postoperative liver remnant and decrease the incidence of postoperative liver failure. In this approach, segment IVa with inflow and venous outflow to the middle hepatic vein is preserved.

Optimal management of T2 tumours

T2 tumours, defined as tumours invading the perimuscular (subserosal) connective tissue without extension beyond the serosa or into the liver, have received a focus since the publication of the current AJCC classification. The reported incidence of nodal metastasis in patients with T2a and T2b tumours has ranged from 15% to 26%, and from 30% to 46%, respectively.[47-50] This is due to the difference in lymphatic vessel density, which is higher on the hepatic side of the GB wall than on its peritoneal side. However, when lymph node metastasis occurs, there is no difference in the anatomical distribution. Hence, a similar extent of lymphadenectomy (standard lymphadenectomy) is recommended in both T2a and T2b tumours.

As T2a tumours are away from the liver, it has been suggested that liver resection may not be required. Lee et al. reported that the survival for peritoneal side T2 GBC was not affected by hepatic resection, which a few other studies have supported. However, it is important to understand that during simple cholecystectomy the risk of bile spillage is greater compared to cholecystectomy with wedge resection of GB due to direct handling of the GB. As bile spillage adversely affects the prognosis in these patients and the addition of small wedge resection of the liver does not significantly increase the morbidity, the current recommendation of a simple cholecystectomy for T2a tumours may not be universally acceptable. Also, visual assessment of T2a and T2b tumours may not be accurate as several tumours may encompass both sides. Further, accurate differentiation of T2 from T3 tumours may not possible without pathological examination. Hence, most centres, including ours, continue to perform liver resection for all T2 tumours. Hepatic resection (wedge or segment IVb/V) is universally recommended for patients with T2b tumours. Similarly, for T2a GB neck tumours, irrespective of their location (hepatic/peritoneal), liver resection is required as the neck of the GB is narrow and close to both the liver and the peritoneal side.

Role of routine bile duct excision

There is some controversy as to whether bile duct excision should be a part of standard radical cholecystectomy. Several Japanese surgeons have advocated routine bile duct excision in all GBC patients with stage T2 disease or above.[71,72] The rationale is to remove occult cancer cells, aid in the clearance of the hepatoduodenal ligament lymph nodes, and address the issue of perineural invasion in patients with advanced-stage disease. However, there is enough evidence in the literature now to suggest that routine bile duct excision does not improve survival and may be linked to an increased risk of early (biliary anastomotic leak and collections) and late sequelae like strictures and cholangitis.[73,74] Current indications for bile duct excision in patients without direct bile duct involvement are gross lymph nodal enlargement close to or involving the common hepatic duct or hilum, inflamed or a fatty hepatoduodenal ligament rendering nodal dissection difficult, positive cystic duct margin on intraoperative frozen section, associated anomalous pancreatobiliary junction abnormality/choledochal cyst, or if an associated vascular resection/reconstruction is needed.

Extrahepatic adjacent organ involvement

The bile duct is the most commonly involved extrahepatic organ by GBC, followed by the gastro-duodenum, pancreas, and colon.[75] Patients with tumours extending to and involving the adjacent viscera may be asymptomatic or present with jaundice, gastric outlet obstruction, or rarely with large bowel obstruction. The algorithmic approach to patients with extrahepatic adjacent organ involvement is depicted in Figure 35.3. In the chapter authors' experience, almost one-third of resectable patients (347 out of 1012) require extrahepatic adjacent visceral resection.

Gastroduodenal and pancreatic involvement

Duodenopancreatic involvement in patients with advanced GBC can occur due to direct infiltration or secondary to infiltration across the hepatoduodenal ligament and bile duct. Also, it can happen secondary to bulky peripancreatic nodal disease. There is marked heterogeneity in the literature regarding the management strategy of GBC patients with duodenopancreatic involvement. While some studies have considered duodenopancreatic involvement in GBC a sign of unresectable disease, others have considered it to be an indication for a more extensive procedure ranging from resection of the part of the stomach and duodenum to a hepatopancreatoduodenectomy (HPD).[76-84]

The surgical options for patients with isolated duodenal involvement are 'sleeve resection' and 'distal gastrectomy with proximal duodenectomy' for more extensive involvement of the gastroduodenum.[83,84] Duodenal sleeve resection is recommended in patients with a small area of duodenal infiltration, where there would be no luminal compromise (Figure 35.4). In the presence of more significant duodenal infiltration without pancreatic involvement, distal gastrectomy with proximal duodenectomy and gastrojejunostomy is recommended (Figure 35.5). Proximal duodenectomy refers to the resection of a variable length of the first and supra-papillary portion of the second part of the duodenum depending upon the extent of duodenal involvement. The presence of symptoms of gastric outlet obstruction, duodenal mural thickening or mucosal irregularity on abdominal CT, and infiltration of the duodenal mucosa on upper gastrointestinal endoscopy significantly reduce the resectability rates; however, these findings do not preclude resection since curative resection may still be performed in a significant proportion of patients.

A few Japanese surgeons perform HPD in all patients with locally advanced disease to complete retropancreatic lymphadenectomy, even when there are no apparent metastatic lymph nodes.[78] However, the survival benefit of this approach has not been proven in the literature.[79-81] Hence HPD is recommended only when there is extensive direct tumour infiltration of the pancreas not amenable to wedge resection and those with bulky retropancreatic lymph nodes, which cannot be cleared without resecting the pancreatic head. The main drawback of doing an HPD is its high morbidity and mortality, especially when it is combined with a major hepatectomy (major HPD). Major HPD in cholestatic liver is associated with significant morbidity and mortality even in high-volume centres. However, morbidity and mortality associated with limited HPD (segment IVb/V resection combined with pancreatoduodenectomy) is comparable with pancreatoduodenectomy. An alternative to HPD, especially in patients with minimal pancreaticoduodenal involvement, is to do a wedge resection of the pancreas. Hirano et al. compared and found no difference in local recurrence or cumulative survival rate between these two procedures.[82]

Colon involvement

The colon though is a less commonly involved extrahepatic adjacent organ in GBC patients, due to its anatomical proximity, the hepatic flexure being the segment of the colon which is frequently infiltrated. Birnbaum et al. reported a 0% 3-year survival rate in GBC patients who required surgical resection of the colon and the authors concluded that the poor outcome casts doubt on the benefits of surgery

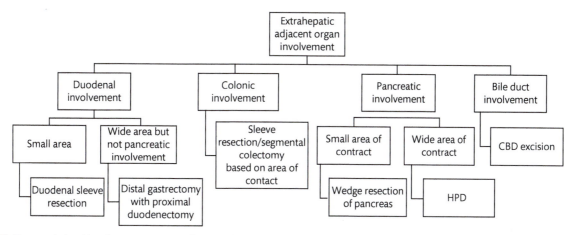

Figure 35.3 Proposed algorithm for management of GBC with extrahepatic adjacent organ involvement. CBD, common bile duct; HPD, hepatopancreatoduodenectomy.

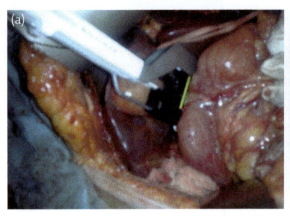
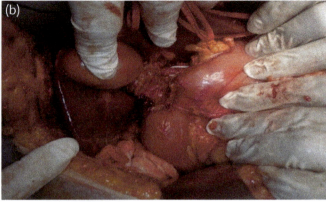

Figure 35.4 Duodenal sleeve resection for a patient with small area of contact with duodenum.

in this group of patients.[85] However, isolated colon involvement is common in patients who have a tumour in the GB fundus and en bloc resection in these patients is associated with an improved survival. In patients with minimal colonic involvement, a colonic sleeve resection can be performed. In those with more extensive colonic infiltration, segmental colonic resection or a right hemicolectomy is usually needed to achieve curative resection (Figures 35.6 and 35.7).

GBC with jaundice/bile duct involvement

Jaundice in GBC is often due to direct infiltration of the bile duct. However, compression of the bile duct by the enlarged nodes at the hilum or retropancreatic region and intraluminal extension of papillary tumours into the bile duct can also cause jaundice. It is essential to remember that occasionally jaundice in GBC may be due to associated common bile duct stones, which can often be managed using an endoscopic approach precluding the need for an extended hepatectomy or bile duct excision. Historically, jaundice in GBC is considered to be a sign of inoperability in many series. Hawkins et al. reported that only six of 82 jaundiced patients underwent resection with curative intent, and all the six patients either died or developed recurrence within 6 months.[86] As the invasion of the bile duct increases the risk of vascular, lymphatic, and perineural invasion, early intervention is required to limit rapid spread to vital structures of the hepatoduodenal ligament. A few small Japanese series have reported the feasibility of surgical resection in patients with bile duct involvement.[87,88] One of this chapter's authors (AKA) had initially documented the oncological benefit of surgical resection in a series of 14 GBC patients with jaundice. While several series from Japan at the time included jaundiced patients, who had a reasonable survival following resection, the chapter authors' publication focusing on GBC patients with biliary obstruction surmised that 'biliary obstruction in GBC is not a sine qua non of inoperability', and a reasonable survival can be achieved after a complete radical resection even in these patients.[89] Recently Nishio et al. in a large series reported a median survival of 18 months and 5-year survival of 23% in 73 patients with pathological extrahepatic duct involvement who underwent curative resection over a period of 30 years.[90] This and other series support the chapter authors' concept that biliary obstruction in GBC is not a sign of inoperability and a reasonable survival can be achieved after a complete radical resection even in these patients. In the chapter authors' centre, more than 150 patients with jaundice have undergone curative surgical resection with acceptable short- and long-term outcomes (unpublished data). Most of the studies have highlighted the need for doing extended liver resections in

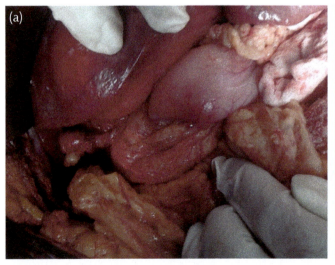
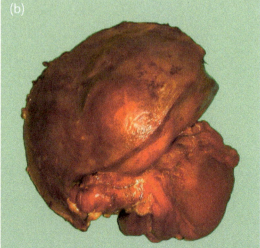

Figure 35.5 Distal gastrectomy with proximal duodenectomy for a patient with wide area of contact with duodenum.

Current management of gall bladder cancer

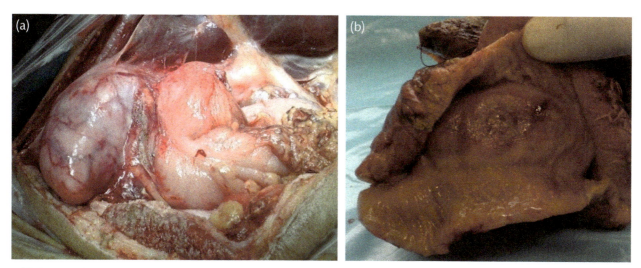

Figure 35.6 GBC with colonic involvement requiring segmental resection.
Reproduced with permission from Agarwal, A., Javid, A., Kalayarasan, R., Sakhuja, P., 'Surgical techniques in the Management of Primary Gallbladder Cancer', In Agarwal, A. and Fong, Y. *Carcinoma of the Gallbladder: The Current Scenario*, Elsevier, 2014, pp.106-29.

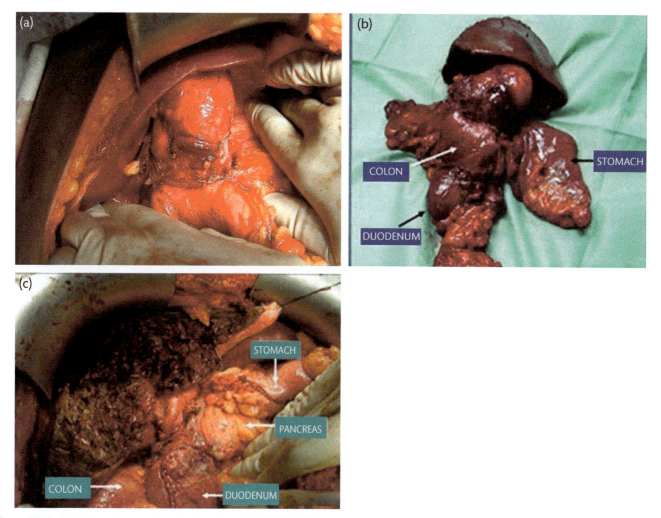

Figure 35.7 GBC with multivisceral involvement (gastroduodenal and colonic involvement).
Reproduced with permission from Agarwal, A., Javid, A., Kalayarasan, R., Sakhuja, P., 'Surgical techniques in the Management of Primary Gallbladder Cancer', In Agarwal, A. and Fong, Y. *Carcinoma of the Gallbladder: The Current Scenario*, Elsevier, 2014, pp.106-29.

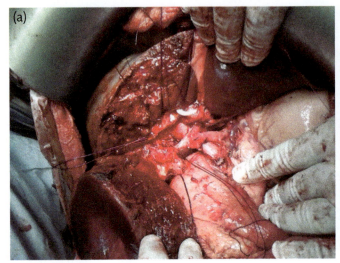 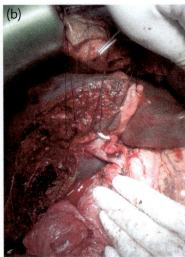

Figure 35.8 GBC with right hepatic artery involvement (arrow).

GBC patients with bile duct involvement and jaundice. While preoperative biliary drainage, portal vein embolization, advancements in surgical technique, and anaesthetic management have reduced mortality associated with major hepatectomy, there is still a mortality of 5–27% and morbidity of 14–53%.[91,92] The feasibility of the parenchyma-preserving approach in the form of segment IVb and V resection in most of the patients without the right portal pedicle involved has been previously reported by us and other authors (**Figure 35.8**). Resection of segment IVb/V exposes the hilar plate and facilitates the accurate assessment of the right anterior and posterior sectoral duct involvement to achieve a tumour-free margin.[89] Even in patients who require extended right hepatectomy, segment IVa is preserved whenever feasible (modified extended right hepatectomy) to reduce postoperative morbidity and mortality (**Figure 35.9**). Alternatively, right portal vein embolization combined with embolization of the segment IV portal vein can be used to increase the remnant liver volume. Biliary drainage is indicated before portal vein embolization. While endoscopic drainage (using endoscopic nasobiliary drainage) is preferred in Japan and some other Eastern centres, percutaneous biliary drainage is preferred in many Western centres. The chapter authors choose to use endoscopic drainage in GBC patients with obstruction below the hepatic confluence and percutaneous route in patients with obstruction involving hepatic confluence with hilar separation. Associating liver partition and portal vein ligation for staged hepatectomy (ALPPS) is not commonly used in GBC patients with jaundice requiring extended right hepatectomy because of increased perioperative complications reported in biliary tumours. While few reports have suggested the feasibility of partial ALPPS in GBC more data are required to define the role of ALPPS in GBC with jaundice.

In the chapter authors' reported experience of 327 GBC patients who underwent curative resection over a period of 6 years, 113 patients had involvement of one (n = 49) or more (n = 64) extrahepatic adjacent organs.[75] Resection of a single extrahepatic adjacent organ improved resection rate from 37.6% (214/569) to 46.2% (263/569) and the addition of more than one extrahepatic adjacent organ resection improved it to 57.5% (327/569). On pathological examination, 38.1% (24/61) of patients who underwent duodenal resection had only serosal involvement while remaining 61.9% (39/61) had mural involvement. Of the 33 patients who underwent colonic resection, 48.5% (16/33) had only serosal involvement and the remaining 51.5% (17/33) had transmural involvement. Pathological transmural bile duct and pancreatic involvement were seen in 68% (51/75) and 76.9% (10/13) of patients, respectively. Non-adenocarcinoma histological types and lymph node involvement were significantly more frequent in patients with extrahepatic adjacent organ involvement. Their median survival was significantly less compared to GBC patients without extrahepatic adjacent organ involvement (33 vs 48 months, p = 0.002). However, there was no significant difference in the median survival of node-negative GBC patients between the two groups (44 vs 49 months, p = 0.413). Among node-positive GBC patients, median survival was significantly less in patients with two or more extrahepatic adjacent organ involvement compared to patients with single or no extrahepatic adjacent organ involvement (30 vs 34 vs 41 months, p <0.0001).

Vascular involvement

Tumours in the GB neck region tend to infiltrate the porta hepatis and may involve the right hepatic artery, common hepatic artery, the main portal vein, or their branches.[93–95] The right hepatic artery is frequently involved, and its involvement is generally considered as an indication for a right hepatectomy. Alternatively, resection and reconstruction of the right hepatic artery have been reported. The safety and feasibility of right hepatic artery ligation without reconstruction has been recently reported by us and other groups. The prerequisites are a patent right portal vein, preservation of the hilar plate with the hilar interlobar artery, and good backflow from the distal arterial stump, confirming the adequacy of collateral flow (**Figure 35.10**). If these criteria are fulfilled, right hepatic artery ligation can be safely combined with parenchyma-preserving liver resection and bile duct excision without the need for major hepatectomy or arterial reconstruction. Limited main portal vein involvement can be managed by a sleeve portal vein resection; more extensive portal infiltration requires either a portal vein resection with end–end anastomosis or an interposition grafting or main portal vein to the left portal vein anastomosis when extended right hepatectomy is required.

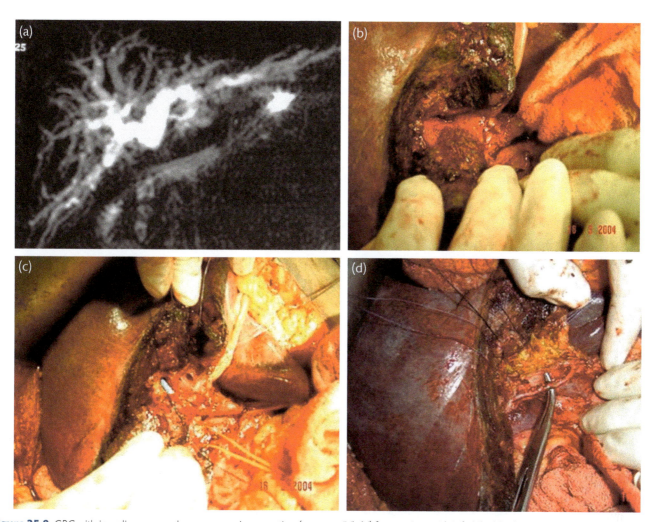

Figure 35.9 GBC with jaundice—parenchyma-preserving resection (segment IVb/V) for a patient with infrahilar block.
Reproduced with permission from Agarwal, A., Javid, A., Kalayarasan, R., Sakhuja, P., 'Surgical techniques in the Management of Primary Gallbladder Cancer', In Agarwal, A. and Fong, Y. *Carcinoma of the Gallbladder: The Current Scenario*, Elsevier, 2014, pp.106–29.

Incidental gall bladder cancer

An IGBC is one that was not suspected before or at operation and is detected for the first time on histopathological examination of the GB removed for a presumed diagnosis of simple gallstone disease. The incidence of IGBC has been reported to be in the range of 0.3–2.1% in various series, with a higher incidence reported following cholecystectomy for empyema of the GB, Mirizzi syndrome, and porcelain GB.[96,97] As mentioned earlier, IGBC is the most common presentation in Western countries and low-incidence areas. While primary GBC is traditionally considered to be an aggressive tumour with a poor prognosis, IGBC is a form of GBC with a good prognosis following appropriate management. However, there is no uniform consensus on the management of the patients with IGBC, and the following issues will be discussed:

1. What is the correct definition of IGBC?
2. Which patients need reoperation?
3. The extent of preoperative evaluation of these patients.
4. Indications and extent of re-resection including informed consent.
5. Role of port-site excision.
6. Timing of surgery after index cholecystectomy.
7. Prevention of unsuspected or missed IGBC.

Definition

A true IGBC is the one which was not suspected before or at operation and even on gross examination of the opened GB specimen by the surgeon and is detected for the first time on histopathological examination of the GB removed for the presumed (clinical, USG, and operative) diagnosis of simple gall stone disease. Ideally, a true IGBC is a histological surprise.[98] However, the term has been loosely applied to all post-cholecystectomy GBCs. The use of various terminologies like inapparent, occult, subclinical, missed, or unsuspected GBC to describe the entity of IGBC highlights this problem. It is important to distinguish true IGBC from other forms of post-cholecystectomy GBC as it has significant prognostic value. True IGBC will be at an early stage of the disease and its appropriate management may offer a chance of long-term survival and even cure. Poor survival following curative resection reported in a few series is a result of the inclusion of all post-cholecystectomy GBC as IGBC that tends to skew the results.

CHAPTER 35 Benign and malignant lesions of the gall bladder

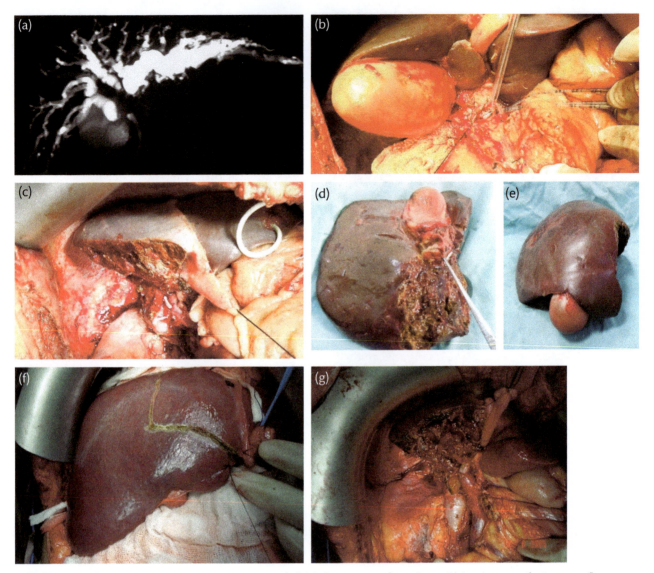

Figure 35.10 GBC with jaundice—segment IVa-preserving extended right hepatectomy for patients with involvement of primary confluence. (f) and (g) Reproduced with permission from Agarwal, A., Javid, A., Kalayarasan, R., Sakhuja, P., 'Surgical techniques in the Management of Primary Gallbladder Cancer', In Agarwal, A. and Fong, Y. *Carcinoma of the Gallbladder: The Current Scenario*, Elsevier, 2014, pp.106-29.

From the chapter authors' experience of managing large numbers of post-cholecystectomy GBC, there are three patient groups that actually represent a continuum of the same disease who have an increasing stage and decreasing prognosis[99,100]:

1. True IGBC: malignancy diagnosed only on histopathology with no suspicion preoperatively or intraoperatively including the examination of opened up GB.
2. Unsuspected GBC: detected perioperatively, that is, malignancy suspected intraoperatively (inspection of the GB after access to the peritoneal cavity or during cholecystectomy) or on the cut section of the removed GB or on frozen section examination (no preoperative suspicion).
3. Missed/overlooked GBC: patients in whom there were some indicators of malignancy on USG but these were missed, misinterpreted, or overlooked by the surgeon. In one of such patients operated on at the authors' centre, the gross pathological examination of the specimen from the referral centre reported a 12 mm polypoid lesion in the GB. This certainly would not have been missed if the removed GB had been cut open and examined by the surgeon in the operation theatre before sending for histopathological examination. Of the 103 patients referred to the authors' centre as IGBC after index cholecystectomy was performed elsewhere, preoperative USG review revealed findings suspicious of malignancy in 40 patients. Also, preoperative CT/MRI was done in 15 patients for suspected malignancy. Intraoperatively, 47 patients had focal thickening or a GB mass suspicious of malignancy. In the overall analysis, 53 (42.7%) patients had preoperative imaging or intraoperative findings suggestive of malignancy and they do not satisfy the criteria of true IGBC. In comparison, true IGBC patients have early-stage disease (96% vs 79.2%), less adjacent organ involvement (10.5% vs 40.9%), a better resectability rate (76% vs 41.5%), and better overall survival (60 vs 28 months) compared to unsuspected or missed GBC.[100]

Preoperative evaluation

While IGBC is frequently an early-stage disease, distant spread is not uncommon. Hence, a complete preoperative evaluation like primary GBC is essential to rule out metastatic disease and select appropriate patients for re-resection. An important component of preoperative evaluation is the careful analysis of the complete perioperative details of the index simple cholecystectomy. It includes symptoms prior to cholecystectomy, preoperative imaging findings, type of surgery (laparoscopic or open), place of surgery (peripheral or referral centre), intraoperative findings, especially with regard to bile spillage, use of a protective bag for GB extraction, the port used for GB extraction, and findings on the cut section of GB (if performed). The GB specimen (if available), paraffin blocks, and slides of the cholecystectomy specimen should be reviewed for the site (fundus, body, or neck/cystic duct), histological type (adenocarcinoma or other), T stage, N stage (if the cystic lymph node was included in the specimen), cystic duct margin, lymphovascular and perineural invasion, and grade of the tumour. However, all this information may not be available in all cases as the majority of the simple cholecystectomy procedures are performed in peripheral centres. Many of these centres do not routinely examine the removed GB or send it for histopathological examination to reduce cost or add burden to the pathologist and this has been a significant roadblock for accurate identification of patients with true IGBC.[101–103]

Management of incidental gall bladder cancer

Indication and extent of re-resection

Management depends upon the T stage of the tumour. For a T1a tumour, simple cholecystectomy is enough for cure provided the cystic duct margin is free of tumour, the cystic lymph node, if included in the cholecystectomy specimen, does not show metastasis, and there is no intraoperative bile spillage. Most series report a 5-year survival of 90–100% with simple cholecystectomy alone.[96,103] Reports of local recurrence in patients with T1a GBC managed by simple cholecystectomy highlight the need for a thorough examination of the specimen. In one of the Japanese series, a patient with a T1a tumour developed metastasis and on review of slides and blocks, the patient was confirmed to have T1b disease.[102] Hence, before recommending observation in T1a GBC patients, especially in those operated elsewhere, it is essential to confirm the T stage by taking multiple sections from the paraffin blocks. Also, an expert pathologist should confirm T1a by scanning through the blocks of the specimen rather than examining a single slide. If blocks are not available for review, re-resection can be considered after explaining the pros and cons of observation to the patients. The chapter authors prefer to reoperate if the requisite information is not available to confirm T1a stage. There is no definite recommendation for a patient with a T1a tumour who had intraoperative bile spillage. Options include close follow-up with serial imaging or chemotherapy.

Patients with T1b and above tumours require re-resection. While some reports suggest that simple cholecystectomy alone is effective in patients with T1b tumours, there is enough evidence in the literature that suggests that simple cholecystectomy alone is not adequate. Ouchi et al. reported recurrences in three of the five cases with pT1b disease within 5 years of simple cholecystectomy.[105] Similar results were reported by Wagholikar et al. in their series of patients with T1b disease treated by simple cholecystectomy alone.[106] The rationale for re-resection in these patients is that about 20% of patients with T1b disease have lymph node metastases, which are not tackled by simple cholecystectomy alone. In a German registry report for IGBC, radical re-resection improved the 5-year survival for T1b IGBC to 72% from 40% for simple cholecystectomy.[107] In a decision-analytical Markov model to estimate and compare T1b IGBC patients' life expectancy who underwent simple cholecystectomy with patients who underwent radical re-resection, radical re-resection provided an additional survival benefit of 3.43 years over simple cholecystectomy alone.[108] All these reports, including the recent National Comprehensive Cancer Network (NCCN) guidelines, support the use of radical cholecystectomy in patients with incidental GBC stage T1b.[109]

While there is a reasonable consensus that the patients with T1b disease require lymphadenectomy, there is still some controversy about whether to add liver resection. You et al. reported that cholecystectomy with hepatoduodenal lymphadenectomy is an effective treatment for T1b GBC as there was no significant difference in locoregional recurrence, metastasis, or survival rate between patients who underwent cholecystectomy and hepatoduodenal lymph node dissection and those who underwent wedge resection of segment IVb and V with hepatoduodenal lymphadenectomy.[110] However, the limitation of their recommendation is it is not easy to diagnose T1b tumours with 100% uncertainty either preoperatively or intraoperatively with frozen section examination. Hence, it is preferable to add liver resection as a part of radical surgery for T1b IGBC. In the IGBC scenario, pathological T staging may not be accurate unless the GB specimen is available for evaluation. Some centres perform PET scanning to decide on the need for reoperation/completion radical cholecystectomy which in our opinion may not be a standard recommendation as completion radical cholecystectomy may address the microscopic disease that cannot be detected on PET scan or even histopathological examination. Also, the addition of small wedge resection of the liver does not significantly increase morbidity and a potential opportunity to cure may be lost.

There is no controversy that patients with T2 and above IGBC without disseminated disease should undergo re-resection. The rationale for re-resection in these patients is that simple cholecystectomy in GBC is likely to transgress tumour-bearing tissue planes as there is no serosal layer on the hepatic surface of the GB. Also, more than 50% of patients with T2 and above tumours have lymph node metastases.

Therefore, our current approach is to perform completion radical cholecystectomy for all T1b and beyond lesions and those when the cystic lymph node (when available) or cystic margin are positive for malignancy irrespective of T stage. Informed consent is essential as often there may not be any residual disease in the resected liver or the lymph nodes, particularly in the early-stage true IGBCs, which have the best prognosis after completion radical cholecystectomy.

Port-site excision

Port-site recurrence has been reported to occur in 14–30% of IGBC patients diagnosed after laparoscopic cholecystectomy.[111] Hence, port-site excision has been considered to be an essential step of the completion radical cholecystectomy. However, recently the role of port-site excision has been questioned.[112,113] In a study by Maker et al., of the 113 IGBC patients diagnosed after laparoscopic cholecystectomy over a period of 17 years and who underwent curative resection, 69 had port-site resection. Port-site metastasis correlated with a higher T stage (T2/T3) and peritoneal metastasis.[112] In patients who underwent curative resection, port-site resection was not associated with overall survival or recurrence-free survival. Based on these results, the authors concluded that port-site resection was not associated with improved survival or disease recurrence and should not be considered mandatory during the definitive surgical treatment. However, the drawbacks of this study were that the selection criteria for port-site excision were not mentioned (only 69 out of 113 patients underwent port-site excision), lack of uniformity in the number of excised ports (mean number of ports removed −2.8), lack of data regarding the incidence of bile spillage, port used for extraction of GB specimen, and the use of endo bags. While port-site metastasis is generally associated with distant metastasis, many reports of isolated port-site recurrence with long-term survival after excision of these recurrences were reported in the literature. These reports underscore that port-site recurrence in GBC does not always indicate disseminated disease and port-site excision can potentially prevent isolated port-site recurrence.[114,115] Port-site recurrence secondary to bile spillage is usually a part of disseminated disease, whereas port-site recurrence secondary to improper extraction technique is usually a localized recurrence. Long-term survival after resection of isolated port-site recurrence has been achieved by the chapter authors.

In our earlier reported experience of 121 IGBC patients, 23 had abdominal wall recurrence (laparoscopic port—16, open cholecystectomy scar site recurrence—7).[116] Of the 16 patients with recurrence in the region of laparoscopic ports, 13 had a single port and three had recurrences in two or more ports. Nineteen patients had evidence of disseminated disease (supraclavicular lymph node metastasis, ascites) on clinical examination (n = 5) or preoperative imaging (n = 14). Three patients with isolated abdominal wall recurrence on preoperative evaluation and one patient with port-site and axillary lymph node metastasis were taken up for surgery. Of the four patients, one had peritoneal metastasis on SL. Surgical procedures performed in the remaining three patients were full-thickness excision of port-site recurrence with axillary lymph node clearance (n = 1), excision of isolated umbilical port recurrence (n = 1), and completion radical cholecystectomy with excision of port-site recurrence (Figure 35.11). Of the three patients, two were free of recurrence at 13- and 38-month follow-up. This report underscores the need to ascertain whether postoperative scar metastasis in IGBC is part of disseminated disease or isolated recurrence.[115] Since information regarding bile spillage and extraction techniques is not always available, and port-site excision does not significantly increase

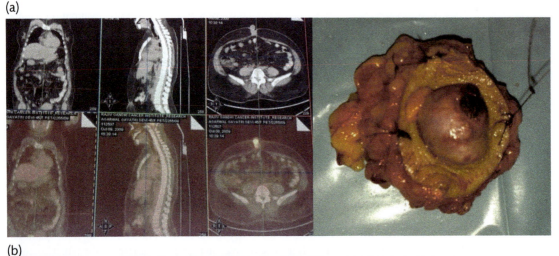
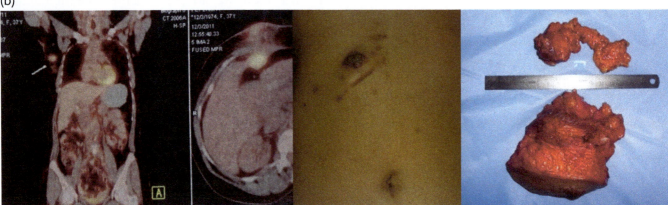

Figure 35.11 Patients with isolated port site recurrence. (a) Isolated port-site recurrence following completion radical cholecystectomy for incidental GBC. (b) Port-site metastasis following port-site excision with axillary lymph node metastasis.

the morbidity of the procedure and the reports of long-term survivors after excision of isolated port-site recurrence, port-site excision is recommended in all IGBC patients who undergo radical re-resection.

Timing of surgery

Re-resection should be offered as soon as IGBC is diagnosed as the interval between the index cholecystectomy and radical re-resection has been implicated as one of the critical factors determining the surgical outcome in these patients.[117,118] In a small retrospective series of 11 patients with T2 IGBC who underwent radical re-resection, Muratore et al. reported that patients who underwent immediate reoperation (mean time of 2.2 months between cholecystectomy and radical resection) had a median survival of 46.7 months.[118] This was significantly better than the patients who underwent late reoperation (mean time of 11.3 months between cholecystectomy and radical resection), where all patients died within 25 months. In the French and German studies, the timing of re-resection was not a significant factor affecting survival.[119,120] However, in both the studies, only a limited number of patients underwent delayed resection and the median times to re-resection in the German and French studies were 11 and 48 days, respectively. In the chapter authors' experience of 170 post-cholecystectomy GBC patients managed over a period of 11 years, patients who presented early (n = 93) after the index cholecystectomy with a histopathology report of GBC had a significantly better resectability rate (69.9% vs 7.8%) and longer survival (54 vs 10 months) compared to patients who presented late (n = 77) with symptoms of recurrence.[24] The median time interval between initial cholecystectomy and reoperation in IGBC patients with resectable and unresectable disease was 25 and 79 days respectively. Therefore, it is important to consider early surgery for IGBC once confirmed on histopathology and worked up to rule out distant metastases. While an increase in the interval between the index cholecystectomy and radical resection increases the risk of dissemination, there is no upper time limit, which precludes radical resection. Hence, irrespective of the time interval after simple cholecystectomy, every patient with IGBC, should be considered for radical re-resection if the preoperative evaluation does not show any evidence of metastatic disease.

Management of suspected gall bladder cancer detected intraoperatively

In a patient planned for simple cholecystectomy, if the intraoperative findings suggest malignancy as a possibility, the treatment options depend upon the centre where the patient is operated and the experience of the surgeon. If the surgical expertise is not available, one should not proceed further for cholecystectomy and refer the patient to a higher centre. Any attempt to perform cholecystectomy should be strongly discouraged as the subserosal plane of a simple cholecystectomy will be going through the tumour, especially if it is T2 and above. The subserosal plane of a simple cholecystectomy also increases the risk of bile spillage and subsequent tumour dissemination. In addition, it is difficult to differentiate postoperative inflammatory changes from recurrent tumour, which can result in an increased incidence of major hepatic resection and extrahepatic adjacent organ resection and its associated morbidity.

If there is a suspicion of GBC on laparoscopy itself, further management is decided by the availability of local expertise of radical resection and index of suspicion. If the local expertise for advanced laparoscopic hepatobiliary surgery is available, one can perform laparoscopic wedge liver resection and frozen section examination or direct segment IVb and V liver resection depending upon the index of suspicion.[121] If the frozen section examination is positive for malignancy, lymphadenectomy should be added, which can be performed laparoscopically or by open technique based on the philosophy and experience of the surgical team. Imprint cytology is a simple and cost-effective alternative in centres where the facility for frozen section examination is not available.

Prevention of unsuspected or missed incidental gall bladder cancer

Patients with early-stage GBC benefit most from radical resection. Hence, every effort should be made to avoid improper management in these patients. Any patient with suspicious findings on USG like focal GB wall thickening or GB mass should be further evaluated with cross-sectional imaging to rule out GBC. A simple cholecystectomy should be avoided in patients with suspected GBC. During a cholecystectomy, every effort should be made to prevent GB perforation and bile spill as it significantly increases the recurrence rate. It is preferable to remove the cholecystectomy specimen using a protective bag, at least in endemic areas. After cholecystectomy, the GB specimen should be cut open and examined for a mass or mucosal irregularity. If suspicious findings are present on macroscopic examination, a frozen section examination should be performed. All GB specimens, irrespective of the findings on macroscopic examination, must be sent for histopathology to detect IGBC. In patients with GBC, radical curative resection is the only hope for a cure. Although a proportion of IGBC patients with T1a disease do not require further treatment, a significant number of IGBC patients have stage Ib or II disease and will benefit from radical resection. Routine histopathological examination of GB specimens would prevent delays in the detection of IGBC.[24]

Laparoscopic radical surgery for gall bladder cancer

In GBC, the role of minimally invasive surgery has been universally accepted for tumour staging (SL), and palliative bypass for a locally advanced or metastatic tumour detected at the time of SL. However, its role in radical surgery for a potentially curable disease is considered to be controversial. While laparoscopic cholecystectomy is one of the most commonly performed minimally invasive procedures, laparoscopic management of GBC has been relatively slow to develop. Although the feasibility of the minimally invasive hepatectomy and hepatoduodenal lymphadenectomy is well documented in the literature, the idea of minimally invasive radical surgery for GBC was vehemently opposed earlier due to reports of tumour recurrence at port sites in up to 48% of patients following laparoscopic cholecystectomy for GBC.[122–124] However, it is crucial to understand the mechanisms of port-site recurrence to decide whether laparoscopic radical surgery for GBC is justified.

Implantation of tumour cells at port sites occurs by both direct and indirect mechanisms[125]:

- Direct implantation of tumour cells occurs when the tumour specimen is forcibly extracted through a small incision or when there is tumour perforation.
- Indirect implantation is due to pneumoperitoneum and both the aerosol theory (dissemination to the port sites during the turbulence of insufflation) and the chimney effect (tumour implantation during episodes of desufflation) were postulated as possible mechanisms.

Experimental studies using solid tumour models instead of intraperitoneal cell culture lines and clinical evidence from laparoscopic colorectal surgery where the use of appropriate preventive measures like careful tumour handling, and use of a wound protector before extraction had reduced the incidence of port-site recurrence to 1% (comparable to open surgery) suggest that mechanical factors like GB perforation with bile spillage and poor specimen extraction techniques play an essential role in port-site recurrence rather than the pneumoperitoneum. The absence of port-site recurrences in all published series with a median follow-up of at least 6 months, the critical period after the index cholecystectomy, is the convincing evidence that LRC does not increase the incidence of port-site recurrence.[126-129]

It is unfair to extrapolate recurrence following cholecystectomy for unsuspected IGBC to laparoscopically performed radical cholecystectomy. The critical technical differences between laparoscopic cholecystectomy performed for unsuspected GBC and a planned laparoscopic radical surgery for GBC highlighted below account for the absence of port-site recurrence:

- The transection breaches the cystic plate (between GB and liver bed) in laparoscopic cholecystectomy performed for unsuspected GBC compared to the planned laparoscopic radical surgery for GBC where it is through the uninvolved liver as the GB is removed with a wedge of segment IVb and V.
- Tumour manipulation is significantly greater as the GB is grasped directly in laparoscopic cholecystectomy performed for unsuspected GBC compared to the LRC where the adjacent liver is grasped to avoid handling the tumour.
- The risk of bile spillage is higher in laparoscopic cholecystectomy performed for unsuspected GBC as it can occur while grasping the GB or dissecting the GB from the liver bed compared to laparoscopic radical surgery for GBC, where the risk is minimized by avoiding these and securely clipping the cystic duct.
- In laparoscopic cholecystectomy performed for unsuspected GBC the specimen is usually removed through the port site without a protective bag compared to the LRC where it is always removed using a retrieval bag.

The innovation of a surgical procedure goes through four stages, as documented by the IDEAL framework. It includes Idea (stage 1), Development (stage 2a), Exploration (stage 2b), Assessment (stage 3), and Long-term study (stage 4).[130] The aim of stage 1 is to provide proof of concept, and for LRC, it was given by Cho et al. from the Bundang Hospital, South Korea, in a series of 18 patients with early-stage GBC.[126] The aim of stage 2a is to document the safety and efficacy of the novel surgical procedure through a small case series (sample size in tens). Reports from high-volume centres have shown that with careful patient selection and proper surgical techniques, safety, and early oncological outcomes comparable to the open procedure could be achieved with LRC in addition to offering the benefits of a minimally invasive procedure to the patients.[127-129] The aim of stage 2b is to document efficacy in a larger group of patients (sample size in hundreds) so that a consensus equipoise can be reached on the new surgical procedure. Based on the available evidence, an expert consensus statement for LRC was published in 2019 to address the risk of port-site recurrence and concerns regarding the oncological adequacy and safety. It stated that early concerns regarding port site/peritoneal metastasis after laparoscopic surgery for GBC have faded with improved preoperative recognition of GBC and preventive measures.[131] Also, the consensus statement asserted that LRC is not associated with decreased survival compared to open surgery in patients with early-stage GBC. The aim of stage 3 is to document how well the novel surgical procedure compares with current standards of care using a randomized controlled trial. Currently, there are no randomized controlled trials comparing open and LRC. However, there is enough evidence in the literature to document the safety and oncological equivalence of LRC compared to open surgery. LRC for GBC has crossed stages 1 and 2 and currently in the assessment phase. Recently, the innovators of LRC (professor Han etal) from the Bundang Hospital have published the long-term outcomes of 45 patients with early-stage GBC managed by the laparoscopic approach. At a median follow-up of 60 months, only two patients developed disease-specific recurrence underscoring the oncological efficacy of LRC.[129] Since the author's initial publication in 2015 comparing laparoscopic and open radical cholecystectomy, minimally invasive (laparoscopic/robotic) radical cholecystectomy with segment IVb and V resection has been performed in more than 200 suspected GBC patients without port-site recurrence and comparable long-term results (unpublished data). In the recent past, selected patients with extrahepatic adjacent organ involvement (bile duct, gastroduodenal, or colon) were resected using the minimally invasive approach (Figure 35.12). Of the 13 patients who required extrahepatic adjacent organ resection, seven underwent bile duct excision, and one patient underwent colonic and duodenal sleeve resection. The remaining patients underwent bile duct excision along with colonic and duodenal sleeve resection. The same procedure has also been performed robotically (five cases in our experience). Like open radical cholecystectomy, LRC is a technically challenging procedure and hence should be restricted to expert centres to achieve comparable long-term outcomes. With accumulating evidence, LRC for early-stage GBC should no longer be considered an experimental procedure and is on the verge of becoming a standard technique for early GBC.

Neoadjuvant and adjuvant therapy for gall bladder cancer

Surgery remains the potential curative therapy for GBC. However, a higher incidence of systemic recurrence after curative resection highlights the need for systemic therapy. Adjuvant chemotherapy with or radiotherapy is indicated to treat micrometastasis. However,

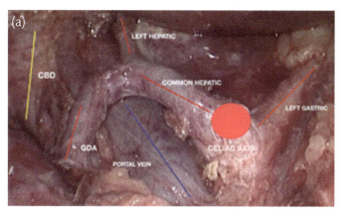 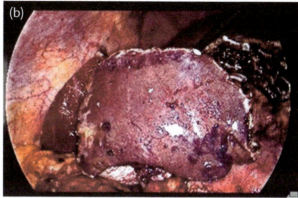

Figure 35.12 Laparoscopic radical cholecystectomy. CBD, common bile duct; GDA, gastroduodenal artery.

the majority of the studies on adjuvant therapy have included other biliary tumours in addition to GBC.[132,133] Also, most are retrospective single-centre studies and have included a smaller number of patients. Hence, there is a lack of high-level evidence on the role of adjuvant therapy for GBC. The current indications for adjuvant therapy are:

- T stage: T2 or more.
- N stage: node-positive disease.
- Resection status: R1 or R2 resection.
- Histological features: poorly differentiated tumour, lymphovascular and perineural invasion.

Gemcitabine alone or with cisplatin or oxaliplatin is the preferred first-line adjuvant chemotherapy. Combination therapy is preferred in good-risk patients. Oral capecitabine is an alternative first-line therapy. Adjuvant chemotherapy should be started within 8–12 weeks after surgery and the usual duration of therapy is 6 months. FOLFOX is the commonly used second-line chemotherapy in patients who do not respond to first-line chemotherapy.[134] Adjuvant radiotherapy in addition to chemotherapy is indicated in patients who underwent R1 resection and those with histological evidence of pericapsular invasion in metastatic lymph nodes.

Neoadjuvant therapy is an emerging concept in the management of GBC. The primary advantage of neoadjuvant therapy is the potential to assess the tumour biology and select appropriate patients for surgery. Patients with progressive disease on neoadjuvant therapy are considered to have biologically aggressive disease.[135] Also, neoadjuvant therapy can potentially downstage the disease and increase resectability rate and overall survival in patients with locally advanced disease. However, a recent systematic review that included six retrospective and two prospective studies concluded that current evidence does not support the routine use of neoadjuvant chemotherapy or neoadjuvant chemoradiotherapy in advanced GBC.[136] Only 40% of patients who received neoadjuvant therapy underwent curative resection. The subsets of patients who could benefit from neoadjuvant therapy are those with borderline resectable tumours. Patients with borderline resectable tumours are at higher risk of perioperative complications due to the complexity of the surgery, elevated risk of systemic recurrence due to the advanced nature of the tumour, and at higher risk of margin positive resection. However, unlike pancreatic cancer, there is no consensus on the definition of borderline resectable GBC as resectability criteria differ significantly between different regions and institutions. Hence, future studies should focus on the consensus definition of borderline resectable GBC and selecting appropriate candidates for neoadjuvant therapy.

Survival outcomes and prognosis in gall bladder cancer

Historically GBC is associated with a dismal prognosis given its propensity for early nodal and distant metastasis, frequent late presentation, and lack of effective systemic therapy. The pessimism towards GBC stemmed from earlier reports, which reported a dismal survival rate of 5–15%.[137,138] However, poor survival rates are mainly due to the use of less radical treatment. With recent reports of improved survival after aggressive surgical resection and chemotherapy in carefully selected patients, there is a shift from nihilism to optimism.

Both locoregional and systemic recurrence are commonly observed after curative resection for GBC.[137] As recurrences are common in the first 3 years after surgery, patients who undergo curative surgical resection should be followed up every 3 months for 1 year, every 6 months for 2 years, and then annually. Follow-up evaluation includes clinical evaluation, liver function tests, tumour markers (carcinoembryonic antigen and CA 19-9) and USG. CT abdomen and PET-CT are indicated in patients with clinical suspicion of recurrence. Survival outcomes and prognosis in patients who underwent curative resection are determined by tumour biology, which in turn are determined by[139,140]:

- T stage: the 5-year survival rates in patients with T1a, T1b, T2, T3a, T3b, T4a, and T4b are 92.5%, 87.2%, 63.7%, 27.0%, 18.8%, 8.2%, and 4.9% respectively.
- N stage: the 5-year survival rate in patients with N0, N1, and N2 disease is 51%, 29%, and 11%, respectively.
- Histological features: lymphovascular, perineural, and pericapsular invasion are associated with worse survival.
- Resection status: as expected, patients who underwent R0 resection have better survival than those who underwent R1 or R2 resection.
- Inflammatory markers: patients with preoperative cholecystitis, cholangitis, and those with elevated neutrophil:lymphocyte ratio have worse survival.

The difference in 5-year survival rate reported in various national databases could be due to differences in the presentation stage, type of GBC, and the treatment philosophy. The reported 5-year survival rate in the Japanese biliary tract registry is more than the survival rate reported in the SEER database.[138,139] The retrospective analysis of 2835 patients from the SEER database reported that only 8.6% of GBC patients underwent an en bloc resection, and lymphadenectomy was performed only in 5.3% of patients.[138] In another report from the US, only 9% of 19,139 resections performed for GBC were radical (extended) cholecystectomy.[141] Also, while comparing the stage-based survival, it is essential to understand the various changes in the different editions of the TNM classification and the implications for survival.

Most Western centres quote a poor 5-year survival rate as a reason for not using the radical surgical treatment for GBC. It is pertinent to note that the 5-year survival rate in pancreatic cancer is comparable to GBC. However, radical surgery is still accepted as the primary treatment for pancreatic cancer, and surgical techniques are constantly refined to improve the R0 resection.[142] Numerous publications from both Eastern and Western centres in the last decade focusing on the surgical techniques of pancreatoduodenectomy underscore the importance given to the surgical treatment in pancreatic cancer. Unfortunately, in the renowned Western centres where radical resection for pancreatic cancer is well accepted, radical surgery for GBC is viewed with scepticism. For an aggressive tumour, like GBC, where the survival is in months for non-operated patients, any survival advantage, even for 2–3 years for an advanced tumour, is worthwhile provided the morbidity and mortality of the surgical procedure are within the acceptable range. With advancements in surgical techniques, perioperative care, and adjuvant treatment, there is a significant improvement in the short- and long-term surgical outcomes from centres routinely performing radical resection for GBC. The scepticism propagated by some based on older results needs to be given a back seat, and nihilism needs to give way to realism.

Conclusion

Advancements in surgical techniques and perioperative management have improved survival and helped to change the nihilistic approach towards GBC. However, poor outcomes reported in a subset of patients highlight the need for more research to identify prognostic and therapeutic biomarkers. The success of precision medicine in a few malignancies like breast cancer and colon cancer underscores the need for future research on genomic profiling-guided targeted therapy in GBC. High-volume centres and funding agencies must focus on molecular research to identify diverse mutations in the GBC genome. Also, large multi-institutional collaborative databases are required to address some of the unanswered questions in the management of GBC.

REFERENCES

1. Are C, Ahmad H, Ravipati A, et al. Global epidemiological trends and variations in the burden of gallbladder cancer. *J Surg Oncol*. 2017;**115**(5):580–590.
2. Torre LA, Siegel RL, Islami F, Bray F, Jemal A. Worldwide burden of and trends in mortality from gallbladder and other biliary tract cancers. *Clin Gastroenterol Hepatol*. 2018;**16**(3):427–437.
3. Paquet KJ. Appraisal of surgical resection of gallbladder carcinoma with special reference to hepatic resection. *J Hepatobiliary Pancreat Surg*. 1998;**5**(2):200–206.
4. Blalock A. A statistical study of 888 cases of biliary tract disease. *Johns Hopkins Hosp Bull*. 1924;**35**:391–409.
5. Ishihara S, Horiguchi A, Miyakawa S, Endo I, Miyazaki M, Takada T. Biliary tract cancer registry in Japan from 2008 to 2013. *J Hepatobiliary Pancreat Sci*. 2016;**23**(3):149–157.
6. Nakamura S, Suzuki S, Konno H, Baba S, Muro H. Ten-year survival after hepatectomy for advanced gallbladder carcinoma: report of two cases. *Surgery*. 1995;**117**(2):232–234.
7. Kondo S, Nimura Y, Kamiya J, et al. Five-year survivors after aggressive surgery for stage IV gallbladder cancer. *J Hepatobiliary Pancreat Surg*. 2001;**8**(6):511–517.
8. Sternby Eilard M, Lundgren L, Cahlin C, Strandell A, Svanberg T, Sandström P. Surgical treatment for gallbladder cancer—a systematic literature review. *Scand J Gastroenterol*. 2017;**52**(5):505–514.
9. Holanda AKG, Lima Júnior ZB. Gallbladder histological alterations in patients undergoing cholecystectomy for cholelithiasis. *Rev Col Bras Cir*. 2020;**46**(6):e20192279.
10. Dilek ON, Karasu S, Dilek FH. Diagnosis and treatment of gallbladder polyps: current perspectives. *Euroasian J Hepatogastroenterol*. 2019;**9**(1):40–48.
11. Lin WR, Lin DY, Tai DI, et al. Prevalence of and risk factors for gallbladder polyps detected by ultrasonography among healthy Chinese: analysis of 34 669 cases. *J Gastroenterol Hepatol*. 2008;**23**(6):965–969.
12. McCain RS, Diamond A, Jones C, Coleman HG. Current practices and future prospects for the management of gallbladder polyps: a topical review. *World J Gastroenterol*. 2018;**24**(26):2844–2852.
13. Aldridge MC, Bismuth H. Gallbladder cancer: the polyp-cancer sequence. *Br J Surg*. 1990;**77**(4):363–364.
14. Mellnick VM, Menias CO, Sandrasegaran K, et al. Polypoid lesions of the gallbladder: disease spectrum with pathologic correlation. *Radiographics*. 2015;**35**(2):387–399.
15. Shapiro RS, Winsberg F. Comet-tail artifact from cholesterol crystals: observations in the postlithotripsy gallbladder and an in vitro model. *Radiology*. 1990;**177**(1):153–156.
16. Kim JH, Lee JY, Baek JH, et al. High-resolution sonography for distinguishing neoplastic gallbladder polyps and staging gallbladder cancer. *AJR Am J Roentgenol*. 2015;**204**(2):W150–W159.
17. Choi JH, Seo DW, Choi JH, et al. Utility of contrast-enhanced harmonic EUS in the diagnosis of malignant gallbladder polyps (with videos). *Gastrointest Endosc*. 2013;**78**(3):484–493.
18. Kim SY, Cho JH, Kim EJ, et al. The efficacy of real-time colour Doppler flow imaging on endoscopic ultrasonography for differential diagnosis between neoplastic and non-neoplastic gallbladder polyps. *Eur Radiol*. 2018;**28**(5):1994–2002.
19. Cheon YK, Cho WY, Lee TH, et al. Endoscopic ultrasonography does not differentiate neoplastic from non-neoplastic small gallbladder polyps. *World J Gastroenterol*. 2009;**15**(19):2361–2366.
20. Lou MW, Hu WD, Fan Y, Chen JH, E ZS, Yang GF. CT biliary cystoscopy of gallbladder polyps. *World J Gastroenterol*. 2004;**10**(8):1204–1207.

21. Irie H, Kamochi N, Nojiri J, Egashira Y, Sasaguri K, Kudo S. High b-value diffusion-weighted MRI in differentiation between benign and malignant polypoid gallbladder lesions. *Acta Radiol.* 2011;**52**(3):236–240.
22. Wiles R, Thoeni RF, Barbu ST, et al. Management and follow-up of gallbladder polyps: joint guidelines between the European Society of Gastrointestinal and Abdominal Radiology (ESGAR), European Association for Endoscopic Surgery and other Interventional Techniques (EAES), International Society of Digestive Surgery - European Federation (EFISDS) and European Society of Gastrointestinal Endoscopy (ESGE). *Eur Radiol.* 2017;**27**(9):3856–3866.
23. Babu BI, Dennison AR, Garcea G. Management and diagnosis of gallbladder polyps: a systematic review. *Langenbecks Arch Surg.* 2015;**400**(4):455–462.
24. Agarwal AK, Kalayarasan R, Singh S, Javed A, Sakhuja P. All cholecystectomy specimens must be sent for histopathology to detect inapparent gallbladder cancer. *HPB (Oxford).* 2012;**14**(4):269–273.
25. Agarwal AK, Javed A, Kalayarasan R, Sakhuja P. Minimally invasive versus the conventional open surgical approach of a radical cholecystectomy for gallbladder cancer: a retrospective comparative study. *HPB (Oxford).* 2015;**17**(6):536–541.
26. Cho JY, Han HS, Yoon YS, Ahn KS, Kim YH, Lee KH. Laparoscopic approach for suspected early-stage gallbladder carcinoma. *Arch Surg.* 2010;**145**(2):128–133.
27. Bray F, Ferlay J, Soerjomataram I, et al. Global cancer statistics 2018: GLOBOCAN estimates of incidence and mortality worldwide for 36 cancers in 185 countries. *CA Cancer J Clin.* 2018;**68**(6):394–424.
28. Shrikhande SV, Barreto SG, Singh S, Udwadia TE, Agarwal AK. Cholelithiasis in gallbladder cancer: coincidence, cofactor, or cause! *Eur J Surg Oncol.* 2010;**36**(6):514–519.
29. Hsing AW, Gao YT, Han TQ, et al. Gallstones and the risk of biliary tract cancer: a population-based study in China. *Br J Cancer.* 2007;**97**(11):1577–1582.
30. Nagaraja V, Eslick GD. Systematic review with meta-analysis: the relationship between chronic Salmonella typhi carrier status and gall-bladder cancer. *Aliment Pharmacol Ther.* 2014;**39**(8):745–750.
31. Mishra RR, Tewari M, Shukla HS. Helicobacter species and pathogenesis of gallbladder cancer. *Hepatobiliary Pancreat Dis Int.* 2010;**9**(2):129–134.
32. Machado NO. Porcelain gallbladder: decoding the malignant truth. *Sultan Qaboos Univ Med J.* 2016;**16**(4):e416–e421.
33. Avgerinos KI, Spyrou N, Mantzoros CS, Dalamaga M. Obesity and cancer risk: emerging biological mechanisms and perspectives. *Metabolism.* 2019;**92**:121–135.
34. Rawla P, Sunkara T, Thandra KC, Barsouk A. Epidemiology of gallbladder cancer. *Clin Exp Hepatol.* 2019;**5**(2):93–102.
35. Kalayarasan R, Javed A, Sakhuja P, Agarwal AK. Squamous variant of gallbladder cancer: is it different from adenocarcinoma? *Am J Surg.* 2013;**206**(3):380–385.
36. Albores-Saavedra J, Tuck M, McLaren BK, Carrick KS, Henson DE. Papillary carcinomas of the gallbladder: analysis of noninvasive and invasive types. *Arch Pathol Lab Med.* 2005;**129**(7):905–909.
37. Higuchi R, Ota T, Araida T, et al. Surgical approaches to advanced gallbladder cancer: a 40-year single-institution study of prognostic factors and resectability. *Ann Surg Oncol.* 2014;**21**(13):4308–4316.
38. Ethun CG, Le N, Lopez-Aguiar AG, et al. Pathologic and prognostic implications of incidental versus nonincidental gallbladder cancer: a 10-institution study from the United States Extrahepatic Biliary Malignancy Consortium. *Am Surg.* 2017;**83**(7):679–686.
39. Chang J, Jang JY, Lee KB, et al. Improvement of clinical outcomes in the patients with gallbladder cancer: lessons from periodic comparison in a tertiary referral center. *J Hepatobiliary Pancreat Sci.* 2016;**23**(4):234–241.
40. Goel S, Aggarwal A, Iqbal A, Gupta M, Rao A, Singh S. 18-FDG PET-CT should be included in preoperative staging of gall bladder cancer. *Eur J Surg Oncol.* 2020;**46**(9):1711–1716.
41. Javed A, Arora A, Kalayarasan R, Sakhuja P, Agarwal AK. Gallbladder cancer management impacted by coexistent tuberculosis. *Trop Gastroenterol.* 2013;**34**(2):87–90.
42. Agarwal AK, Kalayarasan R, Javed A, Sakhuja P. Role of routine 16b1 lymph node biopsy in the management of gallbladder cancer: an analysis. *HPB (Oxford).* 2014;**16**(3):229–34.
43. Edge SB, Byrd DR, Compton CC, Fritz AG, Greene FL, Trotti A, eds. *AJCC Cancer Staging Manual.* 7th ed. New York: Springer; 2010.
44. Amin MB, Edge SB, Greene FL, et al., eds. *AJCC Cancer Staging Manual.* 8th ed. New York: Springer; 2017.
45. Sobin LH, Gospodarowicz MK, Wittekind C. *TNM Classification of Malignant Tumours.* 7th ed. Hoboken, NJ: UICC/Wiley-Blackwell; 2009.
46. Brierley, JD, Gospodarowicz MK, Wittekind C. *TNM Classification of Malignant Tumours.* 8th ed. Hoboken, NJ: UICC/Wiley-Blackwell; 2017.
47. Lee H, Choi DW, Park JY, et al. Surgical strategy for T2 gallbladder cancer according to tumor location. *Ann Surg Oncol.* 2015;**22**(8):2779–2786.
48. Park TJ, Ahn KS, Kim YH, et al. The optimal surgical resection approach for T2 gallbladder carcinoma: evaluating the role of surgical extent according to the tumor location. *Ann Surg Treat Res.* 2018;**94**(3):135–141.
49. Toge K, Sakata J, Hirose Y, et al. Lymphatic spread of T2 gallbladder carcinoma: regional lymphadenectomy is required independent of tumor location. *Eur J Surg Oncol.* 2019;**45**(8):1446–1452.
50. Lee W, Jeong CY, Jang JY, et al. Do hepatic-sided tumors require more extensive resection than peritoneal-sided tumors in patients with T2 gallbladder cancer? Results of a retrospective multicenter study. *Surgery.* 2017;**162**(3):515–524.
51. Chaudhary RK, Higuchi R, Yazawa T, et al. Surgery in node-positive gallbladder cancer: the implication of an involved superior retro-pancreatic lymph node. *Surgery.* 2019;**165**(3):541–547.
52. Wang J, Bo X, Shi X, et al. Modified staging classification of gallbladder carcinoma on the basis of the 8th edition of the American Joint Commission on Cancer (AJCC) staging system. *Eur J Surg Oncol.* 2020;**46**(4 Pt A):527–533.
53. Agarwal AK, Kalayarasan R, Javed A, Gupta N, Nag HH. The role of staging laparoscopy in primary gall bladder cancer—an analysis of 409 patients: a prospective study to evaluate the role of staging laparoscopy in the management of gallbladder cancer. *Ann Surg.* 2013;**258**(2):318–323.
54. Butte JM, Gönen M, Allen PJ, et al. The role of laparoscopic staging in patients with incidental gallbladder cancer. *HPB (Oxford).* 2011;**13**(7):463–472.
55. Kondo S, Nimura Y, Hayakawa N, Kamiya J, Nagino M, Uesaka K. Regional and para-aortic lymphadenectomy in radical surgery for advanced gallbladder carcinoma. *Br J Surg.* 2000;**87**(4):418–422.

56. Ohtani T, Shirai Y, Tsukada K, Muto T, Hatakeyama K. Spread of gallbladder carcinoma: CT evaluation with pathologic correlation. *Abdom Imaging*. 1996;**21**(3):195–201.
57. Noji T, Kondo S, Hirano S, et al. CT evaluation of para-aortic lymph node metastasis in patients withbiliary cancer. *J Gastroenterol*. 2005;**40**(7):739–743.
58. Agarwal A, Saravanan MN, Kalayarasan R. EUS (endoscopic ultrasound) guided FNAC of the interaortocaval lymph node helps in selecting patients for curative surgery in gallbladder cancer. *HPB(Oxford)*. 2014;**18**:e600
59. Mathew J, Kalayarasan R, Javed A, Agarwal A. Inter-aortocaval lymph node biopsy as part of staging laparoscopy for gallbladder cancer: a pilot study. *HPB (Oxford)* 2014;**18**:e287.
60. Sons HU, Borchard F, Joel BS. Carcinoma of the gallbladder: autopsy findings in 287 cases and review of the literature. *J Surg Oncol*. 1985;**28**(3):199–206.
61. Ito M, Mishima Y, Sato T. Lymphatic drainage of gallbladder. *Surg Radiol Anat*. 1991;**13**(2):89–104.
62. Negi SS, Singh A, Chaudhary A. Lymph nodal involvement as prognostic factor in gallbladder cancer: location, count or ratio? *J Gastrointest Surg*. 2011;**15**(6):1017–1025.
63. Ito H, Ito K, D'angelica M, et al. Accurate staging for gallbladder cancer: implications for surgical therapy and pathological assessment. *Ann Surg*. 2011;**254**(2):320–325.
64. Kalayarasan R, Fong Y, Agarwal A.K, Miyazaki M. Standard radical cholecystectomy for T1 and T2 gallbladder cancer. In: Clavien PA, Sarr M, Fong Y, Miyazaki M, eds. *Atlas of Upper Gastrointestinal and Hepato-Pancreato-Biliary Surgery*. Berlin: Springer; 2016: 611–622.
65. Yoshikawa T, Araida T, Azuma T, Takasaki K. Bisegmentectal liver resection for gallbladder cancer. *Hepatogastroenterology*. 1998;**45**(19):14–19.
66. Sasaki R, Takeda Y, Hoshikawa K, et al. Long-term results of central inferior (S4a+S5) hepatic subsegmentectomy combined with extended lymphadenectomy for gallbladder carcinoma with subserous or mild liver invasion (pT2-3) and nodal involvement: a preliminary report. *Hepatogastroenterology*. 2004;**51**(55):215–218.
67. Tsukada K, Hatakeyama K, Kurosaki I, et al. Outcome of radical surgery for carcinoma of the gallbladder according to the TNM stage. *Surgery*. 1996;**120**(5):816–821.
68. Araida T, Higuchi R, Hamano M, et al. Hepatic resection in 485 R0 pT2 and pT3 cases of advanced carcinoma of the gallbladder: results of a Japanese Society of Biliary Surgery survey—a multicenter study. *J Hepatobiliary Pancreat Surg*. 2009;**16**(2):204–215.
69. Reddy SK, Marroquin CE, Kuo PC, Pappas TN, Clary BM. Extended hepatic resection for gallbladder cancer. *Am J Surg*. 2007;**194**(3):355–361.
70. Shimada K, Nara S, Esaki M, Sakamoto Y, Kosuge T, Hiraoka N. Extended right hemihepatectomy for gallbladder carcinoma involving the hepatic hilum. *Br J Surg*. 2011;**98**(1):117–123.
71. Shimizu Y, Ohtsuka M, Ito H, et al. Should the extrahepatic bile duct be resected for locally advanced gallbladder cancer? *Surgery*. 2004;**136**(5):1012–1017.
72. Kosuge T, Sano K, Shimada K, Yamamoto J, Yamasaki S, Makuuchi M. Should the bile duct be preserved or removed in radical surgery for gallbladder cancer? *Hepatogastroenterology*. 1999;**46**(28):2133–2137.
73. Muratore A, Polastri R, Bouzari H, Vergara V, Capussotti L. Radical surgery for gallbladder cancer: a worthwhile operation? *Eur J Surg Oncol*. 2000;**26**(2):160–163.
74. Shukla PJ, Barreto SG. Systematic review: should routine resection of the extra-hepatic bile duct be performed in gallbladder cancer? *Saudi J Gastroenterol*. 2010;**16**(3):161–167.
75. Kalayarasan R, Javed A, Gupta N, et al. Adjacent viscera involvement in gallbladder cancer: is aggressive resection worthwhile? *HPB (Oxford)* 2014;**18**:e317.
76. Singh B, Kapoor VK, Sikora SS, Kalawat TC, Das BK, Kaushik SP. Malignant gastroparesis and outlet obstruction in carcinoma gall bladder. *Trop Gastroenterol*. 1998;**19**(1):37–39.
77. Shimizu H, Kimura F, Yoshidome H, et al. Aggressive surgical approach for stage IV gallbladder carcinoma based on Japanese Society of Biliary Surgery classification. *J Hepatobiliary Pancreat Surg*. 2007;**14**(4):358–365.
78. Yoshikawa T. Clinicopathological study on spreading modes of gallbladder cancer (in Japanese with English abstract). *J Jpn Bil Assoc*. 1988;**2**:34–43.
79. Kokudo N, Makuuchi M, Natori T, et al. Strategies for surgical treatment of gallbladder carcinoma based on information available before resection. *Arch Surg*. 2003;**138**(7):741–750.
80. Ogura Y, Mizumoto R, Isaji S, Kusuda T, Matsuda S, Tabata M. Radical operations for carcinoma of the gallbladder: present status in Japan. *World J Surg*. 1991;**15**(3):337–343.
81. D'Angelica M, Martin RC 2nd, Jarnagin WR, Fong Y, DeMatteo RP, Blumgart LH. Major hepatectomy with simultaneous pancreatectomy for advanced hepatobiliary cancer. *J Am Coll Surg*. 2004;**198**(4):570–576.
82. Hirano S, Tanaka E, Shichinohe T, et al. Feasibility of en-bloc wedge resection of the pancreas and/or the duodenum as an alternative to pancreatoduodenectomy for advanced gallbladder cancer. *J Hepatobiliary Pancreat Surg*. 2007;**14**(2):149–154.
83. Kalayarasan R, Javed A, Puri AS, Puri SK, Sakhuja P, Agarwal AK. A prospective analysis of the preoperative assessment of duodenal involvement in gallbladder cancer. *HPB (Oxford)*. 2013;**15**(3):203–209.
84. Agarwal AK, Mandal S, Singh S, Sakhuja P, Puri S. Gallbladder cancer with duodenal infiltration: is it still resectable? *J Gastrointest Surg*. 2007;**11**(12):1722–1727.
85. Birnbaum DJ, Viganò L, Ferrero A, Langella S, Russolillo N, Capussotti L. Locally advanced gallbladder cancer: which patients benefit from resection? *Eur J Surg Oncol*. 2014;**40**(8):1008–1015.
86. Hawkins WG, DeMatteo RP, Jarnagin WR, Ben-Porat L, Blumgart LH, Fong Y. Jaundice predicts advanced disease and early mortality in patients with gallbladder cancer. *Ann Surg Oncol*. 2004;**11**(3):310–315.
87. Todoroki T, Takahashi H, Koike N, et al. Outcomes of aggressive treatment of stage IV gallbladder cancer and predictors of survival. *Hepatogastroenterology*. 1999;**46**(28):2114–2121.
88. Nakamura S, Suzuki S, Konno H, Baba S, Baba S. Outcome of extensive surgery for TNM stage IV carcinoma of the gallbladder. *Hepatogastroenterology*. 1999;**46**(28):2138–2143.
89. Agarwal AK, Mandal S, Singh S, Bhojwani R, Sakhuja P, Uppal R. Biliary obstruction in gall bladder cancer is not sine qua non of inoperability. *Ann Surg Oncol*. 2007;**14**(10):2831–2837.
90. Nishio H, Ebata T, Yokoyama Y, Igami T, Sugawara G, Nagino M. Gallbladder cancer involving the extrahepatic bile duct is worthy of resection. *Ann Surg*. 2011;**253**(5):953–960.
91. Mizuno T, Ebata T, Yokoyama Y, et al. Major hepatectomy with or without pancreatoduodenectomy for advanced gallbladder cancer. *Br J Surg*. 2019;**106**(5):626–635.
92. Torres OJM, Alikhanov R, Li J, Serrablo A, Chan AC, de Souza M, Fernandes E. Extended liver surgery for gallbladder cancer revisited: is there a role for hepatopancreatoduodenectomy? *Int J Surg*. 2020;**82S**:82–86.

93. Miyazaki M, Ito H, Nakagawa K, et al. Unilateral hepatic artery reconstruction is unnecessary in biliary tract carcinomas involving lobar hepatic artery: implications of interlobar hepatic artery and its preservation. *Hepatogastroenterology.* 2000;**47**(36):1526–1530.
94. Sakamoto Y, Sano T, Shimada K, et al. Clinical significance of reconstruction of the right hepatic artery for biliary malignancy. *Langenbecks Arch Surg.* 2006;**391**(3):203–208.
95. Kalayarasan R, Javed A, Agarwal AK. Gallbladder cancer with right hepatic artery involvement: can the artery be ligated? *HPB (Oxford).* 2014;**16**:258–316.
96. Søreide K, Guest RV, Harrison EM, Kendall TJ, Garden OJ, Wigmore SJ. Systematic review of management of incidental gallbladder cancer after cholecystectomy. *Br J Surg.* 2019;**106**(1):32–45.
97. Aloia TA, Jarufe N, Javle M, et al. Gallbladder cancer: expert consensus statement. *HPB (Oxford).* 2015;**17**(8):681–690.
98. Agarwal AK, Kalayarasan R, Singh S, Javed A, Sakhuja P. All cholecystectomy specimens must be sent for histopathology to detect inapparent gallbladder cancer. *HPB (Oxford).* 2012;**14**:269–273.
99. Singh S, Agarwal AK. Gallbladder cancer: the role of laparoscopy and radical resection. *Ann Surg.* 2009;**250**(3):494–495.
100. Godhi S, Singh S, Kalayarasan R, Javed A, Agarwal A. Incidental gallbladder cancer (IGBC) erroneously includes both true IGBC and pseudo IGBC. *HPB (Oxford).* 2014;**18**:e234.
101. Muszynska C, Lundgren L, Lindell G, et al. Predictors of incidental gallbladder cancer in patients undergoing cholecystectomy for benign gallbladder disease: results from a population-based gallstone surgery registry. *Surgery.* 2017;**162**(2):256–263.
102. Lundgren L, Muszynska C, Ros A, et al. Are incidental gallbladder cancers missed with a selective approach of gallbladder histology at cholecystectomy? *World J Surg.* 2018;**42**(4):1092–1099.
103. Grupo Internacional de Estudos de Câncer Hepatopancreatobiliar—ISG-HPB-Cancer, Coimbra FJF, Torres OJM, et al. Brazilian consensus on incidental gallbladder carcinoma. *Arq Bras Cir Dig.* 2020;**33**(1):e1496.
104. Yamamoto H, Hayakawa N, Kitagawa Y, et al. Unsuspected gallbladder carcinoma after laparoscopic cholecystectomy. *J Hepatobiliary Pancreat Surg.* 2005;**12**(5):391–398.
105. Ouchi K, Sugawara T, Ono H, et al. Diagnostic capability and rational resectional surgery for early gallbladder cancer. *Hepatogastroenterology.* 1999;**46**(27):1557–1560.
106. Wagholikar GD, Behari A, Krishnani N, et al. Early gallbladder cancer. *J Am Coll Surg.* 2002;**194**(2):137–141.
107. Goetze TO, Paolucci V. Immediate re-resection of T1 incidental gallbladder carcinomas: a survival analysis of the German Registry. *Surg Endosc.* 2008;**22**(11):2462–2465.
108. Abramson MA, Pandharipande P, Ruan D, Gold JS, Whang EE. Radical resection for T1b gallbladder cancer: a decision analysis. *HPB (Oxford).* 2009;**11**(8):656–663.
109. Benson AB 3rd, D'Angelica MI, Abbott DE, et al. NCCN guidelines insights: hepatobiliary cancers, version 1.2017. *J Natl Compr Canc Netw.* 2017;**15**(5):563–573.
110. You DD, Lee HG, Paik KY, Heo JS, Choi SH, Choi DW. What is an adequate extent of resection for T1 gallbladder cancers? *Ann Surg.* 2008;**247**(5):835–838.
111. Berger-Richardson D, Chesney TR, Englesakis M, Govindarajan A, Cleary SP, Swallow CJ. Trends in port-site metastasis after laparoscopic resection of incidental gallbladder cancer: a systematic review. *Surgery.* 2017;**161**(3):618–627.
112. Maker AV, Butte JM, Oxenberg J, et al. Is port site resection necessary in the surgical management of gallbladder cancer? *Ann Surg Oncol.* 2012;**19**(2):409–417.
113. Ethun CG, Postlewait LM, Le N, et al. Routine port-site excision in incidentally discovered gallbladder cancer is not associated with improved survival: a multi-institution analysis from the US Extrahepatic Biliary Malignancy Consortium. *J Surg Oncol.* 2017;**115**(7):805–811.
114. Giuliante F, Ardito F, Vellone M, Clemente G, Nuzzo G. Port-sites excision for gallbladder cancer incidentally found after laparoscopic cholecystectomy. *Am J Surg.* 2006;**191**(1):114–116.
115. Povoski SP, Ouellette JR, Chang WW, Jarnagin WR. Axillary lymph node metastasis following resection of abdominal wall laparoscopic port site recurrence of gallbladder cancer. *J Hepatobiliary Pancreat Surg.* 2004;**11**(3):197–202.
116. Kalayarasan R, Javed A, Sakhuja P, Agarwal A. Abdominal wall scar recurrence in incidental gallbladder cancer is not always disseminated disease. *HPB (Oxford).* 2014;**18**:e346.
117. Ethun CG, Postlewait LM, Le N, Pawlik TM, Buettner S, Poultsides G. Association of optimal time interval to re-resection for incidental gallbladder cancer with overall survival. A multi-institution analysis from the US extrahepatic biliary malignancy consortium. *JAMA Surg.* 2017;**152**(2):143–149.
118. Muratore A, Amisano M, Viganò L, Massucco P, Capussotti L. Gallbladder cancer invading the perimuscular connective tissue: results of reresection after prior non-curative operation. *J Surg Oncol.* 2003;**83**(4):212–215.
119. Goetze TO, Paolucci V. Benefits of reoperation of T2 and more advanced incidental gallbladder carcinoma: analysis of the German registry. *Ann Surg.* 2008;**247**(1):104–108.
120. Cubertafond P, Gainant A, Cucchiaro G. Surgical treatment of 724 carcinomas of the gallbladder. Results of the French Surgical Association Survey. *Ann Surg.* 1994;**219**(3):275–280.
121. Agarwal AK, Kalayarasan R, Javed A, Sakhuja P. Mass-forming xanthogranulomatous cholecystitis masquerading as gallbladder cancer. *J Gastrointest Surg.* 2013;**17**(7):1257–1264.
122. Wakabayashi G, Cherqui D, Geller DA, et al. Recommendations for laparoscopic liver resection: a report from the second international consensus conference held in Morioka. *Ann Surg.* 2015;**261**(4):619–629.
123. Chen K, Liu XL, Pan Y, Maher H, Wang XF. Expanding laparoscopic pancreaticoduodenectomy to pancreatic-head and periampullary malignancy: major findings based on systematic review and meta-analysis. *BMC Gastroenterol.* 2018;**18**(1):102.
124. Lundberg O, Kristoffersson A. Port site metastases from gallbladder cancer after laparoscopic cholecystectomy. Results of a Swedish survey and review of published reports. *Eur J Surg.* 1999;**165**(3):215–222.
125. Steinert R, Lippert H, Reymond MA. Tumor cell dissemination during laparoscopy: prevention and therapeutic opportunities. *Dig Surg.* 2002;**19**(4):464–472.
126. Cho JY, Han HS, Yoon YS, Ahn KS, Kim YH, Lee KH. Laparoscopic approach for suspected early-stage gallbladder carcinoma. *Arch Surg.* 2010;**145**(2):128–133.
127. Agarwal AK, Javed A, Kalayarasan R, Sakhuja P. Minimally invasive versus the conventional open surgical approach of a radical cholecystectomy for gallbladder cancer: a retrospective comparative study. *HPB (Oxford).* 2015;**17**(6):536–541.

128. Palanisamy S, Patel N, Sabnis S, et al. Laparoscopic radical cholecystectomy for suspected early gall bladder carcinoma: thinking beyond convention. *Surg Endosc*. 2016;**30**(6):2442–2448.
129. Yoon YS, Han HS, Cho JY, et al. Is laparoscopy contraindicated for gallbladder cancer? A 10-year prospective cohort study. *J Am Coll Surg*. 2015;**221**(4):847–853.
130. Khachane A, Philippou Y, Hirst A, McCulloch P. Appraising the uptake and use of the IDEAL Framework and Recommendations: a review of the literature. *Int J Surg*. 2018;**57**:84–90.
131. Han HS, Yoon YS, Agarwal AK, et al. Laparoscopic surgery for gallbladder cancer: an expert consensus statement. *Dig Surg*. 2019;**36**(1):1–6.
132. Stein A, Arnold D, Bridgewater J, et al. Adjuvant chemotherapy with gemcitabine and cisplatin compared to observation after curative intent resection of cholangiocarcinoma and muscle invasive gallbladder carcinoma (ACTICCA-1 trial)—a randomized, multidisciplinary, multinational phase III trial. *BMC Cancer*. 2015;**15**:564.
133. Primrose JN, Fox RP, Palmer DH, et al. Capecitabine compared with observation in resected biliary tract cancer (BILCAP): a randomised, controlled, multicentre, phase 3 study. *Lancet Oncol*. 2019;**20**(5):663–673.
134. Javle M, Zhao H, Abou-Alfa GK. Systemic therapy for gallbladder cancer. *Chin Clin Oncol*. 2019;**8**(4):44.
135. Nara S, Esaki M, Ban D, et al. Adjuvant and neoadjuvant therapy for biliary tract cancer: a review of clinical trials. *Jpn J Clin Oncol*. 2020;**50**(12):1353–1363.
136. Hakeem AR, Papoulas M, Menon KV. The role of neoadjuvant chemotherapy or chemoradiotherapy for advanced gallbladder cancer—a systematic review. *Eur J Surg Oncol*. 2019;**45**(2):83–91.
137. Jarnagin WR, Ruo L, Little SA, et al. Patterns of initial disease recurrence after resection of gallbladder carcinoma and hilar cholangiocarcinoma: implications for adjuvant therapeutic strategies. *Cancer*. 2003;**98**(8):1689–1700.
138. Coburn NG, Cleary SP, Tan JC, Law CH. Surgery for gallbladder cancer: a population-based analysis. *J Am Coll Surg*. 2008;**207**(3):371–382.
139. Ishihara S, Horiguchi A, Miyakawa S, Endo I, Miyazaki M, Takada T. Biliary tract cancer registry in Japan from 2008 to 2013. *J Hepatobiliary Pancreat Sci*. 2016;**23**(3):149–157.
140. Nagino M, Hirano S, Yoshitomi H, et al. Clinical practice guidelines for the management of biliary tract cancers 2019: the 3rd English edition. *J Hepatobiliary Pancreat Sci*. 2021;**28**(1):26–54.
141. Goussous N, Hosseini M, Sill AM, Cunningham SC. Minimally invasive and open gallbladder cancer resections: 30- vs 90-day mortality. *Hepatobiliary Pancreat Dis Int*. 2017;**16**(4):405–411.
142. Strobel O, Neoptolemos J, Jäger D, Büchler MW. Optimizing the outcomes of pancreatic cancer surgery. *Nat Rev Clin Oncol*. 2019;**16**(1):11–26.

36
Medical and innovative therapies for biliary malignancies

Sudha Kodali, Joy V. Nolte Fong, and R. Mark Ghobrial

Introduction

Cholangiocarcinoma (CCA) is a malignancy arising from the biliary epithelial cells. These tumours arise from varying locations within the biliary tree showing markers of cholangiocyte differentiation. CCA is the second most common primary liver tumour, and the incidence is increasing worldwide.[1] A high mortality is associated with CCA due to late presentation and the aggressive nature of the tumours.[2] Anatomically, they are classified as intrahepatic, perihilar, and distal CCAs.[3] Intrahepatic CCA arises from the bile ducts proximal to the second-degree bile ducts. Intrahepatic CCAs are further divided into mass-forming tumours, periductal-infiltrating types, and intraductal growth types.[4] Perihilar CCA arises from the area between the second-degree bile ducts and the insertion of the cystic duct into the common bile duct. Distal CCA is confined to the area between the origin of the cystic duct and the ampulla of Vater.[3]

With the increasing incidence of CCA, it is important to recognize the risk factors early in the disease process. Some tumours develop sporadically and their incidence varies depending on the geographic areas.[5] In Southeast Asia, hepatobiliary flukes and bile duct disorders are the common risk factors, compared to other aetiologies in Europe and North America.[5] Other important risk factors for CCA include choledochal cysts, cholangitis, inflammatory bowel disease, biliary cirrhosis, cholelithiasis, Thorotrast exposure, alcohol-associated liver disease, and Caroli's disease—characterized by congenital, multifocal, segmental dilatation of the intrahepatic bile ducts.[6,7]

Intrahepatic cholangiocarcinoma

Hepatitis B and C, primary sclerosing cholangitis, and cirrhosis (irrespective of aetiology) have been implicated as potential risk factors for intrahepatic cholangiocarcinoma (iCCA).[7,8] The increasing incidence of obesity, metabolic syndrome, and associated non-alcoholic steatohepatitis may account in part for the increased incidence of primary liver cancer, including CCA, particularly in the Western world.[9] Irrespective of the type, the median survival is 12–24 months without treatment.[10]

Diagnosis

The diagnosis of iCCA needs to be considered if someone with the above-mentioned risk factors presents with cachexia, abdominal pain, night sweats, weight loss, and fatigue, or if a liver lesion is seen on imaging. A good, contrasted imaging study may aid the diagnosis of CCA based on the contrast uptake pattern during the arterial and venous phases of the studies.[11] Magnetic resonance cholangiography and multi-detector computed tomography (CT) are used to assess vascular invasion, tumour size, satellite lesions, regional lymphadenopathy, and volumetric analysis for surgical consideration.[12] The imaging characteristics of iCCA are sometimes difficult to differentiate from hepatocellular carcinoma, especially if there is a rim enhancement because of inflammation at the hepatic parenchyma–tumour interface.

A biopsy is often needed for definitive diagnosis and to guide therapy.[11] Image- or endoscopy-guided biopsy is extremely valuable in tumours that lack typical imaging features or have features of mixed lesions. These mixed tumours have features of CCA and hepatocellular carcinoma based on immunohistochemical analysis for cytokeratins 19 and 7, and are associated with high rates of recurrence and a poor prognosis.[13] Obtaining adequate tissue or samples for biopsies can be challenging because of the intense desmoplastic reaction of these tumours. Detection of aneuploidy using digitized image analysis and fluorescence *in situ* hybridization (FISH) analysis of the brushings aids in diagnosis.[14] Carbohydrate antigen 19-9 (CA 19-9) is a serum marker that is often elevated in patients with iCCA, with a 62% sensitivity and 63% specificity.[15] However, this marker must be critically assessed, as elevations are often seen in patients with primary sclerosing cholangitis as well. A CA 19-9 value greater than 1000 U/mL usually indicates larger tumours and unresectable disease.[16]

Treatment

Several treatment options exist for iCCA including surgery, chemotherapy, and immunotherapy (Figure 36.1).

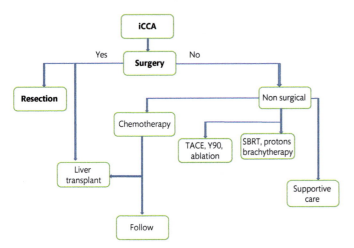

Figure 36.1 Management of iCCA after assessing for surgical candidacy—surgical resection and LT; and transarterial chemoembolization (TACE), yttrium 90 (Y90), short-beam external radiation (SBRT), and proton therapy (protons) for non-surgical candidates.

Surgical resection

Complete resection of the tumour by R0 (negative) margins is desirable and also achievable for smaller lesions. Resection confers excellent post-surgical outcomes in these patients but may not be feasible in larger, multifocal tumours with vascular invasion in the presence of cirrhosis. These patients may be considered for liver transplantation (LT). Post resection, the recurrence rate is higher for multiple tumours with lymph node (LN) metastases compared with single tumours with no LN involvement: 93% versus 47%, respectively.[17] A CA 19-9 level greater than 1000 U/mL perioperatively, multifocal disease, invasion of the liver capsule, positive surgical margins, regional LN metastases, and mass-forming or a periductal infiltrating-type CCA growth are all considered to be poor prognostic factors.[10] If surgical resection is not an option, then various treatment alternatives are available, including chemotherapy, locoregional therapies, and radiation, depending on the patient's functional status and disease burden (Figure 36.1).

Transplantation

LT can be a successful treatment option for unresectable iCCA in selected patients. Previous reports associated LT with a poor 2-year survival of 30% with a 60–84% tumour recurrence at 2 years.[18–20] One study found that LT recipients with incidental iCCA had a 5-year recurrence rate of 70% and a median disease-free survival of 8 months.[13] Several studies showed good outcomes in incidentally discovered iCCA after LT reported with overall 5-year survival of 65% or higher.[21] Conversely, patients with known iCCA prior to LT demonstrated poor outcomes.[22] A large retrospective analysis from the University of California, Los Angeles demonstrated significant improvement in recurrence-free survival with neoadjuvant therapy prior to LT compared to radical bile duct resection and partial hepatectomy.[23] Various centres have now incorporated a protocol-based approach where patients who are not resection candidates undergo a combination of neoadjuvant chemotherapy and liver transplantation. Recent studies have shown that post-LT outcomes for patients with incidental iCCA are comparable to outcomes in patients transplanted for hepatocellular carcinoma for smaller tumours (<2 cm).[24]

Based on the above data, some centres now treat patients with neoadjuvant therapy and advocate LT in those who respond or show stability of disease.[25] In a prospective case series, patients with locally advanced, unresectable iCCA, without extrahepatic disease or vascular involvement, were treated with neoadjuvant chemotherapy followed by LT. Neoadjuvant therapy consisted of gemcitabine-based chemotherapy, such as gemcitabine/cisplatin or gemcitabine/capecitabine, with second-line or third-line therapies given per institutional standards. Patients with a minimum of 6 months of radiographic response or stability were listed for LT. Overall survival (OS) was 100% (95% confidence interval (CI) 100–100%) at 1 year, 83.3% (27.3–97.5%) at 3 years, and 83.3% (27.3–97.5%) at 5 years. Three patients developed recurrent disease at a median of 7.6 months (interquartile range 5.8–8.6 months) after transplantation, with 50% (95% CI 11.1–80.4%) recurrence-free survival at 1, 3, and 5 years. Selected patients with locally advanced iCCA who show pretransplant disease stability on neoadjuvant therapy receive significant benefit from LT.[25]

Chemotherapy

Patients with resected biliary tract cancers should be offered adjuvant capecitabine chemotherapy for a duration of 6 months.[26] These recommendations are based on results of the BILCAP study. This study included 447 patients with iCCA (19%), perihilar CCA (29%), muscle-invasive gallbladder cancer (18%), or CCA of the lower common bile duct (35%). LN involvement was present in 45% of the treatment group and 48% in the control group. R1 resection occurred in 38% of both the treatment and control groups. This study found a significant difference in OS from an intention-to-treat analysis, adjusted for nodal status, disease grade, and sex (hazard ratio (HR) 0.71; 95% CI 0.55–0.92; p <0.01). A per-protocol analysis also found a significant difference in OS (HR 0.75; 95% CI 0.58–0.97; p = 0.028) in favour of capecitabine versus observation.[27]

The Advanced Biliary Cancer (ABC)-02 study was a phase III trial including 410 patients with locally advanced or metastatic CCA, gallbladder cancer, or ampullary cancer. Participants were randomized to receive either cisplatin followed by gemcitabine or gemcitabine alone for up to 24 weeks. The median follow-up time was 8.2 months and 327 deaths occurred. The cisplatin–gemcitabine group achieved a longer median OS of 11.7 months compared to the gemcitabine-alone group of 8.1 months (HR 0.64; 95% CI 0.52–0.80; p <0.001). Similarly, superior median progression-free survival was demonstrated in the cisplatin–gemcitabine group, 8.0 months versus 5.0 months (p <0.001).[28] Combination therapy of cisplatin plus gemcitabine has become the standard-of-care, first-line chemotherapy option for iCCA over gemcitabine alone.[29–31]

The PRODIGE 12 study compared gemcitabine–oxaliplatin therapy to standard surveillance in 194 patients with intrahepatic (46%), perihilar (8%), or distal (27%) CCA or gallbladder adenocarcinoma (20%) after R0 or R1 resection. Equivalent LN involvement was present between groups (63% and 64%). The R0 resection rates in the treatment and control groups were 86% and 88%, respectively, while the remainder were R1 resections. No significant differences between the gemcitabine–oxaliplatin and surveillance groups were found for the recurrence free survival (HR 0.88; 95% CI 0.62–1.25; p = 0.48).[32]

In the ABC-06 trial, participants received FOLFOX and supportive care versus supportive care alone after gemcitabine/cisplatin failure. The study showed positive improvement in the overall 1-year survival (25.9% vs 11.4%) with modest median survival improvement (5.3 to 6.2 months). There was a survival benefit in the iCCA group, though not statistically significant (HR 0.64; 95% CI 0.38–1.06).[33]

Targeted chemotherapy

See **Figure 36.2**.

Fibroblast growth factor receptor 2 (FGFR2) inhibitor

FGFR2 gene signalling is responsible for FGFR2 protein production, which is implicated in cell growth and division. Alterations in FGFR2, including fusions or other rearrangements, can lead to aberrant signalling, which triggers the proliferation and survival of cancer cells.[2,34] *FGFR2* alterations, which occur almost entirely in the intrahepatic subtype, are found in 10–16% of patients with CCA.[34]

Pemigatinib was the first treatment to target *FGFR2* and received US Food and Drug Administration approval in April 2020. It became available for patients with advanced CCA who harbour this biomarker (www.fda.gov/news-events/press-announcements/fda-approves-first-targeted-treatment-patients-cholangiocarcinoma-cancer-bile-ducts).[35] Pemigatinib is a small-molecule kinase inhibitor that targets *FGFR1*, *FGFR2*, and *FGFR3*. Pemigatinib inhibits phosphorylation and signalling along the FGFR1, -2, and -3 pathways, thereby decreasing the proliferation of cancer cells with *FGFR* alterations.[35] The approval was based on the FIGHT-202 study, an open-label, single-arm, phase II clinical trial of 107 patients (median age, 56 years). Participants had locally advanced, unresectable or metastatic CCA associated with *FGFR2* gene fusion or non-fusion rearrangement whose disease progressed with or after one or more previous therapies.[34,35] All participants received 13.5 mg pemigatinib orally once daily in 21-day cycles for 14 consecutive days, followed by 7 days of therapy until disease progression or unacceptable toxicity. The primary efficacy end point was overall response rate; the secondary end point was duration of response.[34] Participants showed an overall response rate of 36% and a median duration of response of 9.1 months. Response was lasting, with 63% exhibiting response to treatment lasting 6 months or longer and 18% with response lasting 12 months or more. The median time to response was 2.7 months.[34,35]

Isocitrate dehydrogenase (IDH) inhibitors

The discovery that there is an increased frequency of isocitrate dehydrogenase 1 and 2 (IDH1 and IDH2) mutations in iCCA led to inhibitors of IDH mutant alleles.[36,37] AG-120 (ivosidenib) is a potent oral inhibitor of mutant IDH1. The ClarIDHy phase III, randomized, double-blind study of ivosidenib at 500 mg versus placebo was performed in 185 participants with advanced CCA with an *IDH1* mutation.[38] Participants randomized to the placebo were allowed to crossover from placebo to ivosidenib if they showed evidence of radiographic progression. There was a favourable trend in OS with ivosidenib: median OS was 10.8 months for ivosidenib versus 9.7 months for placebo (HR 0.69; one-sided p = 0.06). Other IDH1 and IDH2 inhibitors (NCT02273739, NCT02381886, NCT02481154) are now in clinical trials enrolling patients with CCA.

Vascular endothelial growth factor (VEGF) and epidermal growth factor receptor (EGFR) inhibitors

EGFR, VEGF, and VEGF receptor have been implicated in carcinogenesis of iCCA. A randomized phase III trial (n = 133) showed that adding an EGFR inhibitor, erlotinib, to gemcitabine–oxaliplatin (GEMOX) significantly improved response rates versus GEMOX alone in advanced biliary tract cancers. However, improved survival was not demonstrated, with a median OS of 9.5 months in both arms.[30]

Immunotherapy

Approval of immune checkpoint inhibitors that target cytotoxic T lymphocyte-associated antigen (CTLA-4; ipilimumab) and programmed cell death pathway (PD-1; pembrolizumab), has created an increased interest in exploring the role of these agents in CCA.[39] These drugs have primarily been studied in the treatment of other cancers (**Figure 36.3**). However, two phase II trials have examined the effects of ipilimumab with and without nivolumab in patient with biliary tract cancer. The BilT-01 trial compared participants receiving gemcitabine, cisplatin, and nivolumab to participants receiving nivolumab and ipilimumab.[40] This study did not report significant differences in survival between the study cohorts. Conversely, the CA209-538 study of 39 patients receiving a combination of nivolumab and ipilimumab reported a response rate of 23%.[41] Unfortunately, 49% of patients in this study experienced immune-related toxic adverse events.

Pembrolizumab has been studied in conjunction with capecitabine and oxaliplatin in patients with biliary cancer. A recent phase II

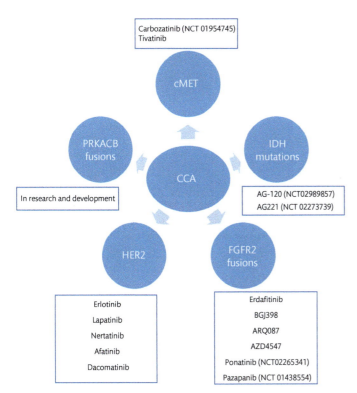

Figure 36.2 Targeted chemotherapy for intrahepatic cholangiocarcinoma, various mutations as potential targets for drug development. cMET, tyrosine-protein kinase Met (or hepatocyte growth factor receptor); FGFR, fibroblast growth factor receptor; HER2, human epidermal growth factor receptor; IDH, isocitrate dehydrogenase; PRKACB, protein kinase CAMP, activated catalytic subunit beta.

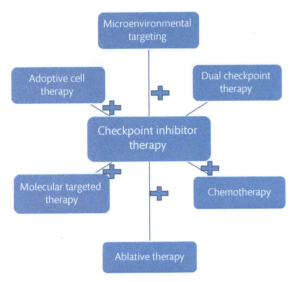

Figure 36.3 Immunotherapy trials for advanced cholangiocarcinoma.

study showed an 81.8% response rate, with median progression-free survival of 4.1 months.[42] Additionally, the KEYNOTE-158 study of pembrolizumab did include some patients with CCA.[43] Of the 233 patients in the study, 34.3% responded to treatment.

Recently, the TOPAZ-1 trial examined outcomes in patients with biliary tract cancer after utilizing a combination of gemcitabine, cisplatin, and durvalumab with or without temelimumab.[44] The combination chemotherapy–immunotherapy regimen led to an objective response in 82 of 124 (66%) chemotherapy- and immunotherapy-naïve patients. None of the study subjects had adverse events that were strong enough to discontinue therapy.

Drugs in the pipeline

IDH1 and IDH2 inhibitors (NCT02273739, NCT02381886, NCT02481154) are now in clinical trials enrolling patients with CCA. Several phase II studies are showing promising results looking at biomarkers in liver-limited iCCA and the role of immunotherapy. Also, combined therapy of CTLA-4/PD-1 inhibitors ipilimumab and nivolumab demonstrated superior efficacy compared to a single-agent anti-PD-1 therapy in patients with advanced melanoma and renal cell carcinoma. The authors aimed to test this combination in patients with metastatic biliary tract cancer. Phase II results showed significant clinical activity in patients with microsatellite stable tumours (NCT02923934). There are several other phase II studies looking at FGFR2 targeting drugs, including futibatinib, and a pan-HER inhibitor drug, vartinilib, in the TREE TOPP trial This study failed to meet the primary and secondary end points of progression-free survival and overall response rate, respectively, as second-line therapy in patients with biliary tract cancer (NCT NCT03093870; http://aslanpharma.com/app/uploads/2019/11/19-11-11-Varlitinib-TreeTopp-Topline_ENG.pdf).

Locoregional options

Locoregional therapies such as ablation and transcatheter arterial chemoembolization (TACE) have been used in patients with iCCA. The most commonly used techniques are conventional TACE, drug-eluting beads TACE, and yttrium-90 radioembolization (Y90).[45] Drug combinations for locoregional therapies consist of doxorubicin, cisplatin, and mitomycin-C, or gemcitabine made into an emulsion with ethiodized oil, which dually functions as a drug carrier as well as an embolic agent. After injection of the oil–drug mix, the occlusion of more proximal arterial blood vessels is achieved by injecting embolic materials, such as Gelfoam, polyvinyl-alcohol particles, or trisacryl gelatin microspheres.[45] Several centres have reported comparable survival in unresectable iCCA with positive margins in patients who received TACE.[46]

Y90 involves intra-arterial administration of small embolic particles (20–40 μm) containing the radio nucleotide ^{90}Y, which emits beta radiation. Much higher local doses are delivered compared to external beam radiation. Hence, Y90 allows maximization of treatment efficacy while sparing the healthy liver parenchyma from radiation-induced injury.[47,48] A systematic review and pooled analysis of 12 studies (n = 5 retrospective, n = 7 prospective) included 298 patients with iCCA who received Y90. Authors report a mean partial response in 28% and stable disease in 54% of patients at 3 months. Successful downstaging occurred by Y90 with subsequent surgery in seven patients. The authors concluded that OS of patients with iCCA after Y90 is higher than historical survival rates and similar to chemotherapy and TACE.[49]

Radiation

Adjuvant radiation

A large, retrospective analysis comparing therapy options for iCCA revealed that adjuvant radiation followed by surgery resulted in the greatest OS benefit (HR 0.40; 95% CI 0.34–0.47). The next highest benefit was found in patients undergoing surgery alone (HR 0.49; 95% CI 0.44–0.54). Patients undergoing radiation therapy alone (HR 0.68; 95% CI 0.59–0.77) also had a lower mortality hazard than patients who did not receive adjuvant treatment.[50]

Definitive radiation

The combination of radiation with chemotherapy offers significantly higher survival than chemotherapy alone in unresectable iCCA.[51] Seventy-nine patients with inoperable iCCA with median tumour size of 7.9 cm (range 2.2–17 cm), with about 89% received chemotherapy prior to radiation, showed that the 3-year OS rate for patients receiving higher dose of external radiation was 73%, compared to 38% for those who received a lower dose. The 3-year local control rate (78%) was also greater after receiving 80.5 Gy therapy than lower doses (45%; p = 0.04).[52]

Proton beam therapy

There has been growing interest in utilizing proton therapy for treatment of inoperable iCAA due to previous studies reporting excellent local control.[53,54] Participants (n = 37) with biopsy-proven iCCA without extrahepatic disease who were determined to be unresectable received 15 fractions of proton beam therapy to a maximum dose of 67.5 Gy. The median follow-up time was 19.5 months, the local control rate at 2 years was 94.1% and OS was 46.5%.[53]

Brachytherapy (BT)

In a propensity score matched pair analysis of patients with unresectable biliary tract cancer, the addition of BT to radiation therapy (RT) did not impact OS (31% (BT alone) vs 40% (BT + RT), p = 0.862), but showed better local control of the disease (35% (BT alone) vs 65% (BT + RT), p = 0.094).[55]

Perihilar cholangiocarcinoma

Extrahepatic CCAs are further divided in to perihilar and distal subtypes. Most cases of perihilar cholangiocarcinoma (pCCA) are sporadic, but known common risk factors consist of primary sclerosing cholangitis, liver fluke infestation (*Clonorchis sinensis* and *Opisthorchis viverrini*), and hepatolithiasis. Approximately 90% of patients present with biliary symptoms, including painless jaundice most commonly. Up to 10% of patients will have concomitant cholangitis.[2]

Diagnosis

Patients presenting with jaundice who have an ultrasound showing intrahepatic biliary ductal dilation and/or hilar mass or stricture should undergo high-resolution magnetic resonance imaging (MRI) or CT scanning. MRI or CT imaging yields the best assessment of size, extent, and resectability of the stricture.[56–58] Most patients require endobiliary drainage for biliary decompression via endoscopic retrograde cholangiopancreatography (ERCP). Brushings at the time of ERCP have a low diagnostic yield of about 40%, given the fibrotic nature of the stricture. However, the addition of FISH can increase the yield to 90%.[59,60] In patients with suspicious appearing regional LNs, endoscopic ultrasound-guided aspiration should be considered. Laparoscopic percutaneous biopsy carries a high risk of tumour cell dissemination and hence is not recommended.[61]

Treatment

Neoadjuvant therapy

In most centres, 5-fluorouracil is administered as a 500 mg/m² daily bolus for 3 days as a part of a pretransplant neoadjuvant protocol. This treatment provides radiosensitization of the tumour. Over a 3-week period, external beam radiotherapy is administered in 30 fractions to achieve a target dose of 4500 cGy. Iridium-192 (2000–3000 cGy) brachytherapy is delivered in conjunction with 2000 mg/m² oral capecitabine per day in two divided doses, 2 out of every 3 weeks, as tolerated until LT.[62] This protocol has been adopted from the Mayo Clinic by several other centres.[63,64] The 5-year disease-free survival of patients with pCCA who underwent LT following neoadjuvant therapy was 65% across 12 US transplantation centres.[65] Several other centres have institution-based protocols for managing patients with pCCA which are similar in the basic approach to these patients (Figure 36.4). The chemotherapy drugs mentioned earlier as treatment for iCCA may also be used for unresectable pCCA.

Liver transplantation

LT following high-dose neoadjuvant radiotherapy with chemosensitization achieves excellent results for patients with early-stage, unresectable pCCA. The Mayo Clinic protocol outlined the selection and treatment of patients with pCCA and no evidence of extrahepatic disease (nodes or metastasis) who are expected to have good outcomes after transplant.[66] Operative staging and transplant are beyond the scope of this chapter.

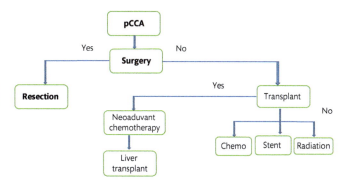

Figure 36.4 Management of pCCA after assessing for surgical candidacy—surgical resection and LT; and chemotherapy, stenting, and short-beam external radiation (SBRT), for non-transplant candidates.

Distal cholangiocarcinoma

Distal cholangiocarcinomas (dCCAs) have the same risk factors as intrahepatic tumours. Patients present with jaundice, dark urine, pale stools, pruritus, malaise, and weight loss. Laboratory tests show obstructive cholestasis with increased alkaline phosphatase and bilirubin.[10]

Diagnosis

Diagnostic modalities remain the same as in other forms of CCA using CT, MRI/magnetic resonance cholangiopancreatography, ERCP, and endoscopic ultrasound plus biopsy.

Treatment

Pancreaticoduodenectomy

Pancreaticoduodenectomy (also called the Whipple procedure) is the surgical procedure of choice for dCCA. In a large series of 564 patients with CCA who underwent surgical resection, 78% of those with dCCA had an R0 resection via the Whipple procedure, with 5-year OS of 27%.[67] Perineural invasion, LN metastasis, resection margin status, and tumour differentiation had prognostic significance in a meta-analysis investigating 5-year OS in patients with dCCA following surgical resection.[68] For patients who have unresectable disease secondary to advanced stage dCCA, chemotherapy in combination with radiation and targeted immunotherapy agents have shown some improvement in OS.

Radiotherapy

In patients with advanced extrahepatic CCA, a dose ranging from 30 to 78 Gy in 1.8–2.0 Gy per fraction (median = 48.25 Gy) along with concurrent chemotherapy with cisplatin and/or 5-fluorouracil showed 1- and 3-year progression-free survival of 38% and 16%, respectively, with disease relapse in 66% patients.[69] Other centres have reported 2-year OS of 27% in patients with unresectable extrahepatic CCA treated with radiotherapy with weekly gemcitabine 100 mg/m² as a 24-hour infusion.[70]

Stereotactic body radiation therapy (SBRT) has been used to treat unresectable dCCA. Patients underwent an initial bilateral biliary drainage with plastic stents before radiotherapy. CyberKnife SBRT with three fractions of 10 Gy was given with weekly gemcitabine and resulted in a median time to progression of 30 months.[71] SBRT has shown improved progression-free survival and OS in many smaller series.[72]

Conclusion

iCCA, pCCA, and dCCA vary in their presentation, natural history, and therapeutic approach to management. Though surgical resection and LT are the definitive treatments for operable cases, they remain a choice for only a small proportion of patients. Various systemic therapy agents and combinations of systemic therapy with radiation have shown improvement in survival in patients with CCA. Genomic analysis and testing has opened up the arena for research and development of biomarker-driven trials. Locoregional options, including TACE, Y90, and ablation help local control of disease. A multidisciplinary approach with a collaboration of various specialists including hepatobiliary surgeons, medical and surgical oncologists, and radiation oncologists has changed the landscape of the management and outcomes of this unique malignancy. A coordinated approach is necessary given the high risk of recurrence and poor prognosis in operable cases, hence the need for close monitoring and surveillance protocols. There remains a need to explore various combination regimens and modalities in prospective trials looking at tailored therapy based on genomic sequencing and combination therapies.

REFERENCES

1. Saha SK, Zhu AX, Fuchs CS, Brooks GA. Forty-year trends in cholangiocarcinoma incidence in the U.S.: intrahepatic disease on the rise. *Oncologist*. 2016;21(5):594–599.
2. Banales JM, Cardinale V, Carpino G, et al. Expert consensus document: cholangiocarcinoma: current knowledge and future perspectives consensus statement from the European Network for the Study of Cholangiocarcinoma (ENS-CCA). *Nat Rev Gastroenterol Hepatol*. 2016;13(5):261–280.
3. Nakeeb A, Pitt HA, Sohn TA, et al. Cholangiocarcinoma. A spectrum of intrahepatic, perihilar, and distal tumors. *Ann Surg*. 1996;224(4):463–473.
4. Yamasaki S. Intrahepatic cholangiocarcinoma: macroscopic type and stage classification. *J Hepatobiliary Pancreat Surg*. 2003;10(4):288–291.
5. Razumilava N, Gores GJ. Cholangiocarcinoma. *Lancet*. 2014;383(9935):2168–2179.
6. Welzel TM, Graubard BI, El-Serag HB, et al. Risk factors for intrahepatic and extrahepatic cholangiocarcinoma in the United States: a population-based case-control study. *Clin Gastroenterol Hepatol*. 2007;5(10):1221–1228.
7. Tyson GL, El-Serag HB. Risk factors for cholangiocarcinoma. *Hepatology*. 2011;54(1):173–184.
8. Burak K, Angulo P, Pasha TM, Egan K, Petz J, Lindor KD. Incidence and risk factors for cholangiocarcinoma in primary sclerosing cholangitis. *Am J Gastroenterol*. 2004;99(3):523–526.
9. Kinoshita M, Kubo S, Tanaka S, et al. The association between non-alcoholic steatohepatitis and intrahepatic cholangiocarcinoma: a hospital based case-control study. *J Surg Oncol*. 2016;113(7):779–783.
10. Lazaridis KN, Gores GJ. Cholangiocarcinoma. *Gastroenterology*. 2005;128(6):1655–1667.
11. Rimola J, Forner A, Reig M, et al. Cholangiocarcinoma in cirrhosis: absence of contrast washout in delayed phases by magnetic resonance imaging avoids misdiagnosis of hepatocellular carcinoma. *Hepatology*. 2009;50(3):791–798.
12. Vilgrain V. Staging cholangiocarcinoma by imaging studies. *HPB (Oxford)*. 2008;10(2):106–109.
13. Sapisochin G, Fidelman N, Roberts JP, Yao FY. Mixed hepatocellular cholangiocarcinoma and intrahepatic cholangiocarcinoma in patients undergoing transplantation for hepatocellular carcinoma. *Liver Transpl*. 2011;17(8):934–942.
14. Rana A, Hong JC. Orthotopic liver transplantation in combination with neoadjuvant therapy: a new paradigm in the treatment of unresectable intrahepatic cholangiocarcinoma. *Curr Opin Gastroenterol*. 2012;28(3):258–265.
15. Blechacz B, Komuta M, Roskams T, Gores GJ. Clinical diagnosis and staging of cholangiocarcinoma. *Nat Rev Gastroenterol Hepatol*. 2011;8(9):512–522.
16. Patel AH, Harnois DM, Klee GG, LaRusso NF, Gores GJ. The utility of CA 19-9 in the diagnoses of cholangiocarcinoma in patients without primary sclerosing cholangitis. *Am J Gastroenterol*. 2000;95(1):204–207.
17. Endo I, Gonen M, Yopp AC, et al. Intrahepatic cholangiocarcinoma: rising frequency, improved survival, and determinants of outcome after resection. *Ann Surg*. 2008;248(1):84–96.
18. Stieber AC, Marino IR, Iwatsuki S, Starzl TE. Cholangiocarcinoma in sclerosing cholangitis. The role of liver transplantation. *Int Surg*. 1989;74(1):1–3.
19. Meyer CG, Penn I, James L. Liver transplantation for cholangiocarcinoma: results in 207 patients. *Transplantation*. 2000;69(8):1633–1637.
20. Ghali P, Marotta PJ, Yoshida EM, et al. Liver transplantation for incidental cholangiocarcinoma: analysis of the Canadian experience. *Liver Transpl*. 2005;11(11):1412–1416.
21. Sapisochin G, Facciuto M, Rubbia-Brandt L, et al. Liver transplantation for 'very early' intrahepatic cholangiocarcinoma: international retrospective study supporting a prospective assessment. *Hepatology*. 2016;64(4):1178–1188.
22. Goss JA, Shackleton CR, Farmer DG, et al. Orthotopic liver transplantation for primary sclerosing cholangitis. A 12-year single center experience. *Ann Surg*. 1997;225(5):472–481.
23. Hong JC, Jones CM, Duffy JP, et al. Comparative analysis of resection and liver transplantation for intrahepatic and hilar cholangiocarcinoma: a 24-year experience in a single center. *Arch Surg*. 2011;146(6):683–689.
24. Gupta R, Togashi J, Akamatsu N, Sakamoto Y, Kokudo N. Impact of incidental/misdiagnosed intrahepatic cholangiocarcinoma and combined hepatocellular cholangiocarcinoma on the outcomes of liver transplantation: an institutional case series and literature review. *Surg Today*. 2017;47(8):908–917.
25. Lunsford KE, Javle M, Heyne K, et al. Liver transplantation for locally advanced intrahepatic cholangiocarcinoma treated with neoadjuvant therapy: a prospective case-series. *Lancet Gastroenterol Hepatol*. 2018;3(5):337–348.
26. Shroff RT, Kennedy EB, Bachini M, et al. Adjuvant therapy for resected biliary tract cancer: ASCO clinical practice guideline. *J Clin Oncol*. 2019;37(12):1015–1027.
27. Primrose JN, Fox RP, Palmer DH, et al. Capecitabine compared with observation in resected biliary tract cancer (BILCAP): a randomised, controlled, multicentre, phase 3 study. *Lancet Oncol*. 2019;20(5):663–673.

28. Valle J, Wasan H, Palmer DH, et al. Cisplatin plus gemcitabine versus gemcitabine for biliary tract cancer. *N Engl J Med.* 2010;**362**(14):1273–1281.
29. Eckmann KR, Patel DK, Landgraf A, et al. Chemotherapy outcomes for the treatment of unresectable intrahepatic and hilar cholangiocarcinoma: a retrospective analysis. *Gastrointest Cancer Res.* 2011;**4**(5–6):155–160.
30. Lee J, Park SH, Chang HM, et al. Gemcitabine and oxaliplatin with or without erlotinib in advanced biliary-tract cancer: a multicentre, open-label, randomised, phase 3 study. *Lancet Oncol.* 2012;**13**(2):181–188.
31. Fiteni F, Jary M, Monnien F, et al. Advanced biliary tract carcinomas: a retrospective multicenter analysis of first and second-line chemotherapy. *BMC Gastroenterol.* 2014;**14**:143.
32. Edeline J, Benabdelghani M, Bertaut A, et al. Gemcitabine and oxaliplatin chemotherapy or surveillance in resected biliary tract cancer (PRODIGE 12-ACCORD 18-UNICANCER GI): a randomized phase III study. *J Clin Oncol.* 2019;**37**(8):658–667.
33. Lamarca A, Ross P, Wasan HS, et al. Advanced intrahepatic cholangiocarcinoma: post hoc analysis of the ABC-01, -02, and -03 clinical trials. *J Natl Cancer Inst.* 2020;**112**(2):200–210.
34. Abou-Alfa GK, Sahai V, Hollebecque A, et al. Pemigatinib for previously treated, locally advanced or metastatic cholangiocarcinoma: a multicentre, open-label, phase 2 study. *Lancet Oncol.* 2020;**21**(5):671–684.
35. Hoy SM. Pemigatinib: first approval. *Drugs.* 2020;**80**(9):923–929.
36. Kipp BR, Voss JS, Kerr SE, et al. Isocitrate dehydrogenase 1 and 2 mutations in cholangiocarcinoma. *Hum Pathol.* 2012;**43**(10):1552–1558.
37. Borger DR, Tanabe KK, Fan KC, et al. Frequent mutation of isocitrate dehydrogenase (IDH)1 and IDH2 in cholangiocarcinoma identified through broad-based tumor genotyping. *Oncologist.* 2012;**17**(1):72–79.
38. Abou-Alfa GK, Macarulla T, Javle MM, et al. Ivosidenib in IDH1-mutant, chemotherapy-refractory cholangiocarcinoma (ClarIDHy): a multicentre, randomised, double-blind, placebo-controlled, phase 3 study [published correction appears in Lancet Oncol. 2020;21(10):e462]. *Lancet Oncol.* 2020;21(6):796–807.
39. Postow MA, Callahan MK, Wolchok JD. Immune checkpoint blockade in cancer therapy. *J Clin Oncol.* 2015;**33**(17):1974–1982.
40. Sahai V, Griffith KA, Beg MS, et al. A randomized phase 2 trial of nivolumab, gemcitabine, and cisplatin or nivolumab and ipilimumab in previously untreated advanced biliary cancer: BilT-01. Cancer. 2022;**128**(19):3523–3530.
41. Klein O, Kee D, Nagrial A, et al. Evaluation of combination nivolumab and ipilimumab immunotherapy in patients with advanced biliary tract cancers: subgroup analysis of a phase 2 nonrandomized clinical trial. JAMA Oncol. 2020;**6**(9):1405–1409.
42. Monge C, Pehrsson EC, Xie C, et al. A phase II Study of pembrolizumab in combination with capecitabine and oxaliplatin with molecular profiling in patients with advanced biliary tract carcinoma. *Oncologist.* 2022;**27**(3):e273–e285.
43. Marabelle A, Le DT, Ascierto PA, et al. Efficacy of pembrolizumab in patients with noncolorectal high microsatellite instability/mismatch repair-deficient cancer: results from the phase II KEYNOTE-158 Study. *J Clin Oncol.* **2020**;38(1):1–10.
44. Oh DY, Lee KH, Lee DW, et al. Gemcitabine and cisplatin plus durvalumab with or without tremelimumab in chemotherapy-naive patients with advanced biliary tract cancer: an open-label, single-centre, phase 2 study. *Lancet Gastroenterol Hepatol.* 2022;**7**(6):522–532.
45. Savic LJ, Chapiro J, Geschwind JH. Intra-arterial embolotherapy for intrahepatic cholangiocarcinoma: update and future prospects. *Hepatobiliary Surg Nutr.* 2017;**6**(1):7–21.
46. Scheuermann U, Kaths JM, Heise M, et al. Comparison of resection and transarterial chemoembolisation in the treatment of advanced intrahepatic cholangiocarcinoma—a single-center experience. *Eur J Surg Oncol.* 2013;**39**(6):593–600.
47. Chakravarty R, Dash A, Pillai MR. Availability of yttrium-90 from strontium-90: a nuclear medicine perspective. *Cancer Biother Radiopharm.* 2012;**27**(10):621–641.
48. Veeze-Kuijpers B, Meerwaldt JH, Lameris JS, van Blankenstein M, van Putten WL, Terpstra OT. The role of radiotherapy in the treatment of bile duct carcinoma. *Int J Radiat Oncol Biol Phys.* 1990;**18**(1):63–67.
49. Al-Adra DP, Gill RS, Axford SJ, Shi X, Kneteman N, Liau SS. Treatment of unresectable intrahepatic cholangiocarcinoma with yttrium-90 radioembolization: a systematic review and pooled analysis. *Eur J Surg Oncol.* 2015;**41**(1):120–127.
50. Shinohara ET, Mitra N, Guo M, Metz JM. Radiation therapy is associated with improved survival in the adjuvant and definitive treatment of intrahepatic cholangiocarcinoma. *Int J Radiat Oncol Biol Phys.* 2008;**72**(5):1495–1501.
51. Kim YI, Park JW, Kim BH, et al. Outcomes of concurrent chemoradiotherapy versus chemotherapy alone for advanced-stage unresectable intrahepatic cholangiocarcinoma. *Radiat Oncol.* 2013;**8**:292.
52. Tao R, Krishnan S, Bhosale PR, et al. Ablative radiotherapy doses lead to a substantial prolongation of survival in patients with inoperable intrahepatic cholangiocarcinoma: a retrospective dose response analysis. *J Clin Oncol.* 2016;**34**(3):219–226.
53. Hong TS, Wo JY, Yeap BY, et al. Multi-institutional phase II study of high-dose hypofractionated proton beam therapy in patients with localized, unresectable hepatocellular carcinoma and intrahepatic cholangiocarcinoma. *J Clin Oncol.* 2016;**34**(5):460–468.
54. Ohkawa A, Mizumoto M, Ishikawa H, et al. Proton beam therapy for unresectable intrahepatic cholangiocarcinoma. *J Gastroenterol Hepatol.* 2015;**30**(5):957–963.
55. Yoshioka Y, Ogawa K, Oikawa H, et al. Impact of intraluminal brachytherapy on survival outcome for radiation therapy for unresectable biliary tract cancer: a propensity-score matched-pair analysis. *Int J Radiat Oncol Biol Phys.* 2014;**89**(4):822–829.
56. Aloia TA, Charnsangavej C, Faria S, et al. High-resolution computed tomography accurately predicts resectability in hilar cholangiocarcinoma. *Am J Surg.* 2007;**193**(6):702–706.
57. Ruys AT, van Beem BE, Engelbrecht MR, Bipat S, Stoker J, Van Gulik TM. Radiological staging in patients with hilar cholangiocarcinoma: a systematic review and meta-analysis. *Br J Radiol.* 2012;**85**(1017):1255–1262.
58. Mollica MP, Mattace Raso G, Cavaliere G, et al. Butyrate regulates liver mitochondrial function, efficiency, and dynamics in insulin-resistant obese mice. *Diabetes.* 2017;**66**(5):1405–1418.
59. Navaneethan U, Njei B, Lourdusamy V, Konjeti R, Vargo JJ, Parsi MA. Comparative effectiveness of biliary brush cytology and intraductal biopsy for detection of malignant biliary strictures: a systematic review and meta-analysis. *Gastrointest Endosc.* 2015;**81**(1):168–176.
60. Gonda TA, Glick MP, Sethi A, et al. Polysomy and p16 deletion by fluorescence in situ hybridization in the diagnosis of indeterminate biliary strictures. *Gastrointest Endosc.* 2012;**75**(1):74–79.

61. Heimbach JK, Sanchez W, Rosen CB, Gores GJ. Trans-peritoneal fine needle aspiration biopsy of hilar cholangiocarcinoma is associated with disease dissemination. *HPB (Oxford)*. 2011;**13**(5):356–360.
62. De Vreede I, Steers JL, Burch PA, et al. Prolonged disease-free survival after orthotopic liver transplantation plus adjuvant chemoirradiation for cholangiocarcinoma. *Liver Transpl*. 2000;**6**(3):309–316.
63. Wong M, Kim J, George B, et al. Downstaging locally advanced cholangiocarcinoma pre-liver transplantation: a prospective pilot study. *J Surg Res*. 2019;**242**:23–30.
64. Duignan S, Maguire D, Ravichand CS, et al. Neoadjuvant chemoradiotherapy followed by liver transplantation for unresectable cholangiocarcinoma: a single-centre national experience. *HPB (Oxford)*. 2014;**16**(1):91–98.
65. Darwish Murad S, Kim WR, Harnois DM, et al. Efficacy of neoadjuvant chemoradiation, followed by liver transplantation, for perihilar cholangiocarcinoma at 12 US centers. *Gastroenterology*. 2012;**143**(1):88–98.
66. Heimbach JK. Successful liver transplantation for hilar cholangiocarcinoma. *Curr Opin Gastroenterol*. 2008;**24**(3):384–388.
67. DeOliveira ML, Cunningham SC, Cameron JL, et al. Cholangiocarcinoma: thirty-one-year experience with 564 patients at a single institution. *Ann Surg*. 2007;**245**(5):755–762.
68. Wellner UF, Shen Y, Keck T, Jin W, Xu Z. The survival outcome and prognostic factors for distal cholangiocarcinoma following surgical resection: a meta-analysis for the 5-year survival. *Surg Today*. 2017;**47**(3):271–279.
69. Moureau-Zabotto L, Turrini O, Resbeut M, et al. Impact of radiotherapy in the management of locally advanced extrahepatic cholangiocarcinoma. *BMC Cancer*. 2013;**13**:568.
70. Autorino R, Mattiucci GC, Ardito F, et al. Radiochemotherapy with gemcitabine in unresectable extrahepatic cholangiocarcinoma: long-term results of a phase II study. *Anticancer Res*. 2016;**36**(2):737–740.
71. Mahadevan A, Dagoglu N, Mancias J, et al. Stereotactic body radiotherapy (SBRT) for intrahepatic and hilar cholangiocarcinoma. *J Cancer*. 2015;**6**(11):1099–1104.
72. Barney BM, Olivier KR, Miller RC, Haddock MG. Clinical outcomes and toxicity using stereotactic body radiotherapy (SBRT) for advanced cholangiocarcinoma. *Radiat Oncol*. 2012;**7**:67.

37

Biliary atresia

Priya Ramachandran

Introduction

Biliary atresia (BA) is a progressive obstructive cholangiopathy which affects the biliary tract in infants causing cholestasis and ultimately cirrhosis. If left untreated, it is fatal, leading to end-stage liver disease requiring liver transplantation (LT). It is a complex disease with a multifactorial aetiology. It is also an unusual disease where the pathological processes may progress even after the initial operation. But with a sequential treatment strategy of a Kasai portoenterostomy (KPE) followed by LT if necessary, a survival of about 90% has been achieved for BA. In the last decade, great inroads have been made in the field of paediatric LT and this has been largely responsible for the high survival rates in these children. However, the quest to identify alternate treatment strategies to reduce the overall morbidity of treatment is by no means over. Challenges which remain include identifying a final common pathway in its pathogenesis which can be pharmacologically targeted to halt and maybe even reverse disease progression. It is also important to identify genetic mutations which cause disease susceptibility with a view to correcting them and preventing the disease altogether. Reversal of the disease process by blocking key pathways has been achieved to some extent in the animal model.[1]

It is important to study and assimilate the current knowledge available on the various aspects of this disease such as its aetiopathogenesis, modalities for early diagnosis, and available treatment options as well as contemplate on futuristic therapies which might make a great difference to the life of these children. It must be mentioned that the disease incidence varies from 1:12,000 live births in North America to as high as 1:3000 live births in East Asia.[2] Hence, finding alternative and less expensive treatment strategies will largely benefit countries which have difficulty coping with the financial burden of LT.

Aetiopathogenesis

The aetiologies proposed for BA include viruses and environmental toxins.[3] Also there is evidence to show that the disease begins *in utero* because of a recent study in which some infants who had a raised conjugated bilirubin level at birth went on to be diagnosed with BA.[3] Therefore it is logical to presume that the liver is affected in the prenatal period by an insult that spares the mother.[3] This insult leads to a cascade of events that includes activation of the immune system. There is also sufficient evidence to show that BA affects genetically susceptible livers.[3] BA occurs only in fetuses and neonates. This time-restricted onset is probably related to the developmental stage of the biliary tract which makes it susceptible to injury.

The only known environmental toxin is biliatresone which is a plant flavinoid that selectively damages extrahepatic bile ducts in experimental models.[3] It is not ingested by humans and is unlikely to cause human BA.[3] However, viruses seem to play a significant role in disease aetiology as evidenced by several studies and deserve close study.

Viral vectors

The morphology of BA was replicated in animal models using cytomegalovirus (CMV) and rotavirus.[2] Although CMV, which is a member of the Herpesviridae family, has a seroprevalence of up to 1–5% in some areas, congenital infections occur in susceptible infants who are premature or immunocompromised. Postnatal CMV is ideally diagnosed within 3 weeks of life to identify congenital infection.[2] Several studies have explored the link between CMV positivity (by polymerase chain reaction (PCR)) and BA. In some of these studies, there is evidence that CMV seropositivity is higher in neonates than mothers and that CMV+ patients were 10–15 days older than CMV− patients at the time of KPE.[2] Therefore it is possible that BA may be secondary to an acquired perinatal CMV infection. Davenport et al. assigned these children into a separate subgroup who had a higher total bilirubin, higher aspartate aminotransferase to platelet index (APRI), and less likelihood of clearing jaundice.[4] In addition to the higher APRI, there was evidence of increased inflammation and fibrosis in the liver on the abdominal ultrasonogram. Although CMV+ has been diagnosed on the basis of CMV immunoglobulin positivity (IgM+), PCR+/pp65+ (CMV immune-dominant phosphoprotein) on liver biopsy is more accurate and unlikely to be falsely negative.[3] CMV+ infants also had a higher incidence of cholangitis after KPE.[3]

Rotavirus which commonly causes gastroenteritis has been investigated for prevalence in BA.[3] Rotavirus A had a prevalence of 0–15% and rotavirus C had a prevalence of 40% in BA but the prevalence was also high in the control group.[3] There is a vaccine for rotavirus and this may affect both prevalence and infection rates. The rhesus rotavirus model (RRV) has been extensively used to study BA and receptors for this virus have been identified in the biliary epithelium.[5] Hence liver tissue testing may provide an additional means of testing for the virus. But diversity among rotaviral strains increases the potential for false positives.[2]

Although studies have explored the role of Epstein–Barr virus and reovirus, there is no conclusive proof of their involvement in BA.[2]

There are limitations to the use of both antibody testing and PCR in identifying viral strains. Also, other limitations which include tissue preservation methods and lack of control groups among the various studies of viruses involved in BA make it difficult to draw conclusions except with regard to CMV+ BA.[2]

Genetic predisposition

Although no single gene has been identified as the cause of BA, multiple genes may play a role in the origin of the disease process and its progression. A high prevalence of a single nucleotide polymorphism has been identified upstream of *ADD3* in a genome-wide association study of a large cohort of Chinese infants.[6] *ADD3* encodes the F-actin binding protein adducin.[6] Although its relevance is not known, the differential expression of *ADD3* in affected livers probably makes it a prime player in disease susceptibility or progression.

In a gene expression analysis of the human liver, a genetic footprint was identified in which genes involved in T-helper (Th)-1 cell response were activated at an early stage of BA with a transient suppression of humoral immunity.[7] The human transcriptome has also been investigated using next-generation sequencing techniques to identify candidate genes that have a high accuracy in the diagnosis of BA. A large number of genes have been identified, some of which are related to inflammation and immunity pathways.[8] Variations in the human glutathione metabolism genes have a potential to cause biliary injury.[9]

Genetic defects may also play a role in non-hepatic anomalies involving the spleen, heart, and intestinal rotation and laterality defects.[5] Whole-exome sequencing of biliary atresia–splenic malformation (*BASM*) syndrome trios (patient and parents) revealed *PKD1L1* variants which produce abnormalities in ciliary function which may contribute to disease susceptibility.[10]

Recently, *MMP7* (matrix metalloproteinase 7) has been featured as a lead biomarker in the serum of infants with BA.[1] *MMP7* expression was increased in the liver and intrahepatic cholangiocytes in BA. Also, transcriptome profiling of the liver in BA has shown that *MMP7* expression is related to the outcome of KPE thereby implying a role for this gene in the progression of disease.[11]

A sequential variation in the candidate genes for T-regulatory (Treg) cells results in their functional immaturity making the liver susceptible to injury by mechanisms detailed below.[5]

Developmental immaturity of the biliary tract

Bile flow reaches the intestine at around 75–85 days of life.[10] The intrahepatic bile ducts arise from a different endoderm than the extrahepatic bile ducts. Cholangiocytes are protected by an apical glycocalyx with a bicarbonate umbrella. Immaturity in the cholangiocyte glycocalyx makes it susceptible to injury which results in bile leakage in neonates. The submucosa in the neonates also lacks the collagen buttress hence making it possible for bile leaks to spread rapidly. This data from the experimental mouse model needs to be validated in human bile ducts to confirm its relevance.[10]

Pathogenic pathways

The innate immune system mounts an immediate response when triggered by a pathogen unlike the adaptive immune response which takes days, sometimes weeks, to respond.[2] The activation of the innate immune system in response to viral vectors in experimental BA leads to the release of proinflammatory cytokines such as tumour necrosis factor alpha (TNFα) and interleukin (IL)-1 and -6.[2] In addition, macrophages, dendritic cells, and natural killer (NK) cells are also activated.[2] The Toll-like receptors (TLR) on these cells recognize the pathogens displayed on the biliary epithelium.[2] Failure to regulate TLR signalling leads to biliary apoptosis.[2] TNFα produced by macrophages also leads to the destruction of biliary epithelium.[2] CD 14 which is a surface glycoprotein on the macrophage recognizes the pathogen and activates TNFα release. NK cells also contribute to the damage of biliary cells by the exaggerated response of the innate immune system.

The response of the adaptive immune system involves effector T cells which may directly release cytokines or activate other immune cells.[2] In BA, effector T-cell response includes Th1 cells which induce the production of IL-2, interferon gamma (IFNγ), and TNFα and Th-17 cells which induce the production of IL-17.[2] IFNγ plays an important role in bile duct injury.[2] Th1 cells and macrophages are elevated in CMV+ BA and are believed to destroy intrahepatic bile ducts.[2] Th17 cells are found in increased numbers in the portal tracts of BA patients and correlate with serum bilirubin levels.[2] It is important to note that unlike Th1 cells, Th17 cells have not been associated with specific viral vectors and hence they may play a role in disease progression.[2] Experimentally, depletion of macrophages, dendritic cells, lymphocytes, and NK cells and inactivation of cytokines such as IL-8, IL-15, IFNγ, and TNFα prevent bile duct injury and maintain duct patency.[10] A transition from a type 1 immune response which is predominantly inflammatory to a mixed type 2 (Th12–Th17) response leads to ongoing liver injury and fibrosis.[10]

Type 2 cytokines such as IL-13, IL-33, and IL-4 have been isolated from the sera in human and experimental BA.[10] In the mouse RRV model, IL-13 induces cholangiocyte proliferation and in the liver IL-13 and IL-33 cause hepatic stellate cell activation from fat-storing cells to myofibroblasts. Th1 lymphocytes also seem to induce this activation.[10] Macrophages also play a role in fibrogenesis by transitioning from a M1 to M2 profile. Also, mediators such as IL-8, PDGF, CXCL1, TLR4, and transforming growth factor beta 1 (TGFβ1) which is a fibrogenic cytokine lead to the ongoing and excessive fibrosis in BA.[10] Hepatic stellate cell activation has been studied using alpha-smooth muscle actin expression.[12] This has positively correlated with stages of fibrosis in the liver thus validating the role of hepatic stellate cell activation in the progression of fibrosis in BA.[12,13] TGFβ1 decreased after successful KPE and the TGFβ superfamily has a role in mediating ongoing fibrosis after a successful KPE.[14]

CD4+ subsets of Treg cells are responsible for controlling T cell response and preventing 'bystander damage' of healthy cells near infected cells.[2] Bystander damage can be directly caused by CD4+ cells or by release of cytokines such as IFNγ, TNFα, lymphotoxin, and nitric oxide.[2] In the murine model, addition of normal Treg cells limits the damage to the bile duct epithelium.[2] Children who are CMV+

and rotavirus+ have significant reduction in Treg cells. All of this suggests that Treg cells may play a role in the pathogenesis of BA.[2]

In summary, exposure to potential environmental toxins and viruses leads to cholangiocyte injury which activates the innate immune system producing chemoattractants to myeloid cells and NK cells which amplify cholangiocyte injury.[5] This is followed by an adaptive immune response with the activation of CD8+ cells and expression of proinflammatory cytokines which target the epithelium and form a luminal plug along with other inflammatory cells.[5] This stops the flow of bile. This is followed by a fibrogenic type 2 immune response. After KPE, there is ongoing transhepatic biliary disease which is attributed to the production of autoantibodies by B cells targeting enolase and other antigens on the cholangiocyte surface.[5]

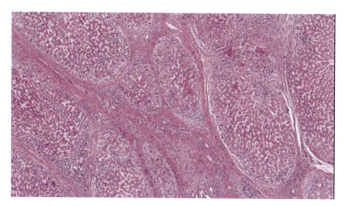

Figure 37.2 Biliary atresia with cirrhosis.

Pathology

The classic features of BA in the liver biopsy are portal tract expansion, ductular proliferation with anastomosing ductules, inflammatory infiltration, and varying degrees of fibrosis (Figure 37.1). Detailed histological studies of the remnants of the bile ducts have been reported with the ducts being replaced by dense fibrotic tissue with inflammatory cell infiltration. In some cases, the liver tissues show circumferential biliary ductular structures within the connective tissue of the portal vein which look like primitive ductular structures known as ductal plate malformations (DPMs). Due to the resemblance to DPMs, these are known as DPM-like arrays. The presence of these structures has been noted to be a poor prognostic factor.[15] Other histological findings identified are portal as well as septal polymorphonuclear and mononuclear inflammation, ductular cholestasis, cholangitis, bile cysts/lakes, foreign body type granulomas, hepatocytes rosetting, syncytial multinucleate giant cells, and hepatocyte ballooning degeneration (giant cell transformation). Extramedullary haematopoiesis is also seen in the liver. Fibrosis progresses with time from local to bridging and finally diffuse fibrosis and micronodular cirrhosis. Fibrosis is defined as mild (grade I), if it ranges from portal fibrous expansion to bridging fibrosis involving less than 50% of portal tracts; moderate (grade II), if bridging fibrosis is greater than 50%; and severe (grade III), if bridging fibrosis involves greater than 50% of portal tracts and is accompanied by nodular architecture (Figure 37.2).

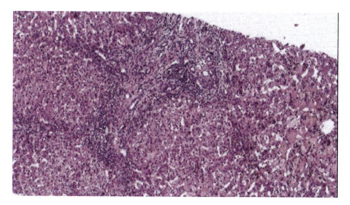

Figure 37.1 Biliary atresia with bridging fibrosis.

Types of biliary atresia

Anatomical classification

Ohi classified BA into three types (Figure 37.3): type 1 atresia of the common bile duct (10%), type II atresia of the hepatic ducts (2%), and type III atresia at the porta hepatis (88%).[16]

Phenotypic classification

In order to evaluate outcomes, it is useful to classify BA clinically as four distinct subtypes.[17] They are:

1. Syndromic BA (7–10%): this includes children with BASM who have laterality defects, splenic malformations, rotation anomalies, an absent retrohepatic cava and a preduodenal portal vein. This form is consistent with early bile duct injury.[5]
2. Cystic BA (8%): this presents with cystic changes in an otherwise obliterated extrahepatic biliary tract. The cystic variant is seen in about 5% of BA. Here, cystic changes are seen in some part of the extrahepatic bile ducts. The cysts may contain mucus or bile and need to be distinguished from congenital choledochal cysts which will be seen to be communicating with the intrahepatic biliary tree on operative cholangiography.
3. CMV-associated BA: here, the infants are CMV+ (IgM+ or PCR+/pp65+). The infection is probably acquired postnatally because they present later.
4. Isolated BA (80%): this is the commonest presentation and includes infants who do not fall into any of the other categories. There is no uniformity of presentation and the disease may be in different stages of progression in this group. A subgroup may have non-hepatic malformations such as cardiovascular abnormalities and intestinal malrotation.

Clinical features

Infants with BA present with jaundice, pale stools, and high-coloured urine. In most cases, there is normal passage of meconium at birth. This may even be followed by passage of pigmented stools in some children with a gradual progression to acholic stools. Some neonates who were considered to have physiological jaundice in the first 14 days of life progress seamlessly to present with conjugated bilirubinaemia later, without having a jaundice-free interval.

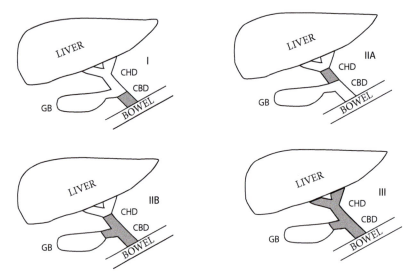

Figure 37.3 Types of biliary atresia. CBD, common bile duct; CHD, common hepatic duct; GB, gall bladder.

Children with BA are generally well nourished and initial clinical examination is unremarkable except for hepatomegaly. With time, the liver becomes hard, the spleen enlarges, and there is onset of ascites. These are signs of advanced liver disease. Without treatment, BA progresses from obstructive jaundice in an otherwise thriving infant to end-stage liver disease and death within 2 years.

Diagnosis

BA must be suspected in all neonates in whom jaundice persists after the first 14 days of life (period of physiological hyperbilirubinaemia). Jaundice is the only symptom in the neonatal age group and hence diagnosis is delayed due to failure to differentiate jaundice due to liver disease from physiological jaundice. Delay in diagnosis is unfortunate since treatment is most effective in this age group (before 30 days of life).

Delay in referral to a specialist centre is because of difficulties in differentiating BA from physiological jaundice and identifying an abnormal stool colour. This is a major problem in developing countries like India, where only 20% of infants are less than 60 days old at presentation.[18] It is vitally important to identify abnormal stool colour and investigate infants in whom pale stools persist for 3 consecutive days. Stool cards, effectively used for screening in Taiwan and Japan, are an economical and practical tool.[19,20]

Since there is no single test available to diagnose BA, a combination of biochemical, radiological, and histological tests are used.

Biochemical tests

A raised serum total bilirubin level with a high conjugated fraction (>50% of the total) with some elevation of transaminases is usually present. However, these findings are common to most forms of neonatal cholestasis. A raised gamma glutamyl transferase level has a high specificity, and is often used to differentiate BA from neonatal hepatitis. There may be an initial coagulopathy with a high international normalized ratio which is responsive to vitamin K injections. Persistent coagulopathy and hypoalbuminaemia are features of advanced disease and signify synthetic dysfunction of the liver.

Perinatal infections that mimic BA can be ruled out by TORCH screening to identify toxoplasmosis, other viruses, rubella, CMV, and herpes simplex virus.

There is a role for next-generation sequencing in the diagnostic algorithm for neonatal cholestasis. This can be used to identify multiple genes and enables a rapid and accurate diagnosis for several disorders.[21]

Radiological tests

Ultrasonogram

The ultrasonogram is used to assess the hepatic architecture, hepatic vasculature, intra- or extrahepatic biliary ductular dilation, and to look for the presence of a gall bladder. The gall bladder in infants is best imaged in the fasting state. More specifically, ultrasound in BA has been used in specialist centres to diagnose the disease with a high degree of sensitivity, specificity, and diagnostic accuracy.[22] The triangular cord sign (which measures the thickness of the fibrotic portal plate), the gall bladder classification, gall bladder length-to-width ratio (LTWR), and hepatic artery and portal vein diameter were studied for their respective sensitivity and specificity in the diagnosis of BA. The fibrotic cord thickness is a measure of the echogenic anterior wall of the anterior branch of right portal vein just distal to the right portal vein without including the right hepatic artery. A normal gall bladder was shown to have a globular or ovoid shape without wall irregularities. An abnormal gall bladder had an irregular lumen and wall outline. The gall bladder classification was as follows:

- Type 1: gall bladder not detected.
- Type 2: gall bladder detected with no lumen, smooth outline, completely or incompletely filled with smooth hyperechogenic mucosal lining.
- Type 3: gall bladder detected with fully filled lumen and lumen length equal to or less than 1.5 cm without wall thickening.
- Type 4: gall bladder detected with fully filled lumen and lumen length more than 1.5 cm without wall thickening.

The LTWR in all type 2, 3, and 4 gall bladders was significantly higher in infants with BA. This study reported that the fibrotic cord thickness was significantly higher in infants with BA and had a specificity of 96%. However, the greatest sensitivity (72%) was the gall bladder LTWR of greater than 4.[1]

Recently, the size of the perihilar lymph nodes and ultrasound shear wave elastography have all been reported to be highly accurate in the diagnosis of BA.[23,24]

A recent study showed that ultrasound shear wave elastography combined with gamma glutamyl transferase levels could distinguish BA from other causes of neonatal cholestasis.[24]

Ultrasonography is also useful in identifying cystic BA and differentiating it from choledochal cysts.

Radionucleotide scintigraphy

The hydroxy iminodiacetic acid (HIDA) scan has a high sensitivity but poor specificity in differentiating BA from other causes of neonatal cholestasis. It requires pretreatment with phenobarbitone for 3–5 days prior to the scan and repeated imaging for up to 24 hours to look for isotope activity in the gut, which may be due to delayed excretion from the liver in cases of advanced liver disease. The technetium-labelled diisopropyl iminodiacetic acid (DISIDA) is more effective in the presence of high bilirubin levels, but is still susceptible to interpretation errors.

The presence of isotope activity in the intestine excludes BA, but the absence of such activity is not diagnostic of BA. Hence, this investigation has limited usefulness and is not recommended because it further delays the diagnosis.

Endoscopic retrograde cholangiopancreatography (ERCP)

ERCP is technically difficult in small infants. However, with the advent of more sophisticated endoscopes, ERCP can be performed as a less invasive alternative to an operative cholangiogram. But ERCP is not routinely performed because of the need for sedation in these infants and also because results are operator dependent. Magnetic resonance cholangiopancreatography is also accurate in the diagnosis of BA, but this is not a cost-effective test.

Liver biopsy

Portal tract expansion with oedematous fibroplasia and proliferation of anastomosing ductules is pathognomonic of BA on a percutaneous liver biopsy. If reported by an experienced pathologist, this investigation is highly accurate. The diagnostic accuracy of the percutaneous needle biopsy was estimated to be 90% with a sensitivity and specificity of 88% and 93%, respectively.[25] Therefore, in countries where the care of these children is not centralized, relying on a liver biopsy to make a conclusive diagnosis may result in a significant number of false negatives. Several portal tracts have to be examined and BA has to be differentiated from non-obstructive cholestasis. In addition to portal tract expansion and ductular proliferation, the presence of bile plugs offers further evidence of BA.

Operative cholangiography

The gold standard for the diagnosis of BA is an operative cholangiogram which has a diagnostic accuracy of 100%. The procedure involves injecting radio-opaque contrast into the gall bladder remnant through a small laparotomy. A diagnosis of BA is made if contrast does not fill the common hepatic duct and intrahepatic ducts. It is important to differentiate BA from the hypoplastic ducts seen in Alagille syndrome, thereby avoiding a potentially damaging and unnecessary operation in the latter.

The operative cholangiogram is performed by placing a stay suture in the gall bladder and exerting traction on it to enable the placement of an angiocath or, size permitting, a small infant feeding tube. Under fluoroscopy, contrast (Gastrografin) is diluted 1:1 with normal saline and gently injected. The flow of contrast is observed and the opacification of the bile ducts at the porta precludes a diagnosis of BA. If the pathways are occluded as in BA, the contrast will leak externally and the surgeon proceeds with a KPE. If the gall bladder and common bile duct are patent, there may be a free flow of bile distally into the duodenum. The common bile duct is then occluded with a soft bulldog clamp and contrast is injected to determine if there is flow into the intrahepatic bile ducts. If these ducts cannot also be delineated, the surgeon proceeds with a KPE.

Management

The management involves a sequential strategy combining KPE as the first-line and LT as the second-line treatment, if the portoenterostomy fails to establish bile flow and/or there is progressive liver disease. The focus of the Kasai operation is to obtain adequate exposure of the porta hepatis and to excise the atretic portal plate up to the level of the Glisson's capsule to establish bile flow from the patent ductules in the porta hepatis into an intestinal conduit. The presence of synthetic liver disease is the only contraindication for a KPE. The presence of ascites, hypoalbuminaemia, and a prolonged international normalized ratio which cannot be corrected by vitamin K injections are signs of liver decompensation. In such cases the Kasai operation is not performed because it can lead to worsening of liver disease and the patient is referred for LT. These signs are usually present in some older children with BA, but rarely can be seen in infants younger than 90 days. As such, it is clear that older age alone is not an absolute cut-off for KPE and it is important to carefully assess the patient and identify signs of liver failure in the absence of which the operation can be performed. Chardot reported jaundice clearance in a 141-day-old infant oldest child who underwent KPE and in Professor Kasai's own series, the survival with native liver (SNL) for infants aged 90–120 days at KPE was 19%.[26,27] Hence, there is a definite benefit in performing KPE in 'seniors' with BA.[28]

Preoperative preparation

The patient is admitted soon after the diagnosis is made and standard preoperative preparation is done which includes one dose of prophylactic intravenous antibiotic prior to surgery. If the coagulation profile is deranged, the patient is given three doses of vitamin K injection. In our centre, during anaesthesia, these children undergo placement of a central line for postoperative parenteral nutrition and an epidural catheter for analgesia.

Surgical technique

Although the standard approach is an open technique, a laparoscopic approach has also been described with a similar success rate. In the open operation, the patient is placed supine on the operating table and a small horizontal incision is made in the right supraumbilical region and the operative cholangiogram is performed through this incision if the gall bladder is present. In some cases, an atretic gall bladder may be seen in which case there is no need to perform the cholangiogram. Once the decision is made to proceed with the KPE, this incision is extended to the left and the underlying muscles are divided including both rectii. The abdominal cavity is inspected for features of BASM including rotational abnormalities of the gut. The liver is almost completely exteriorized by dividing the left triangular ligament. This gives good access to the porta hepatis. The gall bladder is dissected off the gall bladder fossa and the dissection is carried laterally down towards the remnant common bile duct which is divided at the duodenum and retracted up towards the porta. The hepatoduodenal ligament is divided to expose the hepatic artery and portal vein. Cautery is avoided in the dissection and division of the fibrotic elements of the hepatoduodenal ligament to avoid heat injury to microductules at the portal plate. First, the hepatic artery and its branches are exposed. The arterial anatomy is noted looking for replaced and accessory vessels. Special attention is paid to the right hepatic artery which is traced to its bifurcation in the porta. The anterior and posterior branches bifurcate at the right corner of the porta and the space between these vessels is the innominate fossa which is the normal site of entry of the right hepatic duct. Next, the main portal vein and its right and left branches are dissected and small branches from the right and left portal vein to the caudate lobe are carefully ligated and divided to enable the portal vein to be retracted inferiorly to expose the entire portal plate. The left branch of the portal vein is traced to its confluence with the umbilical vein in the Rex recess which is the point of entry of the normal left hepatic duct. To reach this point, it is sometimes necessary to divide the liver bridge which surrounds the umbilical ligament. Branches of the left portal vein to segment 4 can be seen and they mark the limit of dissection at the left corner of the portal plate (Figure 37.4). After retraction of the vessels inferiorly, the portal plate is excised using scissors in continuity with the atretic extrahepatic structures from the right corner (innominate fossa) to the left corner (Rex recess) and down to the Glisson's capsule. Bleeding is controlled by pressure with a surgical gauze soaked in saline adrenaline solution (1:100,000 dilution). Usually bile flow can be observed from the innominate fossa and near the Rex recess and these points must be included in the hepaticojejunostomy.

The next steps involve the creation of a 60 cm Roux loop of jejunum which is brought into the supracolic compartment through a retrocolic window. Biliary drainage is facilitated by an anastomosis extending from the bifurcation of the right hepatic artery into anterior and posterior branches to the Rex confluence of the left portal vein with the obliterated umbilical vein. The lateral-most sutures are placed beyond the presumed entry points of the right and left ducts to avoid damage to microductules. The posterior layer of sutures is placed first. Since the dissection exposes the vessels, some of these sutures can be placed on the adventitia of the artery. The anterior wall of the enterotomy is anchored to the liver parenchyma of the quadrate lobe. Thus, the hepaticojejunostomy forms a funnel around the portal plate. At the end of the operation, the proximal mesenteric defect is closed and the Roux loop is anchored to the defect in the transverse mesocolon to prevent internal bowel herniation. A liver biopsy is done.

Postoperative care

The postoperative care includes the administration of intravenous antibiotics, intravenous fluids, and nasogastric suction for 5 days. In our centre, we start total parenteral nutrition on the second postoperative day which is continued until the establishment of oral feeds on the 5th day. Our antibiotic of choice is piperacillin/tazobactam at a dose of 100 mg/kg four times a day continued for 7 days. In most centres which advocate steroid therapy, oral prednisolone is started on the 6th day after the establishment of oral feeds at a dose of 5 mg/kg, which is tapered weekly to 0.5 mg/kg over a duration of 6 weeks. Patients are discharged after 1 week. Chemoprophylaxis to prevent cholangitis may be given cyclically. In our centre, we use amoxycillin–clavulanic acid (40 mg/kg/day in two divided doses) and cefpodoxime (10 mg/kg/day in two divided doses). Also, fat-soluble vitamins, ursodeoxycholic acid, and formulas rich in medium-chain triglycerides are prescribed for 6–12 months. Bilirubin levels are monitored 1, 3, and 6 months after surgery. Jaundice clearance is defined as a serum direct bilirubin of less than 2 mg/dL in 6 months. A routine upper gastrointestinal endoscopy is performed after 1 year with or without variceal banding. Attention to nutrition in the early postoperative period and the use of special formulas in the long term with monitoring of weight gain, growth and nutritional parameters is important. Growth failure may be an indication for LT.

Complications

With centralization of care of children with BA, there has been a great improvement not only in the outcome of the Kasai operation but also in postoperative morbidity. Complications which occur in the long term are more a consequence of disease progression rather than the operation itself. However, perioperative complications have been reported to be higher in low gestational age patients but these did not impact outcome.[29]

Cholangitis

Postoperatively, the incidence of cholangitis has been reported to range between 40% and 93%.[30] It occurs frequently in the first

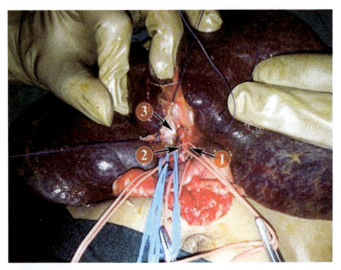

Figure 37.4 Operative photograph of the fibrotic portal plate after lowering of the hilar structures. 1: hepatic artery and branches. 2: portal vein and branches. 3: atretic portal plate.

2 years after the Kasai procedure.[31,32] Repeated attacks of cholangitis can worsen liver fibrosis and must be managed efficiently. Reflux of enteric contents into the biliary tree after hepaticojejunostomy, translocation of bacteria, portal venous infection, and inadequate lymphatic drainage at the porta have been attributed to cause cholangitis. Stasis or poor flow of bile in the newly opened drainage channels may also play a role. The pathogens involved include intestinal flora such as *Escherichia coli*, *Pseudomonas aeruginosa*, and *Enterobacter cloacae*.

Episodes of cholangitis are characterized by fever and pale stools. There may be signs of septicaemia and the C-reactive protein is elevated with leucocytosis and raised serum bilirubin and liver enzymes. However, sometimes fever may be the only symptom and there may be no growth on blood cultures.[30]

Treatment includes broad-spectrum antibiotics and intravenous fluids. Steroids and immunoglobulins have been used to reduce the inflammation and improve bile flow.

Routine use of prophylactic antibiotic regimens reduces the incidence of cholangitis as does a well-constructed Roux loop. Although construction of antireflux valves and revision of hepatic jejunostomy has been tried to prevent reflux of bile and improve drainage from the porta, the results have not been encouraging for these procedures.[33,34]

Portal hypertension

The reported incidence varies from 34% to 76% and patients sometimes present with ascites and variceal bleeding which can be severe and life-threatening.[34] Portal hypertension develops even after jaundice clearance is achieved by KPE and is a sequel of ongoing intrahepatic inflammation and fibrosis or recurrent cholangitis.

Hence surveillance endoscopy and prophylactic banding has been recommended on a yearly basis. This is done not only in the presence of worsening liver disease, but also in asymptomatic patients who have cleared jaundice. In case of massive variceal bleeding, endoscopy and sclerotherapy is performed. Octreotide and beta-blockers are also used to lower the portal pressure. LT is the only recourse for children with recurrent variceal bleeding that does not respond to conventional therapy even though they may not have end-stage liver disease. Hypersplenism due to portal hypertension can further complicate variceal bleeding because of thrombocytopenia. Although treatment options such as splenic embolization and portosystemic shunting have been recommended, LT offers the best solution to this problem.

Factors affecting the outcome of Kasai portoenterostomy

When Professor Kasai reported that his first patient cleared jaundice with a portoenterostomy, it gave new hope to children with BA all over the world.[35] This operation has stood the test of time and despite access to LT, it still remains the first treatment of choice for BA. It was thought initially that a prior KPE may complicate LT and increase the risk of postoperative infection, but a meta-analysis by Wang et al. showed that no major changes in clinical outcomes were observed following LT after a prior portoenterostomy and this had no effect on 1-year or 5-year patient and graft survival rates.[36]

The outcome of portoenterostomy has been correlated with a wide variety of factors:

Age

One of the frequently assessed factors is age at KPE. Earlier studies reported that KPE done at an early age was associated with successful bile drainage and survival with native liver (SNL).[37,38] In 2010, Nio et al. also reported that while age at KPE did have a beneficial effect on jaundice clearance, it did not affect SNL.[39] In 2017, the Japanese Biliary Atresia Registry showed that SNL was better if the KPE was performed within 30 days of birth. Between 30 and 90 days there was no difference in outcome and again if KPE was done after 90 days the outcome was worse.[40] Davenport et al. reported a 40% and 45% 5- and 10-year SNL in children who underwent KPE after 100 days of age and reiterated that age must not be used as a cut off to deny KPE for late presenters.[28] Other studies have shown that there is no association between age at KPE and outcome.[41-44] In a Chinese population-based study with a large number of patients, Qiao et al. showed that KPE after 90 days was associated with poor SNL.[45] There is also evidence to show that if done within the first 45 days of life, KPE is associated with SNL of 65.5% in 2 years and 40.5% in 15 years.[10] Hence, it is clear that some doubts still exist on the effect of age at KPE on jaundice clearance and survival and hence further studies with a larger number of patients is required to clarify the situation.

Bilirubin

Total serum bilirubin is a part of the Model for End-Stage Liver Disease (MELD) score and a high bilirubin indicates increased fibrosis in the liver. A 20% decrease in serum bilirubin on day 7 after portoenterostomy was an indicator of good outcome.[46] Total serum bile acids seems to be a more sensitive bile flow marker and may correlate with long-term outcomes more than the traditional serum bilirubin.[47]

Aspartate aminotransferase-to-platelet index

The APRI was described as an indicator to predict advanced liver fibrosis in chronic hepatitis.[48] In a series of 91 children, pre-KPE APRI score was significantly correlated with liver fibrosis and jaundice clearance after KPE. An APRI of 0.75-0.81 was able to predict significant fibrosis and cirrhosis.[49] This was contradicted by a report from Helsinki which showed no correlation between APRI and Ishak or Metavir scores.[50]

Type of Kasai portoenterostomy

Wada et al. reported their experience with three types of KPE: extended, modified, and laparoscopic. Jaundice clearance was significantly higher after laparoscopic PE.[51] We reported our experience with the extended KPE and this is still our procedure of choice.[52]

Steroids after Kasai portoenterostomy

The use of steroids after KPE is a matter of some dispute. Inflammation either after a viral infection or due to the perinatal leakage of bile leads to the cholangio-destructive pathogenesis of BA.[53] The inflammatory process continues postoperatively and cytokines such as TNFα are increased even after the postoperative period. Hence steroids were thought to be beneficial after KPE. However, the results of the START trial which tested the use of high-dose steroids versus placebo reported an overall non-significant increase in jaundice clearance 6 months after KPE.[54] In a study from King's College Hospital, London, patients were subdivided into cohorts based on age at KPE.[55] The outcome measured was SNL and jaundice clearance at 6 months. Age at KPE had a significant impact on the efficacy of high-dose steroids on the main clinical outcome of jaundice clearance. The authors concluded that the use of high-dose steroids was beneficial in reducing the postoperative bilirubin and that younger age at KPE improved the efficacy of adjuvant therapy. The usual side effects of wound dehiscence and susceptibility to infection is not common in children treated with high-dose steroids after BA.

Liver histology

Histological features such as size of DPM and liver fibrosis have been evaluated for their predictive potential on the outcome of KPE. It has been reported in several studies that the DPM was associated with poor jaundice clearance and SNL.[56,57] We reported in our series of patients who underwent LT for BA that the presence of DPM on explant liver biopsies correlated with a shorter SNL.[15] Sometimes, tissue available from liver biopsy may be inadequate to accurately identify DPM. Hepatic fibrosis has been reported to adversely affect the outcome of KPE and SNL.[56] Another study reported that extent of fibrosis did not correlate with bile flow after KPE.[43] Ductular size in the portal remnants has been shown to impact the outcome of KPE with improved jaundice clearance when the size is greater than 150 μm.[34]

Type of biliary atresia

The poor outcome of KPE in syndromic BA (BASM) has been reported.[58] Poor outcome has also been reported in CMV+ BA which is not treated with antiviral agents. In our centre, we test for CMV urinary PCR and treat with a 3-week course of valganciclovir which is stopped if the subsequent PCR is negative. The outcome of BA is worse in Ohi type 3 atresia compared to the other anatomical variants.[16]

Centralization of care

The England and Wales national study and the French national study reported that the outcome of KPE was better when performed in centres where the operation is performed frequently.[59,60] The highest rates for jaundice clearance and SNL were obtained in centres with the highest caseloads (20/year) as compared to other centers.[60] However, logistically this policy is difficult to implement in most parts of the world.

Genomics

Studies of gene expression in the liver has revealed several factors that play a role in the outcome of KPE. A recent study identified 14 gene expression patterns which were associated with SNL for 2 years.[61] mRNAs coding for proteins that regulate the fibrosis genes were increased in the liver of infants with SNL less than 2 years and mRNAs coding for proteins that regulate glutathione metabolism were increased in infants with longer SNL. The efficacy of N-acetylcysteine which is a precursor to glutathione has been studied for its efficacy in improving bile flow after KPE.[47] In addition to the diagnosis of BA, elevated serum MMP7 levels have been correlated with the need for LT.[62] Increased expression of MMP7 in the liver was also correlated with worse outcome of KPE.[63] This gene seems to reflect the severity of liver fibrosis and disease progression since there is an increase in expression in the liver at the time of transplant compared to the time of diagnosis.[11]

Immune response

Effector CD4+ cells is enhanced in unfavourable outcomes. Inducible T-cell co-stimulator (ICOS)– Treg cells had a protective effect whereas ICOS+ Treg cells were associated with a poor outcome.[64] Liver tissue scoring by histological features and gene expression profiling identified proinflammatory and profibrotic signatures which seem to indicate different stages of the disease with short SNL for patients with fibrotic signatures.[5]

Outcome of Kasai portoenterostomy

The recently published French national study reported that total jaundice clearance was 39%. SNL after KPE was 41% at 5 years and dropped to 22% at 30 years.[65]

Reports from the UK and North America show that at least half of the children will require LT by 2 years of age and ultimately more than 75% will require LT before 20 years of age.[10]

Overall, the patients who cleared jaundice fare well in the long term. The 5-year risk of death/LT reduces 1 year after a successful KPE which achieves stable liver function in the long term. A rapid clearance of jaundice, within 4 weeks of KPE, correlated with a better 5-year SNL.[66]

Some menstruation issues have been reported in adolescent children after KPE. These issues resolve after transplantation.[34] Portal hypertension and progression of liver disease has also been reported during gestation. Hence careful monitoring is recommended during pregnancy.[34]

Future therapies for biliary atresia

Among the anticholestatic and antifibrotic agents being tested in adult liver disease, obeticholic acid which suppress bile acid synthesis and stimulates anticholestatic adaptive responses and norursodeoxycholic acid which reduces cholangiocyte damage may be beneficial in BA.[10] Agents that diminish total bile acid flow through the cholestatic liver, reduce hepatic bile acid retention, and change its composition like the luminally restricted ASBT (ileal bile acid transporter) may also have a role to play.[10] Cenicriviroc is an antifibrotic agent which has improved fibrosis in non-alcoholic steatohepatitis and might benefit a subset of BA patients.[10]

Stem cell technology that drives the differentiation of circulating mononuclear cells and fibroblasts to hepatocytes and cholangiocytes, biliary organoids, and bile ducts generated from collagen-based scaffolds may provide models of human disease which will enable the development of therapies that strategically manipulate disease pathogenesis. These innovations also have the potential to evolve into a patient-specific biliary reconstruction technique.[10]

But for now, a well-performed Kasai operation followed by steroid therapy in the postoperative period and antiviral therapy in CMV+ patients is the best guarantor of outcome.[67] If this strategy fails, LT provides a rescue option for these patients.

REFERENCES

1. Lertudomphonwanit C, Mourya R, Fei L, et al. Large-scale proteomics identifies MMP-7 as a sentinel of epithelial injury and of biliary atresia. *Sci Transl Med*. 2017;**9**:417.
2. Averbukh LD, Wu GY. Evidence for viral induction of biliary atresia: a review. *J Clin Transl Hepatol*. 2018;**6**(4):410–419.
3. Wehrman A, Waisbourd-Zinman O, Wells RG. Recent advances in understanding biliary atresia. *F1000Res*. 2019;**8**:218.
4. Zani A, Quaglia A, Hadžić N, Zuckerman M, Davenport M. Cytomegalovirus-associated biliary atresia: an aetiological and prognostic subgroup. *J Pediatr Surg*. 2015;**50**(10):1739–1745.
5. Asai A, Miethke A, Bezerra JA. Pathogenesis of biliary atresia: defining biology to understand clinical phenotypes. *Nat Rev Gastroenterol Hepatol*. 2016;**12**(6):342–352.
6. Tsai EA. Replication of a GWAS signal in a Caucasian population implicates ADD3 in susceptibility to biliary atresia. *Hum Genet*. 2014;**133**(2):235–243.
7. Bezerra JA, Tiao G, Ryckman FC, et al. Genetic induction of proinflammatory immunity in children with biliary atresia. *Lancet*. 2002;**360**(9346):1653–1659.
8. Xiao J, Xia S-Y, Xia Y, Xia Q, Wang X-R. Transcriptome profiling of biliary atresia from new born infants by deep sequencing. *Mol Biol Rep*. 2014;**41**(12):8063–8069.
9. Zhao X, Lorent K, Wilkins BJ, et al. Glutathione antioxidant pathway activity and reserve determine toxicity and specificity of the biliary toxin biliatresone in zebrafish. *Hepatology*. 2016;**64**(3):894–907.
10. Bezerra JA, Wells RG, Mack CL, et al. Biliary atresia: clinical and research challenges for the 21st century. *Hepatology*. 2018;**68**(3):1163–1173.
11. Ramachandran P, Balamurali D, Peter JJ, et al. RNA-seq reveals outcome-specific gene expression of MMP7 and PCK1 in biliary atresia. *Mol Biol Rep*. 2019;**46**(10):5123–5130.
12. Ramachandran P, Unny AK, Vij M, Safwan M, Balaji MS, Rela M. α-Smooth muscle actin expression predicts the outcome of Kasai portoenterostomy in biliary atresia. *Saudi J Gastroenterol*. 2018;**25**(2):101–105.
13. Shteyer E, Ramm GA, Xu C, White FV, Shepherd RW. Outcome after portoenterostomy in biliary atresia: pivotal role of degree of liver fibrosis and intensity of stellate cell activation. *J Pediatr Gastroenterol Nutr*. 2006;**42**(1):93–99.
14. Kerola A, Lohi J, Heikkilä P, Mutanen A, Jalanko H, Pakarinen MP. Divergent expression of liver transforming growth factor superfamily cytokines after successful portoenterostomy in biliary atresia. *Surgery*. 2019;**165**(5):905–911.
15. Safwan M, Ramachandran P, Vij M, Shanmugam N, Rela M. Impact of ductal plate malformation on survival with native liver in children with biliary atresia. *Pediatr Surg Int*. 2015;**31**(9):837–843.
16. Superina R, Magee JC, Brandt ML, et al. The anatomic pattern of biliary atresia identified at time of Kasai hepatoportoenterostomy and early postoperative clearance of jaundice are significant predictors of transplant-free survival. *Ann Surg*. 2011;**254**(4):577–585.
17. Davenport M. Biliary atresia: clinical aspects. *Semin Pediatr Surg*. 2012;**21**(3):175–184.
18. Ramachandran P, Safwan M, Reddy MS, Rela M. Recent trends in the diagnosis and management of biliary atresia in developing countries. *Indian Pediatr*. 2015;**52**(10):871–879.
19. Lee M, Chen SC, Yang HY, Huang JH, Yeung CY, Lee HC. Infant stool color card screening helps reduce the hospitalization rate and mortality of biliary atresia: a 14-year nationwide cohort study in Taiwan. *Medicine (Baltimore)*. 2016;**95**(12):e3166.
20. Matsui A. Screening for biliary atresia. *Pediatr Surg Int*. 2017;**33**(12):1305–1313.
21. Liu C, Aronow BJ, Jegga AG, et al. Novel resequencing chip customized to diagnose mutations in patients with inherited syndromes of intrahepatic cholestasis. *Gastroenterology*. 2007;**132**(1):119–126.
22. Choochuen P, Kritsaneepaiboon S, Charoonratana V, Sangkhathat S. Is 'gallbladder length-to-width ratio' useful in diagnosing biliary atresia? *J Pediatr Surg*. 2019;**54**(9):1946–1952.
23. Weng Z, Zhou L, Wu Q, et al. Enlarged hepatic hilar lymph node: an additional ultrasonographic feature that may be helpful in the diagnosis of biliary atresia. *Eur Radiol*. 2019;**29**(12):6699–6707.
24. Dillman JR, DiPaola FW, Smith SJ, et al. Prospective assessment of ultrasound shear wave elastography for discriminating biliary atresia from other causes of neonatal cholestasis. *J Pediatr*. 2019;**212**:60–65.
25. Russo P, Magee JC, Anders RA, et al. Key histopathologic features of liver biopsies that distinguish biliary atresia from other causes of infantile cholestasis and their correlation with outcome: a multicenter study. *Am J Surg Pathol*. 2016;**40**(12):1601–1615.
26. Chardot C, Carton M, Spire-Bendelac N, et al. Is the Kasai operation still indicated in children older than 3 months diagnosed with biliary atresia? *J Pediatr*. 2001;**138**(2):224–228.
27. Kasai M, Mochizuki I, Ohkohchi N, Chiba T, Ohi R. Japan: surgical limitation for biliary atresia: indication for liver transplantation. *J Pediatr Surg*. 1989;**24**(9):851–854.
28. Davenport M, Puricelli V, Farrant P, et al. The outcome of the older (≥100 days) infant with biliary atresia. *J Pediatr Surg*. 2004;**39**(4):575–581.
29. Calinescu AM, Wilde JCH, Korff S, McLin VA, Wildhaber BE. Perioperative complications after Kasai hepatoportoenterostomy: data from the Swiss National Biliary Atresia Registry. *Eur J Pediatr Surg*. 2019;**30**(4):364–370.
30. Luo Y, Zheng S. Current concept about postoperative cholangitis in biliary atresia. *World J Pediatr*. 2008;**4**:14–19.
31. Ramachandran P, Safwan M, Balaji MS, et al. Early cholangitis after portoenterostomy in children with biliary atresia. *J Indian Assoc Pediatr Surg*. 2019;**24**(3):185–188.
32. Chen SY, Lin CC, Tsan YT, et al. Number of cholangitis episodes as a prognostic marker to predict timing of liver transplantation in biliary atresia patients after Kasai portoenterostomy. *BMC Pediatr*. 2018;**18**(1):119.
33. Honna T, Tsuchida Y, Kawarasaki H, Utsuki T, Mizuta K. Further experience with the antireflux valve to prevent ascending cholangitis in biliary atresia. *J Pediatr Surg*. 1997;**32**(10):1450–1452.
34. Cowles RA. The jaundiced infant: biliary atresia. In: Coran AG, Caldamone A, Scott Adzich N, Krummel TM, Laberge JM, eds. *Pediatric Surgery*, Volume 2. 7th ed. Oxford: Elsevier Limited; 2012: 1321–1330.
35. Kasai M, Suzuki M. A new operation for non-correctable biliary atresia: hepatic portoenterostomy. *Shujutsu*. 1959;**13**:733–739.
36. Wang P, Xun P, He K, Cai W. Comparison of liver transplantation outcomes in biliary atresia patients with and without prior portoenterostomy: a meta-analysis. *Dig Liver Dis*. 2016;**48**(4):347–352.
37. Serinet MO, Wildhaber BE, Broue P, et al. Impact of age at Kasai operation on its results in late childhood and adolescence: a rational basis for biliary atresia screening. *Pediatrics*. 2009;**123**(5):1280–1286.

38. Chardot C, Buet C, Serinet MO, et al. Improving outcomes of biliary atresia: French national series 1986–2009. *J Hepatol.* 2013;**58**(6):1209–1217.
39. Nio M, Sasaki H, Wada M, Kazama T, Nishi K, Tanaka H. Impact of age at Kasai operation on short- and long-term outcomes of type III biliary atresia at a single institution. *J Pediatr Surg.* 2010;**45**(12):2361–2363.
40. Nio M. Japanese Biliary Atresia Registry. *Pediatr Surg Int.* 2017;**33**(12):1319–1325.
41. Weerasooriya VS, White FV, Shepherd RW. Hepatic fibrosis and survival in biliary atresia. *J Pediatr.* 2004;**144**(1):123–125.
42. Muthukanagarajan SJ, Karnan I, Srinivasan P, Sadagopan P, Manickam S. Diagnostic and prognostic significance of various histopathological features in extrahepatic biliary atresia. *J Clin Diagn Res.* 2016;**10**(6):EC23–EC27.
43. Gupta L, Gupta SD, Bhatnagar V. Extrahepatic biliary atresia: correlation of histopathology and liver function tests with surgical outcomes. *J Indian Assoc Pediatr Surg.* 2012;**17**(4):147–152.
44. Wong KK, Chung PH, Chan IH, Lan LC, Tam PK. Performing Kasai portoenterostomy beyond 60 days of life is not necessarily associated with a worse outcome. *J Pediatr Gastroenterol Nutr.* 2010;**51**(5):631–634.
45. Qiao G, Li L, Cheng W, Zhang Z, Ge J, Wang C. Conditional probability of survival in patients with biliary atresia after Kasai portoenterostomy: a Chinese population-based study. *J Pediatr Surg.* 2015;**50**(8):1310–1315.
46. Chusilp S, Sookpotarom P, Tepmalai K, et al. Prognostic values of serum bilirubin at 7th day post-Kasai for survival with native livers in patients with biliary atresia. *Pediatr Surg Int.* 2016;**32**(10):927–931.
47. Tessier MEM, Shneider BL, Brandt ML, Cerminara DN, Harpavat S. A phase 2 trial of N-acetylcysteine in biliary atresia after Kasai portoenterostomy. *Contemp Clin Trials Commun.* 2019;**15**:100370.
48. Wai CT, Greenson JK, Fontana RJ, et al. A simple noninvasive index can predict both significant fibrosis and cirrhosis in patients with chronic hepatitis C. *Hepatology.* 2003;**38**(2):518–526.
49. Yang LY, Fu J, Peng XF, et al. Validation of aspartate aminotransferase to platelet ratio for diagnosis of liver fibrosis and prediction of postoperative prognosis in infants with biliary atresia. *World J Gastroenterol.* 2015;**21**(19):5893–5900.
50. Suominen JS, Lampela H, Heikkila P, Lohi J, Jalanko H, Pakarinen MP. APRi predicts native liver survival by reflecting portal fibrogenesis and hepatic neovascularization at the time of portoenterostomy in biliary atresia. *J Pediatr Surg.* 2015;**50**(9):1528–1531.
51. Wada M, Nakamura H, Koga H, et al. Experience of treating biliary atresia with three types of portoenterostomy at a single institution: extended, modified Kasai, and laparoscopic modified Kasai. *Pediatr Surg Int.* 2014;**30**(9):863–870.
52. Ramachandran P, Safwan M, Srinivas S, Shanmugam N, Vij M, Rela M. The extended Kasai portoenterostomy for biliary atresia: a preliminary report. *J Indian Assoc Pediatr Surg.* 2016;**21**(2):66–71.
53. Davenport M. Adjuvant therapy in biliary atresia: hopelessly optimistic or potential for change? *Pediatr Surg Int.* 2017;**33**(12):1263–1273.
54. Bezerra JA, Spino C, Magee JC, et al. Use of corticosteroids after hepatoportoenterostomy for bile drainage in infants with biliary atresia: the START randomized clinical trial. *JAMA.* 2014;**311**(17):1750–1759.
55. Tyraskis A, Davenport M. Steroids after the Kasai procedure for biliary atresia: the effect of age at Kasai portoenterostomy. *Pediatr Surg Int.* 2016;**32**(3):193–200.
56. Roy P, Chatterjee U, Ganguli M, Banerjee S, Chatterjee SK, Basu AK. A histopathological study of liver and biliary remnants with clinical outcome in cases of extrahepatic biliary atresia. *Indian J Pathol Microbiol.* 2010;**53**(1):101–105.
57. Shimadera S, Iwai N, Deguchi E, et al. Significance of ductal plate malformation in the postoperative clinical course of biliary atresia. *J Pediatr Surg.* 2008;**43**(2):304–307.
58. Coran AG, Caldamone A, Scott Adzich N, Krummel TM, Laberge JM, eds. *Pediatric Surgery*, Volume 2. 7th ed. Oxford: Elsevier Limited; 2012.
59. Davenport M, Tizzard SA, Underhill J, Mieli-Vergani G, Portmann B, Hadzic N. The biliary atresia splenic malformation syndrome: a 28-year single-center retrospective study. *J Pediatr.* 2006;**149**(3):393–400.
60. Davenport M, Ong E, Sharif K, et al. Biliary atresia in England and Wales: results of centralization and new benchmark. *J Pediatr Surg.* 2011;**46**(9):1689–1694.
61. Chardot C, Buet C, Serinet MO, et al. Improving outcomes of biliary atresia: French national series 1986–2009. *J Hepatol.* 2013;**58**(6):1209–1217.
62. Luo Z, Shivakumar P, Mourya R, Gutta S, Bezerra JA. Gene expression signatures associated with survival times of pediatric patients with biliary atresia identify potential therapeutic agents. *Gastroenterology.* 2019;**157**(4):1138–1152.
63. Wu JF, Jeng YM, Chen HL, Ni YH, Hsu HY, Chang MH. Quantification of serum matrix metallopeptide 7 levels may assist in the diagnosis and predict the outcome for patients with biliary atresia. *J Pediatr.* 2019;**208**:30–37.
64. Zhang S, Goswami S, Ma J, et al. CD4$^+$T cell subset profiling in biliary atresia reveals ICOS$^-$ regulatory t cells as a favorable prognostic factor. *Front Pediatr.* 2019;**7**:279.
65. Fanna M, Masson G, Capito C, et al. Management of biliary atresia in France 1986–2015: long term results. *J Pediatr Gastroenterol Nutr.* 2019;**69**(4):416–424.
66. Wang Z, Chen Y, Peng C, et al. Five-year native liver survival analysis in biliary atresia from a single large Chinese center: the death/liver transplantation hazard change and the importance of rapid early clearance of jaundice. *J Pediatr Surg.* 2019;**54**(8):1680–1685.
67. Parolini F, Hadzic N, Davenport M. Adjuvant therapy of cytomegalovirus IgM +ve associated biliary atresia: prima facie evidence of effect. *J Pediatr Surg.* 2019;**54**(9):1941–1945.

38

Neonatal cholestasis syndrome

Priya Ramachandran

Introduction

The presence of a high conjugated bilirubin concentration in a neonate at birth or within the first few months of life is referred to as neonatal cholestasis. It is the hallmark of a diverse spectrum of diseases termed neonatal cholestasis syndrome (NCS) listed in Table 38.1. Early recognition of decreased bile flow and the consequent cholestasis is of vital importance. Differentiating extrahepatic disease from intrahepatic disease early on helps to identify disorders that require surgical interventions. Among the diseases that result from the obstruction of extrahepatic bile ducts, biliary atresia (BA) is the commonest and this has been considered in another chapter. Other diseases in the NCS spectrum that have relevance to surgical practice are discussed here.

Disorders of the extrahepatic biliary system

Congenital choledochal cysts present as cholestatic jaundice in the neonate. They can also be diagnosed prenatally by ultrasonography. It is imperative to differentiate this from cystic BA and this can be done by magnetic resonance cholangiopancreatography (MRCP). Spontaneous perforation of the bile duct occurs at the junction of the cystic duct with the common hepatic duct and is due to a distal obstruction in the common bile duct. Infants present with pale stools and jaundice and the hallmark clinical feature of ascites. If the operative cholangiogram establishes bile duct continuity and shows contrast flow into the duodenum, the site of perforation can be sutured. However, in most cases, a hepaticojejunostomy is required after excision of the extrahepatic duct system and construction of a Roux loop. Neonatal gallstones leading to cholestasis is rare and is usually secondary to prolonged total parental nutrition or rarely due to ileal resection for acquired disease. Underlying haemolytic conditions may also lead to the formation of gallstones. An abdominal radiography may be useful in the case of radio-opaque haemolytic stones. But ultrasonography has a very high accuracy in the diagnosis of gallstones. It is important to exclude bile transport disorders in these children such as progressive familial intrahepatic cholestasis (PFIC). Stones and sludge can be flushed during an operative cholangiogram but mostly infants who do not have complicated cholelithiasis can be managed conservatively.[1] Surgery is reserved for patients with congenital anomalies and bile duct stenosis.

Extrinsic obstruction of the extrahepatic bile ducts may be caused by tumours such as hepatoblastoma, neuroblastoma, and rhabdomyosarcoma.

Disorders of the intrahepatic biliary system

Paucity of interlobular bile ducts or Alagille syndrome (AGS) is an autosomal dominant disease which is characterized by a dysmorphic facies and affects the liver, heart, kidneys, eyes, and skeleton. It is diagnosed by a mutation in the gene encoding Jagged1 (*JAG1*) and in a minority of patients by a mutation in the gene encoding NOTCH2 (*NOTCH2*), one of the receptors of the Notch signalling pathway. There is a paucity of intrahepatic bile ducts in the liver which leads to cholestasis. Pulmonary stenosis is the commonest lesion in the heart. Butterfly vertebrae and rib defects may be present. Ocular anomalies and vascular anomalies are seen. The facial features are characterized by a triangular facies, deep-set eyes, a prominent forehead, and a small pointed chin. The carriers of the *JAG1* mutation may not have clinical features of AGS and hence this term is reserved only for patients with liver disease in contrast to the broader group referred to as *JAG1* disease. Long-standing liver disease leads to pruritis, ichthyosis, and failure to thrive. Management involves the effective treatment of pruritis, nutritional support, and vitamin supplementation. Liver transplantation is reserved for children who develop cirrhosis.

In neonatal sclerosing cholangitis, infants present with conjugated hyperbilirubinaemia but stools are pigmented and the urine is dark in colour. Endoscopic retrograde cholangiopancreatography demonstrates a patent biliary tree. Histologically, the liver shows features of large duct obstruction. The management is largely medical and involves administration of choleretics and fat-soluble vitamins. If biliary cirrhosis develops, liver transplantation is indicated.

Fibrocystic liver disease includes congenital hepatic fibrosis, Caroli's disease, and Caroli's syndrome. In Caroli's disease, cystic dilation of the intrahepatic bile ducts is seen which may be segmental or lobular. Caroli's disease associated with congenital hepatic fibrosis is termed Caroli's syndrome. In this group of rare disorders, ductal plate

Table 38.1 Mechanistic classification of the aetiologies of neonatal cholestasis

Impaired bile flow	Endocrine
Extrahepatic ducts	Panhypopituitarism
Biliary atresia	Hypothyroidism, cortisol deficiency
Choledochal cyst	McCune–Albright syndrome
Spontaneous bile duct perforation	Donohue syndrome (leprechaunism)
Duct compression (may also be intrahepatic), e.g. hepatoblastoma, neuroblastoma, rhabdomyosarcoma, neonatal leukaemia, systemic juvenile xanthogranuloma, Langerhans cell histiocytosis	**Metabolic**
	Alpha-1-antitrypsin deficiency
Bile duct stenosis	Carbohydrate disorders
Intrahepatic duct obstruction/formation	Galactosaemia
Alagille syndrome	Fructosaemia (hereditary fructose intolerance)
'Non-syndromic paucity of interlobular bile ducts', e.g. Williams syndrome	Glycogen storage disease type IV (Anderson disease)
Cystic fibrosis	Amino acid disorders
Ductal plate malformations: congenital hepatic fibrosis, ARPKD, Caroli's disease; Ivermark, Jeune, Joubert, Bardet–Biedl syndromes	Tyrosinaemia type 1
	Lipid disorders
Neonatal sclerosing cholangitis	Niemann–Pick disease type C
Canalicular membrane transporters	Gaucher disease
PFIC type 1, BRIC, Nielsen syndrome (familial Greenland cholestasis)	Cerebrotendinous xanthomatosis
PFIC type 2	Farber's disease
PFIC type 3	β-Oxidation defects: short- and long-chain acyl-CoA
Neonatal Dubin–Johnson syndrome	Dehydrogenase deficiencies
Villin functional defect	Lysosomal storage disorders
Overload of excretory mechanism capacity: ABO incompatibility with haemolysis	Niemann–Pick disease, type C
Hepatocyte tight junctions	Gaucher disease
Neonatal ichthyosis, sclerosing cholangitis syndrome, claudin-1 protein	Farber disease
Familial hypercholanaemia due to TJP2 (zonulin-2) deficiency	Mucopolysaccharidosis VI (Maroteaux–Lamy syndrome)
Hepato dysfunction	Mucolipidosis II (I-cell disease)
Bile acid synthesis	Urea cycle defects
1°: BASD	Citrin deficiency (formerly type II citrullinaemia)
3-Oxo-Δ4-steroid 5β-reductase deficiency	Mitochondrial respiratory chain disorders
3β-Hydroxy-Δ5-C27-steroid dehydrogenase/isomerase deficiency	Complex deficiencies
Oxysterol 7α-hydroxylase deficiency	Growth retardation, amino aciduria, cholestasis, iron overload, lactic acidosis and early death (GRACILE)
Familial hypercholanaemia due to BAAT deficiency	**Immune meditated**
2°: organelle dysfunction	Gestational alloimmune liver disease
Smith–Lemli–Opitz syndrome (cholesterol formation)	Neonatal lupus erythematosus
Zellweger	Autoimmune haemolytic anaemia with giant cell hepatitis
Peroxisomal disorders: Zellweger, infantile refsum, neonatal ALD	Haemophagocytic lymphohistiocytosis
Infectious	**Hypoxic/ischaemic/vascular**
Bacterial: sepsis (endotoxaemia, e.g., UTI, gastroenteritis)	Shock/hypoperfusion/hypoxia
Listeria	Budd–Chiari syndrome
Syphilis	Cardiac insufficiency (congenital heart disease, arrhythmia)
TB	Multiple haemangiomata
Viral: herpes viruses: CMV, HSV, HHV-6	Sinusoidal obstruction syndrome
Parvovirus B19	**Miscellaneous/unclear mechanism**
Hepatitis A, B, C	ARC syndrome (arthrogryposis-renal tubular dysfunction cholestasis; defective vacuolar protein sorting)
Enterovirus: coxsackieviruses, echoviruses, 'numbered' enteroviruses	
Adenovirus	Chromosomal: trisomy 18, 21
Rubella	Congenital disorders of glycosylation
HIV	Hardikar syndrome
Paramyxovirus	Lymphoedema cholestasis syndrome (Aagenaes syndrome)
Protozoal	Kabuki syndrome
Toxoplasmosis	North American Indian childhood cirrhosis (defective cirhin protein-unknown function)
Toxic	
Parenteral nutrition associated liver disease	Pesudo-TORCH syndrome
Fetal alcohol syndrome	**'Idiopathic neonatal hepatitis'**
Drugs: maternal amphetamines, anticonvulsants; infant antifungals	

ALD, adrenoleukodystrophy; ARPKD, autosomal recessive polycystic kidney disease; BAAT, bile acid coenzyme A: amino acid N-acyltransferase; BRIC, benign recurrent intrahepatic cholestasis; CMV, cytomegalovirus; HHV-6, human herpesvirus type 6; HIV, human immunodeficiency virus; HSV, herpes simplex virus; PFIC, progressive familial intrahepatic cholestasis; UTI, urinary tract infection.

Reproduced with permission from Wyllie R, Hyams JS, Kay M, *Pediatric Gastrointestinal and Liver Disease* 6th Edition, Elsevier 2020, p.745.

malformations are seen in the liver associated with segmental dilatations of the intrahepatic ducts and fibrosis. The disease may be identified incidentally or may present with recurrent cholangitis and septicaemia. Portal hypertension is a feature of congenital hepatic fibrosis. Autosomal recessive polycystic kidney disease (ARPKD) is associated with Caroli's syndrome. If ARPKD presents early, its severity may exceed that of the liver disease. Ultrasonography and MRCP are used to diagnose these disorders. Management of portal hypertension and cholangitis is mandatory. Isolated kidney and liver transplantation may become necessary in some children. A partial hepatectomy has been done for segmental and lobar disease. In liver disease associated with polycystic kidney disease, combined liver kidney transplantation has been performed.[2]

Canalicular membrane transporter defects

Bile is synthesized by hepatocytes and secreted into bile canaliculi from where it reaches the bile ducts. Bile is stored in the gall bladder and drains into the duodenum. Bile is composed of water, bile acids, ions, phospholipids, cholesterol, bilirubin, proteins such as glutathione and peptides, and xenobiotics.[3]

The function of bile is to emulsify lipids facilitating its digestion and absorption. Solute carrier systems on the basolateral membrane of the hepatocytes and ATP-dependent transporters on the canalicular membrane interact with bile acid transporters to form bile. Defects in canalicular membrane transporters leads to cholestatic diseases termed PFIC types I, II, and III. PFIC types I and II are known as low gamma-glutamyl transpeptidase (GGT)-PFIC and type III is known as high GGT-PFIC. But recently this terminology has changed and they are known by their respective gene and transporter defects: PFIC I (*ATP8B1*, also called *F1C1*), PFIC II (*ABCB11*, also called *BSEP*), and PFIC III (*ABCB4*, also called *MDR3*). Patients present with chronic cholestasis in early childhood which progresses to cirrhosis within the first decade of life. Pruritus is present and may be severe enough to cause mutilation of the skin mainly on the extensor surfaces. Pruritus, if not adequately managed, can lead to poor school performance because of lack of sleep and inability to concentrate. Children have growth failure, asthma-like symptoms, and epistaxis. Recently, it was noted that PFIC II (*ABCB11*) patients had more hepatobiliary disease while PFIC I patients had extrahepatic disease involving the pancreas and associated with diarrhoea and a failure to thrive. In PFIC I and II, bile acids are elevated, GGT is low, and serum bile acids are markedly elevated while in PFIC III, the GGT is elevated. Total serum bile acids exceed 200 μmol/L while the total biliary bile acid concentration is low. Hepatocellular and canalicular cholestasis with pseudo-acinar transformation is seen in the liver in PFIC I and II. Giant cell transformation is more common in PFIC II. Apoptosis of biliary epithelium and degeneration of bile ducts may be seen. Lacy lobular fibrosis develops and progresses to portal to central bridging fibrosis. The progression of fibrosis is correlated with the severity of clinical disease. On electron microscopy, coarse granular bile (Byler's bile) is present in the canalicular spaces in PFIC I. Treatment is supportive and consists of fat-soluble vitamin supplementation and ursodeoxycholic acid. Pruritus is managed with cholestyramine and surgical diversion of bile is considered when the medical management of pruritus is ineffective.

Benign recurrent intrahepatic cholestasis (BRIC) has a similar presentation with pruritus, cholestasis, low GGT level, and high serum bile acids. But, unlike PFIC, the onset of disease is late, the cholestasis is intermittent, and it does not progress to liver failure. The mutations in BRIC share the same locus as PFIC I and II (*ATP8B1* and *ABCB11*). The cholestatic episodes have been treated with nasobiliary tube drainage and surgical diversion can be performed in select cases.

Hepatocyte disorders

Bile acid synthetic defects

These are genetic cholestatic diseases in which the mechanism of bile acid generation is impaired. The bile acids are synthesized from cholesterol in the hepatocytes. These disorders are associated with specific gene defects. Hepatocellular cholestasis occurs due to the retention of abnormal bile acid intermediates and low production of normal bile acids. Bile flow is insufficient for normal function and results in progressive liver damage.

Infective hepatitis

Bacteraemia and extrahepatic bacterial infections can cause conjugated hyperbilirubinaemia. Basolateral and canalicular bile acid transport is reduced by the endotoxins and cytokines released by Kupffer cells. Immature bile acid transport mechanisms in newborns make them susceptible to cholestasis in the presence of bacterial infections. The common site of infection is often the urinary tract. *Escherichia coli* is the commonest organism involved. Congenital syphilis transmitted from mother to infant, perinatal tuberculosis, and listeriosis are other bacterial causes of neonatal hepatitis. Viral infections are caused by cytomegalovirus, herpes simplex virus, congenital Rubella, enterovirus, and human immunodeficiency virus (HIV). Hepatotropic viruses such as hepatitis A–E do not play a major role in neonatal hepatitis. Parasitic infections are caused by *Toxoplasma gondii* which crosses the placental barrier and causes chorioretinitis, intracranial calcifications and hydrocephalus, as well as hepatosplenomegaly, jaundice, thrombocytopenia, lymphadenopathy, and a maculopapular rash. The symptoms manifest in infancy and are detected by immunoglobulin M or A levels. Pyrimethamine and sulfadiazine prevents further organ damage.

Idiopathic neonatal hepatitis

There is prolonged cholestasis which does not have an aetiology and the liver biopsy shows the presence of multinuclear giant cells. The familial form can be recurrent unlike the non-familiar form.

Metabolic hepatocyte dysfunction

Alpha-1 antitrypsin deficiency, carbohydrate metabolism disorders such as galactosaemia, fructosaemia, and glycogen storage disorder type IV, lipid metabolism disorders such as Niemann–Pick disease and Gaucher disease, urea cycle defects, and mitochondrial respiratory chain disorders present with cholestasis.

Toxic hepatitis

This includes hepatitis induced by parenteral nutrition, fetal alcohol syndrome, and drugs such as anticonvulsants.

Infants and neonates on parenteral nutrition are susceptible to parenteral nutrition-associated liver disease. It commonly occurs in infants with intestinal failure who require long-term parenteral nutrition. The spectrum of disease in the liver includes biliary sludge, gallstones, and end-stage liver disease. The risk factors are duration of parenteral nutrition, perinatal hypoxia, prematurity, low birth weight, minimal enteral feeds, sepsis from indwelling catheters, and bacterial overgrowth due to short gut. Prevention of risk factors and early establishment of enteral feeds along with administration of ursodeoxycholic acid and the use of fish oil-based parenteral lipid emulsions may reduce the extent of liver damage.

Neonatal hepatitis can be associated with endocrinopathies involving a disturbance of the pituitary–adrenal axis. Hepatitis is also seen in chromosomal disorders such as trisomy 17, 18, and 21 and in autoimmune disorders such as neonatal lupus erythematosus.

Diagnostic evaluation of neonatal cholestasis syndrome

History and physical examination must include a family history and examination of stools is necessary to establish a clinical diagnosis. A biochemical diagnosis can be made from estimation of fractionated bilirubin, liver enzymes, and GGT levels. A genotypic diagnosis can be established by whole-genome sequencing for citrin deficiency, PFIC, and AGS. The Jaundice Chip which includes *SERPINA1*, *JAG1*, *ATP8B1*, *ABCB11*, and *ABCB4* has been used to identify specific genetic disorders. Bacterial cultures, and viral serology establishes the diagnosis in infective hepatitis. Ultrasonography and MRCP when indicated is used to identify extrahepatic bile duct obstruction. An operative cholangiogram also enables this diagnosis. A liver biopsy has a good diagnostic yield in intra- and extrahepatic biliary obstructions as well as for identifying the various PFIC types.

Biliary diversion procedures

Ninety-five per cent of bile acids are reabsorbed in the terminal ileum. Biliary diversion interrupts the enterohepatic circulation resulting in excretion of bile acids. This slowly depletes the total body bile acid pool thereby significantly improving pruritus in PFIC and AGS. The early procedures described involved external diversion of bile. Internal diversion and partial internal diversion procedures have also been described.

In 1988, Whitington et al. described partial external biliary diversion where a cholecystojejunostomy was created to eliminate the accumulated bile acids.[4] This is associated with resolution of pruritus and improved liver function. There is also an improvement in lipid profile after this procedure in PFIC.[5] However, the presence of an external biliary stoma makes it uncomfortable for the children to resume a normal life. An ileal exclusion procedure has also been described wherein 15% of the terminal ileum was excluded from the enterohepatic circulation reducing the total bile acid pool.[6] Although this procedure did not require the creation of a stoma, symptoms recurred in 50% of patients. We reported our experience with partial internal biliary diversion.[7] In this procedure, a 15 cm segment of jejunum was isolated and anastomosed in an isoperistaltic fashion to the fundus of the gall bladder and termino-laterally to the midportion of the ascending colon. Thus, bile acids are diverted to the ascending colon away from the terminal ileum reducing the total bile acid pool.

Although there was relief from pruritus in 75% of patients and serum bile acids reduced significantly from preoperative values, there was no improvement in liver function. An osmotic diarrhoea may occur in these patients which can be controlled with cholestyramine. A laparoscopic cholecystocolostomy has been described with an 85% success rate, good long-term outcomes, and no ascending cholangitis. In this procedure, the transverse colon is anastomosed in a Y-shaped fashion to the gall bladder and mid descending colon.[8] Although biliary diversion procedures have been used for PFIC and AGS, recent reports suggest that they are less efficacious in PFIC II.[9] This has been attributed to more advanced liver disease in these patients.

Conclusion

An infant presenting with prolonged jaundice for more than 2 weeks' duration and conjugated hyperbilirubinaemia must be investigated for diseases falling within the purview of NCS. Timely diagnosis and management are vitally important to reduce the morbidity and mortality of these diseases. More national-level screening programmes will enable early diagnosis. Advances in the development of genetic analysis have resulted in novel diagnostic methods. Liver transplantation was a major step which improved the outcomes in several of these diseases. Hepatocyte transplantation may be the next frontier to be breached in the journey to find less morbid treatment modalities for NCS.[3]

REFERENCES

1. Jeanty C, Derderian SC, Courtier J, Hirose S. Clinical management of infantile cholelithiasis. *J Pediatr Surg*. 2015;**50**(8):1289–1292. doi: 10.1016/j.jpedsurg.2014.10.051.
2. Wyllie R, Hyams JS, Kay M. *Pediatric Gastrointestinal and Liver Disease*. 5th ed. Philadelphia, PA: Elsevier; 2016.
3. Chen H-L, Wu S-H, Hsu S-H, Liou B-Y, Chen H-L, Chang M-H. Jaundice revisited: recent advances in the diagnosis and treatment of inherited cholestatic liver diseases. *J Biomed Sci*. 2018;**25**(1):75.
4. Whitington PF, Whitington GL. Partial external diversion of bile for the treatment of intractable pruritus associated with intrahepatic cholestasis. *Gastroenterology*. 1998;**95**(1):130–136.
5. Jankowska I, Czubkowski P, Wierzbicka A, Pawłowska J, Kaliciński P, Socha P. Influence of partial external biliary diversion on the lipid profile in children with progressive familial intrahepatic cholestasis. *J Pediatr Gastroenterol Nutr*. 2016;**63**(6):598–602.
6. Hollands CM, Rivera-Pedrogo FJ, Gonzalez-Vallina R, Loret-de-Mola O, Nahmad M, Burnwelt CA. Ileal exclusion for Byler's disease: an alternative surgical approach with promising early result for pruritus. *J Pediatr Surg*. 1998;**33**(2):220–224.
7. Ramachandran P, Shanmugam NP, Sinani SA, et al. Outcome of partial internal biliary diversion for intractable pruritus in children with cholestatic liver disease. *Pediatr Surg Int*. 2014;**30**(10):1045–1049. doi: 10.1007/s00383-014-3559-x
8. Diao M, Li L, Zhang JS, Ye M, Cheng W. Laparoscopic cholecystocolostomy: a novel surgical approach for the treatment of progressive familial intrahepatic cholestasis. *Ann Surg*. 2013;**258**(6):1028–1033.
9. Lemoine C, Bhardwaj T, Bass LM, Superina RA, Outcomes following partial external biliary diversion in patients with progressive familial intrahepatic cholestasis. *J Pediatr Surg*. 2017;**52**(2):268–272. doi: 10.1016/j.jpedsurg.2016.11.021

39

Acute cholangitis, recurrent cholangitis, and management of common bile duct calculi

Haitham Triki and Karim Boudjema

Introduction

Cholangitis or biliary tract infection, although a common disease, is not a well-defined clinical condition but rather a spectrum of clinical presentations that any physician may encounter. Its high frequency is related to the high prevalence of its most common aetiology: biliary calculi.

Each step in the management of biliary infection, from diagnosis to treatment, can be challenging and each clinical case can be a subject for discussion. However, time is not always on our side and in some cases, quick decisions must be made to avoid a fatal outcome.

In this chapter, we principally consider acute cholangitis (AC) due to choledocholithiasis and report the most effective and commonly used therapeutic means to handle it.

Acute cholangitis

AC is defined as an acute inflammation and infection in the bile ducts leading to systemic infectious disease. The most common cause is choledocholithiasis. It can be a life-threatening disease making early diagnosis and urgent multidisciplinary management imperative. Advances in critical care, antibiotic treatment, and biliary decompression techniques have significantly improved outcomes. The type and timing of biliary decompression are based on the severity of the disease.

Pathophysiology and microbiology

Several mechanisms are involved to maintain bile sterility including the sphincter of Oddi which prevents the ascent of bacteria from the duodenum, bile flow which flushes the bile duct, and tight junctions between hepatocytes which separate the biliary canaliculi from the hepatic sinusoids preventing bacterial translocation. Kupffer cells, within the hepatic sinusoids, phagocytize microorganisms.[1] Bile itself has antibacterial properties through bile salts and immunoglobulin A secretion.[2,3]

Even when bile is infected, hepatic venous blood and perihepatic lymph remain sterile and AC will not develop unless intraductal pressure is elevated. Conversely, obstruction of the bile duct itself does not result in cholangitis without bacterial infection of the bile. The development of AC requires the presence of both factors: obstruction of the biliary tract leading to increased biliary pressure and infection of the bile.

When biliary pressure exceeds 25 cmH$_2$O, bile ductule permeability increases and results in free translocation of bacteria from the bile into both the lymphatic system (cholangiolymphatic reflux) and the bloodstream (cholangiovenous reflux).[4]

Stagnant bile enhances bacterial infections. Bacteria may enter the bile duct by ascent from the duodenum.[5] Otherwise, the gate might be the portal venous system. Indeed, bacterial translocation from the intestine is increased after biliary obstruction owing to the loss of the detergent effect of bile salts and the decreased capacity of the reticuloendothelial system of the liver.[6]

The microbiology of AC has been changing over the years. The most common bacteria previously identified were *Escherichia coli*, *Klebsiella* species, and *Enterococcus* species. Polymicrobial infections have become more prevalent.[7] Anaerobic bacteria, *Clostridium* or *Bacteroides* species, are commonly isolated in patients with prior biliary surgery and in the elderly. Over the last decade, *Pseudomonas aeruginosa* and *Enterococcus* species have become more common in patients with biliary stents.[8]

Causes

The common cause of biliary obstruction remains choledocholithiasis. Malignant obstruction of the biliary tract remains a very rare cause of AC. However, AC is becoming more and more frequent after biliary stenting for malignant obstruction. Table 39.1 summarizes the most common causes of biliary obstruction resulting in AC.

Table 39.1 The aetiologies of acute cholangitis

Gallstones	Choledocholithiasis Intrahepatic stones Mirizzi syndrome
Benign biliary stricture	Biliary–enteric anastomotic strictures Bile duct injury during cholecystectomy Anastomotic stricture after orthotopic liver transplant Chronic pancreatitis Primary sclerosing cholangitis Autoimmune cholangitis Polycystic liver disease Congenital anomalies (choledochal cysts, biliary atresia)
Endoscopic and percutaneous biliary interventions	Bile duct stent obstruction Endoscopic retrograde cholangiopancreatography Percutaneous transhepatic cholangiography
Parasitic diseases	Ascariasis, clonorchiasis, schistosomiasis, opisthorchiasis Hydatid hepatic cyst rupture into the biliary tree
Malignant biliary stricture	Pancreatic head cancer Cholangiocarcinoma Periampullary tumours Parenchymal liver tumours (primary or secondary) Duodenal neoplasm Gallbladder carcinoma Metastatic lymph nodes
Other	Haemobilia Lemmel syndrome secondary to duodenal diverticulitis Cholangiography in patients with AIDS

Source: data from Bornman PC, Van Beljon JI, Krige JEJ. Management of cholangitis. *J Hepatobiliary Pancreat Surg*. 2003;10(6):406-414; Sulzer JK, Ocuin LM. Cholangitis: causes, diagnosis, and management. *Surg Clin*. 2019;99(2):175-184; Mosler P. Diagnosis and management of acute cholangitis. *Curr Gastroenterol Rep*. 2011;13(2):166-172; and Kochar R, Banerjee S. Infections of the biliary tract. *Gastrointest Endosc Clin*. 2013;23(2):199-218.

Clinical presentation

The classic triad, right upper abdominal pain, fever, and jaundice, was first described by Charcot in 1877.[9] The diagnosis of AC has long been based on these three symptoms. Jaundice is usually mild and intermittent but can be severe in complete obstruction. Fever and chills are the result of bacterial cholangiovenous reflux. In 1959, Reynolds found that confusion and hypotension were signs of severity. Adding these two signs to the classical triad defines the Reynolds pentad.[10] Charcot's triad has high specificity in diagnosing AC but its sensitivity is low.[11] This lack of sensitivity may lead to a delay in diagnosis and treatment especially in elderly patients who often have atypical clinical presentations. Laboratory data and imaging can therefore be essential components to make the diagnosis of AC.

Laboratory data

Typically, the results of laboratory tests show systemic inflammation and cholestasis. Inflammation markers, including leucocytosis and increased C-reactive protein, are often present. Gamma-glutamyl transpeptidase, and alkaline phosphatase are elevated in more than 90% of the patients with AC.[12] Hyperbilirubinaemia is common but the bilirubin level can be normal in incomplete and intermittent biliary obstruction.

Imaging

No single imaging tool exists to definitively diagnose AC. The aim of imaging is to locate the level of the obstacle, to specify its nature and to guide management.

Transabdominal ultrasound (US) can easily identify intrahepatic and extrahepatic biliary dilatation. Normally, the diameter of the common bile duct (CBD) does not exceed 6 mm although it can be slightly increased after cholecystectomy.[13] Intrahepatic biliary dilatation is defined by a diameter greater than 2 mm or greater than 40% of the adjacent portal vein. US is operator dependent and has inadequate sensitivity for the level of biliary obstruction and choledocholithiasis.[14] This lack of accuracy can be explained by a patient's clinical condition, bowel gas interposition, and obstruction location in the retropancreatic segment of the CBD.

The computed tomography (CT) scan has a great advantage in overcoming the technical limitations of US. Compared with US, it can detect stones in the retropancreatic CBD segment. However, iso- or hypodense cholesterol stones are difficult to detect. Intravenous contrast-enhanced CT can reveal the thickness of the bile ducts and peribiliary oedema.[15] The arterial phase may show peripheral or periductal hypervascularization and highlight inhomogeneous liver parenchymal enhancement, so-called transient hyperattenuation differences, which is related to increased arterial blood flow accompanying biliary inflammation.[16] CT can identify other aetiologies such as neoplastic or parasitic obstacles and reveal local complications such as liver abscess and pylephlebitis.

Magnetic resonance cholangiopancreatography (MRCP) has a high sensitivity to detect CBD stones (80–100%), and excellent specificity (90–100%) (**Figure 39.1**).[17] However, it cannot detect stones that are smaller than 5 mm or impacted stones in the ampulla.[18] Magnetic resonance imaging may support the diagnosis of AC by revealing heterogeneous enhancement of the bile duct wall, increased periductal signal on T2-weighted images, and transient enhancement surrounding the dilated intrahepatic duct on dynamic phases, so-called transient periductal signal difference.[19]

Compared with MRCP, endoscopic ultrasonography (EUS) has better diagnostic accuracy and sensitivity and similar specificity.[20] Owing to its exceptional resolution, EUS has great accuracy in detecting small gallstones. It can be combined with fine-needle aspiration and biopsy to confirm suspected malignancy. However, EUS is an invasive technique and requires sedation.

Diagnosis

Considering the low sensitivity of clinical signs, the need for diagnostic criteria using a combination of clinical, biochemical, and imaging data is crucial. These have been established by the Tokyo Guidelines in 2018 (**Box 39.1**), offering high diagnosis rates up to 90%.[11]

Management

Approximately 80% of patients will improve clinically with antibiotics. However, AC can be a life-threatening disease. In 1959, Reynolds and Dragan found that, in patients with severe AC, prolonged resuscitation was ineffective and the mortality risk would only increase over time. They therefore concluded that emergent

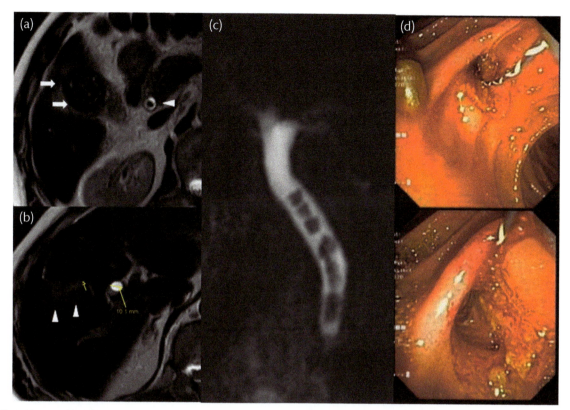

Figure 39.1 A 66-year-old male patient presents with acute cholangitis due to CBD calculi. (a) MRI T2-weighted image shows a stone in the CBD as low-signal-intensity structure (arrow head). The gall bladder is full of stones (white arrows). (b) MRI T2-weighted image shows dilated CBD. An infiltration at the junction of segments V and VIII is related to the beginning of abscess formation. (c) MRCP sequences show multiple stones in the CBD as low-signal-intensity structures. (d) Extraction of stones from the CBD.

biliary decompression was crucial and was the only hope of survival for these critical patients.[10] Since then, remarkable progress has been made and effective and less risky therapeutic procedures compared with surgery have emerged.

Box 39.1 Tokyo Guidelines 2018 for acute cholangitis diagnosis

A. Systemic inflammation
- A-1. Fever >38°C and/or shaking chills.
- A-2. Laboratory data: evidence of inflammatory response:
  - White blood cell counts <4 or >10 (× 1000/μL)
  - CRP ≥1 (mg/dL)

B. Cholestasis
- B-1. Jaundice: total bilirubin ≥2 (mg/dL).
- B-2. Laboratory data: increased liver function tests levels >1.5 × upper limit of normal values: ALP, GGT, AST, and ALT.

C. Imaging
- C-1. Biliary dilatation.
- C-2. Evidence of the aetiology on imaging (stricture, stone, stent, etc.).

Suspected diagnosis
One item in A plus one item in either B or C.

Definite diagnosis
One item in A, one item in B, and one item in C.

ALP, alkaline phosphatase; ALT, alanine aminotransferase; AST, aspartate aminotransferase; CRP, C-reactive protein; GGT, gamma-glutamyl transpeptidase.

Adapted from Kiriyama S, Tokyo Guidelines Revision Committee. New diagnostic criteria and severity assessment of acute cholangitis in revised Tokyo Guidelines. *J Hepatobiliary Pancreat Sci*. 2012;19(5):548–556, under a Creative Commons Attribution 3.0 Unported licence (CC BY 3.0). https://creativecommons.org/licenses/by/3.0/

The management of AC should be based on its severity and three main principles: adequate resuscitation, broad-spectrum parenteral antibiotics, and biliary decompression.

According to the Tokyo Guidelines 2018 for the severity of AC (Box 39.2), patients with mild AC may be treated with antibiotics alone. Biliary decompression is reserved for non-responders to initial treatment. For patients with moderate AC, early biliary decompression within 48–72 hours is indicated. In severe AC patients, emergency biliary drainage should be considered as soon as possible and within 12 hours with appropriate resuscitation. Treatment of the aetiology, if still needed, should be provided after the patient's general condition has improved.[11]

Antibiotics

In routine cases of community-acquired AC, positive cultures do not often provide additional information to change antibiotic therapy. It is therefore not recommended to routinely perform blood cultures except for toxic or immunocompromised patients or in high-severity infections for which the antibiotic therapy and duration of treatment may be modified.[21]

Antibiotics should be given to all patients with suspected AC as early as possible, preferably after blood cultures when indicated. Biliary penetration of antibiotics is limited by increased intraductal pressure. However, the role of an antibiotic is not to sterilize bile, but to control sepsis and inflammation.[22] The choice of broad-spectrum antibiotics is dictated by suspected bacteria, the patient's underlying pathology, and clinical condition.

Community-acquired cholangitis of mild or moderate severity may be treated by several categories of antibiotics targeting

> **Box 39.2** Tokyo Guidelines 2018 for criteria acute cholangitis severity assessment
>
> **Grade III (severe) acute cholangitis**
> Grade III acute cholangitis is defined as acute cholangitis that is associated with the onset of dysfunction at least in any one of the following organs/systems:
> 1. Cardiovascular dysfunction: hypotension requiring dopamine ≥5 μg/kg per min, or any dose of norepinephrine.
> 2. Neurological dysfunction: disturbance of consciousness.
> 3. Respiratory dysfunction: PaO_2/FiO_2 ratio <300.
> 4. Renal dysfunction: oliguria, serum creatinine >2.0 mg/dL.
> 5. Hepatic dysfunction: PT/INR ratio >1.5.
> 6. Haematological dysfunction: platelet count <100,000/mm³.
>
> **Grade II (moderate) acute cholangitis**
> Grade II acute cholangitis is associated with any two of the following conditions:
> 1. Abnormal WBC count (>12,000/mm³, <4000/mm³).
> 2. High fever (≥39°C).
> 3. Age (>75 years old).
> 4. Hyperbilirubinaemia (total bilirubin ≥5 mg/dL).
> 5. Hypoalbuminaemia (<lower limit of normal value × 0.7).
>
> **Grade I (mild) acute cholangitis**
> Grade I acute cholangitis does not meet the criteria of Grade III (severe) or Grade II (moderate) acute cholangitis on initial diagnosis.
>
> PaO_2/FiO_2 ratio, ratio of arterial oxygen partial pressure to fractional inspired oxygen; PT/INR, prothrombin time/international normalized ratio; WBC, white cell count.
>
> Reproduced from Kiriyama S, Tokyo Guidelines Revision Committee. New diagnostic criteria and severity assessment of acute cholangitis in revised Tokyo Guidelines. J Hepatobiliary Pancreat Sci. 2012;19(5):548–556, under a Creative Commons Attribution 3.0 Unported licence (CC BY 3.0). https://creativecommons.org/licenses/by/3.0/

E. coli, *Klebsiella*, and other enteric Gram-negative pathogens. Penicillin and cephalosporin-based therapies are effective in this instance. Because of the current increase in antimicrobial resistance, fluoroquinolones are avoided.[21] Metronidazole is indicated when an anaerobic organism is suspected, such as patients with biliary-enteric anastomosis. For patients with severe cholangitis, empirical antibiotics with wider spectrum and anti-pseudomonal activity such as carbapenems and piperacillin with tazobactam are recommended.[21]

Hospital-acquired cholangitis, after biliary intervention or prolonged hospitalization, is often caused by multiple and resistant bacteria. Carbapenems or piperacillin–tazobactam can be used in association with vancomycin which is recommended to cover *Enterococcus*. Linezolid should be added if suspicion of vancomycin-resistant *Enterococcus* is high.

When blood and/or bile cultures become available, de-escalation should be offered by prescribing selective narrow-spectrum antibiotics to reduce harmful side effects and the emergence of antibiotic resistance for cost-effectiveness.[23]

The Tokyo Guidelines 2018 recommend 4–7 days of antibiotic treatment after verifying the source of infection. If bacteraemia with Gram-positive cocci (*Enterococcus*, *Streptococcus*) is present, a minimum of 2 weeks is recommended owing to the risk of infective endocarditis.[21]

Biliary decompression

When performed in a timely manner, biliary decompression is the most effective way to treat AC. It can be achieved by endoscopic, percutaneous, or surgical means. The preferred method depends on the availability of the technique, local expertise, aetiology, location and severity of obstruction, the patient's anatomy, and his or her clinical condition. Open surgical drainage has the highest mortality rate. Mortality has decreased since the development of endoscopic and percutaneous drainage which has become the most commonly performed method for biliary decompression.

Endoscopic retrograde cholangiopancreatography (ERCP)

ERCP provides CBD clearance and bile drainage at a rate of 98%.[24] It should be considered as the first-line drainage procedure.[25] Two types of drainage can be performed: external drainage with a nasobiliary drain or internal drainage with a biliary stent (**Figure 39.2**). Although endoscopic stenting showed an increased rate of blockage in a prospective randomized study,[26] a recent meta-analysis has demonstrated no statistically significant difference in technical success,

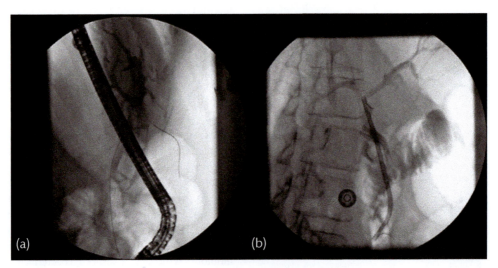

Figure 39.2 (a) A side-viewing scope is used to visualize and cannulate the papilla. Contrast agent is injected into the CBD. Then, a guidewire is pushed across the obstruction. Cholangiogram shows stones in the dilated CBD. (b) Internal drainage with a biliary stent.

clinical success, adverse events, and reinvervention rates between the two procedures.[25] Sphincterotomy can be added in case of difficult biliary cannulation, placement of a larger biliary stent, or removal of bile duct stones. Its most common complications are pancreatitis, bleeding, and retroduodenal perforation. Sphincterotomy is contraindicated in severe AC with coagulopathy or in those on anticoagulant therapy.[27] In severely ill patients, ERCP should be performed in the shortest possible time and in the safest possible manner. Sphincterotomy is therefore not recommended. Nevertheless, in mild to moderate AC, sphincterotomy may be performed to remove bile duct stones with biliary drainage (**Figure 39.1**).[25]

Percutaneous transhepatic cholangiography and drainage (PTCD)

Given its higher morbidity, PTCD is indicated as a second choice. It is useful after failed ERCP in case of altered gastrointestinal anatomy (such as biliary–enteric anastomoses) (**Figure 39.3**) and in hilar obstruction (such as perihilar cholangiocarcinoma).[25,28] In addition, it can be done under local anaesthesia and minimal or no sedation which is a great advantage in septic and critically ill patients. The choice of which side of the liver to drain depends on the aetiology and the location of the obstruction. The success rates of PTCD is 86%.[29] Many interventions including stenting, as performed in ERCP, can be carried out through the catheter.

Endoscopic ultrasound-guided biliary drainage (EUS-BD)

EUS-BD is a relatively recent, useful, and safe alternative to PTCD. This procedure involves the creation of communication between the bile ducts and the gastrointestinal tract under EUS imaging guidance. There are three possible approaches: intrahepatic bile duct drainage by transgastric or transjejunal approach, extrahepatic bile duct drainage by the transduodenal or transgastric approach, and antegrade stenting. Compared with PTCD, it has similar technical and clinical success rates with a significantly lower morbidity. However, EUS-BD is a difficult technique and often performed only in expert and high-volume centres.[25,30]

Surgical management

Emergency laparotomy for biliary decompression in AC carries a high mortality.[31] It should only be used as a last resort when non-surgical modalities have been exhausted or are unavailable.[25] In a severely ill patient, the aim is to decompress the biliary system as rapidly and efficiently as possible using T-tube placement in the CBD above the level of the obstruction to externally drain the biliary system. In patients with mild to moderate AC, treatment of the aetiology can be carried out at the same time as biliary decompression. In these cases, the laparoscopic approach becomes more useful particularly for choledocholithiasis.

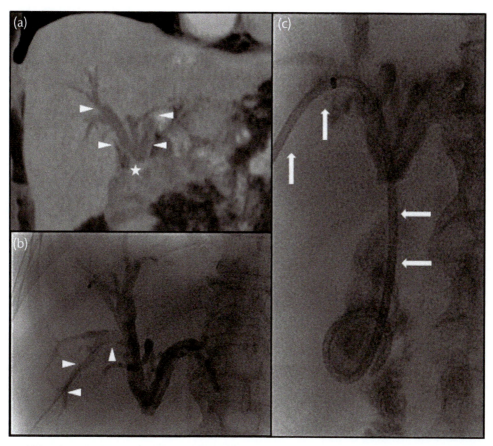

Figure 39.3 A 67-year-old female patient presents with recurrent cholangitis due to biliary–enteric anastomosis stricture 3 months after a Whipple procedure. (a) CT scan (coronal plane) during portal phase with minimum intensity projection shows biliary–enteric anastomosis stricture (star) with upstream dilatation of intrahepatic bile ducts (head arrows). (b, c) Percutaneous transhepatic cholangiography and drainage with internal–external stent.

Recurrent cholangitis

Recurrent cholangitis is due to the relapse of a biliary obstruction mostly due to complex intrahepatic lithiasis which is more difficult to access and remove, and is often associated with intrahepatic biliary strictures. Thus, the risks of treatment failure and recurrence are high. Box 39.3 summarizes the most common causes of recurrent cholangitis. Herein, recurrent pyogenic cholangitis, intrahepatic congenital bile duct dilatation, and recurrent strictures after biliary reconstructive procedure will be highlighted.

Recurrent pyogenic cholangitis is characterized by repeated episodes caused by intra- and extrahepatic bile duct strictures and pigmented biliary stones. It was first described in Hong Kong by Digby in 1930. The prevalence of recurrent pyogenic cholangitis is particularly high in east Asia. It often affects people in the lower socioeconomic classes. The pathogenesis is not yet fully understood. Bowel bacteria reach the small biliary ducts through the portal system during an enteric infection. Infection occurs in bile ducts leading to the formation of pigmented stones.[32] Repeated transmural inflammation causes biliary strictures. Typically, liver atrophy affects the left lobe. Biliary cirrhosis can develop following long-term disease. Chronic inflammation may induce atypical epithelial hyperplasia and cholangiocarcinoma.[33] Partial hepatectomy is indicated for atrophic liver segments, multiple liver abscesses, or segments occupied by stones and biliary strictures. For patients with bilateral intrahepatic stones, hepaticocutaneous jejunostomy facilitates postoperative access to the biliary tree to remove stones and dilate strictures, avoiding repeated procedures.[34]

Intrahepatic congenital bile duct dilatation, first described by Caroli et al. in 1958, is usually characterized by repeated attacks of cholangitis.[35] It corresponds to type V of Todani's classification for congenital bile duct dilatation. It is usually associated with intrahepatic lithiasis.[36] The extension of disease occurs more frequently on the left side of the liver. There is a significant risk of developing cholangiocarcinoma. Imaging tests show multiple cysts arising from dilated intrahepatic bile ducts. For patients with unilobar disease, partial hepatectomy is the treatment of choice. Patients with diffuse bi-lobar disease are candidates for liver transplantation.[36]

Recurrent strictures after biliary reconstructive procedure are significantly more common after bile duct injury repair compared with other surgeries.[37] Management is challenging and requires a multidisciplinary approach. Percutaneous biliary balloon dilatation with placement of an internal–external biliary stent is the best approach for biliary–enteric anastomosis strictures (Figure 39.3). It requires more than one session and has acceptable long-term results. Moreover, the removal of intrahepatic stones percutaneously is feasible and effective.[38] Revision surgery is indicated in case of failed anastomotic balloon dilation. It often requires combined parenchymal resection in order to simplify reconstruction. However, the success rate is lower compared with a successful initial repair.[39] Liver transplantation may be required in patients with recurrent cholangitis who have eventually developed secondary biliary cirrhosis.

Management of common bile duct calculi

The presence of stones in the CBD is most often related to their migration from the gallbladder. Choledocholithiasis can be asymptomatic. However, it may also cause symptoms such as biliary pain and jaundice and it can lead to severe complications including AC and pancreatitis. Although small unsuspected stones can pass spontaneously,[40] once detected, CBD stones should be removed to reduce the risk of complications over time.[41] A conservative approach can be considered especially in asymptomatic elderly patients when the risks of surgical or endoscopic treatment of CBD calculi are higher than the risks of stone complications.[42]

The management of CBD calculi has changed considerably over the past several decades. Whereas laparotomy with CBD exploration was once considered the standard treatment for choledocholithiasis, less invasive endoscopic treatment is now being increasingly adopted. Indeed, the success rate of endoscopic sphincterotomy with CBD stone extraction is 80–90%.[43]

Choledocholithiasis in a patient with previous cholecystectomy is a good indication for ERCP since it provides permanent treatment. However, in patients with gallbladder *in situ*, the management of both CBD and gallbladder stones can be achieved either by a combined endoscopy–surgical approach or by an exclusively surgical approach. The choice between these two approaches remains a matter of debate and should take into account local expertise and resources. When the combined approach is decided, ERCP should be performed first (Figure 39.4).

Endoscopic treatment

Endoscopic extraction of CBD calculi can be carried out using various techniques and tools. During ERCP, adequate access to the biliary tree may be provided by endoscopic sphincterotomy alone, endoscopic papillary balloon dilation alone, or a combination of both.[42] Stone extraction may be achieved by using balloon and basket catheters. Both have similar efficacy and safety.[44]

Difficult stones, which cannot be removed using standard techniques, require additional interventional procedures such as large-balloon dilation, mechanical lithotripsy, cholangioscopy-assisted lithotripsy, or extracorporeal shock wave lithotripsy.[42]

In case of incomplete clearance of CBD, a temporary plastic stent should be placed to relieve the obstruction until a second endoscopic attempt or surgical intervention is performed. It should be

---

Box 39.3 Aetiologies of recurrent cholangitis

- Recurrent pyogenic cholangitis.
- Intrahepatic congenital bile duct dilatation.
- Intrahepatic lithiasis.
- Recurrent strictures after biliary reconstructive procedure.
- Ischaemic type biliary stenosis after liver transplantation.
- Primary sclerosing cholangitis.
- Bile duct stent obstruction.
- Congenital hepatic fibrosis.

Source: data from Chan C, Fan ST, Wong J. Recurrent pyogenic cholangitis. In: Jarnagin W, ed. *Blumgart's Surgery of the Liver, Biliary Tract and Pancreas*. 6th ed. Elsevier; 2017: 725–741; Laurence JM, Greig PD. Recurrent pyogenic cholangitis. In: Dixon E, Vollmer CM Jr, May GR, eds. *Management of Benign Biliary Stenosis and Injury. A Comprehensive Guide*. Springer; 2015: 103–120; and Stain SC, Nigam A. Management of recurrent cholangitis. In: Millis JM, Matthews JB, eds. *Difficult Decisions in Hepatobiliary and Pancreatic Surgery. An Evidence-Based Approach*. Springer; 2016: 227–239.

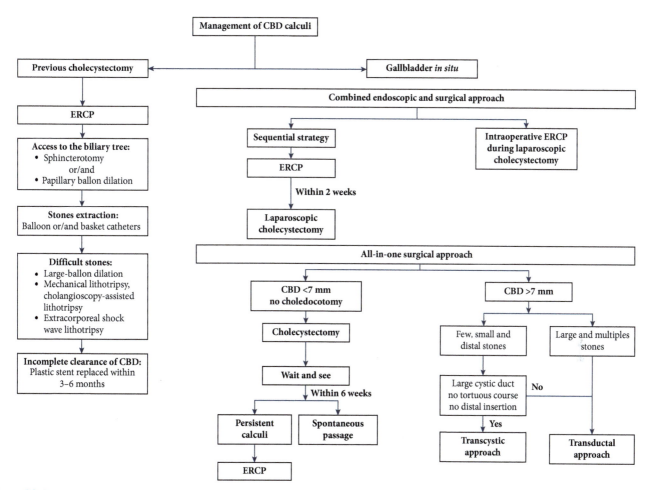

Figure 39.4 Algorithm for management of CBD calculi.

replaced within 3–6 months to reduce the rate of obstruction and subsequent infectious complications.[42]

Combined endoscopic and surgical treatment

In order to treat stones in the gallbladder and the CBD, a sequential strategy can be adopted by performing preoperative ERCP followed by laparoscopic cholecystectomy. The time between the two procedures should not exceed 2 weeks to reduce the risk of biliary events and repeated biliary intervention.[42,45] This strategy enables subsequent surgical exploration if ERCP fails. Intraoperative ERCP during laparoscopic cholecystectomy offers the advantages of a single-stage procedure. Compared with the sequential strategy, it has a similar efficacy, a lower rate of morbidity, including post-ERCP pancreatitis, and shorter hospital stay.[46] However, this approach poses logistical and organizational problems because surgical and endoscopic teams and equipment must be present at the same time and in the same place.

Surgical treatment

Surgical treatment of CBD stones during cholecystectomy offers the opportunity to treat patients in a single-stage procedure. With the development of laparoscopic cholecystectomy in the early 1990s, the use of ERCP has increased in the management of CBD stones, replacing open CBD exploration. However, laparoscopic exploration of the CBD is now a validated technique and remains the technique of choice in some centres. It has a significantly higher efficacy, shorter hospital stay, and similar morbidity compared with the sequential strategy.[47] Small stones detected on intraoperative cholangiography will often pass spontaneously and a wait-and-see approach is reasonable, especially when the CBD is thin.[40]

Laparoscopic CBD exploration can be performed through a transcystic or transductal approach. The transcystic approach does not require opening the CBD. It is appropriate when the cystic duct is large, straight enough, and does not have a very distal insertion. It may include fluoroscopic or choledochoscope-guided techniques. The best indication is the presence of few, small, and distal stones. The transductal approach is generally used as the primary approach. It allows removal of large and multiple stones in almost any location. It should be avoided in a CBD smaller than 7 mm to minimize the risk of ductal stricture. After clearance of the CBD, closing of the choledochotomy around a T-tube is still a common practice. However, choledochotomy can be primarily closed if there is no sign of infection or distal obstruction.[48] Unfortunately, the widespread adoption of a laparoscopic approach remains relatively limited owing to its complexity, prolonged operative time, and the need for sophisticated and expensive instruments as well as surgical expertise.

Open CBD exploration is less frequently performed with the development of endoscopic and laparoscopic techniques. Nevertheless, there are certain circumstances where an open approach is still needed including converted laparoscopic cholecystectomy with choledocholithiasis, Mirizzi syndrome, large common duct stones (>2 cm), the need for a concomitant biliary drainage procedure, such as choledochoduodenostomy, and anatomic alteration precluding the use of ERCP such as long Roux-en-Y limb, peri-ampullary diverticulum, or prior gastroduodenal surgery.[49]

Conclusion

When a diagnosis of AC is made, management should be carried out as soon as possible because its evolution is unpredictable. The progression from mild to severe cholangitis can be rapid. Treatment is based on adequate resuscitation, antibiotics, and biliary decompression.

Recurrent cholangitis could be due to several causes, especially diseases associated with intrahepatic lithiasis. Its management is challenging and aims to reduce the risk of recurrence in order to avoid long-term complications including biliary cirrhosis and cholangiocarcinoma. The management of CBD stones has changed radically over the last few decades. Many options are now available, including endoscopic and laparoscopic techniques. The choice depends on local resources and expertise.

REFERENCES

1. Sung JY, Costerton JW, Shaffer EA. Defense system in the biliary tract against bacterial infection. *Dig Dis Sci*. 1992;**37**(5):689–696.
2. Sung JY, Shaffer EA, Costerton JW. Antibacterial activity of bile salts against common biliary pathogens. Effects of hydrophobicity of the molecule and in the presence of phospholipids. *Dig Dis Sci*. 1993;**38**(11):2104–2112.
3. Reynoso-Paz S, Coppel RL, Mackay IR, Bass NM, Ansari AA, Gershwin ME. The immunobiology of bile and biliary epithelium. *Hepatol*. 1999;**30**(2):351–357.
4. Takada T, Yasuda H, Hanyu F. Pathophysiologic mechanisms in patients with cholangitis or obstructive jaundice: results of a cholangiographic study. *J Hepatobiliary Pancreat Surg*. 1996;**3**(1):17–22.
5. Cetta F. The route of infection in patients with bactibilia. *World J Surg*. 1983;**7**(4):562.
6. Deitch EA, Sittig K, Li M, Berg R, Specian RD. Obstructive jaundice promotes bacterial translocation from the gut. *Am J Surg*. 1990;**159**(1):79–84.
7. Westphal JF, Brogard JM. Biliary tract infections: a guide to drug treatment. *Drugs*. 1999;**57**(1):81–91.
8. Weber A, Schneider J, Wagenpfeil S, et al. Spectrum of pathogens in acute cholangitis in patients with and without biliary endoprosthesis. *J Infect*. 2013;**67**(2):111–121.
9. Charcot M. De la fievre hepatique symptomatique. In: *Comparison avec la fievre uroseptique. Lecons sur les maladies du foie des voies biliaires et des reins*. Paris: Bourneville et Sevestre; 1877: 176–185.
10. Reynolds BM, Dargan EL. Acute obstructive cholangitis; a distinct clinical syndrome. *Ann Surg*. 1959;**150**(2):299–303.
11. Kiriyama S, Kozaka K, Takada T, et al. Tokyo Guidelines 2018: diagnostic criteria and severity grading of acute cholangitis (with videos). *J Hepatobiliary Pancreat Sci*. 2018;**25**(1):17–30.
12. Anciaux ML, Pelletier G, Attali P, Meduri B, Liguory C, Etienne JP. Prospective study of clinical and biochemical features of symptomatic choledocholithiasis. *Dig Dis Sci*. 1986;**31**(5):449–453.
13. Abbitt PL. Ultrasonography of the liver. An update on new applications. *Clin Liver Dis*. 2002;**6**(1):17–28.
14. Pasanen P, Partanen K, Pikkarainen P, Alhava E, Pirinen A, Janatuinen E. Ultrasonography, CT, and ERCP in the diagnosis of choledochal stones. *Acta Radiol*. 1992;**33**(1):53–56.
15. Akaike G, Ishiyama M, Suzuki S, Fujita Y, Ohde S, Saida Y. Significance of peribiliary oedema on computed tomography in diagnosis and severity assessment of acute cholangitis. *Eur J Radiol*. 2013;**82**(9):e429–e433.
16. Arai K, Kawai K, Kohda W, Tatsu H, Matsui O, Nakahama T. Dynamic CT of acute cholangitis: early inhomogeneous enhancement of the liver. *AJR Am J Roentgenol*. 2003;**181**(1):115–118.
17. Håkansson K, Ekberg O, Håkansson H-O, Leander P. MR characteristics of acute cholangitis. *Acta Radiol*. 2002;**43**(2):175–179.
18. Polistina FA, Frego M, Bisello M, Manzi E, Vardanega A, Perin B. Accuracy of magnetic resonance cholangiography compared to operative endoscopy in detecting biliary stones, a single center experience and review of literature. *World J Radiol*. 2015;**7**(4):70–78.
19. Eun HW, Kim JH, Hong SS, Kim YJ. Assessment of acute cholangitis by MR imaging. *Eur J Radiol*. 2012;**81**(10):2476–2480.
20. Meeralam Y, Al-Shammari K, Yaghoobi M. Diagnostic accuracy of EUS compared with MRCP in detecting choledocholithiasis: a meta-analysis of diagnostic test accuracy in head-to-head studies. *Gastrointest Endosc*. 2017;**86**(6):986–993.
21. Gomi H, Solomkin JS, Schlossberg D, et al. Tokyo Guidelines 2018: antimicrobial therapy for acute cholangitis and cholecystitis. *J Hepatobiliary Pancreat Sci*. 2018;**25**(1):3–16.
22. van den Hazel SJ, Speelman P, Tytgat GN, Dankert J, van Leeuwen DJ. Role of antibiotics in the treatment and prevention of acute and recurrent cholangitis. *Clin Infect Dis*. 1994;**19**(2):279–286.
23. Rhodes A, Evans LE, Alhazzani W, et al. Surviving Sepsis Campaign: international guidelines for management of sepsis and septic shock: 2016. *Intensive Care Med*. 2017;**43**(3):304–377.
24. Tantau M, Mercea V, Crisan D, et al. ERCP on a cohort of 2,986 patients with cholelitiasis: a 10-year experience of a single center. *J Gastrointestin Liver Dis*. 2013;**22**(2):141–147.
25. Mukai S, Itoi T, Baron TH, et al. Indications and techniques of biliary drainage for acute cholangitis in updated Tokyo Guidelines 2018. *J Hepatobiliary Pancreat Sci*. 2017;**24**(10):537–549.
26. Zhang R, Cheng L, Cai X, Zhao H, Zhu F, Wan X. Comparison of the safety and effectiveness of endoscopic biliary decompression by nasobiliary catheter and plastic stent placement in acute obstructive cholangitis. *Swiss Med Wkly*. 2013;**143**:w13823.
27. Ito T, Sai JK, Okubo H, et al. Safety of immediate endoscopic sphincterotomy in acute suppurative cholangitis caused by choledocholithiasis. *World J Gastrointest Endosc*. 2016;**8**(3):180–185.
28. Paik WH, Park YS, Hwang J-H, et al. Palliative treatment with self-expandable metallic stents in patients with advanced type III or IV hilar cholangiocarcinoma: a percutaneous versus endoscopic approach. *Gastrointest Endosc*. 2009;**69**(1):55–62.
29. Saad WEA, Wallace MJ, Wojak JC, Kundu S, Cardella JF. Quality improvement guidelines for percutaneous transhepatic cholangiography, biliary drainage, and percutaneous cholecystostomy. *J Vasc Interv Radiol*. 2010;**21**(6):789–795.

30. Sharaiha RZ, Khan MA, Kamal F, et al. Efficacy and safety of EUS-guided biliary drainage in comparison with percutaneous biliary drainage when ERCP fails: a systematic review and meta-analysis. *Gastrointest Endosc*. 2017;**85**(5):904–914.
31. Lai EC, Tam PC, Paterson IA, et al. Emergency surgery for severe acute cholangitis. The high-risk patients. *Ann Surg* 1990;**211**(1):55–59.
32. Nakayama F. Intrahepatic stones: epidemiology and etiology. *Prog Clin Biol Res*. 1984;**152**:17–28.
33. Ohta G, Nakanuma Y, Terada T. Pathology of hepatolithiasis: cholangitis and cholangiocarcinoma. *Prog Clin Biol Res*. 1984;**152**:91–113.
34. Fan ST, Mok F, Zheng SS, Lai EC, Lo CM, Wong J. Appraisal of hepaticocutaneous jejunostomy in the management of hepatolithiasis. *Am J Surg*. 1993;**165**(3):332–335.
35. Caroli J, Couinaud C, Soupault R et al. Une affection nouvelle, sans doute congénitale, des voies biliaires: la dilatation kystique unilobaire des canaux hépatiques. *Sem Hop Paris*. 1958;**34**:136–142.
36. Mabrut J-Y, Kianmanesh R, Nuzzo G, et al. Surgical management of congenital intrahepatic bile duct dilatation, Caroli's disease and syndrome: long-term results of the French Association of Surgery Multicenter Study. *Ann Surg*. 2013;**258**(5):713–721.
37. Quintero GA, Patiño JF. Surgical management of benign strictures of the biliary tract. *World J Surg*. 2001;**25**(10):1245–1250.
38. Cantwell CP, Pena CS, Gervais DA, Hahn PF, Dawson SL, Mueller PR. Thirty years' experience with balloon dilation of benign postoperative biliary strictures: long-term outcomes. *Radiology*. 2008;**249**(3):1050–1057.
39. Pellegrini CA, Thomas MJ, Way LW. Recurrent biliary stricture. Patterns of recurrence and outcome of surgical therapy. *Am J Surg*. 1984;**147**(1):175–180.
40. Collins C, Maguire D, Ireland A, Fitzgerald E, O'Sullivan GC. A prospective study of common bile duct calculi in patients undergoing laparoscopic cholecystectomy: natural history of choledocholithiasis revisited. *Ann Surg*. 2004;**239**(1):28–33.
41. Möller M, Gustafsson U, Rasmussen F, Persson G, Thorell A. Natural course vs interventions to clear common bile duct stones: data from the Swedish Registry for Gallstone Surgery and Endoscopic Retrograde Cholangiopancreatography (GallRiks). *JAMA Surg*. 2014;**149**(10):1008–1013.
42. Manes G, Paspatis G, Aabakken L, et al. Endoscopic management of common bile duct stones: European Society of Gastrointestinal Endoscopy (ESGE) guideline. *Endoscopy* 2019;**51**(5):472–491.
43. Sivak MV. Endoscopic management of bile duct stones. *Am J Surg*. 1989;**158**(3):228–240.
44. Ozawa N, Yasuda I, Doi S, et al. Prospective randomized study of endoscopic biliary stone extraction using either a basket or a balloon catheter: the BasketBall study. *J Gastroenterol*. 2017;**52**(5):623–630.
45. Xu J, Yang C. Cholecystectomy outcomes after endoscopic sphincterotomy in patients with choledocholithiasis: a meta-analysis. *BMC Gastroenterol*. 2020;**20**(1):229.
46. Tan C, Ocampo O, Ong R, Tan KS. Comparison of one stage laparoscopic cholecystectomy combined with intra-operative endoscopic sphincterotomy versus two-stage pre-operative endoscopic sphincterotomy followed by laparoscopic cholecystectomy for the management of pre-operatively diagnosed patients with common bile duct stones: a meta-analysis. *Surg Endosc*. 2018;**32**(2):770–778.
47. Singh AN, Kilambi R. Single-stage laparoscopic common bile duct exploration and cholecystectomy versus two-stage endoscopic stone extraction followed by laparoscopic cholecystectomy for patients with gallbladder stones with common bile duct stones: systematic review and meta-analysis of randomized trials with trial sequential analysis. *Surg Endosc*. 2018;**32**(9):3763–3776.
48. Zhang W-J, Xu G-F, Wu G-Z, Li J-M, Dong Z-T, Mo X-D. Laparoscopic exploration of common bile duct with primary closure versus T-tube drainage: a randomized clinical trial. *J Surg Res*. 2009;**157**(1):e1–e5.
49. Rattner DW. Open common bile duct exploration. In: Santos B, Soper N, eds, *Choledocholithiasis*. Cham: Springer; 2018: 177–185.

40

Cystic diseases of the biliary system

Stefan Heinrich

Introduction

The biliary system comprises the confluence of all lobular canaliculi into segmental and sectoral bile ducts draining into the extrahepatic biliary system and the gall bladder. Accordingly, diseases of the biliary system reveal a major overlap of hepatic and extrahepatic diseases.

Under physiological conditions, bile is excreted by the hepatocytes through the canaliculi into the intra- and then the extrahepatic bile ducts. Due to the sphincter of Oddi, the bile flow is directed upwards into the gall bladder, which resorbs the fluid from the bile. Thus, the bile is concentrated and can be stored in the gall bladder until it is required to digest food in the bowel. Moreover, the sphincter of Oddi prevents influx of pancreatic juice and intestinal bacteria into the bile duct. A hormonal activation triggers the contraction of the gall bladder and relaxation of the sphincter of Oddi. Consequently, the gall bladder is emptied and the bile spills out into the duodenum.

While the physiological diameter of the healthy bile duct is up to 6 mm, a diameter of greater than 8 mm is considered pathological, and a diameter of 6–8 mm is considered borderline.

Cystic diseases of the biliary system are often associated with disturbances of these physiological processes. Such diseases may be congenital or acquired and exhibit different risks of malignancy.

Gall bladder cyst

In general, cysts of the gall bladder and bile ducts are rare. Most often, gall bladder-associated cysts arise from chronic cholecystitis. Due to the low complexity and morbidity of cholecystectomy, such findings are usually dealt with early by operation, and further treatment is given according to the histological diagnosis.

Also, an aberrant embryological development may result in duplicated gall bladders, which may be misinterpreted as gall bladder cysts,[1] ciliated gall bladder cysts containing bronchial epithelium,[2] or cysts of the gall bladder arising from obstruction of glands or sinuses, such as Rokitansky–Ashoff or Luschka sinuses.[3] Also, cystic diseases of the bile ducts (see below) may also affect the gall bladder.

Bile duct diameter

The bile duct diameter increases with age: an increase in the bile duct diameter of 0.4 mm per decade of patient age has been described by several analyses.[4,5] Potential explanations for this incidental finding include connective tissue changes in the bile duct during ageing resulting in a decreased intrabiliary pressure. Also, chronic medication with calcium antagonists or nitroglycerine may increase this effect, and a dysregulation of the sphincter of Oddi may be another explanation (Figure 40.1). However, such an increased bile duct diameter should only be accepted as age-dependent (and physiological) in asymptomatic patients.

The diameter of the common bile duct may also increase postoperatively: it is well known that the diameter of the extrahepatic bile duct increases after a cholecystectomy. The general explanation for this finding is the compensation of the gall bladder capacity by the bile duct after cholecystectomy. In general, a bile duct diameter up to 10 mm is considered normal after a cholecystectomy. Also, a recent analysis revealed increased bile duct diameters of 1.4 mm in patients who underwent gastric bypass procedures independent of a cholecystectomy.[6]

Congenital choledochal malformation

In 1977, Todani et al. reported their experience with *choledochal cysts* or *choledochoceles* and proposed a classification for this group of malformations which is still valid[7]: various cystic anomalies of the intra- or extrahepatic bile ducts are summarized in this classification (Figure 40.2). Due to these variations, the term 'congenital choledochal malformation' (CCM) is currently preferred,[8,9] and these are more frequently seen in Asian than in Western countries, and more females are affected than males.[10]

Some types of CCM are associated with an abnormal junction of the pancreatic and bile ducts as the pancreatic duct drains into the distal bile duct (or vice versa) before the papilla of Vater.[11] The consequence is a *common channel* of both ducts, and pancreatic juice may enter the bile duct and cause chronic (or recurrent) cholangitis with an increased risk of malignancy.[12] Accordingly, aspirates from a choledochal cyst contain amylase/lipase-rich fluid.[13] In

Congenital choledochal malformation 447

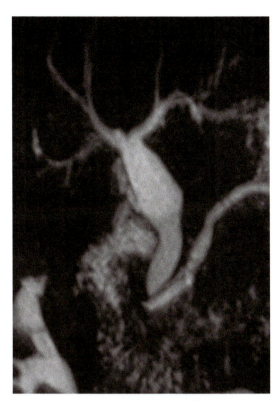

Figure 40.1 MRI scans of a 70-year-old female patient who revealed increased cholestasis parameters after a septic episode following orthopaedic surgery. The laboratory parameters normalized quickly. The MRI scan shows a dilated bile duct. Intrahepatic ducts are normal and a maljunction of the biliary and pancreatic ducts are excluded.

11% developed malignancy, of which 7.5% were diagnosed in the specimen of primary surgery and 3.5% during follow-up.[8] Due to the obvious association of CCM with cancer, longitudinal observational studies have not been performed, and therefore, the true risk of malignancy remains unknown.

Symptoms

Most patients present with right upper quadrant pain, recurrent cholangitis, or a palpable mass in the abdomen. It seems that adults most often present with non-specific pain. Patients may additionally develop cholangitis or pancreatitis. In contrast, children present with two out of the three symptoms: abdominal pain, palpable abdominal mass, and jaundice.[10] For type II CCMs, symptoms appear less specific with cholangitis being a rare symptom.[15]

Imaging

Depending on the type of CCM, the radiological presentation is different. The optimal delineation of the CCM and potentially the abnormal junction of the biliary and pancreatic ducts is achieved by endoscopic retrograde cholangiopancreatography (ERCP) due to the direct opacification of the biliopancreatic system. Non-invasive, high-resolution magnetic resonance imaging (MRI), which adequately depicts the type and extent of the CCM, may also show the abnormal junction of the ducts depending on the resolution of the MRI scanner and the compliance of the patient (Figure 40.3). Moreover, intraductal tumour nodules can sometimes be detected by MRI.

Types I and IV CCMs present with a dilatation of the extrahepatic bile duct and patent hilar bifurcation in contrast to biliary obstruction which is accompanied by a dilatation of the intrahepatic bile ducts. The extent of the bile duct dilatation may vary from a few centimetres up to giant cysts (Figure 40.3).

Simple biliary cysts (types II and III) are usually detected by routine ultrasound or CT scan, but are described best by ERCP or MRI and magnetic resonance cholangiopancreatography (MRCP).

Type V CCM is also known as Caroli syndrome and mainly reveals multiple intrahepatic cysts with intraluminal stone formations. While some patients develop circumscript or unilateral Caroli syndrome, others reveal diffuse and bilateral cystic degeneration.

Management

In the absence of randomized trials for the ideal treatment of the various types of CCM, the best available evidence arises from expert centres and retrospective multicentre analyses. Currently, treatment aims are to treat clinical symptoms and most importantly to prevent malignancy.

contrast, increased biliary pressure has been found in paediatric patients with type I and IV cysts, which positively correlated with bile duct diameter and inversely with amylase concentration in the bile. Histological changes were more severe in patients with higher biliary pressure and lower amylase concentrations.[14] These data suggest a more complex pathophysiology of CCM rather than only a reflux of pancreatic juice into the bile duct.

According to a recent meta-analysis of the literature including 2904 patients, types I and IV are by far the most frequent (90%), while types II and III constitute less than 3% of CCMs, and type V 8.5%.[8] The same analysis revealed that the incidence of malignancy in a CCM increases with age, and malignancy has only been reported for types I and IV (99%) and a single case in type V. Malignant transformation has not been reported for any type II and III CCMs.[8] Among patients with type I and IV CCMs, about

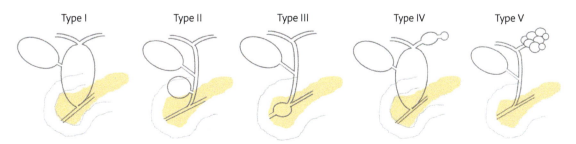

Figure 40.2 Todani classification of CCM.

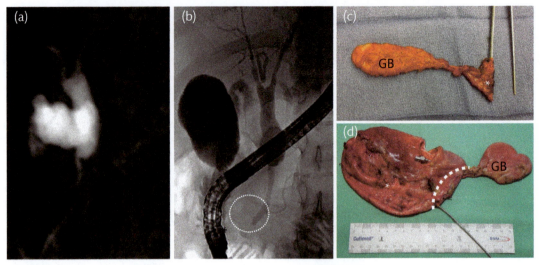

Figure 40.3 A 37-year-old male patient presented with recurrent right upper quadrant pain and a singular episode of cholestasis. MRCP (a) and ERCP (b) demonstrate the maljunction of the pancreatic duct (dotted circle). The resected specimen confirms the dilatation of the mid common bile duct (c). In contrast, a giant type I CCM was resected (d). * CCM; dotted line, bile duct; GB, gall bladder.

Considering the pathophysiology of the abnormal junction of the biliary and pancreatic ducts, the resection of the extrahepatic bile duct down to the intrapancreatic junction is the main treatment concept for types I and IV (**Figure 40.4**).[8] Despite timely surgery in patients with types I and IV CCMs before the development of malignancy, nearly 5% of patients develop cholangiocarcinoma during the follow-up after bile duct resection.[16] The reason for this secondary cancer development may be a genetic disposition, the consequence of previous chronic cholangitis due to the maljunction of the biliary and pancreatic ducts, as well as an incomplete excision of the intrapancreatic duct in a very few patients (**Figure 40.5**).[16] Such secondary malignancies may occur more than 20 years postoperatively and underline the necessity of a complete bile duct resection including the intrapancreatic portion down to the common channel.[16] Moreover, these data suggest that patients who underwent bile duct resection for a CCM should be included in a lifelong surveillance programme to detect secondary malignancy early.

Probably due to the limited size and low risk of malignancy, papillotomy is considered sufficient for types II and III and resection of the cyst is only necessary depending on the symptoms of the patient. However, a European multicentre analysis of CCMs including 19 patients with type II CCMs demonstrated that all patients underwent surgical excision of the bile duct cyst. Depending

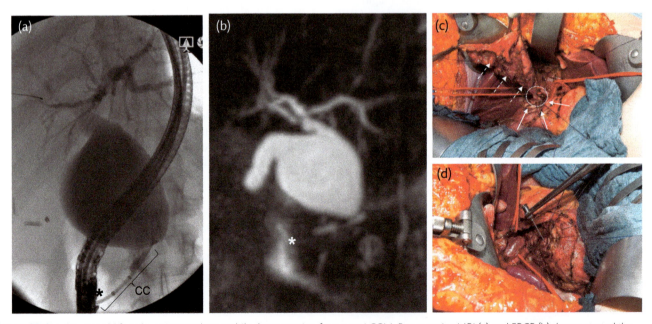

Figure 40.4 A 47-year-old female patient underwent bile duct resection for a type I CCM. Preoperative MRI (a) and ERCP (b) demonstrated the common channel (CC) (* papilla of Vater). (c) Surgery included the resection of the entire bile duct (interrupted arrow) including the intrapancreatic portion (white arrows) down to the junction with the pancreatic duct (dotted circle). Panel (d) reveals the defect in the pancreatic head, the common channel is marked with the probe. The patient had a laparoscopic cholecystectomy 3 years before due to an episode of cholangitis.

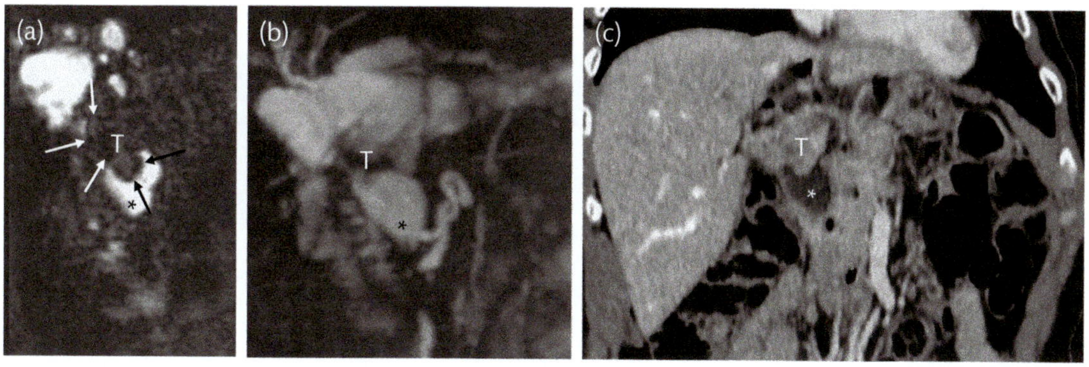

Figure 40.5 A 66-year-old female patient was referred due to recurrent episodes of right upper quadrant pain. She had a cholecystectomy 15 years ago, and required repetitive ERCP for recurrent cholangitis since then. The preoperative imaging revealed a mass within the mid common bile duct, which was enlarged as a type I CCM. A maljunction of the biliary and pancreatic ducts was not proven on the preoperative imaging.

on the localization of the cyst, additional liver or bile duct resections were performed in the majority of the patients. In contrast with the preoperative imaging, intense inflammatory changes around the bile duct cyst necessitated the resection of the extrahepatic bile duct and the frequent conversion from a laparoscopic to an open approach.[15]

In contrast, combined bile duct and liver resections or even orthotopic liver transplantation are adequate procedures for the treatment of types IV and V.[17]

Peribiliary cysts

The incidence of peribiliary cysts is much higher in Asian than in Western countries, and its pathogenesis is unclear. Histologically, peribiliary cysts are dilated peribiliary glands. They may be congenital, associated with syndromes (e.g. adult polycystic kidney disease) or develop due to chronic liver injury (e.g. alcoholic liver cirrhosis). An autopsy study of more than 1000 patients revealed peribiliary cysts in 5% of healthy and 40% of diseased livers.[18] Due to the heterogeneity of this entity, a significant overlap with CCM and simple cysts exists and the differentiation from Caroli tumor or type IV CCM is difficult.

Symptoms

The clinical presentation varies from asymptomatic patients over cholestasis to recurrent episodes of cholangitis with intraductal stone development. Most patients with adult polycystic kidney disease without an underlying liver disease are asymptomatic. An association with malignancy as for CCM has not been demonstrated for peribiliary cysts. However, the incidence of cancer may be increased according to an underlying liver disease.[19]

Imaging

The distribution of the cysts varies widely from solitary to multiple and from perihilar to intrahepatic according to the distribution of the larger and smaller bile ducts. Accordingly, the imaging findings may vary widely. As for all cystic findings, MRI reveals the optimal delineation of the structures (Figure 40.6).

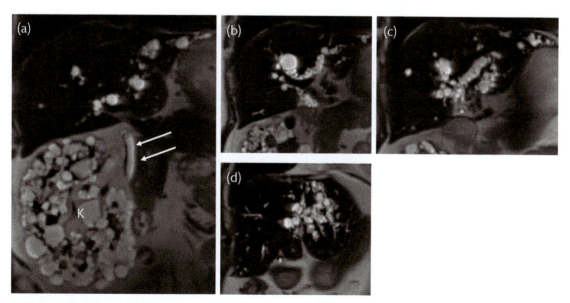

Figure 40.6 A 65-year-old male patient with adult polycystic kidney disease revealed peribiliary cysts upon workup for kidney transplantation. T2-weighted MRIs nicely demonstrate the multiple cysts from the hilar bifurcation along the left bile duct and the ducts to segments 2 and 3 (arrows). The distal bile duct is normal (a, *), the kidneys (K) are polycystic.

Table 40.1 Outcome of patients after surgery for intraductal papillary neoplasm of the bile duct

	N	Invasiveness		Histological subtype				Survival	
		Non-invasive	Invasive	Oncocytic	Pancreatobiliary	Gastric	Intestinal	Median	5 year
Luvira et al., 2017[28]	148	58 (46%)	90 (54%)	-	-	-	-	47.4 months	59.7%*
Lee et al., 2019[29]	120	34 (28%)	86 (72%)	-	-	-	-	-	-
Kubota et al., 2014[30]	119	76 (64%)	43 (36%)	23 (19%)	51 (43%)	12 (10%)	33 (28%)		84%
Jung et al., 2012[31]	93	52 (56%)	41 (44%)	1 (1%)	12 (13%)	24 (26%)	56 (60%)		
Kang et al., 2013[32]	84	9 (11%)	75 (89%)	-	-	-	-	79.7 months**	64%
Choi et al., 2010[33]	55	29 (53%)	26 (47%)	2 (4%)	17 (30%)	12 (22%)	24 (44%)		77.6%***
Rocha et al., 2012[34]	39	10 (26%)	29 (74%)	3 (8%)	23 (69%)	3 (8%)	3 (8%)	49 months	-
Kloeck et al., 2011[35]	20	8 (40%)	12 (60%)	2 (10%)	9 (45%)	5 (25%)	4 (20%)	50 months	24%
	678	275 (41%)	402 (59%)	31 (1%)	112 (35%)	56 (17%)	120 (38%)		

*For R0; ** entire cohort; *** 3-year survival.

Management

Since a malignant potential of peribiliary cysts has not yet been documented, the management of this entity focuses on the symptoms of the patient. In case of recurrent episodes of cholestasis or cholangitis as well as suspected malignancy, liver and/or bile duct resection should be considered according to liver function. Asymptomatic patients should be included in a structured surveillance protocol in order to diagnose malignancy associated with a potentially underlying liver disease early.[19]

Intraductal papillary neoplasms of the bile duct

The exact incidence of intraductal papillary neoplasm of the bile duct (IPNB) is unknown, but it seems to be higher in Eastern countries as for CCM.[20] This entity has been recently described and later on defined by the World Health Organization in 2010.[21] Tumours of this entity develop from the biliary epithelium to papillary neoplasms and produce mucin. IPNB is a rare disease which may occur in the entire hepatobiliary system and has a comparatively high risk for malignancy of about 60% in all resected specimens (Table 40.1).

IPNB occurs with similar frequency intra- and extrahepatically (50%), and are usually analysed together in the literature due to their low incidence. Moreover, it is difficult to distinguish such lesions from each other clinically, since the source of mucin production cannot be identified in a closed system filled with mucin.

Histologically, IPNB shares many similarities with intraductal papillary mucinous neoplasms of the pancreas: several types of IPNB have been identified histologically such as intestinal, pancreaticobiliary, gastric, and oncocytic, of which pancreaticobiliary and intestinal types are most frequent (Table 40.1). Progression to malignancy has been described for all subtypes in a stepwise model from normal biliary epithelium over low-, intermediate-, and high-grade intraepithelial neoplasia to invasive carcinoma. Moreover, these histological steps are associated with molecular changes of the lesions: *KRAS* mutation, overexpression of TP53, and loss of *p16* are present in low-grade intraepithelial neoplasia, while additional loss of SMAD4 as well as increasing overexpression of TP53 were documented in high-grade neoplasia and invasive tumours.[22] As for pancreatic main duct intraductal papillary mucinous neoplasms of the pancreas, all types of IPNB have a high risk of malignancy, of which the pancreaticobiliary subtype has the highest risk.[23]

These data suggest that IPBN are premalignant lesions with a high probability of progression to invasive cancer. Most importantly, the majority of IPNB reveal high-grade neoplasia or even invasive cancer at diagnosis.[24]

Clinical presentation

In addition to the classification based on histological subtypes of IPNB, a clinical classification based on the localization of the tumour has been proposed.[25] This classification differentiates intra- from extrahepatic and diffuse tumours. While the intrahepatic types are most frequent, this subtype exhibits a lower risk of malignancy.[23]

Presenting symptoms depend on the localization of the lesion and the degree of its mucus secretion. The most frequent symptoms of IPNB are non-specific epigastric discomfort. Moreover, many patients suffer from cholestasis and recurrent cholangitis, which are related to the biliary obstruction due to the papillary lesion or mucin excretion into the bile duct (Figure 40.7). Accordingly, changes in the laboratory parameters are mainly related to the degree of biliary obstruction.[20]

Imaging

As the clinical presentation and the tumour characteristics are variable, available imaging modalities may demonstrate different characteristics of IPNB: they may predominantly consist of a papillary tumour with consequent mass formation. Since most IPNBs secrete mucin, a mixed appearance is very frequent: the papillary lesion may cause proximal cholestasis, and the bile duct may reveal cystic dilatation due to the intraductal mucin accumulation (Figure 40.7).[26]

Computed tomography as well as MRI may describe an inhomogeneous mass with intraluminal tumour nodules. Moreover, bile duct dilatation as a consequence of mucus accumulation or secondary to neoplastic bile duct obstruction can be demonstrated. Anatomical delineation of intraluminal nodules and the anatomical associations to the biliary tract are better demonstrated on MRI.

ERCP with papillotomy may demonstrate mucus spilling out of the papilla, and cholangiography often reveals filling defects due to papillary tumour nodules or mucus adhering to the wall of the bile duct. Endoscopic cholangioscopy ('SpyGlass') may demonstrate the

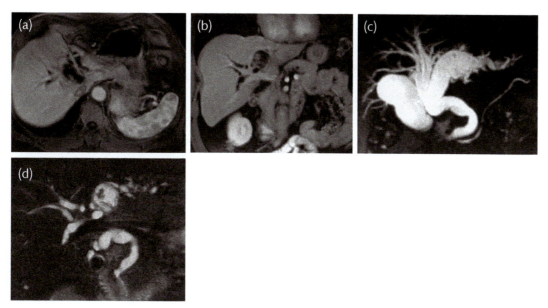

Figure 40.7 A 66-year-old male patient was referred after an ERCP and cholangioscopy had demonstrated mucus accumulation in the bile duct. Upon presentation, the patient was asymptomatic and the liver transaminases and cholestasis parameters were normal. MRI (a) and CT (s) scans as well as MRCP (c) demonstrate the dilatation of the left hepatic and common bile duct. Moreover, soft tissue was visible in a cystic mass in the left liver. (d) Coronal T2-weighed images underlined the papillary nodules within the cystic lesion.

intraluminal mucin accumulation and enables the correct staging of the IPNB regarding histological diagnosis, subtyping, and distribution within the bile duct.[20]

Management

Due to the low incidence of IPNB, evidence-based recommendations on the extent of the resection are lacking.

Considering the high risk of malignancy, resection is generally recommended for all histological subtypes of IPNB in the literature. The aim of surgery is an R0 resection of the IPNB including a hilar lymphadenectomy according to surgery for cholangiocarcinoma, since lymph node metastases, invasive cancer, and positive resection margins have been shown to be prognostic factors for overall survival.[23] Since the exact extent of the disease is difficult to assess on preoperative imaging, intraoperative cholangioscopy and frozen sections of the resection margins may help to define the extent of surgery. It seems reasonable to perform an anatomical resection of the liver for intrahepatic IPNB and to resect the bile duct including the intrapancreatic part in case of extrahepatic IPNB.[20] Whether a resection of the pancreatic head should be added depends on the proximal extent of surgery and the general condition of the patient.

Pseudocystic biliary diseases

According to the pancreatic or hepatic cystic findings, many diseases may present as or similar to cystic diseases of the biliary system: for example, an underlying malignancy may mimic a 'benign' cystic disease of the biliary system, which may present as a cyst or a bile duct dilatation. Bile duct dilatation due to malignant tumours is usually continuous up to the periphery, while cystic diseases of the biliary system may also reveal normal biliary structures proximal and distal to the abnormality. Also, (immunoglobulin G4-associated) autoimmune cholangitis may mimic any benign and malignant disease in the pancreas and the bile ducts.[27]

Conclusion

While hepatic cysts are frequent, cystic diseases of the biliary system are rare diseases particularly in Western countries. Although they present a heterogeneous group of findings, cystic diseases of the biliary system also share some similarities: they are often congenital and associated with malformations or syndromes, and their incidence is highest in Asia, which suggests a genetic background. Also, the clinical presentation is similar and includes cholestasis or cholangitis and an increased risk of cancer.

Most importantly, the differentiation of cystic diseases of the biliary system may be difficult and requires particular experience in this field due to the potential overlap of the respective entities and potential pitfalls of misdiagnosis in cases of cancer. While prophylactic surgery is indicated in some, others require a treatment focused on the patient's complaints. All patients with asymptomatic cystic diseases of the biliary system who have not undergone prophylactic surgery should be included in surveillance programmes in order to detect progression or even malignancy early.

REFERENCES

1. Vezakis A, Pantiora E, Giannoulopoulos D, et al. A duplicated gallbladder in a patient presenting with acute cholangitis. A case study and a literature review. *Ann Hepatol*. 2019;**18**(1):240–245.
2. Giakoustidis A, Morrison D, Thillainayagam A, Stamp G, Mahadevan V, Mudan S. Ciliated foregut cyst of the gallbladder. A diagnostic challenge and management quandary. *J Gastrointestin Liver Dis*. 2014;**23**(2):207–210.

3. Jacobs E, Ardichvili D, D'Avanzo E, Penneman R, Van Gansbeke D. Cyst of the gallbladder. *Dig Dis Sci*. 1991;**36**(12):1796–1802.
4. Bachar GN, Cohen M, Belenky A, Atar E, Gideon S. Effect of aging on the adult extrahepatic bile duct: a sonographic study. *J Ultrasound Med*. 2003;**22**(9):879–882.
5. Itoi T, Kamisawa T, Fujii H, et al. Extrahepatic bile duct measurement by using transabdominal ultrasound in Japanese adults: multi-center prospective study. *J Gastroenterol*. 2013;**48**(9):1045–1050.
6. Mehta N, Strong AT, Stevens T, et al. Common bile duct dilation after bariatric surgery. *Surg Endosc*. 2019;**33**(8):2531–2538.
7. Todani T, Watanabe Y, Narusue M, Tabuchi K, Okajima K. Congenital bile duct cysts: classification, operative procedures, and review of thirty-seven cases including cancer arising from choledochal cyst. *Am J Surg*. 1977;**134**(2):263–269.
8. Ten Hove A, de Meijer VE, Hulscher JBF, de Kleine RHJ. Meta-analysis of risk of developing malignancy in congenital choledochal malformation. *Br J Surg*. 2018;**105**(5):482–490.
9. Mabrut JY, Bozio G, Hubert C, Gigot JF. Management of congenital bile duct cysts. *Dig Surg*. 2010;**27**(1):12–18.
10. Baison GN, Bonds MM, Helton WS, Kozarek RA. Choledochal cysts: similarities and differences between Asian and Western countries. *World J Gastroenterol*. 2019;**25**(26):3334–3343.
11. Lenriot JP, Gigot JF, Segol P, Fagniez PL, Fingerhut A, Adloff M. Bile duct cysts in adults: a multi-institutional retrospective study. French Associations for Surgical Research. *Ann Surg*. 1998;**228**(2):159–166.
12. Park SW, Koh H, Oh JT, Han SJ, Kim S. Relationship between anomalous pancreaticobiliary ductal union and pathologic inflammation of bile duct in choledochal cyst. *Pediatr Gastroenterol Hepatol Nutr*. 2014;**17**(3):170–177.
13. Jeong IH, Jung YS, Kim H, et al. Amylase level in extrahepatic bile duct in adult patients with choledochal cyst plus anomalous pancreatico-biliary ductal union. *World J Gastroenterol*. 2005;**11**(13):1965–1970.
14. Turowski C, Knisely AS, Davenport M. Role of pressure and pancreatic reflux in the aetiology of choledochal malformation. *Br J Surg*. 2011;**98**(9):1319–1326.
15. Ouaissi M, Kianmanesh R, Belghiti J, et al. Todani type II congenital bile duct cyst: European Multicenter Study of the French Surgical Association and literature review. *Ann Surg*. 2015;**262**(1):130–138.
16. Ohashi T, Wakai T, Kubota M, et al. Risk of subsequent biliary malignancy in patients undergoing cyst excision for congenital choledochal cysts. *J Gastroenterol Hepatol*. 2013;**28**(2):243–247.
17. Mabrut JY, Kianmanesh R, Nuzzo G, et al. Surgical management of congenital intrahepatic bile duct dilatation, Caroli's disease and syndrome: long-term results of the French Association of Surgery Multicenter Study. *Ann Surg*. 2013;**258**(5):713–721.
18. Goossens N, Breguet R, De Vito C, et al. Peribiliary gland dilatation in cirrhosis: relationship with liver failure and stem cell/proliferation markers. *Dig Dis Sci*. 2017;**62**(3):699–707.
19. Bazerbachi F, Haffar S, Sugihara T, et al. Peribiliary cysts: a systematic review and proposal of a classification framework. *BMJ Open Gastroenterol*. 2018;**5**(1):e000204.
20. Wan XS, Xu YY, Qian JY, et al. Intraductal papillary neoplasm of the bile duct. *World J Gastroenterol*. 2013;**19**(46):8595–8604.
21. Zen Y, Fujii T, Itatsu K, et al. Biliary papillary tumors share pathological features with intraductal papillary mucinous neoplasm of the pancreas. *Hepatology*. 2006;**44**(5):1333–1343.
22. Schlitter AM, Born D, Bettstetter M, et al. Intraductal papillary neoplasms of the bile duct: stepwise progression to carcinoma involves common molecular pathways. *Mod Pathol*. 2014;**27**(1):73–86.
23. Kim JR, Jang KT, Jang JY, et al. Clinicopathologic analysis of intraductal papillary neoplasm of bile duct: Korean multicenter cohort study. *HPB (Oxford)*. 2020;**22**(8):1139–1148.
24. Ohtsuka M, Shimizu H, Kato A, et al. Intraductal papillary neoplasms of the bile duct. *Int J Hepatol*. 2014;**2014**:459091.
25. Kim JR, Lee KB, Kwon W, Kim E, Kim SW, Jang JY. Comparison of the clinicopathologic characteristics of intraductal papillary neoplasm of the bile duct according to morphological and anatomical classifications. *J Korean Med Sci*. 2018;**33**(42):e266.
26. Park HJ, Kim SY, Kim HJ, et al. Intraductal papillary neoplasm of the bile duct: clinical, imaging, and pathologic features. *AJR Am J Roentgenol*. 2018;**211**(1):67–75.
27. Lee HE, Zhang L. Immunoglobulin G4-related hepatobiliary disease. *Semin Diagn Pathol*. 2019;**36**(6):423–433.
28. Luvira V, Pugkhem A, Bhudhisawasdi V, et al. Long-term outcome of surgical resection for intraductal papillary neoplasm of the bile duct. *J Gastroenterol Hepatol*. 2017;**32**(2):527–533.
29. Lee S, Kim MJ, Kim S, Choi D, Jang KT, Park YN. Intraductal papillary neoplasm of the bile duct: assessment of invasive carcinoma and long-term outcomes using MRI. *J Hepatol*. 2019;**70**(4):692–699.
30. Kubota K, Nakanuma Y, Kondo F, et al. Clinicopathological features and prognosis of mucin-producing bile duct tumor and mucinous cystic tumor of the liver: a multi-institutional study by the Japan Biliary Association. *J Hepatobiliary Pancreat Sci*. 2014;**21**(3):176–185.
31. Jung G, Park KM, Lee SS, Yu E, Hong SM, Kim J. Long-term clinical outcome of the surgically resected intraductal papillary neoplasm of the bile duct. *J Hepatol*. 2012;**57**(4):787–793.
32. Kang MJ, Jang JY, Lee KB, et al. Impact of macroscopic morphology, multifocality, and mucin secretion on survival outcome of intraductal papillary neoplasm of the bile duct. *J Gastrointest Surg*. 2013;**17**(5):931–938.
33. Choi SC, Lee JK, Jung JH, et al. The clinicopathological features of biliary intraductal papillary neoplasms according to the location of tumors. *J Gastroenterol Hepatol*. 2010;**25**(4):725–730.
34. Rocha FG, Lee H, Katabi N, et al. Intraductal papillary neoplasm of the bile duct: a biliary equivalent to intraductal papillary mucinous neoplasm of the pancreas? *Hepatology*. 2012;**56**(4):1352–1360.
35. Kloek JJ, van der Gaag NA, Erdogan D, et al. A comparative study of intraductal papillary neoplasia of the biliary tract and pancreas. *Human Pathol*. 2011;**46**(6):824–832.

Primary sclerosing cholangitis

James Neuberger

Introduction

Primary sclerosing cholangitis (PSC) is a chronic, progressive liver disease characterized by inflammation,[1-3] fibrosis, and destruction of the intra- and/or extrahepatic bile ducts; this leads to bile duct strictures and dilatation, cholestasis, and hepatic fibrosis and may lead to portal hypertension, cirrhosis, liver decompensation, and death. Up to 80% will have inflammatory bowel disease (IBD) (mainly ulcerative colitis (UC)) and up to 25% will have other autoimmune diseases. There is a strong association with cholangiocarcinoma and carcinoma of the colon. There is no definitive medical treatment[4]; liver transplantation is indicated in those with end-stage disease or intractable symptoms but PSC may recur in the graft with an increased risk of graft failure.

Epidemiology

The reported prevalence shows geographical variation with the highest prevalence and incidence in Northern Europe and the US. Studies from Northern Europe and the US suggest the incidence and prevalence rates for PSC range from 0 to 1.3 per 100,000 inhabitants/year and 0–16.2 per 100,000 inhabitants, respectively. Reported rates in Asia and Southern Europe are 10–100-fold less.[5] However, in those with IBD, prevalence rates of 2–4.5% are seen in those with UC and 1–4% in those with Crohn's disease, but only in those with colitis. In those with IBD, the ethnic variation in PSC is much less clear. Conversely, the prevalence of IBD in those with PSC shows a geographical variation, being seen in 60–75% in those in Northern Europe compared with 20–50% in Asia and India. The reported transplant-free survival ranges from 10 to 20 years with a standardized mortality rate of between 2.5 and 4.2.

Several studies suggest that the reported prevalence is rising but it is unclear whether this represents a true increase or is merely a consequence of greater awareness of the condition and greater use of non-invasive techniques (such as magnetic resonance cholangiopancreatography (MRCP)) to diagnose the condition.

Aetiology, genetics, pathogenesis, and pathology

The aetiology of PSC remains unknown: a number of hypotheses have been proposed, including the 'leaky gut' hypothesis (where bacteria or bacterial products released into the portal system activate immune cells in the liver), the aberrant homing hypothesis (where lymphocytes activated in the gut epithelium may be directed to the liver because of shared antigens), and the 'toxic bile' hypothesis where either toxic bile constituents or defective protective systems lead to damage within the biliary cells.

There is a clear genetic component to PSC: siblings of patients with PSC and IBD have a greater risk of developing PSC (12–19-fold and eightfold higher, respectively), offspring of those with PSC have a 11.1-fold higher risk of developing PSC and parents a 2.3-fold higher risk. These rates are comparable to those seen in other autoimmune diseases. Standard human leucocyte antigen (HLA) testing and, more recently, genome-wide association studies have shown the main linkages with related to the HLA complex on chromosome 6 with several other linkages which are predominantly related to other immune-mediated or autoimmune diseases. Risk haplotypes include the ancestral haplotype AH8.1 which includes the B*08 and DRB1*03:01 alleles and DRB3*01:01–DRB1*13:01–DQA1*:03–DQB1*06:03 haplotype. The genome-wide association studies data suggest that class I effects are more important than class II.

More recently, attention has focused on the gut microbiome. *Enterococcus* and *Lactobacillus* levels are increased in PSC patients without liver cirrhosis. A recent study[6] showed that, compared to healthy controls, in those with PSC, new cohort-spanning alterations were identified including an increase of *Proteobacteria* and the bile-tolerant genus *Parabacteroides*. These findings were independent on geographical region. As associated colitis only had minor effects on microbiota composition, the authors suggest that PSC itself drives the faecal microbiota changes observed.

Clinical features

PSC may be diagnosed in children and adults[4,7,8]: the male:female ratio is 2:1 and most patients are diagnosed in their third or fourth decade.

The patient may be asymptomatic at diagnosis (in up to 50%) or may present with abdominal pain, fatigue, or pruritus and, in later stages, with fever, jaundice, and/or weight loss. Depending on the stage at presentation, the patient may be well or present with the signs and symptoms of cirrhosis.

Primary sclerosing cholangitis in children

The distinction between PSC and autoimmune hepatitis (AIH) is much less clear than in adults; many of those children present with features of both conditions and, when treated with corticosteroids, will have a clinical course in the longer term more akin to PSC than AIH. It remains uncertain whether this clinical course represents the natural history of PSC in children, whether this is a sequential syndrome, or even whether the appearance of PSC represents the long-term impact of AIH.

Overlap syndromes

The clinical and pathological significance of overlap syndromes remains controversial. Whether an overlap syndrome merely reflects that the two conditions share some serological and histological features or whether both syndromes occur in the same patient remains unclear. While overlap with primary biliary cholangitis (PBC) may rarely occur, overlap of PSC is most commonly seen with AIH. In adults, PSC/AIH is reported in up to 15% in those diagnosed with PSC and up to 2% in those diagnosed with AIH. In contrast, in children AIH/PSC is more commonly diagnosed, and is discussed below.

Associated features

Inflammatory bowel disease

The strongest association is with IBD, as indicated above. Both with UC and Crohn's colitis associated with PSC, the involvement is usually extensive although rectal sparing and backwash ileitis is more common in IBD associated with PSC. The colitis is often subclinical and may be diagnosed histologically. There is no clear correlation between the severity of the inflammation or date of onset of IBD with PSC. PSC may be diagnosed some time after colectomy and recurrence of PSC after liver transplantation is significantly less common in those without a colon at the time of transplantation and IBD may be diagnosed only after transplantation. Treatment of colitis does not impact the likelihood of developing or the course of PSC.

Other autoimmune diseases

PSC is rarely associated with other organ autoimmune diseases (such as thyroid disease, coeliac disease, autoimmune haemolytic disease, type 1 diabetes mellitus, retroperitoneal fibrosis, and rheumatoid arthritis).

Cholangiocarcinoma

Cholangiocarcinoma (CCA)[9] has become the commonest cause of death in PSC: the lifetime risk is up to 20%, the prevalence between 6% and 15%, and incidence between 0.6% and 1.5%/year. The majority of cancers are located in the perihilar region. Risks factors for the development of CCA include time of diagnosis, with up to half the cases presenting within the first year of diagnosis of PSC and dominant biliary strictures. CCA is rarely seen in association with small duct PSC. The optimal approach for screening and surveillance for CCA is uncertain: the tumour markers carbohydrate antigen (CA) 19-9 and carcinoembryonic antigen have neither the sensitivity nor specificity for routine use. Surveillance using positron emission tomography scanning may be helpful, but its role is not yet defined. There is, at present, no clear evidence that routine surveillance for CCA improves the outcome for patients.

When a diagnosis of CAA is considered, contrast-enhanced cross-sectional imaging should be the first-line investigation. Cholangioscopy may be of value but its use in this situation is unproven at this time. Brush cytology, enhanced by fluorescence *in situ* hybridization, may be of help in improving the sensitivity and specificity of brush cytology. The detailed diagnosis and management of CCA are discussed elsewhere.

Gall bladder cancer

Gall bladder polyps may be seen in those with PSC and these polyps are associated with a greater malignant potential than those without PSC. Annual ultrasound of the gall bladder is recommended. The role of surgery in those with small polyps less than 1 cm in size is uncertain and the risks of cholecystectomy need to be balanced against its advantages.

Hepatocellular carcinoma and pancreatic carcinoma

Hepatocellular carcinoma may be found in association with PSC so standard surveillance should be done in those with cirrhosis. Pancreatic cancer is seen with a greater incidence than in the normal population.

Colon cancer

Current data suggest that the coexistence of PSC in those with UC increases the risk of colon cancer development, with a relative risk of 4.8 compared to those with UC without PSC. Current guidelines recommend that those with PSC and UC should have annual colonoscopy using adjunctive techniques to help detect early dysplasia. The role of colonic surveillance in those with PSC but without UC is uncertain but many clinicians recommend colonoscopy at intervals between 1 and 5 years.

Differential diagnosis

The differential diagnosis of PSC is shown in Box 41.1.

Box 41.1 Differential diagnosis of primary sclerosing cholangitis

- Other causes of cholestatic disease such as PBC, genetic causes, drug-induced liver injury.
- Secondary biliary cholangitis which may be secondary to infection (liver fluke, ascaris, bacterial cholangitis, HIV, cytomegalovirus).
- Ischaemic insults: surgical injury, trauma.
- Autoimmune: IgG4-related disease.
- Malignancy: cholangiocarcinoma, pancreatic cancer.
- Gall stones: choledocholithiasis.
- Congenital: biliary atresia, choledochal cysts, deficiencies in *ABCB4* gene, neonatal sclerosing cholangitis.
- Others including hereditary haemorrhagic cholangiopathy, systemic mastocytosis, histiocytosis X, portal biliopathy, critical illness cholangiopathy, sickle cell disease; drug-associated (such as checkpoint inhibitors).

Clinical investigation

Standard liver tests are not specific for the diagnosis of PSC and may be normal but usually show a typical cholestatic picture, with an elevated serum alkaline phosphatase and gamma-glutamyl transferase; serum aminotransferase activity is usually no more than threefold increased. As liver disease progresses, serum albumin falls, and serum bilirubin rises. Serum amylase may be raised in up to half the patients. Prolonged cholestasis may result in deficiency of fat-soluble vitamins A, D, E, and K.

Immunology

Autoantibodies

There is no disease-specific autoantibody in PSC. The antimitochondrial antibodies are negative, and their presence should suggest the diagnosis of PBC. Other non-specific autoantibodies found in patients with PSC include peripheral antineutrophil cytoplasmic antibody, antinuclear antibodies, anti-smooth muscle antibodies, and, less commonly, anticardiolipin antibodies, rheumatoid factor, and antibodies to thyroid peroxidase and glomerular basement membrane.

Immunoglobulins

Immunoglobulins are often increased with most having a rise in immunoglobulin (Ig)-G. Elevated levels of IgG4 raise the possibility of autoimmune cholangitis. Serum IgG4 may be elevated in those with classic PSC but rarely do levels exceed twice the upper limit of normal. Higher levels should raise the possibility of autoimmune cholangiopathy or IgG4 disease which should be diagnosed by standard means.

Imaging

The characteristic feature of PSC is multiple strictures and dilatations of both the intra- and extrahepatic bile ducts (Figure 41.1). The gall bladder is usually enlarged and cholelithiasis is seen in up to 25%.[10]

Sometimes, in up to 30% cases of PSC, the radiological features of PSC are apparent in just the intrahepatic bile ducts, although it may be difficult to distinguish features of intrahepatic PSC from the normal changes in the intrahepatic biliary tree associated with cirrhosis. PSC affecting just the extrahepatic biliary tree is rare.

MRCP is the principal imaging modality for the diagnosis of PSC and compared to endoscopic retrograde cholangiopancreatography (ERCP) has a sensitivity and specificity approaching 100%. ERCP is indicated only when the diagnosis is not clear on high-quality MRCP or when cytology or endoscopic biliary intervention is required. Because of the risks and consequences of biliary sepsis, patients with PSC undergoing biliary interventions, including ERCP, should be given antimicrobial prophylaxis.

Ultrasound and computed tomography examination are not useful in the diagnosis but may be indicated for monitoring and hepatocellular carcinoma surveillance where indicated. When there is any deterioration in the clinical condition, repeat imaging of the liver and biliary tree should be considered using computed tomography, dynamic magnetic resonance imaging, or MRCP.

Transient elastography correlates well with histological assessment of fibrosis and is useful for monitoring progression of fibrosis and the onset of cirrhosis.

Liver histology

The diagnostic hallmark of PSC is concentric periductal fibrosis, but this finding is not always present on percutaneous liver biopsy specimens. Other characteristic but non-diagnostic features include bile duct proliferation, chronic periportal inflammatory changes, ductopenia, fibrosis, and sometimes cirrhosis. Liver biopsy is rarely indicated to make the diagnosis if the radiological features are diagnostic but may be helpful if there is diagnostic uncertainty such as PSC/AIH overlap syndrome or small duct disease is considered. Small duct disease is diagnosed when the patient has all the clinical and other features of PSC but cholangiographic features are absent and other causes such as genetic causes have been excluded. This variant may be seen in up to 15% of cases.

Criteria for diagnosis

As indicted above, the diagnosis of PSC rests on showing multiple biliary strictures and dilation and exclusion of other causes.

Prognosis and natural history

The natural history is unpredictable and variable although the course is overall deterioration. The average time from diagnosis to death is variable but usually around 20 years. Those who have only small duct disease or who are asymptomatic at diagnosis have a better prognosis. Those associated with UC have a worse prognosis than those with Crohn's colitis. Death is usually due to liver failure or cholangiocarcinoma. For those without known colitis, it is recommended that diagnostic colonoscopy with histology should be done every 5 years and, for those with PSC and UC, screening for colorectal cancer surveillance started from the age of 15 years.

The clinical course is associated with episodes of deterioration—these may be associated with cholangitis and clinicians should have a low threshold for detecting this as the infection may be subclinical, and not always associated with the classical triad of right upper quadrant pain, fever, and jaundice. Treatment is with

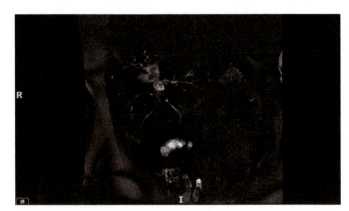

Figure 41.1 MRCP in a 52-year-old, with long-standing UC, who developed cholestatic liver tests, showing features of PSC, showing multiple strictures and dilatation of the biliary tree, diagnostic of PSC; note the cholelithiasis.
Reproduced courtesy of Dr Andrew Holt, Consultant Physician, Queen Elizabeth Hospital, Birmingham, UK.

antimicrobial agents such as ciprofloxacin, and clinicians should consider underlying precipitating factors such as cholelithiasis or even cholangiocarcinoma. Recurrent cholangitis should be treated with rotating antibiotics but if this is ineffective, transplantation may be indicated. Other causes of deterioration include dominant strictures, stones, and malignancy.

Prognosis may be estimated by a variety of scoring systems. Prognostic factors included in these scores include age, type and duration of PSC, serum bilirubin with some including other liver tests, haemoglobin, splenomegaly, and histology.[10,11]

Treatment

Symptomatic

Fatigue

Fatigue is often a major symptom in those with PSC and its presence and severity does not corelate with the degree of liver damage. Fatigue may be associated with a loss of cognitive function including loss of concentration and loss of short-term memory. At present there is no effective treatment for the fatigue associated with PSC. Anecdotal data suggest that a graded programme of exercise may be of benefit. It is important to look for other, treatable causes of fatigue such as depression or myxoedema. Sometimes, occult cholangitis may contribute to the fatigue. The fatigue does not resolve after transplantation, so fatigue is not an indication for liver transplantation.

Pruritus

This should be treated as with other cholestatic diseases. Cholestyramine is the first-line treatment. Those who are intolerant of the drug or where it is ineffective should be considered for naltrexone, sertraline, or rifampicin (unlicensed indications).

Complications of portal hypertension and cirrhosis

These should be managed as for any other patient with cirrhosis. It should be recognized that portal hypertension may develop with advanced fibrosis.

Osteopenia

With cholestatic disease, osteopenia and osteoporosis may occur but is less well studied than in those with PBC. Adults should undergo dual-energy X-ray absorptiometry scanning every 5 years and treatment with calcium and vitamin D considered where indicated with the addition of bisphosphonates as appropriate.

Cholangitis

As indicated above, episodes or suspected or documented cholangitis should be treated promptly with antibiotics. Many clinicians give patients a supply of antibiotics to be started at the onset of symptoms.

Disease specific

Pharmacological

Undertaking clinical trials in PSC is challenging, because of the long and variable natural history and lack of validated surrogate markers; to date, there is no currently recognized treatment for PSC. Despite early reports suggesting ursodeoxycholic acid (UDCA) at the standard dose of 13–15 mg/kg/day may improve liver biochemistry, subsequent studies have failed to show any improvements in histological progression or time to death or transplantation. Indeed, a study at a higher dose of 28–30 mg/kg/day suggested a harmful effect. Other studies suggesting UDCA may be associated with a reduction in the risk of colon cancer or cholangiocarcinoma have not been confirmed. Therefore, UDCA is no longer recommended for newly diagnosed patients. Similarly, there is currently no indication for the use of immunosuppressive agents in classical PSC. Antimicrobials have been advocated but there are no convincing data, as yet, to recommend their use (except in the presence of bacterial cholangitis). Several drugs are being assessed including other immunomodulators, cilofexor (a non-steroidal farnesoid X (FXR) receptor agonist), obeticholic acid (an FXR agonist), nor-UDCA (a side chain-shortened homologue of UDCA), bowel flora-altering treatment (vancomycin, faecal transplant), and inflammatory mediators (such as vedolizumab) and fibrates, including bezafibrate (a pan-peroxisome proliferator-activated receptor (PPAR) agonist), fenofibrate, and statins.[3,4,7,12]

For those with PSC/AIH overlap syndrome, treatment is indicated in those with significantly elevated serum transaminase levels greater than five times upper limit of normal, serum IgG greater than two times upper limit of normal, and AIH-associated autoantibodies such as antinuclear or liver–kidney microsomal antibodies. The treatment regimen should be as for AIH but the response is less than that seen in AIH.

Newer agents being assessed include bile acids (obeticholic acid and norursodeoxycholic acid) and a variety of antifibrotic agents.

Endoscopic

A dominant stricture is present in up to 45% and is defined as a stricture 1.5 mm or less in the common bile duct or 1 mm or less in the hepatic ducts (within 2 cm of the hilum) and should be considered where there are features of a significant stenosis of one of the major bile ducts with dilatation above or worsening liver chemistry. The natural history of a dominant stricture is not clear; endoscopic dilatation or stenting may be helpful in some cases where the deterioration is thought due to the stenosis rather than infection or worsening parenchymal disease. Because of the risks of infection, dilatation is preferred to stenting. When endoscopy is undertaken, investigation or management of a stricture, biliary cytology, or biopsy should always be done to seek evidence for cholangiocarcinoma. ERCP, with or without stenting, is associated with a significant risk of inducing cholangitis so prophylactic antibiotics should be given.

Liver transplantation

The indications for liver transplantation for PSC are similar to those for other chronic liver disease. For those with coexisting cholangiocarcinoma, liver replacement is considered only in highly selected cases because of the very high probability of non-cure. Because of disease in the biliary tree and the possible development of cholangiocarcinoma in the native bile duct, many surgeons use a Roux loop for biliary drainage of the graft. PSC may recur in the graft and is seen in up to 40% cases at 5 years and is a significant cause for graft failure. There is a wide differential diagnosis including infection and ischaemia. It may be difficult to distinguish recurrent PSC from secondary sclerosing cholangitis, especially with ischaemic changes (Figure 41.2). Risk factors for recurrent PSC include an

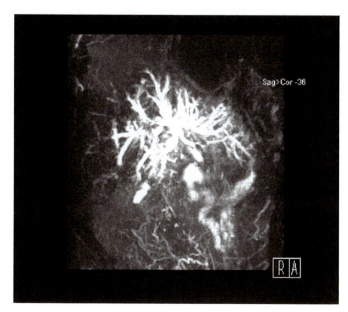

Figure 41.2 MRCP taken 2 years after liver transplant for PSC. It is not possible to differentiate on these images to distinguish recurrent primary PSC from ischaemic changes.

Reproduced courtesy of Dr Andrew Holt, Consultant Physician, Queen Elizabeth Hospital, Birmingham, UK.

intact colon at the time of transplantation and male sex. The implications of the absence of an intact colon on the risk of recurrence is uncertain but there is currently no evidence to recommend prophylactic colectomy to prevent disease recurrence. Immunosuppression should be according to the standard protocol.

Likely developments over the next 5–10 years

The key issues remain that the pathogenesis of PSC remains uncertain and currently there is no effective treatment that halts progression. Liver transplantation remains the only effective treatment for end-stage disease but recurrence of disease in the graft is common and leads to early graft failure. Diagnosis remains difficult in some patients and strategies to detect CCA early need to be developed.

REFERENCES

1. Boonstra K, Beuers U, Ponsioen CY. Epidemiology of primary sclerosing cholangitis and primary biliary cirrhosis: a systematic review. *J Hepatol.* 2012;**56**(5):1181–1188.
2. Karlsen TH, Folseraas T, Thorburn D, Vesterhus M. Primary sclerosing cholangitis—a comprehensive review. *J Hepatol.* 2017;**67**(6):1298–1323.
3. Dyson JK, Beuers U, Jones DEJ, Lohse AW, Hudson M. Primary sclerosing cholangitis. *Lancet.* 2018;**391**(10139):2547–2559.
4. Chapman MH, Thorburn D, Hirschfield GM, et al. British Society of Gastroenterology and UK-PSC guidelines for the diagnosis and management of primary sclerosing cholangitis. *Gut.* 2019;**68**(8):1356–1378.
5. Trivedi PJ, Bowlus CL, Yimam KK, Razavi H, Estes C. Epidemiology, natural history, and outcomes of primary sclerosing cholangitis: a systematic review of population-based studies. *Clin Gastroenterol Hepatol.* 2022;**20**(8):1687–1700.
6. Rühlemann M, Liwinski T, Heinsen FA, et al. Consistent alterations in faecal microbiomes of patients with primary sclerosing cholangitis independent of associated colitis. *Aliment Pharmacol Ther.* 2019;**50**(5):580–589.
7. Lindor KD, Bowlus CL, Boyer J, Levy C, Mayo M. Primary biliary cholangitis: 2021 practice guidance update from the American Association for the Study of Liver Diseases. *Hepatology.* 2022;**75**(4):1012–1013.
8. Bowlus CL, Arrivé L, Bergquist A, et al. AASLD practice guidance on primary sclerosing cholangitis and cholangiocarcinoma. *Hepatology.* 2023;**77**(2):659–702.
9. Song J, Li Y, Bowlus CL, Yang G, Leung PSC, Gershwin ME. Cholangiocarcinoma in patients with primary sclerosing cholangitis (PSC): a comprehensive review. *Clin Rev Allergy Immunol.* 2020;**58**(1):134–149.
10. Goode EC, Clark AB, Mells GF, et al. Factors associated with outcomes of patients with primary sclerosing cholangitis and development and validation of a risk scoring system. *Hepatology.* 2019;**69**(5):2120–2135.
11. Morgan MA, Khot R, Sundaram KM, et al. Primary sclerosing cholangitis: review for radiologists. *Abdom Radiol (NY).* 2023;**48**(1):136–150.
12. Goode EC, Hirschfield GM, Rushbrook SM. Comparison of risk scores in the PSC arena. *Hepatology.* 2020;**71**(1):399–400.

42

Malignant lesions of the extrahepatic biliary system

Philippe Compagnon, Andrea Peloso, and Christian Toso

Introduction

Cholangiocarcinomas (CCAs) are rare tumours arising from the epithelial lining of the biliary tree. Based on their anatomical location, CCAs are classified into intrahepatic (iCCA), and extrahepatic CCA (eCCA). eCCA is further subdivided into perihilar (pCCA; involving the bile duct (BD) confluence in the liver hilum) and distal (dCCA; mid or lower half of the BD, often in the head of the pancreas) subtypes. The latter two subtypes are now considered distinct entities based upon differences in their tumour biology and management. pCCA is the most common subtype (60–70%). The diagnosis requires thoughtful integration of clinical information, serum tumour markers, and high-quality cross-sectional imaging modalities, with cytology/histology when necessary.[1] The treatment of patients with eCCA requires a coordinated, multidisciplinary approach to optimize the chances for both durable survival and effective palliation. The overall prognosis of eCCA is dismal, with median survival of less than 24 months from the time of the diagnosis.[2]

Surgical resection with negative margins offers the only hope for cure, commonly requiring a partial hepatectomy in the case of pCCA and a pancreaticoduodenectomy for dCCA patients. Unfortunately, the majority of patients present with advanced, unresectable disease at the time of diagnosis.[1,3–5] Liver transplantation (LT) in combination with neoadjuvant therapy may be indicated in highly selected patients with unresectable, lymph node-negative pCCA.[6] In case of inoperable metastatic tumours, biliary drainage and palliative systemic chemotherapy represent the primary treatment modality. Recent advances in understanding key molecular pathways of CCA have created a growing interest in identifying novel targeted therapies and immunotherapies. Herein, we provide an overview of the most current principles of management of patients with pCCA and dCCA.

Epidemiology and risk factors

CCA is the second most common primary liver tumour and represents approximately 3–5% of all gastrointestinal malignancies diagnosed worldwide.[7] CCA affects middle-aged and elderly individuals. Although the mean age at the time of presentation worldwide is 50 years, the peak age in Western countries is about 70 years. The male-to-female ratio of CCA is 1:1.2–1.5.[8] eCCA accounts for nearly 90% of all CCAs (pCCA approximately 60–70% and dCCA 20–30%).

There is a wide geographical disparity in the incidence rate of CCA, with a much higher incidence in parts of the Eastern world compared to the West. For instance, Northeast Thailand has reported an age standardized incidence rate of 85/100,000, which is approximately 100-fold greater than North American and European rates (0.6–1.8/100,000).[9] These differences are presumably related to variation in exposure to risk factors as well as genetic determinants.[10] In Western countries, several studies have identified a relatively stable or decreasing incidence of eCCA over the last few decades, in contrast to a rising incidence and mortality of iCCA.[7,10–16]

Although most cases of CCA develop sporadically, well-established risk factors associated with chronic inflammation of the biliary epithelium have been identified.

In the West, primary sclerosing cholangitis (PSC) is the most common known risk factor.[17,18] Unlike sporadic cases, CCAs in these patients tend to present between the ages of 30 and 50 years. The risk does not seem to be correlated to the duration of disease, and nearly half of cases occur within 24 months of diagnosis.[19] In contrast, the hepatobiliary parasites—particularly *Opisthorchis viverrini* and *Clonorchis sinensis*—are mostly responsible for a greater burden of CCA in East Asia.[20] Both parasites increase the susceptibility of cholangiocytes to carcinogens via chronic irritation and an increased cellular turnover.

Other well-described risk factors include congenital biliary tree abnormalities (choledochal cysts, Caroli's disease), viral hepatitis (hepatitis B and C viral infections), hepatolithiasis and choledocholithiasis, and cirrhosis not related to PSC, as well as environmental toxins (dioxin and vinyl chloride).[1,3,7,8,10] Choledochal cysts (i.e. congenital cystic dilatations of BDs) may confer a 10- to 50-fold higher risk of developing eCCA.[7,8] Reflux of pancreatic enzymes, bile stasis, and increased concentration of intraductal bile acids may contribute to malignant transformation of the cyst

Classification and staging

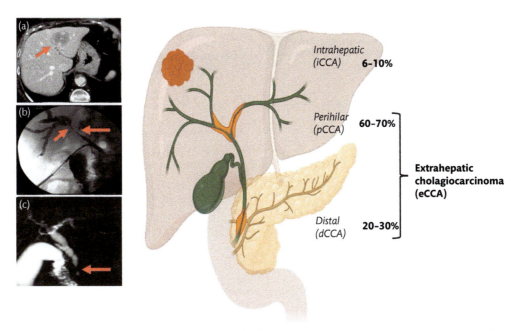

Figure 42.1 CCA classification based on its anatomic location within the biliary tree, with representative sample images of each type of tumour. (a) iCCA (CT scan). (b) pCCA (cholangiography). (c) dCCA (cholangio-MRI).

epithelial cells.[10] Previously inconclusive risk factors (alcohol, inflammatory bowel disease, type 2 diabetes, and smoking) are also associated, albeit to a lesser extent, with the development of eCCA.[7,18]

Classification and staging

Cholangiocarcinomas are generally categorized as either iCCA or eCCA based on their anatomical location with respect to the second-order BDs (Figure 42.1). iCCAs arise from the peripheral BDs within the hepatic parenchyma proximal to the secondary branches of the left and right hepatic ducts and account for 5–10% of cholangiocarcinomas. eCCAs can further be categorized as perihilar (i.e. 'Klatskin' tumours, involving the BD confluence in the liver hilum) or distal (mid or lower half of the BD, often in the head of the pancreas).[3] The latter two subtypes are now considered distinct entities based upon differences in their tumour biology and management.[21] pCCA is the most common subtype (60–70% of biliary tracts malignancies).

Perihilar cholangiocarcinoma

Over the years, various classification and staging systems have been introduced in order to provide a framework for the surgical management of pCCA. The most well-known classification was first described by H. Bismuth and M. B. Corlette in 1975[22] with a subsequent modification in the early 1990s,[23] categorizing lesions into four subtypes based on their relationship to the confluence of the right and left hepatic ducts (Figure 42.2). It is not a staging system

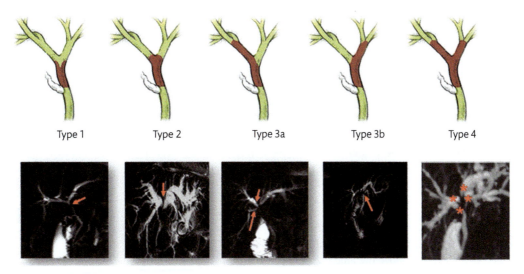

Figure 42.2 Bismuth and Corlette classification system for pCCAs with representative cholangio-MRI sample pictures of each type of tumour.
Adapted from Blechacz B. Cholangiocarcinoma: current knowledge and new developments. *Gut and Liver*. 2017;11(1):13–26, Figure 3, under a Creative Commons Attribution Non-Commercial License (http://creativecommons.org/licenses/by-nc/4.0).

Table 42.1 Memorial Sloan Kettering Cancer Center classification

Stage	Criteria
T1	The tumour involves the biliary confluence with unilateral involvement up to secondary biliary radicles There is no portal vein involvement or liver atrophy
T2	The tumour involves the biliary confluence with unilateral involvement up to secondary biliary radicles There is ipsilateral portal vein involvement or ipsilateral hepatic lobar atrophy
T3	The tumour involves the biliary confluence with bilateral involvement up to secondary biliary radicles, unilateral extension to secondary biliary radicles with contralateral portal vein involvement, unilateral involvement up to secondary biliary radicles with contralateral hepatic lobar atrophy, or main/bilateral portal vein involvement

Adapted with permission from Jarnagin WR, Fong Y, DeMatteo RP, Gonen M, Burke EC, Bodniewicz BJ, et al. Staging, resectability, and outcome in 225 patients with hilar cholangiocarcinoma. *Ann Surg*. 2001;234(4):507-17; discussion 517-519.

Table 42.2 TNM classification according to the UICC staging system for perihilar cholangiocarcinoma (eighth edition)

T–primary tumour	
TX	Primary tumour cannot be assessed
T0	No evidence of primary tumour
Tis	Carcinoma *in situ*
T1	Tumour confined to the bile duct, with extension up to the muscle layer or fibrous tissue
T2a	Tumour invades beyond the wall of the bile duct to surrounding adipose tissue
T2b	Tumour invades adjacent hepatic parenchyma
T3	Tumour invades unilateral branches of the portal vein or hepatic artery
T4	Tumour invades the main portal vein or its branches bilaterally; or the common hepatic artery; or unilateral second-order biliary radicals with contralateral portal vein or hepatic artery involvement

N–regional lymph nodes	
NX	Regional lymph nodes cannot be assessed
N0	No regional lymph node metastasis
N1	Metastases to 1-3 regional lymph nodes
N2	Metastases to 4 or more regional nodes

M–distant metastasis	
M0	No distant metastasis
M1	Distant metastasis

Stage–perihilar bile ducts			
Stage 0	Tis	N0	M0
Stage I	T1	N0	M0
Stage II	T2a, T2b	N0	M0
Stage IIIA	T3	N0	M0
Stage IIIB	T4	N0	M0
Stage IIIC	Any T	N1	M0
Stage IVA	Any T	N2	M0
Stage IVB	Any T	Any N	M1

Reproduced with permission from Brierley, JD, Gospodarowicz MK, and Wittekind C, *TNM Classification of Malignant Tumours*, 8th edition, UICC/Wiley-Blackwell, 2017, pp. 87-88.

per se, but remains widely used in clinical practice to roughly guide the extent of hepatic resection, depending on intraductal tumour extension. This classification is, however, limited by the absence of crucial information such as vascular involvement, lobar atrophy, and spread to the regional lymph nodes.[24,25] Consequently, the decision for laparotomy and potential resectability cannot fully rely on this.

The Memorial Sloan Kettering Cancer Center (MSKCC) introduced different criteria of staging for pCCA according to three factors related to local tumour extent: the level and extent of BD involvement (in agreement with the Bismuth–Corlette system), the presence of portal venous invasion, and the presence of hepatic lobar atrophy.[5] By taking full account of local tumour extent (Table 42.1), the proposed classification provides a good correlation with resectability, likelihood of achieving an R0 resection, as well as overall survival (OS).[5] The accuracy of the MSKCC system has been confirmed in a more recent analysis comparing the different staging systems.[26] pCCA is also frequently staged according to a separate Union for International Cancer Control (UICC) staging system (Table 42.2), which accounts for the degree of local tumour extension (size and vascular invasion), regional lymph node status, and distant metastasis (TNM).[27] This system is simple but mostly appropriate in the post-operative setting, after final pathological determination of the surgical specimen. Although helpful in determining tumour resectability, it may have a lower prognostic accuracy.[28]

More recently, an international working group proposed a new classification system with the aim of increasing simplicity, reproducibility, and consequently applicability.[29] This system introduced criteria in which the BD, hepatic artery, and portal vein are assigned a label depending on local tumour involvement. In addition, tumour biology as well as liver resection-related information (future liver remnant (FLR) volume, underlying liver disease) are also considered (Table 42.3). This international guideline appears relatively complex and still awaits further validation.[30]

Distal cholangiocarcinoma

A dCCA is defined as a tumour arising from the common BD below the confluence of the cystic duct and above the ampulla of Vater and constitutes approximately 20–30% of all diagnosed CCAs. The eighth edition of the UICC (2017) provides the latest staging system for dCCA (Table 42.4). The recent changes in distal CBD cancer designated the T level according to the depth of invasion rather than invaded structures, and N stage would include the number of involved lymph nodes rather than being involved or not. N1 will be given for involvement of one to three lymph nodes and N2 for the involvement of four or more lymph nodes.[31] These changes have improved the survival stratification between the stages based on the TNM stage.[31,32]

Diagnosis

Clinical presentation

Most patients with eCCA present signs of obstructive jaundice. Other symptoms may be apparent, such as vague abdominal

Table 42.3 Consensus classification (European Hepato-Pancreato-Biliary Association)

Bile duct (B)	
B1	Common bile duct
B2	Hepatic duct confluence
B3-R	Right hepatic duct
B3-L	Left hepatic duct
B4	Right and left hepatic duct
Tumour size (T)	
T1	<1 cm
T2	1–3 cm
T3	≥3 cm
Tumour form (F)	
Sclerosing	Sclerosing (or periductal)
Mass	Mass-forming (or nodular)
Mixed	Sclerosing and mass-forming
Polypoid	Polypoid (or intraductal)
Involvement (>180°) of the portal vein (PV)	
PV0	No portal involvement
PV1	Main portal vein
PV2	Portal vein bifurcation
PV3 R	Right portal vein
PV3 L	Left portal vein
PV4	Right and left portal veins
Involvement (>180°) of the hepatic artery (HA)	
HA0	No portal involvement
HA1	Proper hepatic artery
HA2	Hepatic artery bifurcation
HA3 R	Right hepatic artery
HA3 L	Left hepatic artery
HA4	Right and left hepatic artery
Liver remnant volume (V)	
V0	No information on the volume needed (liver resection not foreseen)
V%	Indicate segments Percentage of the total volume of a putative remnant liver after resection
Underlying liver disease (D)	
Fibrosis	
Non-alcoholic steatohepatitis	
Primary sclerosing cholangitis	
Lymph nodes (N)	
N0	No lymph node involvement
N1	Hilar and/or hepatic artery lymph node involvement
N2	Periaortic lymph node involvement
Metastases (M)	
M0	No distant metastases
M1	Distant metastases (including liver and peritoneal metastases)

Adapted with permission from DeOliveira ML, Schulick RD, Nimura Y et al. New staging system and a registry for perihilar cholangiocarcinoma. *Hepatology*. 2011;53(4):1363–1371.

Table 42.4 TNM classification according to the UICC staging system for distal cholangiocarcinomas

Primary tumour (T)	
TX	Primary tumour cannot be assessed
Tis	Carcinoma *in situ*/high-grade dysplasia
T1	Tumour invades the bile duct wall with a depth less than 5 mm
T2	Tumour invades the bile duct wall with a depth of 5–12 mm
T3	Tumour invades the bile duct wall with a depth greater than 12 mm
T4	Tumour involves the coeliac axis, superior mesenteric artery, and/or common hepatic artery
Regional lymph nodes (N)	
NX	Regional lymph nodes cannot be assessed
N0	No regional lymph node metastasis
N1	Metastasis in one to three regional lymph nodes
N2	Metastasis in four or more regional lymph nodes
Distant metastasis (M)	
M0	No distant metastasis
M1	Distant metastasis
Tumour stage	
Stage 0	Tis, N0, M0
Stage I	T1, N0, M0
Stage IIA	T1, N1, M0
Stage IIB	T2, N0, M0
	T2, N1, M0
	T3, N0-1 M0
Stage IIIA	T1-3, N2, M0
Stage IIIB	T4, Any N, M0
Stage IV	Any T, Any N, M1

Reproduced with permission from Brierley, JD, Gospodarowicz MK, and Wittekind C, *TNM Classification of Malignant Tumours*, 8th edition, UICC/Wiley-Blackwell, 2017, pp. 89–90.

discomfort or pain, weight loss, and anorexia. Sometimes patients complain of pruritus, which may precede jaundice by a few weeks.

Blood tests

Serum alkaline phosphatase, gamma-glutamyl transpeptidase, and bilirubin levels are often elevated, reflecting the obstructive pathology. Derangement of liver transaminases and prothrombin time/international normalized ratio usually occurs in the setting of long-standing biliary obstruction and/or cholestatic hepatocellular injury.[33]

There are no specific tumour markers for cholangiocarcinoma. Carbohydrate antigen (CA) 19-9 and carcinoembryonic antigen may be falsely elevated in patients with cholestasis, but may be relevant after biliary decompression. The sensitivity of CA 19-9 levels greater than 100 U/mL in diagnosing cholangiocarcinoma is approximately 53% in patients without PSC, and ranges from 38% to 89% (with a specificity of 50–98%) in patients with PSC.[34] Although the diagnostic accuracy of CA 19-9 is limited, a markedly elevated serum level (i.e. >600 U/mL) may be indicative of a metastatic disease.[35] In case of elevated levels at initial presentation, a rising CA 19-9 level may be the first sign of recurrent disease during the postoperative follow-up.[3,25]

Preoperative radiological evaluation

It is essential to perform all imaging before biliary drainage, because assessment of the tumour extent is more difficult after stent placement. Moreover, the extent of the tumour determines the FLR, which determines the segments to be drained.[36]

Abdominal ultrasound (US) should be the initial diagnostic test in patients with suspected cholangiocarcinoma. It provides preliminary information regarding the level of the biliary duct obstruction and tumour extension. Perihilar CCAs can be suggested by the presence of dilated intrahepatic ducts with an abrupt narrowing or cut-off at the hepatic duct bifurcation. In contrast, distal CCAs present with dilated intrahepatic and extrahepatic ducts.[37] It can identify intrahepatic masses, and suggest other aetiologies, such as choledocholithiasis or Mirizzi syndrome. Duplex US can help to detect vascular involvement or encasement.[38]

Contrast-enhanced computed tomography (CT) scan and magnetic resonance imaging/magnetic resonance cholangiopancreatography (MRI/MRCP) are widely accepted as the most accurate modalities for the diagnosis of pCCA, assessment of tumour ductal extension, and involvement of adjacent vital structures.[28,39] The diagnostic and staging accuracy of both modalities significantly diminish after any biliary tract intervention as a result of decompression and imaging artefacts.[25] The radiographic interpretation should focus on the location and extent of biliary involvement,[22] involvement of vascular structures (hepatic artery, portal vein, superior mesenteric vessels), and evidence of intrahepatic, locoregional (perihilar or portal lymph nodes), or distant metastatic disease.[3,40,41] Cross-sectional imaging for pCCA also provides extremely valuable information regarding liver volumes, caudate lobe involvement, and lobar atrophy. A CT scan frequently does not detect peritoneal metastases.[42] CT scan accuracy for the assessment of BD involvement is 86%, with sensitivity and specificity for portal vein involvement of 89% and 92%, hepatic artery of 83% and 93%, and lymph node involvement of 61% and 88%, respectively.[43] A CT scan has less utility in imaging dCCA because evaluation of tumour spread along and within the BDs is limited. However, lymphadenopathy, vascular invasion, and the presence of metastases are also well characterized using this imaging modality.[44]

MRI can detect intrahepatic spread and its intrinsically high tissue contrast helps to detect hepatic parenchymal invasion and metastatic lesions.[1] MRI with MRCP has an advantage of a better delineation of the intrahepatic spread of the tumour within the BDs.[25,45] MRCP has replaced endoscopic retrograde cholangiopancreatography (ERCP) to determine the intraductal tumoural spread.[46] MRCP can better observe biliary ducts proximal to a lesion that may not adequately fill with ERCP, and its reported accuracy in determining the extent of BD involvement ranges from 71% to 96%.[47] Of note, MRI and MRCP still understage up to 20% of patients with perihilar tumours, require a longer scan time, and are more sensitive to motion artefacts (limiting their usefulness in uncooperative patients).[1] When both are well performed, the accuracy of MRI and CT in predicting resectability exceeds 75%.[25]

Positron emission tomography (PET)-CT should not be routinely used in the diagnostic workup. eCCAs tend not to be fludeoxyglucose avid so PET-CT has low sensitivity for the diagnosing of CCA, and rarely adds to information available from other staging modalities.[3]

Direct cholangiography through either endoscopic retrograde cholangiography (ERC) or percutaneous transhepatic cholangiography (PTC) offers excellent visualization of the biliary tree and usually provides a good understanding of the level of the stricture.[3,48,49] ERCP may be better suited for evaluating more accessible distal lesions, whereas PTC may be required in patients with constricting, perihilar lesions. PTC can also assist in gaining access to strictures not amenable to ERCP.[50] Both approaches allow for tissue sampling by brushings or biopsies, and biliary stenting for the relief of jaundice can be performed at the time of the diagnostic evaluation.[1] The fibrotic nature of CCA often makes it difficult to obtain a pathological diagnosis; endoscopic brushings and washings yield a positive result in only about 40% of eCCA patients.[48,49]

Fluorescence in situ hybridization (FISH) uses fluorescent probes to detect chromosomal aneuploidy. This advanced cytological technique increases the sensitivity up to 46–68% without compromising the specificity.[51]

SpyGlass cholangioscopy provides direct visualization of the biliary system, allowing better sensitivity and specificity (90% and 95.8%, respectively) when compared to ERCP.[52]

Endoscopic ultrasonography (EUS) can be used to evaluate the biliary tree and perform fine-needle aspiration (FNA) of the tumour or suspicious locoregional lymphadenopathy, provided that neoadjuvant protocols are available. FNA is particularly useful for distal lesions. Despite a higher sensitivity than ERCP with brushings, EUS/FNA has the potential for tumour seeding.[53] Consequently, transenteric tissue sampling is not recommended in surgical candidates.

Intraductal ultrasound, endoscopic choledochoscopy, and confocal laser endomicroscopy represent more advanced endoscopic technology that may further enhance the sensitivity for the detection of malignancy as well as diagnostic accuracy, but are not yet used in routine clinical practice.[1,54–56]

The indication for biopsy should always be discussed at a hepatobiliary multidisciplinary meeting that should include a transplant surgeon. Percutaneous or laparoscopic biopsy of the primary tumour is not recommended in patients who may be candidates for resection or transplantation because of the high risk of needle track seeding following these procedures.[25,57] However, pathological confirmation is mandatory prior to chemo- or radiotherapy, or when it is felt that the patient may benefit from neoadjuvant treatment (e.g. presence of suspicious regional lymphadenopathy).[25]

Preoperatively, dCCA is generally difficult to distinguish from pancreatic ductal adenocarcinoma. These tumours are often grouped together and treated as one entity, as 'periampullary tumours'.[58] Final definitive diagnosis is mostly made postoperatively on pathological examination. This is a real concern in determining treatment options in case of unresectable disease or deciding for cholangiocarcinoma-specific neoadjuvant therapy.[44]

Surgical approach

Surgery remains the main potentially curative treatment of eCCA. It is determined by the patient's functional status (i.e. performance status, comorbidity, and nutrition) and their ability to undergo a major procedure, the local extent of the tumour (including vascular and/or parenchymal involvement), and the presence of local or distant metastasis. It should be performed by expert hands and in centres of reference.

Perihilar cholangiocarcinoma

Surgical principles and resectability

The objective of surgery is to remove the entire tumour with negative macro- and microscopic margins (i.e. R0 resection), while maintaining adequate liver remnant volume, vascular inflow/outflow, and biliary drainage. This is often a challenging task, due to the close anatomical contiguity between hilar structures and the spread of the tumour.[36,59]

Careful preoperative staging prior to biliary drainage is crucial in identifying appropriate candidates for attempted curative resection. The disease must be localized and amenable to resection with clear margins. Particular attention should also be paid to the nutritional and performance status of the patient.[1,5] Regardless of staging/classification systems, preoperative assessment of surgical resectability remains a challenge and requires multidisciplinary and multimodal evaluation. But finally, the decision to resect or not can only be made at surgical exploration.

Criteria for resection include the absence of disseminated disease, extrahepatic organ invasion, distant lymph node or metastatic disease, and extensive vascular invasion.[60]

Tumours involving ipsilateral second-order biliary radicals or ipsilateral portal vein branches may be amenable to resection. Also, tumours that result in ipsilateral lobar atrophy would not necessarily preclude resection.[61]

Regional lymph node metastases are no longer an absolute contraindication to surgical resection, although they are associated with worse outcomes compared with patients with negative lymph nodes.[62]

As stated by the 2015 expert consensus meeting, the following situations are classically considered as unresectable[25]:

- Tumour extension to second-order biliary radicals with contralateral vascular involvement.
- Bilateral tumour extension to second-order biliary radicals.
- Lobar atrophy with contralateral tumour extension to second-order biliary radicals *or* contralateral vascular inflow involvement (occlusion/encasement).

Contraindications to surgery can also be due to the presence of severe medical comorbidities, underlying liver disease (especially cirrhosis), or an inadequate FLR as well as metastatic disease (N2 metastases and/or distant metastases).

The conduct of surgery

Surgical resection with curative intent requires most often extrahepatic BD resection with extended hemi-hepatectomy, leaving behind an adequate FLR, and regional lymphadenectomy. Finally, biliary continuity is re-established with a Roux-en-Y hepaticojejunostomy.[63]

Assessment of resectability may start with a selective diagnostic laparoscopy to rule out occult intraperitoneal, locally advanced disease, or liver metastasis (see 'Staging laparoscopy'). The subsequent laparotomy is performed through a Makuuchi incision.

Intraoperative US is used to confirm the preoperative imaging workup, particularly the extent of the tumour and its relationship with important anatomical structures. It may also help to identify unexpected liver metastases. A careful assessment is then performed to exclude distant lymph node metastasis. Surgery is aborted if N2 lymph nodes (i.e. periduodenal, peripancreatic, coeliac, and superior mesenteric artery) are finally invaded. The final step to ascertain resectability requires a systematic evaluation of the local extent of the tumour.[64]

The longitudinal and radial extension of the tumour into the BD is determined by a direct palpation of the main BD confluence. Hilar dissection is carried out to clear all cellulo-lymphatic tissues and to expose the elements of the hepatic pedicle. The main BD is carefully elevated to better assess the main portal vein trunk up to its bifurcation. Depending on the vascular involvement, the surgical procedure may continue and the distal BD is then divided, allowing a better access to the vascular structures. Frozen section analysis of the distal BD should be systematically performed to rule out distal spread along the BD. The hepatic artery and portal vein on the side being resected are ligated and divided extrahepatically, whereas the vessels supplying the future remnant liver are carefully preserved. The proximal BD is sharply transected during liver parenchymal transection.[3] The ipsilateral hepatic vein is also preferentially divided as it enters the inferior vena cava, after inflow control but prior to hepatic parenchymal transection.[4]

The type and extent of resection performed depends on the location of the tumour within the liver or biliary tree and the degree of local invasion.[1] For Bismuth IIIA pCCA, a right trisectionectomy extended to the left hepatic duct is performed, the latter having the advantage of a greater length as compared to the right duct.[65] For Bismuth IIIB tumours, a left hepatectomy or trisectionectomy extended to second-order biliary radicals is needed, often requiring reconstruction of multiple right-sided ducts.[66] With both hemihepatectomies, 'en bloc' resection of the caudate lobe should be carried out.[25]

The need to combine BD resection with major hepatic resection is still controversial for Bismuth types I and II, due to the limited data available.[67,68] Some reports suggest that Bismuth type I/II pCCA may be amenable to extrahepatic BD resection, lymphadenectomy, and bilioenteric anastomosis (especially for aged patients in poor condition), while others recommend a combined central hepatectomy resecting segment 5 and segment 4b only.[69–71] Moreover, some centres of excellence have shown that major liver resection should accompany resection of pCCA to achieve a tumour-negative resection margin and improve long-term survival.[68,72] In these groups, high rates of recurrence were observed if only BD resection is done.

Bismuth type IV pCCAs were initially considered as a contraindication to surgical resection. Recent advances in surgical technique and perioperative management have not only improved clinical outcomes but also allowed an expansion of the indications for resection.[73,74] Consequently, surgery is no longer strictly contraindicated for Bismuth type IV lesions (see 'Extensive resection').

Reconstruction of biliary–enteric drainage is carried out with a retrocolic Roux-en-Y hepaticojejunostomy. To minimize bile reflux, a 70–80 cm Roux limb is made.

Bile duct margin status

Residual high-grade dysplasia/carcinoma *in situ* of the BD margin does not affect the prognosis of patients with eCCA, but it significantly increases the risk of local recurrence compared with R0.[75] Frozen section analysis should be performed to ensure an R0 BD resection margin, but the intraoperative assessment should be carried out with caution. It has been shown that as many as 9% of patients with an intraoperative negative margin actually have a positive margin on final pathology.[76] The initial resection should be performed with the widest margin that is technically feasible, with careful consideration of the potential morbidity and risk for postoperative hepatic insufficiency associated with excessive parenchymal resection.[76] The surgeons should not persist in their attempts to achieve negative ductal resection margins when residual carcinoma *in situ* is diagnosed intraoperatively on frozen sections.[77]

Resection of the caudate lobe

Perihilar CCAs typically extend into this segment via small branches draining into the posterior aspects of the right or left hepatic ducts or the biliary confluence. Hence, caudate lobe involvement has been reported in up to 43–100% of patients.[78,79] Consequently, routine 'en bloc' resection of the caudate lobe is of major importance to carry out negative surgical margins.[5,80–83] In addition, caudate lobectomy minimizes the risk of biliary leak from uncontrolled caudate BDs.[4,25]

Lymphadenectomy

Lymphadenectomy routinely includes N1 lymph nodes (i.e. those along the cystic duct, common BD, hepatic artery, and portal vein), yielding prognostic value.[4,84] For accurate staging, the estimated total lymph node count for pCCA should be seven lymph nodes.[85] Surgical resection can proceed in patients with N1 lymph node metastases.

Only suspicious N2 lymph nodes (i.e. interaortocaval, coeliac axis, and superior mesenteric artery) should be analysed. Any involvement of these nodal basins is considered to be distant metastatic disease and resection should be aborted.[1] N2-positive lymph nodes are associated with a dismal prognosis, 5-year OS rates range between 0% and 2.3%.[86]

Optimization of the future liver remnant

Careful perioperative management is a determining factor for the success of pCCA surgeries. Liver failure remains the most dreaded postoperative complication. It is seldom reversible and represents the main cause of 90-day mortality. To avoid such a fatal complication, patients should be carefully investigated preoperatively with (1) a precise evaluation of the functional capacity of the FLR, (2) aggressive use of preoperative portal vein embolization (PVE), and (3) appropriate biliary drainage.[4,87]

FLR function can be assessed more formally by examining hepatocellular uptake and excretion (indocyanine green clearance), uptake, and biotransformation (^{13}C-methacetin breath test, LiMAx), and uptake (hepatobiliary scintigraphy). These function tests can be combined with single-photon emission computed tomography/CT to differentiate functional from non-functional liver tissue.[88–90]

An inadequate FLR volume and function exposes the patient at risk of post-hepatectomy liver failure. In most studies, cut-offs of the FLR range from 25% to 40%.[36,91] For one of the most experienced centres in the world, PVE should be performed when FLR is below 40%.[73] Patients with pCCA usually present with significant cholestasis and/or required neoadjuvant chemotherapy for locally advanced disease, and it is therefore highly recommended to undertake PVE prior to resection. PVE induces compensatory hypertrophy of the (non-embolized) FLR.[92–94] Minor complications occur in up to 12% of patients, including fever, pain, nausea, or bile leak. Major adverse events, such as major haemorrhage or thrombus propagation into the main or FLR portal vein, occur in only 2% of these patients.[4,95] After PVE, the average increase in the volume of the FLR usually ranges from 8% to 10% over the following 2–3 weeks, and the kinetic growth rate of the FLR seems to reflect the improvement in liver function.[96] The group at the MSKCC has shown that the degree of hypertrophy and kinetic growth rate were highly predictive of postoperative complications and liver failure.[97] In fact, no patient with a growth rate exceeding 2% per week experienced postoperative liver failure in this study.[97] A growth rate of the FLR that does not reach this threshold, or those who do not achieve the expected degree of hypertrophy, should not preclude surgical resection, but a greater risk for postoperative morbidity must be considered.[4]

Associating liver partition and portal vein ligation for staged hepatectomy (ALPPS) is a relatively new procedure in liver surgery.[98] Discouraging outcomes have been reported in patients with pCCA using data from the international ALPPS registry, with a perioperative mortality rate as high as 48%.[99] The authors concluded that PVE should remain the standard approach to augment FLR volumes preoperatively.

There is clear consensus that preoperative biliary drainage (PBD) is indicated in pCCA patients with obstructive cholangitis, those undergoing neoadjuvant chemotherapy, patients with hyperbilirubinaemia-induced malnutrition, hepatic or renal insufficiency, and patients undergoing PVE because of inadequate FLR volume.[25] Additionally, PBD can relieve symptoms such as pruritus in patients who will experience a delay in surgery.[4] Apart from the above-mentioned specific conditions, a selective approach to PBD depending on the size of the FLR may be proposed.[100–102] It can be reasonably recommended to selectively drain the patients with an estimated FLR volume smaller than 40%, because biliary obstruction impairs liver regeneration.[4] Regardless of the patient's condition, the indication for PBD should be systematically evaluated by a hepatobiliary multidisciplinary team.

Strategically, the FLR should be prioritized for drainage, rather than the biliary tree within the proposed parenchymal resection. Decompression of the remnant liver supports the recovery of metabolic and synthetic function on this side and also minimizes the potential for atrophy due to chronic biliary obstruction.[4] Sometimes, additional drainage of the ipsilateral biliary tract may be necessary to alleviate a persistent cholestatic jaundice that may prevent safe liver resection or administration of chemotherapy.

Decompression of the BDs may be performed with percutaneous transhepatic biliary drainage (PTBD), endoscopic biliary drainage (EBD), or endoscopic nasobiliary drainage (ENBD). The rationale for the PTBD includes better delineation of the extent of endobiliary tumour spread within the liver, a higher technical success rate (i.e. significantly less time to achieve the required therapeutic effect, as well as higher patency rates), and the potential for decreasing cholangitis-related complications.[25,100,103–105] Detractors may argue that PTBD is associated with a 1.4–5% risk of tumour seeding of the drain track,[106] while in some experienced centres it is not.[4] A recent multicentre randomized trial comparing PTBD to EBD was stopped due to excess mortality in the PTBD group (41% vs 11%).[107] No clear explanation has been suggested by the authors regarding this disproportionate mortality. This observation is in contrast to the results of previous studies, including other randomized controlled trials (RCTs).[104,108,109]

Due to the reported risk of tumour seeding with PTBD, EBD is increasingly advocated for stent placement. EBD may lead to errant placement of stents, leading to cholangitis and requiring further procedures to optimize drainage.[4,101] To overcome the morbidity of EBD, ENBD has been proposed by others, reporting lower rate of conversion to PTBD.[110] Patient discomfort and the possibility of accidental dislodgment represent the major drawbacks of ENBD. In a more recent work, EBB, ENBD, and PTBD gave comparable results regarding initial technical success rates, complication rates, and surgical outcomes.[111]

There are no clear recommendations with regard to the optimal duration of drainage or the serum bilirubin level that should be reached prior to resection. Some centres suggest delaying surgery until the bilirubin level decreases to less than 2–3 mg/dL, but this is not based on any rigorous assessment of hepatic function.[4,25,112] Based on the current evidence, a reasonable approach would be to carry out biliary drainage of the FLR only in patients presenting with obstructive cholangitis as well as in patients with both a bilirubin level exceeding 4 mg/dL and a FLR below 40%.[36] Drainage of the contralateral liver should be reserved for patients with sepsis and/or persistent jaundice. In the absence of large randomized controlled studies, there is no definitive evidence to recommend PTBD, EBD, or ENBD. For now, modality of choice varies from centre to centre, depending on its experience with a particular technique.[25,36,100]

Staging laparoscopy

Despite extensive evaluation with preoperative imaging, 25–50% of patients thought to benefit from surgical resection are found to have unsuspected unresectable disease at the time of laparotomy.[5,26,73,113] Selective diagnostic laparoscopy to rule out occult intraperitoneal or hepatic metastatic disease may avoid unnecessary laparotomy. Staging laparoscopy is particularly recommended in high-risk patients with long-standing percutaneous stents, advanced disease on preoperative imaging, or markedly elevated serum CA 19-9 levels (i.e. >1000 IU/mL).[35,114–117]

Extensive resection

Trisectionectomy for Bismuth type IV tumours.

The group at Nagoya recently reported the first surgical experience regarding Bismuth type IV tumours, with an impressive series of 216 resections.[74] Combined vascular resection was carried out in 60% of patients. Complications of Clavien–Dindo grade III or greater developed in 42% and the operative mortality was only 1.9%. Such extensive resection allowed better survival rates compared to patients with unresected tumours (32.8 vs 1.5% at 5 years; p <0.001). The 5-year survival rate was as high as 53% in pN0M0 patients. This series shows that in highly experienced hands resection for type IV tumours can be performed with a low mortality, allowing long-term survivals.

Hepatopancreaticoduodenectomy for tumours with extensive longitudinal spread.

In an attempt to improve the R0 resection rate, more extensive resections have been proposed. Liver resection may be combined with a pancreaticoduodenectomy, particularly in patients with (1) diffusely infiltrating tumours of the whole extrahepatic BD, (2) downward superficial spreading, or (3) bulky nodal metastasis of the pancreatoduodenal region.[118,119] While initial experience with HPD for pCCA was discouraging, most recent reports have shown improved postoperative outcomes.[119,120] However, HPD remains associated with a high rate of complications, particularly liver failure and pancreatic fistula. Improvements in perioperative care and surgical techniques are required to increase the benefits of this procedure that is not yet widely accepted.[87]

Vascular resection

Advanced pCCA is likely to involve adjacent vascular structures for hepatic inflow due to the anatomical vicinity between the hilar BD and the portal vein or hepatic artery.[87,121] Recent advances in surgical techniques and knowledge in the era of LT have facilitated the performance of vascular reconstructions. Hence, the need for major vascular resection should not preclude surgical resection if negative margins can be obtained.

Portal vein resection may be necessary to achieve negative margins,[65,118,122,123] but it should not be performed routinely in pCCA. Combined liver and portal vein resection may offer a survival benefit to some patients with advanced pCCA, who would otherwise be considered unresectable. The decision for portal vein resection must be made on an individual patient basis and should be determined intraoperatively in the light of vascular extension.[124–126] This operation should be undertaken by only the most experienced centres with the appropriate hepatobiliary and vascular surgery expertise.

In contrast, invasion of the hepatic artery remains a serious obstacle, and arterial resection (with or without reconstruction) is promoted by a few.[4] Surgical procedures are complex, sometimes requiring alternative hepatic inflow via the gastroduodenal or left hepatic artery or the use of interposition grafts.[127] When all other possible strategies for the reconstruction of the artery have been ruled out, the technique of portal vein arterialization has been described but is associated with the potential for significant portal hypertension and biliary complications.[128–130] Although theoretically appealing and feasible, this salvage procedure should be reserved for critical situations.[128]

The largest experience with arterial resection and subsequent reconstruction comes from the group at Nagoya,[73,131] who recently reported 76 combined hepatic artery resection–reconstructions (13% of the entire series of 574 pCCA patients), with perioperative mortality rates of less than 5% and 5-year survival rates of up to 30%.[73] However, discouraging results with this technically demanding surgical procedure have been reported by other institutions, operative mortality sometimes reaching as high as 56%, without long-term survivors.[132–136] In summary, hepatic artery resection (with or without reconstruction) is being integrated into aggressive resection practices and should be performed only in select patients at experienced centres.

Liver transplantation

The rationale of LT in patients with pCCA is to avoid possible unfavourable outcomes of surgical resection, a positive margin, and an inadequate FLR with post-hepatectomy liver failure. Furthermore, LT is effective in removing any underlying liver disease, such as PSC.[137]

The Mayo Clinic (Rochester, Minnesota, US) initiated the use of neoadjuvant chemoradiotherapy (CRT) followed by LT in carefully selected patients with unresectable tumours.[138,139] Seventy-one patients were treated with external beam radiation (40–45 Gy) followed by transcatheter radiation (20–30 Gy) with iridium wires, intravenous 5-flurouracil administered for chemosensitization during radiation therapy, and capecitabine administered afterwards while waiting for LT. A staging laparoscopy was performed after brachytherapy, and the patients listed for LT if no metastatic and/or lymph node involvement was seen. Overall, 38 (53%)

patients with negative staging operations underwent transplantation and the 5-year survival rate was 84%, which compared favourably with the 5-year survival rate after hepatectomy for pCCA of 21% from the same institution.[139] It is notable that 16 out of 38 explanted livers did not exhibit any evidence of tumour and of these, only one-half of the patients had a cancer diagnosis before treatment, which, as expected, has led to criticism of this study.[140] The Mayo Clinic group updated their experience with 126 pCCA patients transplanted using this protocol, and demonstrated a 5-year OS of 75% in this highly selected group. The survival in PSC patients was 80% compared with 64% for patients with *de novo* pCCA.[141]

More recently, Dawish Murad and colleagues[6] reviewed LT outcomes from 12 high-volume transplant centres in the US. A total of 287 patients with pCCA completed this protocol and the 5-year recurrence-free survival rate was 72% in this large cohort, confirming the efficiency of such a therapeutic approach. Notably, more than two-thirds of the patients had PSC as the underlying disease (compared to about 5% in other pCCA cohorts), while 25% of patients developed progression of their disease while awaiting LT and were dropped-out.[6]

The indications and rationale for LT differ between patients with PSC and those with *de novo* pCCA outside the setting of PSC. The multifocality of the ductal lesions frequently precludes resection as a definitive option in patients with PSC. It explains the good outcomes following LT when combined to a neoadjuvant regimen of chemo- and radiation therapy.[6]

The role of LT in patients with *de novo* pCCA is not well defined. When feasible, resection remains the standard therapy for *de novo* pCCA, after which a 5-year survival of 35–50% is possible in the setting of an R0 resection.[25,142] When patients are not eligible for resection but meet the transplant criteria, enrolling them into a protocol (i.e. neoadjuvant regimen prior to LT) is the best option, given very poor outcomes with margin-positive resections.[137,143]

Clinical outcomes

Five-year OS rates following resection generally range from 20% to 35%[69,72,73,102,112,126,144–146] (Table 42.5). Major liver resection for the treatment of pCCA carries a high risk, with a reported perioperative mortality around 10% in large Western centres.[101,102,144] Most Japanese teams have reported lower rates, not exceeding 5%[72,73,112,145] (Table 42.5). Overall, morbidity rates range from 24% to 57%. Common serious complications after hepatectomy for pCCAs are not specific, including liver failure (post-hepatectomy liver failure), biliary complications (BD leaks), wound sepsis, and intra-abdominal abscess, as well as cardiorespiratory and renal failure.[147] Despite a potentially curative resection, the disease recurrence rate is 50–70%, mostly within 2 years after surgery.

Prognostic factors

Negative margin resection (R0) is one of the strongest determinants of survival,[76] ranging from 67% to 78%.[5,26,70,83,148] Five-year survival is reported at less than 20% in case of positive lymph nodes versus 55% in case of negative lymph nodes, regardless of an R0 resection.[36,146,149] Lymph node involvement is associated with a reduced OS (hazard ratio (HR) = 2.0; 95% confidence interval (CI) 2.1–2.6) and disease-free survival (HR = 4.3; 95% CI 1.89–10.1)[146] and is also an independent determinant of early as well as late recurrence in patients with R0 resection (HR = 2.7; 95% CI 1.4–5.3; p = 0.003).[149] Despite the high proportion of lymph node metastases, there is no evidence to suggest that extended lymph node dissection improves long-term survival.[1,86] Most staging systems consider vascular involvement of the tumour to determine prognosis and resectability, but the available systems differ about which aspect of vascular involvement is most important.[5,27,29] Although not as strong as resection margin status and nodal involvement, the degree of histological differentiation (tumour grade) also represents a significant prognostic factor.[36,146,149–153] Similarly, a tumour with a mucinous component is associated with more aggressive behaviour, advanced stage, a high

Table 42.5 Selected reports of outcomes after resection for perihilar cholangiocarcinoma

Study	N	R0 (%)	Morbidity (%)	Mortality (%)	Overall 5-year survival (%)	R0 5-year survival (%)	N+ 5-year survival (%)
Lee et al.,[72] 2010	302	71	43	1.7	33	47	–
Cho et al.,[69] 2012	105	70.5	–	14.3	34.1	–	–
de Jong et al.,[126] 2012	305	73	–	5.2	20	24	16.5
Nuzzo et al.,[144] 2012	440	77	47.6	10.1	25.5	32	10.7
Song et al.,[112] 2013	230	76.5	–	4.3	33	51	24
Farges et al.,[102] 2013	366	–	27.6	10.7	–	–	–
Nagino et al.,[73] 2013	574	67	57	4.7	33	67	22
Furusawa et al.,[145] 2014	70 (1990-2000) 74 (2001-2012)	70 78	34 24	1.2 0	33 35	41	15
Wiggers et al.,[101] 2016	287	75.6	–	14	–	–	–

rate of recurrence, and a poor prognosis.[152,154–157] Close monitoring is advisable in patients with one or more of the above-mentioned risk factors, even after curative surgery.

It is worth noting that overall worldwide postoperative outcomes in pCCA patients are significantly more favourable in high-volume centres.[25,36,73,158,159] This clearly argues for performing surgery in patients with pCCA only in highly experienced centres, as stated by a recent expert consensus statement.[25]

Distal cholangiocarcinoma

The definitive management of a dCCA is surgical, with chemotherapy and radiotherapy having only a limited role.

Surgical principles

Given their location, pancreatoduodenectomy is the mainstay of treatment of resectable disease, and the only potential for cure. These tumours have the highest resectability rate compared with intrahepatic and perihilar tumours. Very rarely, more proximal tumours may be amenable to a segmental BD resection and hepaticojejunostomy, without compromising the oncological integrity of the operation.

Distant metastatic disease and significant vascular involvement (contact >180° of the hepatic artery or superior mesenteric artery and/or >2 cm involvement of the portal vein or superior mesenteric vein) represent classical contraindications to surgery.[160]

Patients with borderline resectable disease may be considered for neoadjuvant therapy, especially when there are doubts about an ability to achieve a margin-negative resection.[3]

A careful assessment of the BD margin is recommended with intraoperative frozen section as needed. Radical resection should ideally involve removal of at least 11 lymph nodes to be accurately staged.[85]

Pancreaticoduodenectomy with portal vein/superior mesenteric vein resection can be performed at experienced centres. Higher negative margin rates and long-term survival can be achieved with vascular resection.[161,162]

There is a growing consensus that PBD is not needed unless neoadjuvant therapy is planned.[1,3,163]

Clinical outcomes

Survival following curative intent resection for dCCA is superior to that for pancreatic ductal adenocarcinoma and also compares favourably with that reported for resection of pCCA (Table 42.6). Potentially curative operation for dCCA is reported to occur in 67–90% of patients with a median OS of 18–39 months, and an associated 5-year OS rate of 27–52%.[58,164–168] Median survival in patients with unresectable dCCA is poor with most patients living less than a year after diagnosis.[164]

Prognostic factors

Resection margin, lymph node involvement, tumour grade and size, perineural invasion, lymphovascular invasion, vascular invasion, depth of tumour invasion, and pancreatic invasion are important prognostic factors and correlate with survival.[58,85,140,153,162,164–166,169,170–174] The recent changes of the TNM staging system for dCCA (eighth edition of the American Joint Committee on Cancer (AJCC)/UICC) incorporated the depth of invasion in the T level. N stage has been also modified according to the number of involved lymph nodes rather than being involved or not. These changes improved the survival stratification between the stages based on the TNM stage.[31,175]

Given the impact of these factors on survival, specifically that of margin status, patient selection before proceeding with an operation and emphasis on an R0 resection are paramount.[44]

Perioperative therapy

Even after a curative-intent resection, patients remain at a high risk for recurrence. This would suggest that it is necessary to consolidate radical management with some type of additional therapy either in the neoadjuvant or adjuvant setting.

Neoadjuvant therapy

LT for patients with unresectable pCCA provides the largest experience with neoadjuvant therapy for CCA.[6,138,139] A protocol developed at the Mayo Clinic highlights the efficacy of CRT prior to LT for patients with pCCA (see 'Liver transplantation').

The effectiveness of a neoadjuvant therapy prior to surgical resection is not well defined.[176] Neoadjuvant treatment is supposed to increase R0 margin rates, or even to allow radical resection for locally advanced disease. Available data in the setting of eCCA are, however, limited to a few small case series and retrospective studies, with a distinction between pCCA and dCCA not well specified.[177–181] In addition, a clear definition of 'borderline' and 'unresectable' tumours is often lacking, bringing confusion to the interpretation of the results. So far, no formal recommendations for neoadjuvant therapy have been proposed by the National Comprehensive Cancer Network guidelines or American Society of Clinical Oncology clinical practice guidelines.

Regarding more specifically dCCA, retrospective single-institution analyses have also demonstrated a potential benefit for neoadjuvant therapy.[44,176] However, no consensus or RCTs are yet available. Improvement in preoperative discrimination between dCCA and pancreatic ductal adenocarcinoma will ultimately be necessary to provide the best possible care to each distinct group of patients.[44]

Adjuvant therapy

Adjuvant chemotherapy

Traditionally considered chemotherapy resistant, patients with locally advanced or metastatic biliary tract cancer (BTC) have been evaluated in the phase III randomized controlled ABC-02 trial, comparing adjuvant therapy with gemcitabine plus cisplatin versus gemcitabine alone. The combination therapy was associated with an improved median OS (11.7 vs 8 months, $p < 0.001$) and progression-free survival (8 vs 5 months, $p < 0001$).[182]

Later retrospective studies found an improvement in OS after adjuvant chemotherapy, particularly for patients with positive lymph nodes.[183–185] These results were confirmed by multivariate analysis in a multicentre retrospective study of 249 patients with pCCA who underwent resection with curative intent.[186] A systematic review and meta-analysis of 20 studies encompassing 6712 patients with CCAs of all sites (as well as gallbladder cancer), of whom 1797 received adjuvant therapy has also been conducted.[184] The pooled analysis demonstrated a non-significant improvement in survival with the use of any adjuvant therapy compared with surgery alone. However, on

Table 42.6 Selected reports of post-resection outcomes and poor prognostic factors for distal cholangiocarcinoma

Study	N	Surgical mortality (%)	Median survival	5-year survival (%)	Poor prognostic factors
Kwon et al.,[165] 2014	133	–	–	41	R2 margin Lymphovascular invasion High TNM stage
Hong et al.,[170] 2009	147	–	20.3 months	18	Tumour depth >5 mm
Hernandez et al.,[171] 2008	43	9	21 months	–	Staging Adjuvant therapy
Murakami et al.,[166] 2007	43	0	26 months	44	Older age Pathological pancreatic invasion Lymph node metastases Perineural invasion R1/R2 margin TNM stage II and III
De Oliveira et al.,[172] 2007	239	–	–	23	R1/R2 margin Lymph node metastases Tumour >2 cm Poorly differentiated tumours
Jang et al.,[173] 2005	282	4.9	–	32.5	Lymph node metastases AJCC staging Histology
Wakai et al.,[174] 2005	84	3.6	–	42	Lymph node metastases Size and grade of tumour

treatment-specific analysis, patients who received chemotherapy or CRT had improved OS compared with patients who received radiotherapy alone. The effect of adjuvant chemotherapy was especially pronounced in those patients with lymph node-positive disease and in those with R1 resections.[184]

The Bile Duct Cancer Adjuvant Trial (BCAT) was a randomized phase III trial including patients with resected BD cancer, comparing adjuvant chemotherapy with gemcitabine versus surveillance alone.[187] This Japanese work showed no difference in median OS (62.3 vs 63.8 months, p = 0.96) or RFS (36 vs 39.9 months, p = 0.69) between the adjuvant gemcitabine and observation cohorts. This study was, however, underpowered because of its failure to achieve full patient recruitment. The phase III randomized control PRODIGE 12 trial enrolled 194 patients with R0 or R1 resected BTCs (iCCA, pCCA, dCCA, and gallbladder cancers). No survival benefit was associated in patients treated with adjuvant gemcitabine–oxaliplatin (GEMOX) compared with surgery alone, (75.8 vs 50.8 months, p = 0.74), and this trial was deemed a negative trial.[188]

The BILCAP trial was the first randomized controlled, phase III multicentre trial that demonstrated an OS benefit of adjuvant chemotherapy with capecitabine over surveillance alone, among patients with completely resected (R0) BTCs. Although significance was not achieved in the intent-to-treat analysis, patients who received adjuvant capecitabine had an increased median OS compared to the placebo group (51 vs 36 months, respectively; p = 0.028) in the per-protocol analysis.[189] The BILCAP trial has largely contributed to the current consensus guidelines (see below). A possible reason for the differing findings may be attributed to a higher number of patients with positive lymph nodes in the BILCAP trial compared with the PRODIGE 12 trial.

Adjuvant chemoradiotherapy

There are no RCTs demonstrating a benefit of adjuvant CRT after resection; however, retrospective studies indicate a potential benefit, particularly in patients with residual disease (R1) or node-positive eCCA.

Borghero and colleagues[190] showed that resected eCCA patients at high risk for local recurrence (R1 resection and/or pN1) who received adjuvant CRT had an equivalent locoregional recurrence and 5-year OS to patients with standard-risk (R0 resection and pN0) treated with surgery alone: 36% versus 42% and 38% versus 37%, respectively. Kim et al.[191] reported a series of 168 patients with resected eCCA. The use of adjuvant CRT with capecitabine or 5-fluorouracil improved 5-year locoregional control (58.5% vs 44.4%, p = 0.007), disease-free survival (32.1% vs 26.1%, p = 0.041), and OS (36.5% vs 28.2%; p = 0.049) when compared with resection alone. Multivariate analysis indicated an independent beneficial effect of adjuvant CRT (p <0.005) in this study.[191] Additional retrospective series have supported these findings.[178,192] Similarly, a single-arm prospective phase II trial (SWOG0809) demonstrated the feasibility of concurrent CRT after resection of eCCA and gallbladder cancer.[193] Median OS was 35 months, and patients with positive margins had similar outcomes to those with negative margins, suggesting a potential benefit of radiation in patients with positive margins.

Adjuvant radiotherapy

Radiotherapy may be considered for patients with pCCA at high risk of recurrence like those with residual disease (positive margins) or positive nodes, although there are no randomized data to support this strategy.[194,195]

Regarding patients with dCCA, there is a lack of convincing data to recommend adjuvant radiotherapy alone.[44,50]

In summary, the current consensus regarding adjuvant therapy for eCCA is largely based on the BILCAP and SWOG0809 trials. According to the American Society of Clinical Oncology Clinical Practice Guideline, patients with resected eCCA should be offered adjuvant capecitabine chemotherapy for a duration of 6 months.[196]

In addition, patients with eCCA and a microscopically positive surgical margin (R1 resection) may be offered adjuvant CRT.[196] In the latter situation, the experts strongly recommend a shared decision-making approach, considering the risk of harm and potential for benefit associated with radiation therapy.

Palliative management

The vast majority of patients with CCA present with unresectable disease, with a median survival of approximately 3 months (potentially extended to 6 months with biliary drainage).[197] Moreover, a significant percentage of patients treated with resection ultimately die of recurrent disease.[5] Palliative interventions can alleviate symptoms, improve quality of life, and potentially improve survival in a significant percentage of patients.[1]

Management of unresectable disease

Biliary drainage

The goals of biliary decompression are relief of jaundice and related pruritis, prevention of cholangitis and hepatic dysfunction, as well as improvement of quality of life.[53] Before the treatment plan is finalized, plastic or covered self-expandable metal stents should be used. Placement of uncovered self-expandable metal stents, which can be dilated or stented in the future but cannot be removed, is a palliative option.[50] Outcomes of percutaneously versus endoscopically placed biliary metal stents are comparable and the route of placement should be chosen based upon accessibility and comorbidities.[198] A biliary drainage via Roux-en-Y hepaticojejunostomy (for patients with dCCAs) or a segment III cholangio-jejunostomy (for patients with pCCA) may be carried out.[1] Although surgical biliary drainage is more durable, it is associated with greater morbidity and mortality, longer recovery times, and higher costs compared with percutaneous or endoscopic biliary decompression.

Surgical palliation

A gastrojejunostomy is sometimes necessary in case of a large tumour causing duodenal obstruction; rarely, a coeliac plexus block can be indicated to relieve severe epigastric or back pain that is unresponsive to medical treatment.[63]

Systemic therapy

The combination of gemcitabine and cisplatin is the current first-line chemotherapy for patients with advanced-stage CCA not amenable to locoregional and surgical options, irrespective of anatomical disease subtype. The ABC-02 RCT found an increased median OS of 11.7 months with gemcitabine and cisplatin, compared to 8.2 months with gemcitabine alone.[182]

The last targets of therapeutic interest that are expressed in BTCs include the mitogen-activated ERK kinase (MEK) pathway, and the c-MET pathway.[199]

Emerging targeted therapy and immunotherapy

In recent years, genomic and immunoprofiling analyses have provided an insight into the molecular heterogeneity of CCA, opening the way for a multitude of early-phase targeted therapy and immunotherapy trials.[200–202] Molecular therapies currently assessed in BTCs include IDH inhibitors,[203] FGFR inhibitors,[204] BRAF inhibitors,[205] anti-HER2 directed therapies,[206] and immune checkpoint inhibitors (anti-PD-L1)[207] These emerging targeted and immunotherapies have demonstrated favourable safety profiles and clinical responses in patients with advanced disease who do not respond or are intolerant to chemotherapy.[200] There are ongoing phase III clinical trials.[208]

Radiotherapy and stereotactic body radiotherapy

Local progression of unresectable CCA can cause pain and biliary obstruction, leading to liver failure and eventual death. Palliative local radiotherapy may be indicated, allowing improvements in symptoms and survival.[209] Some series have also reported the benefit of stereotactic body radiotherapy, with 85–100% local control rates at 1 year, and acceptable morbidity/mortality.[210,211]

Management of metastatic or locoregional recurrence

The favoured approach in patients with metastatic or locoregional recurrence is systemic chemotherapy with gemcitabine and cisplatin representing first-line chemotherapy agents.[25] Radiotherapy for local recurrence can be associated with significant toxicity to the jejunal limb and generally is not recommended.[4,24]

Prophylactic surgery

Although most cases of CCA develop sporadically, several risk factors have been identified (See 'Epidemiology and risk factors') and prophylactic surgery may be indicated for some patients.

PSC is the most commonly known risk factor, with a reported lifetime risk of developing a CCA estimated to be 5–10%, with nearly 50% of deaths in patients with PSC being due to cancer.[17] No effective medical therapy can contain the progression of the disease or prevent the development of CCA. LT represents the only potentially curative option for advanced PSC, providing excellent long-term outcomes. Therefore, stringent surveillance is needed, though uncertainty remains regarding the best strategy to apply.

Choledochal cysts confer a 10- to 50-fold higher risk of developing CCA, with a lifetime incidence of CCA reaching 30%.[212]

Prophylactic surgery is therefore recommended to avoid malignant transformation in these patients. It implies the complete removal of the dilated biliary duct, with reconstruction by Roux-en-Y hepaticojejunostomy.[213]

Biliary cancers are frequently observed in adult patients with pancreaticobiliary maljunction (PBM).[214] According to a nationwide survey in Japan (n = 2561),[215] extrahepatic BD cancer was detected in 21.6% of PBM patients with congenital biliary dilatation and in 42.4% of PBM patients without biliary dilatation. Once PBM is diagnosed, immediate prophylactic surgery is recommended before malignant changes develop. Resection of the extrahepatic biliary duct must be carried out together with the gallbladder, the latter being the most common cancer site.[216]

REFERENCES

1. Esnaola NF, Meyer JE, Karachristos A, Maranki JL, Camp ER, Denlinger CS. Evaluation and management of intrahepatic and extrahepatic cholangiocarcinoma. *Cancer*. 2016;**122**(9):1349–1369.

2. Everhart JE, Ruhl CE. Burden of digestive diseases in the United States part III: liver, biliary tract, and pancreas. *Gastroenterology*. 2009;**136**(4):1134–1144.
3. Khan AS, Dageforde LA. Cholangiocarcinoma. *Surg Clin North Am*. 2019;**99**(2):315–335.
4. Lidsky ME, Jarnagin WR. Surgical management of hilar cholangiocarcinoma at Memorial Sloan Kettering Cancer Center. *Ann Gastroenterol Surg*. 2018;**2**(4):304–312.
5. Jarnagin WR, Fong Y, DeMatteo RP, et al. Staging, resectability, and outcome in 225 patients with hilar cholangiocarcinoma. *Ann Surg*. 2001;**234**(4):507–519.
6. Darwish Murad S, Kim WR, Harnois DM, et al. Efficacy of neoadjuvant chemoradiation, followed by liver transplantation, for perihilar cholangiocarcinoma at 12 US centers. *Gastroenterology*. 2012;**143**(1):88–98.
7. Clements O EJ, Kim JU, Taylor-Robinson SD, Khan SA. Risk factors for intrahepatic and extrahepatic cholangiocarcinoma: a systematic review and meta-analysis. *J Hepatol*. 2020;**72**(1):95–103.
8. Tyson GL, El-Serag HB. Risk factors for cholangiocarcinoma. *Hepatology*. 2011;**54**(1):173–184.
9. Mosconi S, Beretta GD, Labianca R, Zampino MG, Gatta G, Heinemann V. Cholangiocarcinoma. *Crit Rev Oncol Hematol*. 2009;**69**(3):259–270.
10. Khan SA, Tavolari S, Brandi G. Cholangiocarcinoma: epidemiology and risk factors. *Liver Int*. 2019;**39**(S1):19–31.
11. Khan SA, Taylor-Robinson SD, Toledano MB, Beck A, Elliott P, Thomas HC. Changing international trends in mortality rates for liver, biliary and pancreatic tumours. *J Hepatol*. 2002;**37**(6):806–813.
12. Bertuccio P, Malvezzi M, Carioli G, et al. Global trends in mortality from intrahepatic and extrahepatic cholangiocarcinoma. *J Hepatol*. 2019;**71**(1):104–114.
13. Patel N, Benipal B. Incidence of cholangiocarcinoma in the USA from 2001 to 2015: a US cancer statistics analysis of 50 states. *Cureus*. 2019;**11**(1):e3962–e3962.
14. Shaib Y, El-Serag H. The epidemiology of cholangiocarcinoma. *Semin Liver Dis*. 2004;**24**(02):115–125.
15. Alvaro D, Crocetti E, Ferretti S, Bragazzi MC, Capocaccia R. Descriptive epidemiology of cholangiocarcinoma in Italy. *Dig Liver Dis*. 2010;**42**(7):490–495.
16. Utada M, Ohno Y, Tamaki T, Sobue T, Endo G. Long-term trends in incidence and mortality of intrahepatic and extrahepatic bile duct cancer in Japan. *J Epidemiol*. 2014;**24**(3):193–199.
17. Fung BM, Lindor KD, Tabibian JH. Cancer risk in primary sclerosing cholangitis: epidemiology, prevention, and surveillance strategies. *World J Gastroenterol*. 2019;**25**(6):659–671.
18. Choi J, Ghoz HM, Peeraphatdit T, et al. Aspirin use and the risk of cholangiocarcinoma. *Hepatology*. 2016;**64**(3):785–796.
19. Chapman MH, Webster GJM, Bannoo S, Johnson GJ, Wittmann J, Pereira SP. Cholangiocarcinoma and dominant strictures in patients with primary sclerosing cholangitis: a 25-year single-centre experience. *Eur J Gastroenterol Hepatol*. 2012;**24**(9):1051–1058.
20. Shin H-R, Oh J-K, Masuyer E, et al. Epidemiology of cholangiocarcinoma: an update focusing on risk factors. *Cancer Sci*. 2010;**101**(3):579–585.
21. Blechacz B. Cholangiocarcinoma: current knowledge and new developments. *Gut and liver*. 2017;**11**(1):13–26.
22. Bismuth H, Corlette MB. Intrahepatic cholangioenteric anastomosis in carcinoma of the hilus of the liver. *Surg Gynecol Obstet*. 1975;**140**(2):170–178.
23. Bismuth H, Nakache R, Diamond T. Management strategies in resection for hilar cholangiocarcinoma. *Ann Surg*. 1992;**215**(1):31–38.
24. Poruk KE, Pawlik TM, Weiss MJ. Perioperative management of hilar cholangiocarcinoma. *J Gastrointest Surg*. 2015;**19**(10):1889–1899.
25. Mansour JC, Aloia TA, Crane CH, Heimbach JK, Nagino M, Vauthey J-N. Hilar cholangiocarcinoma: expert consensus statement. *HPB (Oxford)*. 2015;**17**(8):691–699.
26. Rocha FG, Matsuo K, Blumgart LH, Jarnagin WR. Hilar cholangiocarcinoma: the Memorial Sloan-Kettering Cancer Center experience. *J Hepatobiliary Pancreat Sci*. 2010;**17**(4):490–496.
27. Brierley, JD, Gospodarowicz MK, Wittekind C. Perihilar bile ducts. In: *TNM Classification of Malignant Tumours*. 8th ed. Hoboken, NJ: UICC/Wiley-Blackwell; 2017: 87–88.
28. Lewis HL, Rahnemai-Azar AA, Dillhoff M, Schmidt CR, Pawlik TM. Current management of perihilar cholangiocarcinoma and future perspectives. *Chirurgia*. 2017;**112**(3):193.
29. DeOliveira ML, Schulick RD, Nimura Y, et al. New staging system and a registry for perihilar cholangiocarcinoma. *Hepatology*. 2011;**53**(4):1363–1371.
30. Luo Y. A new clinical classification of hilar cholangiocarcinoma (Klatskin tumor). *Open Access J Surg*. 2017;**2**(4):555594.
31. Brierley, JD, Gospodarowicz MK, Wittekind C. Distal extrahepatic bile duct. In: *TNM Classification of Malignant Tumours*. 8th ed. Hoboken, NJ: UICC/Wiley-Blackwell; 2017: 89–90.
32. Jun S-Y, Sung Y-N, Lee JH, Park K-M, Lee Y-J, Hong S-M. Validation of the Eighth American Joint Committee on Cancer Staging System for distal bile duct carcinoma. *Cancer Res Treat*. 2019;**51**(1):98–111.
33. Khan SA, Davidson BR, Goldin RD, et al. Guidelines for the diagnosis and treatment of cholangiocarcinoma: an update. *Gut*. 2012;**61**(12):1657–1669.
34. Patel AH, Harnois DM, Klee GG, LaRusso NF, Gores GJ. The utility of CA 19-9 in the diagnoses of cholangiocarcinoma in patients without primary sclerosing cholangitis. *Am J Gastroenterol*. 2000;**95**(1):204–207.
35. Levy C, Lymp J, Angulo P, Gores GJ, Larusso N, Lindor KD. The value of serum CA 19-9 in predicting cholangiocarcinomas in patients with primary sclerosing cholangitis. *Dig Dis Sci*. 2005;**50**(9):1734–1740.
36. Cillo U, Fondevila C, Donadon M, et al. Surgery for cholangiocarcinoma. *Liver Int*. 2019;**39**(Suppl 1):143–155.
37. Saini S. Imaging of the hepatobiliary tract. *N Engl J Med*. 1997;**336**(26):1889–1894.
38. Bloom CM, Langer B, Wilson SR. Role of US in the detection, characterization, and staging of cholangiocarcinoma. *RadioGraphics*. 1999;**19**(5):1199–1218.
39. Aloia TA, Charnsangavej C, Faria S, et al. High-resolution computed tomography accurately predicts resectability in hilar cholangiocarcinoma. *Am J Surg*. 2007;**193**(6):702–706.
40. Chen HW LE, Pan AZ, Chen T, Liao S, Lau WY. Preoperative assessment and staging of hilar cholangiocarcinoma with 16-multidetector computed tomography cholangiography and angiography. *Hepatogastroenterology*. 2009;**56**(91–92):578–583.
41. Chryssou E, Guthrie JA, Ward J, Robinson PJ. Hilar cholangiocarcinoma: MR correlation with surgical and histological findings. *Clin Radiol*. 2010;**65**(10):781–788.
42. Vilgrain V. Staging cholangiocarcinoma by imaging studies. *HPB (Oxford)*. 2008;**10**(2):106–109.

43. Ruys AT, van Beem BE, Engelbrecht MRW, Bipat S, Stoker J, Van Gulik TM. Radiological staging in patients with hilar cholangiocarcinoma: a systematic review and meta-analysis. *Br J Radiol.* 2012;**85**(1017):1255–1262.
44. Lee RM, Maithel SK. Approaches and outcomes to distal cholangiocarcinoma. *Surg Oncol Clin N Am.* 2019;**28**(4):631–643.
45. Manfredi R, Barbaro B, Masselli G, Vecchioli A, Marano P. Magnetic resonance imaging of cholangiocarcinoma. *Semin Liver Dis.* 2004;**24**(02):155–164.
46. Jhaveri KS, Hosseini-Nik H. MRI of cholangiocarcinoma. *J Magn Reson Imaging.* 2014;**42**(5):1165–1179.
47. Lee SS, Kim M-H, Lee SK, et al. MR cholangiography versus cholangioscopy for evaluation of longitudinal extension of hilar cholangiocarcinoma. *Gastrointest Endosc.* 2002;**56**(1):25–32.
48. Tamada K, Ushio J, Sugano K. Endoscopic diagnosis of extrahepatic bile duct carcinoma: advances and current limitations. *World J Clin Oncol.* 2011;**2**(5):203–216.
49. de Bellis M, Sherman S, Fogel EL, et al. Tissue sampling at ERCP in suspected malignant biliary strictures (part 1). *Gastrointest Endosc.* 2002;**56**(4):552–561.
50. Razumilava N, Gores GJ. Cholangiocarcinoma. *Lancet.* 2014;**383**(9935):2168–2179.
51. Brooks C, Gausman V, Kokoy-Mondragon C, et al. Role of fluorescent in situ hybridization, cholangioscopic biopsies, and EUS-FNA in the evaluation of biliary strictures. *Dig Dis Sci.* 2018;**63**(3):636–644.
52. Dimas ID, Fragaki M, Vardas E, Paspatis GA. Digital cholangioscopy (Spyglass™) in the diagnosis of cholangiocarcinoma. *Ann Gastroenterol.* 2017;**30**(2):253.
53. Abu-Hamda E, Baron T. Endoscopic management of cholangiocarcinoma. *Semin Liver Dis.* 2004;**24**(02):165–175.
54. Stavropoulos S, Larghi A, Verna E, Battezzati P, Stevens P. Intraductal ultrasound for the evaluation of patients with biliary strictures and no abdominal mass on computed tomography. *Endoscopy.* 2005;**37**(8):715–721.
55. Draganov PV, Chauhan S, Wagh MS, et al. Diagnostic accuracy of conventional and cholangioscopy-guided sampling of indeterminate biliary lesions at the time of ERCP: a prospective, long-term follow-up study. *Gastrointest Endosc.* 2012;**75**(2):347–353.
56. Meining A, Chen YK, Pleskow D, et al. Direct visualization of indeterminate pancreaticobiliary strictures with probe-based confocal laser endomicroscopy: a multicenter experience. *Gastrointest Endosc.* 2011;**74**(5):961–968.
57. Heimbach JK, Sanchez W, Rosen CB, Gores GJ. Trans-peritoneal fine needle aspiration biopsy of hilar cholangiocarcinoma is associated with disease dissemination. *HPB (Oxford).* 2011;**13**(5):356–360.
58. Ethun CG, Lopez-Aguiar AG, Pawlik TM, et al. Distal cholangiocarcinoma and pancreas adenocarcinoma: are they really the same disease? A 13-institution study from the US Extrahepatic Biliary Malignancy Consortium and the Central Pancreas Consortium. *J Am Coll Surg.* 2017;**224**(4):406–413.
59. Jo H-S, Kim D-S, Yu Y-D, Kang W-H, Yoon KC. Right-side versus left-side hepatectomy for the treatment of hilar cholangiocarcinoma: a comparative study. *World J Surg Oncol.* 2020;**18**(1):3.
60. Rajagopalan V, Daines WP, Grossbard ML, Kozuch P. Gallbladder and biliary tract carcinoma: a comprehensive update, part 1. *Oncology (Williston Park).* 2004;**18**(7):889–896.
61. Jarnagin W, Winston C. Hilar cholangiocarcinoma: diagnosis and staging. *HPB (Oxford).* 2005;**7**(4):244–251.
62. Nagorney DM, Kendrick ML. Hepatic resection in the treatment of hilar cholangiocarcinoma. *Adv Surg.* 2006;**40**:159–171.
63. Jarnagin W, Shoup M. Surgical management of cholangiocarcinoma. *Semin Liver Dis.* 2004;**24**(02):189–199.
64. Ho J, Curley SA. Diagnosis and management of intrahepatic and extrahepatic cholangiocarcinoma. *Cancer Treat Res.* 2016;**168**:121–163.
65. Neuhaus P, Thelen A, Jonas S, et al. Oncological superiority of hilar en bloc resection for the treatment of hilar cholangiocarcinoma. *Ann Surg Oncol.* 2012;**19**(5):1602–1608.
66. Uesaka K. Left hepatectomy or left trisectionectomy with resection of the caudate lobe and extrahepatic bile duct for hilar cholangiocarcinoma (with video). *J Hepatobiliary Pancreat Sci.* 2011;**19**(3):195–202.
67. van Gulik TM, Kloek JJ, Ruys AT, et al. Multidisciplinary management of hilar cholangiocarcinoma (Klatskin tumor): extended resection is associated with improved survival. *Eur J Surg Oncol.* 2011;**37**(1):65–71.
68. Lim JH, Choi GH, Choi SH, Kim KS, Choi JS, Lee WJ. Liver resection for Bismuth type I and type II hilar cholangiocarcinoma. *World J Surg.* 2013;**37**(4):829–837.
69. Cho MS, Kim SH, Park SW, et al. Surgical outcomes and predicting factors of curative resection in patients with hilar cholangiocarcinoma: 10-year single-institution experience. *J Gastrointest Surg.* 2012;**16**(9):1672–1679.
70. Konstadoulakis MM, Roayaie S, Gomatos IP, et al. Fifteen-year, single-center experience with the surgical management of intrahepatic cholangiocarcinoma: operative results and long-term outcome. *Surgery.* 2008;**143**(3):366–374.
71. Chen XP, Lau WY, Huang ZY, et al. Extent of liver resection for hilar cholangiocarcinoma. *Br J Surg.* 2009;**96**(10):1167–1175.
72. Lee SG, Song GW, Hwang S, et al. Surgical treatment of hilar cholangiocarcinoma in the new era: the Asan experience. *J Hepatobiliary Pancreat Sci.* 2010;**17**(4):476–489.
73. Nagino M, Ebata T, Yokoyama Y, et al. Evolution of surgical treatment for perihilar cholangiocarcinoma. *Ann Surg.* 2013;**258**(1):129–140.
74. Ebata T, Mizuno T, Yokoyama Y, Igami T, Sugawara G, Nagino M. Surgical resection for Bismuth type IV perihilar cholangiocarcinoma. *Br J Surg.* 2018;**105**(7):829–838.
75. Ke Q, Wang B, Lin N, Wang L, Liu J. Does high-grade dysplasia/carcinoma in situ of the biliary duct margin affect the prognosis of extrahepatic cholangiocarcinoma? A meta-analysis. *World J Surg Oncol.* 2019;**17**(1):211.
76. Endo I, House MG, Klimstra DS, et al. Clinical significance of intraoperative bile duct margin assessment for hilar cholangiocarcinoma. *Ann Surg Oncol.* 2008;**15**(8):2104–2112.
77. Ojima H, Kanai Y, Iwasaki M, et al. Intraductal carcinoma component as a favorable prognostic factor in biliary tract carcinoma. *Cancer Sci.* 2009;**100**(1):62–70.
78. Ogura Y, Mizumoto R, Tabata M, Matsuda S, Kusuda T. Surgical treatment of carcinoma of the hepatic duct confluence: analysis of 55 resected carcinomas. *World J Surg.* 1993;**17**(1):85–92.
79. Sugiura Y, Nakamura S, Iida S, et al. Extensive resection of the bile ducts combined with liver resection for cancer of the main hepatic duct junction: a cooperative study of the Keio Bile Duct Cancer Study Group. *Surgery.* 1994;**115**(4):445–451.
80. Cheng QB, Yi B, Wang JH, et al. Resection with total caudate lobectomy confers survival benefit in hilar cholangiocarcinoma of Bismuth type III and IV. *Eur J Surg Oncol.* 2012;**38**(12):1197–1203.

81. Kow AW-C, Wook CD, Song SC, et al. Role of caudate lobectomy in type IIIA and IIIB hilar cholangiocarcinoma: a 15-year experience in a tertiary institution. *World J Surg*. 2012;**36**(5):1112–1121.
82. Wahab MA, Sultan AM, Salah T, et al. Caudate lobe resection with major hepatectomy for central cholangiocarcinoma: is it of value? *Hepatogastroenterology*. 2012;**59**(114):321–324.
83. Nimura Y, Kamiya J, Kondo S, et al. Aggressive preoperative management and extended surgery for hilar cholangiocarcinoma: Nagoya experience. *J Hepatobiliary Pancreat Surg*. 2000;**7**(2):155–162.
84. Turgeon MK, Maithel SK. Cholangiocarcinoma: a site-specific update on the current state of surgical management and multimodality therapy. *Chin Clin Oncol*. 2020;**9**(1):4.
85. Ito K, Ito H, Allen PJ, et al. Adequate lymph node assessment for extrahepatic bile duct adenocarcinoma. *Ann Surg*. 2010;**251**(4):675–681.
86. Kitagawa Y, Nagino M, Kamiya J, et al. Lymph node metastasis from hilar cholangiocarcinoma: audit of 110 patients who underwent regional and paraaortic node dissection. *Ann Surg*. 2001;**233**(3):385–392.
87. Mizuno T, Ebata T, Nagino M. Advanced hilar cholangiocarcinoma: an aggressive surgical approach for the treatment of advanced hilar cholangiocarcinoma: perioperative management, extended procedures, and multidisciplinary approaches. *Surg Oncol*. 2020;**33**:201–206.
88. Imamura H, Sano K, Sugawara Y, Kokudo N, Makuuchi M. Assessment of hepatic reserve for indication of hepatic resection: decision tree incorporating indocyanine green test. *J Hepatobiliary Pancreat Surg*. 2005;**12**(1):16–22.
89. Stockmann M, Lock JF, Riecke B, et al. Prediction of postoperative outcome after hepatectomy with a new bedside test for maximal liver function capacity. *Ann Surg*. 2009;**250**(1):119–125.
90. de Graaf W, van Lienden KP, van Gulik TM, Bennink RJ. 99mTc-mebrofenin hepatobiliary scintigraphy with SPECT for the assessment of hepatic function and liver functional volume before partial hepatectomy. *J Nucl Med*. 2010;**51**(2):229–236.
91. Khan AS, Garcia-Aroz S, Ansari MA, et al. Assessment and optimization of liver volume before major hepatic resection: current guidelines and a narrative review. *Int J Surg*. 2018;**52**:74–81.
92. Kawasaki SMM, Miyagawa S, Kakazu T. Radical operation after portal embolization for tumor of hilar bile duct. *J Am Coll Surg*. 1994;**178**(5):480–486.
93. Abdalla EK, Hicks ME, Vauthey JN. Portal vein embolization: rationale, technique and future prospects. *Br J Surg*. 2001;**88**(2):165–175.
94. Makuuchi M, Thai BL, Takayasu K, et al. Preoperative portal embolization to increase safety of major hepatectomy for hilar bile duct carcinoma: a preliminary report. *Surgery*. 1990;**107**(5):521–527.
95. Glantzounis GK, Tokidis E, Basourakos SP, Ntzani EE, Lianos GD, Pentheroudakis G. The role of portal vein embolization in the surgical management of primary hepatobiliary cancers. A systematic review. *Eur J Surg Oncol*. 2017;**43**(1):32–41.
96. Shindoh J, Truty MJ, Aloia TA, et al. Kinetic growth rate after portal vein embolization predicts posthepatectomy outcomes: toward zero liver-related mortality in patients with colorectal liver metastases and small future liver remnant. *J Am Coll Surg*. 2013;**216**(2):201–209.
97. Leung U, Simpson AL, Araujo RLC, et al. Remnant growth rate after portal vein embolization is a good early predictor of post-hepatectomy liver failure. *J Am Coll Surg*. 2014;**219**(4):620–630.
98. Schnitzbauer AA, Lang SA, Goessmann H, et al. Right portal vein ligation combined with in situ splitting induces rapid left lateral liver lobe hypertrophy enabling 2-staged extended right hepatic resection in small-for-size settings. *Ann Surg*. 2012;**255**(3):405–414.
99. Olthof PB, Coelen RJS, Wiggers JK, et al. High mortality after ALPPS for perihilar cholangiocarcinoma: case-control analysis including the first series from the international ALPPS registry. *HPB (Oxford)*. 2017;**19**(5):381–387.
100. Kennedy TJ, Yopp A, Qin Y, et al. Role of preoperative biliary drainage of liver remnant prior to extended liver resection for hilar cholangiocarcinoma. *HPB (Oxford)*. 2009;**11**(5):445–451.
101. Wiggers JK, Groot Koerkamp B, Cieslak KP, et al. Postoperative mortality after liver resection for perihilar cholangiocarcinoma: development of a risk score and importance of biliary drainage of the future liver remnant. *J Am Coll Surg*. 2016;**223**(2):321–331.
102. Farges O, Regimbeau JM, Fuks D, Le Treut YP, Cherqui D, Bachellier P. Multicentre European study of preoperative biliary drainage for hilar cholangiocarcinoma. *Br J Surg*. 2013;**100**(2):274–283.
103. George C, Byass OR, Cast JEI. Interventional radiology in the management of malignant biliary obstruction. *World J Gastrointest Oncol*. 2010;**2**(3):146–150.
104. Walter T, Ho CS, Horgan AM, et al. Endoscopic or percutaneous biliary drainage for Klatskin tumors? *J Vasc Interv Radiol*. 2013;**24**(1):113–121.
105. Kubota K, Hasegawa S, Iwasaki A, et al. Stent placement above the sphincter of Oddi permits implementation of neoadjuvant chemotherapy in patients with initially unresectable Klatskin tumor. *Endosc Int Open*. 2016;**4**(4):E427–E433.
106. Komaya K, Ebata T, Yokoyama Y, et al. Verification of the oncologic inferiority of percutaneous biliary drainage to endoscopic drainage: a propensity score matching analysis of resectable perihilar cholangiocarcinoma. *Surgery*. 2017;**161**(2):394–404.
107. Coelen R, Roos E, Wiggers JK, et al. Endoscopic versus percutaneous biliary drainage in patients with resectable perihilar cholangiocarcinoma: a multicentre, randomised controlled trial. *Lancet Gastroenterol Hepatol*. 2018;**3**(10):681–690.
108. Al Mahjoub A, Menahem B, Fohlen A, et al. Preoperative biliary drainage in patients with resectable perihilar cholangiocarcinoma: is percutaneous transhepatic biliary drainage safer and more effective than endoscopic biliary drainage? A meta-analysis. *J Vasc Interv Radiol*. 2017;**28**(4):576–582.
109. Saluja S, Gulati M, Garg P, et al. Endoscopic or percutaneous biliary drainage for gallbladder cancer: a randomized trial and quality of life assessment. *Clin Gastroenterol Hepatol*. 2008;**6**(8):944–950.e943.
110. Kawashima H, Itoh A, Ohno E, et al. Preoperative endoscopic nasobiliary drainage in 164 consecutive patients with suspected perihilar cholangiocarcinoma. *Ann Surg*. 2013;**257**(1):121–127.
111. Jo JH, Chung MJ, Han DH, et al. Best options for preoperative biliary drainage in patients with Klatskin tumors. *Surg Endosc*. 2017;**31**(1):422–429.
112. Song SC, Choi DW, Kow AW-C, et al. Surgical outcomes of 230 resected hilar cholangiocarcinoma in a single centre. *ANZ J Surg*. 2013;**83**(4):268–274.

113. Mansfield SD, Barakat O, Charnley RM, et al. Management of hilar cholangiocarcinoma in the North of England: pathology, treatment, and outcome. *World J Gastroenterol.* 2005;**11**(48):7625–7630.
114. Corvera CU, Weber SM, Jarnagin WR. Role of laparoscopy in the evaluation of biliary tract cancer. *Surg Oncol Clin N Am.* 2002;**11**(4):877–891.
115. Jarnagin W. A prospective analysis of staging laparoscopy in patients with primary and secondary hepatobiliary malignancies. *J Gastrointest Surg.* 2000;**4**(1):34–43.
116. Ruys AT, Busch OR, Gouma DJ, van Gulik TM. Staging laparoscopy for hilar cholangiocarcinoma: is it still worthwhile? *Ann Surg Oncol.* 2011;**18**(9):2647–2653.
117. Bird N, Elmasry M, Jones R, et al. Role of staging laparoscopy in the stratification of patients with perihilar cholangiocarcinoma. *Br J Surg.* 2017;**104**(4):418–425.
118. Nimura Y, Hayakawa N, Kamiya J, et al. Combined portal vein and liver resection for carcinoma of the biliary tract. *Br J Surg.* 1991;**78**(6):727–731.
119. Ebata T, Yokoyama Y, Igami T, et al. Hepatopancreatoduodenectomy for cholangiocarcinoma. *Ann Surg.* 2012;**256**(2):297–305.
120. Aoki T, Sakamoto Y, Kohno Y, et al. Hepatopancreaticoduodenectomy for biliary cancer. *Ann Surg.* 2018;**267**(2):332–337.
121. Hoyos S, Navas M-C, Restrepo J-C, Botero RC. Current controversies in cholangiocarcinoma. *Biochim Biophys Acta Mol Basis Dis.* 2018;**1864**(4):1461–1467.
122. Neuhaus P, Jonas S, Bechstein WO, et al. Extended resections for hilar cholangiocarcinoma. *Ann Surg.* 1999;**230**(6):808–819.
123. Ebata T, Nagino M, Kamiya J, Uesaka K, Nagasaka T, Nimura Y. Hepatectomy with portal vein resection for hilar cholangiocarcinoma: audit of 52 consecutive cases. *Ann Surg.* 2003;**238**(5):720–727.
124. Bhardwaj N, Garcea G, Dennison AR, Maddern GJ. The surgical management of klatskin tumours: has anything changed in the last decade? *World J Surg.* 2015;**39**(11):2748–2756.
125. Chen W, Ke K, Chen YL. Combined portal vein resection in the treatment of hilar cholangiocarcinoma: a systematic review and meta-analysis. *Eur J Surg Oncol.* 2014;**40**(5):489–495.
126. de Jong MC, Marques H, Clary BM, et al. The impact of portal vein resection on outcomes for hilar cholangiocarcinoma. *Cancer.* 2012;**118**(19):4737–4747.
127. de Santibañes E, Ardiles V, Alvarez FA, Pekolj J, Brandi C, Beskow A. Hepatic artery reconstruction first for the treatment of hilar cholangiocarcinoma bismuth type IIIB with contralateral arterial invasion: a novel technical strategy. *HPB (Oxford).* 2012;**14**(1):67–70.
128. Bhangui P, Salloum C, Lim C, et al. Portal vein arterialization: a salvage procedure for a totally de-arterialized liver. The Paul Brousse Hospital experience. *HPB (Oxford).* 2014;**16**(8):723–738.
129. Chen Y, Liu Z, Duan W, et al. Modified arterioportal shunting in radical resection of hilar cholangiocarcinoma. *Hepatogastroenterology.* 2014;**61**(129):9–11.
130. Kondo S, Hirano S, Ambo Y, Tanaka E, Kubota T, Katoh H. Arterioportal shunting as an alternative to microvascular reconstruction after hepatic artery resection. *Br J Surg.* 2004;**91**(2):248–251.
131. Nagino M, Nimura Y, Nishio H, et al. Hepatectomy with simultaneous resection of the portal vein and hepatic artery for advanced perihilar cholangiocarcinoma. *Ann Surg.* 2010;**252**(1):115–123.
132. Shimizu H, Kimura F, Yoshidome H, et al. Aggressive surgical resection for hilar cholangiocarcinoma of the left-side predominance. *Ann Surg.* 2010;**251**(2):281–286.
133. Miyazaki M, Kato A, Ito H, et al. Combined vascular resection in operative resection for hilar cholangiocarcinoma: does it work or not? *Surgery.* 2007;**141**(5):581–588.
134. Gerhards MF, van Gulik TM, de Wit LT, Obertop H, Gouma DJ. Evaluation of morbidity and mortality after resection for hilar cholangiocarcinoma—a single center experience. *Surgery.* 2000;**127**(4):395–404.
135. Abbas S, Sandroussi C. Systematic review and meta-analysis of the role of vascular resection in the treatment of hilar cholangiocarcinoma. *HPB (Oxford).* 2013;**15**(7):492–503.
136. van Vugt J, Gaspersz MP, Coelen R, et al. The prognostic value of portal vein and hepatic artery involvement in patients with perihilar cholangiocarcinoma. *HPB (Oxford).* 2018;**20**(1):83–92.
137. Ethun CG, Lopez-Aguiar AG, Anderson, DJ, et al. Transplantation versus resection for hilar cholangiocarcinoma: an argument for shifting treatment paradigms for resectable disease. *Ann Surg.* 2018;**267**(5):797–805.
138. Heimbach J, Gores G, Haddock M, et al. Liver transplantation for unresectable perihilar cholangiocarcinoma. *Semin Liver Dis.* 2004;**24**(02):201–207.
139. Rea DJ, Heimbach, JK, Rosen CB, et al. Liver transplantation with neoadjuvant chemoradiation is more effective than resection for hilar cholangiocarcinoma. *Ann Surg.* 2005;**242**(3):451–461.
140. Boutros C, Somasundar P, Espat NJ. Extrahepatic cholangiocarcinoma: current surgical strategy. *Surg Oncol Clin N Am.* 2009;**18**(2):269–288.
141. Rosen CB, Heimbach JK, Gores GJ. Liver transplantation for cholangiocarcinoma. *Transpl Int.* 2010;**23**(7):692–697.
142. Croome KP, Rosen CB, Heimbach JK, Nagorney DM. Is liver transplantation appropriate for patients with potentially resectable de novo hilar cholangiocarcinoma? *J Am Coll Surg.* 2015;**221**(1):130–139.
143. Anderson B, Doyle MBM. Surgical considerations of hilar cholangiocarcinoma. *Surg Oncol Clin N Am.* 2019;**28**(4):601–617.
144. Nuzzo G. Improvement in perioperative and long-term outcome after surgical treatment of hilar cholangiocarcinoma. *Arch Surg.* 2012;**147**(1):26.
145. Furusawa N, Kobayashi A, Yokoyama T, Shimizu A, Motoyama H, Miyagawa S-I. Surgical treatment of 144 cases of hilar cholangiocarcinoma without liver-related mortality. *World J Surg.* 2014;**38**(5):1164–1176.
146. Tang Z, Yang Y, Zhao Z, Wei K, Meng W, Li X. The clinicopathological factors associated with prognosis of patients with resectable perihilar cholangiocarcinoma: a systematic review and meta-analysis. *Medicine.* 2018;**97**(34):e11999.
147. Sarmiento JM, Nagorney DM. Hepatic resection in the treatment of perihilar cholangiocarcinoma. *Surg Oncol Clin N Am.* 2002;**11**(4):893–908.
148. Lee SG, Lee YJ, Park KM, Hwang S, Min PC. One hundred and eleven liver resections for hilar bile duct cancer. *J Hepatobiliary Pancreat Surg.* 2000;**7**(2):135–141.
149. Hu H-J, Jin Y-W, Shrestha A, et al. Predictive factors of early recurrence after R0 resection of hilar cholangiocarcinoma: a single institution experience in China. *Cancer Med.* 2019;**8**(4):1567–1575.

150. de Jong MC, Hong S-M, Augustine MM, et al. Hilar cholangiocarcinoma: tumor depth as a predictor of outcome. *Arch Surg*. 2011;**146**(6):697–703.
151. Groot Koerkamp B, Wiggers JK, Gonen M, et al. Survival after resection of perihilar cholangiocarcinoma-development and external validation of a prognostic nomogram. *Ann Oncol*. 2015;**26**(9):1930–1935.
152. Lu J, Li B, Li FY, Ye H, Xiong XZ, Cheng NS. Prognostic significance of mucinous component in hilar cholangiocarcinoma after curative-intent resection. *J Surg Oncol*. 2019;**120**(8):1341–1349.
153. Ogino M, Nakanishi Y, Mitsuhashi T, et al. Impact of tumour budding grade in 310 patients who underwent surgical resection for extrahepatic cholangiocarcinoma. *Histopathology*. 2019;**74**(6):861–872.
154. Tang X, Zhang J, Che X, Lan Z, Chen Y, Wang C. The clinicopathological features and long-term survival outcomes of mucinous gastric carcinoma: a consecutive series of 244 cases from a single institute. *J Gastrointest Surg*. 2016;**20**(4):693–699.
155. Viganò L, Russolillo N, Ferrero A, et al. Resection of liver metastases from colorectal mucinous adenocarcinoma. *Ann Surg*. 2014;**260**(5):878–885.
156. Lee DW, Han SW, Lee HJ, et al. Prognostic implication of mucinous histology in colorectal cancer patients treated with adjuvant FOLFOX chemotherapy. *Br J Cancer*. 2013;**108**(10):1978–1984.
157. Chi Z, Bhalla A, Saeed O, et al. Mucinous intrahepatic cholangiocarcinoma: a distinct variant. *Hum Pathol*. 2018;**78**:131–137.
158. Cannon RM, Brock G, Buell JF. Surgical resection for hilar cholangiocarcinoma: experience improves resectability. *HPB (Oxford)*. 2012;**14**(2):142–149.
159. Mehrotra S, Lalwani S, Nundy S. Management strategies for patients with hilar cholangiocarcinomas: challenges and solutions. *Hepat Med*. 2020;**12**:1–13.
160. Schulick RD. Criteria of unresectability and the decision-making process. *HPB (Oxford)*. 2008;**10**(2):122–125.
161. Maeta T, Ebata T, Hayashi E, et al. Pancreatoduodenectomy with portal vein resection for distal cholangiocarcinoma. *Br J Surg*. 2017;**104**(11):1549–1557.
162. Chua TC, Mittal A, Arena J, Sheen A, Gill AJ, Samra JS. Resection margin influences survival after pancreatoduodenectomy for distal cholangiocarcinoma. *Am J Surg*. 2017;**213**(6):1072–1076.
163. van der Gaag NA, Rauws EAJ, van Eijck CHJ, et al. Preoperative biliary drainage for cancer of the head of the pancreas. *N Engl J Med*. 2010;**362**(2):129–137.
164. Dickson PV, Behrman SW. Distal cholangiocarcinoma. *Surg Clin North Am*. 2014;**94**(2):325–342.
165. Kwon HJ, Kim SG, Chun JM, Lee WK, Hwang YJ. Prognostic factors in patients with middle and distal bile duct cancers. *World J Gastroenterol*. 2014;**20**(21):6658–6665.
166. Murakami Y, Uemura K, Hayashidani Y, et al. Prognostic significance of lymph node metastasis and surgical margin status for distal cholangiocarcinoma. *J Surg Oncol*. 2007;**95**(3):207–212.
167. Zhou Y, Liu S, Wu L, Wan T. Survival after surgical resection of distal cholangiocarcinoma: a systematic review and meta-analysis of prognostic factors. *Asian J Surg*. 2017;**40**(2):129–138.
168. Yoshida T. Prognostic factors after pancreatoduodenectomy with extended lymphadenectomy for distal bile duct cancer. *Arch Surg*. 2002;**137**(1):69.
169. Wellner UF, Shen Y, Keck T, Jin W, Xu Z. The survival outcome and prognostic factors for distal cholangiocarcinoma following surgical resection: a meta-analysis for the 5-year survival. *Surg Today*. 2016;**47**(3):271–279.
170. Hong S-M, Pawlik TM, Cho H, et al. Depth of tumor invasion better predicts prognosis than the current American Joint Committee on Cancer T classification for distal bile duct carcinoma. *Surgery*. 2009;**146**(2):250–257.
171. Hernandez J, Cowgill SM, Al-Saadi S, et al. An aggressive approach to extrahepatic cholangiocarcinomas is warranted: margin status does not impact survival after resection. *Ann Surg Oncol*. 2008;**15**(3):807–814.
172. DeOliveira ML, Cunningham SC, Cameron JL, et al. Cholangiocarcinoma: thirty-one-year experience with 564 patients at a single institution. *Ann Surg*. 2007;**245**(5):755–762.
173. Jang JY, Kim, SW, Park, DJ, et al. Actual long-term outcome of extrahepatic bile duct cancer after surgical resection. *Ann Surg*. 2005;**241**(1):77–84.
174. Wakai T, Shirai Y, Moroda T, Yokoyama N, Hatakeyama K. Impact of ductal resection margin status on long-term survival in patients undergoing resection for extrahepatic cholangiocarcinoma. *Cancer*. 2005;**103**(6):1210–1216.
175. Park Y, Hwang DW, Kim JH, et al. Prognostic comparison of the longitudinal margin status in distal bile duct cancer: R0 on first bile duct resection versus R0 after additional resection. *J Hepatobiliary Pancreat Sci*. 2019;**26**(5):169–178.
176. Frosio F, Mocchegiani F, Conte G, et al. Neoadjuvant therapy in the treatment of hilar cholangiocarcinoma: review of the literature. *World J Gastroinest Surg*. 2019;**11**(6):279–286.
177. McMasters KM, Tuttle TM, Leach SD, et al. Neoadjuvant chemoradiation for extrahepatic cholangiocarcinoma. *Am J Surg*. 1997;**174**(6):605–609.
178. Nelson JW, Ghafoori AP, Willett CG, et al. Concurrent chemoradiotherapy in resected extrahepatic cholangiocarcinoma. *Int J Radiat Oncol Biol Phys*. 2009;**73**(1):148–153.
179. Jung JH, Lee HJ, Lee HS, et al. Benefit of neoadjuvant concurrent chemoradiotherapy for locally advanced perihilar cholangiocarcinoma. *World J Gastroenterol*. 2017;**23**(18):3301–3308.
180. Sumiyoshi T, Shima Y, Okabayashi T, et al. Chemoradiotherapy for initially unresectable locally advanced cholangiocarcinoma. *World J Surg*. 2018;**42**(9):2910–2918.
181. Katayose Y, Nakagawa K, Yoshida H, et al. Neoadjuvant chemoradiation therapy for cholangiocarcinoma to improve R0 resection rate: the first report of phase II study. *J Clin Oncol*. 2015;**33**(3 Suppl):402.
182. Valle J, Wasan H, Palmer DH, et al. Cisplatin plus gemcitabine versus gemcitabine for biliary tract cancer. *N Engl J Med*. 2010;**362**(14):1273–1281.
183. Murakami Y, Uemura K, Sudo T, et al. Prognostic factors after surgical resection for intrahepatic, hilar, and distal cholangiocarcinoma. *Ann Surg Oncol*. 2011;**18**(3):651–658.
184. Horgan AM, Amir E, Walter T, Knox JJ. Adjuvant therapy in the treatment of biliary tract cancer: a systematic review and meta-analysis. *J Clin Oncol*. 2012;**30**(16):1934–1940.
185. Kang MJ, Jang J-Y, Chang J, et al. Actual long-term survival outcome of 403 consecutive patients with hilar cholangiocarcinoma. *World J Surg*. 2016;**40**(10):2451–2459.
186. Krasnick BA, Jin LX, Davidson JT, et al. Adjuvant therapy is associated with improved survival after curative resection for hilar cholangiocarcinoma: a multi-institution analysis from the

187. Ebata T, Hirano S, Konishi M, et al. Randomized clinical trial of adjuvant gemcitabine chemotherapy versus observation in resected bile duct cancer. *Br J Surg.* 2018;**105**(3):192–202.
188. Edeline J, Benabdelghani M, Bertaut A, et al. Gemcitabine and oxaliplatin chemotherapy or surveillance in resected biliary tract cancer (PRODIGE 12-ACCORD 18-UNICANCER GI): a randomized phase III study. *J Clin Oncol.* 2019;**37**(8):658–667.
189. Primrose JN, Fox RP, Palmer DH, et al. Capecitabine compared with observation in resected biliary tract cancer (BILCAP): a randomised, controlled, multicentre, phase 3 study. *Lancet Oncol.* 2019;**20**(5):663–673.
190. Borghero Y, Crane CH, Szklaruk J, et al. Extrahepatic bile duct adenocarcinoma: patients at high-risk for local recurrence treated with surgery and adjuvant chemoradiation have an equivalent overall survival to patients with standard-risk treated with surgery alone. *Ann Surg Oncol.* 2008;**15**(11):3147–3156.
191. Kim TH, Han S-S, Park S-J, et al. Role of adjuvant chemoradiotherapy for resected extrahepatic biliary tract cancer. *Int J Radiat Oncol Biol Phys.* 2011;**81**(5):e853–e859.
192. Nakeeb A, Tran KQ, Black MJ, et al. Improved survival in resected biliary malignancies. *Surgery.* 2002;**132**(4):555–564.
193. Ben-Josef E, Guthrie KA, El-Khoueiry AB, et al. SWOG S0809: a phase II intergroup trial of adjuvant capecitabine and gemcitabine followed by radiotherapy and concurrent capecitabine in extrahepatic cholangiocarcinoma and gallbladder carcinoma. *J Clin Oncol.* 2015;**33**(24):2617–2622.
194. Heron DE, Stein DE, Eschelman DJ, et al. Cholangiocarcinoma: the impact of tumor location and treatment strategy on outcome. *Am J Clin Oncol.* 2003;**26**(4):422–428.
195. Cheng Q, Luo X, Zhang B, Jiang X, Yi B, Wu M. Predictive factors for prognosis of hilar cholangiocarcinoma: postresection radiotherapy improves survival. *Eur J Surg Oncol.* 2007;**33**(2):202–207.
196. Shroff RT, Kennedy EB, Bachini M, et al. Adjuvant therapy for resected biliary tract cancer: ASCO clinical practice guideline. *J Clin Oncol.* 2019;**37**(12):1015–1027.
197. Farley DR, Weaver AL, Nagorney DM. 'Natural history' of unresected cholangiocarcinoma: patient outcome after noncurative intervention. *Mayo Clinic Proc.* 1995;**70**(5):425–429.
198. Paik WH, Park YS, Hwang J-H, et al. Palliative treatment with self-expandable metallic stents in patients with advanced type III or IV hilar cholangiocarcinoma: a percutaneous versus endoscopic approach. *Gastrointest Endosc.* 2009;**69**(1):55–62.
199. Faris JE, Zhu AX. Targeted therapy for biliary tract cancers. *J Hepatobiliary Pancreat Sci.* 2012;**19**(4):326–336.
200. Sen S, Shroff RT. Emerging targeted and immunotherapies in cholangiocarcinoma. *Oncol Hematol Rev.* 2019;**15**(2):71.
201. Rizvi S, Khan SA, Hallemeier CL, Kelley RK, Gores GJ. Cholangiocarcinoma—evolving concepts and therapeutic strategies. *Nat Rev Clin Oncol.* 2018;**15**(2):95–111.
202. Simile MM, Bagella P, Vidili G, et al. Targeted therapies in cholangiocarcinoma: emerging evidence from clinical trials. *Medicina (Kaunas).* 2019;**55**(2):42.
203. Lowery MA, Burris HA, Janku F, et al. Safety and activity of ivosidenib in patients with IDH1-mutant advanced cholangiocarcinoma: a phase 1 study. *Lancet Gastroenterol Hepatol.* 2019;**4**(9):711–720.
204. Mazzaferro V, El-Rayes BF, Droz Dit Busset M, et al. Derazantinib (ARQ 087) in advanced or inoperable FGFR2 gene fusion-positive intrahepatic cholangiocarcinoma. *Br J Cancer.* 2019;**120**(2):165–171.
205. Wainberg ZA, Lassen UN, Elez E, et al. Efficacy and safety of dabrafenib (D) and trametinib (T) in patients (pts) with BRAF V600E-mutated biliary tract cancer (BTC): a cohort of the ROAR basket trial. *J Clin Oncol.* 2019;**37**(4 Suppl):187.
206. Javle M, Churi C, Kang HC, et al. HER2/neu-directed therapy for biliary tract cancer. *J Hematol Oncol.* 2015;**8**:58.
207. Arkenau H-T, Martin-Liberal J, Calvo E, et al. Ramucirumab plus pembrolizumab in patients with previously treated advanced or metastatic biliary tract cancer: nonrandomized, open-label, phase I trial (JVDF). *Oncologist.* 2018;**23**(12):1407–1416.
208. Turkes F, Carmichael J, Cunningham D, Starling N. Contemporary tailored oncology treatment of biliary tract cancers. *Gastroenterol Res Pract.* 2019;**2019**:7698786.
209. Kuvshinoff BW, Armstrong JG, Fong Y, et al. Palliation of irresectable hilar cholangiocarcinoma with biliary drainage and radiotherapy. *Br J Surg.* 1995;**82**(11):1522–1525.
210. Barney BM, Olivier KR, Miller RC, Haddock MG. Clinical outcomes and toxicity using stereotactic body radiotherapy (SBRT) for advanced cholangiocarcinoma. *Radiat Oncol.* 2012;**7**:67.
211. Jung DH, Kim M-S, Cho CK, et al. Outcomes of stereotactic body radiotherapy for unresectable primary or recurrent cholangiocarcinoma. *Radiat Oncol J.* 2014;**32**(3):163–169.
212. Søreide K, Körner H, Havnen J, Søreide JA. Bile duct cysts in adults. *Br J Surg.* 2004;**91**(12):1538–1548.
213. Bismuth H, Krissat J. Choledochal cystic malignancies. *Ann Oncol.* 1999;**10**:S94–S98.
214. Li Y, Wei J, Zhao Z, You T, Zhong M. Pancreaticobiliary maljunction is associated with common bile duct carcinoma: a meta-analysis. *ScientificWorldJournal.* 2013;**2013**:618670.
215. Morine Y, Shimada M, Takamatsu H, et al. Clinical features of pancreaticobiliary maljunction: update analysis of 2nd Japan-nationwide survey. *J Hepatobiliary Pancreat Sci.* 2013;**20**(5):472–480.
216. Kamisawa T, Kaneko K, Itoi T, Ando H. Pancreaticobiliary maljunction and congenital biliary dilatation. *Lancet Gastroenterol Hepatol.* 2017;**2**(8):610–618.

Index

For the benefit of digital users, indexed terms that span two pages (e.g., 52–53) may, on occasion, appear on only one of those pages

Tables and boxes are indicated by *t* and *b* following the page number.

abdominal collections 229
abdominal compartment syndrome 121
abscess *see* liver abscess
acetic acid, percutaneous injection 277
acinus 12
actinomycosis (*Actinomyces israeli*) 60
acute bacterial hepatitis 60–61
acute cellular rejection 241
acute cholangitis 307, 437–41
acute liver failure 248
adenofibroma 99–100
adenoma
 bile duct 98
 hepatocellular (hepatic) 87–92
adhesions 289
adrenal insufficiency 31
Alagille syndrome 247–48, 433
alanine 14
alanine aminotransferase (ALT) 42
albumin 43–44
alemtuzumab 243
alkaline phosphatase (ALP) 42–43
alpha-1 antitrypsin deficiency 14
alpha-fetoprotein 187
alveolar echinococcosis (*Echinococcus multilocularis*) 78–80
American Society of Anesthesiologists – Physical Status (ASA-PS) 30, 224–25
amino acid clearance test 47*t*
amino acid metabolism 14
^{14}C-aminopyrine test 47*t*
aminotransferases 42
amoebic liver abscess 62, 76–77
anaesthesia
 anaesthetic drug handling 32
 anaesthetic management 34–35
 liver-directed anaesthesia 225–26
analgesic drug handling 32–33
angiography 55–57
angiomyolipoma 103–4, 294
anticoagulation
 Budd-Chiari syndrome 130–32, 154
 portal vein thrombosis 126, 127–28, 157
antimetabolites 242–43
antithymocyte globulin 243
Armillifer 63
arterialized nodular hyperplasia 97

artificial intelligence 46
Ascaris lumbricoides 64*t*, 319–20
ascites 35, 140–41
aspartate aminotransferase (AST) 42
aspartate aminotransferase-to-platelet index 429
associating liver partition and portal vein ligation for staged hepatectomy (ALPPS) 183, 218–19
ATOM mnemonic 367
atracurium 32
autoimmune cholangiopathy 318–19
autosomal dominant polycystic kidney disease 284
autosomal recessive polycystic kidney disease 433–35
azathioprine 242–43

babesiosis 65
bacterial liver infections 59–62
balloon-occluded retrograde transvenous obliteration 140, 148
balloon-occluded TACE 279
bariatric surgery 316, 351–52
Bartonella henselae 61–62
basiliximab 243
belatacept 243
benign recurrent intrahepatic cholestasis 435
bile acid synthetic defects 435
bile duct
 adenoma 98
 anatomy 8–10
 biopsy/brush 324, 329
 diameter 446
 gall bladder cancer 398–99, 400–2
 injuries 307–8, 332–33
 intraductal papillary neoplasms 82, 304, 320–21, 450–51
 intrahepatic congenital dilatation 442
 percutaneous balloon dilatation 325, 442
 spontaneous perforation 433
bile formation 14–15
bile leak 198, 229, 288, 316
bile salt export pump 14–15
biliary adenofibroma 99–100
biliary atresia 423–32
 aetiology 423–25

biochemical tests 426
bridging fibrosis 425
classification 425
clinical features 425–26
CMV-associated 423, 425
cystic 425
developmental immaturity of biliary tract 424
diagnosis 426–27
DPM-like arrays 425
ERCP 427
genetic factors 424
genomics 430
isolated 425
Kasai portoenterostomy (KPE) 427–30
liver biopsy 427
liver transplantation 247
operative cholangiogram 427
pathology 425
radionuclide scintigraphy 427
syndromic 425
ultrasonogram 426–27
viral vectors 423–24
biliary cystadenocarcinoma 81
biliary cystadenoma 81
biliary cysts 304, 446–52
biliary decompression 440–41
biliary diversion 436
biliary drainage 55, 181, 324–25, 329, 372, 441, 469
biliary embryonal rhabdomyosarcoma 211–12
biliary fistula 376–79
biliary hamartoma 80, 98–99
biliary injury, post-cholecystectomy 366–75
 biliary drainage 372
 biliodigestive anastomosis 370–71
 classification 367
 endoscopy 372
 hepatectomy 372
 liver transplantation 372
 long-term outcome 373–74
 postoperative morbidity 373
 prevention during laparoscopic surgery 369–70
 risk factors 366
 surgical drains 372
 surgical repair 370–72
 therapeutic management 369, 370–72
 vascular injury 366–67

workup 368–69
biliary leak 121, 240, 307
biliary microbiome 351
biliary stents 325–27
biliary stones 442–44
 ERCP 315–16, 442–43
 imaging 304
 percutaneous interventions 330–32
 surgical treatment 443–44
biliary strictures 240, 255–56, 288–89, 307, 316, 330–32
biliary tract
 developmental immaturity 424
 imaging 301–10
biliatresone 423
bilirubin
 metabolism 14
 serum levels 40–42
Billroth II gastrectomy 316–18
biloma 81
biological therapies 243
Bismuth classification 367
Bismuth-Corlette classification 323–24
black fever 62–63
Bordeaux classification 88, 89*t*
brachytherapy 418–19
branched-chain amino acids 142
breast cancer metastases 220, 293
breath tests 47*t*
broncho-biliary fistula 289
brucellosis (*Brucella melitensis*) 59
Budd-Chiari syndrome 130–33, 138, 152–55
Burkholderia pseudomallei 60

caffeine test 47*t*
calcineurin inhibitors 242, 250
canalicular membrane transporter defects 435
capillariasis (*Capillaria hepatica*) 63
carbohydrate antigen 19-9 (CA19-9) 179
carbohydrate metabolism 13
cardiomyopathy, cirrhotic 31
Caroli's disease 80, 433–35
cat scratch disease 61–62
cavernous haemangioma 100–3
checkpoint inhibitors 417–18
chemical ablation 276–77
Child–Turcotte–Pugh (CTP) score 30, 44, 147–48, 224

Index

cholangiocarcinoma 176–86, 458–75
  adjuvant therapy 183–84, 185, 467–69
  ALPPS 183
  anatomical classification 176
  bile duct margin status 463–64
  biliary drainage 181, 469
  blood tests 461
  brachytherapy 418–19
  CA19-9 179
  chemotherapy 416–17, 467–68
  classification 459–60
  clinical presentation 178–79, 184, 460–61
  differential diagnosis 179
  distal 419–20, 460, 467
  epidemiology 176–77, 458–59
  hepatopancreaticoduodenectomy 465
  histology 179
  imaging 51–52, 178–79, 184, 307
  immunotherapy 417–18, 469
  intrahepatic 176, 177, 184–85, 292–93, 415–19
  liver transplantation 183, 185, 416, 419, 465–66
  locoregional options 185, 418
  long-term outcomes 184, 185, 292–93
  lymphadenectomy 464
  metastatic or locoregional recurrence 469
  natural history 176–77
  neoadjuvant therapy 419, 467
  optimization of future liver remnant 464–65
  palliative care 185, 469
  pancreaticoduodenectomy 419
  pathology 177
  perihilar 51–52, 176, 177, 178–84, 419, 459–60, 462–67
  portal vein embolization 182
  preoperative radiology 461–62
  primary sclerosing cholangitis 454
  prophylactic surgery 469
  proton beam therapy 418
  radiation therapy 418–20, 468–69
  risk factors 176–77, 458–59
  staging 177, 459–60
  staging laparoscopy 465
  surgical approach 182–83, 185, 416, 462–67
  systemic therapy 469
  TACE 418
  targeted therapy 469
  therapeutic options 177–78
  trisectionectomy for Bismuth type IV tumours 465
  unresectable disease 469
  vascular resection 183, 465
  yttrium-90 418
cholangiography, intraoperative 364–65, 369–70
cholangioma 98
cholangitis
  acute 307, 437–41
  IgG4-related sclerosing 318–19, 332
  imaging 307
  neonatal sclerosing 433
  post-Kasai portoenterostomy 428–29
  primary sclerosing 307, 332, 453–57
  pyogenic 332
  recurrent 442
cholecardia 31
cholecystectomy
  dome-down 364, 370
  intraoperative cholangiography 364–65, 369–70
  laparoscopic 355–56, 361–64, 369–70
  open approach 364
  open conversion 370
  subtotal 364
  see also biliary injury, post-cholecystectomy
cholecystitis
  cholecystectomy 361–65
  imaging 303
cholecystokinin 350
choledochal cysts 304, 433
choledocholithiasis see biliary stones
cholelithiasis see gallstones
cholesterol
  homeostasis 13
  stones 353–54
cholestyramine 351
choristoma 107
chylomicrons 13
ciclosporin 242, 243
ciliated hepatic foregut duplication cysts 75
cirrhosis
  coagulation system 31–32
  malnutrition 33–34
  pathophysiological changes 31–32
  portal hypertension 138
  portal vein thrombosis 125, 127–28
  timing of non-liver surgery 31
cisatracurium 32
clearance tests 46
Clonorchis sinensis 64t, 319–20
coagulopathy management 35
colon cancer, primary sclerosing cholangitis 454
colorectal liver metastases 54, 219, 229, 283, 290–91, 337
comfrey herb tea 155
computed tomography (CT) 50–53, 223, 301–2
congenital choledochal cysts 433
congenital choledochal malformation 446–49
contrast-enhanced ultrasound 301
corticosteroids 243, 250, 429–30
costimulatory molecules 243
Coxiella burnetii 62
Crohn's disease 350
cryoablation 276
Cryptosporidium 64t
cystadenocarcinoma 81
cystadenoma 81
cystic disease
  benign liver lesions 73–81
  biliary atresia 425
  biliary cystadenoma/cystadenocarcinoma 81
  biliary lesions 304, 446–52
  ciliated hepatic foregut duplication cysts 75
  congenital choledochal cysts 433
  endometrial cysts 80–81
  gall bladder 446
  hepatocellular carcinoma 81–82
  hydatid (echinococcal) cyst 63, 77–78, 283–84
  metastases 82–83
  neoplastic liver lesions 81–83
  peribiliary cysts 449–50
  polycystic liver disease 75, 284
  simple hepatic cysts 73–75, 284
  traumatic cysts 81
cytomegalovirus 423, 425

damage control surgery 119–20
delayed gastric emptying 289
deoxycholate 351
diabetes mellitus 68
diaphragmatic hernia 289
diuretics, ascites therapy 141
DPM-like arrays 425
drug-eluting bead TACE 279
drug handling 32–33
dynamic liver performance 46
dysplastic nodule 97–98

echinococcosis
  alveolar (E. multilocularis) 78–80
  cystic (E. granulosus) 63, 77–78, 283–84
embryonal hepatic sarcoma 82, 209–11
endometrial cysts 80–81
endometriosis 107
endoscopic retrograde cholangiopancreatography (ERCP) 311, 315–16, 427, 440–41, 442–43
endoscopic ultrasound-guided biliary drainage 441
endosonography 311
Entamoeba histolytica 62, 76
enterocytes 13
epidermal growth factor receptor (EGFR) inhibitors 417
epithelioid haemangioendothelioma 204–7
erlotinib 417
erythromycin 351
ethanol, percutaneous injection 276–77
everolimus 243
extrahepatic portal venous obstruction 124–28, 156–58
ex vivo resection and autotransplantation 294

Fasciola hepatica 64t, 319–20
FAST scan 115–16
fatty lesions of liver 103–7
fatty liver 67–72
FDG-PET/CT 54–55, 302
fibroblast growth factor receptor 2 (FGFR2) inhibitor 417
fistula
  biliary 376–79
  broncho-biliary 289
fluids, perioperative 35
focal fatty liver lesions 107
focal nodular hyperplasia 92–94
focused assessment with sonography for trauma (FAST) 115–16
free hepatic venous pressure 137
fungal abscess 80

galactose elimination capacity 47t
gall bladder cancer 391, 392–410
  adjuvant therapy 408–9
  bile duct excision 398–99
  bile duct involvement 400–2
  clinical features 393–94
  colon involvement 399–400
  epidemiology 392–93
  gallstones 354, 392–93
  gastroduodenal involvement 399
  imaging 303–4
  incidental 395–96, 403–7
  inter-aortocaval lymph node 396
  investigations 394
  jaundice 400–2
  laparoscopic surgery 407–8
  liver resection 397–98
  lymphadenectomy 396–97
  missed/overlooked 404
  neoadjuvant therapy 408–9
  outcomes 409–10
  pancreatic involvement 399
  pathology 393
  porcelain gall bladder 392–93
  primary sclerosing cholangitis 454
  prognosis 409–10
  risk factors 392–93
  staging 394–96
  suspected disease detected intraoperatively 407
  T2 tumour management 398
  unsuspected 404
  vascular involvement 402
gall bladder cyst 446
gall bladder drainage 318, 333
gall bladder dysmotility 350–51
gall bladder polyps 391–92
gallstones 348–60
  age factors 348
  asymptomatic 354–55
  bariatric surgery 351–52
  biliary fistula 376–79
  biliary microbiome 351
  cholesterol stones 353–54
  conservative management 355
  epidemiology 348
  gall bladder cancer 354, 392–93
  gall bladder dysmotility 350–51
  gallstone ileus 379–87
  genetic factors 349
  hormone replacement therapy 350
  H. pylori 351
  inflammatory bowel disease 350
  laparoscopic cholecystectomy 355–56
  lifestyle 349
  metabolic syndrome 349
  mixed (brown pigment) stones 354
  natural history 354–56
  neonatal 433
  oral contraceptive pill 349
  parenteral nutrition 350
  pathogenesis 348, 352–54
  pigment stones 354
  pregnancy 349
  risk factors 376–79
  sex differences 349
  statins 350
  symptomatic 355

Index

gamma-glutamyl transferase 43
gastric varices 139
gastrointestinal tumour metastases 220, 221, 293
gastro-oesophageal devascularization 148
Gelfoam 278
global liver function 44–45
glucose homeostasis 13
glucose transporter 1 (GLUT2) 13
graft rejection 241
graft-versus-host disease 241
granulomatous bacterial infection 61–62
gynaecological cancer, liver metastases 220

haemangioendothelioma 204–7
haemangioma 100–3, 283
haemangiopericytoma 207–8
haemangiosarcoma 207
haematoma 81
halothane 32
hamartoma
  biliary 80, 98–99
  mesenchymal 107
hanging manoeuvre 226, 341–42
Helicobacter pylori 351
helminths 63–64
hepatic abscess *see* liver abscess
hepatic adenoma 87–92
hepatic angiomyolipoma 103–4, 294
hepatic artery
  anatomy 7–8
  pseudoaneurysm 239
  stenosis 239
  thrombosis 239, 251–52
hepatic clearance tests 46
hepatic encephalopathy 141–42
hepatic epithelioid haemangioendothelioma 204–7
hepatic haemangiosarcoma 207
hepatic infantile haemangioendothelioma 207
hepatic leiomyoma 107
hepatic lipoma 104–5
hepatic lymphangioma 107
hepatic myelolipoma 105–7
hepatic necrosis 121
hepatico-duodenostomy 318
hepatico-gastrostomy 318
hepatic resection *see* liver resection
hepatic small vessel neoplasm 208
hepatic splenosis 107
hepatic steatosis 67–72
hepatic synthetic function 43–44
hepatic vascular exclusion 226
hepatic vascular malformations 158
hepatic veins
  anatomy 4–6
  embolization 225
  stenosis 240, 253–55
hepatic venous outflow obstruction 130–33
hepatic venous pressure gradient 137, 139*t*
hepatitis
  acute bacterial 60–61
  idiopathic neonatal 435
  infective 435
  syphilitic 61
  toxic 435–36

hepatobiliary iminodiacetic acid (HIDA) tests 225, 427
hepatoblastoma 187–203
  annotation factors 192–93
  bile leak 198
  biopsy 195
  cardiac arrest 198
  chemotherapy 195, 200
  CHIC-HS 187–88
  classification 187–88
  differential diagnosis 188
  genetics 188
  haemorrhage 197–98
  histology 188–90
  ICG-guided surgery 197
  imaging 190
  laparoscopic resection 197
  liver failure 198
  liver transplantation 198–200, 248–50
  metastatic disease 199
  PLTCC 187–88, 189*t*
  POSTEXT 191
  postoperative complications 197–98
  presentation 187
  PRETEXT system 190–93
  recurrence 200
  risk stratification 193–94
  salvage transplantation 199
  serum alpha-fetoprotein 187
  staging 187–88
  surgical resection 196–97
hepatocellular adenoma 87–92
hepatocellular adenomatosis 293–94
hepatocellular carcinoma (HCC)
  ablation with resection 169
  borderline indications for surgery 168–70
  Budd-Chiari syndrome 153
  CT 51–52
  cystic 81–82
  epidemiology of surgical interest 162–64
  guidelines for management 164–66
  laparoscopic liver resection 166–67, 337–38
  liver transplantation 170–74
  living donor transplantation 260–61
  lobar hypertrophy induction 168
  long-term outcomes 291–92
  MRI 53–54
  multinodular 168–69
  non-operative interventional therapies 281–83
  operable 162
  PET-CT 54–55
  portal vein thrombosis 125
  primary sclerosing cholangitis 454
  recurrent 169–70
  risk of postoperative liver failure with chronic liver disease 167–68
  sarcomatous 209
hepatopancreatoduodenectomy 399, 465
hereditary haemorrhagic telangiectasia 158

hernia
  diaphragmatic 289
  incisional 289–90, 344
heterotopic tissue 107
HIDA test 225, 427
high-density lipoprotein 13
high-intensity focused ultrasound 275
HIV cholangiopathy 332
hormone replacement therapy 350
hydatid (echinococcal) cyst 63, 77–78, 283–84
hyperbilirubinaemia 41–42
hyperthermic ablation 274–76
hyponatraemia 31
hypothermic ablation 276

idiopathic neonatal hepatitis 435
idiopathic non-cirrhotic portal hypertension 128–29
IgG4-mediated disease 318–19, 332
immunoregulation 233
immunosuppression 241–43, 250
immunotherapy 417–18, 469
incisional hernia 289–90, 344
indocyanine green-guided surgery 197
indocyanine green test 47*t*, 225
indomethacin 351
infective hepatitis 435
inflammatory bowel disease 350, 454
inflammatory myofibroblastic tumour 109–10
inflammatory pseudotumours 109–10
inhalational anaesthetics 32
insulin 13
international normalized ratio (INR) 43–44
intraductal papillary neoplasms of bile duct 82, 304, 320–21, 450–51
intrahepatic cholangiocarcinoma 176, 177, 184–85, 292–93, 415–19
intrahepatic congenital bile duct dilatation 442
intravenous anaesthetics 32
ipilimumab 417–18
irreversible electroporation 277
isocitrate dehydrogenase (IDH) inhibitors 417, 418
isoflurane 32
ivosidenib 417

Kasai portoenterostomy (KPE) 427–30

lactate 13
lactulose 142
laparoscopic
laparoscopic liver resection 229, 336–47
  benchmarking 337
  bleeding management 343
  caudal approach 338–39
  classification 337
  colorectal liver metastases 337
  conversion to open resection 343–44
  extraction sites 344
  extrafascial approach 341

Glissonian approach 341
hepatoblastoma 197
hepatocellular carcinoma 166–67, 337–38
intrafascial approach 341
learning curve 337
living donor liver transplantation 265, 338
minimization of surgical morbidity 166–67
outcomes 336–37
parenchymal transection 342–43
patient and surgeon positioning 339
pneumoperitoneum 339–40
supra-hilar approach 341
surgical approach 338–39
trocar placement 339–40
vascular control 340–42
laparoscopic surgery
  biliary fistula 377–79
  cholecystectomy 355–56, 361–64, 369–70
  gall bladder cancer 407–8
  gallstone ileus 385–86
  liver resection *see* laparoscopic liver resection
laser-induced thermotherapy 275–76
leiomyoma 107
leiomyosarcoma 211–12
Leishmania donovani 62–63
leptospirosis 61
LIMAX test 225
lipid metabolism 13–14
lipoma 104–5
listeriosis (*Listeria monocytogenes*) 60
liver abscess
  amoebic 62, 76–77
  fungal 80
  liver trauma 121
  pyogenic 59–60, 76
liver acinus 12
liver anatomy 3–11
liver bacterial infections 59–62
liver biochemical tests 40–43, 44, 45–46
liver cysts *see* cystic disease
liver failure
  pathophysiology 232–33
  post-hepatectomy 24–25
  post-hepatoblastoma surgery 198
liver fibrosis 26
liver function assessment 40–48
liver lobule 12
liver metastases *see* metastatic liver disease
liver necrosis 121
liver parasites 62–64, 319–20
liver physiology 12–16
liver regeneration 17–29
liver resection 223–31
  abdominal collections 229
  access 226
  anatomical resections 226–28
  anatomical versus non-anatomical resection 226
  assessment of resectability 223
  bile leak 229
  biliary resection and reconstruction 228–29
  caudate lobectomy 228

Index

liver resection (cont.)
  contraindications 223
  ex vivo resection and autotransplantation 294
  functional assessment 225
  gall bladder cancer 397–98
  haemorrhage 229
  hepatic vein embolization 225
  imaging 223–24
  indications 223
  intraoperative ultrasound 226
  laparoscopic surgery *see* laparoscopic liver resection
  left hemihepatectomy 227
  left lateral sectionectomy 227, 294
  left trisectionectomy 228, 294
  liver-directed anaesthesia 225–26
  liver-first for metastatic rectal cancer 229
  liver function assessment 224–25
  metastatic disease 218–19
  multistage resection 229
  outcomes 229
  parenchymal transection 226
  portal vein embolization 225
  post-cholecystectomy bile duct injury 372
  resection margin 226
  right hemihepatectomy 228, 294
  right posterior sectionectomy 228
  right trisectionectomy 228, 294
  robotic surgery 229
  synchronous versus staged resection for colorectal cancer metastases 229
  three-dimensional reconstruction 57
  timing of surgery 31
  vascular isolation and ischaemia techniques 226
  vascular resection and reconstruction 228–29
  volumetry 225
liver sarcoma *see* sarcoma
liver segmentation 3–4
liver sinusoidal endothelial cells 233
liver steatosis 67–72
liver transplantation
  acute cellular rejection 241
  allograft procurement and preservation 236
  back table allograft preparation 236
  biliary anastomosis 238
  biliary leak 240
  biliary strictures 240, 332
  Budd-Chiari syndrome 133, 155
  candidate evaluation and selection 233
  caval complications 240
  caval replacement implantation 237
  children *see* paediatric liver transplantation
  cholangiocarcinoma 183, 185, 416, 419, 465–66
  chronic rejection 241
  closure 238
  complications 238–41
  contraindications 233–34
  deceased donor 235
  donor selection 236
  graft-versus-host disease 241
  hepatectomy and implantation 236–37
  hepatic artery anastomosis 237–38
  hepatic artery complications 239
  hepatic vein complications 240
  hepatoblastoma 198–200, 248–50
  hepatocellular carcinoma 170–74
  immunosuppression 241–43
  indications 233–34
  infection 241
  live donor *see* living donor liver transplantation
  liver trauma 120
  organ allocation 235
  outcomes 243
  piggyback implantation 237
  portal hypertension 148
  portal vein complications 239–40
  portal vein thrombosis 128, 157
  post-cholecystectomy bile duct injury 372
  post-transplant cholangiopathy 308–9
  post-transplant lymphoproliferative disorder 240
  primary non-function 238–39
  primary sclerosing cholangitis 456–57
  prioritization 233
  recurrence of disease 241
  salvage transplantation 199
  screening 233
  small-for-size syndrome 264–65, 288
  steatotic grafts 69–70
  surgical procedure 236–38
liver trauma 114–23
  abdominal compartment syndrome 121
  angiographic embolization 117
  biliary leak 121
  classification of injury 114–15, 117t
  CT 115–16
  cyst formation 81
  damage control surgery 119–20
  diagnosis 115–16
  extrahepatic biliary injury 120–21
  FAST scan 115–16
  image-guided percutaneous drainage 117–19
  liver abscess 121
  liver necrosis 121
  liver transplantation 120
  non-operative management 116–19
  operative management 119–21
  pathophysiology 114
  planned reoperation 121
  postoperative complications 121
  ultrasound 115–16
living donor liver transplantation 234–35, 259–72
  back table preparation 263–64
  donor evaluation 261–62
  donor hepatectomy 262–63
  ethical issues 260
  fatty liver 69
  hepatic venous outflow management 264–65
  hepatocellular carcinoma 260–61
  history 259–60
  indications 260
  laparoscopic surgery 265, 338
  left lateral segmentectomy 263
  recipient operation 264
  right hepatectomy 263
  robotic surgery 265
  small-for-size syndrome 264–65
long-term outcomes of liver surgery 286–98
L-ornithine-L-aspartate (LOLA) 142
lymphadenectomy 396–97, 464
lymphangioma 107

magnetic resonance cholangiopancreatography (MRCP) 302–3
magnetic resonance imaging (MRI) 53–54, 223–24, 302–3
malarial hepatopathy 62
malignant melanoma 221
malnutrition 33–34
mechanical thrombectomy 157
MEGX tests 47t
melanoma 221
MELD score 30, 44–45, 147–48, 224
  MELD-Na 46b, 233, 235
melioidosis 60
mesenchymal hamartoma 107
mesenterico-left portal venous bypass 148
metabolic liver disease 248, 435
metabolic syndrome 13–14, 349
metastatic liver disease
  aetiology 217
  ALPPS 218–19
  breast primary tumour 220, 293
  clinical features 217–18
  colorectal primary tumour 54, 219, 229, 283, 290–91, 337
  cystic 82–83
  epidemiology 217
  gastrointestinal primary tumour 220, 221, 293
  gynaecological primary tumour 220
  investigations 218
  liver-first in rectal cancer 229
  liver resection 218–19
  melanoma primary tumour 221
  neuroendocrine primary tumour 219–20, 283, 293
  non-operative interventional therapies 283
  sarcomatous primary tumour 221
  treatment principles 218–19
  urological primary tumour 220
Metroticket model 171–72
microbiome 351
microwave ablation 275
Mirizzi syndrome 304, 387–89
Model for End-Stage Liver Disease (MELD) score 30, 44–45, 147–48, 224
  MELD-Na 46b, 233, 235
mTOR inhibitors 243
multidrug resistance-associated protein 2 (MRP2) 14–15
multidrug resistance-associated protein 3 (MRP3) 15

Mycobacterium hepatic tuberculosis 61
mycophenolate 242–43
myelolipoma 105–7

neonatal cholestasis syndrome 433–36
neonatal sclerosing cholangitis 433
neuroendocrine liver metastases 219–20, 283, 293
neuromuscular blockade 32
nodular regenerative hyperplasia 94–96, 126
non-alcoholic fatty liver disease 25–26
non-insulin dependent diabetes 68
non-selective beta-blockers 139, 140
non-steroidal anti-inflammatory drugs (NSAIDs) 32, 351
non-thermal ablation 276–77
nuclear medicine 54–55
5'-nucleotidase 43
nutrition 33–34

obesity, fatty liver 68
octreotide 139, 351
oesophageal transection 148
oesophageal varices 139
opioid drug handling 32–33
Opisthorchis felineus 64t
Opisthorchis viverrini 319–20
oral contraceptive pill 153, 349
organic anion transporting polypeptides (OATPs) 15
overlap syndrome 454

paediatric end-stage liver disease (PELD) score 257
paediatric liver transplantation 247–58
  biliary stricture 255–56
  complications 251–56
  graft size matching 250–51
  hepatic artery thrombosis 251–52
  hepatic vein stenosis 253–55
  hepatoblastoma 198–200, 248–50
  history 247
  immunosuppression 250
  indications 247–50
  outcome 256–57
  PELD score 257
  portal vein thrombosis 252
  timing 257
pancreatic carcinoma 454
pancreaticoduodenectomy 316–18, 419
pancreatitis 332
papillotomy 233
paracetamol 32
parasitic liver disease 62–64, 319–20
parenteral nutrition 13–14, 350, 435–36
PELD score 257
peliosis hepatis 61–62, 107–9
pembrolizumab 417–18
pemigatinib 417
percutaneous imaging and interventions 323–35
  access 324
  acetic acid injection 277
  angioplasty 154
  benign bile duct strictures 330–32

bile duct biopsy/brush 324, 329
bile duct dilatation 325, 442
biliary drainage 55, 324–25, 329, 372
 complications 327–29
 ethanol injection 276–77
 indications and contraindications 324t
 local ablation therapies 274–77
 malignant biliary obstruction 329–30
 planning 323
 stent placement 325–27
 transhepatic cholangiography and drainage 441
peribiliary cysts 449–50
perihilar cholangiocarcinoma 51–52, 176, 177, 178–84, 419, 459–60, 462–67
perioperative care
 anaesthetic management 34–35
 coagulopathy 35
 drug handling 32–33
 fluids 35
 nutrition 33–34
 outcome prediction 30
 pathophysiological considerations 31–32
 risk minimization and optimization 35
 timing of surgery 31
peritonitis, spontaneous bacterial 141
peroral cholangioscopy 312
PET-CT 54–55, 224, 302
PFIC types I, II, and III 435
pigment stones 354
plasma cell granuloma 109–10
Plasmodium falciparum 62
polycystic liver disease 75, 284
polyvinyl alcohol 278
porcelain gall bladder 392–93
portal hypertension
 ascites 140–41
 balloon-occluded retrograde transvenous obliteration 140, 148
 causes 138
 cirrhosis 138
 complications 139–42
 distal splenorenal shunt 148–49
 gastro-oesophageal devascularization 148
 hepatic encephalopathy 141–42
 idiopathic non-cirrhotic 128–29
 intrahepatic 138, 138t
 liver transplantation 148
 measurement 137
 mesenterico-left portal venous bypass (Rex shunt) 148
 natural history 137

oesophageal transection 148
pathophysiology 137
portosystemic shunts 148–50
posthepatic 138, 138t
post-Kasai portoenterostomy 429
prehepatic 138, 138t
schistosomiasis 138
side-to-side portacaval shunt 150
spontaneous bacterial peritonitis 141
TIPS 140, 146–48, 150
variceal haemorrhage 139–40
portal scissura 3–4
portal vein
 anatomy 6–7, 124
 embolization 182, 225, 281
 stenosis 240
 thrombosis 124–28, 139–40, 156–58, 239–40, 252
portosystemic shunts 148–50
positron emission tomography (PET) 54–55
 PET-CT 54–55, 224, 302
POSTEXT 191
post-hepatectomy liver failure 24–25
postoperative outcome prediction 30
post-transplant cholangiopathy 308–9
post-transplant lymphoproliferative disorder 240
pregnancy
 gallstones 349
 hepatocellular adenoma 92
PRETEXT system 190–93
primary sclerosing cholangitis 307, 332, 453–57
priming phase 17, 18–22
Pringle manoeuvre 70, 119, 226, 340–41
probiotics 142
progressive familial intrahepatic cholestasis type 1 15
prostaglandins 351
protein synthesis 14
prothrombin time 43–44
proton beam therapy 418
protozoal infections 62–63
pseudocysts 81, 451
pyogenic cholangitis 332
pyogenic liver abscess 59–60, 76

Q fever 62

radiofrequency ablation 274–75
radiomics 57
rectal metastatic cancer 229
refractory ascites 141
renal failure 31
Rendu–Osler–Weber syndrome 158
respiratory function 31
Rex–Cantlie line 3

Rex shunt 148
rifaximin 142
robotic surgery
 liver resection 229
 living donor liver transplantation 265
rocuronium 32
rotavirus 423–24
R ratio 44

Salmonella enterica 60
salvage transplantation 199
sarcoma
 biliary embryonal rhabdomyosarcoma 211–12
 embryonal hepatic 82, 209–11
 hepatic haemangiosarcoma 207
 hepatocellular carcinoma/ carcinosarcoma 209
 leiomyosarcoma 211–12
 metastatic liver disease 221
schistosomiasis 63, 138
scintigraphy 54
sclerosing cholangitis
 IgG4-related 318–19, 332
 neonatal 433
 primary 307, 332, 453–57
secondary liver neoplasms *see* metastatic liver disease
serum–ascites albumin gradient (SAAG) 140
sevoflurane 32
side-to-side portacaval shunt 150
simple hepatic cysts 73–75, 284
sinusoidal obstruction syndrome 155–56
sirolimus 243
small bowel obstruction 289
small-for-size syndrome 264–65, 288
small vessel neoplasm 208
solitary fibrotic tumour 110
somatostatin 139, 351
sphincterotome 315
spinal injuries 351
splenosis 107
spontaneous bacterial peritonitis 141
SpyGlass 312
statins 350
Strasberg classification 367
sulphobromophthalein test 47t
surgical thrombectomy 127
syphilitic hepatitis 61

tacrolimus 242, 250
terlipressin 139
thermal ablation 274–76
three-dimensional reconstruction 57
thrombolysis
 Budd-Chiari syndrome 132, 154
 portal vein thrombosis 127
thrombophilia 125

toxic hepatitis 435–36
toxocariasis 63
toxoplasmosis (*Toxoplasma gondii*) 63
transaminases 42
transarterial catheter-based therapies 277–81
transarterial chemoembolization (TACE) 55, 278–79, 280–81, 418
transarterial embolization 55
transarterial radioembolization (TARE) 279–81
transcolonic biliary access 328–29
transgastric gall bladder drainage 318
transjugular intrahepatic portosystemic shunts (TIPS)
 Budd-Chiari syndrome 132–33
 portal hypertension 140, 146–48, 150
 portal vein thrombosis 127, 128
 variceal haemorrhage 140
transpleural biliary access 328
transvenous therapy 281
trauma
 bile duct 307–8
 cysts 81
 see also liver trauma
Treponema pallidum 61
Tropheryma whipplei 61
tuberculosis 61
typhoid fever 60

UGT1A1 14
ultrasound 49–50, 301
 intraoperative 50, 226
undifferentiated embryonal liver sarcoma 82, 209–11
urological cancer metastases 220
ursodeoxycholic acid 351–52, 355, 456

variceal haemorrhage 127, 139–40
vascular endothelial growth factor (VEGF) inhibitors 417
vascular liver neoplasms 204–9
vascular malformations 158
vecuronium 32
veno-occlusive disease 155–56
visceral larva migrans 63
visceral leishmaniasis 62–63
von Meyenburg complex 80, 98–99

wedged hepatic venous pressure 137
Whipple's disease 61

yttrium-90 418

zinc, hepatic encephalopathy 142